CHRONIC OBSTRUCTIVE LUNG DISEASES 2

CHRONIC OBSTRUCTIVE LUNG DISEASES 2

NORBERT F. VOELKEL, MD

The E. Raymond Fenton Professor of Pulmonary Research
Director, Victoria Johnson Center for Obstructive Lung Diseases
Virginia Commonwealth University
Richmond, Virginia

WILLIAM MacNEE, MBChB, MD, FRCP(G), FRCP(E)

Honorary Consultant Physician
Lothian University Hospital, NHS Trust
Scotland, United Kingdom

2008
BC Decker Inc
Hamilton

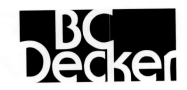

BC Decker Inc
P.O. Box 620, L.C.D. 1
Hamilton, Ontario L8N 3K7
Tel: 905-522-7017; 800-568-7281
Fax: 905-522-7839; 888-311-4987
E-mail: info@bcdecker.com
www.bcdecker.com

08 09 10 11 12 / AOP / 9 8 7 6 5 4 3 2 1
ISBN 978-1-55009-390-2
Printed in India by Ajanta Offset and Packagings Ltd.
Production Editor: Margaret Holmes; Typesetter: DiacriTech; Cover Design: Elizabeth Hayden.

Cover illustrations: Schema of relationship of reticular fibers to capillaries (after Orsos: Die Gerüstsysteme der Lunge und desen physiologische und pathologische Bedeutung. Beitr Klin Tuberk 1936;87:568.) Reproduced with permission from: Taraseviciene-Stewart L; Voelkel NF. Molecular pathogenesis of emphysema. J Clin Invest 2008;118(2):394–402. © American Society for Clinical Investigation. Illustration of lungs reproduced under licence from Shutterstock, "3d organs" by Sebastian Kaulitzki.

Sales and Distribution

United States
BC Decker Inc
P.O. Box 785
Lewiston, NY 14092-0785
Tel: 905-522-7017; 800-568-7281
Fax: 905-522-7839; 888-311-4987
E-mail: info@bcdecker.com
www.bcdecker.com

Canada
McGraw-Hill Ryerson Education
Customer Care
300 Water St.
Whitby, Ontario   L1N 9B6
Tel: 1-800-565-5758
Fax: 1-800-463-5885

Foreign Rights
John Scott & Company
International Publishers' Agency
P.O. Box 878
Kimberton, PA 19442
Tel: 610-827-1640
Fax: 610-827-1671
E-mail: jsco@voicenet.com

Japan
United Publishers Services Limited
1-32-5 Higashi-Shinagawa
Shinagawa-Ku, Tokyo 140-0002
Tel: 03 5479 7251
Fax: 03 5479 7307

UK, Europe, Middle East
McGraw-Hill Education
Shoppenhangers Road
Maidenhead
Berkshire, England SL6 2QL
Tel: 44-0-1628-502500
Fax: 44-0-1628-635895
www.mcgraw-hill.co.uk

Singapore, Malaysia, Thailand, Philippines, Indonesia, Vietnam, Pacific Rim, Korea
McGraw-Hill Education
60 Tuas Basin Link
Singapore 638775
Tel: 65-6863-1580
Fax: 65-6862-3354

Australia, New Zealand
Elsevier Science Australia
Customer Service Department
Locked Bag 16
St. Peters, New South Wales 2044
Australia
Tel: 61 02-9517-8999
Fax: 61 02-9517-2249
E-mail: customerserviceau@elsevier.com
www.elsevier.com.au

Brazil
Tecmedd Importadora E Distribuidora De Livros Ltda.
Avenida Maurílio Biagi, 2850
City Ribeirão, Ribeirão
Preto—SP—Brasil
CEP: 14021-000
Tel: 0800 992236
Fax: (16) 3993-9000
E-mail: tecmedd@tecmedd.com.br

India, Bangladesh, Pakistan, Sri Lanka
CBS Publishers & Distributors
4596/1A-11, Darya Ganj
New Delhi-2, India
Tel: 23271632
Fax: 23276712
E-mail: cbspubs@vsnl.com

To the memory of Norbert J. Völkel, MD
To Elisabeth Völkel, MD, and
Angelika I. Voelkel, MD
                    Norbert Voelkel

To my teachers
                    William MacNee

Preface to the First Edition

...illness for a doctor is always harder to bear than for a patient; the patient only feels, while the doctor, in addition to feeling, knows the process by which his organism is destroyed. — Maxim Gorky

Experiencing feelings of shortness of breath is a frightening thing for a patient; watching a patient fight for the next breath is a dreadful thing for a doctor. It must have been this type of experience that motivated the lung doctors who had seen halls overflowing with shiny tubes filled with polio patients, to explore new treatments for patients with acute and chronic respiratory failure. It was here, in Denver, that I (NV) learned from Dr. Thomas Petty that a ventilator is a machine used to prolong life—not death. I also learned to communicate with my patients suffering from chronic obstructive lung diseases on how to carry out the difficult task of making their final arrangements and following through with their wishes by adding their signed statements to their medical charts, indicating that they would not wish to be intubated when fatal complications arose.

This book on chronic obstructive pulmonary diseases is about our collective knowledge of the process by which the lung is destroyed. The process is likely one where chronic inhalation of xenobiotics stokes the fire of inflammation; eventually lung structure maintenance programs break down in genetically predisposed individuals, with the end result of tissue destruction and the development of neoplasia. This book pays tribute to the early pioneers of chronic obstructive lung disease research and to the notion of a continuum of the pathobiology of the lung's cells from inflammation to lung cancer. Our challenge is very clear: To prevent the development and progression of chronic obstructive lung diseases, and to heal the injured lungs.

Norbert F. Voelkel
William MacNee
November, 2001

PREFACE TO THE SECOND EDITION

The first edition of this book was greeted by many readers with a question: "Obstructive lung diseases—plural?" Since the publication of the first edition, the idea of different phenotypes of chronic obstructive lung disease (COPD), and perhaps of multiple pathobiologies, has taken hold. This second edition is truly an expanded and updated new edition. Some of the chapters that appeared in the first edition have been omitted from this edition, and the reader is referred to the previous edition for this information. The "History of Chronic Obstructive Pulmonary Disease" chapter in this new edition is intended to be complementary to the "Historical Overview of Emphysema" in the first edition. In this edition, many new topics have been added and the majority of the previous chapters have been updated.

The editors' intent in this edition, as in the first, has not been so ambitious as to provide a complete catalogue of COPD-related topics; rather, the emphasis has been on new concepts and ideas, and again efforts were made to identify the frontier of COPD research and to anticipate future developments.

We thank each and all of the contributors for their dedication to the cause of COPD and commend the many talents that they have brought to bear on the analysis and synthesis of a large amount of data. Clearly, COPD remains a group of interesting diseases that has rightfully found a growing number of interested, engaged investigators and readers.

Norbert F. Voelkel, MD
William MacNee, MD
July 2008

CONTRIBUTORS

Kenneth B. Adler, PhD
Professor
Department of Molecular Biomedical Sciences
North Carolina State University
College of Veterinary Medicine
Raleigh, North Carolina
*Mucus and Mucus-Secreting Cells in Chronic
    Obstructive Pulmonary Disease*

Alvar G.N. Agustí, MD, FRCP
Head of Pulmonary Service
HUSD-F. Caubet-Cimera and Ciberes
Hospital Universitario Son Dureta
Palma de Mallorca, Spain
*Muscle Involvement in Chronic Obstructive
    Pulmonary Disease*

Mark V. Avdalovic, MD
Clinical Professor
Division of Pulmonary and Critical Care
Department of Internal Medicine
University of California at Davis
School of Medicine
Davis, California
Chronic Airway Disease in Nonhuman Primates

Joan Albert Barberà, MD
Associate Professor
Department of Medicine
University of Barcelona
Barcelona, Spain
Stem Cells

Alan R. Buckpitt, PhD
Professor
Department of Molecular Biosciences
University of California at Davis
School of Veterinary Medicine
Davis, California
Chronic Airway Disease in Nonhuman Primates

Xavier Busquets, PhD
Professor of Cell Biology
Head, Cell Biology Laboratory
UIB-IUNICS

University of the Balearic Islands
Palma de Mallorca, Spain
*Muscle Involvement in Chronic
    Obstructive Pulmonary Disease*

Matthieu Canuet, MD
Praticien Hospitalier
Division of Pulmonology
Department of Thoracic Diseases
University Hospital
Strasbourg, France
*Pulmonary Hypertension in Chronic
    Obstructive Pulmonary Disease*

Eleonora Cavarra, PhD
Assistant Professor of Pathology
Division of Lung Pathology
Department of Physiopathology
    and Experimental Medicine
University of Siena
Siena, Italy
Small Animal Models of Emphysema

Bartolome R. Celli, MD
Professor
Department of Medicine
Tufts University
School of Medicine
Boston, Massachusetts
*Medical Therapy for Chronic
    Obstructive Pulmonary Disease*

Ari Chaouat, MD
Professor of Respiratory Medicine
University Henri Poincaré
Nancy, France
*Pulmonary Hypertension in Chronic
    Obstructive Pulmonary Disease*

Andrew Churg, MD
Professor of Pathology
University of British Columbia
Vancouver, British Columbia
*Small Airway Obstruction in Chronic
    Obstructive Pulmonary Disease*

Harvey O. Coxson, PhD
Assistant Professor
Department of Radiology
University of British Columbia
Vancouver, British Columbia
Imaging of Chronic Obstructive Pulmonary Disease

Anne L. Crews, MS
Laboratory Supervisor
Department of Molecular Biomedical Sciences
North Carolina State University
College of Veterinary Medicine
Raleigh, North Carolina
*Mucus and Mucus-Secreting Cells in
    Chronic Obstructive Pulmonary Disease*

Jan Dallinga, PhD
Department of Health Risk Analysis
    and Toxicology
Faculty of Health Sciences
University of Maastricht
Maastricht, The Netherlands
*Biomarkers in Chronic Obstructive
    Pulmonary Disease*

Smita Desai, DO
Assistant Professor of Medicine
University of California, San Diego
La Jolla, California
Rehabilitation

Kenneth Donaldson, PhD, DSc, FRCPath, FFOM
Professor of Respiratory Toxicology
Centre for Inflammation Research
University of Edinburgh
Edinburgh, United Kingdom
*Environmental Factors in Chronic Obstructive
    Pulmonary Disease*

Michael J. Evans, PhD
Research Professor
Department of Anatomy, Physiology
    and Cell Biology
University of California at Davis
School of Medicine
Davis, California
Chronic Airway Disease in Nonhuman Primates

Michelle V. Fanucchi, PhD
Associate Professor
Department of Environmental Health Sciences
University of Alabama at Birmingham
School of Public Health
Birmingham, Alabama
Chronic Airway Disease in Nonhuman Primates

Marilyn G. Foreman, MD, MS
Research Fellow in Medicine; Respiratory,
    Environmental and Genetic Epidemiology
Department of Medicine
Channing Laboratory, Brigham and Women's
    Hospital and Harvard Medical School
Boston, Massachusetts
Genetic Risk Factors

Sarah A. Gebb, PhD
Associate Professor
Department of Cell Biology and Neuroscience
University of South Alabama
College of Medicine
Mobile, Alabama
Lung Development

Laurel J. Gershwin, DVM, PhD
Professor
Department of Pathology, Microbiology and Immunology
University of California at Davis
School of Veterinary Medicine
Davis, California
Chronic Airway Disease in Nonhuman Primates

Carlos E. Girod, MD
Associate Professor
Division of Pulmonary and Critical Care Medicine
Department of Internal Medicine
University of Texas Southwestern Medical Center
Dallas, Texas
Other Large-Airway Diseases that Limit Airflow
Diffuse Interstitial Lung Diseases Resulting in Airflow Limitation

Dallas M. Hyde, PhD
Professor, Anatomy, Physiology and Cell Biology
University of California at Davis
School of Veterinary Medicine
Davis, California
Chronic Airway Disease in Nonhuman Primates

Amanda Iglesias, PhD
Member of the Ciberes and Unidad Investigacion
Hospital Universitario Son Dureta
Palma de Mallorca, Spain
*Muscle Involvement in Chronic Obstructive
    Pulmonary Disease*

Jesse P. Joad, MD
Professor
Department of Pediatrics
University of California at Davis
School of Medicine
Davis, California
Chronic Airway Disease in Nonhuman Primates

Sebastian L. Johnston, MBBS, PhD
Professor
Department of Respiratory Medicine
National Heart and Lung Institute
Imperial College
London, United Kingdom
Viral Infections and Chronic Obstructive
   Pulmonary Disease

Steinn Jonsson, MD
Associate Professor
Division of Pulmonary and Critical Care Medicine
University of Iceland
Reykjavik, Iceland
Chronic Obstructive Pulmonary Disease, the
   Final Chapter—Lung Cancer

Radhika Kajekar, PhD
Professor
Department of Molecular, Cellular and
   Integrative Physiology
University of California at Davis
   School of Medicine
Davis, California
Chronic Airway Disease in Nonhuman Primates

Robert L. Keith, MD
Associate Professor
Division of Pulmonary Sciences
   and Critical Care Medicine
University of Colorado at Denver
Denver, Colorado
Chronic Obstructive Pulmonary Disease,
   the Final Chapter—Lung Cancer

Patricia B. Koff, MEd, RRT
Health Program Coordinator
Department of Ambulatory Services
COPD Center
University of Colorado Hospital
Aurora/Denver, Colorado
Telemedicine and Chronic Obstructive Pulmonary Disease

Giuseppe Lungarella, MD
Professor of Pathology
Division of Lung Pathology
Department of Physiopathology
   and Experimental Medicine
University of Siena
Siena, Italy
Small Animal Models of Emphysema

David A. Lynch, MD
Professor
Director of Thoracic Imaging
Department of Radiology

University of Colorado at Denver
Aurora, Colorado
Imaging of Chronic Obstructive Pulmonary Disease

William MacNee, MBChB, MD, FRCP(C), FRCP(E)
Honorary Consultant Physician
Lothian University Hospital,
   NHS Trust
Scotland, United Kingdom
Environmental Factors in Chronic
   Obstructive Pulmonary Disease

Patrick Mallia, MD, MRCP, PhD
Department of Respiratory Medicine
National Heart and Lung Institute
Imperial College
London, United Kingdom
Viral Infections and Chronic Obstructive
   Pulmonary Disease

Piero A. Martorana, DVM
Contract Professor of Pathology
Division of Lung Pathology
Department of Physiopathology
   and Experimental Medicine
University of Siena
Siena, Italy
Small Animal Models of Emphysema

Michael T. McDermott, MD
Professor
Division of Endocrinology, Metabolism
   and Diabetes
Department of Medicine
University of Colorado at Denver
Aurora/Denver, Colorado
Osteoporosis

Lisa A. Miller, PhD
Associate Professor
Department of Anatomy, Physiology & Cell Biology
University of California at Davis
School of Veterinary Medicine
Davis, California
Chronic Airway Disease in Nonhuman Primates

York E. Miller, MD
Thomas L. Petty Chair
Division of Pulmonary Sciences &
Critical Care Medicine
Department of Medicine
University of Colorado
Health Sciences Center
Denver, Colorado
Chronic Obstructive Pulmonary Disease,
   the Final Chapter—Lung Cancer

Montse Morlá, PhD
Member of the Cell Biology Laboratory
University of the Balearic Islands - IUNICS
Palma de Mallorca, Spain
*Muscle Involvement in Chronic Obstructive
    Pulmonary Disease*

Rachel Norwood, MD
Assistant Professor
Department of Psychiatry
University of Colorado at Denver
Health Sciences Center
Denver, Colorado
*Psychosocial Aspects of Chronic
    Obstructive Pulmonary Disease*

Peter D. Paré, MD
Professor of Medicine
Division of Respiratory Medicine
Department of Medicine
University of British Columbia
Vancouver, British Columbia
*Small Airway Obstruction in Chronic
    Obstructive Pulmonary Disease*

Jin-Ah Park, PhD
Research Fellow
Department of Environmental Health
Harvard University
School of Public Health
Boston, Massachusetts
*Mucus and Mucus-Secreting Cells in
    Chronic Obstructive Pulmonary
    Disease*

Victor I. Peinado, PhD
Associate Researcher
Ciber de Enfermedades Respiratorias
University of Barcelona
Barcelona, Spain
Stem Cells

Thomas L. Petty, MD
Professor Emeritus
University of Colorado at Denver
Health Sciences Center
Aurora, Colorado
*History of Chronic Obstructive
    Pulmonary Disease*

Kent E. Pinkerton, PhD
Professor of Anatomy, Physiology
    and Cell Biology
Director, Center for Health and the Environment
University of California at Davis
School of Medicine
Davis, California
Chronic Airway Disease in Nonhuman Primates

Charles G. Plopper, PhD
Professor Emeritus
Department of Anatomy, Physiology
    and Cell Biology
University of California at Davis
School of Veterinary Medicine
Davis, California
Chronic Airway Disease in Nonhuman Primates

Kimberly L. Raiford, PhD
Research Assistant
Department of Molecular Biological Sciences
North Carolina State University
College of Veterinary Medicine
Raleigh, North Carolina
*Mucus and Mucus-Secreting Cells in Chronic
    Obstructive Pulmonary Disease*

David W.H. Riches, PhD
Professor, Departments of Immunology,
    Medicine and Pharmacology
Program in Cell Biology, Departments of Medicine and
    Pediatrics
National Jewish Medical and Research Center
University of Colorado Denver Health Sciences Programs
Denver, Colorado
*Macrophage Involvement in Chronic Obstructive
    Lung Disease*

Andrew L. Ries, MD, MPH
Associate Dean for Academic Affairs
Professor of Medicine & Family Preventive Medicine
University of California, San Diego
La Jolla, California
Rehabilitation

Edward S. Schelegle, PhD
Associate Professor
Department of Anatomy, Physiology & Cell Biology
University of California at Davis
School of Veterinary Medicine
Davis, California
Chronic Airway Disease in Nonhuman Primates

Marvin I. Schwarz, MD
James C. Campbell Professor of Pulmonary Medicine
Division of Pulmonary Sciences & Critical Care Medicine
Department of Medicine
University of Colorado School of Medicine
Denver, Colorado
Other Large-Airway Diseases that Limit Airflow
Diffuse Interstitial Lung Diseases Resulting in
Airflow Limitation

Sanjay Sethi, MD
Professor of Medicine and Division Chief
Division of Pulmonary/Critical Care/Sleep Medicine
Department of Medicine
University at Buffalo, State University of New York
Buffalo, New York
Bacterial Infection in Chronic Obstructive
Pulmonary Disease

Steven D. Shapiro, MD
Jack D. Myers Professor and Chair
Department of Medicine
University of Pittsburgh
Pittsburgh, Pennsylvania
Small Animal Models of Emphysema

Edwin K. Silverman, MD, PhD
Assistant Professor of Medicine
Harvard Medical School
Associate Physician
Brigham and Women's Hospital
Boston, Massachusetts
Genetic Risk Factors

Robert A. Stockley, MD, DSc, FRCP
Professor
Department of Medicine
University of Birmingham
Birmingham, United Kingdom
α_1-*Antitrypsin Deficiency*

Jennifer L. Terry, PhD
Post-Doctoral Fellow
Departments of Medicine and Pediatrics
National Jewish Medical and Research Center
University of Colorado Denver Health Sciences Programs
Denver, Colorado
Macrophage Involvement in Chronic
Obstructive Lung Disease

John Torday, MSc, PhD
Professor of Pediatrics & Ob/Gyn
Director, Perinatal Research Training Program

Los Angeles Biomedical Research Institute at
Harbor-UCLA Medical Center
Torrance, California
Lung Development

Rubin M. Tuder, MD
Director
Division of Pulmonary Pathology
Johns Hopkins University
School of Medicine
Baltimore, Maryland
Pathobiology of Emphysema

Nancy K. Tyler, PhD
Scientist
University of California
School of Medicine
Davis, California
Chronic Airway Disease in Nonhuman Primates

Laura S. Van Winkle, PhD
Associate Professor
Department of Anatomy, Physiology and
Cell Biology
University of California at Davis
School of Veterinary Medicine
Davis, California
Chronic Airway Disease in Nonhuman Primates

Jørgen Vestbo, MD, DMSc
Professor of Respiratory Medicine
Department of Cardiology & Respiratory Medicine
University of Copenhagen
North West Lung Center
Manchester, United Kingdom
Epidemiology

Marc A. Voelkel, MD
Instructor and Physician
Departments of Medicine and Pediatrics
Pulmonary Division
University of Colorado at Denver
Health Sciences Center
National Jewish Medical and Research Center
Denver, Colorado
Macrophage Involvement in Chronic
Obstructive Lung Disease

Norbert F. Voelkel, MD
The E. Raymond Fenton Professor
of Pulmonary Research
Director, Victoria Johnson Center for
Obstructive Lung Diseases
Virginia Commonwealth University

Richmond, Virginia
*History of Chronic Obstructive
    Pulmonary Disease*
Pathobiology of Emphysema
*Vascular Endothelial Growth Factor
    and its Role in Emphysema and Asthma*
*Exacerbation of Chronic Obstructive
    Pulmonary Disease*

Sheryl F. Vondracek, PharmD, FCCP, BCPS
Associate Professor
Department of Clinical Pharmacy
University of Colorado at Denver
Health Sciences Center
Aurora, Colorado
Osteoporosis

Scott Wagers, MD
Fellow, Division of Pulmonary Disease
    and Critical Care Medicine, FAHC
University of Vermont
College of Medicine
Burlington, Vermont
*Biomarkers in Chronic Obstructive
    Pulmonary Disease*

Adam Wanner, MD
Joseph Weintraub Professor of Medicine
Division of Pulmonary/Critical Care
Department of Medicine
University of Miami
Miller School of Medicine
Miami, Florida
*Airway Circulation in Chronic Obstructive
    Pulmonary Disease*

Emmanuel Weitzenblum, MD
Professor of Medicine
Division of Pulmonology
University of Strasbourg
Strasbourg, France
*Pulmonary Hypertension in Chronic
    Obstructive Pulmonary Disease*

John M. Westfall, MD
Associate Professor
Associate Dean, Rural Medicine
Department of Family Medicine
University of Colorado at Denver
Health Sciences Center

Aurora, Colorado
*Telemedicine and Chronic Obstructive
    Pulmonary Disease*

Emile F.M. Wouters, PhD, MD
Department of Pulmonary Disease
University Hospital Maastricht
Maastricht, The Netherlands
*Systemic Manifestations of Chronic
    Obstructive Pulmonary Disease*
*Biomarkers in Chronic
    Obstructive Pulmonary Disease*

Joanne L. Wright, MD, FRCP
Professor
Department of Pathology
University of British Columbia
Vancouver, British Columbia
*Small Airway Obstruction in Chronic
    Obstructive Pulmonary Disease*

Reen Wu, PhD
Professor
Department of Internal Medicine
Division of Pulmonary and Critical Care Medicine
University of California at Davis
School of Veterinary Medicine
Davis, California
Chronic Airway Disease in Nonhuman Primates

Murry W. Wynes, PhD
Instructor
Departments of Pediatrics and Medicine
National Jewish Medical and Research Center
University of Colorado Denver Health Sciences Programs
Denver, Colorado
*Macrophage Involvement in Chronic
    Obstructive Lung Disease*

Martin R. Zamora, MD
Professor of Medicine & Medical Director,
    Lung Transplant Program
Division of Pulmonary Sciences and
    Critical Care Medicine
University of Colorado at Denver
Health Sciences Center
Denver/Aurora, Colorado
*Surgical Therapy for Chronic Obstructive
    Lung Disease*

CONTENTS

CHAPTER 1

History of Chronic Obstructive Pulmonary Disease

Norbert F. Voelkel, MD, and Thomas L. Petty, MD

THE HISTORY OF CHRONIC obstructive pulmonary disease (COPD), as told by recent historians[1–3] and previously reviewed in the first edition of *Chronic Obstructive Lung Diseases,*[4] has, by and large, been a history of emphysema. As historiographers remind us, history writing is highly contextual and seldom without bias but frequently has an agenda. In this regard, our handling of the modern history of COPD makes no exception.

Emphysema and the "Chronic Bronchitis" Syndrome: The Colorado Approach

It is worth going back to the early days of COPD research to the following excerpts from the 1958 first Aspen emphysema conference,[5] which may entice readers belonging to the post–baby boom generation to read the proceedings of this landmark conference. The meeting took place in Aspen, Colorado, June 13–15, 1958, and was launched by several participants, including Richard A. Prindle, chief of the Air Pollution Medical Program, Department of Health Education and Welfare, Washington, DC. He stated that:

> although pulmonary emphysema is a widely applied diagnosis, the condition itself is poorly understood and, even among the experts, there is lack of agreement on almost every point that would characterize the disorder anatomically, functionally and clinically. The need for a universally acceptable concept of pulmonary emphysema has become pressing in recent decades, due to the increased incidence of the disease and the fact that it exhibits an ominous parallel to the progressive pollution of our environment. To some, pulmonary emphysema is already a public health problem in America. Emphysema is, even now, a very serious matter in Great Britain, where it is a prominent feature of the chronic bronchitis syndrome, which has overtaken every other pulmonary disease as the foremost crippler and killer.[5]

At the time—the 1950s—when tuberculosis became a manageable and treatable disease, the "chronic bronchitis syndrome" entered the picture and provided a raison d'etre for academic pulmonary medicine divisions, an opportunity seized in the United States but regretfully not in many parts of Europe. To appreciate the strength of the movement and the degree of enthusiasm, let us return to the 1958 Aspen emphysema conference to review some of the topics and statements that survived in the published proceedings.

The opening talk, "Theories of the Pathogenesis of Emphysema," by Roger S. Mitchell, set the stage for the entire conference. He began by stating, "The Conference Steering Committee has identified three general purposes of this conference: (1) to exchange information on the available knowledge and our lack of knowledge regarding the etiology and pathogenesis of diffuse obstructive pulmonary emphysema, hereinafter called 'emphysema'; (2) to clarify terminology as it pertains to emphysema and related problems; and (3) to endeavor to stimulate interest in research into the etiology and pathogenesis of this obscure and common disorder."[5] He went on to barrage the audience with a large number of questions:

> Why do some patients show carbon dioxide retention and/or polycythemia as an early or predominant manifestation of the disorder, while others do not? Just how frequently does emphysema complicate true bronchial asthma? What is the explanation of the wide variation in the response of the pulmonary circulation and of the right heart to the insult of emphysema in different individuals? How do we account for the wide variations in the course of emphysema? Some become quite ill abruptly, and others very gradually; some progress in a malignant fashion to an early death from respiratory insufficiency and oxygen lack, on the one hand, or right heart failure on the other; while others become disabled gradually and may reach a plateau and live on for many years in a state of moderate chronic disability? Why do most emphysematous persons note marked loss of weight—often from one sixth to one fourth of their total body weight—with the onset of severe pulmonary disability, whereas a few with a comparable disability lose no weight at all? Is emphysema commonly associated with exposure to industrial smog, tobacco smoke and dust? Is "bronchitis" as the British used the term, partially or wholly synonymous with "emphysema" as we use the term? Can emphysema be produced with regularity in an experimental animal? by what method? Is it emphysema

as we know it in man? Is it not true that the term emphysema is a common wastebasket used by clinicians for patients with dyspnea and/or right heart failure that do not fit easily into some standard category? Do we have a simple yet reliable screening test with which to discover emphysema early, and, if so discovered, can we arrest its progress by any means?[5]

He concluded his talk by stating, "It is altogether probable that emphysema may prove to be a *syndrome* with several *different* and probably *overlapping* causes". Nearly 50 years later, it is still humbling to read these sentences and recognize how many of these questions remain unanswered.

Lung Structure and Matrix Proteins

John A. Pierce recently reminisced,

The intricate delicacy of the peripheral lung structure was slightly more fascinating than the strength and toughness of the dried lung skeleton. The well-known and important physical properties of collagen and elastin were generally accepted as responsible for maintenance of lung structure through decades of recurrent stress. Collagen provides the toughness, with 5 times the tensile strength of elastin, but the requirement for long-range extensibility is a property exclusively of elastin. We realized the lung structure could not be remodeled from normal to emphysematous without mechanical interruption of the fibrous network. Our commitment to measuring collagen and elastin in the lung became more resolute because measurements of these critical proteins had never been reported.[6]

Indeed, Pierce did present his first data at the Aspen emphysema conference in June of 1958. During the same session, Vernon E. Krahl discussed the microscopic anatomy of the lungs, referring back to the brilliant depictions of the respiratory elastic framework of the normal lung adapted from Orsos's 1936 article (Figure 1).[7] Krahl paid specific tribute to the elasticity of the lung blood vessels when he stated:

that the pulmonary blood vessels must contribute substantially to total elasticity of the lung is readily appreciated, in view of their rich endowment of elastic and contractile elements…the vessels, intimately connected as they are to adjacent airways through intertwining of respiratory and vascular elastic fibers, are automatically coordinated in their adjustments with those of the bronchioles and other structures to which they lie adjacent…The pulmonary capillaries deserve special mention, because of their rather unique arrangements and relationship. The capillary networks of the inter-alveolar septa are the richest anywhere in the body—cell rich, in fact—that the spaces in the meshwork are often smaller than the diameters of capillaries which surround them.[7]

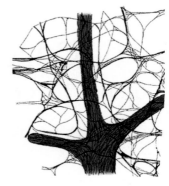

FIGURE 1. Schema of the relationship of reticular fibers to the capillaries. The coarse bundles of fibers are running parallel to the longer vessel and form intercapillary support structures. They give off fine filaments, which form a loosely knit tube around the vessels. Adapted from Orsos, with permission.[7] Reproduced with permission from: Taraseviciene-Stewart L; Voelkel NF. Molecular pathogenesis of emphysema. J Clin Invest 2008;118(2):394–402. © American Society for Clinical Investigation.

He referred again to Orsos, who had shown that "in normal adult lungs, the alveoli are large, and that the capillary plexuses of inter-alveolar septa and the apices of upper lobes have fewer vessels and much wider meshes than those of the caudal parts of the same lobes, or the caudal lobes of the same lungs…. The pulmonary capillaries, therefore, depend entirely for their support upon the fibrous scaffolding upon which they are suspended."[7]

Of course, the discovery of the genetically determined syndrome of α_1-antiprotease insufficiency by Erickson[8] led to the protease/antiprotease hypothesis of emphysema and a framework to understanding lung elastin and lung structure damage.[9] Robert Senior and Steven Shapiro have provided more recent, mechanistic insights with their elegant studies with elastin-derived peptides, demonstrating that elastin fragments attract macrophage and fibroblasts and, again, that macrophage elastase participates in the destruction of the alveolar network (see also Chapter 8).[10]

Hypothesis that Emphysema is a Sequela of Bronchiolitis

Remarkably, Kenneth H. McLean, in his lecture "The Pathology of Emphysema," introduced the term "homeostasis."[5] He stated,

Homeostasis may be defective because of overloading of the mechanisms, or because the mechanisms themselves are deficient. For instance, the overload may be due to excessive mucus or exudate in the respiratory tract… in such circumstances, bronchiolar occlusion occurs more often and plugs tend to remain *in situ* for relatively long periods. Inflammation of this type tends to persist as long as homeostasis remains defective.[5]

Studies of emphysematous lungs were difficult:

Although bronchioles must have been obliterated, search for their remnants was frustrating, and only the remnants of large bronchioles were identified with certainty. Often, this was only possible because a fibrous strand arising from the wall of a damaged bronchiole continued peripherally alongside a pulmonary arterial branch. Observations of this type made it difficult to avoid the conclusion that extensive and inconspicuous obliteration of bronchioles occurs in any lung which is damaged by inflammatory processes: this includes emphysematous lungs.[5]

He concluded with the following: "With repeated inflammatory episodes, each resulting in more obliterated bronchioles, the pattern of air trapping would change repeatedly as more and more lung tissue would be disrupted. The end result is the formation of a new organ which structurally (and functionally) bears only a superficial resemblance to the normal lung."[5]

From here, we can fast-forward to Hogg and colleagues' landmark 2004 article in the *New England Journal of Medicine*, "The Nature of Small-Airway Obstruction in Chronic Obstructive Pulmonary Disease."[11] Paré and colleagues discuss small airway pathology in COPD in their chapter in this book (Chapter 9, "Small Airway Obstruction in Chronic Obstructive Pulmonary Disease").

Emphysema as a Vascular Disease

During the same conference, Averill Liebow picked up this theme and said, "…the interalveolar septa vanish and the process is progressive in that bronchioles and ultimately even bronchi come to communicate with a trabeculated, sometimes multi-locular, and thin-walled cavity that may represent most of the lung. Like the 'chambered nautilus', it comes to consist of more and more stately mansions."[5] The mode of dissolution of the interlobular septa is particularly obscure. Liebow considered several mechanisms leading to atrophy, air trapping, cessation of blood flow to the most distal airspaces, and thrombosis of the small vessels, but he dismissed obliteration of the bronchial arterial supply as he noted that the bronchial arteries do not normally extend beyond the respiratory bronchioles. He concluded his lecture with the following statement:

Most of the pathogenetic factors are often associated with repeated episodes of necrotizing bronchiolitis and pneumonitis, both inter-alveolar and interstitial, but chemical agents and certain dusts can produce similar effects. Vascular changes are occasioned by both functional and organic factors, and these supplement each other. The former seem more significant, as judged by the reversibility upon appropriate treatment of the mild pulmonary hypertension associated with emphysema.

Irreversible organic changes in the vasculature, however, reduce the large reserve of the lung. The most important vasculature lesion appears to be a loss of capillaries.

In the general discussion that followed Dr. Liebow's presentation, Alfred Fishman remarked, "As the assigned discussant, I am happy that Dr. Liebow has extended his remarks beyond the pulmonary vascular changes of emphysema, for there is little to say about these vascular changes…. But, as far as functional significance is concerned, we are on surest ground with the capillary bed, since there is ample physiologic evidence that curtailment of this bed limits the gas exchanging surface of the lung in emphysema."[5]

Animal Models of Emphysema

In Aspen in 1958, there was a short session on animal models. A few of the contributions are worth highlighting here. Dr. Alexander, from the Department of Veterinary Pathology, College of Veterinary Medicine, Colorado State University, Fort Collins, introduced the "heaves," a specific syndrome of chronic alveolar emphysema in horses, characterized by respiratory dyspnea, cough, and lack of endurance to exercise:

The condition is slow in development, prolonged in course, and irreversible in nature. The specific etiology is unknown. The condition has most often been associated with horses that are stabled and fed dusty or moldy hays. In advanced cases, signs of congestive right heart failure may be noted, with development of edematous swelling along the ventral thoracic wall. On autopsy, the lungs are found to be pale in color, rib impressions may be seen and emphysematous bullae may be present. Lesions of bronchitis can be seen throughout the lung. Microscopic examination of involved areas reveals distended and ruptured alveoli, with thin alveolar walls. In these portions stretched capillaries show reduced lumenal diameters and fibrosis is often seen in septal structures and in the peribronchial areas. The most constant finding is that of chronic bronchitis and bronchiolitis.[12]

After the demonstration of the lung histology, Dr. Robert Grover commented that he had had the privilege and opportunity of working with Dr. Alexander and making certain physiologic observations. The emphysematous horse and the normal horse were subjected to cardiac catheterization, which proved to be a surprisingly simple procedure. He stated, "We used a standard human cardiac catheter, with pressure monitoring, and it went directly to the pulmonary artery. There was no question that the emphysematous horse had pulmonary hypertension when compared with a normal animal."[5]

What has happened since then to the "heaves"? It may come as no surprise that the syndrome still exists,[13] but the pathobiology is still not understood.

Dr. Alfred Crowle, from the University of Colorado, School of Medicine, reported on "an attempt to produce emphysema in the guinea pig." Of interest is the concept behind the studies he conducted. He explained:

Emphysema could be due to autoimmunization. Slightly injured lung tissue, due, for example, to inhalation of chemically reactive fumes or large volumes of tobacco smoke, could make it foreign antigenically to the victim's immunologic processes. Many microorganisms can function as adjuvants; molds, spores and bacteria associated with chronic lung diseases are good examples. Thus, with a small amount of injured tissue in proximity with an adjuvant, the victim is primed for autoimmunization. If the affected lung tissue happened to be elastic tissue, for example, emphysema might be its most obvious manifestation.

Today, we find it remarkable that Dr. Crowle presented data based on experiments with only three animals that had been injected subcutaneously with Freund adjuvant, containing guinea pig lung homogenate. In his report, he stated:

Approximately three weeks after their treatment, all the guinea pigs began breathing abnormally, after five weeks two of the three animals died. Major organs, except the lungs, were not obviously abnormal in any of these guinea pigs. The lungs of the two animals that died were larger than normal. Photographs made of whole and sectioned lungs of affected animals showed blebs; in any given section from these lungs about a third of any lobe was affected, arterial muscular walls appeared thickened, and their lumina were often absent.[5]

Interestingly, there was acceptance of the concepts by the audience. Dr. Bukantz stated, "The technique of autoimmunization is perfectly rational…,"[5] and Dr. Jack Reeves commented, "It seems certain that in real circumstances tissue may be destroyed by the animal's own immune response to them. How common a cause of disease in man this is, however, remains to be demonstrated by future work."[5]

This reference to future work is interesting. We can now fast-forward to the hypothesis paper published by Agustí and colleagues.[14]

Dr. Frances Lowell's remarks on the "relationship of allergy to emphysema" also bear on this subject matter.[5] He stated:

A relationship between smoking and emphysema is so firmly fixed in my own mind that it has become quite impossible for me to consider the etiology of emphysema of the type described in terms other than lung damage caused by inhalation of noxious smokes. As a result, I shall limit my discussion of the role of allergy in emphysema to the possibility that the disease is the consequence of some type of allergic reaction to these sub-stances, among which tobacco smoke seems to be far and away the most important.[5]

He then asked, "What do we know about allergy to tobacco smoke? Actually very little. Most of the work has been done by skin testing with extracts of pure tobacco leaf, not extracts of tobacco smoke."[5] It was not until several years later that cigarette smoking was identified as a major cause of emphysema. The reader is referred to reports by Auerbach and colleagues and Mitchell and colleagues.[15–18]

Lung Volume Reduction Surgery

It was at this meeting that Otto Brantigan introduced lung volume reduction surgery:

After eight years of study by trial and error, an operation has evolved designed to restore a well-known physiologic mechanism that has, for the most part, been lost in the patient with idiopathic hypertrophic obstructive pulmonary emphysema. It is an operation directed at restoration of a physiologic principle. It is not concerned with the removal of pathologic tissue. The operation for pulmonary emphysema is directed at a reduction in lung volume and the resection of the most useless and functionless area of lung tissue (see Figure 2). The lung volume is reduced to the capacity that fits the volume of the pleural space on full expiration. Thus, the impaired physiologic mechanism of circumferential pull upon the bronchioles is restored to some degree. It is conceivable that some less diseased areas of lungs that have been held collapsed may be put into use.[5]

He reported that he had performed surgery on 33 patients—the youngest 16 years old, and the oldest 61 years old.

When revisited today, the first Aspen emphysema conference can be seen as a truly prophetic event.

Natural History of Chronic Airflow Obstruction

The *British Medical Journal* published an article with the title above by Charles Fletcher, emeritus professor of clinical epidemiology at Hammersmith Hospital in London, and Richard Peto, reader in cancer studies at Oxford University.[19] This article appeared in 1977 under the rubric "Occasional Reviews" and described the results of a landmark study that began in 1961 when a stratified random sample of men (mostly skilled manual or clerical, aged 30 to 59 years, working in West London) was taken. Of an initial sample of 1,136 men, 792 were seen regularly. Forced expiratory volume (FEV) was measured every 6 months over 8 years; altogether, 9,190 measurements were made and analyzed. The authors summarized their results in four statements:

(1) Firstly, we found that FEV declines continuously and smoothly over an individual's life, the rate of loss seems

to accelerate slightly with aging. (2) Non-smokers lose FEV slowly and almost never developed clinically severe airflow obstruction. (3) Many smokers lose FEV almost as slowly as non-smokers and never develop clinically severe airflow obstruction. They appear to be largely resistant to the effects of smoke on their airflow. Smokers who are more susceptible to those effects develop various degrees of airflow obstruction which in some ultimately becomes disabling or fatal. "Susceptibility" is not an all-or-nothing attribute: rather it appears to be a continuum, where the more susceptible a man is the sooner he will be disabled if he smokes. (4) Stopping smoking will of course make little difference to the FEV of a non-susceptible smoker…but, it may make all the difference to a susceptible smoker. A susceptible smoker who stops smoking will not recover lost FEV but the subsequent rate of loss will revert to normal…. The real effect of smoking on a susceptible smoker may be underestimated by looking only at the mean FEV level in all smokers.[19]

We note that this natural history study involved only men older than 30 years and that the 100% FEV is clearly referenced to the age of 25 years. In a final paragraph, Fletcher and Peto addressed the issue of "susceptibility." Is susceptibility in any way analogous to α-antitrypsin deficiency, or is it due to quantitative differences in leukocyte proteolytic enzymes? Can it be induced by infections in childhood that are associated with impaired lung functions?

Recent studies are beginning to address these questions. For example, Kelleher and colleagues described a functional elastin mutation in a pedigree with severe early-onset COPD.[9]

Nocturnal Oxygen Therapy Trial, National Health and Nutrition Examination Survey, and Global Initiative for Lung Disease

The concept of the treatment of patients with COPD with supplemental oxygen emerged in 1965, and two oxygen treatment trials published in 1980[20] and 1981[21] provide the basis for the chronic oxygen treatment that has been proven to alter the course of the disease in patients with advanced COPD.[22]

Nocturnal Oxygen Therapy Trial

The Nocturnal Oxygen Therapy Trial (NOTT) was a randomized prospective clinical trial in COPD patients and stable hypoxemia, documented over a 3-week stabilization period.[20] Subjects were assigned to receive continuous oxygen therapy (COT) or nocturnal oxygen therapy (NOT) to determine multiple outcomes. These outcomes were survival, quality of life, neuropsychological function, cardiac function, exacerbations, and economic factors. In all, 203 patients were enrolled following screening criteria, including stabilization of their clinical status and the presence of resting hypoxemia of oxygen partial pressure of 55 or less on an oxygen

saturation of 88% or less over a 3-week interval. During this 3-week stabilization phase, the techniques of pulmonary rehabilitation were employed to improve symptoms and exercise tolerance. COT was most commonly given by portable liquid ambulatory systems weighing approximately 10 pounds. Only a few patients received E-cylinders, weighing 22 pounds, for ambulation. Most of the NOT patients received NOT given by concentrators; a few used high-pressure cylinders. Compliance with therapy was judged by carefully maintained diaries and estimates of oxygen use; documentation was good. NOT patients received oxygen for a mean of 11.8 hours and COT patients for a mean of 17.7 hours—a median of 19.4 hours per day. To a statistically significant degree, survival in COT was better after years 2 and 3 of the follow-up, according to the Data Safety Monitoring Board, because of a clear-cut survival outcome. The difference was not apparent after 1 year. This resulted in premature termination of the study.

Better survival was achieved in patients who had improvement in pulmonary artery pressures, but the reduction in pressures was small.[23] A study of the pulmonary vasculature of lungs at autopsy showed changes in the intima and muscular hypertrophy of medium and small pulmonary arteries that did not relate to the level of pulmonary pressure recorded during life or response to oxygen during life.[24] These differences in survival could have been due to the method or the duration of oxygen therapy or both. Exercise results in an increase in cardiac output and increased oxygen delivery to tissues during exercise with oxygen.

There was also a delay in improvement in brain function in the NOTT study,[25] as demonstrated by Wechsler Performance IQ and brain-age quotient. Both of these indicators of mental capacity improved similarly with COT and NOT; however, a continued improvement occurred over the following 12 months with COT (Figures 2 and 3). Probably a more sustained improvement by COT in tissue oxygen delivery led to restoration of oxygen fractions.

This raises the question about the mechanism(s) of delayed improvement. It may be that neurons that are suppressed by hypoxemia have improved function from prolonged improvement in oxygen delivery. This may be akin to "stunned" myocardium.

Both the NOTT study and a study by the British Medical Research Council (MRC), which compared 15 hours of oxygen with no oxygen, showed a delay before a survival benefit was found. In the MRC study, the survival benefit occurred after 500 days of 15 hours per day of oxygen treatment.[21] This again suggests that a slow restoration of function was due to improved oxygen delivery to the organs.

In an attempt to learn more about the factors associated with survival from COT compared with NOT, a retrospective analysis of the NOTT study was undertaken.[22] Daily walking distance, as measured by a calibrated pedometer, was used during the 3 weeks of intensive pulmonary rehabilitation in

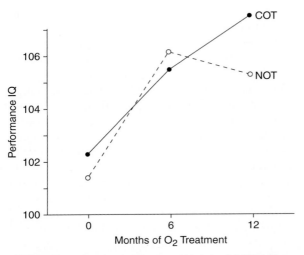

FIGURE 2. Performance IQ from the Wechsler Adult Intelligence Scale in relation to duration of continuous (COT) versus nocturnal (NOT) oxygen therapy in chronic obstructive pulmonary disease patients.

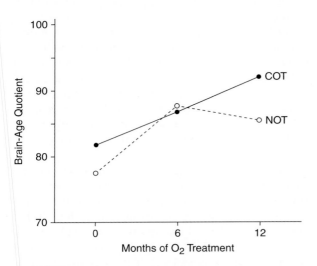

FIGURE 3. Change in "fluid intelligence" (brain-age quotient) in relation to continuous (COT) versus nocturnal (NOT) oxygen treatment in chronic obstructive pulmonary disease patients.

most patients prior to randomization in the NOTT study. Pedometry recordings were available in 157 of the 203 patients randomized. Through reanalysis of the original magnetic data tapes, it was possible to divide patients into a low-walking and a high-walking group by separating the patients at the median walking distance achieved at the end of 3 weeks. The initial division of the patients by walking level was at a median of 3,590 feet, but this yielded groups that were not well matched by age. The low-walking group was approximately 5 years older than the high-walking group. To compensate for this difference, each low-walking patient was manually matched with a high-walking patient of similar age, and treatment group (COT vs NOT) was also matched, including by baseline forced expiratory volume in 1 second (FEV_1).

The 80 matched patients were the subjects of further analysis. The resulting low- and high-walking groups of 40 patients each were further divided into COT and NOT groups. Data from this reexamination were analyzed by the methods of Kaplan and Meier. Statistical significance was detected by the method of Cox. Survival results were analyzed by analysis of variance. This shows that the best survival was in the high-walking NOTT patients compared with the low-walking NOT patients. These differences were statistically significant ($p = .01$) in two other groups, that is, the intermediate survival of low-walking COT and high-walking NOT. The hospital data in the study used both matched and unmatched data and show that the lowest length of stay in admissions per year was in the high walking by oxygen group ($p = .05$ and .01, respectively).

Together, the 1980 NOTT study and its reanalysis provide a scientific basis for the use of ambulatory oxygen to promote conditioning and improve the restoration of function of various tissues throughout the body. These studies also provide the basis for further prospective studies aimed at determining the ideal patient for ambulatory oxygen, taking into account new long-acting bronchodilators and inhaled corticosteroid drugs, which were not available during the conduction of the NOTT.

National Health and Nutrition Examination Survey

The National Center for Health Statistics conducted the first National Health and Nutrition Examination Study (NHANES I) from 1971 to 1975. This was a survey of a probability sample of the civilian noninstitutionalized population of the United States.[26] Spirometric criteria for obstructive and restrictive lung disease in 5,542 subjects in which spirometry was performed were reviewed. Late analysis of outcome of participants followed for up to 22 years revealed that 1,301 deaths occurred in the 5,542 adults in the cohort (23.4%). When adjusted for proportional hazards, the presence of severe and moderate COPD was associated with a higher risk of death than with normal spirometry, with a hazard ratio of 2.7.[27]

In a more recent study designed to estimate the current magnitude of obstructive lung disease in the United States, a second analysis was made of the Third National Health and Nutrition Examination Study (NHANES III). This study aimed to determine the proportion of the population that had obstructive lung disease and respiratory symptoms.[28] Overall, 6.8% of the population had low lung function and 8.5% of the population reported obstructive lung disease (patient report).

Obstructive lung disease was reported in 12.5% of current smokers, 9.4% of former smokers, and 3.1% of pipe smokers. Obstructive lung disease was diagnosed in 5.8% of never-smokers. It was striking that 63.3% of the subjects documented with low lung function had no previous or current reported diagnosis of obstructive lung disease.[28] Thus, this large population had eluded a diagnosis and was not being treated.

These and other studies led to the creation of a national strategy for the prevention, management, and research of COPD, an original initiative of the National Heart, Lung, and Blood Institute.[29] Ultimately, this initiative became known as the National Lung Health Education Program (NLHEP) and focused on early diagnosis and intervention.[30] A spin-off of this workshop led to the establishment of the Global Initiative for Chronic Obstructive Lung Disease (GOLD).[31–33] The GOLD offers guidelines on staging and management of chronic obstructive lung disease and focuses, as its designation states, on the global problem. Collectively, these studies, along with the Lung Health Study, form the basis for efforts in early identification and intervention to prevent or forestall the development of premature morbidity and mortality from COPD,[34–37] soon to be the world's third most common cause of death.

Systemic Effects of COPD

The rather recent recognition of systemic inflammation and peripheral muscle dysfunction as components of COPD[38–40] echoes Roger Mitchell's 1958 remark that "emphysema may prove to be a syndrome with several different and probably overlapping causes."[5] Dr. Celli wrote in a recent editorial, "We are witnessing a change in the COPD paradigm from a simple problem of airflow limitation to a multicomponent disease where the other manifestations may become targets of interventions. Unfortunately, the regulatory agencies, the medical public at large, and many in our midst still cling to the old concept that it is only by changing FEV that we modify the disease."[41] Yet it is clear that COPD patients have cardiovascular comorbidities, which are a major cause of death.[42] Mancini and colleagues recently hypothesized that medications currently associated with cardiovascular risk reduction might impact the clinical outcome of COPD patients.[43] The authors explored this potential impact by interrogating population databases. The first results of these databases examination justify the design and conduct of prospective trials using cardiovascular active drugs.

References

1. Petty TL. The history of COPD. J COPD 2006;1:3–14.
2. Snider GL. Emphysema. The first two centuries and beyond: a historical overview, with suggestions for future research. Part 1. Am Rev Respir Dis 1992;146:1334–44.
3. Snider GL. Emphysema. The first two centuries—and beyond; a historical overview, with suggestions for future research. Part 2. Am Rev Respir Dis 1992;146:1615–22.
4. Voelkel NF. Historical overview of emphysema, In: Voelkel NF, MacNee W, editors. Chronic obstructive lung diseases. Hamilton (ON): BC Decker; 2002. p. 1–6.
5. Symposium on Emphysema and the "Chronic Bronchitis" Syndrome, Aspen, Colorado, June 13-15, 1958. Am Rev Respir Dis 1959;80:1–213.
6. Pierce JA. Lung scleroproteins. In: Schraufnagel DE, editor. "I remember…": reflections on the American Thoracic Society's first century. American Thoracic Society: New York, 2005. p. 40–3.
7. Orsos F. Die Gerüstsysteme der Lunge und desen physiologische und pathologische Bedeutung. Beitr Klin Tuberk 1936;87:568.
8. Eriksson S. Pulmonary emphysema and α-1-antitrypsin deficiency. Acta Med Scand 1964;175:197–205.
9. Kelleher CM, Silverman EK, Broekelmann T, et al. A functional mutation in the terminal exon of elastin in severe, early-onset chronic obstructive pulmonary disease. Am J Respir Cell Mol Biol 2005;33:355–62.
10. Houghton AM, Quintero PA, Perkins DL, et al. Elastin fragments drive disease progression in a murine model of emphysema. J Clin Invest 2006;116:753–9.
11. Hogg JC, Chu F, Utokaparch S, et al. The nature of small-airway obstruction in chronic obstructive pulmonary disease. N Engl J Med 2004;350:2645–53.
12. Alexander AF. Chronic alveolar emphysema in the horse. Am Rev Respir Dis 1959;80 Suppl:141.
13. Foley FD, Lowell FC. Equine centrilobular emphysema. With further observations on the pathology of heaves. Am Rev Respir Dis 1966;93:17–21.
14. Agusti A, MacNee W, Donaldson K, et al. Hypothesis: does COPD have an autoimmune component? Thorax 2003;58:832–4
15. Auerbach O, Stout AP, Hammond EC, et al. Smoking habits and age in relation to pulmonary changes: rupture of alveolar septums; fibrosis and thickening of walls of small arteries and arterioles. N Engl J Med 1963;269:1045–54.
16. Auerbach O, Cuyler Hammond E, Garfinkel L, Benante C. Relation of smoking and age to emphysema. N Engl J Med 1972;300:853–7.
17. Auerbach O, Garfinkel L, Hammond EC. Relation of smoking and age to findings in lung parenchyma: a microscopic study. Chest 1974;65:29–35.
18. Mitchell RS, Vincent TN, Filley GF. Cigarette smoking, chronic bronchitis, and emphysema. JAMA 1964;188:12–6.
19. Fletcher C, Peto R. The natural history of chronic airflow obstruction. Br Med J 1977;1:1645–8.
20. Nocturnal Oxygen Therapy Trial Group. Continuous or nocturnal oxygen therapy in hypoxemic chronic obstruction lung disease: a clinical trial. Ann Intern Med 1980;93:391–8.
21. Report of the Medical Research Council Working Party. Long term domiciliary oxygen therapy in chronic hypoxic cor pulmonale complicating chronic bronchitis and emphysema. Lancet 1981;1(8222):681–6.
22. Petty TL, Bliss PL. Ambulatory oxygen therapy, exercise and survival with advanced chronic obstructive pulmonary disease (The Nocturnal Oxygen Therapy Trial Revisited). Respir Care 2000;45:204–13.
23. Timms RM, Khaja FU, Williams GW. Hemodynamic response to oxygen therapy in chronic obstructive pulmonary disease. Ann Intern Med 1985;102:29–36.
24. Wright JL, Petty TL, Thurlbeck WM. Analysis of the structure of the muscular pulmonary arteries in patients with pulmonary hypertension and COPD: National Institutes of Health Nocturnal Oxygen Therapy Trial. Lung 1992;170:109–24
25. Grant I, Heaton RK, McSweeny AJ, et al. Neuropsychologic findings in hypoxemic chronic obstructive pulmonary disease. Arch Intern Med 1982;142:1470–6.

26. National Center for Health Statistics. Plan and operation of the Health and Nutrition Examination Survey, United States. 1971–1973. Washington (DC): National Center for Health Statistics; 1973.

27. Mannino DM, Gagnon RC, Petty TL, Lydick E. Obstructive lung disease and low lung function in adults in the United States. Arch Intern Med 2000;160:1683–9.

28. Mannino DM, Buist AS, Petty TL, et al. Chronic obstructive pulmonary disease. Lung function and mortality in the United States: data from the First National Health and Nutrition Examination Survey follow up study. Thorax 2003;58:1–6.

29. Petty TL, Weinmann GG. Building a national strategy for the prevention and management of and research in chronic obstructive pulmonary disease. JAMA 1997;277:246–53.

30. Petty TL, editor. Strategies in preserving lung health and preventing COPD and associated diseases. The National Lung Health Education Program (NLHEP). Chest 1998;113:123S–63S.

31. Pauwels RA, Buist AS, Ma P, et al. GOLD Scientific Committee: global strategy for the diagnosis, management, and prevention of chronic obstructive pulmonary disease: National Heart, Lung, and Blood Institute and World Health Organization Global Initiative for Chronic Obstructive Lung Disease (GOLD): executive summary. Respir Care 2001;46:798–825.

32. Global Initiative for Chronic Obstructive Lung Disease. 2004 Global strategy for diagnosis, management of chronic obstructive pulmonary disease. NHLBI workshop report 2003. Available at: <http://www.goldcopd.com> (accessed October 7, 2005).

33. Pauwels RA, Buist AS, Calverley PM, et al. Global strategy for the diagnosis, management, and prevention of chronic obstructive pulmonary disease. NHLBI/WHO Global Initiative for Obstructive Lung Disease (GOLD) workshop summary. Am J Respir Crit Care Med 2001;163:1256–76.

34. Anthonisen NR, Connett JE, Kiley JP, et al. Effects of smoking intervention and the use of an inhaled anticholinergic bronchodilator on the rate of decline of FEV1: the Lung Health Study. JAMA 1994;272:1497–505.

35. Anthonisen NR, Skeans MA, Wise RA, et al. The effect of a smoking cessation intervention on 14.5-year mortality. A randomized clinical trial. Ann Intern Med 2005;142:233–9.

36. Baudiouin SV, Bott J, Ward A, et al. Short term effect of oxygen on renal haemodynamics in patients with hypoxaemic chronic obstructive airways disease. Thorax 1992;47:550–4.

37. Martinez FJ, Foster G, Curtis JL, et al, for the NETT Research Group. Predictors of mortality in patients with emphysema and severe airflow obstruction. Am J Respir Crit Care Med 2006;173:1326–34.

38. Agustì A. Systemic effects of chronic obstructive pulmonary disease. Proc Am Thorac Soc 2005;2:365–9.

39. Sin DD, Man SF. Skeletal muscle weakness reduced exercise tolerance and COPD: is systemic inflammation the missing link? Thorax 2006;61:1–3.

40. Pinto-Plata VM, Livnat G, Girish M, et al. Systemic cytokines, clinical and physiological changes in patients hospitalized for exacerbation of COPD. Chest 2007;131:37–43.

41. Celli BR. Predicting mortality in chronic obstructive pulmonary disease: chasing the "Holy Grail." Am J Respir Crit Care Med 2006;173:1298–9.

42. Sin DD, Authonisen NR, Soriano JB, Agusti AG. Mortality in COPD: role of co-morbidities. Eur Respir J 2006;28:1245–57.

43. Mancini J, Etminan M, Zhang B, et al. Reduction of morbidity and mortality by statins, angiotensin-converting enzyme inhibitors, and angiotensin receptor blockers in patients with chronic obstructive pulmonary disease. J Am Coll Cardiol 2006;47:1–6.

CHAPTER 2

LUNG DEVELOPMENT

SARAH A. GEBB, PHD, AND JOHN TORDAY, MSC, PHD

LUNG ORGANOGENESIS IN THE HUMAN is initiated 4 weeks postconception when the foregut endoderm is induced to push into the surrounding mesenchyme. Thereafter, a series of programmed branching events give rise to the conducting airways, bronchi, and bronchioles and, ultimately, the functional gas exchange unit of the lung, the alveoli. Numerous external stimuli have been shown to disrupt this program, leading to impaired lung development and compromised lung function. This chapter reviews the stages of lung development and our current understanding of the mediators of normal lung growth and development.

Epithelial Branching and Differentiation

Based largely on the characteristic progression of epithelial growth and differentiation, lung development is classically divided into five stages: embryonic, pseudoglandular, canalicular, saccular, and alveolar (Figure 1).[1–3] In humans, the first four stages of lung development normally occur in utero, and the majority of the alveoli are formed postnatally. Rodents, in contrast, are born during the fourth stage, the saccular phase. Despite this difference, both the rat and the mouse serve as important models for lung developmental studies.[4] Early in development, the primitive lung during the embryonic phase appears as an outgrowth from the ventral surface of the foregut endoderm. This primordial lung bud then divides, branching laterally, and gives rise to two epithelial tubules that will ultimately form the mainstem bronchi and the distinct lobular regions of the lung. Thereafter, progressive stereotypic branching of the two primary epithelial tubules forms the bronchi, bronchioles, and terminal bronchioles through the pseudoglandular phase (Figure 2, A and C). In midgestation, the canalicular stage is marked by increased

terminal airway complexity, formation of the respiratory bronchioles, appearance of terminal saccules at the ends of the respiratory bronchioles, and limited differentiation of type I and type II pneumocytes (Figure 3A). Toward the end of this stage (approximately 20 to 22 weeks' gestation), some degree of gas exchange becomes possible. However, the number and efficiency of the gas exchange units increase markedly during the last two stages of lung development, the saccular and alveolar stages, which involve an increase in the

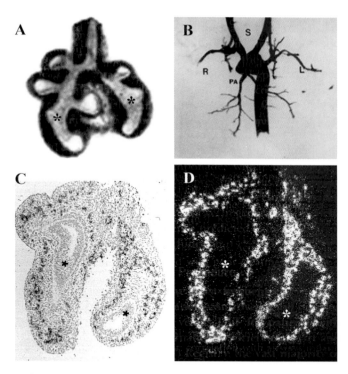

FIGURE 2. Lung epithelial and vascular morphogenesis in the pseudo-glandular lung. (*A*) Photograph of the early pseudoglandular lung (rat, gestational day 13). (*B*) Mercox cast of pseudoglandular lung vasculature (mouse gestational day 12, roughly equivalent to rat gestational day 13). (*C*) and (*D*) Bright- and dark-field images of a lung section localizing developing vascular networks within the pseudoglandular lung (rat, gestational day 13). In situ hybridization, black (bright field) or white (dark field) areas localize cells expressing messenger ribonucleic acid for the endothelial cell–specific vascular endothelial growth factor receptor 2 (VEGFR-2, also known as KDR or Flk-1). The *asterisk* marks the developing airways. Adapted from deMello and colleagues[7] and Gebb and Shannon.[6]

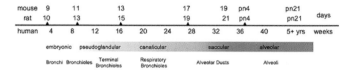

FIGURE 1. Stages of fetal and neonatal lung development in humans and rodents. Human lung development is initiated 4 weeks postconception and continues postnatally for at least 5 years. Although the timing of rodent lung morphogenesis is much shorter, the characteristic branching and differentiation events are similar, making rodent models suitable for general lung development studies.

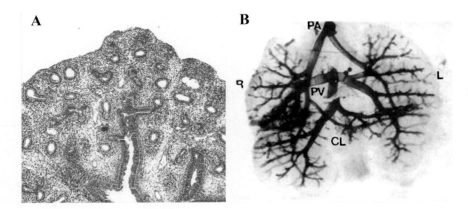

FIGURE 3. Lung epithelial and vascular morphogenesis in the canalicular lung. (*A*) Hematoxylin and eosin–stained lung section (rat, gestational day 16). (*B*) Mercox cast of canalicular lung vasculature (mouse gestational day 14, roughly equivalent to rat gestational day 16). Adapted from deMello and colleagues.[7]

functional gas exchange surface area and maturation of the epithelial and mesenchymal cells within this region.

The saccular phase is marked by an increase in the number of terminal saccules, as well as thinning of the epithelial cells of the distal epithelium (termed type I pneumocytes) and apposition of the endothelial and epithelial cells, which establishes the air-blood barrier (Figure 4A). Type II pneumocytes mature to some extent during the saccular stage and are capable of producing surfactant, although premature neonates born during this stage of development often require exogenous surfactant. The viability and therapeutic requirements of premature neonates vary because the rate of lung development in a given fetus tends to vary slightly. The progression of lung development can be assessed to some extent in utero, and therapies can be designed accordingly. The alveolar stage in humans begins in utero at approximately 32 weeks and extends postnatally well beyond 4 years of age. During this stage, ridge-like projections termed secondary septa extend into the saccule lumen, which further subdivide the saccule and markedly increase the gas exchange surface area of the lung (Figure 5). The type I epithelial cells and interstitial cells that comprise the alveolar walls thin remarkably, and endothelial cells are found in close apposition to the type I cells, which reduces the air-blood barrier to an even greater extent and maximizes the efficiency of gas exchange. Surfactant production by the type II pneumocytes increases exponentially 2 weeks prior to parturition and is maintained in the postnatal lung. At this stage, a fully functional gas exchange unit is present and the lung is well suited to transition normally from the in utero environment to the neonatal state. The end result of this process is a surface area of approximately 70 m^2 for gas exchange.

Pulmonary Vascular Development

Throughout lung development, the branching lung epithelium is surrounded by tissue of mesodermal origin. This mesenchymal tissue compartment gives rise to cells comprising the pulmonary vasculature, including endothelial cells, vascular smooth muscle cells, pericytes, and fibroblasts, as well as airway smooth muscle cells.[5] Endothelial cells and endothelial networks are present in the mesenchyme adjacent to the epithelium, when lung epithelial branching begins.[6] Although somewhat controversial, it is thought that the pulmonary vascular bed arises via two processes, angiogenesis (sprouting of vessels from preexisting vessels) and vasculogenesis (de novo synthesis of vessels from pluripotent mesenchymal precursors).[7] In the pseudoglandular lung, a few primary vessel sprouts extend from the pulmonary artery into the mesenchyme and follow the branching epithelium. At this stage, these central vessels are connected to the heart and are patent, as evidenced by Mercox casting of rodent lungs (Figure 2B). A second population of endothelial cells and/or their precursors are detected in the periphery; however, few seem to be connected to the angiogenic network sprouting from the pulmonary artery (see Figure 2, C and D). The canalicular stage marks a phase of intense vascular proliferation; both central and peripheral vascular networks increase in number and complexity, but flow through the pulmonary circulation remains low owing to shunting through the ductus arteriosus. Despite increased connectivity between the central (angiogenic) and peripheral (vasculogenic) vascular networks, a sparse number of distal networks are perfused (Figure 3B). These data may underestimate the number of distal vessels that are perfused because the casting medium is viscous and may not effectively fill all small peripheral vessels. Despite this fact, later in gestation, as the lung enters the saccular phase, the casting medium fills the vast majority of the peripheral vessels (see Figure 4C). The pulmonary vasculature transforms radically at birth with the first breath, when the pulmonary circulation dilates and the full volume of the right heart ejection fraction is passed through the lungs to be oxygenated. Postnatally, the distal lung vasculature continues to expand exponentially, matching the increase in distal airspace characteristic of alveolarization (Figure 5).

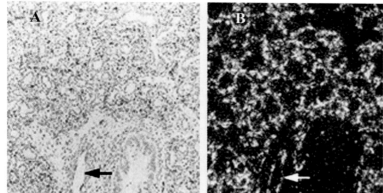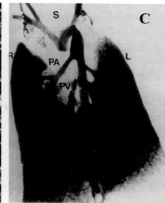

FIGURE 4. Lung epithelial and vascular morphogenesis in the saccular lung. (*A*) and (*B*) Bright- and dark-field images of a lung section localizing developing vascular networks in the lung. In situ hybridization, black (bright field) or white (dark field) areas localize cells expressing messenger ribonucleic acid for the endothelial cell–specific vascular endothelial growth factor receptor 2. The *arrow* indicates endothelial lining of a large muscularized vessel adjacent to an airway. (*C*) Mercox cast of vasculature showing extensive filling of distal pulmonary vasculature. Adapted from deMello and colleagues[7] and Gebb and Shannon.[6]

Whether the central and peripheral lung vascular networks arise from the same or different endothelial precursor populations remains unclear. Endothelial cells isolated from central vessels (large, muscular arteries) versus peripheral vessels (small amuscular arterioles and/or capillaries) display distinct phenotypes, and many of these characteristics are maintained *in vitro*.[8] Although it has been determined that the context or environment in which a cell resides strongly influences cell phenotype, how this information becomes imprinted on the cell and is maintained when the cell is removed from this environment is uncertain. It is clear, however, that the developing lung vasculature is profoundly influenced by environmental cues, including epithelial signaling, cell–cell matrix interactions, and mechanical forces. As with the growth and maturation of the epithelium, the vascular bed is dependent on complex signaling mechanisms that are exquisitely regulated spatially and temporally throughout development (Figure 5).

Tissue Interactions

Interactions between the epithelial and mesenchymal tissue compartments are required for normal lung development, and disruption of these interactions can profoundly alter lung morphogenesis.[9,10] In the absence of mesenchyme, epithelium fails to branch, and expression of lung-specific messenger ribonucleic acids, for example, encoding surfactant protein C, is lost.[11] Conversely, absent of epithelium, mesenchymal cells apoptose, and the once present vascular networks disappear.[6] These epithelial–mesenchymal interactions are critical during all stages of lung development and are certainly important for maintenance of normal lung homeostasis in the adult lung.[12]

Although chronic obstructive pulmonary disease (COPD) is traditionally considered an airways disease, the vasculature is profoundly affected as well.[13] The reciprocal interactions between the airways and vessels established during development continue in the mature lung and serve to maintain normal lung structure and function. It is no surprise then that apoptosis, inflammation, proteolysis, and fibrosis that compromise airway homeostasis also radically alter pulmonary vascular stability and function. In fact, studies designed to target the mature lung vascular endothelium using the vascular endothelial growth factor (VEGF) receptor inhibitor SU5416 caused endothelial cell apoptosis and induced enlargement of the distal air gas exchange units.[14] These studies raise the possibility that the pulmonary vascular dysfunction may lead to compromised airway function in a subpopulation of those suffering from COPD. At the very least, these studies suggest that therapies for COPD should be directed at ameliorating both airway and vascular demise.

Transgenic Mice for Lung Development Studies

Classic developmental biology approaches have shaped the framework of our knowledge of lung development. Traditional anatomic and fate mapping studies provided information on embryonic origins of lung tissue and detailed descriptions of endodermal and mesodermal tissue morphogenesis. Fetal lung explant culture has been used extensively to study factors governing branching, differentiation, proliferation, and epithelial-mesenchymal signaling and has the advantage of maintaining many of the cell–cell and cell–matrix interactions that are present *in vivo* but lost with traditional single-cell culture and coculture approaches. Relatively recent advances in transgenic technology have markedly advanced our understanding of the lung developmental process at the molecular and cellular levels.[15] Isolation and cloning of the surfactant protein C gene promoter have provided the means to express genes of interest in distal lung

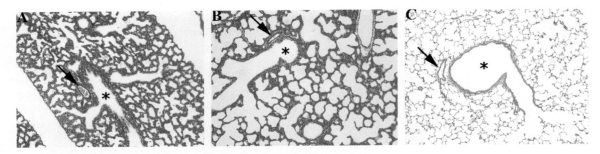

FIGURE 5. Perinatal and neonatal lung development (rodent). Late-gestation lung is fluid filled and characterized by numerous thick-walled septae (*A*). At birth, saccules remain thick walled (*B*) but rapidly transition to thin-walled highly efficient gas exchange units (*C*). *Arrows* mark central blood vessels adjacent to large airways (*asterisk*).

epithelial cells of the developing mouse fetus. Using this transgenic technology, gene expression in the fetal lung can be manipulated; thus, the consequences of ablation or misexpression of a factor can be studied *in vivo*.[16] The promoter region of the Clara cell secretory protein has been used in a similar fashion to express target genes in the proximal airway cells. Bi- and tritransgenic approaches have used these promoters to drive expression of the reverse tetracycline transactivator, in combination with Cre-recombinase (or another gene of choice), driven by the tetracycline operon and cytomegalovirus promoter. Thus, gene ablation or overexpression can be regulated in the lung epithelium in a time-specific manner. Although this technology is not without limitations, our understanding of the molecular signaling events central to lung development have advanced remarkably with the advent of this technology. It is clear that this approach will be used in future studies to investigate the mediators of development and disease.

Transcription Factors

Coordinate regulation of transcription dictates the progression of lung growth and differentiation as well as lung homeostasis and host defense. Transcription factors govern cell form and function by regulating expression of ligands, receptors, extracellular matrix (ECM), cell signaling molecules, and transcription factors themselves. Studies have identified over 100 transcription factors directly involved in one or more aspects of pulmonary growth and development.[17,18] Numerous transcription factors, including those from the homeobox, forkhead box (Fox), zinc finger, SMA/mothers against decapentaplegic (SMAD), and basic helix-loop-helix (bHLH) families, are involved during the early phases of embryogenesis and then again during distinct stages of lung morphogenesis. To date, no lung-specific transcription factor has been identified. Rather, subsets of transcription factors interact cooperatively to specify numerous aspects of lung morphogenesis, such as epithelial branching, epithelial/mesenchymal differentiation, and surfactant protein expression.

Formation of the early lung and other organs derived from the foregut is governed in part by expression of the transcription factors thyroid transcription factor 1 (TTF-1 or Nkx2.1), hepatocyte nuclear factor 3β (HNF-3β), GATA-6, and the forkhead box transcription factor Foxa2 within the endodermally derived epithelium.[19–25] These transcription factors coordinately regulate expression of numerous proteins, which, in turn, act to further modulate growth and differentiation of the developing epithelium and adjacent mesenchyme. It is important to mention that many of the same transcription factors that regulate lung specification also play key roles throughout lung morphogenesis, acting in concert to direct expression of factors that ultimately dictate proximodistal epithelial differentiation and expression of surfactant proteins. Certainly, in the mature adult lung, these transcription factors are also required to maintain normal lung structure and function; thus, perhaps the loss of one or more of these transcription factors may contribute to disrupted lung homeostasis, as in the case of COPD. Further, environmental insults (such as cigarette smoke) can activate stress response and inflammatory transcription elements such as nuclear factor κB (NF-κB), activator protein 1 (AP-1), and the early growth response gene 1 (*Egr1*).[26,27]

Growth Factors

Growth and differentiation factors initiate paracrine and autocrine signaling through their membrane-associated receptors and mediate diverse aspects of lung morphogenesis, including epithelial cell branching and differentiation, vasculogenesis, angiogenesis, and vascular maturation. Growth factors, their receptors, and inhibitors play an important role in epithelial mesenchymal signaling and contribute to the program of lung branching and specification of cell phenotypes in both tissue compartments. Like the transcription factors that function coordinately to direct the program of lung development, complex collections of growth factors signal through broad and varied intracellular cascades to mediate processes such as branching, tube formation, and phenotypes.

The fibroblast growth factor (FGF) family of signaling peptides and cognate transmembrane tyrosine kinase receptors regulate numerous aspects of lung morphogenesis throughout development. More than 20 distinct signaling molecules belong to the FGF family, and at least 6 have definitive roles in lung development. FGF10, through its receptor FGFR2, plays a central role in branching morphogenesis; it is expressed in the distal lung mesenchyme and signals budding and branching in the adjacent epithelium.[28] FGF-induced signaling is negatively regulated by Sprouty2 (Spry2), a signaling molecule that antagonizes FGF signaling by binding FGF effector molecules.[29] In this manner, Spry can limit FGF-induced budding and branching of the epithelium and regulate the pattern of lung branching. FGF1 (acidic FGF) and FGF7 (also known as keratinocyte growth factor [KGF]) appear to stimulate epithelial growth and are important in both the developing lung and lung repair. FGF2, which together with FGF1 was the first of the FGF family to be identified and tested, is an endothelial cell mitogen and a more potent angiogenic factor than either VEGF or platelet-derived growth factor (PDGF). In contrast to the role that FGF10 plays in early lung morphogenesis, FGF18 appears to be important late in gestation and in the postnatal lung. FGF18 is associated with the formation of secondary septae and modulates myo-fibroblast proliferation and elastogenesis.[30] Many members of the FGF family play key roles in lung development and appear to be important mediators of epithelial mesenchymal crosstalk; thus, it is likely that dysregulated signaling within this family of peptides also plays into the pathogenesis of COPD.

The transforming growth factor β (TGF-β) superfamily includes the TGF-β and bone morphogenetic peptide (BMP) subfamilies, important modulators of lung growth and development.[31–33] TGF-β 1, 2, and 3 are all found in the lung throughout development, and balanced regulation of TGF-β signaling is critical for normal lung morphogenesis. Beyond the classic immunosuppressive role of TGF-β, these signaling peptides regulate deposition of ECM proteins such as tenascin-C, collagen, and elastin. TGF-βs also exert an antiproliferative effect on cells of epithelial origin and thus are thought to be important negative regulators of epithelial branching. Null mutations of TGF-β 1, 2, or 3 are lethal at varied developmental time points; however, of these null mutants, TGF-β3 is the only mutant with an overt lung phenotype, and these animals die neonatally with lung dysplasia and cleft palate.[34,35] Lung hypoplasia also results from increased lung TGF-β expression. These studies indicate that TGF-β is keenly regulated, and normal lung morphogenesis is dependent on expression of the proper physiologic quantity and appropriate spatial and temporal patterning.

VEGF regulates endothelial cell differentiation, proliferation, and homeostasis. It is required for normal embryonic growth and development, and loss of a single allele is lethal to the fetus.[36,37] VEGF is expressed in the early lung in both the mesenchyme and the epithelium but is expressed most strongly by the epithelium as lung development progresses. The primary endothelial receptors flk-1 and flt-1 are found in a subpopulation of lung mesenchymal cells at every stage of lung development; acting through these receptors, VEGF mediates vascularization.[38] Overexpression of VEGF in the lung epithelium causes lung dysplasia, suggesting that the quantity of VEGF is critical.[39] VEGF also plays an important role in lung injury repair, and disruption of this pathway leads to alveolar destruction.[14] As indicated previously, it has become apparent that the vasculature is also a target in COPD, and as such, the VEGF signaling cascade is a focal point for investigation.

Extracellular Matrix

Signaling events initiated by the various growth factors, morphogens, and cell–cell interactions mentioned above are further modified locally by the tissue microenvironment, thus providing a means to regulate tissue morphogenesis in a spatially distinct manner.[40] The ECM is an integral part of the local tissue milieu, serving to control cell shape, regulate migration, and modify growth factor and morphogen signaling. The ECM is a complex network of proteins, glycoproteins, and proteoglycans, and its composition varies from tissue to tissue and as a function of specialized cellular response. The ECM contribution to tissue development and homeostasis extends well beyond its traditional role as a passive structural component for tissue organization. The ECM acts dynamically to modulate a wide variety of developmental processes, including cell proliferation, migration, and differentiation. Cell–ECM interactions dictate cell shape and fate and can modify growth factor responses. Further, certain ECM components can engage and signal via specific growth factor receptors. The spectrum of form and functional roles places the ECM centrally in the process of lung morphogenesis.

Expression of numerous ECM components and their integrin receptors has been studied in the developing lung. Redundancies exist in and among the ECM and corresponding cell surface receptors, and null mutations of individual ECM components often yield viable offspring that lack overt pathologic manifestations. Despite this fact, important developmental roles for the ECM have been identified. Collagen, laminin, elastin, and tenascin-C are important for branching, tube formation, septation, and maintenance of tissue interactions.[41,42] Dysregulated ECM catabolism plays a central role in the pathogenesis of COPD, and this has long been appreciated.[43,44] The knowledge gained with regard to the role of the ECM in lung development can be used to design therapies directed at not only preventing further destruction but also regrowth of functional airspaces. Reestablishing an ECM of proper composition and stability should not only stem the tide of lung destruction but will also provide a normal environment for repair and an affable stem cell niche.

Stem Cells

The role of stem cells in lung development and repair is a subject of intense study (see also Chapter 29). Without question, cells with the capacity to proliferate and repopulate the pulmonary epithelium in the setting of lung injury and normal repair reside within certain lung cell populations, as well as possibly in the bone marrow.[45–47] In the adult lung, resident stem cells include the alveolar type II pneumocyte and the Clara cell, as well as a recently described population of primitive adult precursor cells termed the side population cells. Origins of pulmonary vascular stem cells are less well understood, but cells of bone marrow origin can apparently seed the pulmonary vasculature. Because even adult stem cells are of embryonic origin, the possibility exists that stress or injury during the critical period of lung development may damage certain critical stem cell populations. This damage may be manifest in disrupted development or may not be apparent until much later in life when subjected to a "second hit" (chronic inflammation owing to cigarette smoke). Identifying stem cell populations and their susceptibility to fetal and neonatal stressors provides an opportunity to identify individuals most prone to lung developmental disorders, as well as adult lung diseases such as COPD.

Oxygen Tension

The lung develops at low oxygen tension (3–5% O_2, 27 mm Hg) in utero and transitions precipitously at birth to air breathing, whereupon it is required, for the first time, to oxygenate the blood now coursing through the lung vasculature. It is now appreciated that the low oxygen environment of the fetus plays a central role in maintaining normal lung morphogenesis. Recently, van Tuyl and colleagues showed that fetal lung epithelial branching and vascularization are increased at 3% O_2.[48] In this model, inhibition of vascularization markedly reduced hypoxia-induced epithelial branching, suggesting that low oxygen stimulates vascular morphogenesis, and this, in turn, enhances epithelial growth and differentiation. Other *in-vitro* studies further support the notion that the low oxygen environment of the fetus is important for normal lung development. In a similar lung explant model, low oxygen tension suppressed matrix metalloproteinase activity, thereby enhancing deposition of ECM proteins, including tenascin-C.[49] In this case, inhibition of tenascin-C expression reduced the hypoxia-induced lung branching. This normal low oxygen environment is disrupted in infants born prematurely and in some cases may have pathologic consequences. Despite surfactant therapy and improved ventilator regimens, premature neonates often develop bronchopulmonary dysplasia, which is characterized by alveolar simplification, pulmonary capillary dysmorphogenesis, and persistent interstitial hypercellularity.

The Evolving Lung

The theory that ontogeny recapitulates phylogeny was championed by Ernst Haeckel at the turn of the nineteenth century, and although it has been discredited in its strictest form, the central concept remains informative. Today, the idea that an organism's embryologic development reflects its evolutionary history is one of the basic principles of the evolutionary developmental biology approach being used in developmental and evolutionary studies alike. Gene regulatory networks can be compared across phyla and during development, yielding information about the evolutionary origins of embryonic structures such as the lung. Using this approach, the parathyroid hormone–related protein (PTHrP) signaling network has been identified as a model pathway that is conserved evolutionarily and is required for lung development, repair, and homeostasis.[50] PTHrP signals from the epithelium to the mesenchyme and controls alveolar type II cell differentiation and surfactant production. Null mutation of the PTHrP protein disrupts alveolarization and results in an "evolutionarily" immature lung. Across phyla, from the swim bladder in the fish to the mammalian lung, the complexity of the lung increases, reflecting the evolution of the gas exchange unit. By analogy, diseases such as COPD that are characterized by simplification of distal structures may represent a "devolution" of the lung.

Conclusion

A more complete understanding of the complex processes governing lung development will contribute to our understanding of COPD, its causes, and potential therapeutic approaches. The signaling networks involved in development, such as normal injury and repair processes, are exquisitely regulated at multiple levels. Where, when, how, and why these events go awry either during development or repair is unclear; however, we do know that information in one arena sheds light on the dark corners of the other. It is clear that normal lung morphogenesis is dependent on appropriate spatial and temporal expression of transcription factors and paracrine and autocrine signaling cascades. The expression and signaling of these molecules are refined and edited by the local environment (eg, cell–cell and cell–matrix interactions as well as oxygen tension). Lung homeostasis is dependent on similar interactions and on balanced expression of many of the same molecules. With an accurate map of the lung developmental process in hand, we could, in theory, redirect a program of appropriate and balanced lung development (repair) in the chronically injured lung.

References

1. Boyden EA. Development and growth of the airways. In: Hodson WA, editor. Development of the lung. New York: Marcel Dekker;1977. p. 3–35.
2. Harding R. Respiratory system. In: Harding R and Bocking AD, editors. Fetal growth and development. Cambridge (UK): Cambridge University Press;2001. pp. 114–36.
3. Larsen WJ. Human embryology. New York: Churchill Livingstone;1993.
4. Hogan BL, Grindley J, Bellusci S, et al. Branching morphogenesis of the lung: new models for a classical problem. Cold Spring Harb Symp Quant Biol 1997;62:249–56.
5. Hislop A. Developmental biology of the pulmonary circulation. Paediatr Respir Rev 2005;6:35–43.

6. Gebb SA, Shannon JM. Tissue interactions mediate early events in pulmonary vasculogenesis. Dev Dyn 2000;217:159–69.

7. deMello DE, Sawyer D, Galvin N, Reid LM. Early fetal development of lung vasculature. Am J Respir Cell Mol Biol 1997;16:568–81.

8. Gebb S, Stevens T. On lung endothelial cell heterogeneity. Microvasc Res 2004;68:1–12.

9. Minoo P, King RJ. Epithelial-mesenchymal interactions in lung development. Annu Rev Physiol 1994;56:13–45.

10. Shannon JM, Hyatt BA. Epithelial-mesenchymal interactions in the developing lung. Annu Rev Physiol 2004;66:625–45.

11. Shannon JM, Nielsen LD, Gebb SA, Randell SH. Mesenchyme specifies epithelial differentiation in reciprocal recombinants of embryonic lung and trachea. Dev Dyn 1998;212:482–94.

12. Demayo F, Minoo P, Plopper CG, et al. Mesenchymal-epithelial interactions in lung development and repair: are modeling and remodeling the same process? Am J Physiol 2002;283:L510–7.

13. Voelkel NF, Cool CD. Pulmonary vascular involvement in chronic obstructive pulmonary disease. Eur Respir J Suppl 2003;46:28s–32s.

14. Kasahara Y, Tuder RM, Taraseviciene-Stewart L, et al. Inhibition of VEGF receptors causes lung cell apoptosis and emphysema. J Clin Invest 2000;106:1311–9.

15. Whitsett JA, Zhou L. Use of transgenic mice to study autocrine-paracrine signaling in lung morphogenesis and differentiation. Clin Perinatol 1996;23:753–69.

16. Perl AK, Tichelaar JW, Whitsett JA. Conditional gene expression in the respiratory epithelium of the mouse. Transgenic Res 2002;11:21–9.

17. Maeda Y, Dave V, Whitsett JA. Transcriptional control of lung morphogenesis. Physiol Rev 2007;87:219–44.

18. Perl AK, Whitsett JA. Molecular mechanisms controlling lung morphogenesis. Clin Genet 1999;56:14–27.

19. Besnard V, Wert SE, Hull WM, Whitsett JA. Immunohistochemical localization of Foxa1 and Foxa2 in mouse embryos and adult tissues. Gene Expr Patterns 2004;5:193–208.

20. Wan H, Dingle S, Xu Y, et al. Compensatory roles of Foxa1 and Foxa2 during lung morphogenesis. J Biol Chem 2005;280:13809–16.

21. Wan H, Kaestner KH, Ang SL, et al. Foxa2 regulates alveolarization and goblet cell hyperplasia. Development 2004;131:953–64.

22. Wert SE, Dey CR, Blair PA, et al. Increased expression of thyroid transcription factor-1 (TTF-1) in respiratory epithelial cells inhibits alveolarization and causes pulmonary inflammation. Dev Biol 2002;242:75–87.

23. Yang H, Lu MM, Zhang L, et al. GATA6 regulates differentiation of distal lung epithelium. Development 2002;129:2233–46.

24. Zeng X, Yutzey KE, Whitsett JA. Thyroid transcription factor-1, hepatocyte nuclear factor-3beta and surfactant protein A and B in the developing chick lung. J Anat 1998;193 (Pt 3):399–408.

25. Zhou L, Lim L, Costa RH, Whitsett JA. Thyroid transcription factor-1, hepatocyte nuclear factor-3beta, surfactant protein B, C, and Clara cell secretory protein in developing mouse lung. J Histochem Cytochem 1996;44:1183–93.

26. Barnes PJ. Transcription factors in airway diseases. Lab Invest 2006;86:867–72.

27. Reynolds PR, Cosio MG, Hoidal JR. Cigarette smoke-induced Egr-1 upregulates proinflammatory cytokines in pulmonary epithelial cells. Am J Respir Cell Mol Biol 2006;35:314–9.

28. Bellusci S, Grindley J, Emoto H, et al. Fibroblast growth factor 10 (FGF10) and branching morphogenesis in the embryonic mouse lung. Development 1997;124:4867–78.

29. Mailleux AA, Tefft D, Ndiaye D, et al. Evidence that SPROUTY2 functions as an inhibitor of mouse embryonic lung growth and morphogenesis. Mech Dev 2001;102:81–94.

30. Usui H, Shibayama M, Ohbayashi N, et al. Fgf18 is required for embryonic lung alveolar development. Biochem Biophys Res Commun 2004;322:887–92.

31. Massague J, Seoane J, Wotton D. Smad transcription factors. Genes Dev 2005;19:2783–810.

32. Massague J, Wotton D. Transcriptional control by the TGF-beta/Smad signaling system. EMBO J 2000;19:1745–54.

33. McGowan SE. Extracellular matrix and the regulation of lung development and repair. FASEB J 1992;6:2895–904.

34. Warburton D, Bellusci S, De Langhe S, et al. Molecular mechanisms of early lung specification and branching morphogenesis. Pediatr Res 2005;57:26R–37R.

35. Warburton D, Schwarz M, Tefft D, et al. The molecular basis of lung morphogenesis. Mech Dev 2000;92:55–81.

36. Carmeliet P, Ferreira V, Breier G, et al. Abnormal blood vessel development and lethality in embryos lacking a single VEGF allele. Nature 1996;380:435–9.

37. Ferrara N, Carver-Moore K, Chen H, et al. Heterozygous embryonic lethality induced by targeted inactivation of the VEGF gene. Nature 1996;380:439–42.

38. Galambos C, Ng YS, Ali A, et al. Defective pulmonary development in the absence of heparin-binding vascular endothelial growth factor isoforms. Am J Respir Cell Mol Biol 2002;27:194–203.

39. Zeng X, Wert SE, Federici R, et al. VEGF enhances pulmonary vasculogenesis and disrupts lung morphogenesis in vivo. Dev Dyn 1998;211:215–27.

40. Jones FS, Jones PL. The tenascin family of ECM glycoproteins: structure, function, and regulation during embryonic development and tissue remodeling. Dev Dyn 2000;218:235–9.

41. Sannes PL, Wang J. Basement membranes and pulmonary development. Exp Lung Res 1997;23:101–8.

42. Schuger L. Laminins in lung development. Exp Lung Res 1997;23:119–29.

43. Gadek JE, Fells GA, Zimmerman RL, Crystal RG. Role of connective tissue proteases in the pathogenesis of chronic inflammatory lung disease. Environ Health Perspect 1984;55:297–306.

44. Shapiro SD, Senior RM. Matrix metalloproteinases. Matrix degradation and more. Am J Respir Cell Mol Biol 1999;20:1100–2.

45. Giangreco A, Reynolds SD, Stripp BR. Terminal bronchioles harbor a unique airway stem cell population that localizes to the bronchoalveolar duct junction. Am J Pathol 2002;161:173–82.

46. Majka SM, Beutz MA, Hagen M, et al. Identification of novel resident pulmonary stem cells: form and function of the lung side population. Stem Cells 2005;23:1073–81.

47. Reynolds SD, Giangreco A, Hong KU, et al. Airway injury in lung disease pathophysiology: selective depletion of airway stem and progenitor cell pools potentiates lung inflammation and alveolar dysfunction. Am J Physiol 2004;287:L1256–65.

48. van Tuyl M, Liu J, Wang J, et al. Role of oxygen and vascular development in epithelial branching morphogenesis of the developing mouse lung. Am J Physiol 2005;288:L167–78.

49. Gebb SA, Fox K, Vaughn J, et al. Fetal oxygen tension promotes tenascin-C-dependent lung branching morphogenesis. Dev Dyn 2005;234:1–10.

50. Torday JS, Rehan VK. The evolutionary continuum from lung development to homeostasis and repair. Am J Physiol 2007;292:L608–11.

CHAPTER 3

Epidemiology

Jørgen Vestbo, MD, DMSc

Epidemiology deals with the causes, distribution, and control of disease. As this scope is different from studying disease in individual patients, it will come as no surprise that definitions of diseases frequently vary between clinical and epidemiologic settings. Simpler diagnostic criteria are often used in epidemiology, where, for practical reasons, the use of the sophisticated tools available in clinical practice is impossible. However, this is true only to a certain extent for chronic obstructive pulmonary disease (COPD) and has been a problem mainly for the study of emphysema, in which little can be accomplished with the usual available epidemiologic tools. For the study of COPD overall, in which the focus is mainly on measurements of lung function, epidemiology has been well equipped as large sources of data that include measurements of lung function are available. Still, for many measures, epidemiologists have to rely on reported diagnoses from death certificates, hospital discharge forms, and patients' own perception of disease, with all of the expected limitations and potential sources of bias.

Tools in epidemiology include both study design and methodology. Epidemiology basically includes two types of data. Health statistics, which provide large-scale data, enable epidemiologists to look at the impact of the disease on society, make crude comparisons between countries and continents, detect major changes in disease distribution over time, and make qualified predictions for the future. Such data have limited use in establishing anything close to a causal relationship and are often affected by universal and time-dependent biases that can be difficult and sometimes impossible to adjust properly. Population surveys, on the other hand, provide data on a limited number of individuals, but the loss of quantity is made up for by the possibility of information gathered in a standardized way, including questionnaire-derived information (on, for example, symptoms or smoking habits), as well as measurements of lung function. Finally, databases from population surveys, including those with data on repeated screenings, can be merged with locally existing health registers, combining the advantages of the two strategies.

Impact of COPD

COPD is an extremely prominent disease worldwide. Analyses by Murray and Lopez have shown that COPD ranked sixth among causes of death globally in 1990 and is expected to be the third most important cause of death in 2020.[1] This is illustrated in Figure 1, in which the number of deaths from COPD are shown together with the estimated deaths from human immunodeficiency virus (HIV) infection. Furthermore, disability from COPD is believed to be on the increase and will be the fifth leading cause of disability-adjusted life-years lost in 2020. In the United States, age-adjusted COPD mortality rates increased by 17.1% among men from 1979 to 1993, from 96.3 per 100,000 to 112.8 per 100,000.[2] Among women, rates increased 126.1%, from 24.5 per 100,000 in 1979 to 55.4 per 100,000 in 1993. In Canada, the total number of deaths from COPD almost doubled from 1980 to 1995, and this increase is not due merely to a change in the ninth edition of the *International Classification of Disease* (ICD) to ICD-10. The increase was mainly due to the population living longer, although a real increase was seen in women, for whom the age-standardized mortality rate rose from 8.3 to 17.3 per 100,000.[3] In areas of the world where smoking has been prevalent for decades, mortality rates are now higher among women than among men. With the expected increase in female mortality from COPD globally, equal mortality rates are also estimated to occur elsewhere within a decade.[4] It is perhaps important to keep in mind that mortality statistics in COPD, as in other diseases, may be biased.[5] Recent Danish data suggest that COPD is severely underreported on death certificates, that gender differences in degree of underreporting may exist, and that subjects without COPD may be classified as having COPD on the death certificate.[6]

Significant variations exist between countries.[7,8] Differences in smoking habits also exist, and patterns of smoking may vary from one country to another. This may partly explain why differences in COPD mortality cannot be completely explained by differences in crude measures of smoking between countries.[9] It is also difficult to adjust for changes in smoking as the lag time between changes in smoking habits and the impact on society may be as long as 30 to 50 years.[10] Finally, it may also be worthwhile taking into account that although trends in COPD mortality over decades may be valid *within* a country, differences *between* countries may exist solely because of different diagnostic traditions.[11] Trends in subtypes of COPD cannot be ascertained from mortality statistics. There are clear variations in labeling geographically, over time, and (independently of time) owing to revisions in ICD codes.

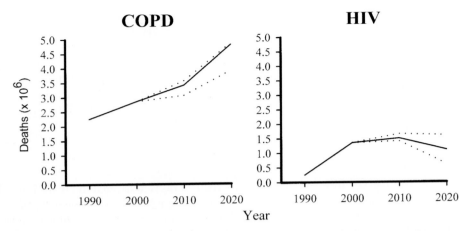

FIGURE 1. The estimated number of deaths from chronic obstructive pulmonary disease (COPD) and human immunodeficiency virus (HIV) infection from 1990 to 2020, based on calculations by Murray and Lopez.[1] The *dotted lines* show the estimated numbers according to best- and worst-case scenarios.

Morbidity data are often regarded as superior to mortality data because of the chronicity of COPD, and there are data suggesting that up to 25% of medical admissions in the United Kingdom are due to respiratory diseases and that half of these are due to COPD.[12] However, there are at least as many sources of diagnostic bias in the available data on morbidity as in the data on mortality. In addition, hospital admissions, contacts with primary care, and costs of medication are all subject to changes independent of changes in the disease. As an example, hospital admissions among US men decreased from 1980 to 1985 in parallel with an increase in outpatient visits,[13] and contacts with general practitioners in the United Kingdom have remained almost constant over 20 years, in spite of obvious changes in the gender distribution of the disease.[14] Data from samples of the random population show that prevalences of COPD vary from 4 to 6.5% and remain relatively stable over time; the high prevalence is reflected in the number of general practice consultations.

The economic burden has recently been the subject of more interest as the costs of COPD are considerable.[15] Burden-of-illness studies have shown significant variations between countries; however, the average cost per COPD patient in the Western world is approximately 1,500 € ($2,300), with a steep increase in costs with increasing severity of the underlying disease.[16] Exacerbations are the major cost drivers and account for 30 to 70% of the direct medical costs, depending on the study and the location.[17,18] Comorbidities are also significant predictors of cost,[19] and they are likely to increase in significance with the increased aging of the population.

All of the above data are, however, merely measures of the impact of the disease on health statistics and costs. It would be of particular interest to be able to provide exact numbers of patients with the disease in different countries around the world. Given the burden of the disease, it is amazing that relatively few good-quality data exist on the prevalence of COPD. Recently, a meta-analysis of population-based prevalence studies found an overall prevalence of COPD of 9.8% based on 26 studies with spirometry-defined disease, most of them from Europe.[20] Many of these studies, however, used different study designs and methodology. For this reason, the Burden of Obstructive Lung Disease (BOLD) program has been established,[21] facilitating the use of standardized study methodology in different countries. A BOLD study group in five Latin American countries found surprisingly high prevalence rates of COPD, ranging from 7.8% in Mexico City to 19.7% in Montevideo.[22]

Natural History of Chronic Bronchitis and Emphysema

Initially, COPD was described as "obstructive bronchitis," in contrast to "simple bronchitis." This was the basis for the testing of "the British hypothesis," which claimed that chronic mucus hypersecretion (CMH), defined as a productive cough for more than 3 months per year for at least 2 years, as a risk factor for recurrent airway infection, was causative in the development of airway obstruction. The seminal work by Fletcher and colleagues clearly rejected this hypothesis by showing that in middle-aged men, CMH and progressive airway obstruction were two separate entities, although they often occurred concomitantly.[23] Following this study, the forced expiratory volume in 1 second (FEV_1) has been established as the key characteristic in the epidemiology of COPD, and interest in mucus has declined considerably until recently. The crucial changes in lung function that define COPD are generally believed to be the results of changes taking place over decades. The model most widely accepted is one showing COPD resulting from decades of a moderately accelerated decline in FEV_1 (Figure 2).

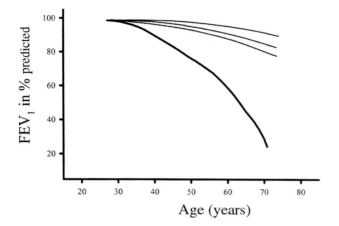

FIGURE 2. The usual model of decline in forced expiratory volume in 1 second (FEV₁) showing the normal variation in smokers not susceptible to the harmful effects of smoking in *thin lines* and the course of decline in susceptible smokers as a *thick line*.

However, it has become apparent that the maximum attained FEV₁ prior to the normal decline from adulthood is at least as important[24] because an abnormally low lung function at age 60 years may have arisen from a number of mechanisms, as shown in Figure 3. This has focused more attention on lung growth. (A more detailed presentation is given in Chapter 2) However, most of the knowledge on risk factors concerns changes taking place in adulthood. Nevertheless, a proper description of the natural history of lung function needs to start at birth.

As in other chronic diseases (such as ischemic heart disease), genetic and nongenetic prenatal factors and perinatal factors may be of importance. Good research in this area is sparse so far, but perinatal factors may contribute by determining lung function at birth and the rate of growth of lung function in childhood and adolescence.[25,26] Altered lung growth—owing to genetic or perinatal factors or environmental factors (eg, to recurrent infections or smoking) during childhood and adolescence—will result in a suboptimal level of lung function in early adulthood (see Chapter 2). Depending on the subsequent lifestyle, this may increase the risk of developing COPD.

Several studies show that there is a plateau phase in lung function from the approximate age of 20 years to the age of 30 to 35 years. Although evidence is also sparse in this area,[27] it seems that the plateau phase in smokers and symptomatic subjects may be shorter or even missing, resulting in an earlier onset of the decline in lung function, which may contribute to the development of COPD.

Undoubtedly, the most significant feature in the natural history of COPD is the excess decline in lung function during adulthood. In normal middle-aged adults, the rate of decline in FEV₁ is approximately 30 mL per year in men and 25 mL per year in women. The rate of decline in FEV₁ shows considerable interindividual variation, and from the literature,

the designation of "rapid decliners" seems justified. It has been suggested that one single measurement (or at least a few measurements) of FEV₁ would be sufficient to identify an individual susceptible to the adverse effects of, for example, tobacco smoke. This assumes that a "tracking" effect is at work, that is, that a low value at any time would predict that the individual would have a subsequent fast decline, thereby staying in his or her own "track." This has been termed the "horse-racing effect,"[23,28] and it indicates that a minor impairment would lead to increasingly lower lung function, disability, and perhaps death from COPD. Although this phenomenon is seen in population studies, it may not be entirely true for individual smokers. First, the initial changes of COPD take place in the small airways and may not be reflected in the FEV₁, which is mainly a measurement of large airway function. As a result, the full effect of these changes may not be reflected in the FEV₁ and in respiratory symptoms until late in middle age. Second, the rates of decline may change over time, which could change the course of the disease considerably. One also needs to take into account that the variation in a single FEV₁ measurement is 175 to 200 mL, which amounts to 5 to 10 years of excess decline in the susceptible smoker. Thus, it is apparent that several measurements, years apart, are necessary to determine the rate of decline in an individual. As an approximation, annual measurements would have to be undertaken for at least 3 to 5 years for an excess decline in FEV₁ to become apparent.

Late in the course of the disease, disability is present as a result of the impaired lung function and the effect of comorbidities. The progressive loss of FEV₁ may be accompanied by a decrease in the diffusion capacity, most often measured as the carbon monoxide (CO) transfer factor (TL$_{CO}$); clearly,

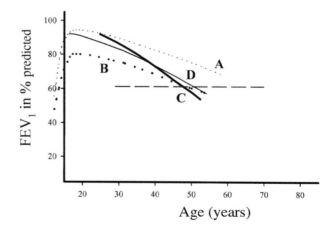

FIGURE 3. Different ways of obtaining an abnormally low forced expiratory volume in 1 second (FEV₁) in middle age. The *thin dotted line* (A) shows the normal age-related decline in FEV₁, the *thick dotted line* (B) shows an abnormal growth rate but normal age-related decline in FEV₁, the *thick line* (C) shows an excessively accelerated decline in FEV₁, and the *thin line* (D) shows a premature and slightly accelerated decline in FEV₁. Adapted from Kerstjens HAM et al.[24]

more data are needed with well-characterized subtypes of COPD followed for years to establish the natural history of change in diffusion capacity. With more advanced reduction in lung function, hypoxemia develops; secondary to this, the pulmonary arterial pressure is increased. In severe COPD, the mean pulmonary arterial pressure increases by approximately 0.5 to 3.0 mm Hg per year, and an elevated pulmonary arterial pressure is a significant predictor of poor prognosis in COPD.[29] As a consequence of the high pressure in the pulmonary vascular bed, right ventricular hypertrophy (cor pulmonale) develops, and this affects survival markedly. Patients with COPD who develop peripheral edema owing to cor pulmonale have a 5-year survival rate of 30 to 40%.[29]

Recent research has focused on the systemic manifestations of COPD and not least the role of systemic inflammation (see also Chapter 23).[30,31] It is well known that patients with COPD lose weight particularly in the severe stages of their disease, and several studies have shown that a low body mass index is a predictor of poor prognosis.[32–35] Recent data indicate that weight loss in milder stages of the disease and even the initial loss of fat-free mass may be a predictor of mortality.[36] These systemic manifestations are generally believed to be the result of systemic inflammation, and studies have shown an association between systemic inflammation and systemic manifestations,[37–40] as well as an independent effect of markers of systemic inflammation and mortality.[41,42] However, it seems too early to properly place these components in the natural history of COPD, and it may even turn out that many of these events are fairly independent of disease progression as measured by FEV_1 and FEV_1 decline. Only future studies that dissect the various subtypes of COPD will be able to enlighten us.

Risk Factors for COPD

Most of our knowledge of risk factors for COPD has been gathered from large surveys. Often a sample of the general population is chosen; this has obvious advantages. An absence of selection bias often means that results can be easily extrapolated. Indeed, studies of COPD in a random population sample are often "translated" into measures of effect in the general population, on which health policy decisions can be based. However, for the purpose of studying potentially hazardous occupational exposures or other rare exposures or aspects of the exposure-disease relationship taking place at a specific point of time, a carefully selected subsample of the population is often more appropriate. On the other hand, the selection of subsamples with particular exposures runs the risk of introducing selection biases. The most well known of these is the "healthy worker effect," which implies that among welders, for example, those with respiratory symptoms or low lung function have been excluded before entering the occupation. Possible selection bias must always be considered when interpreting an epidemiologic study.

When repeated studies are done on the same population sample, these repeated follow-ups are often referred to as constituting a "panel study," with each cross-sectional survey representing a "panel." Epidemiologists have pointed out that conclusions on longitudinal lung function decline based on single cross-sectional surveys may be severely biased.[43] However, it should be noted that panel studies, especially when they include several time points of follow-up, may also be biased because of dropouts and selection owing to competing risks (eg, when heavy smokers dying from ischemic heart disease in a study of the effects of smoking on lung function lead to an excess of "healthy smokers" or smokers presumably less susceptible to the harmful effects of tobacco). Several research tools exist for use in epidemiology. As in clinical work, structured self-reported information is emphasized and is accompanied by various measures, the most important obviously being spirometry. For decades, one of the cornerstones in epidemiologic studies of chronic bronchitis and emphysema has been a questionnaire based mainly on the British Medical Research Council (MRC) questionnaire.[44,45] All such available questionnaires focus on the description and semiquantification of common respiratory symptoms: cough, phlegm, breathlessness, chest tightness, and wheeze. Most questionnaires contain specific questions on familial occurrence of respiratory disease and information on smoking. The most frequently used questionnaires include the MRC questionnaire,[44] the American Thoracic Society questionnaire,[46] and the European Community Coal and Steel questionnaire,[47] all of which have been validated to various degrees. There is general agreement on the need for revision of the questionnaires presently in use; the major obstacle seems to be the ability to update the questionnaires without having to expand the forms considerably in size.

With the establishment of the FEV_1 as the crucial measurement in COPD epidemiology, spirometry plays a central role in epidemiologic surveys; FEV_1, vital capacity, and forced vital capacity (FVC) can be obtained by using simple spirometry, which can be performed in the field with portable equipment if necessary. Guidelines for standardization are continuously being updated, but in contrast to the clinical situation, caution should be used when applying overly strict criteria for spirometry in epidemiology: several studies have shown that subjects with poor spirometric reproducibility or who are unable to produce a technically correct measurement may have a poor prognosis in general and a subsequent excess decline in lung function in particular.[48–50] More complex measures of lung function can be used in epidemiology but with considerably more practical problems and time expenditure. A few decades ago, measurement of small airway function using the single-breath nitrogen test was included in large surveys, but because of a subsequent lack of predictive value,[51–54] this test has been almost abandoned in epidemiology. Measurement of diffusion capacity has also been performed in general population samples[55,56] but with much larger within-subject and between-test variations than those seen for expiratory volumes.[57]

Risk factors for COPD in epidemiology are most convincingly determined from studies showing an association between the risk factor under study and change in FEV_1 (longitudinal assessment). As mentioned previously, a change in FEV_1 often refers to a decline in FEV_1, and there is still an obvious lack of studies that look at changes in lung function related to lung growth associated with well-defined factors or that ideally combine lung function (related to lung growth) and decline with equal assessments or (even) in the same populations. Often longitudinal assessment is not possible, and cross-sectional findings have to be relied on. This may cause bias,[43] but not necessarily. The introduction of statistical models that can simultaneously handle cross-sectional data and longitudinal data on the same population has advanced the capability to assess risk factors.[58] The remainder of this chapter refers to results from studies of lung function and decline in lung function in adults. Some comments on the quality of the available data are given, and some thoughts as to the potential influence of biases are expressed.

Instead of studying the decline in lung function, it may seem tempting to assess the development of the disease, that is, moving from a state of no lung disease to having COPD. This alternative—using the incidence of COPD as a measure of impact of risk—may intuitively seem more straightforward than measuring a change in FEV_1. However, this measure also requires longitudinal studies with the assessment of lung function at baseline and follow-up. In addition, measuring incidence relies on diagnostic criteria that are valid in all age categories, and given the current diagnostic criteria,[59] this may pose problems. Using the fixed ratio of $FEV_1/FVC < 0.7$ may lead to overestimation of COPD incidence in the elderly[60] and underdiagnosis in young adults.[61] The requirement of valid longitudinal data is the explanation for limited data on the incidence of COPD.[62–65]

Although smoking is by far the strongest risk factor for COPD, it is worthwhile to remember that detailed information on this particular risk factor is also the result of the ability (and limitations) of earlier epidemiologic studies to assess the effects of strong risk factors on the decline of FEV_1. Other factors are definitely at work and deserve attention, not only because of their impact but also because several of them can be affected by preventive measures just as smoking cessation can. Risk factors cannot be studied independently of when they exert their effect in the individual's life. Whereas smoking presumably has a profound effect on both lung growth and the decline in FEV_1, other individual features or exposures may have an effect only at limited time intervals and can be overlooked more easily. In subsequent sections of this chapter, each factor believed to be of relevance is discussed. In Table 1, the risk factors for COPD are listed in an approximate descending order of importance.

Tobacco Smoking

By far, the most important cause of COPD is tobacco smoking.[66] Smoking is generally believed to be the cause of 85 to 90% of all COPD in men in the industrialized world,[67] and epidemiologic studies have been crucial in determining this association.[23,68–70] The relationship between smoking and COPD is supported by so many features indicating causality that it is, in fact, often used as a model example of how epidemiology can contribute to elucidating the causes of disease. Knowledge of this cause-and-effect relationship stems from numerous well-conducted population surveys from the last four decades. However, Marsh and colleagues recently suggested that the attributable risk may be severely overestimated,[71] and future studies should include as many other potential risk factors as possible to avoid a bias from existing studies with a more limited field of interest.

Nevertheless, the association between smoking and lung function has been demonstrated in both cross-sectional and longitudinal studies, and the effect of smoking seems to be present from the cradle to the grave. Smoking during pregnancy leads to both low birth weight and decreased lung function at birth.[72,73] The significance of this for the subsequent risk of development of COPD is, of course, difficult to determine. However, it seems highly plausible that decreased lung function at birth may lead to a decreased level of lung function in early adulthood, which would increase the risk of developing COPD, depending on subsequent lifestyle (especially the

Table 1 Risk Factors for Chronic Obstructive Pulmonary Disease*		
External	*Internal*	*Other*
Smoking	Genetic factors	Airway hyperresponsiveness, IgE, and asthma
Socioeconomic status	Gender	Environmental pollution
Occupation	Chronic mucus hypersecretion	Perinatal events and childhood respiratory illness
		Recurrent bronchopulmonary infections
		Diet

IgE = immunoglobulin E.
*In an attempted descending order; external and internal factors presumably have a similar impact.

subject's own smoking career).[24] Evidence of mild airway obstruction and reduced increase of the lung function was found in American adolescents who smoke,[74] and this is in accordance with a previous study showing a slowing of the increment of the FEV$_1$ in adolescent smokers with respiratory symptoms.[75] Although the increment of lung function was slowed by only 1 to 2% on average, the variation was large, and this indicates that susceptible adolescents may suffer substantial lung function impairment owing to smoking. The plateau in the FEV$_1$ in the third decade of life is also shortened considerably by smoking, resulting in the initiation of an FEV$_1$ decline years earlier than in those who have never smoked.[68,75] The effect of smoking on FEV$_1$ decline in adulthood is well documented. Just as in those who have never smoked, the FEV$_1$ decline varies considerably among smokers. Most longitudinal studies have included men, and the FEV$_1$ decline ranges from 45 to 90 mL per year, in contrast to the normal 30 mL per year. As these values are mean values from population studies, a single individual may experience a significantly larger decline, at least temporarily, explaining why COPD may seem to surface within a short period during the fifth or sixth decade. Most studies link COPD to cigarette smoking, mainly because cigarettes are smoked much more often than cigars, cheroots, or pipes. From studies including all types of smokers, it seems that the type of tobacco smoked plays a minor role, if any.[70] The crucial factors seem to be the amount smoked and the extent of inhalation.[76] Cigarettes are generally inhaled more often than other types of tobacco, and this may explain the erroneous notion that cigar and pipe smoking is safe. With regard to the effect on FEV$_1$ decline, filter cigarettes are not significantly different from nonfilter cigarettes, presumably because the substances that cause lung function impairment originate from the volatile components of cigarettes, which is not reduced by filters. Theoretically, low-tar cigarettes should do less harm than ordinary cigarettes, but no convincing studies have demonstrated this. It is possible that more intensive smoking of low-tar products would counteract the beneficial effect of the lowered tar content to some extent.

In several surveys, cessation of smoking has been shown to be favorably associated with both the prevalence of respiratory symptoms and changes in subsequent decline in FEV$_1$.[76–78] With respect to the effect on lung function, the first change seen after cessation of smoking is a small increase in the FEV$_1$, usually between 50 and 100 mL. The favorable effect on the subsequent decline in lung function is seen in younger subjects and in those without apparent COPD, whereas the beneficial effects are less apparent in older subjects with overt COPD.[78] In young and middle-aged subjects, it is a matter of debate whether the decline in FEV$_1$ after cessation of smoking normalizes completely or just approaches the FEV$_1$ decline of those who have never smoked. At present, it seems that, in general, quitters continue to have an FEV$_1$ decline that is slightly larger than that seen in people who have never smoked.[78,79] Whether this is due to a small number of the quitters having continuous respiratory symptoms

(indicating ongoing inflammation in the airways) remains to be seen.

One of the most interesting issues concerning smoking has always been susceptibility. Research in COPD has always been challenged by the "fact" that only 15 to 20% of smokers are susceptible to smoking's harmful effects on FEV$_1$. It is unclear how these 15 to 20% have become a fact; the most direct reference can be found in the book by Fletcher and colleagues, in which they state that "about 13% of a follow-up group derived from an un-stratified sample would have been 'obstructed.'"[23] Clearly, more than 15% of smokers develop COPD.[80] This has been documented in several longitudinal studies of random population samples.[62–64] In fact, approximately 35% of smokers with initially normal lung function developed COPD during a 25-year follow-up of the Copenhagen City Heart Study,[64] as illustrated in Figure 4. Given the fact that this figure is likely to be an underestimate because of selection during follow-up, it seems fair to say that possibly most smokers develop inflammation in their airways that in one way or the other affects measures of lung function.[81] It is, nevertheless, still interesting why the degree of susceptibility varies so markedly.

Occupational Exposures to Dusts and Gases

For decades, it has been generally accepted that occupational dust exposure could lead to cough and sputum production. This association is shown in several occupational cohorts. An association between occupational exposure and excess decline in lung function was previously the topic of heated debates, in particular because of the implications regarding health and safety at work and discussions of workers' compensation. The methodology used to assess the potential deleterious effect of occupational exposures is not simple, and several caveats exist. Among these, the healthy worker effect is the most well known, but other specific problems are almost invariably present.[82] The most important epidemiologic

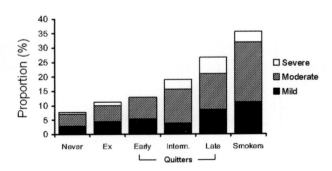

FIGURE 4. Calculated cumulative incidence for chronic obstructive pulmonary disease according to GOLD stages, men and women combined. Ex = stopped smoking before study entry; Never = never-smokers. Adapted from Løkke A et al.[64]

study, which subsequently led to a change in opinion, was a study of Paris-area workers in which working men with exposure to gases, associated with exposure to dust, heat, or both, had an accelerated decline in FEV$_1$.[83] In this study, the effect of different exposures on FEV$_1$ decline was examined; on average, the exposed men had an excess decline in FEV$_1$ of 5 to 15 mL per year owing to the exposure. It should be noted that important information, including data on occupational exposures, has also been gathered from studies of the general population. Although information on occupation in population surveys is less detailed and often more imprecise, the study population is generally less affected by selection biases, especially the healthy worker effect. Findings from several cross-sectional surveys all show an effect of broadly defined occupational exposures on FEV$_1$ decline and COPD incidence.[84–89] In these studies, subjects who described themselves as being exposed to inorganic dust, for example, without describing a level of exposure and giving only a crude number of years for duration, had an FEV$_1$ decline comparable to that of someone who engages in moderate smoking (ie, 5 to 10 cigarettes per day). Findings from very thorough analyses of 1,933 randomly sampled men from Bergen, Norway, have convincingly demonstrated a significant dose-effect relationship between the number of occupational agents to which subjects were exposed and decline in FEV$_1$ (Figure 5).[87] A recent very large Swedish study of construction workers showed an excess mortality from COPD in men exposed to inorganic dust.[89]

Socioeconomic Status

For decades, it has been obvious that the presence of chronic bronchitis and emphysema was strongly associated with

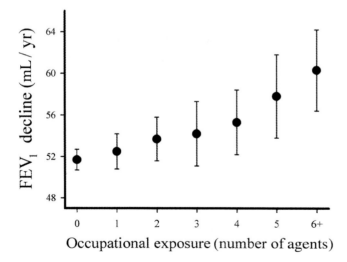

FIGURE 5. Excess forced expiratory volume in 1 second (FEV$_1$) decline in men, according to the number of occupational exposures. Error bars show 95% confidence intervals for the estimated declines. Adapted from Humerfelt S et al.[87]

socioeconomic status, or social class.[90] The association between socioeconomic status and general health has been consistently shown in British studies of social class variations in both doctor consultations and mortality,[91,92] and a recent large European study showed a clear association between the level of education and mortality from COPD.[93] This is not limited to the socioeconomic status of the individual but is probably also an effect of social deprivation in general.[94] For lung cancer, for example, the association between socioeconomic status and both CMH and COPD cannot be explained solely by differences in smoking habits. This is in spite of an obvious association between low socioeconomic status and heavy smoking, an association that seems to have been strengthened in recent decades.[95,96] The differences in attained levels of lung function, which cannot be explained by factors other than socioeconomic status, have been considerable. The association between socioeconomic status and COPD was also shown in a recent Danish cohort study. In spite of relatively small differences between social classes, the study revealed marked associations between education and/or level of income and both lung function and hospitalizations for COPD.[97] The difference in FEV$_1$ between men with long education and high income and those with short education and low income was 400 mL, and the risk of subsequent hospitalization for COPD varied by a factor of 3. The difference was profound in both men and women, suggesting that occupational exposures alone were not to blame. In the article from Paris on occupation and FEV$_1$ decline, unskilled workers had a significantly steeper FEV$_1$ decline than skilled workers after adjustment for smoking and occupational exposures.[83] Similarly, in a community study from Bergen, Norway, education (which is a surrogate marker of socioeconomic status) remained a significant risk factor for obstructive lung disease after adjustment for occupational exposure.[98]

It is unlikely that only a few factors taken together make up the risk factor of socioeconomic status. Most likely, socioeconomic risk factors are multifactorial and may cover an entire range, from intrauterine exposure[99,100] to childhood infections,[25,100] childhood environment,[101] diet,[102–104] housing conditions,[105–107] and occupational[83,87] and (possibly) other lifestyle factors.

α$_1$-Antitrypsin Deficiency

The genetic variant α$_1$-antitrypsin deficiency should perhaps not be included among risk factors as it affects a small proportion of COPD patients and specifically causes disabling emphysema. α$_1$-Antitrypsin deficiency, however, serves as a model for the protease-antiprotease theory of the pathogenesis of emphysema and is described in detail in Chapter 5, "α$_1$-Antitrypsin Deficiency." Several variants of the protein inhibitor system have been described, but, usually, α$_1$-antitrypsin deficiency denotes those homozygous for the Z allele (PiZZ), who have very low levels of α$_1$-antitrypsin in the blood. In recent years, several registers containing both patients with α_1-antitrypsin deficiency and their relatives have been established for the purpose of elucidating the development of emphysema in this subset of COPD patients. Some important points have already emerged. Whereas, owing to an abnormally rapid decline in FEV$_1$, the prognosis is generally poor in subjects identified as COPD patients,[108] subjects identified as nonindex cases—through a Danish register based on family studies—had a much more favorable prognosis.[109,110] Decline in lung function seems well characterized for cohorts of PiZZ subjects,[111,112] whereas the importance of being heterozygous for the Z allele (PiMZ) for decline in FEV$_1$ is more questionable.[113]

Other Genetic Factors

Both family and twin studies have confirmed that a significant genetic contribution to the variance in pulmonary function exists in individuals not selected for respiratory disease.[114–116] In spite of this, few specific genetic factors other than α_1-antitrypsin are known. Genes coding for proteins and proteases associated with increased susceptibility to inhaled toxins have been identified but seem to explain little of the variation in susceptibility.[117] It appears that new paths of research in this area may focus on genes regulating the expression of already known factors of relevance, such as α_1-antitrypsin, α_1-antichymotrypsin, α_2-macroglobulin, and antioxidants. From the results of a recent family study,[118] it seems that an interaction between genetic factors and gender may be important. (The concepts of genetic susceptibility are dealt with in more detail in Chapter 4, "Genetic Risk Factors.")

Chronic Mucus Hypersecretion

As stated earlier, initial epidemiologic studies ruled out CMH, or chronic bronchitis, as an important risk factor for subsequent FEV$_1$ decline[23] and COPD mortality.[119] However, recent findings have somewhat revised our view on the role of CMH. Large longitudinal population-based panel studies have demonstrated an association between CMH and FEV$_1$ decline,[120,121] COPD morbidity,[121,122] overall mortality,[123] and COPD mortality,[124] the latter mainly owing to an association between CMH and death from severe infections.[125] In a Danish population study, the effect of CMH on FEV$_1$ decline was considerable, leading to an excess decline of 10 to 25 mL per year, after adjusting for smoking (Figure 6).[121]

The discrepancy between these results and earlier findings can be explained in different ways. The possibility exists that the prevalence of CMH has changed. Whereas the early studies were conducted mainly in occupational cohorts of men with considerable exposure to airway irritants both at work and in general (owing to higher levels of outdoor particulate pollution), later population studies included subjects with less extensive exposures, reflected in generally lower prevalences of CMH. In the recent studies, CMH may be a marker of airway inflammation, thus leading to a gradual excess loss of lung function. However, it is more likely that the difference relates to the baseline level of lung function. In the study by

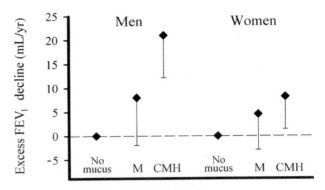

FIGURE 6. Longitudinal excess decline in forced expiratory volume in 1 second (FEV$_1$) owing to mucus hypersecretion, derived from a multivariate model adjusting for age, height, weight change, and smoking. CMH = chronic mucus hypersecretion; M = any mucus reported. Adapted from Vestbo J et al.[121]

Fletcher and colleagues, a working population was included,[23] and when only subjects with normal lung function at baseline were included in the Copenhagen City Heart Study follow-up, CMH was not associated with the development of COPD.[126] A lack of association between early chronic cough or phlegm and subsequent disease progression would fit with the assumption that in COPD, inhaled gases and particles damage the lung's innate defense system and thus reduce mucociliary clearance. This could then produce an ineffective cough, disrupt the epithelial barrier, and initiate an acute or chronic inflammatory process in the airways and lung parenchyma.[127] A recent study using data from the European Community Respiratory Health Survey found an association between CMH and incidence of COPD when looking at young adults only,[65] but more studies in this age group are clearly needed.[61]

Gender

There has been little research on the effect of gender on COPD. The reason for this is obvious: for years, COPD has been a disease of men. This reflects the differences in patterns of smoking in men and women, and in previous textbooks, these differences have led to male gender being considered an "established risk factor" for COPD. The issue is not an easy one to study. A direct comparison of lung function in men and women makes little sense, for obvious physical reasons. More important, it is a difficult task to compare the typical male smoker with the typical female smoker. Such a comparison will invariably be biased by the fact that proper controlling for smoking in terms of gender difference is very difficult, if not impossible. Besides smoking more than women (which is the measurement most often controlled for), men inhale more often, and they previously started smoking at an earlier age.[128] Improper adjustment will often occur since few population studies gather all of the information necessary for proper statistical adjustment for these confounders; insufficient adjustment may actually lead to invalid results. Recent studies indicate that when differences in smoking patterns are correctly controlled for, women show a higher risk of loss in FEV_1 and of subsequent hospitalization for COPD.[129,130] Prescott and colleagues showed that in two populations from Copenhagen, smoking tended to have a larger effect on FEV_1 in women, assessed cross-sectionally, and the risk of hospitalization owing to COPD was increased by a factor of 1.5 to 3.5 in women. In the previously mentioned study on the effects of smoking on the increase of lung function in adolescents, it also seemed that girls were more vulnerable to the harmful effects of smoking than boys.[74] More studies in this area are currently awaited, especially longitudinal studies, although these may prove difficult to interpret because of the relatively rapid gender-specific changes in smoking habits.

Airway Hyperresponsiveness, Immunoglobulin E, and Asthma

For years, it has been hypothesized that susceptibility in the natural history of COPD is determined by an allergic constitution manifest as airway hyperresponsiveness (AHR). Dutch researchers, especially, have favored this hypothesis, which has generally been known as "the Dutch hypothesis."[131,132] Unfortunately, the distinction between asthma and COPD has turned out to be the key in discussions of the Dutch hypothesis. Instead, the principal question to be addressed by pulmonary epidemiology should be does the presence of AHR in smokers predict a subsequent accelerated decline in FEV_1?

This question is, however, not easy to answer. AHR is present in patients with COPD since a significant association between AHR and the level of lung function is found in cross-sectional studies.[133] This is most likely explained by structural or pathologic changes in the airways in COPD. For this reason, longitudinal assessments are crucial. AHR has been shown to be an independent risk factor for an accelerated FEV_1 decline in a number of large cohort studies, including a study from the Groningen group,[133] a study in elderly people by Villar and colleagues,[134] and the Normative Aging Study.[135,136] Furthermore, an association between AHR at baseline and 5-year FEV_1 decline was demonstrated in the Lung Health Study.[137] The impact of AHR on FEV_1 decline has varied between studies, but over the range of studies, the presence of AHR adds approximately 10 mL per year to the decline in FEV_1. For the overall acceptance of AHR as an underlying risk factor, it is disturbing that the effect is by far greater in elderly subjects.[134] A review of the epidemiologic literature on AHR and FEV_1 decline is found elsewhere.[138] AHR is a strong predictor of mortality,[139] and although the Dutch hypothesis has always been subject to criticism, it resonates with the concept that COPD is a complex genetic abnormality in which products of certain genes or groups of genes interact with environmental stimuli to produce an excessive response that results in disease. The identification of disease markers and/or genes capable of predicting the type of response to the inhalation of toxic gases and particles that leads to COPD could lead to more precise studies of the natural history.[140]

Reversibility to a bronchodilator has been regarded as a proxy for AHR, and several studies have assessed reversibility as a predictor of FEV_1 decline. Few of these have adjusted for the actual value of the postbronchodilator FEV_1, but when that is done, little value seems to come from reversibility.[141] At present, reversibility seems to tell us little of value for predicting the decline in lung function.[142,143]

An association between AHR and total immunoglobulin E (IgE) has been shown in many studies, and IgE is crucial in the pathogenesis of extrinsic asthma. Smokers without asthma also have slightly elevated IgE, and it has therefore been suggested that a high IgE level should be included as a risk factor for COPD. Epidemiologic findings are not clear, and it seems that whereas IgE in nonasthmatic individuals may play a role in infancy in determining the growth of lung function and the consequent achieved level of FEV_1, it has little, if any, importance in adulthood.

Asthma is generally regarded as a disease entity that should be separated from COPD; it may thus seem confusing to add asthma to the risk factors for COPD. There is, however, increasing evidence that asthmatic patients have a more rapid decline in FEV_1 than nonasthmatic patients,[144,145] as well as an increased mortality, primarily owing to an increased COPD mortality.[146] It seems likely that asthma that is not properly controlled may lead to airway remodeling and fixed airflow obstruction, fulfilling all of the definitions of COPD. Support for this comes from a recent follow-up study showing that subjects with asthma in general had an excess decline in FEV_1 but that decline in those treated with inhaled corticosteroids was significantly slower.[147,148]

Environmental Pollution

Outdoor air pollution is a risk factor for increased phlegm—and, thus, chronic bronchitis—but is less of a risk factor for the development of airway obstruction or accelerated decline in FEV_1.[149] In patients with established COPD, environmental pollution seems to aggravate symptoms and to increase both admissions to the hospital[150,151] and mortality.[152,153] Whereas the acute effects of air pollution seem firmly established, there is only indirect evidence linking air pollution with progressive airflow obstruction.[149] A number of components of air pollution have been linked to an increase in bronchial responsiveness, and it cannot be excluded that air pollution may have an effect in causing COPD.

Perinatal Events, Childhood Respiratory Illness, and Recurrent Bronchopulmonary Infections

Low birth weight has been shown to predict low lung function in adult life.[25,26] This supports what is generally termed the "Barker theory," which states that the course of many chronic diseases is determined by prenatal and perinatal events. The major problem is to separate the effects of pure perinatal events from those associated with other strong risk factors. In the study by Barker and colleagues, the effect of birth weight was not limited to lung function in adult life but was also related to subsequent death from COPD.[25] The effect of birth weight on FEV1 (Figure 7) was statistically significant, but the difference in FEV1 between those who were small and those who were large at birth was only 250 mL and thus smaller than, for example, those usually found to be the effects of socioeconomic status. Childhood infections (bronchitis, pneumonia, and whooping cough) also had an effect on both lung function and mortality, and the adult level of FEV1 differed by 100 to 150 mL between those with and without childhood infections. The latter finding is in accordance with other cohort studies linking chronic childhood disease to lowered lung function in both early life[154] and late adult life.[155] The mechanism is generally believed to be related to impaired increase in lung function. A major drawback is the uncertainty associated with research in this area. Most studies rely on a combination of lung function measurements and information on childhood respiratory infections, often collected in ways that are unable to preclude significant recall bias and other sources of bias.[156] As the exact mechanisms remain unclear, alternative hypotheses have been sought. A hypothesis linking latent group C adenovirus infection with susceptibility to tobacco smoking and subsequent COPD presently seems to be the most interesting proposed theory[157,158] but is in need of confirmatory studies.

In the 1950s, recurrent bronchopulmonary infections in adulthood were believed to play a major role in the development of chronic bronchitis and emphysema, forming the basis for the British hypothesis. According to this, the presence of chronic phlegm (then labeled chronic bronchitis and later termed chronic mucus hypersecretion) predisposed patients to recurrent bronchopulmonary infections, which would subsequently lead to changes in airways and alveoli, causing progressive chronic airflow limitation (later designated as COPD). As mentioned earlier, this hypothesis was rejected by Fletcher and colleagues since infections caused only temporary impairment of lung function.[23] However, the debate about the impact of CMH and recurrent bronchopulmonary infections continues, especially in established COPD. With increasing severity of airflow obstruction, it is both an epidemiologic and a clinical observation that recurrent bronchopulmonary infections occur with increasing frequency. Several epidemiologic studies have shown that bronchopulmonary infections lead to a temporary decrease in lung function, and one could speculate that recurrent bronchopulmonary infections could, in selected individuals, play a role in the course of the disease.

Diet

As a consequence of the role of oxidative stress in the pathogenesis of COPD, it has been suggested that dietary antioxidants such as vitamins A, C, and E could have a protective effect in smokers. An ecologic analysis using information on baseline diet and the 25-year COPD mortality rate in the Seven Countries Study did indeed reveal an inverse relationship between the baseline intake of fruit and fish and the subsequent COPD mortality.[159] Support for a beneficial effect of vitamin C comes from a Dutch study[160] and from the National Health and Nutrition Examination Survey (NHANES) study[161]; in both studies, COPD is not clearly differentiated from asthma. More convincing data come from two British studies in which COPD was more clearly defined.[162,163] In addition, data have been published that suggest a protective role of fish oil owing to the presence of marine ω-3 fatty acids. Shahar and colleagues found a decreased risk of COPD in subjects with a high intake of ω-3 fatty acids,[164] and at least three other studies have suggested a similar mechanism.[165–167] However, the only longitudinal study to date could not support the hypothesis of a beneficial effect of these nutritional contents.[168]

Conclusion

In conclusion, we have learned much about the natural history of COPD and the risk factors for the disease over the last two to three decades. Future research should include a focus on the development of different clinical subtypes of emphysema and the temporal effects of different risk factors on the natural history of the disease. Importantly, as it is hoped that the concept of "translational science" will expand to include epidemiology, the findings from such studies should be interpreted in parallel with more basic studies assessing the mechanisms through which these risk factors exert their effects.

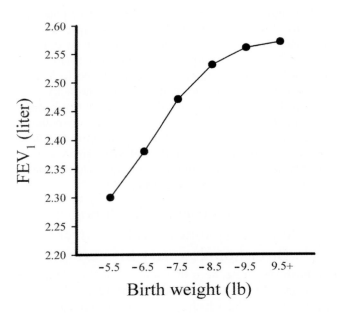

FIGURE 7. The association between birth weight and adult lung function. 1 pound (lb) = 454 g. FEV1 = forced expiratory volume in 1 second. Adapted from Barker DJ et al.[25]

References

1. Murray CJL, Lopez AD. Alternative projections of mortality and disability by cause 1990–2020: Global Burden of Disease Study. Lancet 1997;349:1498–504.

2. Mannino DM, Brown C, Giovino GA. Obstructive lung disease deaths in the United States from 1979 through 1993. An analysis using multiple-cause mortality data. Am J Respir Crit Care Med 1997;156:814–8.

3. Lacasse Y, Brooks D, Goldstein RS. Trends in the epidemiology of COPD in Canada, 1980 to 1995. Chest 1999;116:306–13.

4. Crockett AJ, Cranston JM, Moss JR, Alpers JH. Trends in chronic obstructive pulmonary disease in Australia. Med J Aust 1994;161:600–3.

5. Hansell AL. Lies, damned lies and mortality statistics? Thorax 2006;61:923–4.

6. Jensen HH, Godtfredsen NS, Lange P, Vestbo J. Potential misclassification of causes of death from COPD in a Danish population study. Eur Respir J 2006;28:781–5.

7. European Respiratory Society/European Lung Foundation. The burden of lung disease. In: Loddenkemper R, Gibson GJ, Sibille Y, editors. European lung white book. The first comprehensive survey on respiratory health in Europe. Sheffield (UK): ERSJ; 2003. p.1–182.

8. Hurd S. International efforts directed at attacking the problem of COPD. Chest 2000;117 Suppl:336–8.

9. Brown CA, Crombie IK, Tunstall-Pedoe H. Failure of cigarette smoking to explain international differences in mortality from chronic obstructive pulmonary disease. J Epidemiol Community Health 1994;48:134–9.

10. Wise RA. Changing smoking patterns and mortality from chronic obstructive pulmonary disease. Prev Med 1997;26:418–21.

11. Farebrother MJ, Kelson MC, Heller RF. Death certification of farmer's lung and chronic airway diseases in different countries of the EEC. Br J Dis Chest 1985;79:352–60.

12. Pearson MG, Littler J, Davies PDO. An analysis of medical workload by specialty and diagnosis in Mersey: evidence of a specialist to patient mismatch. J R Coll Physicians Lond 1994;28:230–4.

13. Feinleib M, Rosenberg HM, Cillons JG, et al. Trends in COPD morbidity and mortality in the United States. Am Rev Respir Dis 1989;140:S9–S18.

14. Lung and Asthma Information Agency. Respiratory morbidity in general practice, 1971–1991. Available at <http://www.laia.ac.uk/asthma.htm>, accessed 6 February 2008.

15. Pauwels RA, Rabe KF. Burden and clinical features of chronic obstructive pulmonary disease (COPD). Lancet 2004;364:613–20.

16. Vestbo J. Socioeconomic burden of chronic obstructive pulmonary disease. Eur Respir Mon 2006;38:463–9.

17. Strassels SA, Smith DH, Sullivan SD, Mahajan PS. The costs of treating COPD in the United States. Chest 2001;119:344–52.

18. Andersson F, Borg S, Jansson S-A, et al. The costs of exacerbations in chronic obstructive pulmonary disease (COPD). Respir Med 2002;96:700–8.

19. Mapel DW, McMillan GP, Frost FJ, et al. Predicting the costs of managing patients with chronic obstructive pulmonary disease. Respir Med 2005;99:1325–33.

20. Halbert RJ, Natoli JL, Gano A, et al. Global burden of COPD: systematic review and meta-analysis. Eur Respir J 2006;28:523–32.

21. Buist AS, Vollmer WM, Sullivan SD, et al. The Burden of Obstructive Lung Disease Initiative (BOLD): rationale and design. COPD 2005;2:277–83.

22. Menezes AM, Perez-Padilla R, Jardim JR, et al. Chronic obstructive pulmonary disease in five Latin American cities (the PLATINO study): a prevalence study. Lancet 2005;366:1875–81.

23. Fletcher CM, Peto R, Tinker CM, Speizer FE. The natural history of chronic bronchitis and emphysema. Oxford: Oxford University Press; 1976.

24. Kerstjens HAM, Rijcken B, Schouten JP, Postma DS. Decline of FEV_1 by age and smoking status: facts, figures, and fallacies. Thorax 1997;52:820–7.

25. Barker DJ, Godfrey KM, Fall C, et al. Relation of birth weight and childhood respiratory infection to adult lung function and death from chronic obstructive airways disease. BMJ 1991;303:671–5.

26. Stein CE, Kumaran K, Fall CH, et al. Relation of fetal growth to adult lung function in south India. Thorax 1997;52:895–9.

27. Robbins DR, Enright PL, Sherrill DL. Lung function development in young adults: is there a plateau phase? Eur Respir J 1995;8:768–72.

28. Burrows B, Knudson RJ, Camilli AE, et al. The "horse-racing effect" and predicting decline in forced expiratory volume in one second from screening spirometry. Am Rev Respir Dis 1987;135:788–93.

29. Weitzenblum E, Hirth C, Ducolone A, et al. Prognostic value of pulmonary artery pressure in chronic obstructive pulmonary disease. Thorax 1981;36:752–8.

30. Agusti AG, Noguera A, Sauleda J, et al. Systemic effects of chronic obstructive pulmonary disease. Eur Respir J 2003;21:347–60.

31. Wouters EFM, Schols AMWJ, Celli B. Systemic effects of chronic obstructive pulmonary disease. Eur Respir Mon 2006;38:224–41.

32. Wilson DO, Rogers RM, Wright EC, Anthonisen NR. Body weight in chronic obstructive pulmonary disease: the National Institutes of Health Intermittent Positive-Pressure Breathing Trial. Am Rev Respir Dis 1989;139:1435–8.

33. Gray-Donald K, Gibbons L, Shapiro SH, et al. Nutritional status and mortality in chronic obstructive pulmonary disease. Am J Respir Crit Care Med 1996;153:961–6.

34. Schols AM, Slangen J, Volovics L, Wouters EFM. Weight loss is a reversible factor in the prognosis of chronic obstructive pulmonary disease. Am J Crit Care Med 1998;157:1791–7.

35. Landbo C, Prescott E, Lange P, et al. Prognostic value of nutritional status in chronic obstructive pulmonary disease. Am J Respir Crit Care Med 1999;16:1856–61.

36. Vestbo J, Prescott E, Almdal T, et al. Body mass, fat free body mass and prognosis in COPD patients from a random population sample. Am J Respir Crit Care Med 2006;173:79–83.

37. De Godoy I, Donahoe M, Calhoun WJ, et al. Elevated TNF-alpha production by peripheral blood monocytes of weight-losing COPD patients. Am J Respir Crit Care Med 1996;153:633–7.

38. Di Francia M, Barbier D, Mege JL, Orehek J. Tumor necrosis factor-alpha levels and weight loss in chronic obstructive pulmonary disease. Am J Respir Crit Care Med 1994;150:1453–5.

39. Eid AA, Ionescu AA, Nixon LS, et al. Inflammatory response and body composition in chronic obstructive pulmonary disease. Am J Respir Crit Care Med 2001;164:1414–8.

40. Broekhuizen R, Grimble RF, Howell WM, et al. Pulmonary cachexia, systemic inflammatory profile, and the interleukin 1β–511 single nucleotide polymorphism. Am J Clin Nutr 2005;82:1059–64.

41. Man SFP, Connett JE, Anthonisen NR, et al. C-reactive protein and mortality in mild to moderate chronic obstructive pulmonary disease. Thorax 2006;61;849–53.

42. Dahl M, Vestbo J, Lange P, et al. C-reactive protein as a predictor of prognosis in COPD. Am J Respir Crit Care Med 2006;175:250–5.

43. Glindmeyer HW, Diem JE, Jones RN, Weill H. Non-comparability of longitudinally and cross-sectionally determined annual change in spirometry. Am Rev Respir Dis 1982;125:544–8.

44. Medical Research Council's Committee on the Aaetiology of Chronic Bronchitis. Standardized questionnaires on respiratory symptoms. BMJ 1960;2:1665.

45. Medical Research Council. Instructions for the use of the questionnaire on respiratory symptoms. Devon (UK): W. J. Holman Ltd.; 1966.

46. Ferris BG. Epidemiology standardization project. Am Rev Respir Dis 1978;118:1–53.

47. Minette A. Questionnaire of the European Community for Coal and Steel (ECCS) on respiratory symptoms. 1987 updating of the 1962 and 1967 questionnaires for studying chronic bronchitis and emphysema. Eur Respir J 1989;2:165–77.

48. Eisen EA, Wegman DH, Louis TA. Effects of selection in a prospective study of forced expiratory volume in Vermont granite workers. Am Rev Respir Dis 1983;128:587–91.

49. Eisen EA, Oliver LC, Christiani DC, et al. Effects of spirometry standards in two occupational cohorts. Am Rev Respir Dis 1985;132:120–4.

50. Kellie SE, Attfield MD, Hankinson JL, Castellan RM. Spirometry variability criteria—association with respiratory morbidity and mortality in a cohort of coal miners. Am J Epidemiol 1987;125:437–44.

51. Vestbo J, Knudsen KM, Rasmussen FV. Predictive value of the single breath-nitrogen test for hospitalization due to respiratory disease. Lung 1990;168:93–101.

52. Olofsson J, Bake B, Svärdsudd K, Skoogh B-E. The single breath N_2-test predicts the rate of decline in FEV_1. The study of men born in 1913 and 1923. Eur J Respir Dis 1986;69:46–56.

53. Buist AS, Vollmer WM, Johnson LR, Mccamant LE. Does the single-breath N_2 test identify the smoker who will develop chronic airflow limitation? Am Rev Respir Dis 1988;137:293–301.

54. Stanescu D, Sanna A, Veriter C, Robert A. Identification of smokers susceptible to development of chronic airflow limitation. A 13-year follow-up. Chest 1998;114:416–25.

55. Viegi G, Paoletti P, Prediletto R, et al. Carbon monoxide diffusing capacity, other indices of lung function, and respiratory symptoms in a general population sample. Am Rev Respir Dis 1990;141:1033–9.

56. Sherrill DL, Enright PL, Kaltenborn WT, Lebowitz MD. Predictor of longitudinal change in diffusing capacity over 8 years. Am J Respir Crit Care Med 1999;160:1883–7.

57. Pedersen OF, Miller MR. Lung function. Eur Respir Mon 2000;15:167–98.

58. American Thoracic Society – European Respiratory Society longitudinal data analysis workshop. Am J Respir Crit Care Med 1996;154:S207–84.

59. Pauwels R, Buist A, Calverley P, et al. Global strategy for the diagnosis, management and prevention of chronic obstructive pulmonary disease. NHLBI/WHO Global Initiative for Chronic Obstructive Lung Disease (GOLD) workshop summary. Am J Respir Crit Care Med 2001;163:1256–76.

60. Hardie JA, Buist AS, Vollmer WM, et al. Risk of over-diagnosis of COPD in asymptomatic elderly never-smokers. Eur Respir J 2002;20:1117–22.

61. Vestbo J. Chronic cough and phlegm in young adults. Should we worry? Am J Respir Crit Care Med 2006;175:2–3.

62. Lundbäck B, Lindberg A, Lindström M, et al. Not 15 but 50% of smokers develop COPD? Report from the Obstructive Lung Disease in Northern Sweden Studies. Respir Med 2003;97:115–22.

63. Lindberg A, Jonsson A-C, Rönmark E, et al. Ten-year cumulative incidence of COPD and risk factors for incident disease in a symptomatic cohort. Chest 2005;127:1544–52.

64. Løkke A, Lange P, Scharling H, et al. Developing COPD: a 25 years follow-up study of the general population. Thorax 2006;61:935–9.

65. de Marco R, Accordini S, Cerveri I, et al. Incidence of chronic obstructive pulmonary disease in a cohort of young adults according to the presence of chronic cough and phlegm. Am J Respir Crit Care Med 2007;175:32–9.

66. US Surgeon General. The health consequences of smoking: chronic obstructive lung disease. Washington (DC): US Department of Health and Human Services; 1984. DHHS Publication No.: 84-50205.

67. Davis RM, Novotny TE. The epidemiology of cigarette smoking and its impact on chronic obstructive pulmonary disease. Am Rev Respir Dis 1989;140:S82–4.

68. Tager IB, Segal MR, Speizer FE, Weiss ST. The natural history of forced expiratory volumes. Effect of cigarette smoking and respiratory symptoms. Am Rev Respir Dis 1988;138:837–49.

69. Xu X, Dockery DW, Ware JH, et al. Effects of cigarette smoking on rate of loss of pulmonary function in adults: a longitudinal assessment. Am Rev Respir Dis 1992;146:1345–8.

70. Lange P. Development and prognosis of chronic obstructive pulmonary disease with special reference to the role of tobacco smoking [thesis]. Dan Med Bull 1992;39:30–48.

71. Marsh S, Aldington S, Shirtcliffe P, et al. Smoking and COPD: what really are the risks? Eur Respir J 2006;28:883–4.

72. Hanrahan JP, Tager IB, Segal MR, et al. The effect of maternal smoking during pregnancy on early infant lung function. Am Rev Respir Dis 1992;145:1129–35.

73. Tager IB, Ngo L, Hanrahan JP. Maternal smoking during pregnancy. Effects on lung function during the first 18 months of life. Am J Respir Crit Care Med 1995;152:977–83.

74. Gold DR, Wang X, Wipyj D, et al. Effects of cigarette smoking on lung function in adolescent boys and girls. N Engl J Med 1996;335:931–7.

75. Sherrill DL, Lebowitz MD, Knudson RJ, Burrows B. Smoking and symptom effects on the curves of lung function growth and decline. Am Rev Respir Dis 1991;144:17–22.

76. Lange P, Groth S, Nyboe J, et al. Effects of smoking and changes in smoking habits on the decline of FEV_1. Eur Respir J 1989;2:811–6.

77. Royal College of Physicians of London. Health or smoking? Follow-up report of the Royal College of Physicians. London: Pitman; 1983.

78. Camilli AE, Burrows B, Knudson RJ, et al. Longitudinal changes in forced expiratory volume in one second in adults. Am Rev Respir Dis 1987;135:794–9.

79. Anthonisen NR, Connett JE, Kiley JP, et al. Effects of smoking intervention and the use of an inhaled anticholinergic bronchodilator on the rate of decline of FEV_1: the Lung Health Study. JAMA 1994;272:1497–505.

80. Rennard SI, Vestbo J. COPD: the dangerous underestimate of 15%. Lancet 2006;367:1216–9.

81. Anthonisen NR. "Susceptible"smokers? Thorax 2006;61:924–25.

82. Irwig LM, Groeneveld HT, Becklake MR. Assessing the effect of exposure on lung function loss between two occasions: issues on confounding and measurement error. In: Hensley MJ, Saunders NA, editors. Clinical epidemiology of chronic obstructive pulmonary disease. Basel: Marcel Dekker; 1989.

83. Kauffmann F, Drouet D, Lellouch J, Brille D. Occupational exposure and 12-year spirometric changes among Paris area workers. Br J Ind Med 1982;39:221–32.

84. Krzyzanowski M, Jedrychowski W, Wysocki M. Factors associated with the change in ventilatory function and the development of chronic obstructive pulmonary disease in a 13-year follow-up of the Cracow study. Am Rev Respir Dis 1986;134:1011–9.

85. Korn RJ, Dockery DW, Speizer FE, et al. Occupational exposures and chronic respiratory symptoms. A population-based study. Am Rev Respir Dis 1987;136:298–304.

86. Heederik D, Pouwels H, Kromhout H, Kromhout D. Chronic non-specific lung disease and occupational exposures estimated by means of a job exposure matrix: the Zutphen Study. Int J Epidemiol 1989;18:382–9.

87. Humerfelt S, Gulsvik A, Skjaerven R, et al. Decline in FEV_1 and airflow limitation related to occupational exposures in men of an urban community. Eur Respir J 1993;6:1095–103.

88. Zock JP, Sunjer J, Kogevinas M, et al, and The ECRHS Study Group. Occupation, chronic bronchitis, and lung function in young adults. An international study. Am J Respir Crit Care Med 2001;163:1572–7.

89. Bergdahl IA, Torén K, Eriksson K, et al. Increased mortality in COPD among construction workers exposed to inorganic dust. Eur Respir J 2004;23:402–6.

90. Huisman M, Kunst AE, Bopp M, et al. Educational inequalities in cause-specific mortality in middle-aged and older men and women in eight western European populations. Lancet 2005;365:493–500.

91. Prescott E, Vestbo J. Socioeconomic status and chronic obstructive pulmonary disease. Thorax 1999;54:737–41.

92. Marmot MG, Shipley MJ, Rose G. Inequalities in death—specific explanations of a general pattern? Lancet 1984;i:1003–6.

93. Marmot MG, McDowall ME. Mortality decline and widening in social inequalities. Lancet 1986;i:274–6.

94. Smith GD, Hart C, Blane D, Hole D. Adverse socioeconomic conditions in childhood and cause specific adult mortality: prospective observational study. BMJ 1998;316:1631–5.

95. Osler M, Gerdes LU, Davidsen M, et al. Socioeconomic status and trends in risk factors for cardiovascular diseases in the Danish MONICA population 1982–92. J Epidemiol Community Health 2000;54:108–13.

96. Cavelaars AEJM, Kunst AE, Geurts JJM, et al. Educational differences in smoking: international comparison. BMJ 2000;320:1102–7.

97. Prescott E, Lange P, Vestbo J, and the Copenhagen City Heart Study Group. Socioeconomic status, lung function, and admission to hospital for COPD. Results from the Copenhagen City Heart Study. Eur Respir J 1999;13:1109–14.

98. Bakke PS, Hanoa R, Gulsvik A. Educational level and obstructive lung disease given smoking habits and occupational airborne exposure: a Norwegian community study. Am J Epidemiol 1995;141:1080–8.

99. McCormick MC. The contribution of low birth weight to infant mortality and childhood morbidity. N Engl J Med 1985;312:82–90.

100. Shaheen SO, Barker DJ, Holgate ST. Do lower respiratory tract infections in early childhood cause chronic obstructive pulmonary disease? Am J Respir Crit Care Med 1995;151:1649–51.

101. Coggon D, Barker DJ, Inskip H, et al. Housing in early life and later mortality. J Epidemiol Community Health 1993;47:345–8.

102. Schwartz J, Weiss ST. Relationship between dietary vitamin C intake and pulmonary function in the first National Health and Nutrition Examination Survey (NHANES). Am J Clin Nutr 1994;59:110–4.

103. Sharp DS, Rodriguez BL, Shahar E, et al. Fish consumption may limit the damage of smoking on the lung. Am J Respir Crit Care Med 1994;150:983–7.

104. Sridhar MK. Nutrition and lung health. BMJ 1995;3:1075–6.

105. Rasmussen FV, Borcsenius L, Winslow JB, østergaard ER. Associations between housing conditions, smoking habits and ventilatory lung function in men with clean jobs. Scand J Respir Dis 1978;59:264–76.

106. Comstock GW, Meyer MB, Helsing KJ. Respiratory effects of household exposures to tobacco smoke and gas cooking. Am Rev Respir Dis 1981;124:143–8.

107. Viegi G, Paoletti P, Carozzi L, et al. Effects of home environment on respiratory symptoms and lung function in a general population sample in north Italy. Eur Respir J 1991;4:580–6.

108. Janus ED, Phillips NT, Carrell RW. Smoking, lung function, and alpha-1-antitrypsin deficiency. Lancet 1985;i:152–4.

109. Seersholm N, Wilcke JT, Kok-Jensen A, Dirksen A. Risk of hospital admission for obstructive pulmonary disease in alpha$_1$-antitrypsin heterozygotes of phenotype PiMZ. Am J Respir Crit Care Med 2000;161:81–4.

110. Seersholm N, Kok-Jensen A, Dirksen A. Survival of patients with severe alpha-1-antitrypsin deficiency with special reference to non-index cases. Thorax 1994;49:695–8.

111. Seersholm N, Kok-Jensen A, Dirksen A. Decline in FEV_1 among patients with severe hereditary alpha-1-antitrypsin

deficiency type PiZZ. Am J Respir Crit Care Med 1995;152:1922–5.

112. Piitulainen E, Eriksson S. Decline in FEV$_1$ related to smoking status in individuals with severe alpha-1-antitrypsin deficiency (PiZZ). Eur Respir J 1999;13:247–51.

113. Dahl M, Tybjærg-Hansen A, Lange P, et al. Change in lung function and COPD morbidity in alpha$_1$-antitrypsin MZ heterozygotes: a longitudinal study of the general population. Ann Intern Med 2002;136:270–9.

114. Larson RK, Barman ML, Kueppers F, Fudenberg HH. Genetic and environmental determinants of chronic obstructive pulmonary disease. Ann Intern Med 1970;72:627–32.

115. Kueppers F, Miller RD, Gordon H, et al. Familial prevalence of chronic obstructive pulmonary disease in a matched pair study. Am J Med 1977;63:336–42.

116. Cohen BH, Ball WC Jr, Brashears S, et al. Risk factors in chronic obstructive pulmonary disease (COPD). Am J Epidemiol 1977;105:223–32.

117. Sandford AJ, Weir TD, Pare P. Genetic risk factors for chronic obstructive pulmonary disease. Eur Respir J 1997;10:1380–91.

118. Silverman EK, Chapman HA, Drazen JM, et al. Genetic epidemiology of severe, early-onset chronic obstructive pulmonary disease. Risk to relatives for airflow obstruction and chronic bronchitis. Am J Respir Crit Care Med 1998;157:1770–8.

119. Peto R, Speizer FE, Cochrane AL, et al. The relevance in adults of air-flow obstruction, but not of mucus hypersecretion, to mortality from chronic lung disease. Am Rev Respir Dis 1983;128:491–500.

120. Sherman CB, Xu X, Speizer FE, et al. Longitudinal lung function decline in subjects with respiratory symptoms. Am Rev Respir Dis 1992;146:855–9.

121. Vestbo J, Prescott E, Lange P, and The Copenhagen City Heart Study Group. Association of chronic mucus hypersecretion with FEV$_1$ decline and COPD morbidity. Am J Respir Crit Care Med 1996;153:1530–5.

122. Vestbo J, Rasmussen FV. Respiratory symptoms and FEV$_1$ as predictors of hospitalization and medication in the following 12 years due to respiratory disease. Eur Respir J 1989;2:710–5.

123. Annesi I, Kauffmann F. Is respiratory mucus hypersecretion really an innocent disorder? Am Rev Respir Dis 1986;134:688–93.

124. Lange P, Nyboe J, Appleyard M, et al. The relation of ventilatory impairment and of chronic mucus hypersecretion to mortality from obstructive lung disease and from all causes. Thorax 1990;45:579–85.

125. Prescott E, Lange P, Vestbo J. Chronic mucus hypersecretion in COPD and death from pulmonary infection. Eur Respir J 1995;8:1333–8.

126. Vestbo J, Lange P. Can GOLD stage 0 provide information of prognostic value in chronic obstructive pulmonary disease? Am J Respir Crit Care Med 2002;166:329–32.

127. Vestbo J, Hogg JC. Convergence of the epidemiology and pathology of COPD. Thorax 2006;61:86–8.

128. Prescott E. Tobacco-related diseases: the role of gender. An epidemiologic study based on data from the Copenhagen Centre for Prospective Population Studies [thesis]. Dan Med Bull 2000;47:115–31.

129. Prescott E, Bjerg AM, Andersen PK, et al. Gender differences in smoking effects on lung function and risk of hospitalization for COPD: results from a Danish longitudinal population study. Eur Respir J 1997;10:822–7.

130. Prescott E, Osler M, Vestbo J. Importance of detailed adjustment for smoking when comparing morbidity and mortality in men and women in a Danish population study. Eur J Public Health 1998;8:166–9.

131. Orie NGM, Sluiter HJ, de Vries K, et al. The host factor in bronchitis. In: Orie NGM, Sluiter HJ, editors. Bronchitis: an international symposium. Assen (Netherlands): Royal van Gorcum; 1961.

132. Vestbo J, Prescott E. An update on the Dutch hypothesis and chronic respiratory disease. Thorax 1998;53 Suppl 2:S15–9.

133. Rijcken B, Scouten JP, Xu X, et al. Bronchial hyperresponsiveness to histamine is associated with accelerated decline of FEV$_1$. Am J Respir Crit Care Med 1995;151:1377–82.

134. Villar MT, Dow L, Coggon D, et al. The influence of increased bronchial responsiveness, atopy, and serum IgE on decline in FEV$_1$: a longitudinal study in the elderly. Am J Respir Crit Care Med 1995;151:656–62.

135. Parker DR, O'Connor GT, Sparrow D, et al. The relationship of nonspecific airway responsiveness and atopy to the rate of decline of lung function. The Normative Aging Study. Am Rev Respir Dis 1990;141:589–94.

136. O'Connor GT, Sparrow D, Weiss ST. A prospective study of methacholine airway responsiveness as a predictor of pulmonary function decline: the Normative Aging Study. Am J Respir Crit Care Med 1995;152:87–92.

137. Tashkin DP, Altose MD, Connett JE, et al, for the Lung Health Study Research Group. Methacholine reactivity predicts changes in lung function over time in smokers with early chronic obstructive pulmonary disease. Am J Respir Crit Care Med 1996;153:1802–11.

138. Rijcken B, Weiss ST. Longitudinal analyses of airway responsiveness and pulmonary function decline. Am J Respir Crit Care Med 1996;154:S246–9.

139. Hospers JJ, Postma DS, Rijcken B, et al. Histamine airway hyper-responsiveness and mortality from chronic obstructive pulmonary disease: a cohort study. Lancet 2000;356:1313–7.

140. Postma DS, Boezen HM. The rationale for the Dutch hypothesis. Chest 2004;126:96–104S.

141. Hansen EF, Phanareth K, Laursen LC, et al. Reversible and irreversible airflow obstruction as predictor of overall mortality in asthma and chronic obstructive pulmonary disease. Am J Respir Crit Care Med 1999;159:1267–71.

142. Anthonisen NR, Lindgren PG, Tashkin DP, et al, for the Lung Health Study Research Group. Bronchodilator response in the lung health study over 11 years. Eur Respir J 2005;26:45–51.

143. Hansen EF, Vestbo J. Bronchodilator reversibility in COPD—the roguish but harmless little brother of airway hyperresponsiveness? Eur Respir J 2005;26:6–7.

144. Peat JK, Woolcock AJ, Cullen K. Rate of decline of lung function in subjects with asthma. Eur J Respir Dis 1987;70:171–9.

145. Lange P, Parner J, Vestbo J, et al. A 15-year follow-up of ventilatory function in adults with asthma. N Engl J Med 1998;339:1194–200.

146. Lange P, Ulrik CS, Vestbo J, for The Copenhagen City Heart Study Group. Mortality in adults with selfreported bronchial asthma. A study of the general population. Lancet 1996;347:1285–9.

147. Lange P, Scharling H, Ulrik CS, Vestbo J. Inhaled corticosteroids and decline of lung function in community residents with asthma. Thorax 2006;61:100–4.

148. Dijkstra A, Vonk JM, Jongepier H, et al. Lung function decline in asthma: association with inhaled corticosteroids, smoking and sex. Thorax 2006;61:105–10.

149. Lebowitz MD. Epidemiological studies of the respiratory effects of air pollution. Eur Respir J 1996;9:1029–54.

150. Sunyer J, Saez M, Murillo C, et al. Air pollution and emergency room admissions for COPD: a five year study. Am J Epidemiol 1993;137:701–5.

151. Burnett RT, Dales R, Krewski D, et al. Associations between ambient particulate sulfate and admissions to Ontario hospitals for cardiac and respiratory diseases. Am J Epidemiol 1995;142:15–22.

152. Dockery EW, Schwartz J, Spengler JD. Air pollution and daily mortality: associations with particulates and acid aerosols. Environ Res 1992;59:362–73.

153. Sunyer J, Schwartz J, Tobias A, et al. Patients with chronic obstructive pulmonary disease are at increased risk of death associated with urban particle air pollution: a case-crossover analysis. Am J Epidemiol 2000;151:50–6.

154. Gold DR, Tager IB, Weiss ST, et al. Acute lower respiratory illness in childhood as a predictor of lung function and chronic respiratory symptoms. Am Rev Respir Dis 1989;140:877–84.

155. Shaheen SO, Barker DJ, Shiell AW, et al. The relationship between pneumonia in early childhood and impaired lung function in late adult life. Am J Respir Crit Care Med 1994;149:616–9.

156. Britton J, Martinez FD. The relationship of childhood respiratory infection to growth and decline in lung function. Am J Respir Crit Care Med 1996;154:S240–5.

157. Matsuse T, Hayashi S, Kuwano K, et al. Latent adenoviral infection in the pathogenesis of chronic airways obstruction. Am Rev Respir Dis 1992;146:177–84.

158. Hogg JC. Childhood viral infection and the pathogenesis of asthma and chronic obstructive lung disease. Am J Respir Crit Care Med 1999;160:S26–8.

159. Tabak C, Feskens EJ, Heederik D, et al. Fruit and fish consumption: a possible explanation for population differences in COPD mortality (the Seven Countries Study). Eur J Clin Nutr 1998;52:819–25.

160. Miedema I, Feskens EJM, Heederik D, Kromhout D. Dietary determinants of long-term incidence of chronic nonspecific lung disease. The Zutphen study. Am J Epidemiol 1993;138:37–45.

161. Schwartz J, Weiss ST. Dietary factors and their relation to respiratory symptoms. Am J Epidemiol 1990;132:67–76.

162. Strachan DP, Cox BD, Erzinclioglu SW, et al. Ventilatory function and winter fresh fruit consumption in a random sample of British adults. Thorax 1991;46:624–9.

163. Dow L, Tracey M, Villar A, et al. Does dietary intake of vitamin C and E influence lung function in older people? Am J Respir Crit Care Med 1996;154:1401–4.

164. Shahar E, Folsom AR, Milnick SL, et al. Dietary n-3 polyunsaturated fatty acids and smoking-related chronic obstructive pulmonary disease. N Engl J Med 1994;331:228–33.

165. Sharp DS, Rodriguez BL, Shahar E, et al. Fish consumption may limit the damage of smoking on the lung. Am J Respir Crit Care Med 1994;150:983–7.

166. Schwartz J, Weiss ST. The relationship of dietary fish intake to level of pulmonary function in the first National Health and Nutrition Survey (NHANES I). Eur Respir J 1994;7:1821–4.

167. Tabak C, Smit HA, Rasanen L, et al. Dietary factors and pulmonary function: a cross sectional study in middle aged men from three European countries. Thorax 1999;54:1021–6.

168. Smit HA, Grievink L, Tabak C. Dietary influences on chronic obstructive lung disease and asthma: a review of the epidemiological evidence. Proc Nutr Soc 1999;58:309–19.

CHAPTER 4

GENETIC RISK FACTORS

MARILYN G. FOREMAN, MD, MS, AND EDWIN K. SILVERMAN, MD, PHD

A MAJOR MILESTONE of the modern genetics revolution occurred with the announcement of the initial draft sequence of the human genome in June 2000.[1,2] Other seminal events have included the completion of the high-quality reference sequence of the human genome in April 2003 and the completion of the first phase of the International HapMap Project in 2005, which created a map of common human genetic variation among three ancestral populations (Asian, European, and African).[3–5] This exponential rise in genetic information has paralleled the growth in studies of the genetics of chronic obstructive pulmonary disease (COPD). Although genetic research has yet to reach its full potential, with the prospects of improved genetic testing, gene therapy, individualized medical therapy through pharmacogenetics, and improved understanding of disease pathophysiology, the increased attention to the genetics of COPD is fortuitous as COPD is expected to become the third most common cause of death worldwide by 2020.[6]

Major hypotheses in the pathogenesis of COPD include protease/antiprotease imbalance, oxidant/antioxidant inequity, and the role of inflammation.[7–9] More recent concepts involve the overlap of these pathways and the complex interaction of cellular senescence and apoptosis.[10,11] All of these mechanistic concepts are areas for genetic exploration and are examined in this chapter.

Genetic Epidemiology

Genetic epidemiology is the study of the joint action of genetic and environmental factors in causing disease in human populations.[12] Mendelian disorders, such as sickle cell anemia or cystic fibrosis, are the result of a single major gene. Mendelian diseases typically have predictable, recognizable inheritance patterns, allowing greater ease in establishing a role for genetics.[13] For single-gene diseases, determining how variation in a gene causes disease is relatively straightforward. Complex diseases, such as COPD, hypertension, and obesity, are multifactorial. Complex disorders may result from the modest effects of multiple common genetic variants plus an environmental contribution. Tobacco smoking is the most common environmental risk factor for the development of COPD,[14,15] but all smokers do not possess the same risk. A genetic role in the susceptibility to COPD has been suggested by the fact that COPD occurs only in a subset of smokers.[16] In fact, with similar smoking

exposures, only 15% of the variability in forced expiratory volume in 1 second (FEV_1) is explained by pack-years of smoking.[17] Although Burrows and colleagues demonstrated that mean FEV_1 is significantly reduced with increased smoking intensity, their study also found that the FEV_1 values of many heavy smokers remained in the normal range.[17] The low percentage of variance in pulmonary function explained by smoking is suggestive of a genetic component to smoking–induced airflow obstruction. Heritable factors likely contribute to the propensity to develop COPD at an earlier age, as well as to the velocity of decline in pulmonary function.[18,19] Unlike the situation with monogenic diseases, identifying the genetic determinants in complex disorders is more complicated.

Association analysis assesses the relationship between genotypic information and disease-related phenotypes. If an allele at a polymorphic locus is in linkage disequilibrium (LD) with a disease allele or if the polymorphic variant is the disease mutation itself, the associated allele will be represented disproportionately among affected individuals. LD occurs when alleles occur together more often than can be accounted for by chance. Association studies may be motivated by linkage findings, in which genes relevant to the etiology of the disease are assessed within the linked region. Positional cloning is used to identify genes associated with a disease based on their location on a chromosome. Fine mapping is used to narrow the search using dense panels of markers over the candidate region in unrelated cases and controls or in family units, looking for associations that could reflect LD with the causal genetic variant. Alternatively, association studies may be initiated based on a candidate gene approach, in which the motivation is often based on biologic plausibility. Once a susceptibility gene is identified using one of these approaches, further characterization of the gene is required to determine the function of potential disease-causing variants.

The case-control association study design is widely used. One disadvantage is that this study design may result in false-positive associations owing to population stratification in which subpopulations with different allele frequencies (eg, differences in ethnic composition) are included in the cases and controls.[20] Inclusion of family-based controls obviates the potential for false-positive associations related to population stratification. For example, the transmission/disequilibrium

Table 1   Approaches to Identify Novel Chronic Obstructive Pulmonary Disease Susceptibility Genes

Method	Status	Study
Association analysis of candidate genes	Frequently used; inconsistent results	Hersh et al, 2005[111]
Linkage analysis followed by association analysis of candidate genes	Infrequently used; *TGFB1* has been reported	Celedón et al, 2004[50]
Linkage analysis followed by association analysis of gene expression candidate genes	Infrequently used; *SERPINE2* has been reported	DeMeo et al, 2006[134]
Linkage analysis followed by dense fine mapping	No published reports	—
Rare variant analysis	Infrequently used; elastin variant has been reported	Kelleher et al, 2005[182]
Animal model quantitative trait locus analysis followed by association analysis in humans	No published reports	Shapiro et al, 2004[169]
Genome-wide association analysis	No published reports	—

Adapted from Sliverman EK.[29]

test, which typically employs genotypic data from affected individuals and their parents, provides a test of linkage and association without bias from population stratification or admixture.[20] An alternative approach, which is especially pertinent for late-onset diseases such as COPD, is to assess for population stratification in cases and controls by genotyping random single nucleotide polymorphisms (SNPs) unlinked to the disease of interest or by genotyping ancestry informative markers (AIMs).[21] Failure to demonstrate association to these unrelated SNPs demonstrates that significant population stratification is likely not present, and case-control genetic association studies can be performed with amelioration of the risk of biased results owing to population stratification. It remains unclear whether random SNPs or AIMs are preferential, but AIMs are especially useful for admixed populations such as African Americans. If population stratification is demonstrated between the case and control populations, methods to detect significant disease-gene associations have been developed based on correction for the degree of stratification.[22] Principal components analysis approaches have also been reported to correct for population stratification in genome-wide association studies.[23] Disagreement about the risk of population stratification still remains as some authors believe that the potential is low in studies of non-Hispanics of European descent.[22] Data are limited on other ethnicities. Although the case-control design is frequently used for genetic association studies, the method has been faulted for the lack of replication.[24] As a result, recommendations for performing, reporting, and evaluating case-control studies have been published.[25–27]

There are multiple approaches to identify novel candidate genes and elucidate the genetic determinants in the pathogenesis of COPD. These were recently discussed and reviewed (Table 1).[28,29]

Evidence for Familial Clustering of COPD

Genetic epidemiology can involve methods based exclusively on phenotypic data in which deoxyribonucleic acid (DNA) is not needed, such as familial aggregation studies, which confirm that diseases tend to run in families, and segregation analysis, which tests hypotheses about modes of inheritance. One of the primary characteristics of a genetic trait is that it aggregates, or clusters, within families. The risk to relatives is estimated by comparing the risk of a disease phenotype in relatives of affected subjects with the risk in the general population. Twin studies are useful in genetic analyses because they may be used to compare disease rates between monozygotic twins, who share 100% of their genes, and dizygotic twins, who share an average of 50% of their genes. An increased concordance of disease in monozygotic twins is consistent with a genetic effect. Analysis of other pairs of relatives such as sib-sib pairs or parent-child pairs may also be used to assess for familial aggregation. Additionally, segregation analysis is a modeling tool that determines whether a phenotype observed in families is compatible with a specific mode of inheritance.

Familial clustering, however, may not necessarily be genetic in nature. Alternative explanations for clustering include shared environmental influences. Other evidence to substantiate a genetic cause for familial clustering may be provided by family histories,[30] calculation of an attributable fraction, and the use of correlation coefficients from scatterplots.[13] Heritability, h^2, is the percentage of phenotypic variation that is due to genetic factors. Heritability, however, may be overestimated from twin studies for quantitative phenotypes such as lung function because of the increased environmental sharing among monozygotic twins that begins *in utero*. In twin studies, heritability estimates for FEV_1 have ranged from 0 to 0.77.[31,32] An additional caveat in the comparison of heritability estimates for pulmonary function among studies is the inconsistent inclusion of environmental exposures such as tobacco smoking, which may impact the heritability estimates, particularly in the setting of a gene-by-environment interaction.[33] Therefore, accurate comparison across studies requires assessment of the covariates and the models.

Twin studies and studies of relatives with airflow obstruction have suggested that genetic factors other than α_1-antitrypsin (A1AT) deficiency may contribute to the susceptibility to develop COPD or influence variation in pulmonary function.[34–38] Familial aggregation for COPD and COPD-related phenotypes has been demonstrated.[19,39] In a study of 44 patients with severe (FEV_1 <40% predicted) early-onset (age 52 years or less) COPD, Silverman and colleagues demonstrated that the risk of airflow obstruction in smoking first-degree relatives of early-onset COPD probands was threefold higher than in smokers from the general population.[19] McCloskey and colleagues confirmed this increased familial risk in a study in which 111 current or former smoking siblings of COPD subjects were compared with matched controls from the European Prospective Investigation of Cancer (EPIC)-Norfolk cohort.[40] The prevalence of airflow obstruction was significantly higher in the current or former smoking siblings of COPD patients compared with controls (odds ratio [OR] 4.70; 95% confidence interval [CI] 2.63–8.41), demonstrating a significant, quantifiable risk for airflow obstruction in the relatives of COPD subjects who smoke. DeMeo and colleagues reported that both smoking and nonsmoking first-degree relatives of early-onset COPD probands manifested significantly lower midflow lung function parameters, forced expiratory flow (FEF)$_{25–75}$ and FEF$_{25–75}$/forced vital capacity (FVC), than population-based controls.[39] An h^2 of 0.38 for FEF$_{25–75}$ and an h^2 of 0.45 for FEF$_{25–75}$/FVC were similar to the heritability estimates for FEV_1 and FEV_1/FVC. Heritability estimates have also been published in studies evaluating longitudinal decline in pulmonary function, such as the Tucson Epidemiological Study of Airway Obstructive Diseases and the Framingham Heart Study.[41,42] In these studies, correlations and heritability estimates were higher in smoking concordant siblings.

Evidence for Linkage

One approach to localize causative genes is linkage analysis, in which DNA samples from potentially informative members of affected families are typed for genetic markers at known locations to provide evidence for the general chromosomal location of the susceptibility gene. Genome scan

linkage studies often use approximately 400 short tandem repeat (STR) markers, which are spaced approximately 10 cM apart across the genome. STRs are more polymorphic than SNPs, so SNP-based linkage studies require a larger number of markers. A statistical estimate of whether two loci, the marker and the purported causal genetic locus, are likely to lie near one another on the same chromosome and are likely to be concomitantly inherited is calculated as the logarithm of the odds of linkage (to the base 10) or LOD. Linkage analysis is a technique to determine whether the recombination frequency between two loci is significantly different from 0.5 (random assortment).[43,44] An LOD score of ≥3 was initially proposed as significant evidence and indicates that the odds are 1,000 to 1 in favor of genetic linkage. The level for a significant LOD score with genome-wide significance varies depending on the study design. At a genome-wide alpha level of 5% ($p = .05$), a significant LOD score for a family study is ≥3.3 when the method of inheritance is specified (parametric linkage analysis) and ≥3.6 in studies of sib pairs in which the method of inheritance is not specified (nonparametric).[43,45] An LOD score of at least 1.9 is considered suggestive of linkage in parametric linkage analysis in pedigrees[45] and may still be relevant as linkage studies may be underpowered.

The only reported linkage study in COPD was performed in the Boston Early-Onset COPD Study, in which quantitative and qualitative phenotypes were analyzed.[46–48] Genome-wide linkage analysis was performed on 585 members of 72 extended pedigrees with 377 STR markers. Improvement in the LOD scores in several genomic regions occurred with the analysis of postbronchodilator quantitative spirometric phenotypes compared with prebronchodilator measurements.[46] Postbronchodilator spirometric phenotypes have been suggested to have the ability to provide more robust evidence for linkage owing to amelioration of the day-to-day variability in the level of baseline lung function.[29]

Genome-wide linkage analysis of FEV_1 and FEV_1/FVC was performed with multipoint variance component analysis using sequential oligogenic linkage analysis routines (SOLAR) for the postbronchodilator spirometric values, with adjustment for pack-years of smoking and other relevant covariates.[48] Postbronchodilator FEV_1 was linked to several regions, with the most significant evidence for linkage found on chromosome 8p (LOD = 3.30) and chromosome 1p (LOD = 2.24). Analysis of the postbronchodilator FEV_1/FVC ratio was also linked to multiple loci, with the most significant evidence for linkage found on chromosome 2q (LOD = 4.42) and chromosome 1p (LOD = 2.52). After the initial genome-wide study was completed, additional flanking markers were genotyped to enhance the evidence for linkage. Analyses limited to smokers resulted in a reduced sample size but selected for genetic determinants influenced by gene–by–smoking interactions.[49,50] The addition of flanking markers and stratification by smoking status increased the evidence for linkage on chromosomes 2q, 12p, and 19q.

Population-based cohorts have also been analyzed for linkage to spirometric measures. In a 10 cM genome-wide scan of 1,578 members of 330 families from the Framingham cohort, a five-decade longitudinal study of Caucasians, loci most strongly associated with FEV_1 and FVC were found on chromosomes 4, 6, and 21.[51] The highest LOD of 2.6 for FVC was found on chromosome 21. The strongest evidence for FEV_1 (LOD 2.4) was found on chromosome 6. This area was followed up with a fine mapping study using additional markers.[52] Using GENEHUNTER (<http://www.broad. mit.edu/ftp/distribution/software/genehunter/>) for variance component linkage analysis, a maximum multipoint LOD score of 5.0 was observed for FEV_1 at 184.5 cM. LOD scores above 1 were found in this region for FEV_1/FVC ratio and FVC, supporting the potential for a gene influencing pulmonary function to exist on the q-terminal region of chromosome 6. The linkage findings on chromosome 6 stimulated this group to perform a candidate gene investigation of secreted modular calcium binding protein 2 (SMOC2), located at 168.6 Mb.[53] Twenty SNPs in or adjacent to this gene were genotyped in 1,734 individuals. The minor allele of rs1402 was associated with higher mean FEV_1 ($p = .003$) and FVC ($p = .02$). In never-smoking subjects, the minor allele of rs747995 was associated with higher measures for FEV_1 ($p = .0006$) and FVC ($p = .0008$). These two SNPs are in different haplotype blocks within intron 4. A two-SNP, G-T haplotype (rs747995-rs1402) was detected in 77% of never-smoking participants in the Framingham Heart Study. This haplotype was associated with a reduction in FEV_1 ($p = .0002$) and FVC ($p = .0002$) and was replicated in never-smoking participants from the Family Heart Study ($p = .03$, for FEV_1 and FVC, respectively).

In a study of 264 members of 26 Utah Genetic Reference pedigrees originally collected for the Centre d'Etude du Polymorphisme Humain (CEPH) genetic mapping project, suggestive evidence for linkage was found for FEV_1/FVC on chromosome 2q (LOD 2.36, dominant model), similar to the findings of Silverman and colleagues,[48] as well as on chromosome 5 (LOD 2.23, recessive model). Using spirometric data obtained from the National Heart, Lung, and Blood Institute Family Heart Study, a multicenter study of the genetic and nongenetic determinants of cardiovascular events and risk factors, a genome wide linkage scan delineated regions on chromosomes 4 and 18 with LOD >2.5, supporting linkage to FEV_1/FVC.[54] Genotyping more markers in these areas led to an increase in the LOD score to 3.5 on chromosome 4. The LOD score for FEV_1/FVC on chromosome 4 was 2.0 when the FEV_1 to FVC ratio was transformed for non-normality.

Evidence for Candidate Genes from Association Studies
Xenobiotic Metabolizing Enzymes
MICROSOMAL EPOXIDE HYDROLASE (EPHX1)

Mainstream tobacco smoke is composed of thousands of compounds: particulates, gases, and carcinogens. Microsomal epoxide hydrolase (EPHX1) functions in the metabolism of highly reactive xenobiotic epoxide metabolites resulting from the degradation of procarcinogenic polyaromatic compounds to substances that can be conjugated and excreted. SNPs in exon 3 (Tyr113His) (slow) and exon 4 (His139Arg) (fast) are associated with alteration of enzyme activity levels.[55,56] These two common polymorphisms confer slow and fast enzyme activity. Enzyme activity is reduced by at least 50% with the "slow" allele and increased by at least 25% with the "fast" allele in comparison with normal activity with the wild-type alleles.[55] Since these variants result only in modest changes in enzymatic activity levels, variation in the gene's regulatory regions may also be important.[57]

Individuals with COPD were four times more likely to be homozygous for the Tyr113His variant (OR 4.1; 95% CI 1.8–9.7) in a Scottish study (Table 2).[58] In the same study, individuals with a pathologic diagnosis of emphysema from tissue specimens were five times more likely to be homozygous for this allele (OR 5.0; 95% CI 2.3–10.9). Two studies did not find differences in the genotypes for EPHX1 in cases and controls, but the frequency of the homozygous Tyr113His variant was higher in patients with FEV_1 <35%.[59,60] A haplotype analysis for EPHX1 found an association with accelerated lung function decline in the presence of a family history for COPD.[61] Another report found associations between EPHX1 variants and measures of functional status.[62] Other studies have not concurred.[63,64] A protective effect for the Tyr113His polymorphism was demonstrated in an association analysis and meta-analysis.[65] Although the preponderance of evidence seems to support a role for this biologically plausible candidate gene, the divergent study results may be explained by the differences in study design, ethnic origins of the study populations, and the phenotype definitions employed.

GLUTATHIONE-S-TRANSFERASES

Glutathione-S-transferases are members of a family of enzymes that conjugate multiple electrophilic substances with glutathione, resulting in detoxification, metabolism, and excretion. As a modifier of oxidative stress through detoxification of some of the injurious contents of tobacco smoke,[66] the genes coding for these enzymes are biologically plausible candidates in the pathogenesis of COPD. These enzymes are categorized as alpha (GSTA), mu (GSTM), pi (GSTP), theta (GSTT), sigma, and kappa. Potentially functional variants reported in GSTP1 include isoleucine (Ile) 105 valine (val) in exon 5 and alanine (Ala) 114 valine (Val) in exon 6.[67,68] The most widely studied GSTM1 variant is a large deletion known as a null allele; homozygosity for the null allele results in no measurable GSTM1 activity. The strongest evidence for association with COPD lies with GSTP1 and GSTM1.

Ishii and colleagues reported an association of GSTP1 with COPD susceptibility in a Japanese cohort in which homozygosity for the GSTP1/Ile105 allele conferred an OR of 3.5 (95% CI 2.7–4.6) (Table 3).[69] The same authors also reported that underexpression of GSTP1 induced apoptosis in human lung fibroblasts without affecting glutathione levels[70] and

Table 2 Evidence for Microsomal Epoxide Hydrolase (EPHX1) as a Genetic Determinant of Chronic Obstructive Pulmonary Disease

Study	Study Population	Analysis	Comments	Results
Smith and Harrison, 1997[58]	Caucasian subjects, 203 blood donor controls, 57 asthmatics, 50 lung cancer patients, 94 emphysema patients, 68 COPD patients, A1AT excluded	Case-control association analysis for COPD susceptibility	Scottish study Emphysema was diagnosed pathologically COPD patients were from a respiratory failure clinic Proportion of the genotypes in the asthma and cancer cohorts was not different from controls	COPD patients were 4 times more likely to be homozygous for the Tyr113His variant
Yoshikawa et al, 2000[59]	40 COPD patients, 71 lung cancer patients, 247 controls	Case-control association analysis Authors felt their findings reflected risk for advanced COPD rather than COPD susceptibility	Japanese study in which the frequency of codon 113 variant is higher than in Caucasians A novel SNP was detected 20 bp downstream of the codon 113 SNP with strong LD with the wild-type allele for codon 113	Tyr113His significant only where $FEV_1 < 35\%$
Yim et al, 2000[63]	83 COPD cases, 76 healthy smoking controls	Case-control association analysis	Korean study	Negative
Takeyabu et al, 2000[64]	79 COPD cases (CT confirmed), 58 smoking controls, 114 general population controls	Case-control association analysis	Japanese study	Negative
Sandford et al, 2001[61]	283 Lung Health Study participants with rapid FEV_1 decline 308 non-decliners	Association analysis of rapid lung function decline vs no decline		Haplotype frequencies significantly differed, $p = .03$ Family history of COPD plus His[113]/His[139] haplotype associated with decline, OR 4.9, $p = .04$
Cheng et al, 2004[60]	184 COPD patients, 212 asymptomatic current or former smoking controls	Case-control association analysis for COPD susceptibility	Taiwanese study	Significant for Tyr113His only where $FEV_1 < 35\%$
Hersh et al, 2005[111]	Boston Early-Onset COPD Study and NETT participants vs NAS controls	Family-based and case-control studies	EPHX1 did not replicate across both study designs	His139Arg significant in an additive model in the case-control study, $p = .03$
Brøgger et al, 2006[65]	Self-reported Caucasian 248 COPD cases, 244 controls, A1AT excluded	Case-control association analysis and meta-analysis of 16 studies	Norwegian study Reduced frequency of Tyr113His homozygotes in the COPD cases compared with controls	Reduced risk for COPD in Tyr113His homozygotes, OR 0.5, $p = .02$ (codominant model), adjusted OR 0.51, $p = .06$
Hersh et al, 2006[62]	304 Caucasian NETT subjects with replication analysis in the Boston Early-Onset COPD Study	Test-replication association analyses of candidate genes with functional impairment phenotypes		Tyr113His significant for reduction in maximum work (watts) His139Arg associated with increased DL_{CO}

A1AT = α_1-antitrypsin; COPD = chronic obstructive pulmonary disease; CT = computed tomography; DL_{CO} = carbon monoxide diffusing capacity; FEV_1 = forced expiratory volume in 1 second; LD = linkage disequilibrium; NAS = Normative Aging Study; NETT = National Emphysema Treatment Trial; OR = odds ratio; SNP = single nucleotide polymorphism.

Table 3 Evidence for Glutathione-S-Transferase pi (*GSTP1*) as a Genetic Determinant of Chronic Obstructive Pulmonary Disease

Study	Study Population	Analysis	Comments	Results
Ishii et al, 1999[69]	53 COPD patients, 50 controls	Case-control association analysis of two exonic *GSTP1* SNPs (Ile105Val and Ala114Val) with COPD susceptibility	Japanese study	Homozygous *GSTP1* (Ile105) associated with COPD (OR 3.5; CI 2.7–4.6)
Çalikoglu et al, 2006[73]	149 COPD subjects, 150 healthy controls	Case-control association analysis for COPD susceptibility and gene-gene interactions	Turkish study	Homozygous *GSTP1* (Ile/Ile) genotype was higher in COPD patients (61.1%) than in controls (38%) *GSTP1* Val/Val genotype (OR 0.25; CI 0.12–0.5; *p* = .0001) and *GSTP1* Ile/Val genotype (OR 0.47; CI 0.28–0.8; *p* = .005) were associated with reduced susceptibility Combined genotypes were associated with increased odds of COPD
He et al, 2002[72]	Caucasian subset of the Lung Health Study 286 rapid decliners, 308 non-decliners	Multigene study of susceptibility to lung function	*GSTP1* *GSTM1* *GSTT1*	None of the variants independently associated with rapid decline in lung function
Cheng et al, 2004[60]	184 COPD patients, 212 asymptomatic current or former smoking controls	Case-control association analysis of 3 GST genes for COPD susceptibility	Taiwanese study *GSTP1* *GSTM1* *GSTT1*	Association of *GSTM1*-null genotype with COPD (OR 2.2; CI 1.3–3.5) Combination of at least one *EPHX1* (Tyr113His) allele and *GSTM1*-null associated with COPD (OR 3.6; CI 1.9–8.6) OR 6.8 (CI 1.6–17) when the combined genotypes included the homozygous *GSTP1* wild-type genotype (Ile105/Ile105)

CI = 95% confidence interval; COPD = chronic obstructive pulmonary disease; GST = glutathione-S-transferase; OR = odds ratio; SNP = single nucleotide polymorphism.

that *GSTP1* provided a protective effect in human lung fibroblasts against tobacco smoke extract *in vitro*.[71] In a study of Caucasian participants in the Lung Health Study that investigated the relationship of several genes with rapid decline in lung function, *GSTP1* was associated with rapid lung function deterioration only when polymorphisms in *GSTP1*, *GSTM1*, and *GSTT1* were simultaneously present (OR 2.83; *p* = .03) or in the presence of *GSTP1* 105Ile/Ile plus a family history of COPD (OR 2.2; *p* = .01).[72] A Russian report of 149 patients and 150 healthy controls found a higher genotype frequency for *GSTP1* Ile/Ile in cases compared with controls and a protective effect of the Ile/Val and Val/Val genotypes.[73]

HEME OXYGENASE

Heme oxygenase 1 (HMOX1) is the inducible isoform of heme oxygenase. HMOX1 functions in the metabolism of heme, resulting in the release of biliverdin, iron, and carbon monoxide.[74] These by-products of heme metabolism are metabolically active in that they are purported to mediate the antioxidant, antiproliferative, vasodilatory, antiapoptotic, and anti-inflammatory properties of HMOX1.[75] HMOX1 is found in higher concentrations in the lungs of smokers, where it may be upregulated owing to increased oxidative stress from smoking or inflammatory cells,[76] but COPD subjects have been shown to have reduced levels of HMOX1 in alveolar macrophages isolated from bronchoalveolar

Table 4   Evidence for Heme Oxygenase 1 as a Genetic Determinant of Chronic Obstructive Pulmonary Disease

Study	Study Population	Analysis	Comments	Results
Yamada et al, 2000[80]	101 COPD cases with CT scans showing low-attenuation areas and 100 smoking controls	Case-control association analysis of COPD susceptibility and measurement of promoter activities of different [GT]n repeats (n = 16–20, 29, 38) analyzed by transient-transfection assay in cultured cell lines	Japanese study, [GT]n repeats were classified as short (<25), middle (25–29), and long (≥30) because of a trimodal distribution in the peaks of repeats	The L-class allele frequencies (L/L, L/M, L/S) were higher in COPD cases (OR 2.4; CI 1.3–5.7) H_2O_2 exposure upregulated promoter/luciferase fusion in [GT]16 or [GT]20 but not in the longer alleles
He et al, 2002[72]	Caucasian subset of the Lung Health Study with 286 rapid decliners and 308 non-decliners	Multigene study of susceptibility to lung function decline Rapid decline defined as a decrease of 152 ± 2.5 mL/yr in FEV_1 Non-decliners defined as 15 ± 1.5 mL/yr gain in FEV_1		No association with *HMOX* [GT]n alleles
Budhi et al, 2003[81]	235 heavy smokers: 63 with CT-confirmed emphysema; 172 without CT-confirmed emphysema	Multigene case-control analysis of genetic susceptibility to emphysematous changes detected by CT	Japanese study	No allele frequencies were statistically different between the two study groups Combination of the genotype with very slow activity (homozygous variant for codon 114) for *EPHX1* and at least one large size [GT]n repeat in the *HMOX1* gene promoter region was higher in the CT-confirmed emphysema group (p = .03; OR 2.8; CI .07–7.5)
Nakayama et al, 2006[83]	101 COPD subjects	Longitudinal study of lung function decline Rapid decline was defined as a mean annual decrease of ≥ 3% predicted in FEV_1)	Japanese study, Class S (< 27 repeats), M (27–32 repeats), L (≥ 33 repeats)	28 L-allele carriers, 73 without the L-allele The mean annual FEV_1 decline was higher in L-allele carriers than in non-carriers (2.74% vs −0.57%; p = .044) The proportion of rapid decliners was higher among L-allele carriers (43% vs 18%; p = .009) The adjusted odds of L-allele carriers for rapid decline was 3.9 (CI 1.4–10.6; p = .009)
Guénégou et al, 2006[82]	749 subjects	General population study of level of lung function and FEV_1 and FEV_1/FVC decline in smokers	French study, Class L (≥ 33 repeats) was pooled with any genotype containing the L-allele vs noncarriers	The L-allele carriers had significantly more rapid decline in FEV_1/FVC The decline was steeper in heavy smokers (≥20 cigarettes daily) with the L-allele than without for both FEV_1 and FEV_1/FVC The gene–smoking interaction for heavy smokers was p = .009 and p = 0006 respectively

COPD = chronic obstructive pulmonary disease; CT = computed tomography; FVC = forced vital capacity; FEV_1 = forced expiratory volume in 1 second.

lavage.[77] Its importance in mediating cellular stress has been underscored in that HMOX1 is uniquely proposed to be directly regulated by four distinct stress-responsive transcription factors, including heat shock factor, nuclear factor-erythroid 2, activator protein-1 families, and nuclear factor κB.[78]

The most comprehensively studied *HMOX1* variant is a dinucleotide repeat polymorphism, [GT]*n*, located within the proximal promoter.[79] The length of this microsatellite may vary from [GT]10 to [GT]40.[79] The threshold for dichotomizing the repeat length in classes of long or short has not been consistent across studies, but [GT]25 has often been used as a cutoff, resulting in repeat lengths above 26 being classified as long (L) and <25 considered short (S) alleles. Further complicating the comparison of studies is the occasional use of a middle (M) allele length designation. Longer alleles have been associated with less effective induction of HMOX1 by oxidative stress and increased risk of COPD (Table 4).[80,81] Longer alleles were associated with accelerated loss of lung function in a French study[82] and a Japanese study[83] but not confirmed in a report from the Lung Health Study.[72]

Inflammatory Mediators

VITAMIN D BINDING PROTEIN (GC)

Vitamin D binding protein is a serum α_2-globulin, a major plasma carrier protein of vitamin D that is officially termed group-specific component (vitamin D binding protein). Vitamin D binding protein has undergone several name changes over several decades (group-specific component, vitamin D binding protein, macrophage-activating factor), often as new biologic functions were discovered.[84] The official Human Genome Organisation (HUGO) symbol is *GC*. *GC* is highly polymorphic, with three major isotypes (Gc1S, slow electrophoretic migration; Gc1F, fast electrophoretic migration; and Gc2) and more than 120 rare variants.[85,86] GC belongs to a family of genes composed of albumin, α-fetoprotein, and α-albumin/afamin that are predominantly synthesized in the liver. Although its major function is transport, binding, and solubilization of vitamin D and its metabolites, macrophage activation and chemotaxis, fatty acid transport, and actin scavenging are other attributed physiologic functions. Biologic functions related to inflammation include conversion to a potent macrophage-activating factor (MAF)[87,88] and interaction with neutrophils to increase chemotaxis to the C5a peptide during activation of complement.[89–92] Functional differences between the alleles have not yet been described.

Significant racial and geographic differences in allelic distribution exist. The approximate frequency of each isotype in Caucasians is 0.56 Gc1S, 0.16 Gc1F, and 0.28 Gc2.[93,94] White populations have a comparatively lower frequency of the Gc1F allele and a higher frequency (50–60%) of the Gc1S allele compared with African Americans and Africans.[85] Africans and African Americans have a higher frequency of the Gc1F allele.[85] Caucasians have a markedly higher Gc2 allele frequency in comparison with blacks.[85]

Several studies have demonstrated a protective role for the Gc2 allele in COPD.[34,93,95] The study by Schellenberg and colleagues differed from other early studies in that genotyping was used in comparison with serologic methodologies employed in other studies.[93] This protective effect was not confirmed in other reports.[96,97] The viability of the Gc2 allele as a potential explanation for reduction in the risk of airflow obstruction is suggested by the fact that only 10% of this isoform is converted to MAF,[43] but no differences in neutrophil chemotaxis were demonstrated in functional assays by genotype.[93]

Studies have also reported that the Gc1F allele is seen with increased frequency in COPD cases in comparison with controls.[95,97] Ito and colleagues also demonstrated increased frequency of this allele in COPD cases in addition to association of this allele with rapidity of lung function decline in another Japanese cohort that included physiologic and radiologic phenotyping (computed tomography score, low-attenuation area percentage [LAA%]).[98] Homozygous Gc1F was associated with a higher frequency of LAA% >60% ($p = .01$). The increased risk for the Gc1F allele in Caucasians reported by Horne and colleagues[95] was not replicated in the study by Schellenberg and colleagues,[93] but the homozygous Gc1F genotype was rare in the latter study and therefore underpowered to test this hypothesis. Racial variation in gene associations has also been offered as another explanation for the discordant results.[43]

TUMOR NECROSIS FACTOR

Tumor necrosis factor (TNF)-α is a potent cytokine with the ability to maintain neutrophilic inflammation and to stimulate apoptosis and cellular differentiation. Murine studies of TNF overexpression demonstrated the development of elements of pulmonary fibrosis and emphysema,[99] resulting in less clarity for its role in the pathogenesis of COPD. A variant in the promoter region of TNF (−308) has been associated with high TNF production[100] and has been studied in multiple populations for association with COPD, with mixed results. The −308 G/A variant has been found to be associated with COPD susceptibility in studies of Taiwanese[101] and Japanese COPD subjects[102] but not replicated in an additional Japanese study,[103] a Thai study,[104] or a Chinese study (Table 5).[105] Other than an association study that found the +489 G/A variant associated with COPD susceptibility in a Dutch population[106] and an Australian population-based study of the association of the −308 G/A variant with a reduced FEF$_{25–75}$,[107] several studies in Caucasian populations have not found a significant relationship to COPD susceptibility[108–112] or a rapid decline in lung function.[61]

TRANSFORMING GROWTH FACTOR β

In mammalian organisms, the transforming growth factor (TGF) superfamily includes approximately 30 members.[113] TGF-β is a member of this family of growth and differentiation

Table 5 Evidence for Tumor Necrosis Factor (TNF) as a Genetic Determinant of Chronic Obstructive Pulmonary Disease

Study	Study Population	Analysis	Comments	Results
Huang et al, 1997[101]	42 male subjects with chronic bronchitis, 42 matched controls, 99 schoolchildren	Case-control association analysis	Taiwanese study	Association of −308 G/A (OR 11.1; CI 2.89-42.57)
Higham et al, 2000[108]	86 Caucasian COPD subjects, 63 asymptomatic smokers, 99 population controls	Case-control association analysis of the −308 (G _ A) promoter SNP	British study	Negative
Keatings et al, 2000[183]	106 COPD subjects, 99 controls	A cross-sectional case-control analysis of the −308 (G _ A) promoter SNP on COPD susceptibility with 2-year follow-up for mortality	Irish study	Negative study AA homozygotes had less reversible airflow obstruction (p <.05) and increased mortality (p <.001)
Küçükaycan et a, 2002[106]	169 Caucasian COPD patients, 358 population controls	Case-control analysis of −376 G/A, −308 G/A, −238 G/A, +489 G/A	Dutch study	+489 G/A associated with COPD (OR 1.9; p = .009) and in COPD subjects without CT-confirmed emphysema compared with controls (Bonferroni adjusted p <.025)
Sandford et al, 2001[61]	283 Lung Health Study participants with rapid FEV1 decline, 308 non-decliners	Association analysis of rapid lung function decline vs no decline		No association with −308 G/A
Sakao et al, 2001[102]	106 COPD patients, 110 current or former smoking controls, 129 population controls	Association analysis of COPD susceptibility	Japanese study	Significant association of −308 G/A with COPD (OR 2.58)
Ferrarotti et al, 2003[109]	63 Caucasian COPD subjects, 86 healthy smokers	Association analysis of −308	Italian study	Negative
Seifart et al, 2005[110]	113 Caucasian COPD subjects with chronic bronchitis, 113 hospitalized coronary heart disease patients, 243 healthy controls	Association analysis of TNF for COPD susceptibility	German study	Negative for −308 G/A
Jiang et al, 2005[105]	111 COPD patients, 97 controls	Case-control association analysis of −308 G/A for COPD susceptibility	Chinese study	Negative for COPD susceptibility
Hegab et al, 2005[103]	88 Japanese COPD patients, 61 controls, 106 Egyptian COPD patients, 72 controls	Case-control association analysis of TNF for COPD susceptibility		None of the variants were associated with COPD susceptibility
Chierakul et al, 2005[104]	57 COPD patients, 116 controls	Case-control association analysis for COPD susceptibility	Thai study	Negative
Matheson et al, 2006[107]	828 participants (after exclusion of 404 with current asthma and bronchial hyperreactivity)	Population-based study of lung function and respiratory symptoms	Unselected, 94% Caucasian, community-based Australian study	−308 G/A associated with a reduced FEF_{25-75} (p = .03)

(Continued)

Table 5(Cont.) Evidence for Tumor Necrosis Factor (*TNF*) as a Genetic Determinant of Chronic Obstructive Pulmonary Disease

Study	Study Population	Analysis	Comments	Results
Ruse et al, 2007[112]	220 COPD cases, 141 controls	Case-control association analysis of −308 G/A for COPD susceptibility	United Kingdom study	No differences in the genotype distributions for either variant of COPD susceptibility
Brøgger et al, 2006[65]	Self-reported Caucasian, 248 COPD cases, 244 controls, A1AT excluded	Case-control association analysis of 3 genes and meta-analysis of 16 studies	Norwegian study	Negative for the three TNF variants studied

A1AT = α₁-antitrypsin; CI = 95% confidence interval; COPD = chronic obstructive pulmonary disease; CT = computed tomography; FEF = forced expiratory flow; FEV₁ = forced expiratory volume in 1 second; OR = odds ratio; SNP = single nucleotide polymorphism; TNF = tumor necrosis factor.

Table 6 Evidence for Transforming Growth Factor β (*TGFB1*) as a Genetic Determinant of Chronic Obstructive Pulmonary Disease

Study	Study Population	Analysis	Comments	Results
Celedón et al, 2004[50]	Boston Early-Onset COPD Study, predominantly Caucasian subjects; 304 Caucasian NETT participants; 441 Caucasian smokers from the NAS	Family-based association analysis; Case-control association analysis	Families ascertained through probands with severe, early-onset COPD; All NAS participants are male; Similar but slightly attenuated results in the males-only analysis from NETT	Significant association of rs2241712, rs2241718, and rs6957 with pre- and postbronchodilator FEV1 in the families (p <.05); Significant association with rs2241712, rs1800469, and rs1982073 for COPD susceptibility in the case-control study (*p* ≤ .02)
Wu et al, 2004[122]	165 subjects with COPD, 140 healthy blood donors, and 76 healthy smokers; All Caucasian subjects	Case-control association study for COPD susceptibility	No information on smoking in the blood donors	Significantly increased frequency of the proline allele at codon 10
Su et al, 2005[123]	84 Chinese COPD patients, 97 age- and gender-matched controls	Case-control study of a promoter variant with COPD susceptibility		Reduced frequency of carriers for the −509T allele in COPD patients, rs1800469 (*p* = .018)
Yoon et al, 2006[124]	102 male Korean COPD patients; 159 age-, gender-, smoking-matched controls	Case-control study of three previously associated SNPs	Although ethnically homogeneous, no formal testing for population stratification	No association for rs2241713, rs1800469, rs1982073
van Diemen et al, 2006[126]	1,390 subjects from the Vlagtwedde/Vlaardingen cohort	Population-based study of *TGFB1*		Higher prevalence of the minor allele of rs6957 in patients with COPD (*p* = .001); Lower prevalence of the haplotype with the major allele of rs6957 and minor alleles of rs1800469 and rs1982073 in patients with COPD (*p* = .03)

factors. It exists in three isoforms (β_1, β_2, β_3) that share 60 to 80% sequence homology.[114] Each isoform is encoded by a different gene. *TGFB1* maps to chromosome 19q13.1-q13.3.[115] *TGFB2β* maps to chromosome 1q41.[116] *TGFB3β* has been mapped to chromosome 14q23-24.[116] Physiologic functions attributed to TGF-β have included cell proliferation, differentiation, matrix deposition, and apoptosis.[117–120] COPD studies have largely focused on *TGFB1*. The precise role of TGF-β in COPD remains to be elucidated. Despite the lack of clear delineation of precise mechanisms, the relationship between TGF-β and lung inflammation and repair is likely important in the pathogenesis of COPD.[121]

In a follow-up study to the first genome-wide linkage analysis of COPD susceptibility and COPD phenotypes, Celedón and colleagues used linkage analysis analyzing additional STR markers on chromosome 19, followed by a case-control association analysis of SNPs in *TGFB1* (Table 6).[47,48,50] Among current and former smokers in pedigrees from the Boston Early-Onset COPD Study, there was significant evidence of linkage, with a LOD score of 3.30 between chromosome 19q STR markers and prebronchodilator FEV_1, as well as suggestive evidence of linkage with other COPD phenotypes. In these families, three SNPs in *TGFB1* were significantly associated with pre- and postbronchodilator FEV_1: rs2241712 in the promoter region in addition to rs2241718 and rs6957 in the 3′ genomic region. In an association study comparing COPD patients from the National Emphysema Treatment Trial (NETT) with smoking controls from the Normative Aging Study (NAS), three SNPs were significantly associated with COPD: rs2241712 and rs1800469 in the promoter region of *TGFB1* and rs1982073 in exon 1 of *TGFB1*. In a previous candidate gene association study, Wu and colleagues analyzed a single nonsynonymous coding SNP in *TGFB1* (rs1982073) at exon 1 nucleotide position 29 (T → C) that produces a substitution at codon 10 (Leu → Pro).[122] In this analysis for association with COPD susceptibility, the genotypes were nearly identical for the two control groups. The proline allele at codon 10 was significantly less common in COPD individuals than in controls. The fact that this allele is associated with increased production of *TGFB1* suggested that individuals who produce more *TGFB1* might be less prone to develop COPD despite similar or greater smoking histories. Studies in Chinese and Korean cohorts have had divergent results.[123,124] Su and colleagues found significantly fewer carriers of the −509T allele of rs1800469 in Chinese COPD patients, consistent with the findings of Celedón and colleagues in NETT cases and NAS controls, and more carriers of the −800A allele.[50,123] Yoon and colleagues did not find an association with three previously associated SNPS, −10807G/A (rs2241712), −509T/C (rs1800469), or 29T/C (rs1982073), in a Korean cohort.[124] No association was found between −509 (C → T), +869 (T → C), or +915 (G → C) and airway responsiveness or lung function decline in smokers from the Lung Health Study.[125] Another study with a significantly larger sample size also did not find an association of *TGFB1*

SNPs with accelerated lung function decline.[126] In this large Dutch cohort however, there was a significant association of the minor allele of rs6957, an SNP in the 3′ untranslated region (UTR) of *TGFB1*, with COPD ($p = .001$). There was also a statistically significant decrease in the prevalence of the haplotype with the major allele of rs6957 and minor alleles for rs1800469 and rs1982073 in *TGFB1* in subjects with COPD ($p = .03$). This study finds further substantiation for a role of variants in *TGFB1* in COPD, similar to the findings of Celedón and colleagues[50]; however, further studies will be required to confirm whether *TGFB1* is a genetic determinant of COPD susceptibility.

Protease/Antiprotease Imbalance
Intermediate A1AT Deficiency

The predominant action of A1AT (encoded by the *SERPINA1* gene) is to inhibit neutrophil elastase. Classified by their speed of migration on gel electrophoresis, there are three common variants of A1AT: M (medium), slow (S), and very slow (Z). The Pi ZZ homozygous state, discussed in detail in Chapter 5, "α_1-Antitrypsin Deficiency," is associated with severe deficiency of the enzyme inhibitor. Pi MZ heterozygotes also have reduced A1AT levels in comparison with Pi MM individuals, but the risk for lung disease is controversial. In a meta-analysis of 16 studies that reported COPD as a categorical outcome, the combined OR for Pi MZ versus Pi MM was 2.31 (95 % CI 1.60–3.35).[127] The summary OR was higher in case-control studies (OR 2.97; 95% CI 2.08–4.26) than in cross-sectional studies (OR 1.5; 95% CI 0.97–2.31). In studies that controlled for smoking, the OR was attenuated (OR 1.61; 95% CI 0.92–2.81). However, in population-based studies that compared FEV_1 values in Pi MZ and Pi MM subjects, no differences were observed. Thus, it remains unclear whether Pi MZ subjects are at increased risk; more research will be required to demonstrate this definitively.

Matrix Metalloproteinases

Matrix metalloproteinases (MMPs) are capable of degrading many components of lung extracellular matrix and likely function in tissue remodeling.[128] Murine studies have provided substantiation for a role in COPD pathogenesis,[129] but less clear evidence has been demonstrated in humans. *MMP-1* (G-1607GG) and *MMP-12* (Asn357Ser) haplotypes have been associated ($p = .0007$) with decline in lung function in Caucasian participants in the Lung Health Study who were segregated into groups with fastest annual decline ($n = 284$) versus slowest decline ($n = 306$).[130] The *MMP-1* −1607GG allele was negatively associated with a fast rate of decline, $p = .02$. Although Joos and colleagues found no relationship with *MMP-9* to lung function decline, a Chinese study and a Japanese study found an association of a promoter SNP in *MMP-9* (−1562 C/T) with COPD susceptibility.[131,132] This SNP has also been associated with upper lung zone–predominant emphysema.[133]

SERPINE2

Assessment of gene expression in relevant tissues is one strategy for identifying candidate genes for genetic association studies. These genes may be prioritized by mapping them to published genomic regions of linkage. This strategy was used by DeMeo and colleagues, who analyzed 48 SERPINE2 SNPs with COPD-related phenotypes in 949 individuals from 127 pedigrees in the Boston Early-Onset COPD Study.[134] Using the PBAT program (http:// www.biostat. harvard.edu/~clange /default.htm) with an additive model of inheritance in models that included an interaction term for a gene-by-environment effect (SNP-by-smoking), 18 SERPINE2 SNPs were significantly associated with quantitative and/or qualitative spirometric phenotypes ($p < .05$).

To replicate these findings, a case-control analysis of 304 NETT cases and 441 NAS smoking controls was performed. In the case-control study, seven SERPINE2 SNPs were significantly associated ($p < .05$). Five of these SNPs demonstrated a significant association in both the family-based analysis and the case-control study. With a sliding window approach, adjacent two-, four-, and six-SNP haplotypes were analyzed. This analysis localized the most significant association to a haplotype of two SNPs, rs1866153 and rs6747096, with $p = .004$. These SNPs are located in or near the boundary of exon 3. SERPINE2 is a protease inhibitor, but it is an inhibitor of plasmin, thrombin, and urokinase rather than elastase[135,136]; thus, its role in protease/antiprotease balance is uncertain in COPD pathogenesis. Because none of these associated SNPs have a known functional effect, the functional variant or variant is likely in LD with the significantly associated SNPs in SERPINE2.

Genetic Determinants for COPD-Related Phenotypes

COPD is complex and heterogeneous. Multiple COPD-related phenotypes are of clinical interest. COPD-related phenotypes may differ between different genetic subtypes of COPD. Alternatively, genes in other pathways may modify the expression of a COPD-related phenotype among individuals with the same COPD genetic subtype.

Emphysema Distribution

Many genetic association studies for COPD have failed to be replicated. False-positive results owing to population stratification, false-negative results owing to a lack of power to detect true associations of a modest effect, and true differences between populations have been proposed as explanatory mechanisms.[24] Population differences may occur as a result of different genetic subtypes, different environmental exposures, or genetic modifiers. COPD has inherent increased complexity because it is a heterogeneous disease composed of small airway disease, chronic bronchitis, and emphysema in which all or varying proportions of these three pathologies may contribute to the disease in any one individual. Reilly argued that this heterogeneity has limited the progress in the understanding of the pathogenesis of the disease, the development of therapies, and the identification of genetic susceptibility factors.[137] Computed tomographic (CT) assessment of emphysema and airway disease may provide more accurate phenotyping of COPD patients.[138–140] The data that may be obtained from quantitative CT scans in the evaluation of COPD have been reviewed.[137]

Measuring the percentage of low lung attenuation areas (LAA%), the emphysematous areas of the lung,[17,141,142] Sakao and colleagues analyzed the association of the −308 promoter region polymorphism in TNF with a CT-derived emphysema score.[143] Japanese patients with COPD were classified based on the median visual score as having severe emphysema (score ≥11) compared with mild to moderate emphysema (score < 11). The distribution of the TNF-308 genotypes did not differ between the two groups ($p = .2$), but the frequency of the TNF-α-308*2 rare allele tended toward a higher frequency in the severe emphysema group ($p = .09$; OR 2.15; 95% CI 0.87–5.30). Ito and colleagues studied 84 COPD patients and 85 healthy Japanese smokers for association of an allele of MMP-9, 1562 C/T, for COPD susceptibility and CT-confirmed emphysema.[133] No association was found with susceptibility for COPD, but an association was demonstrated for upper lobe–predominant emphysema. Individuals with a T allele (C/T or T/T) exhibited larger percentages of low attenuation areas (LAA%) on CT scans ($p = .04$) and smaller average CT densitometry, the average of the densitometry values in Hounsfield units (HU) of all pixels in both lungs, in the upper lung fields ($p = .04$) compared with individuals without T alleles (C/C). These findings implicate a role for the T allele in the progression of emphysema. DeMeo and colleagues recently evaluated CT densitometry phenotypes for association with 77 SNPs in 20 candidate genes in 282 individuals from the NETT.[144] Using computerized density mask quantitation of emphysema at a threshold of −950 HU, GSTP1, EPHX1, and MMP1 polymorphisms were associated with the apical predominant distribution of emphysema (p range = .001–.05). For the apical predominant phenotype determined by the radiologist scoring method, GSTP1 and EPHX1 SNPs were significantly associated. Limited to the densitometric upper lobe–predominant cases, the His139Arg SNP in EPHX1 was significant in the case-control analysis of COPD susceptibility ($p = .005$).

COPD Exacerbations

COPD exacerbations may result in accelerated decline in lung function[145] and increased mortality.[146] A genetic predisposition for susceptibility to develop COPD exacerbations is suggested by the variable frequency of exacerbations in individuals exhibiting the same level of lung function. Although highly important in determining patient outcomes, the genetic determinants of COPD exacerbations are less well studied compared with COPD susceptibility.

Table 7 Genetic Determinants of Exacerbations of Chronic Obstructive Pulmonary Disease

Study	Study Population	Analysis	Gene	Comments	Results
Yang et al, 2003[147]	200 COPD subjects (all Caucasian except 1), 104 healthy smokers, Australian study	Case-control association analysis of a variant in *MBL2* (codon 54) for COPD susceptibility, measurement of MBL levels, and correlation of MBL levels to hospitalization for infective COPD exacerbations	MBL2 (chromosome 10q11.2–q21)	MBL levels were measured as serum mannan binding activity in 82 patients Exacerbations were measured in the 82 patients with MBL levels Retrospective data with abstraction for admissions No microbiologic confirmation	No association with COPD susceptibility Median mannan binding activity was nearly 10-fold lower in A/B or B/B genotypes, $p < .001$ 49% had hospitalizations for exacerbations OR 4.9 (CI 1.7-14.4) for ≤1 admission for infective COPD exacerbation with A/B or B/B genotypes
Takabatake et al, 2006[148]	276 male Japanese COPD patients	2-year retrospective analysis of exacerbation frequency and 30-month prospective study of severity of AEs	*CCL11, CCL1, CCL5* (chromosome 17q11.2–q12)	Clinical AE definition confirmed by two physicians (82% concordance) Only rs2282691 was analyzed against severity of the AE (end point death) in the prospective study 47 patients died, 48.9% from AEs	In the retrospective study, rs2282691 of *CCL1* was associated with exacerbations in a dominant model (OR 3.06; CI 1.46–6.41; $p = .003$) In the prospective study, Cox proportional hazards model (A allele dominant), OR 4.73 (CI 1.11–20.18)

AE = acute exacerbation; CI = 95% confidence interval; COPD = chronic obstructive pulmonary disease; MBL = mannose binding lectin; OR = odds ratio.

Yang and colleagues studied the relationship of variants in mannose binding lectin 2 (*MBL2*) to infective exacerbations in COPD, COPD susceptibility, and mannose binding lectin levels.[147] MBL2 is a pattern recognition receptor important in the innate immune response to pathogens. Over a 2-year retrospective period of study, the MBL2 codon 54 B allele was associated with an increased frequency of hospital admissions (OR 4.9; 95% CI 1.7–14.4; $p = .011$) for COPD exacerbations and reduced mannose binding lectin levels, $p < .001$ (Table 7).[147] There was no association with COPD susceptibility. In contrast to the event-based definition used by Yang and colleagues, Takabatake and colleagues evaluated 276 Japanese males with COPD using a symptomatic definition of exacerbations.[148] In this study of four SNPs in *CCL11, CCL1*, and *CCL5*, the clinical definition of an exacerbation included three components: (1) change in sputum volume, texture, or color; (2) one additional symptom among increased dyspnea, cough, or fever; and (3) evidence of exacerbation severity, such as an unscheduled hospital visit or prescription of antibiotics. Additional objective confirmation was obtained through the use of an increased C-reactive protein or an increased leukocyte count and new radiographic findings, such as a pneumonic infiltrate. In the retrospective analysis of exacerbation frequency over a 2-year period, an SNP in *CCL1* was associated with exacerbations in a dominant model of inheritance, OR 3.06 (95% CI 1.46–6.41), $p = .03$. In the prospective survival analysis of the association of the *CCL1* SNP with acute exacerbations, the OR from a Cox proportional hazards model was 5.93 (95% CI 1.28–27.48).

Functional Impairment

There is poor correlation between disabling respiratory symptoms and airflow obstruction in COPD subjects. Hersh and colleagues analyzed 304 subjects from the NETT for association with COPD-related phenotypes such as exercise capacity, pulmonary function, and respiratory symptoms using 80 markers in 22 positional or biologically plausible candidate genes.[62] Using a test-replication approach to decrease the risk of false-positive associations, variants in microsomal epoxide hydrolase (*EPHX1*), latent transforming growth factor β binding protein 4 (*LTBP4*), *TGFB1*, and surfactant protein B (*SFTPB*) were significantly associated with COPD-related phenotypes. Specifically, SNPs in *EPHX1* ($p \le .03$) and *LTBP4* ($p \le .03$)

were associated with maximal output on cardiopulmonary exercise testing; SNPs in *LTBP4* ($p \leq .05$) and SFTPB ($p = .005$) were associated with 6-minute walking distance; and SNPs in *EPHX1* were associated with carbon monoxide diffusion capacity ($p \leq .04$). Three polymorphisms in *TGFB1* were associated with dyspnea ($p \leq .002$). One of the *TGFB1* SNPs associated with dyspnea replicated in families from the Boston Early-Onset COPD Study. Thus, polymorphisms in several genes were associated with phenotypes other than lung function. The authors suggested that since these genes may be classified into different physiologic pathways, *EPHX1* (xenobiotic metabolism),[149] inflammation and cellular signaling (*TGFB1*),[114] and extracellular matrix properties (*LTBP4*),[150] these associations might reflect the underlying heterogeneity of COPD.

Rare Syndromes
Cutis Laxa

Cutis laxa is an inherited or acquired connective tissue disorder with substantial genotypic and phenotypic variation. As a result of improper elastic fiber processing, emphysema in childhood and adolescence may occur in cutis laxa.[151] The disease is characteristically manifested by the presence of loose, redundant, inelastic skin. Other associated abnormalities include hernias, intestinal diverticuli, genital prolapse, pulmonary artery stenosis, aortic dilation and tortuousity, and bronchiectasis.[152]

Different inheritance patterns underlie the various forms of this heterogeneous disorder. X-linked cutis laxa can be caused by mutations in the ATP7A Cu^{2+} transporter and is categorized in the copper transport diseases.[153] The autosomal recessive form is the most frequent and most severe form in the United States and can be caused by a serine-to-proline substitution in the fibulin 5 (*FBLN5*) gene.[154] Another report has documented that mutations in fibulin 4, another member of the fibulin gene family, cause a severe, recessive disease associated with cutis laxa, bone fragility, vascular tortuousity and aneurysm, diaphragmatic and inguinal hernia, and developmental emphysema.[155] Other studies have reported frameshift mutations in exon 30 or 32 of the elastin gene in the autosomal dominant form of the disease.[156–158] Urban and colleagues reported that a partial tandem duplication in the elastin locus can cause autosomal dominant cutis laxa with severe COPD.[152] Severe emphysematous lung disease is frequently associated with the autosomal recessive forms of the disease with significantly increased infant mortality.[159] Although the inherited forms of the disease are more common than acquired disease, the most common cause of death in the acquired form is emphysema.[160] There are no specific treatments that alter disease progression. Smoking cessation is an integral component in reducing the complications of lung involvement.

Hypocomplementic Urticarial Vasculitis

COPD is a common complication of hypocomplementemic urticarial vasculitis. Although panacinar emphysema is most common, basilar hyperlucency has also been reported.[161] The lung disease may be severe, and airflow obstruction may be rapidly progressive.[162] Women are far more commonly affected, with eight times the incidence seen in males.[163] Urticaria is the most common initial manifestation, with angioedema, conjunctivitis, episcleritis, pericarditis, and nondeforming arthritis or synovitis as other systemic modes of involvement.[164]

Animal Models

Animal models of COPD have been instrumental in discerning essential pathways for the pathogenesis of COPD. Murine experimental models provide the ability to alter gene expression, but assessment of lung function is more difficult. The development of emphysema-like lesions is strain dependent, suggesting that there are differences in genetic susceptibility to develop emphysema between strains.[165,166] Future research to identify the genetic determinants responsible for these strain-dependent effects could lead to the identification of human COPD susceptibility genes. Mice differ anatomically from humans in that they are obligate nose breathers without a cough reflex, have fewer cilia and Clara cells, and have submucosal glands only in the trachea.[165] Among their advantages is the ability to tolerate at least two cigarettes daily without a substantial change in carboxyhemoglobin levels or body weight,[165] genomic similarity to humans,[167] and availability of inbred strains and genetic maps with more than 10,000 markers.[168] Gene-targeted ("knockout") mice and transgenic mice provide opportunities to study gene absence or overexpression.[169]

Murine experimental approaches in COPD have included inhalation of tobacco smoke and other environmental pollutants, tracheal instillation of tissue-degrading enzymes simulating protease/antiprotease imbalance, and genetic manipulation. MMP-12 knockout mice were protected from the development of emphysema in a long-term cigarette smoke exposure model.[170] The expression of MMP-12 in human alveolar macrophages and partial inhibition of the emphysematous lesions with MMP inhibitors adds evidence to the contribution of MMPs in lung tissue damage.[171] Transgenic mice overexpressing interleukin-13 in the adult lung develop emphysema, mucus hyperplasia, and inflammation.[172] Induced overexpression of interferon-γ in the lungs of mice also results in an emphysema-like phenotype.[173] Spontaneous emphysema has also developed in mice lacking surfactant protein D.[174,175] Recent extensive reviews of genetically manipulated and naturally occurring murine emphysema have been published. [168,176]

Future Directions
Genome-Wide Association Studies

Technological innovations in genotyping have made genome-wide association studies feasible; they provide an exciting alternative to linkage studies, which have generally provided disappointing results in complex disorders. The lack of success for genome-wide linkage studies has been attributed to (1) the occurrence of multiple genetic determinants of modest effect; (2) imprecise phenotype definitions; and (3) inadequately powered study designs and sample sizes.[177] Several commercial entities now provide genome-wide association SNP platforms with 100 to 500K multiplex arrays, with costs below $0.01 per genotype.[178] Genome-wide association studies may focus on genes and their regulatory regions (the sequence-based approach) or spatially cover the genome without regard to gene content (the map-based approach).[178] Marker selection may use the missense approach, in which nonsynonymous SNPs are targeted, but this approach would miss mutations outside the coding region. Marker selection may be based on conveniences such as ease and cost of genotyping; however, providing adequate LD coverage is a primary goal to avoid missing key disease susceptibility loci.[177]

It is estimated that a few hundred thousand carefully chosen SNPs should provide adequate information concerning most of the common variation in the human genome.[177] An increased number of LD-based markers would be needed in studies of populations of African ancestry in which LD is typically narrower and variation is increased. Multistage designs have been proposed in which a full set of SNPs is analyzed in a relatively small population with a liberal p value prior to progressing to a second stage or subsequent stages in which a larger population is used with progressively more restrictive p values required for achieving statistical significance. Unresolved issues include adequate correction for multiple testing in which prodigious amounts of information are analyzed and thresholds for significance in multistage designs.[179] Although some issues remain to be resolved, general medical studies highlighting the promise of genome-wide association studies include the results found by Herbert and colleagues in detecting a role for *INSIG2* in obesity[180] and complement factor H in age-related macular degeneration.[181]

Rare Variant Analysis

Rare genetic variants may be paramount in a subset of individuals predisposed to COPD. Linkage and association studies are typically underpowered to detect such variants. One approach to identify rare functional variants is to analyze genes that have been implicated in monogenic disorders that have emphysema-like pathology or manifestations. Such an approach was used by Kelleher and colleagues.[182] In their study, variation in the terminal exon of human elastin was assessed in 116 probands from the Boston Early-Onset COPD study. Resequencing of the distal six exons of the elastin gene resulted in the identification of a mutation in the first base of the last exon in a single early-onset COPD proband. Transfection studies with elastin complementary DNAs confirmed that the c.2318 G > A variant resulted in a glycine 773 to aspartate (G773D) substitution. This molecular change rendered a mutant protein that was unable to undergo normal elastin assembly, altered the proteolytic susceptibility of

the C-terminal region, and reduced interaction of the exon 36 sequence with matrix receptors on cells. There was reasonable but not complete concordance with airflow obstruction in the extended pedigree of this individual. Although this variant was detected in 1.2% of NETT COPD cases, providing evidence that this mutation was not a private mutation limited to one early-onset COPD pedigree, the significance of this variant in COPD susceptibility could not be confirmed with genetic association analysis because this mutation was also seen in 0.6% of control subjects. The functional molecular experiments in this report did, however, demonstrate structural and physiologic effects pertinent to the pathogenesis of COPD.

Conclusions

Methodologic and technological advances are converging to provide innovative insight into the pathogenesis of COPD, a complex and heterogeneous disorder. Elucidation of causal mechanisms, specific pathways, and improved discrimination of COPD-related phenotypes and subtypes may lead to cogent, targeted therapies.

References

1. Lander ES, Linton LM, Birren B, et al. Initial sequencing and analysis of the human genome. Nature 2001;409:860–921.
2. Venter JC, Adams MD, Myers EW, et al. The sequence of the human genome. Science 2001;291:1304–51.
3. The International HapMap Project. Nature 2003;426:789–96.
4. A haplotype map of the human genome. Nature 2005;437:1299–320.
5. Thorisson GA, Smith AV, Krishnan L, Stein LD. The International HapMap Project Web site. Genome Res 2005;15:1592–3.
6. Murray CJ, Lopez AD. Alternative projections of mortality and disability by cause 1990–2020: Global Burden of Disease study. Lancet 1997;349:1498–504.
7. Turino GM. The origins of a concept: the protease-antiprotease imbalance hypothesis. Chest 2002;122:1058–60.
8. MacNee W. Pathogenesis of chronic obstructive pulmonary disease. Proc Am Thorac Soc 2005;2:258–66; discussion 290–51.
9. Ito K, Ito M, Elliott WM, et al. Decreased histone deacetylase activity in chronic obstructive pulmonary disease. N Engl J Med 2005;352:1967–76.
10. Tuder RM, Yoshida T, Arap W, et al. State of the art. Cellular and molecular mechanisms of alveolar destruction in emphysema: an evolutionary perspective. Proc Am Thorac Soc 2006;3:503–10.
11. Demedts IK, Demoor T, Bracke KR, et al. Role of apoptosis in the pathogenesis of COPD and pulmonary emphysema. Respir Res 2006;7:53.
12. Thomas DC. Statistical methods in genetic epidemiology. Oxford: Oxford University Press; 2004.
13. Ashley-Koch A. Determining the genetic component of a disease. In: Haines JL, Pericak-Vance MA, editors. Genetic analysis of complex disease. 2nd ed. Hoboken (NJ): Wiley; 2006. p. 91–115.

14. Doll R, Peto R, Boreham J, Sutherland I. Mortality in relation to smoking: 50 years' observations on male British doctors. BMJ 2004;328:1519.

15. Mannino DM. COPD: epidemiology, prevalence, morbidity and mortality, and disease heterogeneity. Chest 2002;121 (5 Suppl):121S–6S.

16. Cigarette smoking and health. American Thoracic Society. Am J Respir Crit Care Med 1996;153:861–5.

17. Burrows B, Knudson RJ, Cline MG, Lebowitz MD. Quantitative relationships between cigarette smoking and ventilatory function. Am Rev Respir Dis 1977;115:195–205.

18. Warburton D, Gauldie J, Bellusci S, Shi W. Lung development and susceptibility to chronic obstructive pulmonary disease. Proc Am Thorac Soc 2006;3:668–72.

19. Silverman EK, Chapman HA, Drazen JM, et al. Genetic epidemiology of severe, early-onset chronic obstructive pulmonary disease. Risk to relatives for airflow obstruction and chronic bronchitis. Am J Respir Crit Care Med 1998;157 (6 Pt 1):1770–8.

20. Spielman RS, McGinnis RE, Ewens WJ. Transmission test for linkage disequilibrium: the insulin gene region and insulin-dependent diabetes mellitus (IDDM). Am J Hum Genet 1993;52:506–16.

21. Pritchard JK, Rosenberg NA. Use of unlinked genetic markers to detect population stratification in association studies. Am J Hum Genet 1999;65:220–8.

22. Reich DE, Goldstein DB. Detecting association in a case-control study while correcting for population stratification. Genet Epidemiol 2001;20:4–16.

23. Price AL, Patterson NJ, Plenge RM, et al. Principal components analysis corrects for stratification in genome-wide association studies. Nat Genet 2006;38:904–9.

24. Hirschhorn JN, Altshuler D. Once and again—issues surrounding replication in genetic association studies. J Clin Endocrinol Metab 2002;87:4438–41.

25. Silverman EK, Palmer LJ. Case-control association studies for the genetics of complex respiratory diseases. Am J Respir Cell Mol Biol 2000;22:645–8.

26. Hirschhorn JN, Lohmueller K, Byrne E, Hirschhorn K. A comprehensive review of genetic association studies. Genet Med 2002;4:45–61.

27. Lohmueller KE, Pearce CL, Pike M, et al. Meta-analysis of genetic association studies supports a contribution of common variants to susceptibility to common disease. Nat Genet 2003;33:177–82.

28. Cookson WO. State of the art. Genetics and genomics of chronic obstructive pulmonary disease. Proc Am Thorac Soc 2006;3:473–5.

29. Silverman EK. Progress in chronic obstructive pulmonary disease genetics. Proc Am Thorac Soc 2006;3:405–8.

30. Khoury MJ, Beaty TH, Cohen BH. Fundamentals of genetic epidemiology. New York: Oxford University Press; 1993.

31. Hubert HB, Fabsitz RR, Feinleib M, Gwinn C. Genetic and environmental influences on pulmonary function in adult twins. Am Rev Respir Dis 1982;125:409–15.

32. Ghio AJ, Crapo RO, Elliott CG, et al. Heritability estimates of pulmonary function. Chest 1989;96:743–6.

33. DeMeo DL, Hersh CP, Silverman EK. Linkage analysis of spirometric phenotypes and chronic obstructive pulmonary disease. In: Postma DS, Weiss ST, editors. Genetics of asthma and chronic obstructive pulmonary disease. New York: Taylor & Francis; 2006. p. 211–22.

34. Kueppers F, Miller RD, Gordon H, et al. Familial prevalence of chronic obstructive pulmonary disease in a matched pair study. Am J Med 1977;63:336–42.

35. Redline S, Tishler PV, Lewitter FI, et al. Assessment of genetic and nongenetic influences on pulmonary function. A twin study. Am Rev Respir Dis 1987;135:217–22.

36. Larson RK, Barman ML, Kueppers F, Fudenberg HH. Genetic and environmental determinants of chronic obstructive pulmonary disease. Ann Intern Med 1970;72:627–32.

37. Rybicki BA, Beaty TH, Cohen BH. Major genetic mechanisms in pulmonary function. J Clin Epidemiol 1990;43:667–75.

38. Tishler PV, Carey VJ, Reed T, Fabsitz RR. The role of genotype in determining the effects of cigarette smoking on pulmonary function. Genet Epidemiol 2002;22:272–82.

39. DeMeo DL, Carey VJ, Chapman HA, et al. Familial aggregation of FEF(25–75) and FEF(25–75)/FVC in families with severe, early onset COPD. Thorax 2004;59:396–400.

40. McCloskey SC, Patel BD, Hinchliffe SJ, et al. Siblings of patients with severe chronic obstructive pulmonary disease have a significant risk of airflow obstruction. Am J Respir Crit Care Med 2001;164(8 Pt 1):1419–24.

41. Kurzius-Spencer M, Sherrill DL, Holberg CJ, et al. Familial correlation in the decline of forced expiratory volume in one second. Am J Respir Crit Care Med 2001;164:1261–5.

42. Gottlieb DJ, Wilk JB, Harmon M, et al. Heritability of longitudinal change in lung function. The Framingham study. Am J Respir Crit Care Med 2001;164:1655–9.

43. Wood AM, Stockley RA. The genetics of chronic obstructive pulmonary disease. Respir Res 2006;7:130.

44. Morton NE. Sequential tests for the detection of linkage. Am J Hum Genet 1955;7:277–318.

45. Lander E, Kruglyak L. Genetic dissection of complex traits: guidelines for interpreting and reporting linkage results. Nat Genet 1995;11:241–7.

46. Palmer LJ, Celedon JC, Chapman HA, et al. Genome-wide linkage analysis of bronchodilator responsiveness and post-bronchodilator spirometric phenotypes in chronic obstructive pulmonary disease. Hum Mol Genet 2003; 12:1199–210.

47. Silverman EK, Mosley JD, Palmer LJ, et al. Genome-wide linkage analysis of severe, early-onset chronic obstructive pulmonary disease: airflow obstruction and chronic bronchitis phenotypes. Hum Mol Genet 2002;11:623–32.

48. Silverman EK, Palmer LJ, Mosley JD, et al. Genomewide linkage analysis of quantitative spirometric phenotypes in severe early-onset chronic obstructive pulmonary disease. Am J Hum Genet 2002;70:1229–39.

49. DeMeo DL, Celedón JC, Lange C, et al. Genome-wide linkage of forced mid-expiratory flow in chronic obstructive pulmonary disease. Am J Respir Crit Care Med 2004;170:1294–301.

50. Celedón JC, Lange C, Raby BA, et al. The transforming growth factor-beta1 (TGFB1) gene is associated with chronic obstructive pulmonary disease (COPD). Hum Mol Genet 2004;13:1649–56.

51. Joost O, Wilk JB, Cupples LA, et al. Genetic loci influencing lung function: a genome-wide scan in the Framingham study. Am J Respir Crit Care Med 2002;165:795–9.

52. Wilk JB, DeStefano AL, Joost O, et al. Linkage and association with pulmonary function measures on chromosome 6q27 in the Framingham Heart Study. Hum Mol Genet 2003;12:2745–51.

53. Wilk JB, Herbert A, Shoemaker CM, et al. Secreted modular calcium-binding protein 2 haplotypes are associated with pulmonary function. Am J Respir Crit Care Med 2007;175:554–60.

54. Wilk JB, DeStefano AL, Arnett DK, et al. A genome-wide scan of pulmonary function measures in the National Heart, Lung, and Blood Institute Family Heart Study. Am J Respir Crit Care Med 2003;167:1528–33.

55. Hassett C, Aicher L, Sidhu JS, Omiecinski CJ. Human microsomal epoxide hydrolase: genetic polymorphism and functional expression in vitro of amino acid variants. Hum Mol Genet 1994;3:421–8.

56. Hosagrahara VP, Rettie AE, Hassett C, Omiecinski CJ. Functional analysis of human microsomal epoxide hydrolase genetic variants. Chem Biol Interact 2004;150:149–59.

57. Raaka S, Hassett C, Omiencinski CJ. Human microsomal epoxide hydrolase: 5′-flanking region genetic polymorphisms. Carcinogenesis 1998;19:387–93.

58. Smith CA, Harrison DJ. Association between polymorphism in gene for microsomal epoxide hydrolase and susceptibility to emphysema. Lancet 1997;350:630–3.

59. Yoshikawa M, Hiyama K, Ishioka S, et al. Microsomal epoxide hydrolase genotypes and chronic obstructive pulmonary disease in Japanese. Int J Mol Med 2000;5:49–53.

60. Cheng SL, Yu CJ, Chen CJ, Yang PC. Genetic polymorphism of epoxide hydrolase and glutathione S-transferase in COPD. Eur Respir J 2004;23:818–24.

61. Sandford AJ, Chagani T, Weir TD, et al. Susceptibility genes for rapid decline of lung function in the Lung Health Study. Am J Respir Crit Care Med 2001;163:469–73.

62. Hersh CP, Demeo DL, Lazarus R, et al. Genetic association analysis of functional impairment in chronic obstructive pulmonary disease. Am J Respir Crit Care Med 2006;173:977–84.

63. Yim JJ, Park GY, Lee CT, et al. Genetic susceptibility to chronic obstructive pulmonary disease in Koreans: combined analysis of polymorphic genotypes for microsomal epoxide hydrolase and glutathione S-transferase M1 and T1. Thorax 2000;55:121–5.

64. Takeyabu K, Yamaguchi E, Suzuki I, et al. Gene polymorphism for microsomal epoxide hydrolase and susceptibility to emphysema in a Japanese population. Eur Respir J 2000;15:891–4.

65. Brøgger J, Steen VM, Eiken HG, et al. Genetic association between COPD and polymorphisms in TNF, ADRB2 and EPHX1. Eur Respir J 2006;27:682–8.

66. Mannervik B. The isoenzymes of glutathione transferase. Adv Enzymol Relat Areas Mol Biol 1985;57:357–417.

67. Johansson AS, Stenberg G, Widersten M, Mannervik B. Structure-activity relationships and thermal stability of human glutathione transferase P1-1 governed by the H-site residue 105. J Mol Biol 1998;278:687–98.

68. Sundberg K, Johansson AS, Stenberg G, et al. Differences in the catalytic efficiencies of allelic variants of glutathione transferase P1-1 towards carcinogenic diol epoxides of polycyclic aromatic hydrocarbons. Carcinogenesis 1998;19:433–6.

69. Ishii T, Matsuse T, Teramoto S, et al. Glutathione S-transferase P1 (GSTP1) polymorphism in patients with chronic obstructive pulmonary disease. Thorax 1999;54:693–6.

70. Ishii T, Fujishiro M, Masuda M, et al. Depletion of glutathione S-transferase P1 induces apoptosis in human lung fibroblasts. Exp Lung Res 2003;29:523–36.

71. Ishii T, Matsuse T, Igarashi H, et al. Tobacco smoke reduces viability in human lung fibroblasts: protective effect of glutathione S-transferase P1. Am J Physiol Lung Cell Mol Physiol 2001;280:L1189–95.

72. He JQ, Ruan J, Connett JE, et al. Antioxidant gene polymorphisms and susceptibility to a rapid decline in lung function in smokers. Am J Respir Crit Care Med 2002;166:323–8.

73. Çalikoglu M, Tamer L, Ates Aras N, et al. The association between polymorphic genotypes of glutathione S-transferases and COPD in the Turkish population. Biochem Genet 2006;44:307–19.

74. Tenhunen R, Marver HS, Schmid R. The enzymatic conversion of heme to bilirubin by microsomal heme oxygenase. Proc Natl Acad Sci U S A 1968;61:748–55.

75. Fredenburgh LE, Perrella MA, Mitsialis SA. The role of heme oxygenase-1 in pulmonary disease. Am J Respir Cell Mol Biol 2007;36:158–65.

76. Maestrelli P, El Messlemani AH, De Fina O, et al. Increased expression of heme oxygenase (HO)-1 in alveolar spaces and HO-2 in alveolar walls of smokers. Am J Respir Crit Care Med 2001;164(8 Pt 1):1508–13.

77. Slebos DJ, Kerstjens HA, Rutgers SR, et al. Haem oxygenase-1 expression is diminished in alveolar macrophages of patients with COPD. Eur Respir J 2004;23:652–3.

78. Alam J, Cook JL. How many transcription factors does it take to turn on the heme oxygenase-1 gene? Am J Respir Cell Mol Biol 2007;36:166–74.

79. Exner M, Minar E, Wagner O, Schillinger M. The role of heme oxygenase-1 promoter polymorphisms in human disease. Free Radic Biol Med 2004;37:1097–104.

80. Yamada N, Yamaya M, Okinaga S, et al. Microsatellite polymorphism in the heme oxygenase-1 gene promoter is associated with susceptibility to emphysema. Am J Hum Genet 2000;66:187–95.

81. Budhi A, Hiyama K, Isobe T, et al. Genetic susceptibility for emphysematous changes of the lung in Japanese. Int J Mol Med 2003;11:321–9.

82. Guénégou A, Leynaert B, Benessiano J, et al. Association of lung function decline with the heme oxygenase-1 gene promoter microsatellite polymorphism in a general population sample. Results from the European Community Respiratory Health Survey (ECRHS), France. J Med Genet 2006;43:e43.

83. Nakayama K, Kikuchi A, Yasuda H, et al. Heme oxygenase-1 gene promoter polymorphism and decline in lung function in Japanese men [letter]. Thorax 2006;61:921.

84. Gomme PT, Bertolini J. Therapeutic potential of vitamin D– binding protein. Trends Biotechnol 2004;22:340–5.

85. Speeckaert M, Huang G, Delanghe JR, Taes YE. Biological and clinical aspects of the vitamin D binding protein (Gc-globulin) and its polymorphism. Clin Chim Acta 2006;372:33–42.

86. Svasti J, Kurosky A, Bennett A, Bowman BH. Molecular basis for the three major forms of human serum vitamin D

binding protein (group-specific component). Biochemistry 1979;18:1611–7.

87. Yamamoto N, Homma S, Haddad JG, Kowalski MA. Vitamin D3 binding protein required for in vitro activation of macrophages after alkylglycerol treatment of mouse peritoneal cells. Immunology 1991;74:420–4.

88. Yamamoto N, Naraparaju VR. Role of vitamin D3-binding protein in activation of mouse macrophages. J Immunol 1996;157:1744–9.

89. Perez HD. Gc globulin (vitamin D-binding protein) increases binding of low concentrations of C5a des Arg to human polymorphonuclear leukocytes: an explanation for its cochemotaxin activity. Inflammation 1994;18:215–20.

90. Piquette CA, Robinson-Hill R, Webster RO. Human monocyte chemotaxis to complement-derived chemotaxins is enhanced by Gc-globulin. J Leukoc Biol 1994;55:349–54.

91. Kew RR, Webster RO. Gc-globulin (vitamin D-binding protein) enhances the neutrophil chemotactic activity of C5a and C5a des Arg. J Clin Invest 1988;82:364–9.

92. Kew RR, Fisher JA, Webster RO. Co-chemotactic effect of Gc-globulin (vitamin D binding protein) for C5a. Transient conversion into an active co-chemotaxin by neutrophils. J Immunol 1995;155:5369–74.

93. Schellenberg D, Pare PD, Weir TD, et al. Vitamin D binding protein variants and the risk of COPD. Am J Respir Crit Care Med 1998;157(3 Pt 1):957–61.

94. Gaensslen RE, Bell SC, Lee HC. Distributions of genetic markers in United States populations: III. Serum group systems and hemoglobin variants. J Forensic Sci 1987;32:1754–74.

95. Horne SL, Cockcroft DW, Dosman JA. Possible protective effect against chronic obstructive airways disease by the GC2 allele. Hum Hered 1990;40:173–6.

96. Kauffmann F, Kleisbauer JP, Cambon-De-Mouzon A, et al. Genetic markers in chronic air-flow limitation. A genetic epidemiologic study. Am Rev Respir Dis 1983;127:263–9.

97. Ishii T, Keicho N, Teramoto S, et al. Association of Gc-globulin variation with susceptibility to COPD and diffuse panbronchiolitis. Eur Respir J 2001;18:753–7.

98. Ito I, Nagai S, Hoshino Y, et al. Risk and severity of COPD is associated with the group-specific component of serum globulin 1F allele. Chest 2004;125:63–70.

99. Lundblad LK, Thompson-Figueroa J, Leclair T, et al. Tumor necrosis factor-alpha overexpression in lung disease: a single cause behind a complex phenotype. Am J Respir Crit Care Med 2005;171:1363–70.

100. Wilson AG, Symons JA, McDowell TL, et al. Effects of a polymorphism in the human tumor necrosis factor alpha promoter on transcriptional activation. Proc Natl Acad Sci U S A 1997;94:3195–9.

101. Huang SL, Su CH, Chang SC. Tumor necrosis factor-alpha gene polymorphism in chronic bronchitis. Am J Respir Crit Care Med 1997;156:1436–9.

102. Sakao S, Tatsumi K, Igari H, et al. Association of tumor necrosis factor alpha gene promoter polymorphism with the presence of chronic obstructive pulmonary disease. Am J Respir Crit Care Med 2001;163:420–2.

103. Hegab AE, Sakamoto T, Saitoh W, et al. Polymorphisms of TNFalpha, IL1beta, and IL1RN genes in chronic obstructive pulmonary disease. Biochem Biophys Res Commun 2005;329:1246–52.

104. Chierakul N, Wongwisutikul P, Vejbaesya S, Chotvilaiwan K. Tumor necrosis factor-alpha gene promoter polymorphism is not associated with smoking-related COPD in Thailand. Respirology 2005;10:36–9.

105. Jiang L, He B, Zhao MW, et al. Association of gene polymorphisms of tumour necrosis factor-alpha and interleukin-13 with chronic obstructive pulmonary disease in Han nationality in Beijing. Chin Med J (Engl) 2005;118:541–7.

106. Küçükaycan M, Van Krugten M, Pennings HJ, et al. Tumor necrosis factor-alpha +489G/A gene polymorphism is associated with chronic obstructive pulmonary disease. Respir Res 2002;3:29.

107. Matheson MC, Ellis JA, Raven J, et al. Association of IL8, CXCR2 and TNF-alpha polymorphisms and airway disease. J Hum Genet 2006;51:196–203.

108. Higham MA, Pride NB, Alikhan A, Morrell NW. Tumour necrosis factor-alpha gene promoter polymorphism in chronic obstructive pulmonary disease. Eur Respir J 2000;15:281–4.

109. Ferrarotti I, Zorzetto M, Beccaria M, et al. Tumour necrosis factor family genes in a phenotype of COPD associated with emphysema. Eur Respir J 2003;21:444–9.

110. Seifart C, Dempfle A, Plagens A, et al. TNF-alpha-, TNF-beta-, IL-6-, and IL-10-promoter polymorphisms in patients with chronic obstructive pulmonary disease. Tissue Antigens 2005;65:93–100.

111. Hersh CP, Demeo DL, Lange C, et al. Attempted replication of reported chronic obstructive pulmonary disease candidate gene associations. Am J Respir Cell Mol Biol 2005;33:71–8.

112. Ruse CE, Hill MC, Tobin M, et al. Tumour necrosis factor gene complex polymorphisms in chronic obstructive pulmonary disease. Respir Med 2007;101:340–4.

113. Camoretti-Mercado B, Solway J. Transforming growth factor-beta1 and disorders of the lung. Cell Biochem Biophys 2005;43:131–48.

114. Bartram U, Speer CP. The role of transforming growth factor beta in lung development and disease. Chest 2004;125:754–65.

115. Fujii D, Brissenden JE, Derynck R, Francke U. Transforming growth factor beta gene maps to human chromosome 19 long arm and to mouse chromosome 7. Somat Cell Mol Genet 1986;12:281–8.

116. Barton DE, Foellmer BE, Du J, et al. Chromosomal mapping of genes for transforming growth factors beta 2 and beta 3 in man and mouse: dispersion of TGF-beta gene family. Oncogene Res 1988;3:323–31.

117. Massague J. The TGF-beta family of growth and differentiation factors. Cell 1987;49:437–8.

118. Sporn MB, Roberts AB. Transforming growth factor-beta: recent progress and new challenges. J Cell Biol 1992;119:1017–21.

119. Kulkarni AB, Huh CG, Becker D, et al. Transforming growth factor beta 1 null mutation in mice causes excessive inflammatory response and early death. Proc Natl Acad Sci U S A 1993;90:770–4.

120. Grande JP. Role of transforming growth factor-beta in tissue injury and repair. Proc Soc Exp Biol Med 1997;214:27–40.

121. Rennard SI. Inflammation and repair processes in chronic obstructive pulmonary disease. Am J Respir Crit Care Med 1999;160(5 Pt 2):S12–6.

122. Wu L, Chau J, Young RP, et al. Transforming growth factor-beta1 genotype and susceptibility to chronic obstructive pulmonary disease. Thorax 2004;59:126–9.

123. Su ZG, Wen FQ, Feng YL, et al. Transforming growth factor-beta1 gene polymorphisms associated with chronic obstructive pulmonary disease in Chinese population. Acta Pharmacol Sin 2005;26:714–20.

124. Yoon HI, Silverman EK, Lee HW, et al. Lack of association between COPD and transforming growth factor-beta1 (TGFB1) genetic polymorphisms in Koreans. Int J Tuberc Lung Dis 2006;10:504–9.

125. Ogawa E, Ruan J, Connett JE, et al. Transforming growth factor-beta1 polymorphisms, airway responsiveness and lung function decline in smokers. Respir Med 2007;101(5):938–43.

126. van Diemen CC, Postma DS, Vonk JM, et al. Decorin and TGF-beta1 polymorphisms and development of COPD in a general population. Respir Res 2006;7:89.

127. Hersh CP, Dahl M, Ly NP, et al. Chronic obstructive pulmonary disease in alpha1-antitrypsin PI MZ heterozygotes: a meta-analysis. Thorax 2004;59:843–9.

128. Belvisi MG, Bottomley KM. The role of matrix metalloproteinases (MMPs) in the pathophysiology of chronic obstructive pulmonary disease (COPD): a therapeutic role for inhibitors of MMPs? Inflamm Res 2003;52:95–100.

129. Shapiro SD. Proteinases in chronic obstructive pulmonary disease. Biochem Soc Trans 2002;30:98–102.

130. Joos L, He JQ, Shepherdson MB, et al. The role of matrix metalloproteinase polymorphisms in the rate of decline in lung function. Hum Mol Genet 2002;11:569–76.

131. Zhou M, Huang SG, Wan HY, et al. Genetic polymorphism in matrix metalloproteinase-9 and the susceptibility to chronic obstructive pulmonary disease in Han population of south China. Chin Med J (Engl) 2004;117:1481–4.

132. Minematsu N, Nakamura H, Tateno H, et al. Genetic polymorphism in matrix metalloproteinase-9 and pulmonary emphysema. Biochem Biophys Res Commun 2001; 289:116–9.

133. Ito I, Nagai S, Handa T, et al. Matrix metalloproteinase-9 promoter polymorphism associated with upper lung dominant emphysema. Am J Respir Crit Care Med 2005;172:1378–82.

134. DeMeo DL, Mariani TJ, Lange C, et al. The SERPINE2 gene is associated with chronic obstructive pulmonary disease. Am J Hum Genet 2006;78:253–64.

135. Baker JB, Low DA, Simmer RL, Cunningham DD. Protease-nexin: a cellular component that links thrombin and plasminogen activator and mediates their binding to cells. Cell 1980;21:37–45.

136. Scott RW, Bergman BL, Bajpai A, et al. Protease nexin. Properties and a modified purification procedure. J Biol Chem 1985;260:7029–34.

137. Reilly J. Using computed tomographic scanning to advance understanding of chronic obstructive pulmonary disease. Proc Am Thorac Soc 2006;3:450–5.

138. Fabbri LM, Luppi F, Beghe B, Rabe KF. Update in chronic obstructive pulmonary disease 2005. Am J Respir Crit Care Med 2006;173:1056–65.

139. Cerveri I, Dore R, Corsico A, et al. Assessment of emphysema in COPD: a functional and radiologic study. Chest 2004;125:1714–8.

140. Lapperre TS, Snoeck-Stroband JB, Gosman MM, et al. Dissociation of lung function and airway inflammation in chronic obstructive pulmonary disease. Am J Respir Crit Care Med 2004;170:499–504.

141. Goddard PR, Nicholson EM, Laszlo G, Watt I. Computed tomography in pulmonary emphysema. Clin Radiol 1982;33:379–87.

142. Kuwano K, Matsuba K, Ikeda T, et al. The diagnosis of mild emphysema. Correlation of computed tomography and pathology scores. Am Rev Respir Dis 1990;141:169–78.

143. Sakao S, Tatsumi K, Igari H, et al. Association of tumor necrosis factor-alpha gene promoter polymorphism with low attenuation areas on high-resolution CT in patients with COPD. Chest 2002;122:416–20.

144. DeMeo DL, Hersh CP, Hoffman EA, et al. Genetic determinants of emphysema distribution in the National Emphysema Treatment Trial. Am J Respir Crit Care Med 2007;176(1):42-8.

145. Donaldson GC, Seemungal TA, Bhowmik A, Wedzicha JA. Relationship between exacerbation frequency and lung function decline in chronic obstructive pulmonary disease. Thorax 2002;57:847–52.

146. Donaldson GC, Wedzicha JA. COPD exacerbations .1: Epidemiology. Thorax 2006;61:164–8.

147. Yang IA, Seeney SL, Wolter JM, et al. Mannose-binding lectin gene polymorphism predicts hospital admissions for COPD infections. Genes Immun 2003;4:269–74.

148. Takabatake N, Shibata Y, Abe S, et al. A single nucleotide polymorphism in the CCL1 gene predicts acute exacerbations in chronic obstructive pulmonary disease. Am J Respir Crit Care Med 2006;174:875–85.

149. Koyama H, Geddes DM. Genes, oxidative stress, and the risk of chronic obstructive pulmonary disease. Thorax 1998;53 Suppl 2:S10–4.

150. Shapiro SD. Evolving concepts in the pathogenesis of chronic obstructive pulmonary disease. Clin Chest Med 2000;21:621–32.

151. Corbett E, Glaisyer H, Chan C, et al. Congenital cutis laxa with a dominant inheritance and early onset emphysema. Thorax 1994;49:836–7.

152. Urban Z, Gao J, Pope FM, Davis EC. Autosomal dominant cutis laxa with severe lung disease: synthesis and matrix deposition of mutant tropoelastin. J Invest Dermatol 2005;124:1193–9.

153. Das S, Levinson B, Vulpe C, et al. Similar splicing mutations of the Menkes/mottled copper-transporting ATPase gene in occipital horn syndrome and the blotchy mouse. Am J Hum Genet 1995;56:570–6.

154. Loeys B, Van Maldergem L, Mortier G, et al. Homozygosity for a missense mutation in fibulin-5 (FBLN5) results in a severe form of cutis laxa. Hum Mol Genet 2002;11:2113–8.

155. Hucthagowder V, Sausgruber N, Kim KH, et al. Fibulin-4: a novel gene for an autosomal recessive cutis laxa syndrome. Am J Hum Genet 2006;78:1075–80.

156. Tassabehji M, Metcalfe K, Hurst J, et al. An elastin gene mutation producing abnormal tropoelastin and abnormal elastic fibres in a patient with autosomal dominant cutis laxa. Hum Mol Genet 1998;7:1021–8.

157. Zhang MC, He L, Giro M, et al. Cutis laxa arising from frameshift mutations in exon 30 of the elastin gene (ELN). J Biol Chem 1999;274:981–6.

158. Rodriguez-Revenga L, Iranzo P, Badenas C, et al. A novel elastin gene mutation resulting in an autosomal dominant form of cutis laxa. Arch Dermatol 2004;140:1135–9.

159. Beighton P. The dominant and recessive forms of cutis laxa. J Med Genet 1972;9:216–21.

160. Hogan DJMolis T, May J. Cutis laxa (elastolysis). Available at: <http://www.emedicine.com/derm/topic93.htm> (date accessed 2/4/08)

161. Ghamra Z, Stoller JK. Basilar hyperlucency in a patient with emphysema due to hypocomplementemic urticarial vasculitis syndrome. Respir Care 2003;48:697–9.

162. Schwartz HR, McDuffie FC, Black LF, et al. Hypocomplementemic urticarial vasculitis: association with chronic obstructive pulmonary disease. Mayo Clin Proc 1982;57:231–8.

163. Lee P, Gildea TR, Stoller JK. Emphysema in nonsmokers: alpha 1-antitrypsin deficiency and other causes. Cleve Clin J Med 2002;69:928–9, 933, 936 passim.

164. Wisnieski JJ, Baer AN, Christensen J, et al. Hypocomplementemic urticarial vasculitis syndrome. Clinical and serologic findings in 18 patients. Medicine (Baltimore) 1995;74:24–41.

165. Groneberg DA, Chung KF. Models of chronic obstructive pulmonary disease. Respir Res 2004;5:18.

166. Guerassimov A, Hoshino Y, Takubo Y, et al. The development of emphysema in cigarette smoke-exposed mice is strain dependent. Am J Respir Crit Care Med 2004;170:974–80.

167. Waterston RH, Lindblad-Toh K, Birney E, et al. Initial sequencing and comparative analysis of the mouse genome. Nature 2002;420:520–62.

168. Brusselle GG, Bracke KR, Maes T, et al. Murine models of COPD. Pulm Pharmacol Ther 2006;19:155–65.

169. Shapiro SD, Demeo DL, Silverman EK. Smoke and mirrors: mouse models as a reflection of human chronic obstructive pulmonary disease. Am J Respir Crit Care Med 2004;170:929–31.

170. Hautamaki RD, Kobayashi DK, Senior RM, Shapiro SD. Requirement for macrophage elastase for cigarette smoke-induced emphysema in mice. Science 1997;277:2002–4.

171. Shapiro SD. Elastolytic metalloproteinases produced by human mononuclear phagocytes. Potential roles in destructive lung disease. Am J Respir Crit Care Med 1994;150 (6 Pt 2):S160–4.

172. Zheng T, Zhu Z, Wang Z, et al. Inducible targeting of IL-13 to the adult lung causes matrix metalloproteinase- and cathepsin-dependent emphysema. J Clin Invest 2000;106:1081–93.

173. Wang Z, Zheng T, Zhu Z, et al. Interferon gamma induction of pulmonary emphysema in the adult murine lung. J Exp Med 2000;192:1587–600.

174. Wert SE, Yoshida M, LeVine AM, et al. Increased metalloproteinase activity, oxidant production, and emphysema in surfactant protein D gene-inactivated mice. Proc Natl Acad Sci U S A 2000;97:5972–7.

175. Wert S, Jones T, Korfhagen T, et al. Spontaneous emphysema in surfactant protein D gene-targeted mice. Chest 2000;117(5 Suppl 1):248S.

176. Mahadeva R, Shapiro SD. Chronic obstructive pulmonary disease. 3: experimental animal models of pulmonary emphysema. Thorax 2002;57:908–14.

177. Hirschhorn JN, Daly MJ. Genome-wide association studies for common diseases and complex traits. Nat Rev Genet 2005;6:95–108.

178. Moffatt MF, Cookson WO. Fine mapping and whole genome association studies in asthma and chronic obstructive pulmonary disease. In: Postma DS, Weiss ST, editors. Genetics of asthma and chronic obstructive pulmonary disease. New York: Taylor & Francis; 2006. p. 223–37.

179. Thomas DC, Haile RW, Duggan D. Recent developments in genomewide association scans: a workshop summary and review. Am J Hum Genet 2005;77:337–45.

180. Herbert A, Gerry NP, McQueen MB, et al. A common genetic variant is associated with adult and childhood obesity. Science 2006;312:279–83.

181. Klein RJ, Zeiss C, Chew EY, et al. Complement factor H polymorphism in age-related macular degeneration. Science 2005;308:385–9.

182. Kelleher CM, Silverman EK, Broekelmann T, et al. A functional mutation in the terminal exon of elastin in severe, early-onset chronic obstructive pulmonary disease. Am J Respir Cell Mol Biol 2005;33:355–62.

183. Keatings VM, Cave SJ, Henry MJ, et al. A polymorphism in the tumor necrosis factor-alpha gene promoter region may predispose to a poor prognosis in COPD. Chest 2000;118:971–5.

CHAPTER 5

α_1-ANTITRYPSIN DEFICIENCY

ROBERT A. STOCKLEY, MD, DSc, FRCP

α_1-ANTITRYPSIN DEFICIENCY (A1ATD) was first recognized in the early 1960s, presenting as an absent α_1 band on paper electrophoresis of serum. Subsequent studies indicated that this protein band represented the major serum inhibitor of trypsin, and although the main function of the protein is not to inhibit this enzyme, the name has become generally accepted. Clinical evaluation of the initial patients indicated that several of them had severe early-onset emphysema,[1] and subsequent studies showed that the severe deficiency appeared to run through families phenotypically in an autosomal recessive manner.[2] However, it was also recognized that the heterogeneous state could be identified by finding intermediate low levels of α_1-antitrypsin.

α_1-Antitrypsin is a 54 kDa serine proteinase inhibitor. It is the major serum inhibitor of serine proteinases and is coded for on chromosome 14 at q32.1. The gene consists of four translated exons, and the active site (coded for in exon 5) consists of a critical methionine-serine (Met^{358}-Ser^{359}) amino acid sequence that gives the protein its specificity against serine proteinases. This active site interacts specifically with the Ser^{173}-His^{41}-Asp^{88} triad of the active site of neutrophil elastase, which is its major target enzyme. The paired alleles on chromosome 14 are coexpressed, therefore, from a genetic point of view, the protein is inherited in a codominant manner. To date, over 120 different mutations have been identified, although the vast majority consist of variations on the normal M gene with single amino acid substitutions that do not influence the level or function of the protein.

The protein is defined by its characteristics on isoelectric focusing, and individual bands are labeled alphabetically (in the Pi system). The most common variant is labeled Pi M and accounts for approximately 93% of the alleles in subjects of Northern European descent. As indicated above, however, this phenotype has its own variants, including M1 (Ala^{213}), M3 (Val^{213} + Glu^{376} to Asp), and M2 (M3 + Arg^{101} to His). Other common variants include the S allele (M1 Val^{213} + Glu^{264} to Val), which is associated with a serum protein level of approximately 60% of that produced by the M allele. The incidence of the S allele varies widely, being most common around the Mediterranean, and results in the United Kingdom (obtained by screening spouses of our patients) suggest that the allele is present in approximately 6% of individuals. The slight reduction in the protein level is related to instability in the endoplasmic reticulum and increased catabolism. However, the function of the intact protein (once released) is essentially normal.

The most common allele associated with marked deficiency of α_1-antitrypsin is referred to as Pi Z. This deficiency allele originated in Scandinavia and is most common around the Baltic coasts, with an incidence of Z homozygotes as high as 1 in 1,600 in Denmark. The Z allele results in a marked reduction in secretion, releasing approximately 20% of the equivalent produced by the M allele. The Z defect is related to a single point mutation at position 342, where the nucleotide sequence for this codon is changed from GAG to AAG, resulting in an amino acid change from glutamic acid to lysine. This change leads to a very slight reduction in the association rate constant with its major target neutrophil elastase.[3] However, there is also a resultant increase in the mobility of the active site and a slight opening of the beta sheets, resulting in spontaneous protein polymerization within hepatocytes.[4] This leads to the characteristic periodic acid-Schiff-positive inclusion bodies in hepatocytes that represent accumulation of the α_1-antitrypsin polymers in the endoplasmic reticulum. Since the gene is translated normally, this accumulation is the mechanism whereby a major reduction in protein secretion takes place.

There are many other rare α_1-antitrypsin defects that lead, for instance, to intrahepatic accumulation, as in Pi Mmalton,[5] production of nonfunctional protein (Pi F), or nonexpression owing to frame shift mutations, including insertions[6] or deletions,[7] which produce premature stop codons and even total gene deletion.[8]

Detection of Deficiency

The first and key step in the detection of deficiency is to be aware of it. Because of the association, particularly with pulmonary emphysema, current World Health Organization guidelines suggest that all patients with a diagnosis of chronic obstructive pulmonary disease (COPD) or even adult-onset asthma should be tested.[9] This latter group is highlighted as many patients with COPD owing to A1ATD are initially misdiagnosed as asthmatic. The first and simplest test is to measure the serum level that relates to the Pi typing, as indicated in Figure 1 for the most common alleles. It should be noted that there is some overlap between the α_1-antitrypsin level for the common MM subjects and even subjects with the MZ heterozygote state. This largely relates to the fact that

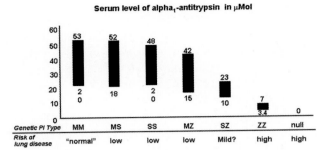

FIGURE 1. The range of α_1-antitrypsin levels is indicated for each phenotype. Current studies indicate that only the Pi Z or null patients are clearly at increased risk for developing lung disease.

α_1-antitrypsin is an acute-phase protein and the normal M allele can rapidly double its α_1-antitrypsin production during acute inflammatory episodes. However, protein levels also increase in line with the menstrual cycle and therapies such as the contraceptive pill. Nevertheless, it should be noted that patients with severe deficiency of the Pi Z type have distinct low levels that are separate from other phenotypes.

Once the serum level has been measured, the next step in characterization is to phenotype the α_1-antitrypsin using isoelectric focusing. This technique, although relatively simple, does require care not only in performing the assay but also its interpretation. However, it should be noted that even with careful phenotyping, it is not always possible to identify or be sure of heterozygote or homozygote states. This largely relates to the fact that other deficiency genes or null genes may be present, producing weak or, in the case of null genes, no α_1-antitrypsin bands on isoelectric focusing. These rarer alleles can be identified only by inference from family studies (Figure 2) or by direct genotyping. This latter approach is usually carried out as a two-stage procedure. First, simple polymerase chain reaction (PCR) specific for the common deficiency alleles (S and Z) can be combined with PCR specific for the M allele. This will correctly identify S, Z, and M alleles based on whether the point mutations for the S or Z allele are present or absent (implying that the sequence relates to that of the M protein). However, it should be noted that with the many other deficiency alleles, the S and Z sequences will also be absent; hence, it is either necessary to develop a multitude of primers specifically aimed at other known variants or to consider progressing to the second stage of complete gene sequencing to detect the other mutations. At present, the incidence of these rarer deficiency alleles is largely unknown, although studies of a large group of Pi Z samples have indicated that up to 8% of these patients may be heterozygote with another deficiency or null allele (E. Campbell, personal communication, 2004).

Whom to Test?

Because of the inherited nature of the deficiency, a typical family cohort is illustrated in (Figure 3). Deficient patients are usually the offspring of heterozygotes, and all offspring of

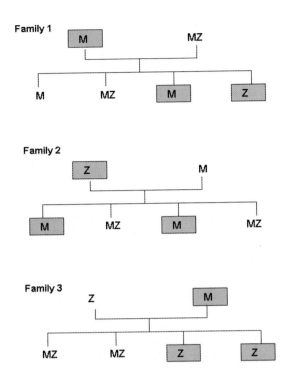

FIGURE 2. Examples of the inheritance patterns in which a null gene is present (as indicated by the boxes around the phenotypes). As null genes do not lead to secreted protein, they are not detected by isoelectric focusing. In family 1, the children should be phenotypically M or MZ if the parent was an M homozygote. The presence of a phenotypically Z child suggests that the parent was genotypically M null, and there should be a reduced serum concentration (50%) of α_1-antitrypsin in the absence of an acute-phase rise. In addition, any children who are phenotypically M should be genotyped to confirm the presence of any null genes. In family 2, the presence of children who are phenotypically M suggests that the parent was genotypically Z null. Finally, in family 3, the presence of children who are phenotypically Z suggests that the parent was genotypically M null.

such parents would stand a 1 in 4 chance of inheriting severe deficiency. Thus, there is a 1 in 4 chance of finding a further deficient patient among all siblings and a 2 in 4 chance of finding other heterozygotes. It is usual clinical practice therefore to start by screening any siblings of the identified patient.

It is well recognized that finding affected homozygous siblings usually identifies individuals with a lesser degree of lung function impairment compared with the index case (Figure 4). This enables preventive strategies such as cigarette smoking advice to be introduced at an earlier stage.

The next step is to confirm (where possible) the phenotype/genotype of the patient's partner to determine risks to their offspring. When there is a likelihood that a Pi Z child would be present, early detection should be undertaken to instigate long-term preventive measures such as smoking advice and occupational advice.

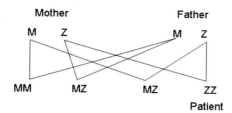

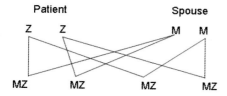

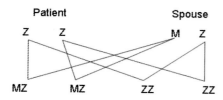

FIGURE 3. In the absence of null genes, a typical family is shown in which both parents are heterozygotes and all siblings have a 1 in 4 chance of inheriting a Pi Z homozygote state. Patient partners are usually Pi M, and all children will therefore be MZ heterozygotes. By chance (approximately 1 in 30), the partner will be Pi MZ, and the offspring have a 50% chance of being Z homozygotes.

The heterozygote state is not, in general, a specific risk factor in the development of lung disease, although recent epidemiologic evidence suggests that there may be a small risk[10] or that once COPD has developed, there is a slightly greater risk for hospitalization.[11] In practice, therefore, little intervention needs to be undertaken following the discovery of a heterozygote patient, although it would be of importance to check any partner as there is a 3% chance, for instance, in the

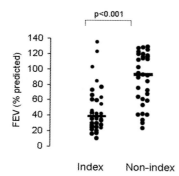

FIGURE 4. Lung function (forced expiratory volume in 1 second [FEV₁] % predicted) is shown for a series of index cases and their siblings (nonindex) identified by family screening. The *line* indicates the median value.

United Kingdom that the partner would also be heterozygote. If so, this should lead to early assessment of the α₁-antitrypsin phenotype of any offspring. If, on the other hand, the partner has a normal M phenotype, all of the children should be heterozygote, and the general principle is not to test these individuals unless or until they are thinking of having children themselves, when it is appropriate to check their partner and hence determine any likelihood of homozygous deficiency in the next generation.

The ultimate testing would be to carry out α₁-antitrypsin measurement in all infants in the neonatal period when screening takes place for other metabolic deficiencies. At present, however, the implication of such screening remains uncertain. Identification of A1ATD potentially has implications for future insurance, although in many countries this is not yet the case, particularly as the overall natural history remains largely unknown and many individuals remain healthy. Indeed, the Swedish cohort that was identified some 30 years ago has been followed up and so far seems to remain relatively healthy.[12] There were concerns about the implications of such screening from a psychological point-of-view that reflected a feeling of guilt probably related to a lack of understanding.[13] However, individuals identified have been less likely to start smoking in their teens or early adult life.

Relationship to Lung Disease

There now seems to be a general acceptance that A1ATD is related to an increased susceptibility to developing lung disease. Of the first five cases identified, three were young patients with severe lower-zone emphysema. It was therefore believed that A1ATD predisposed individuals to the early onset of lower-zone emphysema, and for this reason, further patients who presented in a similar way were tested for A1ATD and more cases were identified. This led to a continuing belief that the deficiency of α₁-antitrypsin was specific for early-onset lower-zone emphysema (see below).

As indicated previously, α₁-antitrypsin is an inhibitor of serine proteinases, and although neutrophil elastase is generally considered to be its major target enzyme, α₁-antitrypsin is also an efficient inhibitor of cathepsin-G and proteinase 3. All three of these enzymes are preformed and stored in the azurophil granule of the mature neutrophil and have been shown by a series of *in-vivo* and *in-vitro* experiments to produce all of the major pathophysiologic features of COPD. Neutrophil elastase and proteinase 3 have been shown to produce pathologic changes in the airways of experimental animals that resemble human emphysema.[14] In addition, neutrophil elastase and cathepsin-G have been shown to produce mucous gland hyperplasia (which is also a feature of human COPD). Finally, these enzymes have been shown to have a major effect on mucociliary clearance. Neutrophil elastase and cathepsin-G are major secretogogues, and neutrophil elastase reduces ciliary beat frequency and can cause significant direct damage to ciliated epithelium.[14]

Thus, it is generally believed that the pathologic changes in the lungs of patients with A1ATD are a direct result of the release of these neutrophil granule proteins into an environment in which there is insufficient α_1-antitrypsin to tightly control the activity of the enzymes. The resultant, persistent enzyme activity is thus able to interact with lung tissues, producing the typical pathologic changes. However and interestingly, despite this concept, it has been very difficult to identify the presence of free elastase activity in the peripheral airways of patients with α_1-antitryspin, with a few exceptions (see below).

The exact mechanism of predisposition in A1ATD has been elucidated in recent years following both theoretical and experimental data indicating that lung tissue damage is the result of a process called quantum proteolysis.[15,16] The serine proteinases are released from the azurophil granules of an activated neutrophil in high concentrations. As the enzyme diffuses away from the granule, its concentration drops in an exponential manner. This means that even in the presence of normal α_1-antitrypsin, there is an area of obligate proteolysis occurring close to the azurophil granule as the initial high concentrations of neutrophil elastase (and possibly other proteinases) are released, and this may be necessary for the normal function and migration of the neutrophil.

Nevertheless, in the presence of normal α_1-antitrypsin, this area of obligate proteolysis is very tightly limited. As the α_1-antitrypsin level decreases, released neutrophil elastase can remain active at a greater distance from the granule. However, once the concentration of α_1-antitrypsin falls below 10 μM, there is an exponential increase in the area of persistent enzyme activity. Subjects with the Pi ZZ genotype have α_1-antitrypsin levels between 2 and 5 μM in the plasma, whereas those with the SZ phenotype who have little risk from lung disease have levels generally between 11 and 18 μM.[17] This difference in the concentration of α_1-antitrypsin relative to the released enzymes at differing distances from the granule[15] therefore helps explain the potential for and extent of damage likely to occur and fits with what is known about the susceptibility.

It is, however, uncertain what the concentration of α_1-antitrypsin is in the interstitium of the lung, where destruction of lung connective tissue (particularly elastin) is believed to be central to the development of emphysema. Nevertheless, it is known that albumin (which has the same molecular size as α_1-antitrypsin) diffuses relatively freely into the interstitium, with concentrations approximately 80% of that of plasma.[18] Thus, it can be predicted that α_1-antitrypsin levels at this site would be approximately 80% of that occurring in serum. However, albumin and hence α_1-antitrypsin levels on the surface epithelium of the lung are much reduced because of the tight epithelial junctions necessary to restrict fluid movements into the airspaces.[18] This results in approximately a 10-fold drop in α_1-antitrypsin concentration between plasma and the lung

secretions, and this has important consequences for therapy (see below).

With this as a background, the current concepts of the development of lung disease in α_1-antitrypsin relate to two factors: first, the low levels of protection against proteolytic enzymes that occur in A1ATD and, second, the increased neutrophil traffic that is seen in these individuals. Indeed, the two may act synergistically. Even in health, there is some neutrophil traffic into the lung. In the presence of A1ATD, the inhibition of neutrophil elastase released by these "normal" migrating neutrophils would be decreased, and this would result in an increased zone of neutrophil elastase activity in the lungs. Evidence has shown that elastase can stimulate resident alveolar macrophages to release neutrophil chemoattractants, including leukotriene B4 (LTB4),[19] and this would, in turn, attract more neutrophils, perpetuating the cycle (Figure 5). In the presence of cigarette smoking or a chest infection, this whole process would be amplified further by even greater attraction of neutrophils as part of the secondary host response.

These data are consistent with the identification of an excessive number of neutrophils in bronchoalveolar lavage,[20] airway tissues,[21] and the higher levels of LTB4 in comparison with nondeficient patients with COPD.[22] More recently, others have suggested that the propensity for the Pi Z protein to polymerize plays a role either in promoting inflammation or by directly causing chemotaxis.[23] The relative contribution of this latter mechanism is unknown.

Studies of the neutrophils themselves have indicated that they have normal migratory function in A1ATD,[24] suggesting that the above proposed mechanism of increased chemotactic factor alone accounts for the amplified neutrophilic response seen in A1ATD. These concepts have implications for current and future therapeutic management (see below).

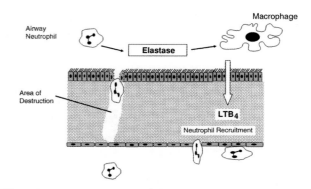

FIGURE 5. Recruitment of neutrophils to the airway results in elastase release. Deficiency of α_1-antitrypsin in the alveolar region prevents inactivation of this enzyme that stimulates alveolar macrophages to release leukotriene B4 (LTB4). This chemoattractant leads to further neutrophil recruitment and connective tissue destruction during cell migration. The deficiency of α_1-antitrypsin results in more extensive tissue degradation than results from normal levels of α_1-antitrypsin.

Patient Characteristics

Although patients with A1ATD have an increased incidence of liver cirrhosis, hepatic cell carcinoma, vasculitis, and panniculitis, the lung disease seems to predominate. In general, the condition presents like usual COPD, although the tendency is to present at an earlier age than in those without A1ATD. Indeed, many patients do present in their thirties with symptoms of exercise-induced breathlessness, often leading to a possible erroneous diagnosis of asthma. However, there are studies that suggest that asthma may be more common in patients with A1ATD,[25,26] and, indeed, bronchodilator reversibility in this group of patients is often greater than that seen in usual COPD (see below).

The initial patients who were identified had severe panlobular basal emphysema, and in view of this, testing has been more commonly undertaken in patients who present with this distribution, particularly at a young age. This has also led to a largely erroneous assumption that most patients with A1ATD have severe lower lobe emphysema. Subsequent studies have shown that in more random testing, approximately two-thirds of the patients have lower lobe emphysema, with the remainder having a predominance of apical and mid-lung zone emphysema,[27] which may be centrilobular in nature, as in usual COPD. This distribution of emphysema has been shown to reflect the physiologic impairment in A1ATD.[27]

Figure 6 demonstrates the relationship between forced expiratory volume in 1 second (FEV$_1$, a measure of airway diameter) and coefficient of carbon monoxide (Kco, a measure of gas exchange); although there is a general relationship between the two measurements in A1ATD, some subjects have relatively discordant lung function. There are subjects who have predominantly airflow obstruction and no defect in gas exchange, whereas others have a defect in gas exchange but no airflow obstruction. Studies by Parr and colleagues suggested that this disparity is related to the distribution of emphysema.[27] Those with an apical distribution have relatively impaired gas transfer but relatively normal FEV$_1$, whereas those with a more basal distribution are more likely to have an impaired FEV$_1$ with relatively preserved gas transfer. This raises the issue that monitoring progression in A1ATD should include a more comprehensive physiologic testing than just the FEV$_1$ (see "Monitoring Progression" below).

Bronchiectasis

The relationship between A1ATD and bronchiectasis is unclear. Individual case studies had reported patients with bronchiectasis alone, but in more extensive studies using high-resolution computed tomography (CT), severe bronchiectasis appears to be relatively uncommon, although tubular or varicose bronchiectasis is present in 26% of patients,[28] which is similar in incidence to that seen in usual COPD.[29] However, patients do suffer from bronchial disease, and approximately 40% have chronic cough and mucus production, again similar in incidence to normal COPD. Such patients may be colonized with bacteria and, if so, have more evidence of inflammation than patients with usual COPD.[30] Patients nevertheless suffer from recurrent exacerbations, and the number is related to the decline in lung function,[31] again reflecting pathophysiologic processes seen in ordinary COPD.

Self-reported exacerbations have been documented as increased in A1ATD but reduced with augmentation therapy, suggesting that patients with A1ATD experience more episodes than in usual COPD.[32] However, in a more direct study, exacerbations did not appear to be more frequent in most patients with A1ATD.[33] Indeed, approximately 50% of patients have no exacerbations year to year, and the remainder have, on average, 2.5 exacerbations per year. Although usually of the Anthonisen type I, these episodes are associated with detection of free elastase activity in the upper airways to a much greater extent than in usual COPD,[34] and this may in part account for the more rapid progression of lung function decline seen in deficient individuals.

Siblings

Siblings of patients with A1ATD are usually less affected. This may reflect reporting bias in that the first patient who presents to health services is likely to be the most symptomatic. However, it has been recognized that even when corrections are made for age and smoking habit, there is a degree of discordance between the FEV$_1$ for sibling pairs (Figure 7). This in itself suggests that other gene-environment interactions play a role in the development of lung disease in A1ATD, and such genetic studies are currently under way. Interestingly, despite the discordance of FEV$_1$ between siblings, there is a greater degree of concordance between gas transfer in siblings (see Figure 7). This suggests that the pathophysiologic factors influencing the development of emphysema and airflow obstruction in A1ATD may differ. Again, this is a feature of ongoing research, and such studies may cast light on the overall discordance between FEV$_1$ and Kco mentioned above.

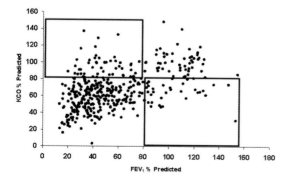

FIGURE 6. The relationship of forced expiratory volume in 1 second (FEV$_1$) to Kco (% predicted) is shown for a cohort of patients. The two boxes enclose patients with a normal FEV$_1$ and reduced gas transfer and vice versa.

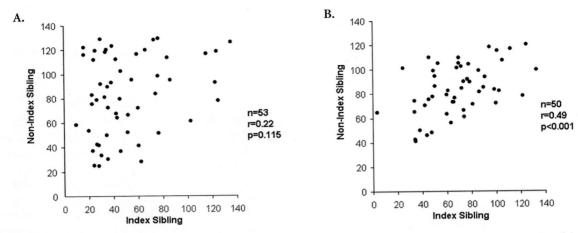

FIGURE 7. The relationship between forced expiratory volume in 1 second (FEV$_1$) (*A*) and Kco (*B*) is shown (expressed as % predicted) for sibling pairs. Note the lack of correlation for FEV$_1$ but not for Kco.

Monitoring Progression

Inflammation is thought to be central to the pathophysiology and progression of COPD. Indeed, recent data have demonstrated that measures of neutrophilic airway inflammation can predict the subsequent deterioration in lung function and increase in emphysema in non-A1ATD COPD.[35] Where comparisons have been made, studies have shown that these markers of inflammation are greater in A1ATD than in COPD, not only in the stable clinical state[22] but also during acute exacerbations.[34] These data are entirely consistent with the role of neutrophilic inflammation in the progression of disease in A1ATD and the more rapid progression seen in these patients. Whether such biomarkers have a role in monitoring disease progression remains uncertain.

The conventional method for monitoring progression in COPD in general and in A1ATD has been sequential measurement of the FEV$_1$. It is well recognized that this parameter has a degree of daily variability inherent in its measurement but that it does predict health status[36] and mortality.[37] For these reasons, it has remained the measure of choice, and compared with usual COPD, the overall decline in FEV$_1$ is increased in A1ATD. Nevertheless, FEV$_1$ decline does not predict or identify progression early in the disease or indeed late in the disease, although the latter may reflect a survival effect. The FEV$_1$ seems to decline most in patients who already have mild or moderate impairment (Figure 8).

An alternative way of monitoring progression is the use of gas transfer, and the carbon monoxide diffusing capacity corrected for alveolar volume (Kco) is the most specific physiologic measure of emphysema. Indeed, gas transfer also shows a relationship to health status[38] that is comparable with that for FEV$_1$ and similarly relates to the likelihood of mortality.[39] However, the decline in gas transfer is most notable in those with more severe disease (see Figure 8), perhaps reflecting the fact that the disease is predominantly a lower lobe disease to begin with, but as it progresses, it spreads more toward the apical regions of the lung, which reflect measures of gas transfer more than the basal regions.[28]

High-resolution CT is the most direct measure of emphysema in life. The measure is highly reproducible and shows progression with time irrespective of the severity of lung function impairment.[40] However, at present, there is a significant controversy concerning the best way to analyze the scans as three potential measurements from the density output can be obtained. These include the density mask in which the proportion of low-attenuation voxels are obtained either at fixed sites or for the whole lung; the percentile 15, which is the density below which 15% of the voxels occur; or the mean lung density, which averages the density of the individual voxels for the whole lung. Each measurement has its benefit and drawback, but the former two in particular correlate well with FEV$_1$ decline,[40] suggesting that either may be appropriate for long-term monitoring.

Further studies are ongoing to determine the signal to noise ratio and, therefore, the appropriate sensitivity of individual parameters for determining progression. Nevertheless, at present, CT is gaining increasing support as the primary outcome measure in future clinical trials. Studies have shown that CT correlates well with lung function, health status, and exercise capacity; can monitor progression; and is the best independent predictor of mortality in A1ATD.[39]

Finally, health status is known to show decline with time in usual COPD. Indeed, some studies in A1ATD have also indicated that health status declines with time and correlates with the change in CT.[41] Nevertheless, in our own studies in a specialist clinic with long-term follow-up and monitoring, the decline in health status has not occurred, and in many cases, improvements in the overall impact of the disease occur over a 3-year period.[33] This may reflect a variety of complex factors, including optimization of therapy, education, and reassurance.

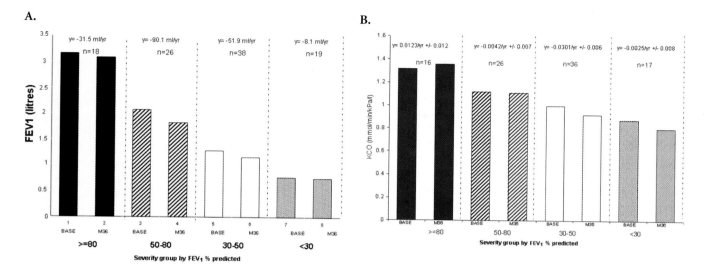

FIGURE 8. The annual decline in forced expiratory volume in 1 second (FEV₁) (*A*) is shown for a UK cohort of Pi Z patients grouped according to their baseline FEV₁. The most rapid decline occurs in subjects with mild to moderate impairment. The decline in Kco (*B*) is greatest in those with moderate to severe FEV₁ impairment.

Treatment

Treatment in general for patients with A1ATD should follow lines similar to those for usual COPD. The patient group as a whole has a degree of reversible airflow obstruction, and in many instances, the change is consistent with that describing "asthma" rather than COPD.[26] Indeed, evidence from our own cohort suggests that the use of a β_2-agonist and anticholinergic agents together has an overall additive effect on simple measures of lung function (Figure 9). Inhaled corticosteroids should be introduced for patients with multiple exacerbations in line with management for usual COPD. However, probably more importantly, bacterial exacerbations in A1ATD are associated with increased elastase activity in the airway, and as this is the putative mediator of the destructive lung disease, such episodes should be identified and treated rapidly and appropriately if the sputum has a purulent nature.

Indications for long-term oxygen therapy and rehabilitation are the same as those in usual COPD. However, in view of their general younger age and thus decreased likelihood of comorbidity, patients with A1ATD are often more suitable for surgical interventions. In selected patients, lung volume reduction surgery may be beneficial, although in the limited studies that have been undertaken, the magnitude and duration of the benefits seem to be inferior and shorter than in patients with nondeficient emphysema,[42] perhaps reflecting disease distribution (bases compared with apices in usual COPD) and the more rapid progression in A1ATD.

Transplantation has almost a 70% 1-year survival in A1ATD, and in long-term follow-up, the overall 10-year survival has been 22%, which is inferior to that seen in usual COPD.[43] The question of whether augmentation therapy can improve this outcome remains unanswered (see below).

Change in FEV₁ % predicted post dual bronchodilation

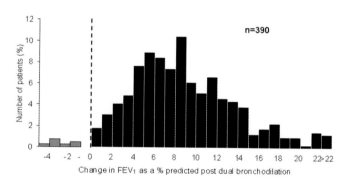

FIGURE 9. The response of forced expiratory volume in 1 second (FEV₁) to treatment with a β_2-agonist and anticholinergic agents is shown together. The response is shown as the increase expressed as a percentage of the predicted value.

Augmentation Therapy

The role of augmentation therapy still remains controversial. From our understanding of the pathophysiology, augmentation therapy seems logical. Low serum levels are related to low levels of α_1-antitrypsin in the interstitium and the airways. In view of the relationship between elastase concentrations released from the neutrophil azurophil granule and the subsequent diffusion gradient, it seems logical that raising α_1-antitrypsin levels in the interstitium would reduce the area of connective tissue destruction during neutrophil infiltration. It is possible, however, that rather than preventing lung function decline, augmentation therapy may reduce lung function decline closer to that seen in ordinary COPD, in which subjects have normal serum and, hence by implication, normal interstitial and airway α_1-antitrypsin levels.

Whether inhaled augmentation therapy can raise levels sufficiently high in the airway to be protective in the interstitium remains unknown, particularly since a marked diffusion gradient occurs across the epithelial lining of the airways. However, local deposition in the airways may interfere with the proposed pathophysiologic process outlined in Figure 5, breaking the proinflammatory cycle. The neutrophil traffic would be reduced and less damage would ensue, meaning that the interstitium would need less protection.

However, the problem of alveolar deposition of α_1-antitrypsin remains a challenge. On the other hand, more central deposition may prove effective in reducing the elastase burden (and hence its effects in the airway) both in the stable state and particularly during exacerbations in patients specifically with bronchial inflammation and damage.

The evidence that IV α_1-antitrypsin augmentation therapy is beneficial remains, at best, indirect:

1. In the large National Institutes of Health study, patients who received augmentation therapy for at least 6 months had a better outcome in terms of overall survival and FEV_1 decline in the midrange than subjects who never received augmentation therapy.[44] However, differences in social class and exposure to health care services as part of the treatment may have influenced the outcome.

2. A comparison of FEV_1 decline in two populations from Denmark (where no augmentation therapy is available) and Germany (where augmentation therapy is available) demonstrated that the decline in German patients was less than that seen in Denmark,[45] although this could reflect cultural or environmental differences.

3. A further study in Germany indicated that patients who had a rapid FEV_1 decline had a much less rapid decline in FEV_1[46] once started on augmentation therapy. Clearly, this sequential study may reflect the natural history of FEV_1 decline in A1ATD (see Monitoring Progression).

4. The closest to a controlled clinical trial was carried out by Dirksen and colleagues comparing monthly infusions of α_1-antitrypsin over a 3-year period versus an albumin placebo.[47] Although no difference in the decline of lung function was seen, there appeared to be a trend toward reduced progression of emphysema as quantified by CT, although this failed to achieve conventional statistical significance.

5. In a retrospective survey, Lieberman found that the number of exacerbations self-reported by A1ATD patients was greater prior to augmentation than after augmentation therapy.[32] Since exacerbations are related to the subsequent decline in lung function,[31] this survey provides further indirect support for augmentation therapy.

6. Finally, in a short-term study, Stockley and colleagues demonstrated that airway inflammation and particularly the key chemoattractant LTB_4 were reduced during augmentation therapy in a small number of patients.[48] This provides biochemical plausibility of the potential efficacy of augmentation in reducing the central pathophysiologic process of inflammation.

Augmentation therapy is available in many countries. Nevertheless, there is still a reluctance to embark on augmentation therapy, which is not only costly but still awaits proof of efficacy. The focus of the regulatory authorities on FEV_1 as the primary outcome in COPD and hence A1ATD has meant that the power to detect a beneficial effect requires far too many patients over too long a time period to be feasible. However, the recent validation of high-resolution CT as a primary outcome measure has changed this view, and, currently, a preliminary study in Europe involving a placebo-controlled trial of augmentation in 76 patients over 30 months is nearing completion, with high-resolution CT as the primary outcome. This methodology varies between scanners and centres and hence requires rigorous standardization. Nevertheless, its use is now seen as central to future studies of specific interventions in A1ATD in particular and perhaps also emphysema in usual COPD.

The process of clinical trials has been facilitated by the establishment of central registries for A1ATD, including the Alpha One Foundation self-reported registry in the United States and the Alpha-1-Antitrypsin International Registry centralized in Europe.[49] The latter registry, including over 3,000 patients with a confirmed diagnosis of A1ATD of the Z genotype on its database, has enabled not only the controlled augmentation pilot study to be undertaken but also the delivery of a significant controlled trial of a retinoic acid receptor γ-agonist that has the potential for alveolar regrowth. Again, the results of this study should be forthcoming early in 2008.

In summary, a renewed interest in A1ATD and the accompanying increase in research funding have led to greatly increased understanding of the condition and its progression. International collaboration has facilitated the delivery of controlled clinical trials, which should further our ability to understand and manage the condition.

References

1. Laurell C-B, Eriksson S. The electrophoretic α_1-globulin pattern of serum in α_1-antitrypsin deficiency. Scand J Clin Lab Invest 1963;15:132–40.
2. Eriksson S. Studies in α_1 antitrypsin deficiency. Acta Med Scand 1965;432 Suppl:1–85.
3. Ogushi F, Fells GA, Hubbard RC, et al. Z-type α_1 antitrypsin is less competent than M1-type α_1 antitrypsin as an inhibitor of neutrophil elastase. J Clin Invest 1987;80:1366–74.
4. Lomas DA, Evans DL, Finch JT, Carrell RW. The mechanism of Z α_1 antitrypsin accumulation in the liver. Nature 1992;357:605–7.
5. Fabbretti G, Sergi C, Consales G, et al. Genetic variants of alpha-1-antitrypsin (AAT). Liver 1992;12(4 Pt 2):296–301.

6. Curiel D, Brantly M, Curiel E, et al. α_1 Antitrypsin deficiency caused by the α_1 antitrypsin null subset mattawa gene. J Clin Invest 1989;83:1144–52.

7. Takahashi H, Crystal RG. α_1 Antitrypsin null subset. Isolade d procida: an alpha-1-antitrypsin deficiency allele caused by deletion of all alpha-1-antitrypsin coding exona. Am J Hum Genet 1990;47:403–13.

8. Poller W, Faber JP, Fiedinger S, Olek K. DNA polymorphism associated with a new α_1 antitrypsin Pi QO variant (Pi QO Reidenburg). Hum Genet 1991;86:522–4.

9 Alpha-1-antitrypsin deficiency: memorandum from a WHO meeting. Bull World Health Organ 1997;75:397–415.

10. Hersh CP, Dahl M, Ly NP, et al. Chronic obstructive pulmonary disease in alpha-1-antitrypsin Pi MZ heterozygotes: a meta-analysis. Thorax 2004;59:843–9.

11. Seersholm N, Wilcke JT, Kok-Jensen A, Dirksen A. Risk of hospital admission for obstructive pulmonary disease in alpha-1 antitrypsin heterozygotes of phenotype MZ. Am J Respir Crit Care Med 2000;161:81–4.

12. Piitulainen E, Carlson J, Ohlsson K, Sveger T. Alpha-1-antitrypsin deficiency in 26-year old subjects: lung, liver and protease/protease inhibitor studies. Chest 2005;128:2076–81.

13. Sveger T, Thelin T. 4-Year old children with alpha-1-antitrypsin deficiency clinical follow-up and parental attitudes towards neonatal screening. Acta Paediatr Scand 1981;70:171–7.

14. Stockley RA. New approaches to the management of COPD. Chest 2000;117:58S–62S.

15. Liou TJ, Campbell EJ. Quantum proteolysis resulting from release of single granules by human neutrophils. J Immunol 1996;157:2624–31.

16. Campbell EJ, Campbell MA, Boukedes SS, Owen CA. Quantum proteolysis by neutrophils; implications for pulmonary emphysema and alpha-1-antitrypsin deficiency. J Clin Invest 1999;104:337–44.

17. Seersholm N, Kok-Jensen A. Intermediate alpha-1 antitrypsin deficiency Pi SZ: a risk factor for pulmonary emphysema? Respir Med 1998;92:241–5.

18. Gorin AB, Stewart PA. Differential permeability of endothelial and epithelial barriers to albumin flux. J Appl Physiol 1979;47:114–24.

19. Hubbard RC, Fells G, Gadek J, et al. Neutrophil accumulation in the lung in alpha-1-antitrypsin deficiency: spontaneous release of leukotriene B4 by alveolar macrophages. J Clin Invest 1991;88:891–7.

20. Morrison HM, Kramps JA, Burnett D, Stockley RA. Lung lavage fluid from patients with α_1-protease inhibitor deficiency or chronic obstructive bronchitis: anti-elastase function and cell profile. Clin Sci 1987;72:373–81.

21. Mahadeva R, Atkinson C, Li Z, et al. Polymers of Z alpha1-antitrypsin co-localize with neutrophils in emphysematous alveoli and are chemotactic in vivo. Am J Pathol 2005;166:377–86.

22. Hill AT, Bayley DL, Campbell EJ, et al. Airway inflammation in chronic bronchitis: the effects of smoking an alpha-1-antitrypsin deficiency. Eur Respir J 2000;15:886–90.

23. Parmar JS, Mahadeva R, Reed BJ, et al. Polymers of alpha-1-antitrypsin chemotactic for human neutrophils: a new paradigm for the pathogenesis of emphysema. Am J Respir Cell Mol Biol 2002;26:723–30.

24. Woolhouse IS, Bayley DL, Lalor P, et al. Endothelial interaction of neutrophils under flow in chronic obstructive pulmonary disease. Eur Respir J 2005;25:612–7.

25. Piitulainen E, Tornling G, Eriksson S. Effect of age and occupational exposure to airway irritants on lung function in non-smoking individuals with α_1-antitrypsin deficiency (Pi ZZ). Thorax 1997;52:244–8.

26. Eden E, Hammel J, Rouhani FN, et al. Asthma features in severe alpha-1-antitrypsin deficiency. Experience of the National Heart, Lung and Blood Institute Registry. Chest 2003;123:765–71.

27. Parr DG, Stoel BC, Stolk J, Stockley RA. Patterns of emphysema distribution in α_1 antitrypsin deficiency influences lung function impairment. Am J Respir Crit Care Med 2004;170:1172–8.

28. Dowson LJ, Guest PJ, Stockley RA. The relationship of chronic sputum expectoration to physiologic, radiologic and health status characteristics in α_1 antitrypsin deficiency (Pi Z). Chest 2002;122:1247–55.

29. O'Brien C, Guest PJ, Hill SL, Stockley RA. Physiological and radiological characterisation of patients diagnosed as chronic obstructive pulmonary disease in primary care. Thorax 2000;55:635–42.

30. Stockley RA, Hill AT, Hill SL, Campbell EJ. Bronchial inflammation, its relationship to colonising microbial load and α_1 antitrypsin deficiency. Chest 2000;117:291S–3S.

31. Dowson LJ, Guest PJ, Stockley RA. Longitudinal changes in physiological, radiological and health status measurements in α_1-antitrypsin deficiency and factors associated with decline. Am J Respir Crit Care Med 2001;164:1805–9.

32. Lieberman J. Augmentation therapy reduces frequency of lung infections in antitrypsin deficiency: a new hypothesis with supporting data. Chest 2000;118:1480–5.

33. Needham M, Stockley RA. Exacerbations in α_1 antitrypsin deficiency. Eur Respir J 2005;25:992–1000.

34. Hill AT, Campbell EJ, Bayley DL, et al. Evidence for excessive bronchial inflammation during an acute exacerbation of chronic obstructive pulmonary disease in patients with α_1-antitrypsin deficiency (Pi Z). Am J Respir Crit Care Med 1999;160:1968–75.

35. Parr DG, White AJ, Bayley DL, et al. Inflammation in sputum relates to progression of disease in subjects with COPD: a prospective descriptive study. Respir Res 2006;7:136:1–11.

36. Ketelaars CA, Schlosser MA, Mastert R, et al. Determinants of health related quality of life in patients with chronic obstructive pulmonary disease. Thorax 1996;51:39–43.

37. Ebi-Kryston KL. Respiratory symptoms and pulmonary function as predictors of 10 year mortality from respiratory disease, cardiovascular disease and all causes in the Whitehall study. J Clin Epidemiol 1988;41:251–60.

38. Dowson LJ, Guest PJ, Hill SL, et al. High resolution computed tomography scanning in α_1 antitrypsin deficiency (Pi Z): relationship to lung function and health status. Eur Respir J 2001;17:1097–104.

39. Dawkins PA, Dowson LJ, Guest PJ, Stockley RA. Predictors of mortality in α_1 antitrypsin deficiency. Thorax 2003;58:1020–6.

40. Parr DG, Stoel BC, Stolk J, Stockley RA. Validation of computed tomographic lung densitometry for monitoring emphysema in α_1 antitrypsin deficiency. Thorax 2006;61:485–90.

41. Stolk J, Ng WH, Bakker ME, et al. Correlation between annual change in health status and computer tomography derived lung density in subjects with alpha-1 antitrypsin deficiency. Thorax 2003;58:1027–30.

42. Tutic M, Bloch KE, Lardinois D, et al. Long-term results after lung volume reduction surgery of patients with alpha-1 antitrypsin deficiency. J Thorac Cardiovasc Surg 2004;128:408–13.

43. De Perrot M, Chaparro C, McRae K, et al. Twenty-year experience of lung transplantation at a single center: influence of recipient diagnosis on long-term survival. J Thorac Cardiovasc Surg 2004;127:1493–501.

44. Alpha-1-Antitrypsin Deficiency Registry Study Group: survival and FEV1 decline in individuals with severe deficiency of α_1 antitrypsin. Am J Respir Crit Care Med 1998;158:49–59.

45. Seersholm N, Wencker M, Banik N, et al. Does α_1 antitrypsin augmentation therapy slow the annual decline in FEV1 in patients with severe hereditary α_1 antitrypsin deficiency? Eur Respir J 1997;10:2260–3.

46. Wencker M, Fuhrmann B, Banik N, Konietzko N. Longitudinal follow-up of patients with alpha (1) protease inhibitor deficiency before and during therapy with IV alpha (1) protease inhibitor. Chest 2001;119:737–44.

47. Dirksen A, Dijkman JH, Madsen F, et al. A randomised clinical trial of α_1 antitrypsin augmentation therapy. Am J Respir Crit Care Med 1999;160:1468–72.

48. Stockley RA, Bayley DL, Unsal I, Dowson LJ. The effect of augmentation therapy of bronchial inflammation in α_1 antitrypsin deficiency. Am J Respir Crit Care Med 2002;165:1494–8.

49. Stockley RA, Luisetti M, Miravitlles M, et al. Ongoing research in Europe: Alpha One International Registry (AIR) objectives and development. Eur Respir J 2007;29:582–6.

CHAPTER 6

PATHOBIOLOGY OF EMPHYSEMA

RUBIN M. TUDER, MD, AND NORBERT F. VOELKEL, MD

EMPHYSEMA OF THE LUNG is defined as a destructive and irreversible airspace enlargement without a significant component of fibrosis, resulting in a loss of alveolar gas exchange units.[1] Emphysema is part of the chronic obstructive pulmonary disease (COPD) syndrome, which, in turn, is characterized by only partially reversible airflow limitation.[2] Although this definition portends to distinguish between COPD and "asthma," there may be a continuum between the two diseases, as pointed out by Gelb and Zamel, who described "unexpected pseudophysiological emphysema in chronic persistent asthma."[3]

Whereas the small airway component of COPD is discussed in Chapter 9, "Small Airway Obstruction in Chronic Obstructive Pulmonary Disease," we focus on the pathobiology of emphysema. The precise relationship between small airways disease and emphysema in COPD remains unclear. As apparent in this chapter, exposure to cigarette smoke or environmental toxins, inflammation, and cellular damage by oxidative stress are common to both entities. However, emphysema and small airways disease involve two clearly distinct anatomic regions of the lung, each with its own molecular and cellular signatures. Perhaps the most striking difference between these manifestations of COPD is that in emphysema, the alveolar septal structures are destroyed and literally disappear, leaving little ground for tissue remodeling. Recent genomic studies have stressed that the molecular profiles between the involved airways and lung parenchyma are distinct. These differences reflect the anatomic, cellular, and molecular diversity between these lung compartments. Although most patients with COPD have varying degrees of small airway involvement and emphysema, there are patients with emphysema without airflow limitation who demonstrate a reduction in the diffusion capacity only.[4]

The evolution of chest computed tomographic (CT) scanning technology allowed for accurate regional and quantitative assessments of emphysema (see Chapter 18). The accuracy of the CT technology continues to be improved against the diagnostic benchmark reliant on gross and microscopic histomorphometry of the alveolar space. Given that alveolar morphometry depends on proper inflation and random sampling of lung explants or autopsy material, CT assessment of emphysema allows for the assessment of the extent of disease and correlation with pathogenetic parameters and, most importantly, may provide a valuable tool to monitor therapeutic interventions.

An ever-growing number of genetically engineered, developmentally triggered, or pharmacologically induced rodent models support the concept that airway disease and alveolar septal compartments can be dissociated, that is, the development of airspace enlargement can certainly occur unrelated to small airways disease. In fact, the most remarkable insight is that emphysema may occur unrelated to exposure to cigarette smoking.[5] Given the large amount of specific molecular information derived from these animal models (see Chapter 16), it remains to be elucidated whether genetic or signaling events that cause emphysema are indeed part of the pathway of disease relevant to cigarette smoke–induced disease or whether these events are unrelated to cigarette smoke but trigger relevant and shared molecular pathways involved in alveolar destruction. Emphysema appears to represent a prototypic lung disease phenotype compromising genetically susceptible individuals exposed to environmental challenges. Although cigarette smoke inhalation and air pollutants[6,7] are widely regarded as the most frequent causes of emphysema, it is important to keep an open mind and consider additional environmental causes associated with alveolar destruction.

The present discussion proposes that the conceptual framework for emphysema relies on the existence of a "Lung Structure Maintenance Program," which, under most conditions, successfully responds to the various environmental stressors and organizes the homeostatic maintenance of the lung structure.[5] We propose this maintenance program as the sum total of redundant molecular and cellular mechanisms, encompassing those residing within or outside the lung, that contribute to the orderly and accurate replacement of injured and senescent cells and maintenance of the matrix scaffold of the alveolar spaces. As apparent from the discussion that follows, the so-called traditional concepts of inflammation and protease/antiprotease imbalance fulfill the premises that alveolar integrity, including homeostatic control of inflammatory cell processes, relies on alveolar septal maintenance. Novel concepts of the interplay among oxidative stress and cell signaling, alveolar cell apoptosis, and extracellular matrix remodeling, among others, can now be critically reassessed, offering novel insights about the disease.

Lung Structure Maintenance Program

We introduced the concept of emphysema as a failure of the lung structure maintenance program in the first edition of this book.[5] This alternative hypothesis to explain lung tissue destruction and disappearance was derived from the realization that the protease-antiprotease hypothesis of emphysema could not fully explain how cigarette smoke inhalation causes emphysema in susceptible individuals. In fact, alveolar inflammation and excessive alveolar matrix proteolysis are seen in several lung diseases not associated with emphysema. Alveolar maintenance is based on the proposal that the adult lung requires constant trophic signals required for cell survival, replacement, and differentiation and that interruption of these trophic signals results in apoptosis of the lung's septal cells.[8] The traditional protease-antiprotease model of emphysema is intricately embedded in the larger concept of inflammation. In short, inflammatory cells produce the proteases, which destroy the alveolar structures. Although several elements of this classic paradigm are supported by abundant data, these data characterize a complex disease. More telling is the realization that the inflammation/protease imbalance has not provided any significant inroads into treatment of emphysema. What do we miss as we focus mostly on inflammation?

In the following, we frame inflammation within the paradigm of the lung structure maintenance program. One point of departure is the fact that virtually every smoker has chronic or persistent respiratory bronchiolitis, but only a minority of these smokers develop severe and progressive emphysema. Furthermore, it is unclear whether the inflammation seen early or late in the disease plays pathogenetically similar roles. Thus, the genetic susceptibility to tissue destruction (mediated or not by inflammation) encompasses the central role for a dysfunctional maintenance program in emphysema caused by cigarette smoke inhalation. We propose that disruption of this program is complex and progressive and that tissue destruction relies on multiple hits, which leave "marks" of damage. The lung, as such, acts as a memory bank, which stores information that relates to childhood infectious diseases, exposure to environmental toxins, and allergen exposures. It is conceivable that the alveolar maintenance reflects a person's nutritional history, with the program being shaped to some degree by dietary habits, which protect the lung against oxidants and proteases and facilitate resolution of inflammation (Figure 1).[9–11]

As we recognize that we argue for the teleology of a robust system, which is molecularly designed to limit and resolve inflammation, we also realize that the two cardinal functions of the alveolar septal spaces, namely gas exchange and endothelial cell input and output functions,[12] must be maintained. In simple terms, the gas exchanger must remain dry (hence the constant work of ion channels and molecular pumps), and septal endothelial cell dysfunction, or loss of endothelial cell numbers, is undesirable. We also realize that this program is also complex because it probably draws from

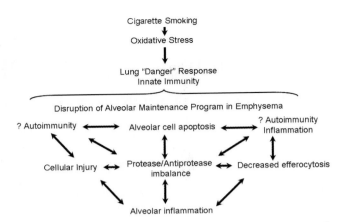

FIGURE 1. Cigarette smoking induces a "danger"-like response in the lung, with a resetting of the injury threshold by oxidative stress. Disruption of alveolar maintenance is directly affected by abnormal inflammation, potentially leading to autoimmune responses. Protease/antiprotease imbalance and inflammation may lead to dysfunctional efferocytosis. These processes are mutually interactive and may lead to self-propagating alveolar injury despite the interruption of smoking.

the support from resources provided by the bone marrow and the integrated immune system (including the spleen) to defend itself.

Innate and Adaptive Immunity

Innate (inborn) immunity is activated by microbial or viral proteins and viral deoxyribonucleic acid (DNA) and ribonucleic acid, by bacterial lipopolysaccharide and glycolipids through Toll-like receptors (TLRs), which are cell surface and intracellular compartment pattern recognition receptors.[13] The immune system scans tissues for infectious threats, detects infectious agents, and gathers information about infections to rapidly limit the spread and pathogenicity of infections. Built into this highly effective system of early pathogen recognition and containment is the ability to fend off future infections and, by extension, perhaps subsequent environmental threats or stresses. TLRs are abundantly expressed on innate immune cells such as macrophages and dendritic cells and have recently been found to be expressed by T-lymphocytes, including regulatory T-cells.[14,15] A subset of TLR-induced signals is dedicated to the control of the adaptive immune response[16] and host-derived nucleic acids, generated in the course of apoptosis, and in the setting of impaired efferocytosis (removal of apoptotic bodies).[17] Chromatin-immunoglobulin G complexes can activate B cells through ligation of B-cell antigen receptors and TLR-9, a mechanism that can lead to development of autoimmunity.[18] Autoantigens are cleaved by granzyme B and other granule proteases. Granzyme B activates CD8+ lymphocytes and dendritic cells, driving the development of granzyme B+ CD8+ cells. Vernooy and colleagues recently reported granzyme A expression in lymphocytes within alveolar septal structures, alveolar macrophages, and type II pneumocytes in lung tissue samples from patients with end-stage COPD. Granzyme B was also expressed in lymphoid aggregates.[19]

The important finding here is that the expression of granzyme A and B in lung *structural* cells (such as alveolar type II cells) directs our attention away from the fixed viewpoints of inflammatory cells and suggests alternative mechanisms of apoptotic septal cell destruction (see above) and a mechanism for the development of autoimmunity.

A highly interesting study by Zhang and colleagues demonstrated that TLR-4 knockout mice spontaneously develop emphysema as they age.[13] Remarkably, the lungs of these mice were characterized by overexpression of Nox 3 (a novel reduced nicotinamide adenine dinucleotide oxidase) and elastin breakdown without the presence of inflammation that is without neutrophils or macrophages. We are tempted to speculate that the environmental organ lung experiences a chronic low-level activation of TLR, leading to a TLR "tone," which is part of the adult lung structure maintenance program by activating protective mechanisms or stimulating cell growth. Jiang and colleagues showed that hyaluronan oligomers, which can signal through TLR-4 in endothelial cells, can protect cells against apoptosis, in part through activation of nuclear factor κB (NF-κB).[20]

Taken together, the data from different groups and experimental models illustrate the complex nature of lung tissue inflammation and the activation or survival of lung structure cells, which, if abnormal, may lead to autoimmunity. In addition, a new level of complexity is generated by the overlapping signals of inflammation and hypoxia. Patients with severe COPD become hypoxemic, leading to a decrease in oxygen supply at the cellular level. Not only hypoxia but also interleukin (IL)-1, endothelin, and angiotensin II stimulate hypoxia-inducible factor 1 (HIF-1) protein abundance and/or HIF-1 transactivation activity.[21] Although the number of HIF-1-inducible genes is large, (including vascular endothelial growth factor [VEGF], telomerase, CXCR4, the proto-oncogene *met*, connective tissue growth factor, and genes encoding glycolytic enzymes, among many others), it is peculiar that the expression of VEGF is decreased in the lungs from patients with end-stage COPD[22] and that apoptosis dominates over cell proliferation. The gene expression analysis of lung tissue samples from patients with end-stage COPD is characterized by and large by a global downregulation of genes, in particular mitochondrial genes, encoding proteins involved in energy metabolism.[23] The paradox of decreased VEGF expression in the setting of hypoxia can perhaps be explained by oxidative damage to the VEGF promoter, preventing effective HIF transactivation.[24] In addition, hypoxia also has an immunomodulating effect on dendritic cell and T-lymphocyte functions.[25]

Inflammation in Emphysema

In COPD, there are complex interactions between resident and migrating cells. Like the skin and the gastrointestinal tract, which are continuously challenged by the environment, lung tissue homeostasis requires vigilance and protection against environmental stress. These stress responses require migration and specialized functions of inflammatory cells, particularly lymphocytes (part of the bronchial associated lymphoid tissue), and of alveolar macrophages. These cellular processes involve highly coordinated molecular signaling events, orchestrated by all cells involved in the inflammatory cell response. Most importantly, the fate of incoming inflammatory cells relies on modulation of the inflammatory cell response by lung epithelial and endothelial cells and dendritic cells. Responses to injury are tightly regulated, with positive and negative feedback loops, such as recently demonstrated with regard to an initial decrease in active transforming growth factor β (TGF-β) in the lung matrix via downregulation of $\alpha_v\beta_6$ integrin (in type II cells) after a bacterial infection, followed by macrophage-led matrix metalloprotease (MMP) activation of TGF-β and reexpression of $\alpha_v\beta_6$ integrin, causing resolution of the inflammatory response.[26] Abnormalities of these signaling mechanisms and disruption of negative feedback mechanisms underlie the alterations in lung tissue and cell responses during acute lung injury.[27] However, our understanding of how the deregulation of alveolar cell crosstalk with inflammatory cells results in emphysema remains rudimentary. Teleologically, lung inflammation has been evolutionarily designed to protect organisms against infectious agents.[8] Cigarette smoke exposure of rodents and the effects of smoking on the airways and the lung parenchyma have been studied for years,[28–30] and the pathologic changes in the airways of smokers and the effects on human lung cells have been reported (Table 1).

There is no evidence that cigarette smoke directly and specifically activates inflammation as primarily mediated by infectious agents, which apparently is the evolutionary reason for the survival advantage of inflammation and immunity. We have proposed an alternative hypothesis that cigarette smoke induces a "danger" signal, which amplifies oxidative stress and oxidative stress-dependent cell injury, manifesting itself through alveolar inflammation and alveolar cell apoptosis.[8] RTP801, a HIF-transduced gene that amplifies oxidative stress and inhibits mammalian target of rapamycin (mTOR) and protein translation, may be centrally positioned as a switch of cell stress signaling.[31]

Acute cigarette smoke exposure of rodents generates an acute inflammatory response, characterized by an increase in neutrophils and, most prominently, macrophages. There are limited data regarding the nature of the targets of neutrophil and macrophage influx after short-term exposure to cigarette smoke. Activated neutrophils are retained in the lungs of humans after inhalation of cigarette smoke,[32] and short-term exposure causes increased desmosine detectable in bronchoalveolar lavage fluid (BALF), indicative of elastin fiber breakdown in mouse lungs.[33] We have documented that exposure of mice to acute cigarette smoke (up to 7 days) leads to inflammation (as assessed by an increased cellularity in the BALF) at days 1 and 4, with relative quiescence at days 2 and 7. These alterations in cellularity suggested that cigarette

Table 1 Effects of Cigarette Smoking

Tissue	Cellular and Molecular Actions		Studies
Small airways	Goblet cell metaplasia airway wall inflammation and wall fibrosis	Human	Wright JL et al, 1983[30]
Small airways	Respiratory bronchiolitis	Human	Niewoehner D et al, 1974[28]
Vascular remodeling	Intima thickening Increased elastin and collagen	Human	Santos S et al, 2002[29]
Lung parenchyma	Emphysema, loss of capillaries	Guinea pigs	Yamato H et al, 1996[138]
Vascular muscularization	Increased expression of endothelin, VEGF, eNOS	Guinea pigs	Wright JL et al, 2002[66]
Lung tissue change in gene expression	Upregulation of metallothionein, arginase 1, cathepsin K	Rat	Gebel S et al, 2006[139]
Lung immune cells	Increased gamma/delta T cells and B-cell follicles Increased cytokine production by splenocytes	Mice	Guerrassimov A et al, 2004[140]
Lung B cells	—	Mice	Van der Strate BWA et al, 2006[141]
Spleen	—	Mice	Robbins C et al, 2005[142]

eNOS = endothelial nitric oxide synthase; VEGF = vascular endothelial growth factor.

smoke–induced inflammation is not persistent (in the acute stage) but that it follows a cyclical pattern owing to the potential activation of dampening mechanisms (that may be part of the lung structure maintenance program). This process may serve the purpose of counteracting potentially life-threatening persistent inflammation after cigarette smoke inhalation. Whether these acute oscillations in inflammatory cells and cytokines play a role in chronic lung tissue damage remains unknown. It is conceivable that the pathobiologic responses of the early inflammation may be different from the chronic inflammation in the setting of a progressive failure of the alveolar maintenance program.

Chronic cigarette smoke exposure increases the inflammatory cell numbers in the BALF and lung tissue of humans and experimental models.[5] Of all inflammatory cells, an increase in CD8+ T-cells has been linked to a worse prognosis and heightened lung tissue destruction in patients with COPD.[34] However, neutrophils and eosinophils predominate with the progression of COPD, particularly during exacerbations, and may participate in accelerated tissue destruction or airway disease.[35] That inflammatory cells are required for emphysematous alveolar destruction resulting from cigarette smoke exposure was supported by experimental studies showing that depletion of macrophages prevents emphysema development (see Chapter 8).

The enhanced infiltration of inflammatory cells in COPD has been attributed to either cigarette smoke or pollutants or to oxidative stress as the result of exposure to environmental hazards, causing enhanced recruitment of inflammatory cells. Chemokines and cytokines mediate the attraction of inflammatory cells owing to cigarette smoke exposure. Healthy human smokers show increased levels of BALF IL-1β, IL-6, IL-8, IL-10, IL-12p70, and tumor necrosis factor (TNF)-α when compared with nonsmokers in BALF, and all cytokines

were increased during COPD (Global Initiative for Chronic Obstructive Lung Disease [GOLD] stages III and IV) exacerbations when compared with patients with stable COPD.[36] The functional relevance of these chemokines is best illustrated by the protection afforded by the deletion of the TNF-α receptor[37] and emphysema observed in transgenic mice with TNF-α overexpression.[38]

The role of chemokines was substantiated by the partial protection against emphysema observed in CCR5 knockout mice (from a mean chord length of approximately 45 μm in wild-type animals versus 37 μm in the lungs from knockout animals; room air = 35 μm[39]) and in CCR6 knockout mice (from a mean linear intercept of approximately 47 μm in wild-type versus 44 μm in knockout lungs; room air = 42 μm).[40] CCR5 binds macrophage inflammatory protein (MIP-1α, MIP-1β, and RANTES, and CCR6 is the receptor for MIP)[40]-3α. Perhaps the strongest indication that inflammatory cells are intimately involved with alveolar structure maintenance is the finding that CCR5 knockout mice not only have decreased inflammation but also a significantly lower number of apoptotic alveolar septal cells.[39] The data on CCR5 are of interest since lymphocytes obtained from advanced emphysematous lungs (following lung volume reduction surgery) are strongly polarized toward a so-called TH-1 phenotype, with enhanced secretion of interferon (IFN)-γ, CCR5, and CXCR3 and increased expression of CXCR3 ligands, monokine-induced + interferon (MIG) and IP10.[41]

Given the data of the role of inflammation in emphysema, the specific roles of alveolar inflammation in emphysematous tissue destruction remain to be elucidated. We have proposed that the alveolar tissue destruction requires the convergence of inflammatory cell responses and a faulty alveolar maintenance program.[8] The aggregate of data from the group of Elias and collaborators support the contention that alveolar inflammation caused by cigarette smoke exposure of transgenic mice overexpressing IL-13 or IFN-γ is intimately linked to alveolar cell apoptosis.[43] How does inflammation cause alveolar cell death and airspace enlargement? One explanation is that the excessive matrix proteolysis drives alveolar cell apoptosis, yet data from Elias and colleagues using MMP-9/MMP-12 knockout mice suggest the existence of two separate pathogenetic pathways of emphysema, one associated with apoptosis and another dependent on matrix proteolysis.[42]

The pathogenetic role of specific inflammatory cells remains unclear. Experimental evidence has not substantiated the notion that neutrophils are necessary and sufficient to cause emphysema. Neutrophil elastase contributes to about 60% of airspace enlargement based on experiments with neutrophil elastase-null mice.[43] However, neutrophils may induce macrophage influx and elastin fragments, originating from neutrophil influx, and neutrophil elastase could be critical for the attraction of macrophages (see below).[44] Careful time course studies of inflammatory responses and elastolytic activity for up to 6 months of cigarette smoke exposure revealed an increase in rat BALF but not lung *tissue* neutrophils from 2 to 6 months of cigarette smoke exposure (when alveolar enlargement starts in this model), despite a temporary increase after 1 month of exposure.[45] Nevertheless, neutrophil elastase knockout mice are protected only by 50% when chronically exposed to cigarette smoke.[43]

Macrophages are the predominant inflammatory cells in smokers, COPD patients, and animal models of emphysema (see Chapter 16) and are thought to represent the effector cells of alveolar destruction. Time course studies revealed increased macrophage numbers in rat BALF and lung tissue during 2 and 6 months of cigarette smoke exposure and, most importantly, that BALF and lung tissue elastolytic activity, BALF desmosine, and alveolar morphometry correlated closely with the interstitial macrophage infiltrates.[46] The corollary of this experiment is that macrophages are required for cigarette smoke–induced emphysema in rats since depletion of macrophages (by 50%), but not neutrophil depletion, significantly protected against an increase in elastin peptide levels, BALF desmosine levels, and alveolar size owing to chronic cigarette smoke inhalation.[46] These findings are in line with a central role of macrophage metalloprotease 12 in mouse emphysema models.[47] Manipulations of in cigarette smoke–induced cytokines, chemokines, and chemokines, such as IL-1, TNF-α, IFN-γ, IL-13, CCR5, and CCR6, led to closely paralleled numbers of alveolar macrophage and the degree of experimental emphysema. Given that normal lungs have large numbers of alveolar macrophages with immunosuppressive functions and that lung tissue macrophages are conspicuous in inflammatory lung disease, the pathogenetic function of macrophages in emphysema might be framed in the context of disruption of the alveolar maintenance program. Abnormal alveolar cell signaling, a decrease in the activity of antiproteases, and abnormalities of the extracellular matrix may all render the infiltrating macrophages the

actor of alveolar destruction. The link between macrophages and alveolar cell apoptosis has not been addressed in the context of chronic lung diseases. A fascinating link between developmental apoptosis of endothelial cells lining the temporary hyaloid artery (which is destined to disappear immediately after birth) and macrophages was uncovered,[48] in which macrophages lining the target artery mediate endothelial cell apoptosis via wnt 7B secretion and paracrine signaling via endothelial cell frizzle receptors.[49]

As mentioned, the reasons underlying the attraction of inflammatory cells by cigarette smoke remain unknown. Oxidative stress leading to activation of proinflammatory signaling such as NF-κB might represent one mechanism of activation of inflammation, although acute exposure to cigarette smoke leads to upregulation of antioxidants,[50] which contribute to the reestablishment of the oxidative balance. Furthermore, NF-κB signaling contains several negative counterregulatory feedback loops, some involved in short-term inflammation, controlled by MKK3/IκK/IκBα, whereas long-term tonic activation is controlled by MKK2/IKK/IκBβ.[51] Built into the termination of NF-κB-mediated inflammation are components of this signaling pathway, such as IκBα for short-term shutoff and IκBβ.[52]

Despite the compelling theoretical evidence supporting abnormalities of NF-κB activation in cigarette smoke–induced emphysema, we know little about the role of the members of this signaling pathway in cigarette smoke–induced inflammation. IκBα proteosomal degradation and NF-κB DNA binding is significantly increased in healthy smokers and current smokers with moderate COPD compared with healthy nonsmokers. The degree of NF-κB DNA binding is similar in ex-smokers with COPD and in healthy smokers. Evidence of NF-κB activation in experimental models of emphysema is limited. Acute (5 hour) cigarette smoke exposure of guinea pigs caused increased NF-κB expression in alveolar macrophages, which correlated with enhanced neutrophil influx and IL-8 expression.[53] Interestingly, these effects are blocked by pretreatment with superoxide dismutase. The complexity of manipulating NF-κB activation *in vivo* led to investigations to control NF-κB-dependent inflammatory cytokines by means of decreasing histone acetylation.[54,55]

The recent groundbreaking studies revealing that oligoclones of T cells exist in advanced emphysematous lungs may have a significant impact on how to interpret the nature of inflammation in COPD.[56,57] These findings may imply that specific lung antigens participate in the selection of these T-cell clones, including potential autoantigens. This forms the basis of the recent autoimmune hypothesis of emphysema,[58] in which the authors postulated that autoreactive T cells might be selected against alveolar cell self-antigens revealed by chronic injury caused by cigarette smoke or superimposed infections. Adenovirus latent infection antigen might be targeted by infiltrating lymphocytes, therefore amplifying the inflammatory responses to cigarette smoke in the guinea pig model.[59] Latent adenovirus expression was enhanced in the lung tissue from patients with advanced emphysema when compared with milder forms of emphysema.[60] As stated, it has been proposed that COPD or emphysema could in some patients take the form of an autoimmune disorder.[58] This concept was supported by the demonstration that rat immunization with endothelial cells triggered an antibody-cellular response against alveolar cells, leading to apoptosis and emphysema.[61] It is of interest that tolerizing strategies (eg, pretreatment of rats with lipid A, a component of endotoxin that activates TLR-4) protect against this form of experimental autoimmune emphysema.[135]

In summary, inflammation is an essential element of the pathobiology of emphysema. Alveolar structural damage may reveal autoantigenic sites responsible for some of the inflammatory reactions, particularly after chronic cigarette smoke inhalation and in advanced disease states. The nature of the acute inflammatory cell reaction owing to cigarette smoke inhalation might represent a preinnate immune response owing to cellular danger signals caused by cigarette smoke, potentiating inflammatory lung responses owing to oxidative stress. Furthermore, hypersensitivity to tobacco antigens has been suggested as an initiator of lung inflammation.[62] Interestingly, the breakdown of negative regulatory feedback loops of inflammation and of dampening mechanisms of inflammatory cell responses in COPD might be seen in the context of the disruption of the alveolar maintenance program. This concept applies not only to structural alveolar cells but also to the homeostatic role of inflammation in the lung. In short, good and bad elements (destructive and protective) may be contained within the inflammatory response following the inhalation of noxious volatile compounds or particles.[17]

Protease/Antiprotease Imbalance

The lung's architectural scaffold is composed predominantly of elastin, collagen, and matrix glycoproteins. This scaffold has a central role during lung morphogenesis (see Chapter 2), during preservation of adult lung function, and in lung disease. Emphysema is associated with the breakdown of the elastin scaffold, documented histologically by fragmentation of elastin fibrils and by detection of its associated amino acid desmosine in BALF or urine. The evidence that disrupted elastin leads to disrupted fetal lung growth, resulting in a simplified and emphysematous-like lung,[63] and that mice lacking tissue inhibitor of metalloproteinase-3 (TIMP-3) develop emphysema highlights the potential of alveolar structure disruption as a consequence of an abnormal extracellular matrix. The discovery of α_1-antitrypsin deficiency as a leading genetic cause of emphysema[64] propelled the protease-antiprotease hypothesis of emphysema[64] as necessary and sufficient for alveolar destruction. This hypothesis rests heavily on the infiltrating inflammatory cells as the contributing source of matrix proteases, particularly of neutrophil elastase and macrophage metalloproteases (MMPs).

The role of neutrophil elastase was initially supported by the tracheal elastase instillation model of emphysema,[65] still a useful model of the disease. Although this model has provided important data regarding some aspects related to cigarette smoke–induced disease, the functional role of neutrophil elastase has been further uncovered in the past 15 years. As discussed previously, there is no conclusive evidence that neutrophils or neutrophil-derived proteases are *required* for experimental emphysema in rats exposed acutely or chronically to cigarette smoke.[46] Mice with a knockout of the neutrophil elastase provide only partial protection against chronic exposure to cigarette smoke (see above), which is associated with a decrease in the MMP-12 to TIMP-1 ratio.[43] Furthermore, treatment with a synthetic neutrophil elastase inhibitor ZD0892 reduces BALF neutrophil number, desmosine, and hydroxyproline levels to levels similar to those found in control lungs. Elastase inhibition also reduces the levels of MIP-2, macrophage chemotactic protein-1 (MCP-1), and TNF-α and decreases airspace enlargement by 45%.[66] Recent data demonstrate that elastase fragmentation of lung elastin contributes to macrophage chemotaxis[44] and that a peptide N-acetyl-proline-glycine-proline derived from the extracellular collagen matrix breakdown has structural homology with α-chemokines and activates neutrophil accumulation by binding to the chemokine receptor CXCR4.[67] These data suggest that the breakdown of the lung extracellular matrix *induces* inflammation, particularly macrophage infiltration, and that neutrophils alone cannot account for the alveolar destruction in emphysema. Macrophages contribute with a significant component of extracellular matrix degradation, mostly by producing MMPs (see Chapter 8).

MMPs comprise at least 20 proteolytic enzymes that play an essential role in tissue remodeling and repair associated with development and inflammation by degrading collagen, laminin, and elastin. Depending on the substrate specificity, amino acid similarity, and identifiable sequence modules, the MMP family can be divided into distinct subclasses as collagenases (MMP-1, -8, -13), gelatinases (MMP-2, -9), stromelysins (MMP-3, 10, -11), membrane-type MMP (MMP-14 to MMP-25), matrilysin (MMP-7), and macrophage metalloelastase (MMP-12). The major physiologic *in vivo* inhibitors of the MMPs are α2-macroglobulin and the TIMP family, which are naturally occurring proteins specifically inhibiting these proteases and produced by different cell types. The TIMP family at present comprises four structurally related members: TIMP-1, -2, and -3 and the recently discovered TIMP-4.

MMP-12 knockout mice are protected against cigarette smoke–induced emphysema and therefore provide compelling evidence for the role of this macrophage MMP in the pathogenesis of emphysema.[47] MMP-12 has been detected in sputum, BALF, bronchial biopsies,[68,69] and peripheral lung tissue samples from patients with advanced disease.[70] Patients with COPD caused by cigarette smoke, as well as wood smoke exposure (indoor pollution), showed higher expression levels of MMP-2, -9, and -12 transcripts in BALF macrophages when compared with samples from control patients.[71] MMP-12 immunoreactivity can be demonstrated in alveolar macrophages and septal macrophages after cigarette smoke exposure in male C57BL/6 mice.[72] Chronic inhalation of cigarette smoke for 1, 3, and 6 months causes a significant increase in MMP-12 messenger ribonucleic acid (mRNA) and protein in the lungs and mRNA in BALF cells of male C57BL/6 mice, with no differences in the expression levels of TIMP-1 and -2, indicating an increase in the MMP-12 to TIMP ratio.[73] MMP-12 also acts as a TNF-α-converting enzyme, promoting the release of active TNF-α for subsequent endothelial activation, neutrophil influx, and elastase release in cigarette smoke–induced acute pulmonary injury.[33] These acute lung changes are not dependent on NF-κB activation since both MMP-12-null mice and wild-type mice showed a rapid increase in NF-κB DNA binding activity.

Despite evidence of MMP-9 and -2 (which also degrade elastin) expression in COPD lungs, there is no conclusive evidence that either MMP has a central role in the emphysema pathogenesis. MMP-9 knockout mice were not protected against emphysema.[74] On the other hand, experimental emphysema caused by lung overexpression of IL-13 or deletion of surfactant protein D involved both MMP-9 and MMP-12[75,76] as surfactant D-deficient mice expressed high levels of MMP-9 and -12.[31,77] However, surfactant D-deficient mice lacking MMP-9 or -12 develop airspace enlargement similar to surfactant D-deficient mice.[76]

Collagenases, particularly of MMP-1, might have a significant role in emphysema. MMP-1 expression is increased in COPD lungs when compared with control lungs.[78] Furthermore, there is solid evidence that lung expression of human MMP-1 caused emphysema.[79,80] Interestingly, despite the suggested lack of significant fibrosis in emphysema,[1] lungs with advanced emphysema exhibit a complex pattern of collagen deposition, which eventually replaces the elastin framework.[81]

In summary, excessive degradation of the lung extracellular matrix is part of the process of lung tissue destruction. However, recent paradigms have weakened the proposed exclusive role of the protease/antiprotease imbalance in emphysema. Instead, the protease/antiprotease hypothesis needs to be integrated within the larger context of inflammation (as defined above), apoptosis and failure of efferocytosis, and oxidative stress. Indeed, oxidative stress can activate MMPs, as shown with MMP-9 in brain ischemia.[82] Furthermore, the role of protease/antiprotease imbalance in emphysema was supported by the finding that TIMP-3 knockout mice have spontaneous and progressive emphysema,[83] consistent with the critical role of extracellular matrix homeostasis in lung morphogenesis, development, and maintenance.

Apoptosis and Efferocytosis

Apoptosis, or programmed cell death, has now been recognized as a feature of human emphysema[22,84] and is mechanistically linked to the disease in many animal models of emphysema.[85,86]

Teleologically, apoptosis is part of normal organismal life and homeostasis. For example, circulating neutrophils undergo apoptosis every day.[87–93] We initially demonstrated an enhanced rate of alveolar cell apoptosis as part of the disrupted alveolar lung cell maintenance program owing to VEGF receptor blockade.[94] The potential role of alveolar cell apoptosis in emphysema was further documented by other investigators, including transgenic and cigarette smoke models of emphysema.[95–97] We also documented that apoptosis interacts with oxidative stress in the process of airspace enlargement caused by VEGF receptor blockade,[98] potentially leading to feedforward loops, causing disruption of alveolar maintenance. Endogenous signaling mediators can then amplify alveolar tissue destruction, even with the cessation of the main factor causing lung injury, such as cigarette smoke. This hypothesis led us to demonstrate that ceramide, a second-messenger lipid involved in oxidative stress and apoptosis, was upregulated by VEGF receptor blockade and mediated alveolar cell apoptosis and oxidative stress in this model of emphysema. Importantly, emphysematous lungs have increased levels of ceramide, mostly of medium-size carbon side chain, whereas smokers have a predominance of long-chain ceramides.[99] Ceramide may therefore not only enhance alveolar cell apoptosis but may also affect endothelial cell survival, disrupt efferocytosis, and lead to enhanced senescence and inflammation.

Peter Henson has pointed out that failure of phagocytosis of apoptotic cells (called "efferocytosis" and initially termed "physiologic inflammation") is more critical than apoptosis per se for tissue homeostasis. Effective efferocytosis causes the release of TGF-β, leading to an anti-inflammatory and anti-immunogenic microenvironment.[17] Ingestion of apoptotic cells by macrophages increases production of prostaglandin E2 and induces intracellular prostaglandin synthases.[100] Furthermore, efferocytosis leads to the synthesis and release of growth factors[23] and can induce compensatory cell proliferation through the JNK pathway.[101] There is an intriguing interplay not only between extracellular protease action and apoptosis[95,102] but also between proteases and ineffective cell removal. Excessive elastase activation inhibits efferocytosis, whereas effective dead cell removal results in production of antiproteases.[103] Aoshiba and colleagues demonstrated in mice that intratracheal instillation of active caspase caused emphysema and possibly activation of cathepsin in apoptotic epithelial cells.[104] Although the authors did not investigate phagocyte- and nonphagocyte-mediated removal of apoptotic cells, it is possible that apoptotic cell clearance was indeed overwhelmed by excessive apoptosis. In contrast to the results of Aoshiba and colleagues, our own studies (Lee JH et al, unpublished data, 2008) indicate that massive apoptotic alveolar septal cell loss after intratracheal caspase instillation is not spontaneously repaired and that emphysema persists.

Deficient apoptotic cell removal clearly leads to inflammation, autoimmunity, and tissue damage.[105] A recent report described impaired neutrophil chemotaxis in patients with

COPD,[106] which warrants the question of whether impaired in situ neutrophil apoptosis or impaired neutrophil clearance is involved in neutrophilic airway inflammation. At this juncture, we propose at least two important mechanisms for the persistence of emphysema. One mechanism relates to an apoptosis/repair imbalance (see the discussion below), and the other mechanisms are related to dysfunctional apoptotic cell clearance. Both mechanisms, either alone or in combination, will jeopardize the lung structural maintenance program, but only the latter mechanism would perpetuate inflammation. The detailed interactions between apoptotic cells and professional or nonprofessional phagocytes are complex, require "eat me" signals, and are under intense investigation.[86] A better understanding of the mechanisms of efferocytosis failure will likely lead to new treatment strategies for COPD. It is already known that "statins," macrolide antibiotics, and Rho kinase inhibitors all can improve efferocytosis and perhaps can "cool off" inflammation because of enhanced removal of dead cells.

Emphysema—Also a Vascular Disease

The observations of involvement of the lung microcirculation in emphysema were developed many decades ago, and they are discussed in the first edition of this book. Here we can expand on the mechanisms of microvessel loss in the context of endothelial cell biology. As mentioned above, the lung capillary endothelial cells depend on the presence of the endothelial growth and maintenance factor VEGF and on effective signaling through its receptors. Lung capillary endothelial cells generate and secrete VEGF in culture,[107] and, if confirmed in vivo in the lung microcirculation, then VEGF may have an autocrine endothelial cell maintenance role in the lung. Different experimental approaches by several investigators support the thesis that disturbance of VEGF signaling leads to endothelial cell loss and emphysema[108] and to loss of capillaries in the skeletal muscle of mice.[88] Effective efferocytosis by professional phagocytes leads to secretion of growth factors, which cause proliferation of endothelial cells and epithelial cells.[109] Because phagocytic clearance of apoptotic cells is impaired in COPD,[110] alveolar septal repair via secretion of growth factors from phagocytes is likely impaired. In addition to a lack of growth factors and impaired growth factor actions, we also need to consider destruction of lung capillary endothelial cells by anti-endothelial cell antibodies[61] and endothelial cell-lymphocyte interactions.[111] Lastly, there is the possibility of impairment of mobilization of precursor cells from the bone marrow or failure of integration of circulating growth factors into the residual lung structure, with its damaged matrix protein scaffold.

There is no a priori reason why the vascular damage in COPD should be restricted to the lung microvessels, yet systematic studies of systemic vessels or microvessels of other organs are lacking. Only a small number of studies address the issue of endothelial cell dysfunction in patients with COPD and in smokers.[112–115]

Cellular Senescence in Emphysema

We have illustrated that a failure of alveolar structural maintenance is characterized by inappropriate inflammatory responses, excessive apoptosis, deficient efferocytosis, abnormal extracellular matrix remodeling, and excessive oxidative stress. A novel insight into the manifestation of this process is the accumulation of cellular and molecular markers of senescence. In this regard, there is a close relationship between alveolar cell senescence and lung aging, as we recently proposed.[116]

The aged lung shows a progressive airspace enlargement, which has been considered the result of a nondestructive process (versus the destruction that is characteristic of centrilobular emphysema). This process parallels a progressive decrease in forced ventilatory capacity, with little or no clinical relevance.[117] However, this process may not be "physiological" as elastin fiber fragmentation and loss of elasticity are seen in the aged lungs. Furthermore, there are shared molecular signatures of aging in the emphysematous lungs and in COPD patients. Peripheral blood mononuclear cells from patients with COPD have decreased telomere length, a hallmark of senescing cells in vitro, when compared with normal individuals.[118] This observation has been extended to lung cells as alveolar epithelial and endothelial cells of emphysema patients exhibited enhanced expression of markers of cell senescence, including $p16^{Ink4a}$ and $p21^{CIP1/WAF1/Sdi1}$ and telomere shortening when compared with smokers without emphysema and normal individuals.[119] Lung fibroblasts from emphysema patients express the senescence-associated β-galactosidase (SA-β-Gal), along with the upregulation of senescence-associated insulin-like growth factor binding protein III (IGFBP-III) and IGFBP-related protein 1 (which are HIF-1 α-dependently induced), all of this in support of a senescent lung phenotype.[120] Senescing cells had increased production of cytokines and chemokines and enhanced matrix protease activity, which can stimulate active tissue destruction.[8]

The senescent changes in emphysema lungs could be related to oxidative stress originating from cigarette smoke exposure. Increased ceramide levels in the smoker's lung may also contribute to aging as ceramide promoted senescence in cultured cells.[121] With age, neutrophils and macrophages reduce superoxide production, accompanied by an impairment of chemotaxis, cytokine production, and signal transduction.[122]

Animals prone to premature aging have been used to study the link between aging and cigarette smoke–induced emphysema, including the senescence-accelerated mice,[123] the klotho knockout mouse, and the FGF23-null mouse.[124]

Based on studies of the senescence marker protein 30 (SMP-30) knockout mouse, which develops aging-related changes in the lung, including alveolar enlargement that resembled emphysema,[125,126] there is an enhanced cigarette smoke–induced phenotype associated with increased alveolar cell apoptosis and oxidative stress. This synergistic effect between cigarette smoke and SMP-30 deficiency might be explained by the interaction of shared pathophysiologic events, leading to enhanced alveolar destruction (Figure 1).

Therefore, the accumulation of alveolar injury and failure of alveolar maintenance lead to the emergence of molecular signatures of prolonged damage, such as cell senescence. These are important considerations with regard to the ability of the organ to regenerate as attempted with all-*trans* retinoic acid supplementation,[127] or lung-specific increases in hepatocyte growth factor engineered in adipose cells,[128] or overexpression of adrenomedullin.[127]

Summary and Conclusions

For the time being, it may be more productive to consider the small airways disease (bronchiolitis) and the emphysematous parenchyma destruction as distinct, that is, pathobiologically independent manifestations of COPD. At the time of this writing, it is apparent that there is no unifying hypothesis that can explain whether or how small airway remodeling and loss of alveolar septal structures are mechanistically linked. Although inflammation remains at the center of all discussions of the pathobiology of emphysema, we like to adopt Carl Nathan's concept of "informmation as a system of information flow."[128] This concept is all-inclusive and would be useful for the exploration of the systemic COPD manifestations.

Accordingly, the "informmatory information" imposes on the lung structure maintenance program "go/no go" decisions. This inflammatory information is processed by the lung and passes through a series of checkpoints,[128] requiring ongoing verification and initially highly localized responses. Activation of antigen-presenting cells carries the potential for the inflammatory response to turn into an (auto)immune response. The inflammation includes not only the effectors of inflammatory response but also, importantly, holding patterns and resolution programs. If we can accept this inflammation as a system of information flow idea, the challenge will now be to determine which components of the inflammatory response destroy or protect and which of the inflammatory gene products are "essential effectors of homeostasis."[130]

As the emphysematous lung is characterized by loss of vasculature, in particular by loss of alveolar capillaries, it follows that emphysema is also a vascular disease, requiring an extended understanding of capillary endothelial cell biology. This point is perhaps illustrated by an observed association of emphysema and pulmonary capillaritis.[130] Again, this viewpoint is appropriately holistic. Beyond that, many mysteries remain and invite investigation.

Outlook

How will the new concepts of "lung structure maintenance" and "inflammatory information flow" determine the future treatment of emphysema? At present, we can separate strategies that could prevent emphysema development from strategies designed to repair the emphysema, that is, to rebuild the destroyed lung.

Possibly effective prevention strategies may rest on dietary adjustments. Animal studies have already shown that tomato juice,[132] resveratrol,[133] and *N*-acetylcysteine[134] can prevent emphysema development. Prospective studies in human smokers will be needed. Disease arrest strategies, using adjuvants, may be considered. In this case, causing inflammation by using adjuvants may paradoxically halt disease progression, perhaps by dampening the adaptive immune response. Hanaoka and colleagues demonstrated in rats that pristane, which is widely used as an adjuvant, can protect against emphysema development.[135] Whether end-stage COPD or emphysema, "the vanishing lung syndrome," is amenable to such therapy is unclear.

Rebuilding an utterly destroyed lung remains a dream, at least for the foreseeable future, and we want to emphasize that it is questionable whether experiments with rodents, designed to explore the capacity of the emphysematous lung to repair itself, can be translated to the situation of the long-time susceptible and aged smoker.

The lungs of rodents, which live in an environmentally challenging and polluted habitat, may have developed a mechanism that allows lifelong repair and cell growth, which adult humans may not possess. Nevertheless, ongoing studies exploring lung repair mechanisms based on use of bone marrow-derived precursor cells and experiments that investigate the growth and repair potential of lung-specific stem cells are of great interest.[136,137]

References

1. Snider GL, Kleinerman LJ, Thurlbeck WM, Bengali ZH. The definition of emphysema: report of a National, Heart, Lung and Blood Institute Division of Lung Diseases workshop. Am Rev Respir Dis 1985;131:182–5.
2. Buist AS. Similarities and differences between asthma and chronic obstructive pulmonary disease: treatment and early outcomes. Eur Respir J Suppl 2003;39:30s–5s.
3. Gelb AF, Zamel N. Unsuspected pseudophysiologic emphysema in chronic persistent asthma. Am J Respir Crit Care Med 2000;162:1778–82.
4. Aduen JF, Zisman DA, Mobin SI, et al. Retrospective study of pulmonary function tests in patients presenting with isolated reduction in single-breath diffusion capacity: implications for the diagnosis of combined obstructive and restrictive lung disease. Mayo Clin Proc 2007;82:48–54.
5. Tuder RM, Voelkel NF. The pathobiology of chronic bronchitis and emphysema. In Voelkel NF, MacNee W, editors. Chronic obstructive lung disease. Hamilton (ON): BC Decker; 2002. p. 90–113.
6. Abbey DE, Burchette RJ, Knutsen SF, et al. Long-term particulate and other air pollutants and lung function in nonsmokers. Am J Respir Crit Care Med 1998;158:289–98.
7. Karakatsani A, Andreadaki S, Katsouyanni K, et al. Air pollution in relation to manifestations of chronic pulmonary disease: a nested case-control study in Athens, Greece. Eur J Epidemiol 2003;18:45–53.
8. Tuder RM, Yoshida T, Arap W, et al. Cellular and molecular mechanisms of alveolar destruction in emphysema: an evolutionary perspective. Proc Am Thorac Soc 2006;3:503–10.

9. Tabak C, Smit HA, Heederik D, et al. Diet and chronic obstructive pulmonary disease: independent beneficial effects of fruits, whole grains, and alcohol (the MORGEN study). Clin Exp Allergy 2001;31:747–55.

10. Sharp DS, Rodriguez BL, Shahar E, et al. Fish consumption may limit the damage of smoking on the lung. Am J Respir Crit Care Med 1994;150:983–7.

11. Machowetz A, Poulsen HE, Gruendel S, et al. Effect of olive oils on biomarkers of oxidative DNA stress in Northern and Southern Europeans. FASEB J 2007;21:45–52.

12. Aird WC. Mechanisms of endothelial cell heterogeneity in health and disease. Circ Res 2006;98:159–62.

13. Zhang X, Shan P, Jiang G, et al. Toll-like receptor 4 deficiency causes pulmonary emphysema. J Clin Invest 2006;116:3050–9.

14. Sutmuller RP, den Brok MH, Kramer M, et al. Toll-like receptor 2 controls expansion and function of regulatory T cells. J Clin Invest 2006;116:485–94.

15. Peng G, Guo Z, Kiniwa Y, et al. Toll-like receptor 8-mediated reversal of CD4+ regulatory T cell function. Science 2005;309:1380–4.

16. Barton GM, Medzhitov R. Control of adaptive immune responses by Toll-like receptors. Curr Opin Immunol 2002;14:380–3.

17. Henson PM. Dampening inflammation. Nat Immunol 2005;6:1179–81.

18. Colonna M. Toll-like receptors and IFN-alpha: partners in autoimmunity. J Clin Invest 2006;116:2319–22.

19. Vernooy JH, Moller GM, van Suylen RJ, et al. Increased granzyme A expression in type II pneumocytes of patients with severe chronic obstructive pulmonary disease. Am J Respir Crit Care Med 2007;175:464–72.

20. Jiang D, Liang J, Fan J, et al. Regulation of lung injury and repair by Toll-like receptors and hyaluronan. Nat Med 2005;11:1173–9.

21. Wenger RH, Stiehl DP, Camenisch G. Integration of oxygen signaling at the consensus HRE. Sci Signal 2005: Oct.18(306). p. re12.

22. Kasahara Y, Tuder RM, Cool CD, et al. Endothelial cell death and decreased expression of vascular endothelial growth factor and vascular endothelial growth factor receptor 2 in emphysema. Am J Respir Crit Care Med 2001;163:737–44.

23. Golpon HA, Coldren CD, Zamora MR, et al. Emphysema lung tissue gene expression profiling. Am J Respir Cell Mol Biol 2004;31:595–600.

24. Ziel KA, Grishko V, Campbell CC, et al. Oxidants in signal transduction: impact on DNA integrity and gene expression. FASEB J 2005;19:387–94.

25. Lukashev D, Klebanov B, Kojima H, et al. Cutting edge: hypoxia-inducible factor 1alpha and its activation-inducible short isoform I.1 negatively regulate functions of CD4+ and CD8+ T lymphocytes. J Immunol 2006;177:4962–5.

26. Takabayshi K, Corr M, Hayashi T, et al. Induction of a homeostatic circuit in lung tissue by microbial compounds. Immunity 2006;24:475–87.

27. Pittet JF, Griffiths MJ, Geiser T, et al. TGF-beta is a critical mediator of acute lung injury. J Clin Invest 2001;107:1537–44.

28. Niewoehner DE, Kleinerman J, Rice DB. Pathologic changes in the peripheral airways of young cigarette smokers. N Engl J Med 1974;291:755–8.

29. Santos S, Peinado VI, Ramirez J, et al. Characterization of pulmonary vascular remodelling in smokers and patients with mild COPD. Eur Respir J 2002;19:632–8.

30. Wright JL, Lawson LM, Pare PD, et al. Morphology of peripheral airways in current smokers and ex-smokers. Am Rev Respir Dis 1983;127:474–7.

31. Yoshida T, Rangasamy T, Biswal S, et al. Role of RTP801, a suppressor of the mTOR pathway, in cigarette smoke–induced pulmonary injury in mice. Proc Am Thorac Soc 2006;3:551a–2.

32. MacNee W, Wiggs B, Belzberg AS, Hogg JC. The effect of cigarette smoking on neutrophil kinetics in human lungs. N Engl J Med 1989;321:924–8.

33. Churg A, Wang RD, Tai H, et al. Macrophage metalloelastase mediates acute cigarette smoke–induced inflammation via tumor necrosis factor-alpha release. Am J Respir Crit Care Med 2003;167:1083–9.

34. Finkelstein R, Fraser RS, Ghezzo H, Cosio MG. Alveolar inflammation and its relation to emphysema in smokers. Am J Respir Crit Care Med 1995;152:1666–72.

35. Papi A, Luppi F, Franco F, Fabbri LM. Pathophysiology of exacerbations of chronic obstructive pulmonary disease. Proc Am Thorac Soc 2006;3:245–51.

36. Gessner C, Scheibe R, Wotzel M, et al. Exhaled breath condensate cytokine patterns in chronic obstructive pulmonary disease. Respir Med 2005;99:1229–40.

37. Churg A, Wang RD, Tai H, et al. Tumor necrosis factor-alpha drives 70% of cigarette smoke–induced emphysema in the mouse. Am J Respir Crit Care Med 2004;170:492–8.

38. Fujita M, Shannon JM, Irvin CG, et al. Overexpression of tumor necrosis factor-alpha produces an increase in lung volumes and pulmonary hypertension. Am J Physiol Lung Cell Mol Physiol 2001;280:L39–49.

39. Ma B, Kang MJ, Lee CG, et al. Role of CCR5 in IFN-gamma-induced and cigarette smoke–induced emphysema. J Clin Invest 2005;115:3460–72.

40. Bracke KR, D'hulst AI, Maes T, et al. Cigarette smoke–induced pulmonary inflammation and emphysema are attenuated in CCR6-deficient mice. J Immunol 2006;177:4350–9.

41. Grumelli S, Corry DB, Song LZ, et al. An immune basis for lung parenchymal destruction in chronic obstructive pulmonary disease and emphysema. PLoS Med 2004;1:75–83.

42. Elias JA, Kang MJ, Crouthers K, et al. State of the art. Mechanistic heterogeneity in chronic obstructive pulmonary disease: insights from transgenic mice. Proc Am Thorac Soc 2006;3:494–8.

43. Shapiro SD, Goldstein NM, Houghton AM, et al. Neutrophil elastase contributes to cigarette smoke–induced emphysema in mice. Am J Pathol 2003;163:2329–35.

44. Houghton AM, Quintero PA, Perkins DL, et al. Elastin fragments drive disease progression in a murine model of emphysema. J Clin Invest 2006;116:753–9.

45. Ofulue AF, Ko M, Abboud RT. Time course of neutrophil and macrophage elastinolytic activities in cigarette smoke–induced emphysema. Am J Physiol 1998;275:L1134–44.

46. Ofulue AF, Ko M. Effects of depletion of neutrophils or macrophages on development of cigarette smoke–induced emphysema. Am J Physiol 1999;277:L97–105.

47. Hautamaki RD, Kobayashi DK, Senior RM, Shapiro SD. Requirement for macrophage elastase for cigarette smoke–induced emphysema in mice. Science 1997; 277:2002–4.

48. ez-Roux G, Lang RA. Macrophages induce apoptosis in normal cells in vivo. Development 1997;124:3633–8.

49. Lobov IB, Rao S, Carroll TJ, et al. WNT7b mediates macrophage-induced programmed cell death in patterning of the vasculature. Nature 2005;437:417–21.

50. Rahman I, MacNee W. Lung glutathione and oxidative stress: implications in cigarette smoke–induced airway disease. Am J Physiol 1999;277:L1067–88.

51. Schmidt C, Peng B, Li Z, et al. Mechanisms of proinflammatory cytokine-induced biphasic NF-kB activation. Mol Cell 2003;12:1287–300.

52. Liu SF, Ye X, Malik AB. Inhibition of NF-kappaB activation by pyrrolidine dithiocarbamate prevents in vivo expression of proinflammatory genes. Circulation 1999;100:1330–7.

53. Nishikawa M, Kakemizu N, Ito T, et al. Superoxide mediates cigarette smoke–induced infiltration of neutrophils into the airways through nuclear factor-kappaB activation and IL-8 mRNA expression in guinea pigs in vivo. Am J Respir Cell Mol Biol 1999;20:189–98.

54. Ito K, Ito M, Elliott WM, et al. Decreased histone deacetylase activity in chronic obstructive pulmonary disease. N Engl J Med 2005;352:1967–76.

55. Marwick JA, Kirkham PA, Stevenson CS, et al. Cigarette smoke alters chromatin remodeling and induces proinflammatory genes in rat lungs. Am J Respir Cell Mol Biol 2004; 31:633–42.

56. Sullivan AK, Simonian PL, Falta MT, et al. Oligoclonal CD4+ T cells in the lungs of patients with severe emphysema. Am J Respir Crit Care Med 2005;172:590–6.

57. Korn S, Wiewrodt R, Walz YC, et al. Characterization of the interstitial lung and peripheral blood T cell receptor repertoire in cigarette smokers. Am J Respir Cell Mol Biol 2005;32:142–8.

58. Agusti A, MacNee W, Donaldson K, Cosio M. Hypothesis: does COPD have an autoimmune component? Thorax 2003;58:832–4.

59. Meshi B, Vitalis TZ, Ionescu D, et al. Emphysematous lung destruction by cigarette smoke-the effects of latent adenoviral infection on the lung inflammatory response. Am J Respir Cell Mol Biol 2002;26:52–7.

60. Retamales I, Elliott WM, Meshi B, et al. Amplification of inflammation in emphysema and its association with latent adenoviral infection. Am J Respir Crit Care Med 2001;164:469–73.

61. Taraseviciene-Stewart L, Scerbavicius R, Choe KH, et al. An animal model of autoimmune emphysema. Am J Respir Crit Care Med 2005;171:734–42.

62. Becker CG, Dubin T, Wiedemann HP. Hypersensitivity to tobacco antigen. Proc Natl Acad Sci U S A 1976;73:1712–6.

63. Wendel DP, Taylor DG, Albertine KH, et al. Impaired distal airway development in mice lacking elastin. Am J Respir Cell Mol Biol 2000;23:320–6.

64. Shapiro SD. The pathogenesis of emphysema: the elastase:antielastase hypothesis 30 years later. Proc Assoc Am Physicians 1995;107:346–52.

65. Senior RM, Tegner H, Kuhn C, et al. The induction of pulmonary emphysema with human leukocyte elastase. Am Rev Respir Dis 1977;116:469–75.

66. Wright JL, Farmer SG, Churg A. Synthetic serine elastase inhibitor reduces cigarette smoke–induced emphysema in guinea pigs. Am J Respir Crit Care Med 2002;166:954–60.

67. Weathington NM, van Houwelingen AH, Noerager BD, et al. A novel peptide CXCR ligand derived from extracellular matrix degradation during airway inflammation. Nat Med 2006;12:317–23.

68. Demedts IK, Morel-Montero A, Lebecque S, et al. Elevated MMP-12 protein levels in induced sputum from patients with COPD. Thorax 2006;61:196–201.

69. Molet S, Belleguic C, Lena H, et al. Increase in macrophage elastase (MMP-12) in lungs from patients with chronic obstructive pulmonary disease. Inflamm Res 2005;54:31–6.

70. Caramori G, Di Gregorio C, Carlstedt I, et al. Mucin expression in peripheral airways of patients with chronic obstructive pulmonary disease. Histopathology 2004;45:477–84.

71. Montano M, Beccerril C, Ruiz V, et al. Matrix metalloproteinases activity in COPD associated with wood smoke. Chest 2004;125:466–72.

72. Valenca SS, da Hora K, Castro P, et al. Emphysema and metalloelastase expression in mouse lung induced by cigarette smoke. Toxicol Pathol 2004;32:351–6.

73. Bracke K, Cataldo D, Maes T, et al. Matrix metalloproteinase-12 and cathepsin D expression in pulmonary macrophages and dendritic cells of cigarette smoke-exposed mice. Int Arch Allergy Immunol 2005;138:169–79.

74. Atkinson JJ, Senior RM. Matrix metalloproteinase-9 in lung remodeling. Am J Respir Cell Mol Biol 2003;28:12–24.

75. Lanone S, Zheng T, Zhu Z, et al. Overlapping and enzyme-specific contributions of matrix metalloproteinases-9 and -12 in IL-13-induced inflammation and remodeling. J Clin Invest 2002;110:463–74.

76. Wert SE, Yoshida M, LeVine AM, et al. Increased metalloproteinase activity, oxidant production, and emphysema in surfactant protein D gene-inactivated mice. Proc Natl Acad Sci U S A 2000;97:5972–7.

77. Hawgood S, Ochs M,. Jung AJ, et al. Sequential targeted deficiency of SP-A and -D leads to progressive alveolar lipoproteinosis and emphysema. Am J Physiol Lung Cell Mol Physiol 2002;283:L1002–10.

78. Imai K, Dalal SS, Chen ES, et al. Human collagenase (matrix metalloproteinase-1) expression in the lungs of patients with emphysema. Am J Respir Crit Care Med 2001;163:786–91.

79. Darmiento J, Dalal SS, Okada Y, et al. Collagenase expression in the lungs of transgenic mice causes pulmonary-emphysema. Cell 1992;71:955–61.

80. Foronjy RF, Okada Y, Cole R, D'Armiento J. Progressive adult-onset emphysema in transgenic mice expressing human MMP-1 in the lung. Am J Physiol Lung Cell Mol Physiol 2003;284:L727–37.

81. Finlay GA, O'Donnell MD, O'Connor CM, et al. Elastin and collagen remodeling in emphysema. A scanning electron microscopy study. Am J Pathol 1996;149:1405–15.

82. Gu Z, Kaul M, Yan B, et al. S-Nitrosylation of matrix metalloproteinases: signaling pathway to neuronal cell death. Science 2002;297:1186–90.

83. Leco KJ, Waterhouse P, Sanchez OH, et al. Spontaneous air space enlargement in the lungs of mice lacking tissue inhibitor of metalloproteinases-3 (TIMP-3). J Clin Invest 2001;108:817–29.

84. Demedts IK, Demoor T, Bracke KR, et al. Role of apoptosis in the pathogenesis of COPD and pulmonary emphysema. Respir Res 2006;7:53.

85. Vandivier RW, Henson PM, Douglas IS. Burying the dead: the impact of failed apoptotic cell removal (efferocytosis) on chronic inflammatory lung disease. Chest 2006;129:1673–82.

86. Henson PM, Hume DA. Apoptotic cell removal in development and tissue homeostasis. Trends Immunol 2006;27:244–50.

87. Coxson HO, Chan IH, Mayo JR, et al. Early emphysema in patients with anorexia nervosa. Am J Respir Crit Care Med 2004;170:748–52.

88. Tang K, Breen EC, Gerber HP, et al. Capillary regression in vascular endothelial growth factor-deficient skeletal muscle. Physiol Genom 2004;18:63–9.

89. Hunt DP, Weil R, Nicholson AG, et al. Pulmonary capillaritis and its relationship to development of emphysema in hypocomplementaemic urticarial vasculitis syndrome. Sarcoidosis Vasc Diffuse Lung Dis 2006;23:70–2.

90. Thet LA, Delaney MD, Gregorio CA, Massaro D. Protein metabolism by rat lung: influence of fasting, glucose, and insulin. J Appl Physiol 1977;43:463–7.

91. Harkema JR, Mauderly JL, Gregory RE, Pickrell JA. A comparison of starvation and elastase models of emphysema in the rat. Am Rev Respir Dis 1984;129:584–91.

92. Shapiro SD. Vascular atrophy and VEGF R2 signaling: old theories of pulmonary emphysema meet new data. J Clin Invest 2000;106:1309–10.

93. Massaro D, Massaro GD, Baras A, et al. Calorie-related rapid onset of alveolar loss, regeneration, and changes in mouse lung gene expression. Am J Physiol Lung Cell Mol Physiol 2004;286:L896–906.

94. Kasahara Y, Tuder RM, Taraseviciene-Stewart L, et al, Inhibition of vascular endothelial growth factor receptors causes lung cell apoptosis and emphysema. J Clin Invest 2000;106:1311–9.

95. Tang K, Rossiter HB, Wagner PD, Breen EC. Lung-targeted VEGF inactivation leads to an emphysema phenotype in mice. J Appl Physiol 2004;97:1559–66.

96. Zheng T, Kang MJ, Crothers K, et al. Role of cathepsin S-dependent epithelial cell apoptosis in IFN-g-induced alveolar remodeling and pulmonary emphysema. J Immunol 2005;174:8106–15.

97. Bartalesi B, Cavarra E, Fineschi S, et al. Different lung responses to cigarette smoke in two strains of mice sensitive to oxidants. Eur Respir J 2005;25:15–22.

98. Tuder RM, Zhen L, Cho CY, et al. Oxidative stress and apoptosis interact and cause emphysema due to vascular endothelial growth factor receptor blockade. Am J Respir Cell Mol Biol 2003;29:88–97.

99. Petrache I, Natarajan V, Zhen L, et al. Ceramide upregulation causes pulmonary cell apoptosis and emphysema-like disease in mice. Nat Med 2005;11:491–8.

100. Freire-de-Lima CG, Xiao YQ, Gardai SJ, et al. Apoptotic cells, through transforming growth factor-beta, coordinately induce anti-inflammatory and suppress pro-inflammatory eicosanoid and NO synthesis in murine macrophages. J Biol Chem 2006;281:38376–84.

101. Ryoo HD, Gorenc T, Steller H. Apoptotic cells can induce compensatory cell proliferation through the JNK and the wingless signaling pathways. Dev Cell 2004;7:491–501.

102. Henson PM, Vandivier RW, Douglas IS. Cell death, remodeling, and repair in chronic obstructive pulmonary disease? Proc Am Thorac Soc 2006;3:713–7.

103. Vandivier RW, Fadok VA, Hoffmann PR, et al. Elastase-mediated phosphatidylserine receptor cleavage impairs apoptotic cell clearance in cystic fibrosis and bronchiectasis. J Clin Invest 2002;109:661–70.

104. Aoshiba K, Yokohori N, Nagai A. Alveolar wall apoptosis causes lung destruction and emphysematous changes. Am J Respir Cell Mol Biol 2003;28:555–62.

105. Takemura Y, Ouchi N, Shibata R, et al. Adiponectin modulates inflammatory reactions via calreticulin receptor-dependent clearance of early apoptotic bodies. J Clin Invest 2007;117:375–86.

106. Yoshikawa T, Dent G, Ward J, et al. Impaired neutrophil chemotaxis in chronic obstructive pulmonary disease. Am J Respir Crit Care Med 2007;175:473–9.

107. Stevens T, Kasper M, Cool C, Voelkel NF. Pulmonary ciruclation and pulmonary hypertension. In: Aird WC, editor. Endothelial cells in health and disease. 1st ed. Boca Raton (FL): Taylor and Francis; 2005. p. 417–38.

108. Kang K, Wagner PD, Breen EC. Lung-specific inactivation of VEGF in adult mice leads to emphysema like changes. Am J Respir Crit Care Med 2002;A165:B54.

109. Golpon HA, Fadok VA, Taraseviciene-Stewart L, et al. Life after corpse engulfment: phagocytosis of apoptotic cells leads to VEGF secretion and cell growth. FASEB J 2004;18:1716–8.

110. Hodge S, Hodge G, Scicchitano R, et al. Alveolar macrophages from subjects with chronic obstructive pulmonary disease are deficient in their ability to phagocytose apoptotic airway epithelial cells. Immunol Cell Biol 2003;81:289–96.

111. Biedermann BC, Sahner S, Gregor M, et al. Endothelial injury mediated by cytotoxic T lymphocytes and loss of microvessels in chronic graft versus host disease. Lancet 2002;359:2078–83.

112. Peinado VI, Barbera JA, Ramirez J, et al. Endothelial dysfunction in pulmonary arteries of patients with mild COPD. Am J Physiol 1998;18:L908.

113. Dinh-Xuan AT, Higenbottam TW, Clelland CA, et al. Impairment of endothelium-dependent pulmonary-artery relaxation in chronic obstructive lung disease. N Engl J Med 1991;324:1539–47.

114. Beckman JA, Liao JK, Hurley S, et al. Atorvastatin restores endothelial function in normocholesterolemic smokers independent of changes in low-density lipoprotein. Circ Res 2004;95:217–23.

115. Barua RS, Ambrose JA, Eales-Reynolds LJ, et al. Heavy and light cigarette smokers have similar dysfunction of endothelial vasoregulatory activity: an *in vivo* and *in vitro* correlation. J Am Coll Cardiol 2002;39:1758–63.

116. Tuder RM. Aging and cigarette smoke: fueling the fire. Am J Respir Crit Care Med 2006;174:490–1.

117. Janssens JP, Pache JC, Nicod LP. Physiological changes in respiratory function associated with ageing. Eur Respir J 1999;13:197–205.

118. Morla M, Busquets X, Pons J, et al. Telomere shortening in smokers with and without COPD. Eur Respir J 2006;27:525–8.

119. Tsuji T, Aoshiba K, Nagai A. Alveolar cell senescence in pulmonary emphysema patients. Am J Respir Crit Care Med 2006;174:886–93.

120. Muller KC, Welker L, Paasch K, et al. Lung fibroblasts from patients with emphysema show markers of senescence in vitro. Respir Res 2006;7:32–40.

121. Obeid LM, Hannun YA. Ceramide, stress, and a "LAG" in aging. Sci Aging Knowledge Environ 2003:(39)PE27.

122. Solana R, Pawelec G, Tarazona R. Aging and innate immunity. Immunity 2006;24:491–4.

123. Teramoto S. Age-related changes in lung structure and function in the senescence-accelerated mouse (SAM): SAM-P/1 as a new model of senile hyperinflation of lung. Am J Respir Crit Care Med 1997;156:1361.

124. Razzaque MS, Sitara D, Taguchi T, et al. Premature aging-like phenotype in fibroblast growth factor 23 null mice is a vitamin D-mediated process. FASEB J 2006;20:720–2.

125. Ishigami A, Fujita T, Handa S, et al. Senescence marker protein-30 knockout mouse liver is highly susceptible to tumor necrosis factor-alpha- and Fas-mediated apoptosis. Am J Pathol 2002;161:1273–81.

126. Mori T, Ishigami A, Seyama K, et al. Senescence marker protein-30 knockout mouse as a novel murine model of senile lung. Pathol Int 2004;54:167–73.

127. Massaro GD, Massaro D. Retinoic acid treatment abrogates elastase-induced pulmonary emphysema in rats. Nat Med 1997;3:675–7.

128. Shigemura N, Okumura M, Mizuno S, et al. Lung tissue engineering technique with adipose stromal cells improves surgical outcome for pulmonary emphysema. Am J Respir Crit Care Med 2006;174:1199–205.

129. Murakami S, Nagaya N, Itoh T, et al. Adrenomedullin regenerates alveoli and vasculature in elastase-induced pulmonary emphysema in mice. Am J Respir Crit Care Med 2005; 172:581–9.

130. Nathan C. Points of control in inflammation. Nature 2002;420:846–52.

131. Schwarz MI, Mortenson RL, Colby TV, et al. Pulmonary capillaritis. The association with progressive irreversible airflow limitation and hyperinflation. Am Rev Respir Dis 1993;148:507–11.

132. Kasagi S, Seyama K, Mori H, et al. Tomato juice prevents senescence-accelerated mouse P1 strain from developing emphysema induced by chronic exposure to tobacco smoke. Am J Physiol Lung Cell Mol Physiol 2006;290:L396–404.

133. Culpitt SV, Rogers DF, Fenwick PS, et al. Inhibition by red wine extract, resveratrol, of cytokine release by alveolar macrophages in COPD. Thorax 2003;58:942–6.

134. Demura Y, Taraseviciene-Stewart L, Scerbavicius R, et al. N-Acetylcysteine treatment protects against VEGF-receptor blockade-related emphysema. COPD 2004;1:25–32.

135. Hanaoka M, Kraskausas D, Burns N, et al. Immune tolerance in a rat model of emphysema. Amer J Resp Crit Care Med 2007;175:A650.

136. Suratt BT, Cool CD, Serls AE, et al. Human pulmonary chimerism after hematopoietic stem cell transplantation. Am J Respir Crit Care Med 2003;168:318–22.

137. Majka SM, Beutz MA, Hagen M, et al. Identification of novel resident pulmonary stem cells: form and function of the lung side population. Stem Cells 2005;23:1073–81.

138. Yamato H, Sun JP, Churg A, Wright JL. Cigarette smoke-induced emphysema in guinea pigs is associated with diffusely decreased capillary density and capillary narrowing. Lab Invest 1996;75:211–9.

139. Gebel S, Gerstmayer B, Kuhl P, et al. The kinetics of transcriptomic changes induced by cigarette smoke in rat lungs reveals a specific program of defense, inflammation, and circadian clock gene expression. Toxicol Sci 2006;93:422–31.

140. Guerassimov A, Hishino Y, Takubo Y, et al. The development of emphysema in cigarette smoke-exposed mice is strain dependent. Am J Respir Crit Care Med 2004;170:974–80.

141. Van der Strate BWA, Postma DS, Brandsma C, et al. Cigarette smoke-induced emphysema: A role for the B cell? Am J Respir Crit Care Med 2006;173:751–8.

142. Robbins CS, Poulaid MA, Fattouh R, et al. Mainstream cigarette smoke exposure attenuates airway immune inflammatory responses to surrogate and common environmental allergens in mice, despite evidence of increased systemic sensitization. J Immunol 2005;1;175:2834–42.

Vascular Endothelial Growth Factor and its Role in Emphysema and Asthma

Norbert F. Voelkel, MD

Asthma is functionally defined as reversible airway obstruction. It presents with a wide spectrum of etiologies, trigger factors, and clinical manifestations, which include chronic cough, dyspnea, status asthmaticus, and sudden death.[1] Areas of intense research in the last decade have been the immune response of the lung, mechanisms of chronic inflammation, and remodeling of the airways in chronic asthma.[2–10] A reactive, often asthma-like component of airway disease (reversible obstruction) is also present in some patients with chronic obstructive pulmonary disease (COPD). Thus, whereas patients with asthma usually have no emphysema, patients with COPD and emphysema can have asthma-like symptoms. A new hypothesis is that vascular endothelial growth factor (VEGF) plays a central role in chronic asthma and that this growth and permeability factor may be involved in the remodeling of the airways and in lung parenchymal changes. COPD and asthma can perhaps be seen as opposites of a wide spectrum of obstructive airway diseases if one considers the vascular components of these two presentations; in short, asthma may (also) be a "pulmonary hyperperfusion syndrome," and VEGF may participate in the immune response in asthma. If so, then VEGF may be at the crossroads of asthma and emphysema since decreased VEGF expression and impaired VEGF receptor signaling have been associated with the pathobiology of emphysema.[11,12]

Traditionally, and understandably, asthma has been considered to be purely an airway disease, and the tendency to compartmentalize lung diseases and to focus on classic concepts of inflammation and mediators of asthma (such as histamine and, more recently, leukotrienes) has perhaps obstructed the view of an integrated lung tissue response in the pathobiology of asthma and prevented an examination of the role of the lung vessels in the pathogenesis of asthma. However, recently in mouse models, a link between airway inflammation and angiogenic growth of bronchial microvessels has been shown,[2] and substantial airway mucosa hypervascularity was demonstrated bronchoscopically in patients with newly diagnosed asthma.[13] Others have considered that the "vascular compartment" plays a role in chronic airway remodeling.[14–17]

Studies of bronchial mucosa vessels in asthma have begun only recently; however, it has been recognized for decades that patients with asthma frequently show a supernormal diffusion capacity, which can be as much as 130% of the predicted value or even greater (Table 1), whereas patients with emphysema demonstrate a reduction in their diffusion capacity. The classic explanation of this phenomenon has been the recruitment of "reserve capillaries" in the hyperinflated asthmatic lung.[18] Here it is proposed that the supernormal diffusion capacity of carbon monoxide (DL_{CO}) is explained rather by *a real increase in the number of lung capillaries* (alveolar septal capillaries) *driven by the angiogenic actions of VEGF.* Thus, asthma and emphysema may mark the ends of a spectrum on which emphysema is characterized by loss of alveolar capillaries (significantly decreased DL_{CO}) and decreased lung tissue expression of VEGF and vascular endothelial growth factor receptor 2 (VEGFR-2) messenger ribonucleic acid (mRNA) and protein,[11] whereas chronic asthma is characterized by overexpression of VEGF and, possibly, an increased number of alveolar capillaries.

VEGF in the Lung

VEGF, the obligatory endothelial cell survival factor[19–23] and vascular permeability factor, is abundantly expressed in the adult lung that is believed not to grow any longer and is produced by many different cell types[24–26] (including microvascular endothelial cells[27]) and released from platelets.[28] VEGF and VEGFR-2 kinase insert domain-containing receptor (KDR) expression is increased by hypoxia, and VEGF gene transcription is under the control of hypoxia-inducible factor 1 (HIF-1α) but can also be increased by cytokines.[29,30] VEGF causes increased production of prostacyclin and nitric oxide in endothelial cells,[31] and, until proven otherwise, the assumption is made that VEGF participates in the generation of any hypervascular condition, not only in tumor angiogenesis.[32,33] How VEGF affects nonendothelial cells, in particular cells that participate in immune responses (such as lymphocytes and macrophages), is largely unexplored (Figure 1).[34–36]

VEGF levels are increased in lung edema fluid;[37] lung overexpression of the VEGF gene caused pulmonary edema[38] and chronic VEGFR inhibition caused emphysema in adult rats.[39,40]

Demoly and colleagues in France reasoned that VEGF "is a multifunctional cytokine which plays a role in chronic

	Prebronchodilator		
Values	*Actual*	*Predicted*	*% Predicted*
Lung mechanics	—	—	—
FVC (L)	1.89	4.47	42
FEV_1 (L)	1.28	3.53	36
$FEF_{25-75\%}$ (L/s)	0.84	3.42	25
PEF (L/s)	3.73	—	—
FEV_1/FVC (%)	68	79	—
Lung volumes	—	—	—
Vtg (L)	5.10	3.41	150
RV (L)	4.38	2.12	207
TLC (L)	6.54	6.61	99
RV/TLC (%)	67	32	—
Raw (cmH_2O/L/s)	2.70	1.33	203
Lung diffusion	—	—	—
DL_{CO} (mL/mm Hg/min)	38.2	32.7	117
VA (L)	4.61	—	—
DL_{CO}/VA (mL/mm Hg/min/L)	8.30	5.07	164

Table 1 Spirometry, Lung Volumes, and Diffusion Capacity for Carbon Monoxide of a Patient with Asthma

DL_{CO} = diffusion capacity of carbon monoxide; FEF = forced expiratory flow; FEV_1 = forced expiratory volume in 1 second; FVC = forced vital capacity; PEF = peak expiratory flow; RV = residual volume; TLC = total lung capacity; VA = alveolar volume.

Note the supernormal DL_{CO}, in particular if corrected for alveolar volume.

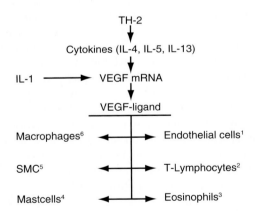

FIGURE 1. T-helper 2 (Th2) cells are a source of the pluripotent mediator vascular endothelial growth factor (VEGF). They may be involved in (1) endothelial cell growth and maintenance; (2) natural killer cell adhesion to endothelium; (3) Flt-dependent chemotaxis and release of eosinophil cationic protein[78]; (4) production of VEGF[69] 5-lipoxygenase (5-LO) dependently?); (5) smooth muscle cell (SMC) migration; and (6) phagocytosis and migration. IL = interleukin; mRNA = messenger ribonucleic acid.

inflammation" and measured VEGF in bronchoalveolar fluid lavage; no clear differences in asthma patients when compared with normals were found.[41] In contrast, Kanazawa and colleagues found increased VEGF levels in induced sputum of patients with asthma and patients with exercise-induced asthma.[42,43] Hoshino and colleagues used immunohistochemistry to show increased VEGF protein expression in bronchial biopsy specimens from patients with asthma (in CD34+ cells, eosinophils and macrophages),[44] and increased VEGF mRNA by in situ hybridization (apparently macrophage and T cells expressed both VEGFRs (Figure 2).[45] Bradykinin increases VEGF secretion from human airway smooth muscle cells via B2 receptors,[25] and budesonide inhibits *in-vitro* VEGF secretion from airway and A549 epithelial cells.[24] In a murine isocyanate asthma model, VEGF inhibitors, indicative perhaps of a functional role of VEGF in this model,[46] reduced inflammation and hyperresponsiveness, whereas low-dose allergen exposure significantly increased sputum VEGF in allergic nonasthmatic patients.[47]

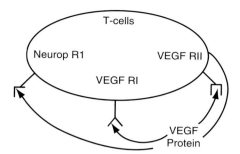

FIGURE 2. T cells; autocrine effects of vascular endothelial growth factor (VEGF). T cells express neuropilin 1 receptor on natural killer cells,[72] VEGF RI (flt), and VEGF RII (KDR).

VEGF and Lymphocytes

Peripheral blood T lymphocytes and tumor-infiltrating T cells express VEGF mRNA and secrete VEGF.[33,48] Blood CD4[+] cells secrete VEGF in response to tuberculin.[49] T- helper 2 (Th2) cytokines (interleukin [IL]-4, IL-5, IL-13) enhance VEGF production in airway smooth muscle cells.[29] VEGF can increase natural killer (NK) cell adhesion to microvascular endothelial cells[34] and matrix metalloproteinase 9 production of splenic T cells.[35] Splenic T cells express both VEGFR-1 and VEGFR-2.[35] IL-1α has been shown to increase VEGF production of peripheral blood mononuclear cells and cause VEGFR-2-dependent angiogenesis,[50] and bradykinin can synergize with IL-1 to induce angiogenesis.[51,52] VEGF may promote T-cell infiltration in acute allograft rejection.[53,54] Remarkably, VEGF infusion in mice has been shown to increase B lymphocytes sixfold and impair dendritic cell maturation.[55]

Angiogenesis and Lymphocytes, Interactions between T Cells and Endothelial Cells

Angiogenesis is a complex interaction between several cell types and growth factors, leading in the context of a conducive microenvironment to vessel sprouting and formation of a vascular network. This vascular network is either maintained by vascular survival factors or removed because of endothelial cell apoptosis. Lymphocytes are present in the tissue undergoing angiogenesis[56,57] and produce and release VEGF.[35,48,49] Yet no molecular theory that causally connects immunosurveillance and angiogenesis exists today. Possibly, successful tumor growth, which critically depends on VEGF, requires an impairment of immunosurveillance, and, again, possibly VEGF accomplishes this, and VEGF-driven angiogenesis and VEGF-driven impairment of immunosurveillance are, in fact, flip sides of the same coin. Impairment of immunosurveillance would, in this context, amount to a reprogramming of the local immune response (of T-lymphocyte activities) to serve angiogenesis. Indeed, there is abundant evidence that T cells can support (initiate) angiogenesis, and experimental data demonstrating a synergy between tumor immunotherapy and antiangiogenic therapy in the treatment of cancers appear to support this concept. What is unknown is whether VEGF is indeed an all-important protein that joins angiogenesis and immune response. Interestingly, NK T cells can repress tumor immunosurveillance via IL-13 and the IL-4R-STAT-6 pathway[9] and can inhibit angiogenesis via IL-12,[58] and tumor-infiltrating T cells can inhibit angiogenesis via interferon-γ.[59] Lastly, antitumor therapy has been engineered based on cytotoxic T cells targeting VEGFRs.[60,61]

Of note, CD4 knockout mice have an impaired angiogenic response after hind limb ischemia[62]; on the other hand, extensive lymphocyte infiltration can be documented in vascularized tumor tissue[33,63] and, for that matter, in the lungs from asthma patients. Retinal vessel growth and remodeling, which are critically VEGF dependent, are also T cell dependent.[64] Importantly, the antiapoptotic protein Mcl-1 plays a critical role in B- and T-cell maintenance via inhibition of the proapoptotic protein BIM,[65] and in endothelial cells, the antiapoptotic effect of Mcl-1 is enhanced by VEGF.[66] If asthma is a "high VEGF state," one would expect nonsmoking asthma patients to have a higher risk of developing cancer; there are studies that suggest this.[67]

VEGF, β-Adrenergic Receptor Agonists, and Steroids

Isoprenaline activates the transcription of VEGF mRNA, which is blocked by propranolol.[68] Possibly, inhaled β-adrenergic agonists could increase VEGF expression in the lungs of asthma patients. Prostaglandin E$_2$ induces VEGF production in mast cells[69] and prostacyclin in smooth muscle cells.[70] The effects of steroid treatment on VEGF expression are not uniform and seem to differ between in-vitro cell studies and integrated lung tissue responses. For example, steroids inhibit VEGF expression in human airway and alveolar epithelial cells[24] and smooth muscle cells[25] and induce emphysema in rats,[40] but they increase VEGF expression in human fetal lung explants.[71] Inhaled steroids did not reduce the increased number of mucosa vessels in asthma patients.[16]

As far as high doses of steroids are also lymphocytotoxic, this effect may well involve impaired VEGF signaling.

T cells express VEGF receptors and neuropilin-1 receptors,[72] which bind VEGF. The antiapoptotic protein Mcl-1 is critically important for B- and T-cell development and maintenance,[64] and the Th2 cytokine IL-5 inhibits apoptosis via Mcl-1.[73] If there is an autocrine role for VEGF produced by T cells, it may include upregulation of T-cell Mcl-1 by VEGF.

The number of experiments one can think of to explore the effects of VEGF on lymphocytes in the context of either asthma or emphysema (see Chapter 6) is certainly large, in particular if B lymphocytes and NK T cells are included, which are abundant in the spleen and in the lung. Recent data indicate that the development of airway hyperreactivity after allergen exposure requires activation of NK T cells that produce IL-4 and IL-13.[9] NK T cells also may be responsible for repression of tumor immunosurveillance.[74,75] Elimination of T cells involves induction of apoptosis, and Fas–Fas ligand interactions induce apoptosis after T-cell activation.[8]

Relevance to Asthma

A VEGF-centric, vascular hypothesis of asthma transcends present concepts of the pathobiology of asthma since it may allow one to "see" the involvement of the entire lung, not only airway changes. If verified, such a hypothesis could explain aspects of the chronicity of asthma and steroid resistance. A link between T lymphocytes and VEGF, with its consequences for angiogenesis and inhibition of T-cell apoptosis, would provide the rationale for new (nonsteroid) treatment possibilities. Beyond that, such a link may also provide a concept for the synchronization of angiogenesis and impaired immunosurveillance in tumor biology. In asthma, a VEGF-based treatment would make sense given the pleiotropic nature of this protein. This, however, implies that targeting VEGF receptors in asthma would have to be a measured strategy because chronic inhibition of VEGF signal transduction may shift the lung biology to the other side of the obstructive lung disease spectrum and lead to alveolar septal cell apoptosis and emphysema.[76] Of associated interest is that a connection between asthma and obesity has been observed for some time. This topic was discussed at a recent workshop of the National Heart, Lung, and Blood Institute,[77] and the question was raised whether leptin and estrogen could be a causal link between asthma and obesity.[78] If one considers the "vascular paradigm" of this proposal and remembers that both leptin and estrogen are endothelial cell growth factors, an obesity-angiogenesis-asthma hypothesis emerges.

Conclusion

The pathobiology of asthma may not play out only in the compartment of the airways. In fact, as in many chronic inflammatory lung diseases, several of the lung's compartments may be involved. A novel hypothesis is being presented that sets the vascular endothelial permeability and growth factor centerstage. Increased expression of VEGF[79] may be responsible for the hypervascularity of the lung in asthma, which can manifest itself in the form of increased submucosal airway vessel density[80] and in a higher than normal DL_{CO}. Avdalovic and colleagues recently reported increased VEGF gene expression in a primate model of house dust mite allergen exposure of chronic asthma,[80] and

Bhandari and colleagues reported that VEGF overexpression generated nitric oxide–dependent angiogenesis, edema, mucus gland metaplasia, airway hyperresponsiveness, lymphocyte accumulation, and dendritic cell hyperplasia in mice.[81]

Autocrine actions of VEGF on naive and antigen-specific T lymphocytes and paracrine actions of VEGF on pulmonary microvascular endothelial cells may occur in asthma, and VEGF may alter the cytokine profile of T cells. In contrast, a decrease in lung or lung microvascular VEGF and/or impaired VEGF signaling may affect the behavior of the lung lymphocyte population and lead to alveolar septal endothelial cell apoptosis and emphysema. Thus, VEGF may indeed be one of the factors that "decides" whether the chronic obstructive disease takes on the form of an asthmatic/hypervascular or an emphysematous/hypovascular response. T lymphocytes may control lung microvascular growth or loss of microvessels, again in a VEGF-dependent fashion. To what degree VEGF affects dendritic cell maturation and T-cell and B-cell proliferation is a subject for future explorations.

References

1. Drazen JM. Bronchial asthma. In: Baum GL, Crapo JD, Celli BR, Karlinsky J, editors. Text book of pulmonary diseases. New York: Lippincott-Raven, 1998. p. 791–805.
2. Elias JA, Lee CG, Zheng T, et al. New insights into the pathogenesis of asthma. J Clin Invest 2003;111:291–7.
3. Bousquet J, Jeffery PK, Busse WW, et al. Asthma. From bronchoconstriction to airways inflammation and remodeling. Am J Respir Crit Care Med 2000;161:1720–45.
4. McDonald DM. Angiogenesis and remodeling of airway vasculature in chronic inflammation. Am J Respir Crit Care Med 2001;164(10 Pt 2):S39–45.
5. Elias JA, Lee CG, Zheng T, et al. Interleukin-13 and leukotrienes: an intersection of pathogenetic schema. Am J Respir Cell Mol Biol 2003;28:401–4.
6. Hoshino M, Aoike N, Takahashi M, et al. Increased immunoreactivity of stromal cell-derived factor-1 and angiogenesis in asthma. Eur Respir J 2003;21:804–9.
7. Zimmermann N, King NE, Laporte J, et al. Dissection of experimental asthma with DNA microarray analysis identifies arginase in asthma pathogenesis. J Clin Invest 2003;111:1863–74.
8. Akdis M, Trautmann A, Klunker S, et al. T helper (Th) 2 predominance in atopic diseases is due to preferential apoptosis of circulating memory/effector Th1 cells. FASEB J 2003;17:1026–35.
9. Akbari O, Stock P, Meyer E, et al. Essential role of NKT cells producing IL-4 and IL-13 in the development of allergen-induced airway hyperreactivity. Nat Med 2003;9:582–8.
10. Umetsu DT, McIntire JJ, Akbari O, et al. Asthma: an epidemic of dysregulated immunity. Nat Immunol 2002;3:715–20.
11. Kasahara Y, Tuder RM, Cool CD, et al. Endothelial cell death and decreased expression of vascular endothelial growth factor and vascular endothelial growth factor receptor 2 in emphysema. Am J Respir Crit Care Med 2001;163 (3 Pt 1):737–44.

12. Tang K, Rossiter HB, Wagner PD, Breen EC. Lung-targeted VEGF inactivation leads to an emphysema phenotype in mice. J Appl Physiol 2004;97:1559–66.

13. Tanaka H, Yamada G, Saikai T, et al. Increased airway vascularity in newly diagnosed asthma using a high-magnification bronchovideoscope. Am J Respir Crit Care Med 2003;168:1495–9.

14. Wilson J. The bronchial microcirculation in asthma. Clin Exp Allergy 2000;30 Suppl 1:51–3.

15. Hogg JC. Vascularity in asthmatic airways: relation to inhaled steroid dose. Thorax 1999;54:283.

16. Orsida BE, Li X, Hickey B, et al. Vascularity in asthmatic airways: relation to inhaled steroid dose. Thorax 1999;54:289–95.

17. Thurston G, Rudge JS, Ioffe E, et al. Angiopoietin-1 protects the adult vasculature against plasma leakage. Nat Med 2000;6:460-3.

18. Bates DV. Respiratory function in disease. 1st ed. Philadelphia: W.B. Saunders;1971.

19. Dvorak HF, Brown LF, Detmar M, Dvorak AM. Vascular permeability factor/vascular endothelial growth factor, microvascular hyperpermeability, and angiogenesis. Am J Pathol 1995;146:1029–39.

20. Zhang HT, Craft P, Scott PA, et al. Enhancement of tumor growth and vascular density by transfection of vascular endothelial cell growth factor into MCF-7 human breast carcinoma cells. J Natl Cancer Inst 1995;87:213–9.

21. Voelkel NF, Cool C, Taraceviene-Stewart L, et al. Janus face of vascular endothelial growth factor: the obligatory survival factor for lung vascular endothelium controls precapillary artery remodeling in severe pulmonary hypertension. Crit Care Med 2002;30(5 Suppl):S251–6.

22. Bhatt AJ, Pryhuber GS, Huyck H, et al. Disrupted pulmonary vasculature and decreased vascular endothelial growth factor, Flt-1, and TIE-2 in human infants dying with bronchopulmonary dysplasia. Am J Respir Crit Care Med 2001;164(10 Pt 1):1971–80.

23. Mayo LD, Kessler KM, Pincheira R, et al. Vascular endothelial cell growth factor activates CRE-binding protein by signaling through the KDR receptor tyrosine kinase. J Biol Chem 2001;276:25184–9.

24. Bandi N, Kompella UB. Budesonide reduces vascular endothelial growth factor secretion and expression in airway (Calu-1) and alveolar (A549) epithelial cells. Eur J Pharmacol 2001;425:109–16.

25. Knox AJ, Corbett L, Stocks J, et al. Human airway smooth muscle cells secrete vascular endothelial growth factor: up-regulation by bradykinin via a protein kinase C and prostanoid-dependent mechanism. FASEB J 2001;15:2480–8.

26. Ishida A, Murray J, Saito Y, et al. Expression of vascular endothelial growth factor receptors in smooth muscle cells. J Cell Physiol 2001;188:359–68.

27. Tuder RM, Flook BE, Voelkel NF. Increased gene expression for VEGF and the VEGF receptors KDR/Flk and Flt in lungs exposed to acute or to chronic hypoxia. Modulation of gene expression by nitric oxide. J Clin Invest 1995;95:1798–807.

28. Maloney JP, Silliman CC, Ambruso DR, et al. In vitro release of vascular endothelial growth factor during platelet aggregation. Am J Physiol 1998;275(3 Pt 2):H1054–61.

29. Wen FQ, Liu X, Manda W, et al. TH2 cytokine-enhanced and TGF-beta-enhanced vascular endothelial growth factor production by cultured human airway smooth muscle cells is attenuated by IFN-gamma and corticosteroids. J Allergy Clin Immunol 2003;111:1307–18.

30. Corne J, Chupp G, Lee CG, et al. IL-13 stimulates vascular endothelial cell growth factor and protects against hyperoxic acute lung injury. J Clin Invest 2000;106:783–91.

31. He H, Venema VJ, Gu X, et al. Vascular endothelial growth factor signals endothelial cell production of nitric oxide and prostacyclin through flk-1/KDR activation of c-Src. J Biol Chem 1999;274:25130–5.

32. Senger DR, Galli SJ, Dvorak AM, et al. Tumor cells secrete a vascular permeability factor that promotes accumulation of ascites fluid. Science 1983;219:983–5.

33. Freeman MR, Schneck FX, Gagnon ML, et al. Peripheral blood T lymphocytes and lymphocytes infiltrating human cancers express vascular endothelial growth factor: a potential role for T cells in angiogenesis. Cancer Res 1995;55:4140–5.

34. Chen WS, Kitson RP, Goldfarb RH. Modulation of human NK cell lines by vascular endothelial growth factor and receptor VEGFR-1 (FLT-1). In Vivo 2002;16:439–45.

35. Owen JL, Iragavarapu-Charyulu V, Gunja-Smith Z, et al. Up-regulation of matrix metalloproteinase-9 in T lymphocytes of mammary tumor bearers: role of vascular endothelial growth factor. J Immunol 2003;171:4340–51.

36. Ohm JE, Shurin MR, Esche C, et al. Effect of vascular endothelial growth factor and FLT3 ligand on dendritic cell generation in vivo. J Immunol 1999;163:3260–8.

37. Ware LB, Kaner R, Crystal R, et al. Vascular endothelial growth factor (VEGF) levels in the alveolar compartment do not distinguish between patients with pulmonary edema from inflammatory and non-inflammatory causes. Am J Respir Crit Care Med 2004;169:A157.

38. Kaner RJ, Ladetto JV, Singh R, et al. Lung overexpression of the vascular endothelial growth factor gene induces pulmonary edema. Am J Respir Cell Mol Biol 2000;22:65764.

39. Bhatt AJ, Amin SB, Chess PR, et al. Expression of vascular endothelial growth factor and Flk-1 in developing and glucocorticoid-treated mouse lung. Pediatr Res 2000;47:606–13.

40. Choe KH, Taraseviciene-Stewart L, Scerbavicius R, et al. Methylprednisolone causes matrix metalloproteinase-dependent emphysema in adult rats. Am J Respir Crit Care Med 2003;167:1516–21.

41. Demoly P, Maly FE, Mautino G, et al. VEGF levels in asthmatic airways do not correlate with plasma extravasation. Clin Exp Allergy 1999;29:1390–4.

42. Kanazawa H, Hirata K, Yoshikawa J. Involvement of vascular endothelial growth factor in exercise induced bronchoconstriction in asthmatic patients. Thorax 2002;57:885–8.

43. Asai K, Kanazawa H, Kamoi H, et al. Increased levels of vascular endothelial growth factor in induced sputum in asthmatic patients. Clin Exp Allergy 2003;33:595–9.

44. Hoshino M, Takahashi M, Aoike N. Expression of vascular endothelial growth factor, basic fibroblast growth factor, and angiogenin immunoreactivity in asthmatic airways and its relationship to angiogenesis. J Allergy Clin Immunol 2001;107:295–301.

45. Hoshino M, Nakamura Y, Hamid QA. Gene expression of vascular endothelial growth factor and its receptors and angiogenesis in bronchial asthma. J Allergy Clin Immunol 2001;107:1034–8.

46. Lee YC, Kwak YG, Song CH. Contribution of vascular endothelial growth factor to airway hyperresponsiveness and inflammation in a murine model of toluene diisocyanate-induced asthma. J Immunol 2002;168:3595–600.

47. Boulay ME, Boulet LP. Airway response to low-dose allergen exposure in allergic nonasthmatic and asthmatic subjects: eosinophils, fibronectin, and vascular endothelial growth factor. Chest 2003;123(3 Suppl):430S.

48. Lummen G, Blass-Kampmann S, Rubben H, et al. Tumor-infiltrating lymphocytes express vascular endothelial growth factor in renal cell carcinomas. Onkologie 2000;23:458–62.

49. Matsuyama W, Kubota R, Hashiguchi T, et al. Purified protein derivative of tuberculin upregulates the expression of vascular endothelial growth factor in T lymphocytes in vitro. Immunology 2002;106:96–101.

50. Salven P, Hattori K, Heissig B, Rafii S. Interleukin-1alpha promotes angiogenesis in vivo via VEGFR-2 pathway by inducing inflammatory cell VEGF synthesis and secretion. FASEB J 2002;16:1471–3.

51. Miura S, Matsuo Y, Saku K. Transactivation of KDR/Flk-1 by the B2 receptor induces tube formation in human coronary endothelial cells. Hypertension 2003;41:1118–23.

52. Hu DE, Fan TP. [Leu8]des-Arg9-bradykinin inhibits the angiogenic effect of bradykinin and interleukin-1 in rats. Br J Pharmacol 1993;109:14–7.

53. Briscoe DM, Alexander SI, Lichtman AH. Interactions between T lymphocytes and endothelial cells in allograft rejection. Curr Opin Immunol 1998;10:525–31.

54. Reinders ME, Sho M, Izawa A, et al. Proinflammatory functions of vascular endothelial growth factor in alloimmunity. J Clin Invest 2003;112:1655–65.

55. Gabrilovich D, Ishida T, Oyama T, et al. Vascular endothelial growth factor inhibits the development of dendritic cells and dramatically affects the differentiation of multiple hematopoietic lineages in vivo. Blood 1998;92:4150–66.

56. Naldini A, Pucci A, Bernini C, Carraro F. Regulation of angiogenesis by Th1- and Th2-type cytokines. Curr Pharm Des 2003;9:511–9.

57. Ruddell A, Mezquita P, Brandvold KA, et al. B lymphocyte-specific c-Myc expression stimulates early and functional expansion of the vasculature and lymphatics during lymphomagenesis. Am J Pathol 2003;163:2233–45.

58. Yao L, Sgadari C, Furuke K, et al. Contribution of natural killer cells to inhibition of angiogenesis by interleukin-12. Blood 1999;93:1612–21.

59. Beatty G, Paterson Y. IFN-gamma-dependent inhibition of tumor angiogenesis by tumor-infiltrating CD4+ T cells requires tumor responsiveness to IFN-gamma. J Immunol 2001;166:2276–82.

60. Niederman TM, Ghogawala Z, Carter BS, et al. Antitumor activity of cytotoxic T lymphocytes engineered to target vascular endothelial growth factor receptors. Proc Natl Acad Sci U S A 2002;99:7009–14.

61. Gabrilovich DI, Ishida T, Nadaf S, et al. Antibodies to vascular endothelial growth factor enhance the efficacy of cancer immunotherapy by improving endogenous dendritic cell function. Clin Cancer Res 1999;5:2963–70.

62. Stabile E, Burnett MS, Watkins C, et al. Impaired arteriogenic response to acute hindlimb ischemia in CD4-knockout mice. Circulation 2003;108:205–10.

63. Melder RJ, Koenig GC, Witwer BP, et al. During angiogenesis, vascular endothelial growth factor and basic fibroblast growth factor regulate natural killer cell adhesion to tumor endothelium. Nat Med 1996;2:992–7.

64. Ishida S, Yamashiro K, Usui T, et al. Leukocytes mediate retinal vascular remodeling during development and vaso-obliteration in disease. Nat Med 2003;9:781–8.

65. Opferman JT, Letai A, Beard C, et al. Development and maintenance of B and T lymphocytes requires antiapoptotic MCL-1. Nature 2003;426:671–6.

66. Vinci MC, Visentin B, Cusinato F, et al. Effect of vascular endothelial growth factor and epidermal growth factor on iatrogenic apoptosis in human endothelial cells. Biochem Pharmacol 2004;67:277–84.

67. Vandentorren S, Baldi I, Annesi MI, et al. Long-term mortality among adults with or without asthma in the PAARC study. Eur Respir J 2003;21:462–7.

68. Fredriksson JM, Lindquist JM, Bronnikov GE, Nedergaard J. Norepinephrine induces vascular endothelial growth factor gene expression in brown adipocytes through a beta-adrenoreceptor/cAMP/protein kinase A pathway involving Src but independently of Erk1/2. J Biol Chem 2000;275:13802–11.

69. Abdel-Majid RM, Marshall JS. Prostaglandin E2 induces degranulation-independent production of vascular endothelial growth factor by human mast cells. J Immunol 2004;172:1227–36.

70. Hoper MM, Voelkel NF, Bates TO, et al. Prostaglandins induce vascular endothelial growth factor in a human monocytic cell line and rat lungs via cAMP. Am J Respir Cell Mol Biol 1997;17:748–56.

71. Acarregui MJ, Penisten ST, Goss KL, et al. Vascular endothelial growth factor gene expression in human fetal lung in vitro. Am J Respir Cell Mol Biol 1999;20:14–23.

72. Romeo PH, Lemarchandel V, Tordjman R. Neuropilin-1 in the immune system. Adv Exp Med Biol 2002;515:49–54.

73. Huang HM, Huang CJ, Yen JJ. Mcl-1 is a common target of stem cell factor and interleukin-5 for apoptosis prevention activity via MEK/MAPK and PI-3K/Akt pathways. Blood 2000;96:1764–71.

74. Marincola FM, Jaffee EM, Hicklin DJ, Ferrone S. Escape of human solid tumors from T-cell recognition: molecular mechanisms and functional significance. Adv Immunol 2000;74:181–273.

75. Nair S, Boczkowski D, Moeller B, et al. Synergy between tumor immunotherapy and antiangiogenic therapy. Blood 2003;102:964–71.

76. Demura Y, Taraseviciene-Stewart L, Scerbavicius R, et al. N-Acetylcysteine treatment protects against VEGF-receptor blockade-related emphysema. COPD 2004;1:25–32.

77. Weiss ST, Shore S. Obesity and asthma: directions for research. Am J Respir Crit Care Med 2004;169:963–8.

78. Feistritzer C, Kaneider NC, Sturn DH, et al. Expression and function of the vascular endothelial growth factor receptor FLT-1 in human eosinophils. Am J Respir Cell Mol Biol 2004;30:729–35.

79. Feltis BN, Wignarajah D, Zheng L et al. Increased vascular endothelial growth factor and receptors: relationship to angiogenesis in asthma. Am J Respir Crit Care Med 2006;173:1201–7.

80. Avdalovic MV, Putney LF, Schlegele ES, et al. Vascular remodeling is airway generation-specific in a primate model of chronic asthma. Am J Respir Crit Care Med 2006;174:1069–76

81. Bhandari V, Choo-Wing R, Chapoval SP, et al. Essential role of nitric oxide in VEGF-induced, asthma-like angiogenic, inflammatory and physiologic responses in the lung. Proc Natl Acad Sci U S A 2006;103:11021–6.

Macrophage Involvement in Chronic Obstructive Pulmonary Disease

Marc A. Voelkel, MD, Jennifer L. Terry, PhD, David W.H. Riches, PhD, and Murry W. Wynes, PhD

Chronic obstructive pulmonary disease (COPD) is a chronic lung disorder that affects both the conducting airways and the lung parenchyma. The clinical course of COPD is associated with marked changes in lung pathology that are characterized by (1) loss of alveolar septal tissue and capillaries, leading to emphysema (airspace enlargement); (2) mucous cell hyperplasia, increased airway hyperresponsiveness, and fibrosis of the airways, resulting in chronic bronchitis; and (3) subpleural fibrosis. By far, the leading cause of COPD is current or former cigarette smoking, although other causes include occupational exposure to wood smoke, benzene, agricultural products, nitrogen dioxide, air pollution, sidestream (secondhand) tobacco smoke, and specific genetic deficiencies, especially α_1-antitrypsin deficiency.[1–3] Since current or former cigarette smoking is the most important environmental factor in the development of COPD, this chapter primarily focuses on smoking-related COPD.

Bronchoalveolar lavage (BAL) and biopsy studies show that leukocytes, especially neutrophils, macrophages, and CD4+ and CD8+ T cells, are detected in the airspaces and the lumen and walls of small- and medium-sized airways. B cells, eosinophils, and natural killer cells are also detected in variable numbers and in different anatomic locations in the lung in COPD.[4–10] Recent studies in mice and translational studies in COPD patients have begun to tease apart the relative roles of the innate and adaptive limbs of the immune system in the development of smoking-induced COPD. To investigate the requirement for adaptive immunity, D'Hulst and colleagues exposed CB.17*scid* mice, which are genetically deficient in both T cells and B cells, to mainstream cigarette smoke.[11] Although these mice are incapable of developing antigen-specific immune responses, the development of emphysema was indistinguishable from the control BALB/c mice. Although this study needs to be confirmed and extended to include controls of the appropriate genetic background, it provides some support to the notion that T cells and B cells are dispensable for the development of cigarette smoke–induced emphysema in mice. Similarly, emphysema develops in human patients infected with human immunodeficiency virus (HIV).[12] Other studies, however, have provided compelling data to suggest that the development of COPD is associated with the activation of the adaptive immune system. For example, disease severity in COPD patients correlates more with pulmonary CD8+ than CD4+ T-cell numbers in the airways of chronic bronchitis patients.[6,7,13] Another study suggests that the number of CD4+ T cells correlates most with severe emphysematous lesions and the number of CD8+ T cells corresponds with only mild emphysematous areas.[14] Recent studies also revealed the presence of oligoclonal expansions of both CD4+ T cells and B cells in explants of lung tissue obtained from patients with emphysema.[15,16] Work reported by Taraseviciene-Stewart and colleagues further suggests that the development of emphysema may involve a breach in tolerance to an as yet undefined antigen.[17,18] These provocative findings provide preliminary support to the novel concept that COPD may be an autoimmune disease.

Unlike the lack of consensus about the role of cells of the adaptive immune system in the development of COPD, there is broad agreement that innate immune cells, especially neutrophils and macrophages, play a fundamental role in the development of both chronic bronchitis and emphysema. Neutrophils are the dominant inflammatory cell type of the airway lumen in chronic bronchitis and are abundant in the distal airspaces in emphysema.[5,9,10] Similarly, macrophages are present in the airway wall and lumen in chronic bronchitis, as well as in the distal airspaces and alveoli in emphysema.[5–10] However, unlike neutrophils, which tend to be absent from pulmonary tissues and airspaces of normal individuals, macrophages are ubiquitously present at these locations in both normal individuals and in COPD, although their numbers are markedly increased in the latter (Figure 1).[19,20]

Evaluating the relative contribution of macrophages to the pathogenesis of COPD (and experimental animal models of COPD) is difficult, primarily because COPD is a chronic disease that becomes established over an extended time frame. However, several important points have emerged. Abundant numbers of macrophages are detected in the earliest lesions of young smokers who develop COPD, in early centrilobular emphysema, and in the respiratory bronchioles of cigarette smokers.[21] Studies reported by Finkelstein and colleagues found a positive relationship between macrophage numbers in resected lung tissues and emphysema disease severity, as quantified by point counting of cell subsets (neutrophils, macrophages, and T cells) and comparison with the alveolar area.[22] This was in contrast to neutrophils,

Normal   COPD

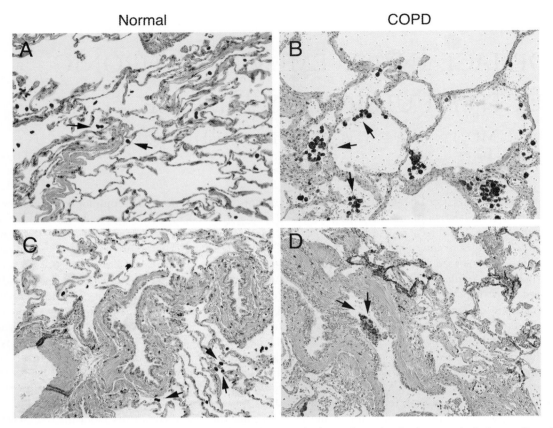

FIGURE 1. 25X images of lung tissue. Macrophages, identified by CD68 staining (*arrows*), are abundantly present in the lumen of bronchioles and distal airspaces in chronic obstructive pulmonary disease (COPD) compared with normal lung tissue. Additionally, there is mucus accumulation, thickening of the airway walls, and extensive airspace enlargement (emphysema) in COPD. *A* and *C*, Normal parenchyma and airways, respectively. *B* and *D*, COPD parenchyma and airways, respectively.

which had a negative correlation with disease severity. Macrophages are abundantly present in experimental models of emphysema induced by exposing mice and rats to sidestream and mainstream cigarette smoke.[23,24] Further, to directly evaluate the role of macrophages in emphysema initiation and progression, Ofulue and Ko treated rats with rabbit polyclonal antimacrophage or antineutrophil antibodies for up to 2 months during the course of daily exposure to cigarette smoke via "head-only" exposure chambers.[25] Control rats that received nonimmune rabbit immunoglobulin G (IgG) developed a robust inflammatory response in the airspaces and interstitium and significant airspace enlargement. Rats receiving antineutrophil antibodies showed a partial reduction in the development of smoke–induced pulmonary inflammation and emphysema. However, rats receiving antimacrophage antibodies were completely protected against the development of pulmonary inflammation and emphysema. Although questions remain about (1) the specificity of the antimacrophage antibody used in this study and (2) the consequences of the ensuing immune response against the injected rabbit IgG during the 2 months of exposure to cigarette smoke, these findings, combined with

those of other studies, support the view that macrophages play a fundamental role in the airway inflammation and the airspace enlargement in this model.

Although multiple cell types of both the innate and adaptive immune systems have been implicated in the development of COPD, here we review the functional properties of macrophages in the context of COPD. In particular, we discuss how these cells contribute to both airway disease and emphysema through their effects on inflammation, tissue remodeling, and apoptotic cell removal. Finally, we attempt to synthesize information about the phenotypes and functions of macrophages to develop an integrated model defining the roles of macrophages in the pathogenesis of this disease.

Macrophage Function, Classification, and the Modifying Effects of Smoke Exposure

Macrophages are well-established pluripotent members of the innate immune system. Their functions range from (1) phagocytosis of foreign particles, bacteria, viruses, and apoptotic cells (efferocytosis); (2) antigen processing and presentation; and (3) release of cytokines and chemokines

Table 1 General Macrophage Functions
Phagocytosis
Efferocytosis
Pinocytosis
Antibody-dependent cell-mediated cytotoxicity
Antigen processing/presentation
Respiratory burst
Granuloma formation/giant cell formation
Metalloproteinase release
Cytokine release
Chemokine release

that function to modulate and regulate other cells of the adaptive and innate immune systems. Table 1 lists some of the varied functions of macrophages. The roles of macrophages in COPD, although still evolving, include (1) phagocytosis of the components of cigarette smoke; (2) regulation of matrix metalloproteinases (MMP-1, -9, and -12) and protease inhibitors (tissue inhibitor of matrix metalloproteinase 1 [TIMP-1] and secretory leukocyte peptidase inhibitor (SLPI)); (3) regulation of oxidant (hydrogen peroxide [H_2O_2], nitric oxide [NO], reactive oxygen species [ROS], and reactive nitrogen species [RNS]) and antioxidant (super-oxide dismutase [SOD] and hydroxide [HO]) release; and (4) release of cytokines (tumor necrosis factor α[TNF-α], interleukin [IL]-1β, IL-8, macrophage-colony stimulating factor [M-CSF], and granulocyte-macrophage colony-stimulating factor [GM-CSF]) and chemokines (monocyte chemoattractant protein [MCP]-1, macrophage inflammatory protein MIP-1α, MIP-1β, MIP-2, IL-8, growth-related protein GRO-α, and thymus and activated regulatory chemokine [TARC]). Thus, in COPD, the function of macrophages involves the activation of the adaptive and innate immune systems; recruitment of T cells, B cells, macrophages, neutrophils, and eosinophils; and modulating the repair of the damaged lung via regulation of fibroblasts and extracellular matrix deposition and degradation.

Classification of Macrophages Based on Activation and Typified Behavior

Macrophages are part of the monocyte lineage and can differentiate into organ-specific macrophage types (eg, Kupffer cells, microglia, Langerhans cells, and alveolar macrophages), as well as dendritic cells (Figure 2). Macrophages play numerous roles and have multiple functions, likely in response to the diverse stimuli they encounter.[26–29] Because of these heterogeneous functions of macrophages, some of which are just beginning to be understood, it has been difficult to categorize macrophages simplistically. Past approaches have been to classify macrophages based on their activation state, and we expand on that here.[29,30]

Although not universally agreed on, macrophages can be classified into five different functional phenotypes based on their activation state from various stimuli (Figure 3). Effectively, these five macrophage phenotypes comprise (1) panactivated, (2) classically activated, (3) alternatively activated, (4) immune complex-activated, and (5) suppressor-activated macrophages. Along with these, an immunologically naive macrophage phenotype (M_0) type is postulated.[30,31] These macrophage phenotypes have some degree of overlap, and there is likely some degree of fluidity between the phenotypes. For instance, there is evidence of conversion from a classically activated phenotype to an alternatively activated or suppressor-activated phenotype, in vitro.[32] However, reverse conversion is still controversial.

Panactivated, or innate-activated, macrophages are stimulated by, for example, bacterial cell products. Lipopolysaccharide (LPS), flagellin, peptidoglycans, and unmethylated CpG deoxyribonucleic acid (DNA) can induce a panactivated macrophage via ligation of the appropriate Toll-like receptor (TLR) or, possibly, triggering-receptor expressed on myeloid cells (TREM) pathways. Activation through these pathways leads to upregulation of global inflammatory responses, such as release of cytokines (IL-1β, IL-6, TNF-α, IL-12, and type I interferons [IFNs]) and chemokines (IL-8, MCPs, and MIPs) and activation of inducible nitric oxide synthase (iNOS) and arginase I.[30,33,34] TLRs, most of which interact with the adapter protein MyD88, activate nuclear factor κ (NFκB) through inhibitor of kappa B kinase (IKKs) and activator protein-1 (AP-1) through mitogen-activated protein (MAP) kinases, which results in increased expression of TNF-α, IL-1, IL-6, and IL-8.[35,36] TREM-1 associates with the immunoreceptor tyrosine-based activation motif (ITAM)-containing molecule DAP12 and, following activation and multiple signal transduction events, including phosphatidylinositol 3-kinase (PI3K), phospholipase C (PLC), protein kinase B(Akt), and MAP kinase, induces the expression of IL-8, MCP-1, MCP-3, and MIP-1α.[37] Additionally, IFN-γ costimulated pan-activated macrophages display a synergistic response to increased respiratory bursts, phagocytic activity, and cytokine production,[38] whereas pan-activated macrophages that are costimulated with immune complexes or IL-4 will produce high levels of IL-10.[32,39]

The classically activated macrophage is arguably the prototypical macrophage and probably has been the most studied. These macrophages are usually activated by T-helper 1 (Th1)-like cytokines (such as, and especially, IFN-γ but also TNF-α, IL-12, and IL-18), as well as by direct stimulation by Th1 T cells via cell-to-cell contact.[30,40–42] Classically activated macrophages typically produce high levels of IL-12 and IL-23 but low levels of IL-10.[43] These cells exert inflammatory and cytotoxic activities, resulting partly from their ability to secrete moderate levels of reactive nitrogen and oxygen species, proinflammatory cytokines (TNF-α, IL-1β, IL-6, IL-12, and type I IFNs), and inflammatory chemokines (GRO-α, monokine induced by interferon

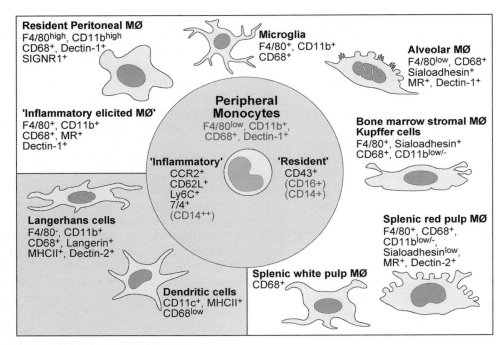

FIGURE 2. Phenotypic markers of organ- and tissue-specific monocyte-derived macrophage and dendritic cell lineages. Reproduced with permission from Taylor PR et al.[34]

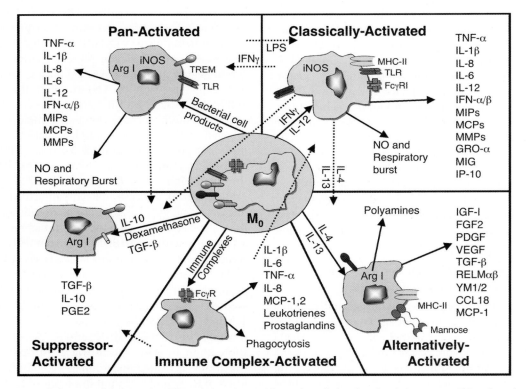

FIGURE 3. Exposure to distinct stimuli induces the differentiation of macrophages into distinct functional phenotypes. Although each phenotype exhibits overlap in its pattern of gene expression, the expression of some genes is specific to a given phenotype and may be used as markers. CCL18 = AMAC-1; FGF2 = fibroblast growth factor 2; GRO-α =growth related protein; IFN = interferon; IGF-1 = insulinlike growth factor 1; IL = interleukin; iNOS = inducible nitric oxide synthase; IP-10 = interferon γ-inducible protein of 10 kD; LPS = lipopolysaccharide; MCP = monocyte chemoattractant protein; MHC = major histocompatibility complex; MIG = monokine-induced and interferon; MIP = macrophage inflammatory protein; MMP = matrix metalloproteinase; NO = nitric oxide; PDGF = platelet-derived growth factor; PGE2 = prostaglandin E$_2$; RELM$\alpha\beta$ = resistin-like molecule/FiZZ; TGF-β = transforming growth factor β; TLR = Toll-like receptor; TNFα = tumor necrosis factor α; TREM triggering -receptor expressed on myeloid cells = ; VEGF = vascular endothelial growth factor; YM1/2 = chitinase 3 like 3.

(MIG), IL-8, interferon-inducible protein-10(IP-10), MCP-1, MIP-1α, MIP-1β, regulated upon activation normal t-cell expressed and secreted (CCL-5/RANTES), eotaxin, and TARC).[43–49] IFN-γ stimulation leads to a marked increase in FcγR1 (CD64) and moderate increases in FcγIII (CD16) and FcγRII (CD32) on macrophages.[49] Increased levels of TLR-2 and -4, B7-1 (CD80), and B7-2 (CD86) are also observed, along with the replacement of the constitutive proteasome subunits β_1, β_2, and β_5 with latent membrane protein-2 (LMP2), multicatalytic endopeptidase complex like-1 (MECL-1), and low molecular mass polypeptide-7 which has been suggested to increase the diversity of peptides available for the major histocompatibility complex (MHC) class I cleft.[50] Similarly, IFN-γ induces upregulation of MHC class II proteins, as well as cathepsins B, H, and L, lysosomal proteases implicated in the production of antigenic peptides for the cleft of MHC class II.[51,52]

Often the responses seen with classic activation are difficult to separate from panactivation, and, many times, classically and panactivated macrophages are grouped together because of iNOS activation and ROS and RNS release. Moreover, classic activation frequently occurs in combination with (pre, post, or concurrent) TLR ligation, and priming with IFN-γ is necessary to get a "good" LPS response and vice versa; that is, there is a synergistic effect between LPS and IFN-γ.[53] In response to IFN-γ and LPS, macrophages downregulate arginase, macrosialin, and the mannose receptor[54] but upregulate iNOS, oxidants involved in the classic respiratory burst, and inflammatory cytokines and chemokines, more than seen with either stimulus alone.[55] Expression of TLR-2, -4, and -9 is increased,[56–58] and a change in B7 receptor profile, from the B7-2 to a more B7-1 phenotype, has been observed.[59,60] Also, with high doses of a panactivator (LPS) that induces an endogenous primer (IFN-β), there appears to be an increase in the cell-mediated killing response, whereas phagocytosis is decreased.[61]

In contrast to the classic state, an alternatively activated macrophage phenotype, as currently understood, is macrophage activated (1) by Th2-like cytokines, prototypically IL-4 or IL-13 (but potentially IL-21)[30,62]; (2) by parasites or parasite degradation products; or (3) by Th2 T cells via a cell-to-cell contact-mediated mechanism. Alternatively activated macrophages upregulate arginase,[63] matrix metalloproteinase-1 (MMP-1), MMP-9,[30] and several distinct products: found in inflammatory zone / resistin-like molecule (FIZZ1/RELMα) (in mice), RELMβ/HIMF (in humans),[64–66] and chitinase-like protein-3 (YM1/2) (in mice).[67,68] These macrophages downregulate inducible nitric oxide synthase (iNOS), by a so far incompletely understood mechanism,[69] and display a uniquely patterned release of cytokines (IL-1, IL-6, transforming growth factor [TGF]-β, and IL-10, as well as lower levels of TNF-α).[70,71] The increased expression of the alternatively activated macrophage associated chemokine-1 (AMAC-1/CCL-18) chemokine and secretion of other chemokines (MDC, TARC, MCP-1) are characteristic of these macrophages.[72–75] Finally, these macrophages alter their receptor repertoire by

upregulation of mannose receptors and a change in MHC II receptors.[34,54]

Immune complex–activated macrophages result from the binding of IgG with FcγRI, FcγRIIA, FcγRIIB, or FcγRIIIB. FcγRI binding sets in motion the clustering of the receptors with other receptors containing an ITAM, followed by activation of *src* and *syk* tyrosine kinases, protein kinase C, PI3 kinases, and Rho kinase.[76] FcγRI-mediated activation leads to (1) the activation of prostaglandin and lipo-oxygenase pathways, (2) membrane depolarization, and (3) spreading, actin polymerization, and pseudopod motor extension that results in phagocytosis or engulfment of the cell or particle. A respiratory burst is delivered into the phagolysosome, which initiates microbe killing.[76,77] Immune complex activation also provides for humoral activation, antigen processing and presentation, degranulation, antibody-dependent cell-mediated cytotoxicity (ADCC), and release of cytokines (IL-1β, IL-6, and TNF-α), chemokines (IL-8, MCP-1, MCP-2, and eotaxin), growth factors, leukotrienes, and prostaglandins that can signal and recruit other cells of the innate and adaptive immune system.[76,78,79] Ligation of the FcγRIIB receptor can lead to phagocytosis but is thought to be inhibitory with regard to cell activation and the inflammatory response.[79] Fc receptor activation alone may not cause a dramatic inflammatory response but may potentiate other responses via TLRs, IFN-γ, or IL-4/IL-13 receptors. IFN-γ priming produces a strong classic response, with substantial upregulation of FcγRI and possibly higher affinity binding via the phosphorylated FcγRI.[80] IL-4 priming results in lower FcγRI expression but a marked increase in FcγRIIB expression and loss or reduced ADCC, respiratory burst, and iNOS expression.[81] Thus, IFN-γ and IL-4 might work as amplifiers to trigger other more patterned behaviors seen with classically or alternatively activated macrophages or provide possible synergy with other inflammatory stimuli.

Suppressor-activated macrophages are typically classified as macrophages that are suppressive toward surrounding immune responses. They are activated by ligation of the IL-10 receptor, glucocorticoid receptor, IFN-α and IFN-β receptors, scavenger receptors, CD200R, CD47, and some integrins.[30] In response to these stimuli, a suppressor-activated macrophage upregulates arginase activity[82] and functionally acts to decrease immune responses[83,84] by downregulating cytokine (IL-1β, TNF-α, IFN-γ, and IL-12)[85] and chemokine production (MIPs and MCPs), decreasing MHC class II receptors and releasing TGF-β, IL-10, and prostaglandin (E2),[34,82] thus resulting in restoration of localized homeostasis. The anti-inflammatory cascade is initiated by Janus kinase-1 (JAK-1) (in the absence of JAK-2) recruitment and signal transducer and activator of transcription-3 (STAT-3) activation.[86] Although IL-6 also activates this JAK/STAT pathway in the presence of LPS, immune complex activation seems to affect different downstream signals[87] and functionally acts to suppress a subset of TLR- and IL-6-stimulated genes, by an unknown mechanism. A similar response is seen to dexamethasone stimulation of the glucocorticoid receptor.[88] Because there appears to be incomplete suppression of TLR, IFN-γ, or IL-4/13 signaled responses, it is unclear what the role of the macrophage may be in chronic inflammation. However, it has been speculated that many tumors, as well as bacteria, hijack the IL-10R-STAT-3 axis to escape macrophage-mediated killing, and this may implicate tumor escape by chronic suppressor-activated macrophage activity.[71,89]

The roles that these macrophage phenotypes, and their varied immune responses, play in COPD and other lung diseases are not well understood.

Effects of Cigarette Smoke on Macrophage Clearance and Killing of Pathogens

The alveolar macrophage has been studied in its acute response to cigarette smoke in both humans and animal models. An important feature of the lung macrophage is its ability to phagocytose and kill pathogens. In contrast to the normally functioning lung, the antimicrobial function of macrophages in smokers is suppressed, as evidenced by decreased clearance of bacteria (*Pseudomonas*)[90] and decreased killing of intracellular microbes (*Haemophilus influenzae*, *Mycoplasma*, and *Candida*).[91] Although not entirely clear, this may be explained by reduced levels of surfactant protein-A (SP-A) and surfactant protein-D (SP-D) in the lung owing to smoking and worsening emphysema.[92,93] SP-A and SP-D, in conjunction with activation of the mannose receptor, enhance opsonization, internalization, and bacteria killing by alveolar macrophages.[94–97]

Smoke Provokes Macrophages to Secrete Elastases

Since the initial discovery of α₁-antitrypsin in 1963[3,98] and evidence of papain-induced lung injury in animal models,[99–101] the predominant theory of COPD pathogenesis has been the protease-antiprotease hypothesis. A large number of proteases, such as the metalloproteinases, collagenases, and bacterial enzymes (brinase, thermolysin and pronase), are implicated.[102–106] Historically, the role of macrophages in cigarette smoke–induced lung injury revolved around their ability to function as an elastase-secreting cell. Macrophage elastase (MMP-12) levels have been measured in smokers and compared with those of nonsmokers. Elastolytic activity is at least 20-fold higher in smokers' alveolar macrophages than in those of nonsmokers, and these results are also observed in mouse macrophages.[107] MMP-12$^{-/-}$ mice do not develop emphysema when exposed to cigarette smoke,[108] thus demonstrating a necessity for MMP-12 in emphysema development. MMP-9 (gelatinase B) levels also appear to increase in mouse lungs following cigarette smoke exposure.[109]

Cigarette Smoke Effects on Macrophage Oxidants and Antioxidants

Oxidative stress, which is defined as a shift in the balance between cellular oxidants and antioxidants in favor of oxidants, is important in the pathogenesis of cigarette smoke–induced lung damage.[110–112] The potential role of the macrophage in this oxidative stress is in the regulation and release of oxidants and antioxidants.[101,113] For example, MonoMac6 cells, a macrophage cell line, stimulated with cigarette smoke extract have depleted levels of glutathione but secrete elevated levels of ROS and activate NFκB, a redox-sensitive transcription factor that regulates the expression of many inflammatory genes, including TNF-α and IL-8. Consistent with this, MonoMac6 cells also express elevated levels of TNF-α and IL-8 on cigarette smoke extract exposure. Pretreatment of MonoMac 6 cells with antioxidants results in a reduction in these responses.[114] Additionally, when a transcription factor, Nrf2, that regulates induction of phase 2 detoxifying and antioxidant enzymes via the antioxidant response element is knocked out in mice, the mice develop progressive emphysema when exposed to cigarette smoke, unlike the wild-type controls.[115,116] This effect is apparently due not only to decreases in the antioxidants heme oxygenase 1, peroxiredoxin I, and reduced nicotinamide adenine dinucleotide phosphate (NAD(P)H):quinone oxidoreductase 1 but also to a decrease in the macrophage-derived antiprotease SLPI, an inhibitor of neutrophil elastase that is equally as effective as α₁-antitrypsin. These observations may potentially tie the protease and oxidant pathways together.[117]

Smoke Induces Cytokine Release from Macrophages

The macrophage-derived cytokines most likely associated with COPD include TNF-α, IL-1β, IL-6, IL-8, TGF-β, and IL-10.[118] In a study measuring breath condensate, patients with stable COPD have elevated levels of TNF-α, IL-1β, IL-6, and IL-8 compared with volunteers. COPD patients with more frequent exacerbations have even higher levels of these cytokines. In contrast, there is a tendency for stable COPD patients to express less IL-10 than volunteers.[119] Additionally, sputum macrophages from smokers produce more TNF-α at baseline than controls,[120] and IL-6 and IL-8 levels in bronchoalveolar lavage fluid (BALF) are positively correlated with pack-years of smoking and diminished forced expiratory volume in 1 second (FEV₁).[121] However, more direct evidence of cigarette smoke–induced release of cytokines from macrophages comes from *in vitro* studies. Macrophages exposed to either cigarette smoke or cigarette smoke extract express elevated levels of IL-8, TNF-α, IL-1β, and IL-6 compared with controls.[122–126]

Role of Macrophages in Chronic Bronchitis and Airway Hyperreactivity

Chronic bronchitis is a clinical syndrome associated with airway thickening, chronic mucus secretion by bronchial glands, and airway hyperresponsiveness (AHR). The major risk factor for its development is cigarette smoking. Histologic evaluation of bronchial biopsy specimens from patients with chronic bronchitis have revealed goblet cell hyperplasia and mucus hypersecretion. They have also consistently shown the presence of active inflammation associated with neutrophil, macrophage, and CD8[+] T-cell accumulation in the airway lumen and walls and in bronchial mucus-secreting glands.[7,127] To address the potential role of macrophages in airway inflammation, Borchers and colleagues chronically exposed mice to acrolein and studied airway cell accumulation and mucin gene expression and found a correlation between monocytic cell accumulation and mucus hypersecretion.[128] Although these collective findings suggest that macrophages contribute to the development of chronic bronchitis, little is known about their functional activities or phenotypes at these sites. Although many studies have been conducted with macrophages isolated from BAL, these cell populations consist of variable mixtures of cells derived from both the distal airspaces (ie, alveoli) and airways. Hence, it is not possible to discriminate what genes and other products are expressed by the macrophages from the airway lumen versus those from the alveoli. It is clear that studies are needed in which macrophage phenotypic markers are used to query the activation state of macrophages in bronchial biopsies and postmortem specimens to further understand the functional role of macrophages in chronic bronchitis.

AHR is a common characteristic of patients with allergic asthma, cystic fibrosis, and, to some degree, COPD. Since many studies examining AHR have been conducted with asthma patients or models, the remainder of this section emphasizes AHR in the context of asthma; however, it is viewed that many elements that regulate AHR in asthma also exist in COPD.[129] A correlation exists between the extent of inflammation in the airways and the severity of AHR,[130] although structural alterations and airway remodeling also contribute to the development of AHR.[131] Macrophage-derived mediators, especially when abnormally expressed, have the potential to contribute to the excessive bronchoconstrictive response observed in AHR. Interestingly, the defective clearance of apoptotic cells by macrophages is also linked to AHR, demonstrating that macrophages may contribute to AHR in a variety of ways.

Macrophage-Derived Cytokines and AHR

Many cytokines are integral to the initiation of the early stages of AHR and to the maintenance of the chronic inflammatory processes that perpetuate the condition. Macrophages are the principal source of TNF-α in the lung. TNF-α can amplify inflammation by (1) stimulating epithelial cells to release cytokines (eg, GM-CSF) and chemokines (eg, RANTES and IL-8); (2) upregulating the adhesion molecule intercellular adhesion molecule 1 (ICAM-1) on endothelial cells; (3) increasing the expression of vascular cell adhesion molecule 1 (VCAM-1) on endothelial cells, promoting adhesion and entry of more inflammatory cells; (4) enhancing MHC class II expression on antigen-presenting cells (including macrophages); and (5) augmenting the release of IL-1β and more TNF-α from macrophages.[132] A link

between macrophage- and monocyte-derived TNF-α and allergic inflammation in studies of both patients with asthma and rodent models of asthma has been well documented. The increased levels of TNF-α in the exhaled breath condensate of asthmatic patients are significantly correlated to methacholine threshold and peak expiratory flow.[133] TNF-α levels in the BALF of severe corticosteroid-dependent asthmatics are increased,[134] and patients with refractory asthma have increased TNF-α, tumor necrosis factor receptor (TNF-R)1, and TNF-α-converting enzyme in peripheral blood monocytes compared with patients with mild to moderate asthma and controls.[135] In addition, higher levels of TNF-α, GM-CSF, and IL-6 have been found in BAL from symptomatic versus asymptomatic asthmatics,[136] and monocytes and macrophages derived from asthmatic individuals produce more TNF-α, IL-1β, and GM-CSF after LPS stimulation than normal subjects.[137] In two studies, patients with severe and refractory asthma demonstrated an improvement in AHR, lung function, and quality of life after treatment with etanercept, a recombinant human soluble TNF-R1 that binds to TNF-α and inhibits its effects.[134,135] Finally, TNF-α knockout mice exhibit reduced AHR in response to methacholine challenge, along with a decreased number of BALF inflammatory cells; decreased IL-4, IL-5, and IL-17 in the lung; and reduced pulmonary inflammation by histology compared with wild-type mice.[138]

The macrophage-derived inflammatory cytokine IL-1β exerts very similar effects as TNF-α in AHR, and increased IL-1β has been detected in the BALF of symptomatic asthmatics.[136] The signaling pathways of these cytokines closely interact, and just like TNF-α, many cytokines will increase the production of IL-1β, including TNF-α, GM-CSF, and IL-1β itself.[132] TNF-α and IL-1β both can regulate fibroblast/myofibroblast proliferation and matrix production, two hallmarks of airway fibrosis and remodeling in asthma.[131]

Another macrophage-derived cytokine, GM-CSF, stimulates the proliferation and function of most hematopoietic cells and especially primes eosinophils for respiratory bursts on arrival in the lung. BALF from asthmatic patients enhances the survival of eosinophils compared with BALF from healthy controls, an effect that is inhibited by the immunodepletion of GM-CSF.[139] GM-CSF was found in the BALF of the same asthmatic subjects that had increased TNF-α and IL-1β.[136] Alveolar macrophages from asthmatic patients that have shown symptomatic improvement after inhaled corticosteroid treatment produce significantly less GM-CSF than asthmatics taking placebo.[140] In a study that used an adenoviral vector to introduce GM-CSF into the murine lung, the overexpression of GM-CSF caused the accumulation of eosinophils and macrophages in BALF and lung tissue sections at early stages and, at later stages, resulted in irreversible fibrosis rich in fibroblasts, collagen, elastin, and pigmented macrophages.[141] GM-CSF induces the synthesis and release of IL-1β and TNF-α from monocytes and macrophages, demonstrating that these three cytokines feed back to amplify the inflammatory response.[142]

The selective recruitment of leukocytes into the lung during airway inflammation and AHR is mediated by chemotactic cytokine and chemokine expression. Monocytes and tissue macrophages are generally abundant sources of CC chemokines.[132] Common CC chemokines include RANTES; MIP-1α; MCP-1, -2, -3, and -4; and eotaxin, and all cause eosinophil migration to the lung, with eotaxin being a strong activator of eosinophil degranulation.[130] RANTES and MIP-1αare also chemotactic for lymphocytes; MCP-1, -2, -3, and -4 are potent monocyte/macrophage and lymphocyte attractants; and MCP-1 induces the activation and aggregation of mast cells.[143,144] After allergen challenge, RANTES, MIP-1α, and MCP-1 are all found to be significantly elevated in the BALF of asthmatic patients compared with normal controls.[145] In cryostat sections of bronchial biopsies analyzed by immunohistochemistry and in situ hybridization, macrophages are a major source of increased eotaxin, RANTES, MCP-3, and MCP-4 in atopic and nonatopic asthmatics.[146] In another study of asthmatics, the inhalation of corticosteroids significantly reduced the expression and secretion of MIP-1α from alveolar macrophages.[140] Macrophages and monocytes also release CXC cytokines, such as IL-8. Alveolar macrophages from asthmatic subjects constitutively release IL-8, and after stimulation with TNF-α or IL-1β, the expression of IL-8 increased.[147] IL-8 is a major neutrophil chemoattractant and activator.

With so many cytokines involved in the development and maintenance of AHR, it is difficult to differentiate the mediators of an acute inflammatory response from mediators of a chronic response that leads to remodeling. However, macrophage-derived growth factors such as TGF-β1 and insulin-like growth factor I (IGF-I) contribute directly to fibrosis and remodeling.[131] TGF-β1 contributes to airway remodeling and AHR by (1) inducing airway smooth muscle cell hyperplasia and hypertrophy; (2) causing subepithelial fibrosis through increasing fibroblast survival, fibroblast to myofibroblast differentiation, and fibroblast/myofibroblast proliferation; (3) enhancing goblet cell proliferation and mucus secretion; and (4) aiding vascular remodeling.[148,149] The levels of TGF-β1 in exhaled breath condensate are significantly greater in asthmatics and correlate with methacholine threshold and peak expiratory flow.[133] The alveolar macrophages of patients with mild atopic asthma express TGF-β at higher levels compared with healthy controls.[150] Parenthetically, alternatively activated macrophages may be responsible for TGF-β1 production in the airways since IL-4-treated macrophages release significantly more TGF-β1 than macrophages that were activated with LPS or IFN-γ.[41] Like TGF-β1, IGF-1 is likely to cause airway remodeling owing to its ability to induce fibroblast survival, proliferation, and collagen release. In a mouse model of asthma, IGF-I expression is detected in the BALF and the airway after allergen challenge. If an aerosolized IGF-I neutralizing antibody is administered before challenge, airway resistance, inflammation, and wall thickening are diminished.[151] When bone marrow-derived macrophages are alternatively activated with IL-4 or IL-13, IGF-I is expressed and secreted into the media, and this macrophage-derived IGF-I protects myofibroblasts from apoptosis.[152,153]

Macrophages can also contribute to a Th2-skewed cytokine milieu often associated with AHR. In a recent study, patients with atopic disease, compared with healthy controls, had an increase in an IL-10-secreting monocyte population in peripheral blood that differentiated into alternatively activated macrophages. These cells triggered increased IL-4 and IL-13 production in naive T cells, which, in turn, can induce the secretion of IL-10 from macrophages, thus reinforcing the Th2 environment.[154] Alveolar macrophages isolated from allergy-susceptible rats were shown to express IL-13 itself,[155] and macrophages, through an IL-4-dependent mechanism, upregulate cell surface MHC class II expression, enhancing antigen presentation to and activation of Th2 CD4+ T cells.[132] Alveolar macrophages from atopic subjects with asthma, post-allergen inhalation, have increased expression of the CD86 T cell costimulatory molecule, which can also facilitate T-cell proliferation.[156] Obviously, similar studies in patients with COPD and AHR are lacking.

Other Macrophage-Derived Mediators of AHR

An imbalance of MMPs and their inhibitors, TIMPs, in the lung may play a role in AHR by contributing to tissue remodeling. In addition, the release of these mediators affects leukocyte extravasation, which is important for the initiation and maintenance of inflammation.[157,158] In the BALF of asthmatic patients, both MMP-9 and TIMP-1 levels are increased; however, the molar ratio of MMP-9 to TIMP-1 is lower than in the BALF of controls.[159] This decreased ratio of MMP-9 to TIMP-1 is positively correlated with reduced FEV1 values.[160] Macrophages are thought to be directly involved in the tissue remodeling and destruction that cause AHR through the regulation of MMP and TIMP expression. Alveolar macrophages from untreated asthmatic patients are a source of both the increased MMP-9 and TIMP-1.[161,162] Immunohistochemical investigation of lungs from a rat model of asthma revealed alveolar macrophages to be the source of increased MMP-12.[163] MMP-9 expression is induced in macrophages by TNF-α and IL-1 β,[164] whereas TIMP-1 expression is regulated by IL-6.[165,166] Since macrophages are also a source of these cytokines, autocrine feedback mechanisms may enforce the imbalance. Additionally, the imbalance of MMPs and TIMPs in the lung may be the result of a Th2-like cytokine environment. IL-4 can suppress the expression of MMP-9 in macrophages[165] and can induce MMP-1 production in differentiated monocytes,[167] whereas IL-10 suppresses MMP-9 and induces TIMP-1 in macrophages.[168]

MMPs may also function as inducers of cytokines and chemokines, thus influencing inflammation. In MMP-12-deficient mice, there was a significant reduction in allergen-induced inflammatory lung injury concomitant with a reduction in the BALF levels of IL-5, MIP-1α, MCP-1, and TNF-α.[169] In MMP-9-deficient mice, lung inflammation was enhanced and levels of IL-4, IL-5, IL-13, and eotaxin were increased.[170] These studies in genetically deficient mice demonstrate the potential complexity of MMP and TIMP regulation in the development of AHR.

The precise regulation of NO is important for normal airway homeostasis, and the dysregulation of NO is implicated in airway disease and AHR. Common allergens implicated in the development of asthma stimulate the production of NO in a rat alveolar macrophage cell line.[171] Primary alveolar macrophages from allergen-sensitive (Brown-Norway) rats generate more NO after sensitization and challenge than macrophages from allergy-resistant (Sprague-Dawley) rats.[172] A study examining the effectiveness of iNOS inhibitors in a rat model of allergic asthma found that short-term administration of iNOS inhibitors completely suppresses AHR, whereas persistent inhibition of iNOS results in more severe airway inflammation than that induced by allergen alone.[173] NO can normally be detected in the exhaled air of healthy individuals. However, increased levels of NO are found in patients with inflammatory airway diseases.[174] Although, compared with rodent alveolar macrophages, the NO production in human alveolar macrophages is much more tightly regulated and limited, human macrophages can and will generate NO in response to a variety of stimuli and also readily respond to NO.[175] It is hypothesized that NO can tip the Th1/Th2 balance by suppressing Th1 cells, thus enhancing the Th2 environment in the lung. Alternatively activated macrophages may play a role in NO regulation by increasing the production and activity of arginase following IL-4 and IL-13 stimulation (M. Voelkel, unpublished observations, 2004). Arginase, in addition to iNOS, competitively uses arginine as a substrate. Therefore, when arginase activity is elevated, less substrate is available for NO synthesis. Downstream products of the arginase pathway may also have direct inhibitor control on iNOS.[69]

Macrophage Clearance of Apoptotic Cells and AHR

Macrophages may also influence the development of AHR if they are unable to remove apoptotic cells from the lung. In some chronic inflammatory lung diseases, such as asthma, the number of apoptotic cell bodies observed in the lung is increased.[176] Alveolar macrophages from ovalbumin (OVA)-sensitized rats demonstrate decreased phagocytosis of fluorescent beads compared with macrophages from un-sensitized rats.[177] Alveolar macrophages from patients with severe asthma demonstrate defective apoptotic cell clearance compared with patients with mild to moderate asthma and healthy controls.[176] When macrophages are ineffective in the uptake of apoptotic cells, continued inflam-

mation will occur. For example, apoptotic neutrophils and eosinophils that are not rapidly cleared will undergo secondary necrosis and release inflammatory intracellular contents. In addition, if macrophages do not engulf apoptotic cells, they will not secrete anti-inflammatory mediators.[178]

Macrophages, although sentinels and key regulatory cells in the normal lung, play different roles in the development of chronic bronchitis and asthma through the release of cytokines, chemokines, growth factors, MMPs, MMP inhibitors, and NO. In addition, defective clearance of apoptotic cells by macrophages has the potential to affect the development of chronic bronchitis and COPD, but, again, such studies are lacking in COPD patients.

Association of the Macrophage with Emphysema, Vascular Remodeling, and Fibrosis

Macrophages are one of the main orchestrators of the chronic inflammation and tissue destruction seen in emphysema (Figure 4). According to one study, macrophages are increased approximately 13-fold in both the tissue and airspaces of smokers with severe emphysema compared with those with mild or no evidence of emphysema.[179] Other groups have found that the destruction of the lung associated with emphysema is directly related to the number of alveolar macrophages in the lung.[22,180] There are many postulated mechanisms by which macrophages contribute to the specific airspace changes that lead to emphysema: 1) macrophages are responsible for the cytokine milieu in, and inflammatory cell recruitment to, the lung; (2) macrophages directly cause airspace enlargement, destruction of lung parenchyma, and loss of lung elasticity by releasing or causing other cells to release proteolytic enzymes or by inhibiting the production and release of antiproteases; (3) macrophages generate free radical oxidants, which can damage alveolar cells; (4) the defective clearance of apoptotic cells by macrophages disrupts lung homeostasis and leads to emphysema; (5) macrophages contribute to vascular homeostasis, which is disrupted, if after endothelial damage; and (6) macrophages contribute to fibrosis, which can occur in conjunction with emphysema.

Macrophage-Derived Cytokines and Chemokines in Emphysema

As has been seen in asthma, macrophages are responsible for the recruitment, activation, and survival of inflammatory cells that contribute to the generation of emphysema. Macrophage-derived cytokines (eg, TNF-α, IL-1β, TGF-β, and GM-CSF) and chemokines (eg, IL-8, GRO-α, MCP-1, and MIP-1α) are all involved in the pathogenesis of emphysema.[181] Cigarette smoke has been shown to suppress histone deacetylase expression in human alveolar macrophages, thus allowing enhanced and unregulated expression of macrophage-derived mediators.[182]

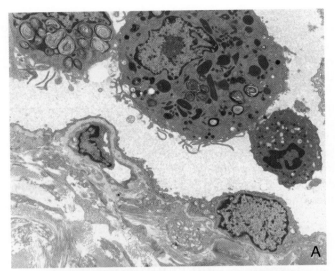

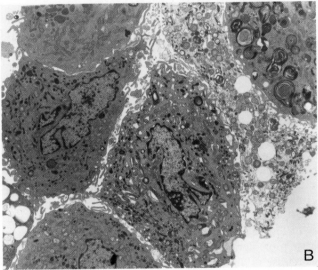

FIGURE 2. Electron micrographs illustrating the localization of alveolar macrophages to the distal airspaces in emphysema. Both electron micrographs were taken from a lung section from a patient with chronic obstructive pulmonary disease who received a lung allograft. (*A*) shows a large macrophage (*upper center*) in apposition to a neutrophil (*right center*). Note the alveolar type II epithelial cell (*upper left corner*), airspace edema, and collagen deposition in the alveolar septum. (*B*) shows a cluster of alveolar macrophages located in the distal airspace. Note the disintegrated macrophage juxtaposed between a viable macrophage and an alveolar type II epithelial cell. Macrophages engulf a variety of material, including pulmonary surfactant and inhaled particulate matter. (Electron micrograph X 9,000. Heavy metal staining for the EM tissues with 2% aqueous uranyl acetate and Reynold's lead stain.) Courtesy of Jan Henson, National Jewish Medical and Research Center.

Alveolar macrophages are not only the primary source of the proinflammatory cytokine TNF-α, they also potently respond to it. TNF-α stimulates a range of inflammatory responses, including the activation of many genes encoding inflammatory mediators in several cell types in the lung. Airway macrophages from smokers release more TNF-α than macrophages from nonsmokers.[120] In addition, patients with severe disease and cachexia have increased TNF-α in serum and TNF-α production is elevated in peripheral blood monocytes.[183] In a murine model of smoking, both TNF-R1- and TNF-R2-deficient mice exhibit a lower degree of emphysema compared with wild-type animals after 6 months of smoke exposure. The lungs of these smoke-exposed TNF-R-null mice do not have the characteristic influx of macrophages, have 65% fewer neutrophils, and have reduced MMP-2, MMP-9, MMP-12, and MMP-13 expression when compared with the wild-type animals.[184]

The IL-1β released from alveolar macrophages has a role similar to that of TNF-α in emphysema; it is a potent activator of alveolar macrophages. Macrophages are a prime source of IL-1β in the lung. In a murine model of elastase-induced emphysema, combined IL-1β and TNF-R-deficient mice show a significant reduction in disease compared with each single null strain.[185] Although GM-CSF is crucial for neutrophil survival, unlike asthma, there is no difference between the basal and induced secretion of GM-CSF from macrophages in smokers versus nonsmokers.[124] Another cytokine, IL-10, is more highly expressed by airway macrophages from smokers than by macrophages from nonsmokers.[120] Monocyte- and macrophage-derived IL-10 can suppress the release of MMP-9 and increase the release of the MMP inhibitor TIMP-1 from monocytes obtained from emphysema patients.[168]

The expression of TGF-β1, a growth factor that has both anti-inflammatory and profibrotic properties, in addition to chemotactic activity for both macrophages and mast cells, is increased in small airway alveolar macrophages of smokers compared with nonsmokers and is released at higher levels from COPD patients' monocytes.[186,187] However, the role of TGF-β1 produced by alveolar macrophages in emphysema may be more complicated. Contrary to the above, it has been reported that there is less TGF-β1 produced by macrophages from smokers with COPD, compared with smokers without disease or nonsmokers, after LPS stimulation.[188] Of interest, Morris and colleagues demonstrated that mice unable to activate latent TGF-β1 because of loss of the β6 subunit of the αvβ6 integrin spontaneously develop progressive pulmonary emphysema attributable to uncontrolled MMP-12 expression by macrophages. Emphysema or airspace enlargement is not detected when these mice are crossed with MMP-12−/− mice or when active TGF-β1 is expressed through an inducible transgene.[189] This is consistent with the observation that TGF-β1 inhibits the expression of MMP-12, in a Smad3- and AP-1-dependent manner.[190] Thus, the timing and location of TGF-β1 expression, release, or activation may play an important role in the development, or lack of development, of emphysema.

The chemokine IL-8, a neutrophil chemotactic factor, is secreted at higher levels by alveolar macrophages from emphysema patients than by macrophages from nondiseased smokers.[124] Human monocyte-derived macrophages are also found to be more likely to release IL-8 on cigarette smoke stimulation than lymphocytes and neutrophils.[191] GRO-α, a neutrophil and monocyte chemotractant that also activates neutrophils, monocytes, basophils, and T cells, is secreted by alveolar macrophages in response to TNF-α, and BAL cells from smokers released higher levels of GRO-α compared with those from nonsmokers. This suggests that increased GRO-α plays a role in the abnormal influx of macrophages into the lungs of patients with emphysema.[118] However, alveolar macrophage-derived MCP-1 and MIP-1α are also monocyte and lymphocyte chemoattractants and may contribute to the intense recruitment of macrophages to the lung.[192]

Macrophage-Derived Elastases and Emphysema

The long-held dogma that neutrophils and neutrophil elastase are the critical agents that cause emphysema has recently been challenged. A new evolving theory states that alveolar macrophages and macrophage-derived proteases are the main players in the development of emphysema, a hypothesis that is supported by the increased presence of macrophages in the lung of COPD patients (discussed above).[22,157] This influx of macrophages into the lungs of patients with emphysema may result in the production of excessive amounts of proteases that cannot be controlled by α1-antitrypsin and other antiproteases. Indeed, alveolar macrophages cultured from the BALF of emphysema patients have elevated elastolytic and collagenolytic activities.[193] Interestingly, macrophages have even been shown to internalize neutrophil elastase and hold the active enzyme for subsequent release.[194,195] Alveolar macrophages isolated from patients with COPD show reduced degradation of elastin in the presence of either a cysteine protease inhibitor, an MMP inhibitor, or a serine protease inhibitor.[109] Thus, macrophages contribute to the lung elastolytic load via the release of cysteine proteases (cathepsins), MMPs, and serine proteases.

Although the cathepsins are normally located in acidic endosomal/lysosomal compartments, macrophages can secrete active cathepsins D, L, and S, which have elastolytic activity.[196] Cathepsin L has been shown to cleave and inactivate α1-antitrypsin, whereas cathepsins B, L, and S can cleave SLPI, thereby diminishing total lung antiproteases and promoting emphysema.[197] Macrophages isolated from lung tissue of mice exposed to smoke for 1, 3, and 6 months produce more cathepsin D and macrophage elastase (MMP-12) than macrophages isolated from control mice.[198] Immunohistochemical analysis of lung tissue from smoke-exposed mice demonstrates alveolar localization of MMP-12-expressing macrophages.[199] In contrast to wild-type mice, MMP-12-deficient mice do not develop emphysema after cigarette smoke exposure and do not demonstrate the characteristic influx of macrophages. These MMP-12-null mice also

revealed a role for MMP-12 in the degradation and inactivation of α1-antitrypsin.[108] Alveolar macrophages from COPD patients and healthy smokers secrete more MMP-9 but less TIMP-1 in response to stimulation compared with alveolar macrophages from nonsmokers.[109] This disparity in expression contributes to the imbalance of proteases and antiproteases in the lung, thus favoring the development of emphysema.

The pulmonary proteases discussed above also contribute to emphysema in ways other than alveolar destruction. For example, in a study involving MMP-12-deficient mice, MMP-12 was found to be necessary for the cigarette smoke-induced cleavage of membrane-bound TNF-α from macrophages, thus resulting in soluble TNF-α release.[157] In another study, MMP-9 was reported to induce the cleavage of latent TGF-β, causing the release of active TGF-β, thereby linking elastolysis to fibrosis.[200] Taken together, it is evident that the action of many macrophage-derived proteases contributes to the development of emphysema.

Macrophage-Derived Free Radicals and Emphysema

Oxidative stress is implicated in the pathogenesis of COPD and emphysema. ROS that cause oxidative stress are produced by activated macrophages in the lung. The oxidant burden in the lung, which is enhanced in smokers, can decrease the activities of many antiproteases and skew the protease/antiprotease balance in favor of tissue destruction. Alveolar macrophages from smokers release increased amounts of oxidizing agents, such as superoxide anion (O2($^-$)) and H_2O_2, which may interact with a free ion to form the reactive hydroxyl radical (OH)).[201,202] In transgenic mice with emphysema caused by the lack of surfactant protein D, H_2O_2 production from alveolar macrophages is increased 10-fold.[203] These macrophage-derived oxidants can inactivate α1-antitrypsin, thus enabling neutrophil elastase to act unchecked in the lung to cause cellular damage.[204] Oxidative stress, potentially created by macrophages, also activates histone acetyltransferase activity, which causes a relaxation of chromatin structure, allowing increased transcription of genes encoding inflammatory mediators in macrophages.[205] Oxidants can also increase direct macrophage cytotoxicity toward normal lung parenchymal cells.[206]

Oxidants generated by macrophages can regulate inflammatory processes and, contrary to the above, protect against lung tissue destruction. For example, oxidants promote inflammation by activating the redox-sensitive transcription factor NFκB, which regulates the expression of many inflammatory genes important in the pathogenesis of emphysema, such as IL-8 and TNF-α. With regard to protection, MMP-12 is inactivated in the presence of the reactive intermediates O2.− and H_2O_2.[207] Additionally, whereas mice lacking gp91(phox), a phagocyte-specific component of nicotinamide adenin dinucleotide phosphate (NADPH) oxidase used by macrophages to generate ROS, spontaneously develop severe emphysema and have higher MMP-12 activity, mice with both MMP-12 and NADPH oxidase genes ablated are protected from peripheral airway destruction.[207] These results suggest that, in some cases, oxidants may protect against the development of emphysema, underscoring the importance of proper temporal and spatial regulation of macrophage oxidant generation.

Macrophages and Apoptosis in Emphysema

Excessive proteolysis, oxidative stress, and cellular apoptosis all interact to promote the lung destruction characteristic of emphysema.[208] Cell damage caused by proteolysis or ROS initiates apoptosis, but the clearance of apoptotic cells by alveolar macrophages is necessary to prevent more tissue damage owing to the release of necrotic and inflammatory cellular products. Additionally, clearance of apoptotic cells by macrophages is necessary to initiate the repair process. However, the proteolytic environment in the emphysematous lung may prevent macrophages from recognizing and efferocytosing apoptotic bodies, as evidenced by the increased presence of apoptotic cells in the alveolar septa of lungs from patients with emphysema compared with normal lungs.[209] Indeed, alveolar macrophages isolated from the BALF of COPD patients less effectively ingest apoptotic airway epithelial cells than normal controls, a defect that is specific to the epithelial cells since the deficiency is not noted with the ingestion of polystyrene beads.[210] Additionally, neutralization of vascular endothelial growth factor (VEGF) in macrophage cultures inhibits efferocytosis. Since VEGF is decreased in the lungs of patients with emphysema[211] and is critical for endothelial cell survival,[212] the decreased availability of VEGF in the lung would cause not only increased endothelial cell apoptosis but also defective clearance of apoptotic cells.[212] This suggests that the disruption of proper VEGF expression and signaling disturbs normal lung homeostasis by affecting apoptosis and clearance of apoptotic cells.

Macrophages in Vascular Remodeling and Hypertension

The mechanisms leading to the development of pulmonary hypertension in some patients with emphysema are not well understood, although hypertension is most likely caused by a loss of vascular homeostasis. The severity of emphysema in smokers lungs is correlated with the early pathology of pulmonary artery intimal thickening, increased medial smooth muscle, and blood vessel narrowing.[213] The role of macrophages in the vascular remodeling associated with pulmonary hypertension also remains unclear; however, perivascular inflammatory infiltrates in human pulmonary arterial hypertension include macrophages and monocytes.[214] Localized hypoxia, lung injury from cigarette smoking, or emphysema itself may have a direct effect on the recruitment and activation of macrophages, which contribute to the endothelial hyperplasia and perivascular fibrosis characteristic of pulmonary hypertension. FIZZ1 (RELMα/HIMF), a macrophage-derived hypoxia-induced gene that causes neovascularization of pulmonary vessels and increases both pulmonary arterial pressure and vascular resistance,[65] is produced and secreted by alternatively activated alveolar

macrophages in the lung. FIZZ1 can also promote cell proliferation and migration, induce murine endothelial cells to produce localized VEGF and MCP-1, and cause monocytes and macrophages to produce ROS.[64] Additionally, macrophages themselves have the capacity to produce VEGF in response to hypoxia and TGF-β, both of which are present in the emphysematous lung.[215–217] Paradoxically, decreased VEGF production from macrophages in the lung may lead to defective repair of the vasculature and contribute to hypertension. As discussed above, VEGF is decreased in the lungs of patients with emphysema,[211] and the expression of VEGF in alveolar macrophages from older, lifelong smokers and patients with emphysema is significantly reduced compared with alveolar macrophages from lifelong nonsmokers.[218] In addition, transgenic mice that overexpress TNF-α demonstrate the characteristics of emphysema and pulmonary hypertension,[219] which are associated with decreased VEGF, perivascular fibrosis, and adventitial thickening.[220] Perhaps this provides an explanation as to why some patients with COPD develop pulmonary hypertension; that is, abnormally increased expression of TNF-α reduces VEGF. These examples demonstrate that the proper regulation of macrophage mediators, especially VEGF, is integral in maintaining vasculature homeostasis.

Contribution of Macrophages to Fibrosis

Many patients with emphysema of the apical lung areas and diffuse parenchymal disease also present with fibrosis of the lower lung areas, although the mechanisms that cause this combined disease are unknown.[221] Many animal models of emphysema show alveolar septal fibrosis as a pathologic feature.[158,222,223] Most of our understanding of the mechanism by which macrophages contribute to lung fibrosis is derived from the bleomycin-induced model of lung injury. We recently observed the presence of alternatively activated macrophages in regions of bleomycin-induced fibrosis (M. Voelkel, unpublished observation, 2005). This macrophage phenotype produces FIZZ1, which can induce fibroblast differentiation into myofibroblasts and cause secretion of extracellular matrix proteins.[66] Alternative activation of macrophages results from the presence of IL-13/IL-4 in specific microenvironments of the lung, and IL-13/IL-4, although having a direct effect on fibroproliferation itself, also induces macrophages to produce TGF-β, another cytokine implicated in the fibrosis.[224] The neutralization of IL-13/IL-4 signaling is found to attenuate the development of bleomycin-induced pulmonary fibrosis.[225–227] Other investigations into the role of macrophages in pulmonary fibrosis reveal that macrophages, alternatively activated by IL-4 and IL-13, produce and secrete IGF-I, which promotes myofibroblast survival, proliferation, and extracellular matrix deposition, leading to fibrosis.[152,153,228] CCL-18, a chemokine that stimulates fibroblast production of collagen, is constitutively expressed in human alveolar macrophages isolated from BALF and is increased in the BALF from patients with fibrosis.[229] Again, in addition, alveolar macrophages that are activated by IL-13, IL-4, and IL-10 express more CCL-18, thus setting up an interactive cycle of alternative macrophage activation and fibroblast collagen production.[229] In conclusion, macrophages can simultaneously participate directly and indirectly in the development of both pulmonary fibrosis and emphysema depending on the local microenvironment created by endothelial cells, fibroblasts, and macrophages themselves.

Conclusion

Macrophages very likely play a fundamental role in the pathogenesis of COPD. Their "activation" appears to be not only necessary but also potentially sufficient in the pathology of emphysema and chronic bronchitis; however, as mentioned in the introduction, many other cell types have been found in COPD. At present, many of the studies examining the role of pulmonary macrophages in COPD have been descriptive (either *in-vitro* models of macrophages exposed to cigarette smoke extract or analysis of BALF or BAL macrophages). Meticulous studies to elucidate the exact phenotype(s) of the macrophages responsible for the observations in patients with COPD have so far not been conducted, nor has a comprehensive model been proposed that includes multiple macrophage phenotypes. We therefore offer a model based on the activation of specific macrophage phenotypes in particular locations of the lung that may serve as an outline for future studies examining the pathogenesis of cigarette smoke–induced COPD. Any model of macrophage function needs to take into account the fact that macrophages likely play a role throughout the pathobiology, for example, initiation of inflammation, progression, tissue destruction, remodeling, lack of efferocytosis, fibrosis, and revascularization. Parenthetically, the concept of a cigarette smoke exposure-driven selection of specific macrophage phenotypes may explain why cigarette smoking appears to be protective in some lung diseases.

Our macrophage-centric model of COPD has many components, with the first being pulmonary filtering. The lung has an extremely large surface area of bronchial and alveolar epithelial cells. This surface area is convoluted into a complex shape to provide numerous gas-exchange units but at the same time effectively creates a progressively smaller particulate filter. Interspersed in the alveolar airspaces, as well as along the airway surfaces, are macrophages, which function to clear pathogens and foreign particles. In the nondiseased state, macrophages and epithelial cells may provide mutual survival and supportive signals via receptor crosstalk. Stereotypically, it is thought that when a macrophage (a naive or, more likely, suppressor-activated macrophage) encounters a pathogen or foreign particle in the lung, it is activated and becomes a panactivated or classically activated macrophage, depending on whether the pathogen interacts directly with the macrophage or epithelium, respectively. In the process of activation, inflammatory cytokines and chemokines are released, MMPs are expressed, and oxidants are produced.

Other leukocytes are likely recruited to the area, and phagocytosis of the pathogen or particle may occur. As the inflammation progresses, classically activated macrophages clear apoptotic cells and provide an anti-inflammatory environment. Subsequently, recruited or phenotypically differentiated macrophages become suppressor-activated macrophages owing to feedback mechanisms. Alternatively activated macrophages appear late in the process and promote wound healing, neovascularization, and repair, all culminating in the resolution of inflammation and the return to homeostasis.

The second component is that cigarette smoke, in addition to its ability to directly damage the epithelium by oxidative stress, has thousands of components, including LPS and LPS-like materials, acrolein, tar, clay dusts, hydrocarbons, partially burned hydrocarbon fragments, ethylenediaminetetraacetic acid (EDTA), and gases such as CO_2, CO, alcohols, and aryl-hydrocarbons. Each of these may be carried along the bronchial tree into different levels of the lung. For example, lighter or more gaseous substances, such as LPS, CO, CO_2, and EDTA (an inhibitor of arginase), may be carried into the proximal and distal airspaces, whereas heavier materials, such as clay, dust, partially burned hydrocarbons, and wood dust, may be carried less far and deposit in the small and medium-sized airways, sparing the distal airspaces (Figure 5).

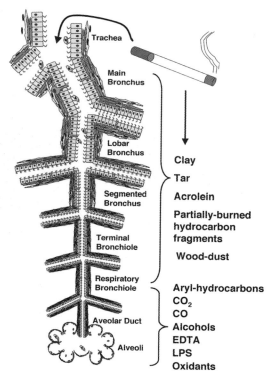

FIGURE 5. The multitude of components in cigarette smoke are proposed to travel to different levels of the bronchial tree owing to the physical characteristics of the compounds and the increasingly smaller airways from the trachea to the alveoli. EDTA = ethylenediaminetetraacetic acid; LPS = lipopolysaccharide.

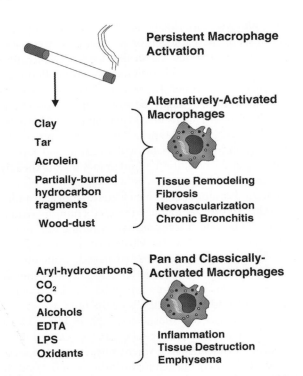

Persistent Macrophage Activation

Alternatively-Activated Macrophages

Clay
Tar
Acrolein
Partially-burned hydrocarbon fragments
Wood-dust

Tissue Remodeling
Fibrosis
Neovascularization
Chronic Bronchitis

Pan and Classically-Activated Macrophages

Aryl-hydrocarbons
CO_2
CO
Alcohols
EDTA
LPS
Oxidants

Inflammation
Tissue Destruction
Emphysema

FIGURE 6. The compounds in cigarettes are thought to assiduously activate distinct macrophage functional phenotypes, resulting in the pathophysiology seen in chronic obstructive pulmonary disease. EDTA = ethylenediaminetetraacetic acid; LPS = lipopolysaccharide.

The final component is that cigarette smoke exposure interrupts the normal sequence of macrophage-orchestrated initiation and resolution of inflammation by selecting and perpetually activating specific macrophage phenotypes (Figure 6). This is thought to occur not only in those individuals continually exposed to the multitude of cigarette compounds but also in former smokers, as evidenced by disease progression in some individuals after smoking cessation. Thus, macrophage activation never resolves to the inactivated or suppressive state, and restoration to homeostasis is never achieved.

Putting all of the components together, we speculate that the lighter components of cigarette smoke travel to the airspaces and induce unrelenting panactivated macrophages and classically activated macrophages in the alveolar spaces. These macrophages chronically release cytokines and chemokines such as TNF-α, IL-1β, IL-8, GRO-α, MCP-1, MIP-1α, and eotaxin, which leads to continued recruitment of more inflammatory cells, which have a deleterious effect on lung structure. Furthermore, persistent macrophage activation in the airspaces leads to increased expression of tissue-degrading proteases such as MMP-9 and -12 and decreased expression of antiproteases such as TIMP-1 and SLPI, which results in progressive damage and breakdown of the lung parenchyma, loss of lung elasticity, and airspace enlargement. These macrophages will also (1) produce oxidants that directly affect alveolar cells and decrease the activity of antipro-

teases and (2) decrease expression of antioxidants, including heme oxygenase 1. Apoptotic neutrophils will not be cleared properly owing to decreased VEGF expression and because panactivated macrophages, being constantly costimulated with IFN-γ from recruited Th1 T cells, phagocytose poorly. Decreased efferocytosis will result in neutrophil necrosis and release of inflammatory intracellular contents. The decreased expression of VEGF, probably caused by abundant TNF-α in the lung, will not only cause reduced efferocytosis but will also lead to defective vasculogenesis and angiogenesis. These states will continue in perpetuity, and injury repair and resolution will fail.

The heavier components of cigarette smoke are thought to deposit in the medium and small airways and induce alternatively activated macrophages. Because of the abundance of Th2-like cytokines, the alternatively activated macrophages will chronically make FIZZ1, a molecule known to increase pulmonary artery pressure and vascular resistance. FIZZ1 also induces MCP-1 and VEGF expression by endothelial cells, which will recruit more macrophages and stimulate both vasculogenesis and angiogenesis, respectively. The relentless alternative activation of macrophages will also result in fibrosis and remodeling of the airways because of continued expression of profibrogenic molecules, including IGF-I, TGF-β, FIZZ1, and CCL-18. Both FIZZ1 and TGF-β stimulate myofibroblast differentiation and smooth muscle α-actin expression, whereas IGF-I, TGF-β, FIZZ1, and CCL-18 all increase collagen expression in myofibroblasts and fibroblasts. CCL-18, also known as pulmonary and activation-regulated cytokine, is an accepted marker of the alternatively activated macrophage. CCL18 expression is inverse to that of MIP-1α and is a strong chemoattractant for T cells, which may explain the preponderance of IL-4- and IL-13-expressing T cells. IL-4 and IL-13 are suspects in mucus hypersecretion, a hallmark of chronic bronchitis. Alternatively activated macrophages have been associated with the production of specific growth factors (fibroblast growth factor, IGF-I, platelet-derived growth factor, VEGF, and polyamines), which support tumor growth and may therefore explain the increased cancer incidence within the bronchial tree of patients with COPD. Considering the autoimmune component of COPD, immune complex-activated macrophages may reside in the airways, and when stimulated in the presence of IL-4, these macrophages would exhibit decreased ADCC, respiratory burst, and iNOS expression but, in contrast, will have increased arginase expression and activity. Some suppressor-activated macrophages may be present in the airways, as evidenced by the presence of TGF-β, but there may not be enough TGF-β or IL-10 to move the response from the repair to the resolution stage. However, the TGF-β that is produced may be enough to maintain the fibroproliferative response.

In summary, it has become clear that macrophages are critically important cells invested in the health of the lung. It is likewise clear that we have only begun to understand the various macrophage functions required for lung homeostasis. The approach of categorizing macrophages into activation phenotypes based on characterized responses and functions will increase our understanding of lung diseases and repair. A focus on lung macrophage biology may even invite new therapeutic modalities; for instance, etanercept (an anti-TNF agent used in rheumatoid arthritis), marimastat (an inhibitor of MMP-12), or agmatine (an iNOS and possibly arginase inhibitor, currently in use as an anti-multiple sclerosis agent) could potentially attenuate the disease process. It is hoped that a better understanding of the complete roles of the various macrophage phenotypes in COPD will lead the future therapies that will prevent the worsening of the disease in both current and former smokers and possibly provide insights into other areas of lung injury and repair.

References

1. Doll R, Peto R, Wheatley K, et al. Mortality in relation to smoking: 40 years' observations on male British doctors. BMJ 1994;309:901–11.

2. Turino GM, Rodriguez JR, Greenbaum LM, Mandl I. Mechanisms of pulmonary injury. Am J Med 1974;57:493–505.

3. Laurell CB, Eriksson S. Scand J Clin Lab Invest 1963;15:132–40.

4. Grashoff WF, Sont JK, Sterk PJ, et al. Chronic obstructive pulmonary disease: role of bronchiolar mast cells and macrophages. Am J Pathol 1997;151:1785–90.

5. Peleman RA, Rytila PH, Kips JC, et al. The cellular composition of induced sputum in chronic obstructive pulmonary disease. Eur Respir J 1999;13:839–43.

6. Saetta M, Di Stefano A, Maestrelli P, et al. Activated T-lymphocytes and macrophages in bronchial mucosa of subjects with chronic bronchitis. Am Rev Respir Dis 1993;147:301–6.

7. Saetta M, Turato G, Facchini FM, et al. Inflammatory cells in the bronchial glands of smokers with chronic bronchitis. Am J Respir Crit Care Med 1997;156:1633–9.

8. Saetta M, Di Stefano A, Turato G, et al. CD8+ T-lymphocytes in peripheral airways of smokers with chronic obstructive pulmonary disease. Am J Respir Crit Care Med 1998;157:822–6.

9. Di Stefano A, Capelli A, Lusuardi M, et al. Severity of airflow limitation is associated with severity of airway inflammation in smokers. Am J Respir Crit Care Med 1998;158:1277–85.

10. Majo J, Ghezzo H, Cosio MG. Lymphocyte population and apoptosis in the lungs of smokers and their relation to emphysema. Eur Respir J 2001;17:946–53.

11. D'Hulst AI, Maes T, Bracke KR, et al. Cigarette smoke–induced pulmonary emphysema in scid-mice. Is the acquired immune system required? Respir Res 2005;6:147.

12. Yearsley MM, Diaz PT, Knoell D, Nuovo GJ. Correlation of HIV-1 detection and histology in AIDS-associated emphysema. Diagn Mol Pathol 2005;14:48–52.

13. O'Shaughnessy TC, Ansari TW, Barnes NC, Jeffery PK. Inflammation in bronchial biopsies of subjects with chronic bronchitis: inverse relationship of CD8+ T lymphocytes with FEV1. Am J Respir Crit Care Med 1997;155:852–7.

14. Aoshiba K, Koinuma M, Yokohori N, Nagai A. Differences in the distribution of CD4+ and CD8+ T cells in emphysematous lungs. Respiration 2004;71:184–90.

15. van der Strate BW, Postma DS, Brandsma CA, et al. Cigarette smoke–induced emphysema: a role for the B cell? Am J Respir Crit Care Med 2006;173:751–8.

16. Sullivan AK, Simonian PL, Falta MT, et al. Activated oligoclonal CD4+ T cells in the lungs of patients with severe emphysema. Proc Am Thorac Soc 2006;3:486.

17. Taraseviciene-Stewart L, Burns N, Kraskauskas D, et al. Mechanisms of autoimmune emphysema. Proc Am Thorac Soc 2006;3:486–7.

18. Taraseviciene-Stewart L, Douglas IS, Nana-Sinkam PS, et al. Is alveolar destruction and emphysema in chronic obstructive pulmonary disease an immune disease? Proc Am Thorac Soc 2006;3:687–90.

19. McLaughlin RF, Tueller EE. Anatomic and histologic changes of early emphysema. Chest 1971;59:592–9.

20. Rutgers SR, Timens W, Kaufmann HF, et al. Comparison of induced sputum with bronchial wash, bronchoalveolar lavage and bronchial biopsies in COPD. Eur Respir J 2000;15:109–15.

21. Niewoehner DE, Kleinerman J, Rice DB. Pathologic changes in the peripheral airways of young cigarette smokers. N Engl J Med 1974;291:755–8.

22. Finkelstein R, Fraser RS, Ghezzo H, Cosio MG. Alveolar inflammation and its relation to emphysema in smokers. Am J Respir Crit Care Med 1995;152:1666–72.

23. D'Hulst A I, Vermaelen KY, Brusselle GG, et al. Time course of cigarette smoke–induced pulmonary inflammation in mice. Eur Respir J 2005;26:204–13.

24. Ofulue AF, Ko M, Abboud RT. Time course of neutrophil and macrophage elastinolytic activities in cigarette smoke–induced emphysema. Am J Physiol 1998;275:L1134–44.

25. Ofulue AF, Ko M. Effects of depletion of neutrophils or macrophages on development of cigarette smoke–induced emphysema. Am J Physiol 1999;277:L97–105.

26. Stein M, Keshav S, Harris N, Gordon S. Interleukin 4 potently enhances murine macrophage mannose receptor activity: a marker of alternative immunologic macrophage activation. J Exp Med 1992;176:287–92.

27. Laszlo DJ, Henson PM, Remigio LK, et al. Development of functional diversity in mouse macrophages. Mutual exclusion of two phenotypic states. Am J Pathol 1993;143:587–97.

28. Lake FR, Noble PW, Henson PM, Riches DW. Functional switching of macrophage responses to tumor necrosis factor-alpha (TNF alpha) by interferons. Implications for the pleiotropic activities of TNF alpha. J Clin Invest 1994;93:1661–9.

29. Riches DW. Signalling heterogeneity as a contributing factor in macrophage functional diversity. Semin Cell Biol 1995;6:377–84.

30. Gordon S. Alternative activation of macrophages. Nat Rev Immunol 2002;3:23–35.

31. Gordon S, Taylor PR. Monocyte and macrophage heterogeneity. Nat Rev Immunol 2005;5:953–64.

32. Edwards JP, Zhang X, Frauwirth KA, Mosser DM. Biochemical and functional characterization of three activated macrophage populations. J Leukoc Biol 2006;80:1298–307.

33. Curran CS, Demick KP, Mansfield JM. Lactoferrin activates macrophages via TLR4-dependent and -independent signaling pathways. Cell Immunol 2006;242:23–30.

34. Taylor PR, Martinez-Pomares L, Stacey M, et al. Macrophage receptors and immune recognition. Annu Rev Immunol 2005;23:901–44.

35. Medzhitov R, Preston-Hurlburt P, Janeway CA Jr. A human homologue of the Drosophila Toll protein signals activation of adaptive immunity. Nature 1997;388:394–7.

36. Akira S, Uematsu S, Takeuchi O. Pathogen recognition and innate immunity. Cell 2006;124:783–801.

37. Bouchon A, Dietrich J, Colonna M. Cutting edge: inflammatory responses can be triggered by TREM-1, a novel receptor expressed on neutrophils and monocytes. J Immunol 2000;164:4991–5.

38. Lorsbach RB, Murphy WJ, Lowenstein CJ, et al. Expression of the nitric oxide synthase gene in mouse macrophages activated for tumor cell killing. Molecular basis for the synergy between interferon-gamma and lipopolysaccharide. J Biol Chem 1993;268:1908–13.

39. Sironi M, Martinez FO, D'Ambrosio D, et al. Differential regulation of chemokine production by Fcgamma receptor engagement in human monocytes: association of CCL1 with a distinct form of M2 monocyte activation (M2b, type 2). J Leukoc Biol 2006;80:342–9.

40. Burger D. Cell contact-mediated signaling of monocytes by stimulated T cells: a major pathway for cytokine induction. Eur Cytokine Netw 2000;11:346–53.

41. Song E, Ouyang N, Horbelt M, et al. Influence of alternatively and classically activated macrophages on fibrogenic activities of human fibroblasts. Cell Immunol 2000;204:19–28.

42. Watkins SK, Egilmez NK, Suttles J, Stout RD. IL-12 rapidly alters the functional profile of tumor-associated and tumor-infiltrating macrophages in vitro and in vivo. J Immunol 2007;178:1357–62.

43. Verreck FA, de Boer T, Langenberg DM, et al. Human IL-23-producing type 1 macrophages promote but IL-10-producing type 2 macrophages subvert immunity to (myco)bacteria. Proc Natl Acad Sci U S A 2004;101:4560–5.

44. Van Ginderachter JA, Movahedi K, Hassanzadeh Ghassabeh G, et al. Classical and alternative activation of mononuclear phagocytes: picking the best of both worlds for tumor promotion. Immunobiology 2006;211:487–501.

45. Mytar B, Siedlar M, Woloszyn M, et al. Induction of reactive oxygen intermediates in human monocytes by tumour cells and their role in spontaneous monocyte cytotoxicity. Br J Cancer 1999;79:737–43.

46. Stuehr DJ, Nathan CF. Nitric oxide. A macrophage product responsible for cytostasis and respiratory inhibition in tumor target cells. J Exp Med 1989;169:1543–55.

47. Bonnotte B, Larmonier N, Favre N, et al. Identification of tumor-infiltrating macrophages as the killers of tumor cells after immunization in a rat model system. J Immunol 2001;167:5077–83.

48. Urban JL, Shepard HM, Rothstein JL, et al. Tumor necrosis factor: a potent effector molecule for tumor cell killing by activated macrophages. Proc Natl Acad Sci U S A 1986;83:5233–7.

49. Mantovani A, Sica A, Sozzani S, et al. The chemokine system in diverse forms of macrophage activation and polarization. Trends Immunol 2004;25:677–86.

50. Schroder K, Hertzog PJ, Ravasi T, Hume DA. Interferon-gamma: an overview of signals, mechanisms and functions. J Leukoc Biol 2004;75:163–89.

51. Lafuse WP, Brown D, Castle L, Zwilling BS. IFN-gamma increases cathepsin H mRNA levels in mouse macrophages. J Leukoc Biol 1995;57:663–9.

52. Lah TT, Hawley M, Rock KL, Goldberg AL. Gamma-interferon causes a selective induction of the lysosomal proteases, cathepsins B and L, in macrophages. FEBS Lett 1995;363:85–9.

53. Schroder K, Sweet MJ, Hume DA. Signal integration between IFNgamma and TLR signalling pathways in macrophages. Immunobiology 2006;211:511–24.

54. Mokoena T, Gordon S. Human macrophage activation. Modulation of mannosyl, fucosyl receptor activity in vitro by lymphokines, gamma and alpha interferons, and dexamethasone. J Clin Invest 1985;75:624–31.

55. Xie QW, Cho HJ, Calaycay J, et al. Cloning and characterization of inducible nitric oxide synthase from mouse macrophages. Science 1992;256:225–8.

56. Mita Y, Dobashi K, Shimizu Y, et al. Surface expression of Toll-like receptor 4 on THP-1 cells is modulated by Bu-Zhong-Yi-Qi-Tang and Shi-Quan-Da-Bu-Tang. Methods Find Exp Clin Pharmacol 2002;24:67–70.

57. Bosisio D, Polentarutti N, Sironi M, et al. Stimulation of Toll-like receptor 4 expression in human mononuclear phagocytes by interferon-gamma: a molecular basis for priming and synergism with bacterial lipopolysaccharide. Blood 2002;99:3427–31.

58. Ahmad-Nejad P, Hacker H, Rutz M, et al. Bacterial CpG-DNA and lipopolysaccharides activate Toll-like receptors at distinct cellular compartments. Eur J Immunol 2002;32:1958–68.

59. Pace JL, Russell SW, Torres BA, et al. Recombinant mouse gamma interferon induces the priming step in macrophage activation for tumor cell killing. J Immunol 1983;130:2011–3.

60. Russell SW, Pace JL. The effects of interferons on macrophages and their precursors. Vet Immunol Immunopathol 1987;15:129–65.

61. De Whalley CV, Riches DW. Influence of the cytocidal macrophage phenotype on the degradation of acetylated low density lipoproteins: dual regulation of scavenger receptor activity and of intracellular degradation of endocytosed ligand. Exp Cell Res 1991;192:460–8.

62. Pesce J, Kaviratne M, Ramalingam TR, et al. The IL-21 receptor augments Th2 effector function and alternative macrophage activation. J Clin Invest 2006;116:2044–55.

63. Munder M, Eichmann K, Moran JM, et al. Th1/Th2-regulated expression of arginase isoforms in murine macrophages and dendritic cells. J Immunol 1999;163:3771–7.

64. Yamaji-Kegan K, Su Q, Angelini DJ, et al. Hypoxia-induced mitogenic factor has proangiogenic and proinflammatory effects in the lung via VEGF and VEGF receptor-2. Am J Physiol Lung Cell Mol Physiol 2006;291:L1159–68.

65. Teng X, Li D, Champion HC, Johns RA. FIZZ1/RELMalpha, a novel hypoxia-induced mitogenic factor in lung with vasoconstrictive and angiogenic properties. Circ Res 2003;92:1065–7.

66. Liu T, Dhanasekaran SM, Jin H, et al. FIZZ1 stimulation of myofibroblast differentiation. Am J Pathol 2004;164:1315–26.

67. Welch JS, Escoubet-Lozach L, Sykes DB, et al. TH2 cytokines and allergic challenge induce Ym1 expression in macrophages by a STAT6-dependent mechanism. J Biol Chem 2002;277:42821–9.

68. Loke P, MacDonald AS, Robb A, et al. Alternatively activated macrophages induced by nematode infection inhibit proliferation via cell-to-cell contact. Eur J Immunol 2000;30:2669–78.

69. Satriano J. Agmatine: at the crossroads of the arginine pathways. Ann N Y Acad Sci 2003;1009:34-43.

70. Mantovani A, Locati M, Vecchi A, et al. Decoy receptors: a strategy to regulate inflammatory cytokines and chemokines. Trends Immunol 2001;22:328–36.

71. Mantovani A, Sozzani S, Locati M, et al. Macrophage polarization: tumor-associated macrophages as a paradigm for polarized M2 mononuclear phagocytes. Trends Immunol 2002;23:549–55.

72. Bonecchi R, Sozzani S, Stine JT, et al. Divergent effects of interleukin-4 and interferon-gamma on macrophage-derived chemokine production: an amplification circuit of polarized T helper 2 responses. Blood 1998;92:2668–71.

73. Imai T, Nagira M, Takagi S, et al. Selective recruitment of CCR4-bearing Th2 cells toward antigen-presenting cells by the CC chemokines thymus and activation-regulated chemokine and macrophage-derived chemokine. Int Immunol 1999;11:81–8.

74. Gu L, Tseng S, Horner RM, et al. Control of TH2 polarization by the chemokine monocyte chemoattractant protein-1. Nature 2000;404:407–11.

75. Gu L, Tseng SC, Rollins BJ. Monocyte chemoattractant protein-1. Chem Immunol 1999;72:7–29.

76. Aderem A, Underhill DM. Mechanisms of phagocytosis in macrophages. Annu Rev Immunol 1999;17:593–623.

77. Unkeless JC, Scigliano E, Freedman VH. Structure and function of human and murine receptors for IgG. Annu Rev Immunol 1988;6:251–81.

78. Gerber JS, Mosser DM. Reversing lipopolysaccharide toxicity by ligating the macrophage Fc gamma receptors. J Immunol 2001;166:6861–8.

79. Loegering DJ, Lennartz MR. Signaling pathways for Fc gamma receptor-stimulated tumor necrosis factor-alpha secretion and respiratory burst in RAW 264.7 macrophages. Inflammation 2004;28:23–31.

80. Daeron M. Structural bases of Fc gamma R functions. Int Rev Immunol 1997;16:1–27.

81. Tridandapani S, Siefker K, Teillaud JL, et al. Regulated expression and inhibitory function of Fcgamma RIIb in human monocytic cells. J Biol Chem 2002;277:5082–9.

82. Lang R, Patel D, Morris JJ, et al. Shaping gene expression in activated and resting primary macrophages by IL-10. J Immunol 2002;169:2253–63.

83. Murray PJ. The primary mechanism of the IL-10-regulated antiinflammatory response is to selectively inhibit transcription. Proc Natl Acad Sci U S A 2005;102:8686–91.

84. Bogdan C, Vodovotz Y, Nathan C. Macrophage deactivation by interleukin 10. J Exp Med 1991;174:1549–55.

85. Riley JK, Takeda K, Akira S, Schreiber RD. Interleukin-10 receptor signaling through the JAK-STAT pathway. Requirement for two distinct receptor-derived signals for anti-inflammatory action. J Biol Chem 1999;274:16513–21.

86. Weber-Nordt RM, Riley JK, Greenlund AC, et al. Stat3 recruitment by two distinct ligand-induced, tyrosine-phosphorylated docking sites in the interleukin-10 receptor intracellular domain. J Biol Chem 1996;271:27954–61.

87. Murray PJ. STAT3-mediated anti-inflammatory signalling. Biochem Soc Trans 2006;34:1028–31.

88. Ogawa S, Lozach J, Benner C, et al. Molecular determinants of crosstalk between nuclear receptors and toll-like receptors. Cell 2005;122:707–21.

89. Levy DE, Lee CK. What does Stat3 do? J Clin Invest 2002;109:1143–8.

90. Drannik AG, Pouladi MA, Robbins CS, et al. Impact of cigarette smoke on clearance and inflammation after *Pseudomonas aeruginosa* infection. Am J Respir Crit Care Med 2004;170:1164–71.

91. Vecchiarelli A, Dottorini M, Puliti M, et al. Defective candidacidal activity of alveolar macrophages and peripheral blood monocytes from patients with chronic obstructive pulmonary disease. Am Rev Respir Dis 1991; 143:1049–54.

92. Betsuyaku T, Kuroki Y, Nagai K, et al. Effects of ageing and smoking on SP-A and SP-D levels in bronchoalveolar lavage fluid. Eur Respir J 2004;24:964–70.

93. Honda Y, Takahashi H, Kuroki Y, et al. Decreased contents of surfactant proteins A and D in BAL fluids of healthy smokers. Chest 1996;109:1006–9.

94. van Iwaarden F, Welmers B, Verhoef J, et al. Pulmonary surfactant protein A enhances the host-defense mechanism of rat alveolar macrophages. Am J Respir Cell Mol Biol 1990;2:91–8.

95. Ofek I, Mesika A, Kalina M, et al. Surfactant protein D enhances phagocytosis and killing of unencapsulated phase variants of *Klebsiella pneumoniae*. Infect Immun 2001;69:24–33.

96. Kostina E, Ofek I, Crouch E, et al. Noncapsulated *Klebsiella pneumoniae* bearing mannose-containing O antigens is rapidly eradicated from mouse lung and triggers cytokine production by macrophages following opsonization with surfactant protein D. Infect Immun 2005;73:8282–90.

97. Balagopal A, MacFarlane AS, Mohapatra N, et al. Characterization of the receptor-ligand pathways important for entry and survival of *Francisella tularensis* in human macrophages. Infect Immun 2006;74:5114–25.

98. Ganrot PO, Laurell CB, Eriksson S. Obstructive lung disease and trypsin inhibitors in alpha-1-antitrypsin deficiency. Scand J Clin Lab Invest 1967;19:205–8.

99. Johanson WG Jr, Pierce AK. Effects of elastase, collagenase, and papain on structure and function of rat lungs *in vitro*. J Clin Invest 1972;51:288–93.

100. Johanson WG Jr, Reynolds RC, Scott TC, Pierce AK. Connective tissue damage in emphysema. An electron microscopic study of papain-induced emphysema in rats. Am Rev Respir Dis 1973;107:589–95.

101. Janoff A, White R, Carp H, et al. Lung injury induced by leukocytic proteases. Am J Pathol 1979;97:111–36.

102. Parra SC, Gaddy LR, Takaro T. Early ultrastructural changes in papain-induced experimental emphysema. Lab Invest 1980;42:277–89.

103. Snider GL. The pathogenesis of emphysema-twenty years of progress. Am Rev Respir Dis 1981;124:321–4.

104. Takaro T, Chapman WE, Burnette R, Cordell S. Acute and sub-acute effects of injury on the canine alveolar septum. Chest 1990;98:724–32.

105. Mass B, Ikeda T, Meranze DR, et al. Induction of experimental emphysema. Cellular and species specificity. Am Rev Respir Dis 1972;106:384–91.

106. Blackwood CE, Hosannah Y, Perman E, et al. Experimental emphysema in rats: elastolytic titer of inducing enzyme as determinant of the response. Proc Soc Exp Biol Med 1973;144:450–4.

107. White R, White J, Janoff A. Effects of cigarette smoke on elastase secretion by murine macrophages. J Lab Clin Med 1979;94:489–99.

108. Hautamaki RD, Kobayashi DK, Senior RM, Shapiro SD. Requirement for macrophage elastase for cigarette smoke–induced emphysema in mice. Science 1997;277:2002–4.

109. Russell RE, Culpitt SV, DeMatos C, et al. Release and activity of matrix metalloproteinase-9 and tissue inhibitor of metallo-proteinase-1 by alveolar macrophages from patients with chronic obstructive pulmonary disease. Am J Respir Cell Mol Biol 2002;26:602–9.

110. Repine JE, Bast A, Lankhorst I. Oxidative stress in chronic obstructive pulmonary disease. Oxidative Stress Study Group. Am J Respir Crit Care Med 1997;156:341–57.

111. Macnee W, Rahman I. Oxidants and antioxidants as therapeutic targets in chronic obstructive pulmonary disease. Am J Respir Crit Care Med 1999;160:S58–65.

112. Rahman I, MacNee W. Lung glutathione and oxidative stress: implications in cigarette smoke–induced airway disease. Am J Physiol 1999;277:L1067–88.

113. Cohen AB. Lung cell biology. Fed Proc 1979;38:2635–6.

114. Yang SR, Chida AS, Bauter MR, et al. Cigarette smoke induces proinflammatory cytokine release by activation of NF-kappaB and posttranslational modifications of histone deacetylase in macrophages. Am J Physiol Lung Cell Mol Physiol 2006;291:L46–57.

115. Itoh K, Chiba T, Takahashi S, et al. An Nrf2/small Maf heterodimer mediates the induction of phase II detoxifying enzyme genes through antioxidant response elements. Biochem Biophys Res Commun 1997;236:313–22.

116. Ishii T, Itoh K, Takahashi S, et al. Transcription factor Nrf2 coordinately regulates a group of oxidative stress-inducible genes in macrophages. J Biol Chem 2000;275:16023–9.

117. Iizuka T, Ishii Y, Itoh K, et al. Nrf2-deficient mice are highly susceptible to cigarette smoke–induced emphysema. Genes Cells 2005;10:1113–25.

118. Barnes PJ. Mediators of chronic obstructive pulmonary disease. Pharmacol Rev 2004;56:515–48.

119. Gessner C, Scheibe R, Wotzel M, et al. Exhaled breath condensate cytokine patterns in chronic obstructive pulmonary disease. Respir Med 2005;99:1229–40.

120. Lim S, Roche N, Oliver BG, et al. Balance of matrix metallo-protease-9 and tissue inhibitor of metalloprotease-1 from alveolar macrophages in cigarette smokers. Regulation by interleukin-10. Am J Respir Crit Care Med 2000;162:1355–60.

121. Soler N, Ewig S, Torres A, et al. Airway inflammation and bronchial microbial patterns in patients with stable chronic obstructive pulmonary disease. Eur Respir J 1999;14:1015–22.

122. Castro P, Legora-Machado A, Cardilo-Reis L, et al. Inhibition of interleukin-1beta reduces mouse lung inflammation induced by exposure to cigarette smoke. Eur J Pharmacol 2004;498:279–86.

123. Culpitt SV, Rogers DF, Fenwick PS, et al. Inhibition by red wine extract, resveratrol, of cytokine release by alveolar macrophages in COPD. Thorax 2003;58:942–6.

124. Culpitt SV, Rogers DF, Shah P, et al. Impaired inhibition by dexamethasone of cytokine release by alveolar macrophages from patients with chronic obstructive pulmonary disease. Am J Respir Crit Care Med 2003;167:24–31.

125. Dubar V, Gosset P, Aerts C, et al. *In vitro* acute effects of tobacco smoke on tumor necrosis factor alpha and interleukin-6 production by alveolar macrophages. Exp Lung Res 1993;19:345–59.

126. Wang S, Lantz RC, Vermeulen MW, et al. Functional alterations of alveolar macrophages subjected to smoke exposure and antioxidant lazaroids. Toxicol Ind Health 1999;15:464–9.

127. Saetta M, Turato G, Baraldo S, et al. Goblet cell hyperplasia and epithelial inflammation in peripheral airways of smokers with both symptoms of chronic bronchitis and chronic airflow limitation. Am J Respir Crit Care Med 2000;161:1016–21.

128. Borchers MT, Wesselkamper S, Wert SE, et al. Monocyte inflammation augments acrolein-induced Muc5ac expression in mouse lung. Am J Physiol 1999;277:L489–97.

129. Guerra S. Overlap of asthma and chronic obstructive pulmonary disease. Curr Opin Pulm Med 2005;11:7–13.

130. Blease KL, NW, Hoagboam, CM, Kunkel SL. Chemokines and their role in airway-hyper-reactivity. Respir Res 2000;1:54–61.

131. Elias JA, Zhu Z, Chupp G, Homer RJ. Airway remodeling in asthma. J Clin Invest 1999;104:1001–6.

132. Chung KF, Barnes PJ. Cytokines in asthma. Thorax 1999;54:825–57.

133. Matsunaga K, Yanagisawa S, Ichikawa T, et al. Airway cytokine expression measured by means of protein array in exhaled breath condensate: correlation with physiologic properties in asthmatic patients. J Allergy Clin Immunol 2006;118:84–90.

134. Howarth PH, Babu KS, Arshad HS, et al. Tumour necrosis factor (TNFalpha) as a novel therapeutic target in symptomatic corticosteroid dependent asthma. Thorax 2005;60:1012–8.

135. Berry MA, Hargadon B, Shelley M, et al. Evidence of a role of tumor necrosis factor alpha in refractory asthma. N Engl J Med 2006;354:697–708.

136. Broide DH, Lotz M, Cuomo AJ, et al. Cytokines in symptomatic asthma airways. J Allergy Clin Immunol 1992;89:958–67.

137. Hallsworth MP, Soh CP, Lane SJ, et al. Selective enhancement of GM-CSF, TNF-alpha, IL-1 beta and IL-8 production by monocytes and macrophages of asthmatic subjects. Eur Respir J 1994;7:1096–102.

138. Nakae S, Lunderius C, Ho LH, et al. TNF can contribute to multiple features of ovalbumin-induced allergic inflammation of the airways in mice. J Allergy Clin Immunol 2007;119:680–6.

139. Park CS, Choi YS, Ki SY, et al. Granulocyte macrophage colony-stimulating factor is the main cytokine enhancing

survival of eosinophils in asthmatic airways. Eur Respir J 1998;12:872–8.

140. John M, Lim S, Seybold J, et al. Inhaled corticosteroids increase interleukin-10 but reduce macrophage inflammatory protein-1alpha, granulocyte-macrophage colony-stimulating factor, and interferon-gamma release from alveolar macrophages in asthma. Am J Respir Crit Care Med 1998;157:256–62.

141. Xing Z, Ohkawara Y, Jordana M, et al. Transfer of granulocyte-macrophage colony-stimulating factor gene to rat lung induces eosinophilia, monocytosis, and fibrotic reactions. J Clin Invest 1996;97:1102–10.

142. Plater-Zyberk C, Joosten LA, Helsen MM, et al. GM-CSF neutralisation suppresses inflammation and protects cartilage in acute streptococcal cell wall arthritis of mice. Ann Rheum Dis 2007;66:452–7.

143. Campbell EM, Charo IF, Kunkel SL, et al. Monocyte chemoattractant protein-1 mediates cockroach allergen-induced bronchial hyperreactivity in normal but not CCR2−/− mice: the role of mast cells. J Immunol 1999;163:2160–7.

144. Conti P, Boucher W, Letourneau R, et al. Monocyte chemotactic protein-1 provokes mast cell aggregation and [3H]5HT release. Immunology 1995;86:434–40.

145. Holgate ST, Bodey KS, Janezic A, et al. Release of RANTES, MIP-1 alpha, and MCP-1 into asthmatic airways following endobronchial allergen challenge. Am J Respir Crit Care Med 1997;156:1377–83.

146. Ying S, Meng Q, Zeibecoglou K, et al. Eosinophil chemotactic chemokines (eotaxin, eotaxin-2, RANTES, monocyte chemoattractant protein-3 (MCP-3), and MCP-4), and C-C chemokine receptor 3 expression in bronchial biopsies from atopic and nonatopic (intrinsic) asthmatics. J Immunol 1999;163:6321–9.

147. Mazzarella G, Grella E, D'Auria D, et al. Phenotypic features of alveolar monocytes/macrophages and IL-8 gene activation by IL-1 and TNF-alpha in asthmatic patients. Allergy 2000;55 Suppl 61:36–41.

148. Makinde T, Murphy RF, Agrawal DK. Immunomodulatory role of vascular endothelial growth factor and angiopoietin-1 in airway remodeling. Curr Mol Med 2006;6:831–41.

149. Makinde T, Murphy RF, Agrawal DK. The regulatory role of TGF-beta in airway remodeling in asthma. Immunol Cell Biol 2007; 85:348–56.

150. Prieto J, Lensmar C, Roquet A, et al. Increased interleukin-13 mRNA expression in bronchoalveolar lavage cells of atopic patients with mild asthma after repeated low-dose allergen provocations. Respir Med 2000;94:806–14.

151. Yamashita N, Tashimo H, Ishida H, et al. Role of insulin-like growth factor-I in allergen-induced airway inflammation and remodeling. Cell Immunol 2005;235:85–91.

152. Wynes MW, Riches DW. Induction of macrophage insulin-like growth factor-I expression by the Th2 cytokines IL-4 and IL-13. J Immunol 2003;171:3550–9.

153. Wynes MW, Frankel SK, Riches DW. IL-4-induced macrophage-derived IGF-I protects myofibroblasts from apoptosis following growth factor withdrawal. J Leukoc Biol 2004;76:1019–27.

154. Prasse A, Germann M, Pechkovsky DV, et al. IL-10-producing monocytes differentiate to alternatively activated

macrophages and are increased in atopic patients. J Allergy Clin Immunol 2007;119:464–71.

155. Sirois J, Bissonnette EY. Alveolar macrophages of allergic resistant and susceptible strains of rats show distinct cytokine profiles. Clin Exp Immunol 2001;126:9–15.

156. Lensmar C, Katchar K, Eklund A, et al. Phenotypic analysis of alveolar macrophages and lymphocytes following allergen inhalation by atopic subjects with mild asthma. Respir Med 2006;100:918–25.

157. Churg A, Wang RD, Tai H, et al. Macrophage metalloelastase mediates acute cigarette smoke–induced inflammation via tumor necrosis factor-alpha release. Am J Respir Crit Care Med 2003;167:1083–9.

158. Elias JA, Kang MJ, Crouthers K, et al. State of the art. Mechanistic heterogeneity in chronic obstructive pulmonary disease: insights from transgenic mice. Proc Am Thorac Soc 2006;3:494–8.

159. Mautino G, Henriquet C, Jaffuel D, et al. Tissue inhibitor of metalloproteinase-1 levels in bronchoalveolar lavage fluid from asthmatic subjects. Am J Respir Crit Care Med 1999;160:324–30.

160. Vignola AM, Riccobono L, Mirabella A, et al. Sputum metalloproteinase-9/tissue inhibitor of metalloproteinase-1 ratio correlates with airflow obstruction in asthma and chronic bronchitis. Am J Respir Crit Care Med 1998;158:1945–50.

161. Mautino G, Oliver N, Chanez P, et al. Increased release of matrix metalloproteinase-9 in bronchoalveolar lavage fluid and by alveolar macrophages of asthmatics. Am J Respir Cell Mol Biol 1997;17:583–91.

162. Mautino G, Henriquet C, Gougat C, et al. Increased expression of tissue inhibitor of metalloproteinase-1 and loss of correlation with matrix metalloproteinase-9 by macrophages in asthma. Lab Invest 1999;79:39–47.

163. Chiba Y, Yu Y, Sakai H, Misawa M. Increase in the expression of matrix metalloproteinase-12 in the airways of rats with allergic bronchial asthma. Biol Pharm Bull 2007;30:318–23.

164. Saren P, Welgus HG, Kovanen PT. TNF-alpha and IL-1beta selectively induce expression of 92-kDa gelatinase by human macrophages. J Immunol 1996;157:4159–65.

165. Lacraz S, Nicod L, Galve-de Rochemonteix B, et al. Suppression of metalloproteinase biosynthesis in human alveolar macrophages by interleukin-4. J Clin Invest 1992;90:382–8.

166. Sato T, Ito A, Mori Y. Interleukin 6 enhances the production of tissue inhibitor of metalloproteinases (TIMP) but not that of matrix metalloproteinases by human fibroblasts. Biochem Biophys Res Commun 1990;170:824–9.

167. Chizzolini C, Rezzonico R, De Luca C, et al. Th2 cell membrane factors in association with IL-4 enhance matrix metalloproteinase-1 (MMP-1) while decreasing MMP-9 production by granulocyte-macrophage colony-stimulating factor-differentiated human monocytes. J Immunol 2000;164:5952–60.

168. Lacraz S, Nicod LP, Chicheportiche R, et al. IL-10 inhibits metalloproteinase and stimulates TIMP-1 production in human mononuclear phagocytes. J Clin Invest 1995;96:2304–10.

169. Warner RL, Lukacs NW, Shapiro SD, et al. Role of metalloelastase in a model of allergic lung responses induced by cockroach allergen. Am J Pathol 2004;165:1921–30.

170. McMillan SJ, Kearley J, Campbell JD, et al. Matrix metalloproteinase-9 deficiency results in enhanced allergen-induced airway inflammation. J Immunol 2004;172:2586–94.

171. Peake HL, Currie AJ, Stewart GA, McWilliam AS. Nitric oxide production by alveolar macrophages in response to house dust mite fecal pellets and the mite allergens, Der p 1 and Der p 2. J Allergy Clin Immunol 2003;112:531–7.

172. Careau E, Sirois J, Bissonnette EY. Characterization of lung hyperresponsiveness, inflammation, and alveolar macrophage mediator production in allergy resistant and susceptible rats. Am J Respir Cell Mol Biol 2002;26:579–86.

173. Abe M, Hayashi Y, Murai A, et al. Effects of inducible nitric oxide synthase inhibitors on asthma depending on administration schedule. Free Radic Biol Med 2006;40:1083–95.

174. Curran AD. The role of nitric oxide in the development of asthma. Int Arch Allergy Immunol 1996;111:1–4.

175. Thomassen MJ, Kavuru MS. Human alveolar macrophages and monocytes as a source and target for nitric oxide. Int Immunopharmacol 2001;1:1479–90.

176. Huynh ML, Malcolm KC, Kotaru C, et al. Defective apoptotic cell phagocytosis attenuates prostaglandin E2 and 15-hydroxyeicosatetraenoic acid in severe asthma alveolar macrophages. Am J Respir Crit Care Med 2005;172:972–9.

177. Careau E, Proulx LI, Pouliot P, et al. Antigen sensitization modulates alveolar macrophage functions in an asthma model. Am J Physiol Lung Cell Mol Physiol 2006;290: L871–9.

178. Haslett C. Granulocyte apoptosis and its role in the resolution and control of lung inflammation. Am J Respir Crit Care Med 1999;160:S5–S11.

179. Retamales I, Elliott WM, Meshi B, et al. Amplification of inflammation in emphysema and its association with latent adenoviral infection. Am J Respir Crit Care Med 2001;164:469–73.

180. Abboud RT, Ofulue AF, Sansores RH, Muller NL. Relationship of alveolar macrophage plasminogen activator and elastase activities to lung function and CT evidence of emphysema. Chest 1998;113:1257–63.

181. Barnes PJ. Alveolar macrophages as orchestrators of COPD. Copd 2004;1:59–70.

182. Ito K, Lim S, Caramori G, et al. Cigarette smoking reduces histone deacetylase 2 expression, enhances cytokine expression, and inhibits glucocorticoid actions in alveolar macrophages. FASEB J 2001;15:1110–2.

183. de Godoy I, Donahoe M, Calhoun WJ, et al. Elevated TNF-alpha production by peripheral blood monocytes of weight-losing COPD patients. Am J Respir Crit Care Med 1996;153:633–7.

184. Churg A, Wang RD, Tai H, et al. Tumor necrosis factor-alpha drives 70% of cigarette smoke–induced emphysema in the mouse. Am J Respir Crit Care Med 2004;170:492–8.

185. Lucey EC, Keane J, Kuang PP, et al. Severity of elastase-induced emphysema is decreased in tumor necrosis factor-alpha and interleukin-1beta receptor-deficient mice. Lab Invest 2002;82:79–85.

186. de Boer WI, van Schadewijk A, Sont JK, et al. Transforming growth factor beta1 and recruitment of macrophages and mast cells in airways in chronic obstructive pulmonary disease. Am J Respir Crit Care Med 1998;158:1951–7.

187. Takizawa H, Tanaka M, Takami K, et al. Increased expression of transforming growth factor-beta1 in small airway epithelium from tobacco smokers and patients with chronic obstructive pulmonary disease (COPD). Am J Respir Crit Care Med 2001;163:1476–83.

188. Pons AR, Sauleda J, Noguera A, et al. Decreased macrophage release of TGF-beta and TIMP-1 in chronic obstructive pulmonary disease. Eur Respir J 2005;26:60–6.

189. Morris DG, Huang X, Kaminski N, et al. Loss of integrin alpha(v)beta6-mediated TGF-beta activation causes Mmp12-dependent emphysema. Nature 2003;422:169–73.

190. Feinberg MW, Jain MK, Werner F, et al. Transforming growth factor-beta 1 inhibits cytokine-mediated induction of human metalloelastase in macrophages. J Biol Chem 2000;275:25766–73.

191. Karimi K, Sarir H, Mortaz E, et al. Toll-like receptor-4 mediates cigarette smoke–induced cytokine production by human macrophages. Respir Res 2006;7:66.

192. Traves SL, Culpitt SV, Russell RE, et al. Increased levels of the chemokines GROalpha and MCP-1 in sputum samples from patients with COPD. Thorax 2002;57:590–5.

193. Finlay GA, O'Driscoll LR, Russell KJ, et al. Matrix metalloproteinase expression and production by alveolar macrophages in emphysema. Am J Respir Crit Care Med 1997;156:240–7.

194. Campbell EJ, Wald MS. Fate of human neutrophil elastase following receptor-mediated endocytosis by human alveolar macrophages. Implications for connective tissue injury. J Lab Clin Med 1983;101:527–36.

195. McGowan SE, Stone PJ, Snider GL, Franzblau C. Alveolar macrophage modulation of proteolysis by neutrophil elastase in extracellular matrix. Am Rev Respir Dis 1984;130:734–9.

196. Punturieri A, Filippov S, Allen E, et al. Regulation of elastinolytic cysteine proteinase activity in normal and cathepsin K-deficient human macrophages. J Exp Med 2000;192: 789–99.

197. Taggart CC, Lowe GJ, Greene CM, et al. Cathepsin B, L, and S cleave and inactivate secretory leucoprotease inhibitor. J Biol Chem 2001;276:33345–52.

198. Bracke K, Cataldo D, Maes T, et al. Matrix metalloproteinase-12 and cathepsin D expression in pulmonary macrophages and dendritic cells of cigarette smoke-exposed mice. Int Arch Allergy Immunol 2005;138:169–79.

199. Valenca SS, da Hora K, Castro P, et al. Emphysema and metalloelastase expression in mouse lung induced by cigarette smoke. Toxicol Pathol 2004;32:351–6.

200. Yu Q, Stamenkovic I. Cell surface-localized matrix metalloproteinase-9 proteolytically activates TGF-beta and promotes tumor invasion and angiogenesis. Genes Dev 2000;14: 163–76.

201. Davis WB, Pacht ER, Spatafora M, Martin WJ 2nd. Enhanced cytotoxic potential of alveolar macrophages from cigarette smokers. J Lab Clin Med 1988;111:293–8.

202. Hoidal JR, Fox RB, LeMarbe PA, et al. Altered oxidative metabolic responses *in vitro* of alveolar macrophages from asymptomatic cigarette smokers. Am Rev Respir Dis 1981;123:85–9.

203. Wert SE, Yoshida M, LeVine AM, et al. Increased metalloproteinase activity, oxidant production, and emphysema in surfactant protein D gene-inactivated mice. Proc Natl Acad Sci U S A 2000;97:5972–7.

204. Hubbard RC, Ogushi F, Fells GA, et al. Oxidants spontaneously released by alveolar macrophages of cigarette smokers can inactivate the active site of alpha 1-antitrypsin, rendering it ineffective as an inhibitor of neutrophil elastase. J Clin Invest 1987;80:1289–95.

205. Tomita K, Barnes PJ, Adcock IM. The effect of oxidative stress on histone acetylation and IL-8 release. Biochem Biophys Res Commun 2003;301:572–7.

206. Dekhuijzen PN. Antioxidant properties of N-acetylcysteine: their relevance in relation to chronic obstructive pulmonary disease. Eur Respir J 2004;23:629–36.

207. Kassim SY, Fu X, Liles WC, et al. NADPH oxidase restrains the matrix metalloproteinase activity of macrophages. J Biol Chem 2005;280:30201–5.

208. Tuder RM, Petrache I, Elias JA, et al. Apoptosis and emphysema: the missing link. Am J Respir Cell Mol Biol 2003;28:551–4.

209. Kasahara Y, Tuder RM, Taraseviciene-Stewart L, et al. Inhibition of VEGF receptors causes lung cell apoptosis and emphysema. J Clin Invest 2000;106:1311–9.

210. Hodge S, Hodge G, Scicchitano R, et al. Alveolar macrophages from subjects with chronic obstructive pulmonary disease are deficient in their ability to phagocytose apoptotic airway epithelial cells. Immunol Cell Biol 2003;81:289–96.

211. Santos S, Peinado VI, Ramirez J, et al. Enhanced expression of vascular endothelial growth factor in pulmonary arteries of smokers and patients with moderate chronic obstructive pulmonary disease. Am J Respir Crit Care Med 2003;167:1250–6.

212. Voelkel NF, Vandivier RW, Tuder RM. Vascular endothelial growth factor in the lung. Am J Physiol Lung Cell Mol Physiol 2006;290:L209–21.

213. Hale KA, Niewoehner DE, Cosio MG. Morphologic changes in the muscular pulmonary arteries: relationship to cigarette smoking, airway disease, and emphysema. Am Rev Respir Dis 1980;122:273–8.

214. Tuder RM, Groves B, Badesch DB, Voelkel NF. Exuberant endothelial cell growth and elements of inflammation are present in plexiform lesions of pulmonary hypertension. Am J Pathol 1994;144:275–85.

215. Yu AY, Frid MG, Shimoda LA, et al. Temporal, spatial, and oxygen-regulated expression of hypoxia-inducible factor-1 in the lung. Am J Physiol 1998;275:L818–26.

216. Yu M, Pinkerton KE, Witschi H. Short-term exposure to aged and diluted sidestream cigarette smoke enhances ozone-induced lung injury in B6C3F1 mice. Toxicol Sci 2002;65:99–106.

217. Iyer NV, Kotch LE, Agani F, et al. Cellular and developmental control of O2 homeostasis by hypoxia-inducible factor 1 alpha. Genes Dev 1998;12:149–62.

218. Nagai K, Betsuyaku T, Ito Y, et al. Decrease of vascular endothelial growth factor in macrophages from long-term smokers. Eur Respir J 2005;25:626–33.

219. Fujita M, Shannon JM, Irvin CG, et al. Overexpression of tumor necrosis factor-alpha produces an increase in lung volumes and pulmonary hypertension. Am J Physiol Lung Cell Mol Physiol 2001;280:L39–49.

220. Fujita M, Mason RJ, Cool C, et al. Pulmonary hypertension in TNF-alpha-overexpressing mice is associated with decreased VEGF gene expression. J Appl Physiol 2002;93:2162–70.

221. Cottin V, Nunes H, Brillet PY, et al. Combined pulmonary fibrosis and emphysema: a distinct underrecognised entity. Eur Respir J 2005;26:586–93.

222. Frasca JM, Auerbach O, Parks VR, Jamieson JD. Electron microscopic observations on pulmonary fibrosis and emphysema in smoking dogs. Exp Mol Pathol 1971;15:108–25.

223. Lundblad LK, Thompson-Figueroa J, Leclair T, et al. Tumor necrosis factor-alpha overexpression in lung disease: a single cause behind a complex phenotype. Am J Respir Crit Care Med 2005;171:1363–70.

224. Fichtner-Feigl S, Strober W, Kawakami K, et al. IL-13 signaling through the IL-13alpha2 receptor is involved in induction of TGF-beta1 production and fibrosis. Nat Med 2006;12:99–106.

225. Belperio JA, Dy M, Burdick MD, et al. Interaction of IL-13 and C10 in the pathogenesis of bleomycin-induced pulmonary fibrosis. Am J Respir Cell Mol Biol 2002;27:419–27.

226. Liu T, Jin H, Ullenbruch M, et al. Regulation of found in inflammatory zone 1 expression in bleomycin-induced lung fibrosis: role of IL-4/IL-13 and mediation via STAT-6. J Immunol 2004;173:3425–31.

227. Jakubzick C, Choi ES, Joshi BH, et al. Therapeutic attenuation of pulmonary fibrosis via targeting of IL-4- and IL-13-responsive cells. J Immunol 2003;171:2684–93.

228. Goldstein RH, Poliks CF, Pilch PF, et al. Stimulation of collagen formation by insulin and insulin-like growth factor I in cultures of human lung fibroblasts. Endocrinology 1989;124:964–70.

229. Prasse A, Pechkovsky DV, Toews GB, et al. A vicious circle of alveolar macrophages and fibroblasts perpetuates pulmonary fibrosis via CCL18. Am J Respir Crit Care Med 2006;173:781–92.

Small Airway Obstruction in Chronic Obstructive Pulmonary Disease

Peter D. Paré, MD, Joanne L. Wright, MD, FRCP, and Andrew Churg, MD

There are a variety of pulmonary diseases and exposures that are characterized predominantly by narrowing of the "small airways" (Table 1). Collectively, these conditions are called bronchiolitis, and they share narrowing of the lumen of "small" airways owing to pathologic processes that involve inflammation, repair, and remodeling. Small airway obstruction is also a principal feature of chronic obstructive pulmonary disease (COPD), and it is mainly this form of "bronchiolitis" that is discussed in this chapter. COPD can be defined broadly to encompass any of the variety of clinical conditions that manifest by decreased expiratory flow from the lung, or it can be defined narrowly in reference to the common condition of decreased expiratory flow caused predominantly by inhalation of cigarette smoke. It is in this narrow sense that we use COPD in this chapter. To retain any usefulness, the term should exclude specific well-defined entities characterized by persistent airway obstruction, such as asthma, bronchiectasis, and cystic fibrosis, as well as the many forms of obstructive bronchiolitis that have clearly defined etiologies, clinical characteristics, and/or pathologic findings. Although "small airways disease" is important in these conditions, we concentrate on the "small airways disease"* associated with COPD (narrow sense definition).[1]

COPD, or its synonyms chronic airflow obstruction and chronic airflow limitation, can be caused by either loss of lung elasticity or intrinsic narrowing of the small airways owing to remodeling. The process that causes loss of lung elasticity also causes the pathologic lesion of emphysema. Although the site of airflow limitation during maximal expiratory flow is the small airways, whether the predominant pathology is emphysema or airway remodeling, this chapter is devoted to a discussion of the pathogenesis, pathology, detection, and functional consequences of the small airway narrowing component of COPD. Emphysema is discussed at length in several chapters of this book.

Because irreversible airway obstruction cannot be easily attributed solely to loss of elastic recoil or airway narrowing in the vast majority of patients, use of the term COPD or its synonyms has increased. In fact, a combination of intrinsic airway narrowing and loss of lung elasticity coexists in most patients who have COPD. Although a number of investigators have reported that there are associations between the degree of small airway abnormalities and the severity of emphysema in patients who have COPD,[2] many patients have airway obstruction and small airway abnormalities on histologic examination and no emphysema. In addition, membranous and respiratory bronchiolitis tends to be more severe in the lower lobes, whereas centriacinar emphysema is more severe in the upper lobes.[3] Small airway remodeling (SAR) is more severe in patients who have centiacinar as opposed to panacinar emphysema.[4]

Despite the frequent concordance of emphysema and small airway narrowing, it is important to try to separate the relative contribution of the two processes in individual patients. It is clear that some individuals are preferentially susceptible to one or other of the processes, and it is likely that the mechanisms leading to the two pathologies are distinct. Ultimately, novel therapeutic interventions may be developed that target one or other of the lesions, and it is possible that the appropriate therapy for one process could be contraindicated in the other and vice versa.

The definition of small airways is an arbitrary one but generally refers to airways that have an internal diameter less than ≈2 to 3 mm.[5] Airways of this size may be anywhere from the fourth to the twelfth generation from the trachea[6] and may be small cartilaginous bronchi or membranous bronchioles. Normally, these airways contribute relatively little to total airway resistance, not because the resistance of individual airways is small but because there are so many airways of this size in parallel. The total cross-sectional area of the tracheobronchial tree at the eighth generation is at least an order of magnitude greater than at its narrowest point in the mainstem bronchi. Thus, airways smaller than 2 to 3 mm internal diameter normally contribute less than 30% of total airway resistance,[7–9] and considerable narrowing of these airways can occur before pulmonary function becomes impaired and symptoms develop. Despite this, it is narrowing of these airways that contributes the major increase in airway resistance in many obstructive lung diseases, including cigarette smoke–induced COPD, asthma, and bronchiectasis.[7,10,11] In children, the small airways normally contribute a larger fraction of

---

*The term "small airway disease" has been used to refer to a distinct clinical presentation that is seen in a small number of patients who have a "specific" clinical-radiologic-pathologic form of COPD.[1] We believe that the use of the term in the latter context should be abandoned, to prevent confusion. Disease of the small airways is one of the abnormalities that leads to airway obstruction in COPD; it is not a disease in its own right.

Table 1 Exposures and Clinical Conditions Associated with Bronchiolitis
Inhalation of gases, fumes, and dusts
Cigarette smoke
Irritant gases (NO_2, SO_2, ammonia, chlorine, phosgene, HCl)
Mineral dust fumes (eg, from welding)
Mineral dust particles (eg, asbestos, silica)
Grain dust
Infection
Viruses (respiratory syncytial virus, parainfluenza, adenovirus, influenza, rhinovirus, and human immunodeficiency virus [HIV])
Fungi (*Aspergillus* species and *Pneumocystis carinii*)
Bacteria (eg, *Bordetella pertussis*)
Parasites (malaria, *Cryptosporidium* species and *Microsporida*)
Miscellaneous organisms (*Mycoplasma pneumoniae* and *Chlamydia* species)
Drugs and chemicals
Hexamethonium, L-tryptophan, busulfan, bleomycin, methotrexate, lomustine, penicillamine, gold, free-base cocaine, sulfasalazine, naproxen, amiodarone, amphotericin B, acebutolol, sulindac, paraquat
Immunologic disease
Organ transplantation (bone marrow, heart-lung, lung)
Mixed connective tissue disease
Rheumatoid arthritis
Systemic lupus erythematosus
Dermatomyositis
Eosinophilic fasciitis
Sjögren syndrome
Progressive systemic sclerosis
Polymyalgia rheumatica
Miscellaneous conditions
Idiopathic pulmonary fibrosis
Extrinsic allergic alveolitis
Acute and chronic eosinophilic pneumonia
Wegener granulomatosis
Ulcerative colitis
Aspiration
Primary biliary cirrhosis
Neoplasia
Carcinoid tumor

Adapted from King TE,[125] Costabel U et al,[126] and Fraser RS et al.[127]

total airway resistance, possibly owing to a delay in airway maturation relative to lung maturation, and it has been proposed that this explains why acute infectious bronchiolitis is a more frequent and serious illness in children than in adults.[12]

It is not clear why the small airways are the most important site of increased resistance in disease. One possibility is that inhaled toxic particles are preferentially deposited in these generations of airways; this has been demonstrated for model particles with aerodynamic diameters less than 5 microns and presumably is true of smoke particles as well.[13]

Alternatively, there may be relatively slower clearance of toxic substances owing to anatomic differences such as a lower density of ciliated epithelial cells. The walls of airways of this size are relatively thick compared with their luminal diameter, and it is possible that inflammatory repair processes that affect the whole tracheobronchial tree preferentially narrow these airways. Tiddens and colleagues showed that thickening of the cartilaginous airway wall also occurs in cigarette smoke–induced COPD, and the degree of thickening in the large airways correlates with estimates of inflammation in the membranous bronchioles, which are the site of predominant obstruction.[14] More recently, Nakano and colleagues found that thickening of the apical segmental bronchus of the right upper lobe was associated with airflow obstruction in COPD, suggesting that large airway thickening may be a surrogate for the functionally important small airway narrowing.[15]

Pathogenesis of Small Airway Narrowing in COPD

The mechanism responsible for the narrowing of the small airways in COPD is incompletely understood. It is related to one or more of several processes and abnormalities, including (1) loss of elastic recoil in the peribronchiolar alveolar interstitial tissue;[16] (2) loss of the alveolar attachments to the outer wall of the small airways;[17] (3) increased bronchiolar surface tension owing to a protein-rich inflammatory exudate, resulting in an alteration of the relationship between pressure and cross-sectional area of the airways; this is comparable to the change in the pressure-volume curve of the lung, which occurs in the presence of pulmonary edema; (4) competition for space between the terminal bronchiole and the dilated centrilobular emphysematous space;[18] (5) accumulation of mucus in the airway lumen secondary to goblet cell hyperplasia and impaired mucociliary clearance;[19] (6) an inflammatory cell infiltrate within the airway wall;[20] and (7) fibrosis of the airway wall, resulting in thickening of the wall at the expense of the lumen (small airway remodeling—SAR).[19,21]

Among these mechanisms, the role of SAR is well established; however, remarkably little is known about the pathogenesis of this lesion. The usual assumption is that SAR is a reflection of cigarette smoke–induced inflammation,[22–25] but this idea is largely an unproven extrapolation from the extensive evidence for a role for inflammation in the development of emphysema. More recently, it has been suggested that

inflammation and airway remodeling in SAR may be independent events.[22,26]

In many senses, such a conclusion would not be surprising since airway wall fibrosis with subsequent luminal narrowing and distortion appears to be central to cigarette smoke–induced SAR, and there is increasing evidence in the literature that, at least for interstitial fibrosis, inflammation and fibrosis are separate and often (depending on the model) unrelated events in which fibrosis is actually caused by injury to and/or repeated stimulation of the epithelium and subsequent epithelial production and release of growth factors that influence underlying mesenchymal cells.[27–29]

Role of Growth Factors in Cigarette Smoke–Induced SAR

The most detailed literature on the pathogenesis of SAR concerns the role of growth factors, especially transforming growth factor β (TGF-β). TGF-β is a powerful profibrotic cytokine that causes, among other effects, collagen production by fibroblasts, smooth muscle cell hyperplasia, and differentiation of fibroblasts to myofibroblasts, cells that are important in both matrix production and extracellular matrix contraction.

Studies on biopsies or resected lung specimens from humans have consistently shown the presence of TGF-β in large and small airway epithelial cells and other airway wall cells.[30–33] Takizawa and colleagues found that cultured human small airway cells spontaneously release TGF-β_1.[32] However, proof of a role for TGF-β based on human material is elusive, and the data have sometimes been contradictory. de Boer and colleagues found a significant negative correlation between forced expiratory volume in 1 second (FEV$_1$) and the level of expression of TGF-β assessed by immunostaining and in situ reverse transcriptase–polymerase chain reaction (RT-PCR) in bronchial biopsies. However, Vignola and colleagues reported a positive correlation between the number of airway cells expressing TGF-β and basement membrane thickness in chronic bronchitis.[31] Such studies, which rely on biopsies of large airways, are based on the assumption that large airway growth factor expression correlates with the expression level in small airways. Takizawa and colleagues used a special, very fine, bronchoscope to obtain cells from the small airways.[32] They found that gene expression levels for TGF-β_1 correlated with pack-years of smoking and severity of airflow obstruction. However, protein levels of TGF-β and release of active TGF-β from cultured airway epithelial cells did not differ between smokers with and without COPD. Aubert and colleagues demonstrated expression of *TGF-β1* in small airway epithelial and wall cells using in situ hybridization and immunochemistry, but they were unable to show differences among asthmatics, smokers with COPD, and smokers without COPD.[33]

Interpretation of studies of expression of *TGF-β* by measurement of messenger ribonucleic acid (mRNA) or by immunohistochemistry is complicated by the fact that TGF-β is produced with the active TGF-β moiety complexed to a latency-associated peptide (LAP) that prevents biologic activity, and this "small latent complex" is itself complexed to the latent TGF-β binding protein, which binds the inactive cytokine to matrix components. Thus, gene expression at the message or protein level does not necessarily correlate with TGF-β activity. Furthermore, detection of active versus latent TGF-β by immunochemistry is extremely difficult, and almost all studies report only the presence of latent protein. Taken together, these studies support the conclusion that TGF-β certainly exists in the airway epithelium and wall and thus is potentially available to exert fibrotic effects. However, the human data do not really shed light on when and how this occurs.

More direct evidence supporting a role for TGF-β in SAR has come from animal experiments and studies of tracheal explants. Kenyon and colleagues showed that intratracheal instillation of recombinant TGF-β1 to BALB/C mice resulted in increased expression of type I and type III collagen and greater total collagen content in the subepithelial layer of lobar bronchi and more distal airways.[34] Of particular note, this process occurred without any inflammatory response.

Churg and colleagues showed that mice exposed to cigarette smoke daily for 6 months develop SAR.[35] The most prominent feature of the remodeling was an increase in collagen. Using laser capture microdissection of small airways and real-time RT-PCR, they found abrupt but transient upregulation of *TGF-β1* and its downstream mediator, connective tissue growth factor (*CTGF*), as well as procollagen type I after a single smoke exposure. (*CTGF*, stimulated by TGF-β1, is believed to be the growth factor responsible for actual activation of collagen-producing genes in fibroblasts.) Following a single smoke exposure, upregulation of gene expression was most marked at 2 hours and declined to control values by 24 hours, exactly the opposite time course of that found for lavaged inflammatory cells.[36] This observation suggests that, at least initially, inflammation is not required for SAR.

With repeated daily smoke exposure for 6 months, there was persistent upregulation of *CTGF* and procollagen type I.[35] Phospho-Smad 2, a direct mediator of TGF-β effects, was also elevated over 6 months, but, paradoxically, *TGF-β1* expression itself decreased. Since there was evidence of persistent TGF-β signaling (elevated *CTGF* gene expression and phospho-Smad 2 staining) throughout this period, it is possible that there had been increases in the total amount of latent TGF-β over this period. This could come about if TGF-β1 mRNA was stabilized or if there were posttranscriptional modifications of the protein after smoke exposure.

Churg and colleagues also showed that *PDGF-A* and *-B* gene expression levels were transiently elevated after a single smoke exposure and that *PDGF-B* levels remained markedly elevated throughout the 6 months of exposure.[35] Aubert and colleagues also detected *PDGF*-producing cells in the wall of small airways in human lung using immunochemistry.[37] PDGF can cause increased collagen production by fibroblasts, but its most important role is as a stimulator of fibroblast

proliferation, and the combination of PDGF and TGF-β can upregulate collagen production manyfold.

In aggregate, these findings provide strong support for the idea that smoke induces growth factor production in the small airway walls. Some data also exist concerning the mechanism that causes TGF-β production and activation. Wang and colleagues used rat tracheal explants as an inflammatory cell-free model of the airway wall, with the acknowledged limitation that the explants are of a large airway.[38,39] The explants were exposed to whole smoke in air and then maintained for various periods in an air-exposed organ culture system with basal feeding. Twenty-four hours after a 15-minute exposure to smoke, there was an increase in both procollagen gene expression and hydroxyproline, a marker of collagen content. Smoke exposure caused release of active TGF-β1, measured by a specific enzyme-linked immunosorbent assay, and release was prevented by the oxidant scavenger tetramethythiourea. Within 1 hour after the beginning of smoke exposure, immunostaining for phospho-Smad2 was present, largely in the airway epithelial cells. Over the next hour, the staining appeared to shift to the underlying mesenchymal cells. *CTGF* gene expression was elevated within 2 hours of smoke exposure. Figure 1 shows a schematic that summarizes the potential pathways involving TGF-β signaling in the genesis of SAR.

To investigate how smoke caused TGF-β release, a cell-free system was used in which recombinant human TGF-β LAP was exposed to smoke-conditioned medium. This exposure led to oxidation of the LAP and release of active TGF-β.[40–42]

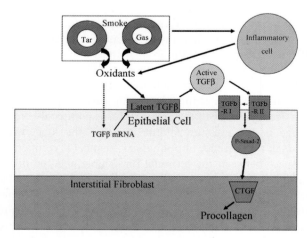

FIGURE 1. This schematic shows possible pathways of transforming growth factor β (TGF-β) activation and signaling in small airway remodeling. Oxidants in cigarette smoke activate latent TGF-β on the epithelial cell surface (or TGF-β attached to the matrix), leading to TGF-β signaling through TGF-β receptors I and II and the phosphorylation of Smads. This causes increased release of connective tissue growth factor (CTGF), which stimulates increased production of collagen by interstitial fibroblasts and myofibroblasts. Smoke-evoked inflammatory cells may play a similar role by releasing oxidants that activate latent TGF-β.

Oxidation of LAP is known to release active TGF-β, and when the same experiment was carried out using recombinant latent TGF-β, the release of active TGF-β was blocked by the addition of an oxidant scavenger. These experiments suggest that direct, smoke-mediated, oxidant-driven induction of growth factor (at least TGF-β) signaling in the airway wall may be important in the pathogenesis of SAR and that SAR does not necessarily require exogenous inflammatory cells.

Role of Matrix Metalloproteinases

Although the matrix metalloproteinases (MMPs) were originally described as enyzmes that break down matrix proteins, they are now known to have a much broader role, and it has been suggested that their principal function is to act on or release chemokines and cytokines in such a way as to increase their activity.[43]

There is little direct evidence concerning the role of MMPs in SAR in smokers; however, MMPs have been examined as potential mediators of remodeling in the airways in asthma. In particular, MMP-9 has generally been found to be increased in both human airway biopsies and the airways in animal models of asthma. Although some studies have not confirmed this, blockade of MMP-9 activity or use of MMP-9 knockout mice reduce airway remodeling in these models.[44–47] Since MMP-9 can activate latent TGF-β and act directly to increase fibroblast collagen production,[44] involvement of MMP-9 in airway remodeling makes intuitive sense. Atkinson and Senior suggested that it is actually the ratio of MMP-9 to tissue inhibitor of metalloproteinase 1 that drives the deposition or removal of collagen in the airways, with low ratios favoring collagen deposition.[44] Postma and Timens proposed that the balance of the proteolytic capacity of MMPs and the fibrogenic activity of TGF-β might be responsible for the different responses observed in the airways and parenchyma in cigarette smokers.[26] In a recent study, two of us found that a selective dual MMP-9–MMP-12 inhibitor not only ameliorated emphysema but completely prevented SAR in smoke-exposed guinea pigs.[48]

Role of Smoke-Evoked Inflammation

An increase in lavage inflammatory cells is a consistent finding in cigarette smokers, and, as noted above, "inflammation" is usually assumed to be the cause of SAR, despite the lack of direct evidence. One possible mechanism by which inflammatory cells could produce or augment SAR stems from the observation just described that smoke oxidatively activates TGF-β. Since activated inflammatory cells release oxidants, and cells from smokers release more oxidants than those from nonsmokers,[49] inflammatory cells might act to cause even more growth factor release and thus potentiate the formation of active TGF-β.

Direct effects of cytokine mediators in SAR are also possible. Interleukin (IL)-1β levels are increased in cigarette smokers, and Lappalainen and colleagues reported that transgenic mice that overexpress IL-1β develop both emphysema and SAR, manifest as increased small airway collagen.[50] Of particular interest is the observation that these mice also have elevated levels of MMP-12, MMP-2, and MMP-9, providing additional support for a possible role of MMPs in releasing TGF-β.

Vascular endothelial growth factor (VEGF) is an inflammatory cell chemoattractant, and levels of both VEGF and its receptors are increased in large and small airways in COPD.[25] Immunohistochemically determined levels of VEGF appear to correlate positively with immunohistochemical staining for TGF-β and inversely with FEV_1.

Role of Collagen Remodeling

We have observed that the collagen in the small airways in guinea pigs chronically exposed to smoke differs from that in air-exposed control animals (JLW, unpublished observations, 2007). The collagen fibers appear thicker in the smoke-exposed animals and on circular polarization appear both more mature and more coherently aligned. Such "dense" collagen should be stiffer than normal and may thus be associated with rigid and distorted airways.

Role of Mechanical Strain

Milic-Emili recently proposed an additional potential mechanism that could contribute to the development of SAR in smokers.[51] In the early stages of smoke–induced lung damage, premature airway closure occurs at low lung volumes; later airway closure and dynamic collapse accompanied by flow limitation occur during tidal breathing. Airway closure and collapse distort the airway wall, and, at least in theory, this mechanical strain could injure the airway and accelerate remodeling.[51] Choe and colleagues recently reported that a model airway consisting of bronchial epithelial cells cultured on a matrix of collagen and fibroblasts and exposed to dynamic mechanical strain demonstrated "remodeling," manifest as increased production of MMP-2, MMP-9, collagen III, and collagen IV.[52] Collagen III colocalized with myofibroblasts near the epithelial cells, suggesting epithelial control of the fibrotic response. Their model system was primarily designed to mimic the effects of increased mechanical strain on the epithelium as occurs in asthma during airway smooth muscle contraction, but similar effects might apply in smoke–induced SAR as well since this lesion is also characterized by increased collagen in the subepithelial airway compartment.

Pathology of Small Airway Narrowing in COPD

The pathology of the small airways in COPD can be broadly described as a mucosa-based chronic inflammatory process with evidence of repeated cycles of injury and repair.[53] The severity of different aspects of the inflammatory/repair reaction in membranous bronchioles can be measured using semiquantitative grading schema. Bronchioles are examined microscopically and scored for pathologic features, including inflammatory cell infiltration, hyperplasia of goblet cells, squamous metaplasia, fibrosis, smooth muscle hyperplasia, and pigment deposition (Figure 2). The earlier grading methods scored pathologic features as either present or absent,[54,55] modified to indicate the percentage of airways affected.

Since these schema could not provide information concerning the severity of the individual lesions, more elaborate systems were developed,[56,57] which involve assigning each airway a separate score (0–3) for a variety of parameters, based on comparison with a series of standard images. To provide an estimation of overall severity for each parameter, all of the airway scores are added and then expressed as a percentage of the maximal possible score (number of airways times 3). Addition of the scores for all parameters provides a total pathologic score for that individual. Using such methods, it was found that assessment of a single lobe was relatively representative of the lung as a whole.[58–60] Such grading schema allowed investigators to extend their qualitative descriptions in a semiquantitative fashion[61] and to test how these morphologic findings relate to airflow obstruction.[62,63] A valuable contribution of this type of analysis was the demonstration that young smokers characteristically develop collections of macrophages in the lumen of the respiratory bronchioles.[64] Other studies have shown that the membranous and respiratory bronchioles in cigarette smokers have an increase in mural and luminal inflammation, accompanied by an increased amount of fibrous tissue and goblet cell metaplasia.[65,66] More quantitative morphometric estimates of airway abnormalities can also be used, such as measurements of the number of inflammatory cells per square millimeter of airway wall, the thickness of the airway wall,[60] the ratio of airway size to the size of the accompanying pulmonary artery,[67] and the number of airways per unit of lung area or volume.[68] Smokers and ex-smokers have been shown to have increased numbers of neutrophils and mononuclear cells in the airway walls,[69] and CD8+ lymphocytes are increased in the smokers who develop airflow obstruction.[70–74] In some studies, the numbers of inflammatory cell types also correlated with the severity of airflow obstruction.[70,74]

More recently, Hogg and his colleagues developed rigorous methods based on the multilevel cascade design of Cruz-Orive and Weibel that allow a quantitative estimate of specific microscopic abnormalities for the whole lung.[19,75] Using this approach, the cut surface of the lung or a computed tomographic image of the lung is used as the reference, and all measurements at higher magnification are ultimately expressed with this "volume" as the denominator.[75] They conducted a comprehensive and quantitative morphometric examination of the dimensions and cellular changes in the membranous bronchioles of smokers and related these changes to the degree of airway obstruction. They found that the degree of airflow limitation was strongly associated with an increase in the volume of tissue in the wall and to the presence of an inflammatory mucus exudate in the lumen of the small airways. Airflow obstruction was related to an accumulation of polymorphonuclear

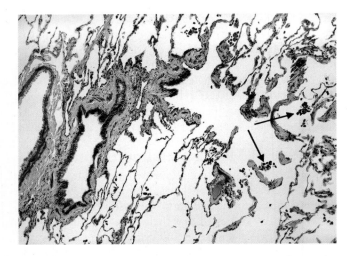

FIGURE 2. Abnormal membranous bronchiole and subtending respiratory bronchiole, both showing thickened and distorted walls. Note the increased numbers of macrophages in and surrounding the respiratory bronchiole (*arrows*) (Masson trichrome stain; original magnification, 35 ×).

leukocytes, macrophages, CD4+ and CD8+ lymphocytes, and B lymphocytes and the presence of lymphoid follicles. In obstructed individuals, all components of the airway wall (epithelium, lamina propria, smooth muscle, and adventitial tissue) were increased relative to the length of the basement membrane.

The significance of the presence of lymphoid follicles (Figure 3) in the peripheral airways of the most obstructed individuals is unknown. This finding indicates the development of a local adaptive immune response, but it is unclear what antigen(s) is driving this response. Possibilities include an autoimmune response to altered lung proteins[76,77] or a robust immune response to the microbial colonization and infection known to occur in the later stages of COPD.[78]

Although repeated injury and repair can cause thickening of the airway wall, airway wall thickening by itself does not lead to an increase in resistance or a decrease in maximal expiratory flow unless it causes narrowing of the lumen of the airways. Airway resistance is inversely related to the fourth power of the radius according to Poiseuille's law. This means that a 10% decrease in the radius of an airway causes a ≈50% increase in resistance, and a halving of the radius causes a 16-fold increase in resistance. Thus, even if airway remodeling causes relatively minor degrees of luminal encroachment, substantial increases in resistance can be produced. The potential impact of airway remodeling on the total resistance of the tracheobronchial tree has been demonstrated using computational models.[79,80] These models illustrate the potential interaction of the multiple factors that contribute to airway narrowing in COPD; the combination of relatively minor degrees of airway wall thickening, increased luminal content, smooth muscle contraction, increased surface tension, and loss of elasticity of the surrounding parenchyma can interact to have substantial effects on airway resistance.

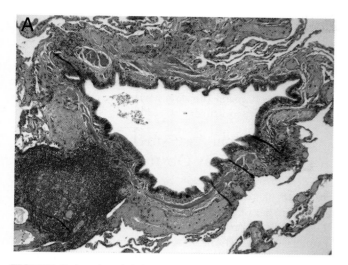
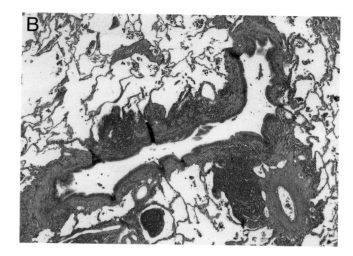

FIGURE 3. Lymphocytic inflammation in a small bronchus and a bronchiole from a patient with Global Initiative for Chronic Obstructive Lung Disease (GOLD) stage III chronic obstructive pulmonary disease. In the larger airway (*A*), the lymphoid tissue forms a distinct germinal center. In the membranous bronchiole (*B*), there are multiple lymphoid follicles within the thickened wall (hematoxylin-eosin stain; original magnification, 60 ×).

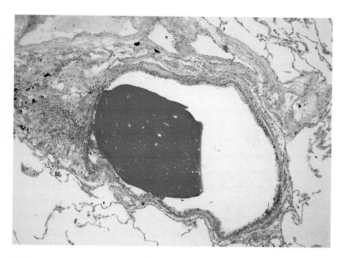

FIGURE 4. A membranous bronchiole in the lung of a patient with chronic obstructive pulmonary disease demonstrating goblet cell metaplasia of the epithelium and abundant intraluminal mucus. Note also the thickened airway wall and increased numbers of chronic inflammatory cells within the wall (periodic acid-Schiff stain; original magnification, 60 ×).

There is evidence for increased intraluminal mucus and an exudate containing inflammatory cells and mucus in both the central and peripheral airways of subjects with COPD (Figure 4). Aikawa and colleagues calculated that in the peripheral airways, 19.6% of the available lumen was occupied by "mucus" in patients with severe COPD (FEV$_1$ ≈46% predicted) compared with 0.6% in normal lungs.[81] In more recent work, Hogg and colleagues found that an increased ratio of mucus to luminal area correlated with airflow obstruction in subjects with a range of airflow obstruction (GOLD stages 0–IV) and that the relationship was independent of measures of airway wall remodeling in a multivariate analysis.[19]

The original method used to assess peripheral airway narrowing was the determination of the internal bronchiolar diameter, with the measurement taken on cross sections, or as the short axes of elliptically sectioned airways.[82] Using this methodology, it was shown that the airways of current and ex-smokers are thickened or have decreased internal diameter and/or a shift in size distribution toward the smaller sizes. This method assumes that the airways in the fixed tissues were inflated with a transmural pressure similar to that which distends the airway *in vivo*, which is problematic since excised or postmortem lungs are rarely inflated with fixative to *in-vivo* volume. This potential artifact can be circumvented if true cross sections, rather than elliptical sections, are obtained. In these airways, the internal lumen perimeter (Pi) can be used as an index of size by assuming that in life the airway was circular (ie, Pi = circumference).[83] However, this method is also subject to artifact in that the narrowed airway in COPD may never conform to a circular profile *in vivo*. However, if one makes the assumption that the airway internal perimeter or basement membrane perimeter remain constant as airways narrow, these measurements can be employed as convenient "yardsticks" to compare the area occupied by various airway wall constituents. The data collected can be expressed as a mean or median value or by construction of histograms or as cumulative distribution curves.[84] The findings of a thickened airway wall and a shift toward decreased luminal area have been confirmed using these techniques in the lungs of subjects who have mild to moderate emphysema or decreased airflow without emphysema.[84,85] It should be remembered that these methods are valid only if standard morphometric random techniques are employed to prevent sample bias since airway luminal diameter will vary according to airway generation. An alternate method to assess airway size is by comparison with the size of the adjacent pulmonary artery; the ratio of the airway diameter to the diameter of the accompanying pulmonary artery should be roughly 1.[67]

In addition to measuring total bronchial wall thickness, it is possible to measure the thickness of the various constituents of the wall. The bronchiolar wall can be divided into three compartments: (1) an inner wall, consisting of epithelium, basement membrane, and lamina propria; (2) an outer wall, consisting of the connective tissue between the muscle layer and the surrounding parenchyma (the adventitia); and (3) the smooth muscle layer.[86] By using the basement membrane length as a yardstick of airway size, the area occupied by the tissue in the different compartments can be quantified.[83] The results of several such studies have shown that all components of the airway wall are thickened in smokers who develop COPD compared with smokers who do not.[19,84,85] The wall thickness measured morphometrically in these lungs correlated significantly with the semiquantitative pathology score,[84] with airway responsiveness to inhaled methacholine,[87] and with measures of airflow obstruction.

Opazo Saez and colleagues measured the amount and function of airway smooth muscle from peripheral airways of obstructed and nonobstructed smokers.[88] The airways of the obstructed smokers contained more smooth muscle, and the muscle was able to generate more force and stress (force/cross-sectional area) than in nonobstructed smokers.

In addition to being narrower, the small airways of subjects who have COPD are irregular and distorted. Bronchial casts have demonstrated widespread airway stenoses of variable length with either an eccentric or a concentric arrangement. Three-dimensional reconstruction of the peripheral airways from serial sections has revealed areas of stenosis, dilatation, and tortuosity, as well as rough and irregular airway lumina.[89,90] A simpler method to estimate small airway distortion is determination of the conformity/deformity index. This index is based on the assumption that airways approximate cylinders and that sections through the cylinders should therefore be round or elliptical.[91–93] Deviations from these shapes provide a quantitative measurement of airway distortion that improves on simple descriptions.[93–99] Although this index indicates that the airways in patients who have COPD are irregular and distorted, it does not provide any information as to whether the distortion is intrinsic to the airway, secondary to emphysematous loss of support, or some combination of both.

The small airways are imbedded in the lung parenchyma and rely for patency on the distending force applied by the tensed alveolar walls that attach to the adventitial layer of the airway. A morphologic estimate of this force can be determined by counting the number of intact alveolar walls that insert into the outer perimeter of membranous airways per unit length. Loss of the alveolar attachments was noted in the early descriptions of emphysema,[94] but its importance was not fully appreciated until quantitative estimates of the number of attachments were compared with lung function tests.[100,101] Various investigations have demonstrated a decreased number of attachments in emphysema[102–106] and

in smokers compared with nonsmokers,[107,108] as well as correlations between the loss of attachments and airflow limitation.[106–108] Although loss of alveolar attachments can accompany emphysema and the pathogenesis of the lesion is probably very similar, it causes decreased expiratory flow by a different mechanism (airway narrowing as opposed to decreased driving pressure).

Functional Assessment of Small Airway Obstruction

The demonstration in 1968 by Hogg and colleagues that airways smaller than 3 mm in internal diameter are the most important sites of increase in resistance in patients who have COPD led to the development of tests to detect abnormalities of small airway function.[7,109–111] The hope was that a test that could detect abnormal function in the airways prior to the onset of a decrease in FEV_1 would allow the identification of a subset of smokers who had preclinical COPD and were therefore at risk for the development of symptomatic disease. It was hoped that intensive interventions in such subjects, such as smoking cessation campaigns, might be more efficacious than a program targeting all smokers.

The so-called small airway tests that were developed included the measurement of the frequency dependence of dynamic compliance (Cdyn), the single-breath nitrogen washout ($\Delta N_2/L$, closing volume and closing capacity), the density dependence of maximal expiratory flow, and flows at lower lung volumes (FEF_{25-75} and the instantaneous forced expiratory flow rates at 50% and 25% of vital capacity). Other than the FEF_{25-75} and $\dot{V}max_{50}$, which are measured on spirometric tracings and flow-volume curves, these tests are no longer performed on a routine or even an experimental basis. However, for the historical record, we include a brief description of these tests and the rationale behind them. Frequency dependence of Cdyn is a decrease in compliance with increasing frequency of breathing. In normal individuals, compliance remains constant as the frequency of breathing increases up to 60 to 90 breaths per minute. Cdyn decreases as frequency increases if there are substantially different time constants in peripheral parallel lung units. In the presence of heterogeneous small airway narrowing, Cdyn decreases with increasing respiratory frequency; in fact, some smokers who do not have a significant decline in maximal expiratory flow do show frequency dependence of Cdyn.[112]

Because the small airways close at low lung volumes,[113] the single-breath nitrogen washout, which allows the measurement of closing volume and closing capacity, was an attractive test for the detection of early abnormalities in COPD. The single-breath test also gives a measure of the evenness of lung emptying. The slope of the alveolar plateau (phase 3) would be flat if all lung units emptied homogeneously. Sequential emptying occurs if there are regional differences in small airway resistance and/or airspace compliance and the concentration of nitrogen increases progressively as exhalation progresses. Both closing volume and the slope of phase 3 are abnormal in some smokers.[109] However, these tests of "small airway function" may be abnormal even when the decrease in maximal expiratory flow is caused by loss of lung elasticity.[114]

Density dependence of maximal expiratory flow should theoretically decrease in patients who have small airway narrowing because the equal pressure point moves from large to small airways, where the flow more closely conforms to laminar conditions than the turbulent flow regimens, which dominate in the larger airways. The less dense helium-oxygen mixture used to test density dependence has a beneficial effect only if the flow regimen is turbulent. However, in practice, the density dependence of maximal expiratory flow did not prove to be an effective screening test and did not appear to relate to pathologic abnormalities in small airways.[115]

Decreased expiratory flow at low lung volumes should also reflect small airway narrowing. During most of the FEV_1 maneuver, flow either is not limited or is limited at choke points in central airways. Because the equal-pressure point and choke points move peripherally in the lung at lower lung volumes, flow at these volumes ($\dot{V}max_{50}, \dot{V}max_{25}*$, and FEF_{25-75}) is influenced to a greater extent by narrowing at these sites.

The basic premise behind the hypothesis that small airway tests would predict later decline in FEV_1 was that they are more sensitive than simple spirometry; however, there is considerable evidence that this is incorrect. Changes in FEV_1 and FEV_1/forced vital capacity (FVC) parallel those in the small airway tests,[116–118] and although the absolute changes in FEV_1 may be less than those in small airway test values, they are of equal or greater significance because the coefficients of variation of FEV_1 and FVC are much smaller. The results of longitudinal studies have, in general, not confirmed the hypothesis that abnormalities in small airway tests will predict longitudinal decline in FEV_1.[119,120] In fact, alterations in spirometry that occur in some young smokers probably identify those at risk.[121] Because spirometry is easier and cheaper to perform, it remains the most valuable test in the clinical management and epidemiologic investigation of patients who have or at risk of developing small airway obstruction and COPD.[122]

Imaging of Small Airways

Although the resolution of high-resolution computed tomography (HRCT) is not sufficient to accurately measure the dimensions of 2 mm diameter airways, there is increasing evidence that the dimensions of larger airways, easily visible on CT, provide a surrogate estimate of small airway dimensions (Figure 5). The fact that the thickness and wall area to lumen area ratio of the apical segmental bronchus of the right upper lobe measured on CT were shown to be associated with airflow

obstruction in smokers, independently of the degree of emphysema, was the first observation to suggest this.[123] Subsequently, Nakano and colleagues compared the dimensions of all airways

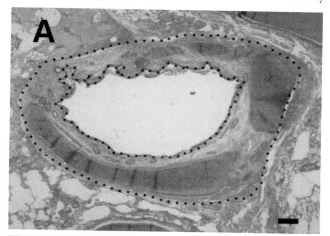

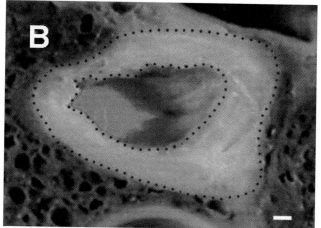

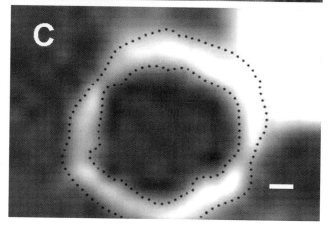

FIGURE 5. This three-part image shows the same small bronchus microscopically (*A*), macroscopically (*B*), and on a high-resolution computed tomographic (CT) image (*C*). To do this comparison, a resected lung was sectioned in the same plane as the CT images, and the corresponding lung and CT slices were matched using anatomic markers such as airways and blood vessels. High-resolution CT images have been shown to provide reliable estimates of the airway wall dimensions, although actual airway wall area and thickness tends to be overestimated in smaller airways. The dotted lines indicate the luminal and adventitial border of the airway.

---

*$\dot{V}max_{50}$ and $\dot{V}max_{25}$ are abbreviations for maximal expiratory flow at 50 and 25% of vital capacity respectively. FEF 25–75 is the average expiratory flow between 25 and 75% of expired volume during a maximal expiratory maneuver.

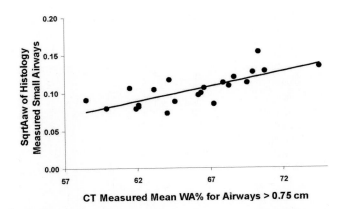

FIGURE 6. The mean wall area percentage (WA%) measured on computed tomography (CT) for all airways with an internal perimeter > 0.75 cm for each of 21 subjects is plotted against the mean square root of the wall area measured microscopically on membranous bronchioles in the same subjects. The mean internal perimeter of the membranous bronchioles was 4 mm, which corresponds to an internal diameter ≈1.3 mm). The R^2 value for this relationship was .56, and the p value was < .01. These data suggest that the dimensions of the small bronchi that can be adequately visualized and measured on CT scans serve as a valid surrogate for the dimensions of the bronchioles, which are the primary site of increased resistance in chronic obstructive pulmonary disease. WA% is calculated as wall area/wall area + lumen area × 100.

visible on CT with the dimensions of the membranous bronchioles measured morphometrically in the excised lungs of 21 smokers.[15] Although the CT overestimated airway wall area and underestimated lumen area, the wall area percentage (wall area/lumen area + wall area × 100) was related to the mean wall area/lumen perimeter of 1 to 3 mm diameter airways in the same lungs (Figure 6).

The independent relationship between the degree of airflow obstruction and CT estimates of airway remodeling and emphysema has been confirmed in a much larger (>1,100 individuals) study of the genetics of COPD.[124] Since this was a family-based study, the authors were able to estimate the familial concordance of these phenotypes. They found that the siblings of subjects who had predominant emphysema on CT were also more likely to have emphysema on CT, and, similarly, the siblings of subjects who had more severe airway remodeling were more likely to have airway remodeling. This suggests that shared genes (and/or environmental factors other than cigarette smoking) contribute to the predominant pathophysiologic process in individual subjects with COPD.

Acknowledgments

We would like to acknowledge the support of the Canadian Institutes of Health Research (grants 42539 and 81407) and GlaxoSmithKline, which supported the studies investigating the use of HRCT for measuring airway dimensions.

References

1. Macklem PT, Thurlbeck WM, Fraser RG, et al: Chronic obstructive disease of small airways. Ann Intern Med 1971;74:167–77.

2. Linhartova A, Anderson AE Jr. Small airways in severe panlobular emphysema: mural thickening and premature closure. Am Rev Respir Dis 1983;127:42–5.

3. Wright JL, Wiggs BJ, Hogg JC. Airway disease in upper and lower lobes in lungs of patients with and without emphysema. Thorax 1984;39:282–5.

4. Kim WD, Ling SH, Coxson HO, et al. The association between small airway obstruction and emphysema phenotypes in chronic obstructive pulmonary disease. Chest 2007; 131:1372–8.

5. Macklem P, Mead J. Resistance of central and peripheral airways measured by a retrograde catheter. J Appl Physiol 1967;22:395–401.

6. Weibel ER. Morphometry of the human lung. New York: Academic Press; 1963.

7. Hogg JC, Macklem PT, Thurlbeck WM. Site and nature of airway obstruction in chronic obstructive lung disease. N Engl J Med 1968;268:1355–60.

8. Van Brabandt H, Cauberghs M, Verbeken E, et al. Partitioning of pulmonary impedance in excised human and canine lungs. J Appl Physiol 1983;55:1733–42.

9. Yanai M, Sekizawa K, Ohrui T, et al. Site of airway obstruction in pulmonary disease: direct measurement of intrabronchial pressure. J Appl Physiol 1992;72:1016–2.

10. Wagner EM, Liu MC, Weinmann GG, et al. Peripheral lung resistance in normal and asthmatic subjects. Am Rev Respir Dis 1990;141:584–8.

11. Roberts HR, Wells AU, Milne DG, et al. Airflow obstruction in bronchiectasis: correlation between computed tomography features and pulmonary function tests. Thorax 2000;55:198–204.

12. Hogg JC, Williams J, Richardson JB, et al. Age as a factor in the distribution of lower-airway conductance and in the pathologic anatomy of obstructive lung disease. N Engl J Med 1970;282:1283–7.

13. Gerrity TR, Lee PS, Hass FJ, et al. Calculated deposition of inhaled particles in the airway generations of normal subjects. J Appl Physiol 1979;47:867–73.

14. Tiddens HA, Paré PD, Hogg JC, et al. Cartilaginous airway dimensions and airflow obstruction in human lungs. Am J Respir Crit Care Med 1995;152:260–6.

15. Nakano Y, Muro S, Sakai H, et al. Computed tomographic measurements of airway dimensions and emphysema in smokers. Correlation with lung function. Am J Respir Crit Care Med 2000;162(3 Pt 1):1102–8.

16. Petty TL, Silvers GW, Stanford RE, et al. Radial traction and small airway disease in excised human lungs. Am Rev Respir Dis 1986;133:132–5.

17. Cosio MG, Shiner RJ, Saetta M, et al. Alveolar fenestrae in smokers: relationship with light microscopic and functional abnormalities. Am Rev Respir Dis 1986;133:126–31.

18. Verbeken EK, Cauberghs M, van de Woestijne KP. Membranous bronchioles and connective tissue network of normal and emphysematous lungs. J Appl Physiol 1996;81:2468–80.

19. Hogg JC, Chu F, Utokaparch S, et al. The nature of small-airway obstruction in chronic obstructive pulmonary disease. N Engl J Med 2004;350:2645–53.

20. Hogg JC. Pathophysiology of airflow limitation in chronic obstructive pulmonary disease. Lancet 2004;364:709–21.

21. Verbeken EK, Cauberghs M, Lauweryns JM, van de Woestijne KP. Anatomy of membranous bronchioles in normal, senile and emphysematous human lungs. J Appl Physiol 1994;77:1875–84.

22. Jeffery PK. Remodeling in asthma and chronic obstructive lung disease. Am J Respir Crit Care Med 2001;164:S28–S38.

23. Molfino NA, Jeffery PK. Chronic obstructive pulmonary disease: histopathology, inflammation and potential therapies. Pulm Pharmacol Ther 2007;20:462–72

24. Papi A, Luppi F, Franco F, Fabbri LM. Pathophysiology of exacerbations of chronic obstructive pulmonary disease. Proc Am Thorac Soc 2006;3:245–51.

25. Barnes PJ, Shapiro SD, Pauwels RA. Chronic obstructive pulmonary disease: molecular and cellular mechanisms. Eur Respir J 2003;22:672–88.

26. Postma DS, Timens W. Remodeling in asthma and chronic obstructive pulmonary disease. Proc Am Thorac Soc 2006;3:434–9.

27. Gauldie J, Kolb M, Sime PJ. A new direction in the pathogenesis of idiopathic pulmonary fibrosis? Respir Res 2002;3:1.

28. Chapman HA. Disorders of lung matrix remodeling. J Clin Invest 2004;113:148–57.

29. Selman M, King TE, Pardo A. Idiopathic pulmonary fibrosis: prevailing and evolving hypotheses about its pathogenesis and implications for therapy. Ann Intern Med 2001;134:136–51.

30. de Boer WI, van Schadewijk A, Sont JK, et al. Transforming growth factor-β_1 and recruitment of macrophages and mast cells in airways in chronic obstructive pulmonary disease. Am J Respir Crit Care Med 1998;158:1951–7.

31. Vignola AM, Chanez P, Chiappara G, et al. Transforming growth factor-β expression in mucosal biopsies in asthma and chronic bronchitis. Am J Respir Crit Care Med 1997;156:591–9.

32. Takizawa H, Tanaka M, Takami K, et al. Increased expression of transforming growth factor-β_1 in small airway epithelium from tobacco smokers and patients with chronic obstructive pulmonary disease (COPD). Am J Respir Crit Care Med 2001;163:1476–83.

33. Aubert JD, Dalal BI, Bai TR, et al. Transforming growth factor-β_1 gene expression in human airways. Thorax 1994;49:225–32.

34. Kenyon NJ, Ward RW, McGrew G, Last JA. TGF-β_1 causes airway fibrosis and increased collagen I and III mRNA in mice. Thorax 2003;58:772–7.

35. Churg A, Tai H, Coulthard T, et al. Cigarette smoke drives small airway remodeling by induction of growth factors in the airway wall. Am J Respir Crit Care Med 2006;15;174:1327–34.

36. Dhami R, Gilks B, Xie C, et al. Acute cigarette smoke–induced connective tissue breakdown is mediated by neutrophils and prevented by α-1-antitrypsin. Am J Respir Cell Mol Biol 2000;22:244–52.

37. Aubert JD, Hayashi S, Hards J, et al. Platelet-derived growth factor and its receptor in lungs from patients with asthma and chronic airflow obstruction. Am J Physiol 1994;266:L655–63.

38. Wang RD, Tai H, Xie C, et al. Cigarette smoke produces airway wall remodeling in rat tracheal explants. Am J Respir Crit Care Med 2003;168:1232–6.

39. Wang RD, Wright JL, Churg A. TGFβ_1 drives airway remodeling in cigarette smoke-exposed tracheal explants. Am J Respir Cell Mol Biol 2005;33:387–93.

40. Barcellos-Hoff MH, Dix TA. Redox-mediated activation of latent transforming growth factor-β_1. Mol Endocrinol 1996;10:1077–83.

41. Pociask DA, Sime PJ, Brody AR. Asbestos-derived reactive oxygen species activate TGFβ. Lab Invest 2004;84:1013–23.

42. Annes JP, Munger JS, Rifkin DB. Making sense of latent TGFα activation. J Cell Sci 2003;116(Pt 2):217–24.

43. Parks WC, Wilson CL, Lopez-Boado YS. Matrix metalloproteinases as modulators of inflammation and innate immunity. Nat Rev Immunol 2004;4:617–29.

44. Atkinson JJ, Senior RM. Matrix metalloproteinase-9 in lung remodeling. Am J Respir Cell Mol Biol 2003;28:12–24.

45. Lim DH, Cho JY, Miller M, et al. Reduced peribronchial fibrosis in allergen-challenged MMP-9-deficient mice. Am J Physiol Lung Cell Mol Physiol 2006;291:L265–71.

46. Hoshino M, Nakamura Y, Sim J, et al. Bronchial subepithelial fibrosis and expression of matrix metalloproteinase-9 in asthmatic airway inflammation. J Allergy Clin Immunol 1998;102:783–8.

47. Kelly EA, Busse WW, Jarjour NN. Increased matrix metalloproteinase-9 in the airway after allergen challenge. Am J Respir Crit Care Med 2000;162:1157–61.

48. Churg A, Wang R, Wang X, et al. An MMP-9/-12 inhibitor prevents smoke–induced emphysema and small airway remodeling in guinea pigs. Thorax 2007;62:706–13.

49. MacNee W. Oxidants/antioxidants and COPD. Chest 2000;117:303S–17S.

50. Lappalainen U, Whitsett JA, Wert SE, et al. Interleukin-1beta causes pulmonary inflammation, emphysema, and airway remodeling in the adult murine lung. Am J Respir Cell Mol Biol 2005;32:311–8.

51. Milic-Emili J. Does mechanical injury of the peripheral airways play a role in the genesis of COPD in smokers? COPD 2004;1:85–92.

52. Choe MM, Sporn PH, Swartz MA. Extracellular matrix remodeling by dynamic strain in a three-dimensional tissue-engineered human airway wall model. Am J Respir Cell Mol Biol 2006;35:306–13.

53. Kumar V, Abbas AK, Fausto N (eds). Robbins and Cotran: Pathologic Basis of Disease, 7e. Philadelphia: Elsevier, 2005.

54. Niewoehner DE, Kleinerman J, Rice DB. Pathologic changes in the peripheral airways of young cigarette smokers. N Engl J Med 1974;291:755–8.

55. Mitchell RS, Stanford RE, Johnson JM, et al. The morphologic features of the bronchi, bronchioles, and alveoli in chronic airway obstruction: a clinicopathologic study. Am Rev Respir Dis 1976;114:137–45.

56. Cosio MG, Ghezzo H, Hogg JC, et al. The relations between structural changes in small airways and pulmonary function tests. N Engl J Med. 1978 ;298:1277–81.

57. Wright JL, Cosio M, Wiggs BJ, et al. A morphologic grading scheme for membranous and respiratory bronchioles. Arch Pathol Lab Med 1985;109:163–5.

58. Cosio MG, Hale KA, Niewoehner DE. Morphologic and morphometric effects of prolonged cigarette smoking on the small airways. Am Rev Respir Dis 1980;122:265–71.

59. Wright JL, Wiggs BR, Hogg JC. Airway disease in upper and lower lobes in lungs of patients with and without emphysema. Thorax 1984;39:282–5.

60. Wright JL. Airway inflammatory cells in upper and lower lobes in lungs of patients with and without emphysema. Pathol Res Pract 1988;183:297–300.

61. Berend N, Wright JL, Thurlbeck WM, et al. Small airways disease: reproducibility of measurements and correlation with lung function. Chest 1981;79:263–8.

62. Wright JL, Hobson J, Wiggs BR, et al. Effect of cigarette smoking on structure of the small airways. Lung 1987165:91–100.

63. Bosken CH, Hards J, Gatter K, Hogg JC. Characterization of the inflammatory reaction in the peripheral airways of cigarette smokers using immunocytochemistry. Am Rev Respir Dis 1992;145:911–7.

64. Niewoehner DE, Kleinerman J, Rice DB. Pathologic changes in the peripheral airways of young cigarette smokers. N Engl J Med 1974;291:755–8.

65. Berend N, Thurlbeck WM. Correlations of maximum expiratory flow with small airway dimensions and pathology. J Appl Physiol 1982;52:346–51.

66. Wright JL, Lawson LM, Paré PD, et al. Morphology of peripheral airways in current smokers and ex–smokers. Am Rev Respir Dis 1983;127:474–7.

67. Berend N, Woolcock AJ, Marlin GE. Relationship between bronchial and areterial diameters in normal human lungs. Thorax 1979;34:353–8.

68. Matsuba K, Thurlbeck WM. Disease of the small airways in chronic bronchitis. Am Rev Respir Dis 1973;107: 552–8.

69. Wright JL, Hobson JE, Wiggs BR, et al. Investigation of airway inflammation and peribronchiolar attachments in the lungs of nonsmokers, current and ex-smokers. Lung 1988;166:277–86.

70. Di Stefano A, Capelli A, Lusuardi M, et al. Severity of airflow limitation is associated with severity of airway inflammation in smokers. Am J Respir Crit Care Med 1998;158:1277–85.

71. Bosken CH, Hards J, Gatter K, Hogg JC. Characterization of the inflammatory reaction in the peripheral airways of cigarette smokers using immunocytochemistry. Am Rev Respir Dis 1992;145:911–7.

72. Saetta M, Di Stefano A, Turato G, et al. CD8+ T-lymphocytes in peripheral airways of smokers with chronic obstructive pulmonary disease. Am J Respir Crit Care Med 1998;157:822–6.

73. Saetta M, Turato G, Maestrelli P, et al. Cellular and structural bases of chronic obstructive pulmonary disease. Am Rev Respir Dis 2001;163:1304–9.

74. Saetta M, Baraldo S, Corbino L, et al. CD8+ve cells in the lungs of smokers with chronic obstructive pulmonary disease. Am J Respir Crit Care Med 1999;160:711–7.

75. Cruz-Orive LM, Weibel ER. Sampling designs for stereology. J Microsc 1981;122:235–57.

76. Cosio MG. Related autoimmunity, T-cells and STAT-4 in the pathogenesis of chronic obstructive pulmonary disease. Eur Respir J 2004;24:3–5.

77. Taraseviciene-Stewart L, Douglas IS, Nana-Sinkam PS, et al. Is alveolar destruction and emphysema in chronic obstructive pulmonary disease an immune disease? Proc Am Thorac Soc 2006;3:687–90.

78. Veeramachaneni SB, Sethi S. Pathogenesis of bacterial exacerbations of COPD. COPD 2006;3:109–15.

79. Wiggs BR, Moreno R, Hogg JC, et al. A model of the mechanics of airway narrowing. J Appl Physiol 1990;69:849–60.

80. Wiggs BR, Bosken CH, Paré PD, et al. A model of airway narrowing in asthma and in chronic obstructive pulmonary disease. Am Rev Respir Dis 1992;145:1251–8.

81. Aikawa T, Shimura S, Sasaki H, et al. Morphometric analysis of intraluminal mucus in airways in chronic obstructive pulmonary disease. Am Rev Respir Dis 1989;140:477–82.

82. Matsuba K Thurlbeck WM. The number and dimensions of small airways in nonemphysematous lungs. Am Rev Respir Dis 1971;104:516–24.

83. James AL, Hogg JC, Dunn LA, Paré PD. The use of the internal perimeter to compare airway size and to calculate smooth muscle shortening. Am Rev Respir Dis 1988;138:136–9.

84. Bosken CH, Wiggs BR, Paré PD, Hogg JC. Small airway dimensions in smokers with obstruction to airflow. Am Rev Respir Dis 1990;142:563–70.

85. Kuwano K, Bosken CH, Paré PD, et al. Small airways dimensions in asthma and in chronic obstructive pulmonary disease. Am Rev Respir Dis 1993;148:1220–5.

86. Bai A, Eidelman DH, Hogg JC, et al. Proposed nomenclature for quantifying subdivisions of the bronchial wall. J Appl Physiol 1994;77:1011–4.

87. Finkelstein R, Ma HD, Ghezzo H, et al. Morphometry of small airways in smokers and its relationship to emphysema type and hyperresponsiveness. Am J Respir Crit Care Med 1995;152: 267–76.

88. Opazo Saez AM, Seow CY, Paré PD. Peripheral airway smooth muscle mechanics in obstructive airways disease. Am J Respir Crit Care Med 2000;161:910–7.

89. Linhartova A, Anderson AE, Foraker AG. Topology of nonrespiratory bronchioles of normal and emphysematous lungs. Hum Pathol 1974;5:729–35.

90. Linhartova A, Anderson AE, Foraker AG. Further observations on luminal deformity and stenosis of nonrespiratory bronchioles in pulmonary emphysema. Thorax 1977;32:53–9.

91. Nagai A, West WW, Paul JL, Thurlbeck WM. The National Institutes of Health intermittent positive-pressure breathing trial: pathology studies. 1. Interrelationship between morphologic lesions. Am Rev Respir Dis 1985;132:937–45.

92. Nagai A, West WW, Thurlbeck WM. The National Institutes of Health intermittent positive-pressure breathing trial: pathology studies II. Correlation between morphologic findings, clinical findings, and evidence of expiratory airflow obstruction. Am Rev Respir Dis 1985;132:946–53.

93. Spain DM Kaufman G. The basic lesion in chronic pulmonary emphysema. Am Rev Respir Dis 1953;68:24–30.

94. Leopold JG, Gough J. The centrilobular form of hypertrophic emphysema and its relation to chronic bronchitis. Thorax 1957;12:219–35.

95. McLean KH. The histology of generalized pulmonary emphysema. The genesis of the early centrilobular lesion: focal emphysema. Aust Ann Med 1957;6:124–40.

96. McLean KH. The histology of generalized pulmonary emphysema. Diffuse emphysema. Aust Ann Med 1957;6:203–17.

97. McLean KH. The histology of localized emphysema. Aust Ann Med 1957;6:282–94.

98. McLean KH. The pathogenesis of pulmonary emphysema. Am J Med 1958;25:62–74.

99. McLean KH. The pathology of emphysema. Am Rev Respir Dis 1959;80:58–64.
100. Pratt PC, Jutabha O, Klugh GA. Quantitative relationship between structural extent of centrilobular emphysema and postmortem volume and flow characteristics of lungs. Med Thorac 1965;22:197–208.
101. Pratt PC, Haque A, Klugh GA. Correlation of postmortem function and structure in normal and emphysematous lungs. Am Rev Respir Dis 1961;83:856–65.
102. Anderson AE, Foraker AG. Relative dimensions of bronchioles and parenchymal spaces in lungs from normal subjects and emphysematous patients. Am J Med 1962;32:218–26.
103. Petty TL, Silvers GW, Stanford RE. Radial traction and small airways disease in excised human lungs. Am Rev Respir Dis 1986;133:132–5.
104. Petty TL, Silvers GW, Stanford RE. Mild emphysema is associated with reduced elastic recoil and increased lung size but not with air-flow limitation. Am Rev Respir Dis 1987;136:867–71.
105. Linhartova A, Anderson AE, Foraker AG. Radial traction and bronchiolar obstruction in pulmonary emphysema. Arch Pathol Lab Med 1971;92:384–91.
106. Nagai A, Yamawaki I, Takizawa T, Thurlbeck WM. Alveolar attachments in emphysema of human lungs. Am Rev Respir Dis 1991;144:888–91.
107. Saetta M, Ghezzo H, King M, et al. Loss of alveolar attachments in smokers: a morphometric correlate of lung function impairment. Am Rev Respir Dis 1985;132:894–900.
108. Willems LNA, Kramps JA, Stijnen T, et al. Relation between small airways disease and parenchymal destruction in surgical lung specimens. Thorax 1990;45:89–94.
109. Buist AS, Ghezzo H, Anthonisen NR, et al. Relationship between the single-breath N₂ test and age, sex and smoking habit in three North American cities. Am Rev Respir Dis 1979;120:305.
110. Becklake MR, Leclerc M, Strobach H, et al. The N₂ closing volume test in population studies: sources of variation and reproducibility. Am Rev Respir Dis 1975;111:141–7.
111. Becklake MR, Permutt S. Evaluation of tests of lung function for "screening" for early detection of chronic obstructive lung disease. In: Macklem PT, Permutt S, editors. The lung in the transition between health and disease. New York, Marcel Dekker1979. p. 345.
112. Martin RR, Lindsay D, Despas P, et al. The early detection of airway obstruction. Am Rev Respir Dis 1975;111:119–25.
113. Murtagh PS, Proctor DF, Permutt S, et al. Bronchial closure with mecholyl in excised dog lobes. J Appl Physiol 1971;31:409–15.
114. Demedts M, Cosemans J, De Roo M, et al. Emphysema with minor airway obstruction and abnormal tests of small airway disease. Respiration 1978;35:148–57.
115. Paré PD, Brooks LA, Coppin CA, et al. Density dependence of maximal expiratory flow and its correlation with small airway disease in smokers. Am Rev Respir Dis 1985;131:521–6.
116. Detels R, Tashkin DP, Simmons MS, et al. The UCLA population studies of chronic obstructive respiratory disease. 5. Agreement and disagreement of tests in identifying abnormal lung function. Chest 1982;82:630–8.
117. Dosman JA, Cotton DJ, Graham BL, et al. Sensitivity and specificity of early diagnostic tests of lung function in smokers. Chest 1981;79:6–11.
118. Nemery B, Moavero NE, Brasseur L, et al. Significance of small airway tests in middle-aged smokers. Am Rev Respir Dis 1981;124:232–8.
119. Olofsson J, Bake B, Svardsudd K, et al. The single breath N₂-test predicts the rate of decline in FEV₁. Eur J Respir Dis 1986;69:46–56.
120. Buist AS, Vollmer WM, Johnson LR, McCamant LE. Does the single-breath N₂ test identify the smoker who will develop chronic airflow limitation? Am Rev Respir Dis 1988;137:293–301
121. Walter S, Nancy NR, Collier CR, et al. Changes in the forced expiratory spirogram in young male smokers. Am Rev Respir Dis 1979;119:717–24.
122. Solomon DA. Clinical significance of pulmonary function tests: are small airways tests helpful in the detection of early airflow obstruction? Chest 1978;74:567–9.
123. Nakano Y, Muro S, Sakai H, et al. Computed tomographic measurements of airway dimensions and emphysema in smokers. Correlation with lung function. Am J Respir Crit Care Med 2000;162(3 Pt 1):1102–8.
124. Coxson HO, Lake S, Muller NL, et al. Heritability of quantitative emphysema phenotypes in chronic obstructive pulmonary disease. Am J Respir Crit Care Med 2005; A44.
125. King TE. Overview of bronchiolitis. Clin Chest Med 1993;14:607–10.
126. Costabel U, Guzman J, Teschler H. Bronchiolitis obliterans with organizing pneumonia: outcome. Thorax 1995;50:S59–64.
127. Fraser RS, Paré PD, Colman NC, Muller NL. Diagnosis of diseases of the chest. Vol 3. 4th ed. Philadelphia: WB Saunders; 1999.

CHAPTER 10

Environmental Factors in Chronic Obstructive Pulmonary Disease

William MacNee, MBChB, MD, FRCP(G), FRCP(E), and
Kenneth Donaldson, PhD, DSc, FRCPath

The production of energy in the form of heat and light requires the combustion of biologic fossil fuel, a process that leads to the release of products of this combustion and the pollution of the air. Recognition of the harmful effects of air pollution has been present for centuries. One of the first publications in the English literature recognizing the adverse health effects of air pollution and calling for its reduction is the booklet of John Evelyn, a fellow of the Royal Society, *Fumifugium or The Inconvenience of the Aer and Smoak of London Dissipated* (1661).[1,2]

The industrial revolution in Western Europe in the eighteenth century, which led to the growth of cities to house workers, and the industrial and domestic use of coal as a source of power had a major effect on the impact of air pollution on health. At this time, major cities developed smoky fogs or smogs, particularly during the winter, and the effects of these on the lungs of city dwellers were increasingly recognised: "'Twas a misery to hear the retching Londoners wheezing and coughing and gasping for breath as they walked the streets, and I myself was a fellow-sufferer for the fogs and damps and night air by no means suit my lungs."[2] The nineteenth century saw the growth in population of the cities, leading to the recognition of increased mortality in urban areas.[3,4] In 1895, Russell drew attention to the many deaths in London from bronchitis, which, among other things, he attributed to the smoky fogs.[3] In the early part of the twentieth century, a report of the relationship between fog and mortality from respiratory diseases was published.[5] However, increasing awareness of the effects of air pollution resulted from the study of three severe air pollution episodes: the Meuse Valley, Belgium (1930), Donora, Pennsylvania, United States (1948), and London, United Kingdom (1952).

These studies showed associations between the levels of air pollutants and mortality, as shown most clearly by the sharp rise in black smoke and sulfur dioxide (SO_2) levels during the London smog in the second week of December 1952, when London experienced a period of stagnant weather when the wind speed fell to virtually zero for almost 3 days. The attendant accumulation of fog and air pollution produced a smog containing principally particles and SO_2 that reached extremely high airborne concentrations. From December 5 to 9, hospital admissions rose by 50% and respiratory admissions by 160%, associated with an increase in the daily death rate, resulting in more than 4,000 extra deaths (Figure 1).[6,7] Between 80 and 90% of these deaths were from cardiorespiratory causes, and the greatest relative increase was in deaths from bronchitis, which rose by a factor of 9. Although it was more than 20 years until the term *chronic obstructive pulmonary disease* (COPD) was to be adopted, many of those who died or became ill were in the category of "chronic bronchitis" and no doubt had COPD. Such was the severity of the pollution that cattle at an agricultural show died, and theater performances were cancelled because the audience could not see the stage.

In Los Angeles around the same time, a new type of air pollution was first documented. Effluent from the large number of road vehicles, together with intense sunlight, led to the formation of photochemical smog. Release of nitrogen oxides from vehicles during the morning rush hour is followed by the formation of nitrogen dioxide (NO_2). This then reacts, in a complex series of reactions, with polluting hydrocarbons in sunlight to form ozone, among other potentially harmful compounds. Atmospheric pollutants accumulate and become concentrated when air movement is stopped by a temperature inversion, as was the case in the London smogs. Usually, the air is warmer at the earth's surface and colder above, but during a temperature inversion, a layer of warm air forms above and holds down a layer of cool air at the ground.

The recognition of the adverse health effects of these very high levels of air pollution (the average black smoke level during the 1952 London smog was 1,600 $\mu g/m^3$, 4 times the normal values) led to worldwide legislation that dramatically decreased the emissions of air pollutants from the use of coal as a domestic and industrial source of fuel and the abolition of winter smogs.[8]

Until recently, it was perceived that the problem of air pollution had largely been solved. Modern cities such as London suffer much less from air pollution than they did in the 1950s, and this downward change in the quantity of air pollution has been accompanied by a qualitative change.

With the decrease in the levels of the traditional air pollutants of black smoke, SO_2, and acid aerosols, there has been a relative increase in air pollutants, associated with the second important social change in the twentieth century relevant to air pollution: the increase in motor vehicle traffic. Although air pollution from motor vehicles contains less black or visible

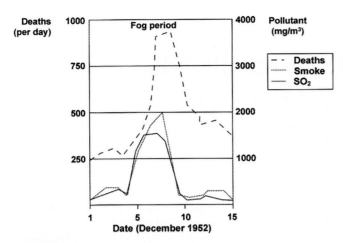

FIGURE 1. Increase in deaths associated with increased smoke and sulfur dioxide (SO_2) levels during a 5-day period of London fog in December 1952.

particles and less SO_2 than that produced by the burning of fossil fuels, there is a relative increase in the generation of nitrogen oxides and small particulates and the generation of secondary pollutants by the photochemical production of ozone. There is now overwhelming epidemiologic evidence of associations between adverse health effects and present-day levels of air pollutants such as ozone, NO_2, and particles, and this is particularly true for adverse health effects in susceptible individuals, such as those with COPD. It is also recognized that indoor air pollution, such as pollutants derived from the burning of gas appliances in developed countries or wood smoke in less developed areas, may also have important adverse health effects. This chapter deals with the major air pollutants and their effects on the respiratory system, specifically in relation to COPD and the proposed mechanisms of these effects.

Major Air Pollutants

Indoor versus Outdoor Air Pollution

Most people spend the majority of their time, up to 95%, indoors, so the indoor environment is likely to be most important in the genesis of respiratory disease. Health effects research uses outdoor sampling sites to monitor air pollution. Outdoor air pollution permeates rather readily indoors, where it is added to by the local pollutants generated inside, for example, gas cookers. There may also be a risk from specific indoor air pollution, such as fungal spores and fungal products, environmental tobacco smoke, or radon.

The main sources of major air pollutants are shown in Table 1.

Sulfur Dioxide

SO_2 is released into the atmosphere when coal and oil, which contain significant amounts of sulfur, are burnt or during industrial processes, as well as from natural sources, such as volcanoes and sulfur springs. Emissions from motor vehicles, using either petrol or diesel fuel, are a relatively minor source of SO_2. Although a minor source of SO_2 at a national level, road traffic can produce significant levels of SO_2 alongside busy roads, but this should be reduced by the introduction in the mid-1990s in the United States and the European Union of regulations to control the sulfur levels in motor fuels. SO_2 is the main pollutant associated with acid aerosols in the atmosphere. Although the concentrations of SO_2 have declined over the past 50 years in the United States and in many European countries, owing to the reduction in the use of coal as a means of domestic heating, significant concentrations of SO_2 do occur still in Eastern European countries. In the atmosphere, SO_2 can form acidic particles or react with cloud droplets, producing acid rain. SO_2, like other pollutant gases, readily enters the lungs and penetrates according to their solubility, with the most soluble compounds dissolving high in the pulmonary tree and the less soluble ones penetrating more deeply. When it interacts with water in lung-lining fluid, it forms sulfite (SO_3^{2-}) and bisulfite (HSO_3^-) ions, along with some other compounds. Both HSO_3^- and SO_3^{2-} have a lone pair of electrons and so are readily oxidized by biologic molecules forming and consuming free radicals, such as superoxide anion, hydroxyl radical, and sulfoxyl radical. Thus, SO_2 exposure can result in free radical production and oxidative stress in lungs.[9]

Table 1 Major Components of Modern Air Pollution	
Pollutant	*Sources*
Sulfur dioxide	Domestic homes and power stations burning fossil fuels; industry
Nitrogen dioxide	Burning of fossil fuels; automobile fuel combustion
Ozone	Formed in sunlight by the photochemical reaction of nitrogen oxides and hydrocarbons released by motor vehicles and industry
Particles	Motor vehicles, industry, burning of fossil fuels, large scale bush/forest fires
Other air pollutants less likely to be involved in COPD	Volatile organic compounds, heavy metals, polycyclic aromatic hydrocarbons, etc.

COPD = chronic obstructive pulmonary disease.

Oxides of Nitrogen

NO_2 is the most important oxide of nitrogen (NOx) (which includes nitric oxide [NO]) with respect to adverse effects on human health. NO_2 is produced directly as a primary pollutant, released by the oxidation of atmospheric nitrogen during high-temperature fuel combustion in vehicles and in industrial processes. NO_2 is also produced indirectly, as a secondary pollutant, as a result of the spontaneous conversion of NO to NO_2 in the presence of ozone. Among the most important sources of NO are lightening, forest fires, volcanoes, and bacterial activity in the soil. Although these are the most important sources in global terms, the dominant sources in Western Europe and North America are anthropogenic. In Europe, road transport produces about 50% of all emissions, and in the United States, about half of all emissions are contributed by industrial combustion. Other sources of NO_2 are the burning of domestic gas as an indoor pollutant and cigarette smoke.

Since NO_2 concentrations in the air are derived largely from NO by the action of ozone, NO_2 concentrations are therefore dependent on the ambient ozone level. Concentrations may also increase in cold still weather as a result of trapping of pollutants in a layer of cold air close to the ground. In general, NO_2 levels are higher in urban areas owing to the effects of traffic. The levels of NO_2 in indoor air are largely determined by the outdoor concentrations, except if there is an indoor source of NO, such as gas appliances, which can produce very high levels during cooking.

In the lung-lining fluid, NO and NO_2 dissolve to form nitrate, nitrite, and nitrous acid. If there is a coexposure to cigarette smoke or smog, both of which contain hydrogen peroxide, then hydroxyl radical forms from the reaction of H_2O_2 with NOx. Thus, NOx can also lead to free radical generation and oxidative stress in the lungs.

Carbon Monoxide

Carbon monoxide is largely generated from the incomplete combustion of fossil fuel. The principal source is from motor vehicles. The majority of carbon in motor vehicle fuel is oxidized to carbon dioxide, whereas a small fraction is incompletely oxidized to carbon monoxide. Carbon monoxide is also an important source of indoor air pollution as a result of faulty domestic heating systems, which cause many deaths each year, and is also an important component of the gas phase of tobacco smoke.

Ozone

Ozone occurs naturally in the lower atmosphere, in low concentrations, as a result of reactions involving volatile organic compounds (VOCs) produced by plants and as a result of compounds entering the lower atmosphere from the upper atmosphere during certain meteorologic conditions, such as thunderstorms. Ozone can also be produced indirectly by the action of sunlight on NO_2 to form monoatomic oxygen, which reacts with molecular oxygen to form ozone (triatomic

oxygen). Thus, the rate of ozone production by this process is dependent on the intensity of sunlight and the concentration of the compounds required for its formation. Atmospheric hydrocarbons such as acetylene, benzene, butane, ethane, and hexane accelerate the reaction between NO_2 and sunlight through the formation of peroxyl radicals and hydroxyl radicals. Ozone is short-lived in the lower atmosphere and is removed indoors and at night by its reaction with surfaces. The photochemical reduction of NO_2 to NO uses an oxygen radical that combines with oxygen to form ozone. NO itself reacts with ozone to reform NO_2 and oxygen. Thus, under certain circumstances, an equilibrium exists between oxygen, ozone, and NO_2. An increase in VOCs may shift the balance toward greater production of ozone. The intensity of sunlight is clearly important to the production of ozone, which is therefore a more important air pollutant in southern climates in summer. In cities, where concentrations of oxides of nitrogen are higher, ozone may be consumed in oxidizing NO. Thus, concentrations of ozone tend to be higher in rural rather than in urban areas. Ozone can also travel large distances and can cross national boundaries. Background concentrations of ozone have doubled over the last 100 years.

On dissolving in lung-lining fluid, ozone forms hydrogen peroxide, hydroxylhydroperoxides, and reactive aldehydes by a process known as ozonolysis; malondialdehyde may also be produced.[10] In addition to ozone, photochemical smog contains a number of other harmful secondary pollutants such as peroxyacetyl nitrate and aldehydes, which are severe irritants. Thus, ozone and other components of photochemical smog also cause oxidative stress in lung tissue following its deposition.

Particles

Particles of sea salt and dust from volcanic eruptions arise naturally in the atmosphere. Motor vehicles and industry, however, add significantly to the concentration of particles in the atmosphere in cities, where many people can be exposed. The particle cloud (aerosol) is a complex mixture comprising organic matter, elemental carbon or soot, metals, sea salt, sulfates, nitrates, and dust. Particles are divided into those that are primary, that is, formed immediately, such as diesel particles, and secondary, those particles that form from chemical reactions in the atmosphere, for example, ammonium nitrate. Particles can be heterogeneous, such as diesel particles that have a carbon core coated with metals, polyaromatic hydrocarbons (PAHs), and sulfates. Particles deposit in the lung depending on their aerodynamic diameter, but the sampling conventions that quantify environmental particulate collect all particles that enter the bronchial tree (PM_{10}) or those that can reach the nonciliated airspaces ($PM_{2.5}$). Once they deposit, the particles may dissolve if they are salts, such as nitrate and sulfate, or if they release transition metals that undergo Fenton chemistry; then hydroxyl radicals may be produced. If the ubiquitous bacterial product endotoxin is present in association with the particles, then lung cells may be stimulated to produce inflammation. All of these effects may lead to oxidative stress.

Particles have a special problem of nomenclature because they are always measured by a sampling convention that collects some fraction of the material suspended in the air. For the purposes of risk assessment, the fraction of particles that enters the lungs is clearly the preferred index:

- *Total suspended particulate (TSP)*. As the name suggests, these particles can be collected regardless of size; this means that it is not necessarily representative of the particles that will enter the lungs since large particles that do not enter the respiratory tract can be measured;
- *Black smoke*. This is the system that was used in the United Kingdom and in other countries until the end of the 1980s. Air was drawn through a size-selective filter onto a white paper, and the blackness of the "smudge" was measured. This method obviously is biased toward black, that is, carbon-based, particles; there is a variable relationship between particles as measured by black smoke and PM_{10}.
- *PM_{10}*. This is a size-selective sampling convention that captures particles of 10 μm with 50% efficiency; it roughly corresponds to the thoracic fraction of particles.
- *$PM_{2.5}$*. This is a size-selective sampling convention that captures particles of 2.5 μm with 50% efficiency; it roughly corresponds to the respirable fraction of particles.

It has therefore been suggested that measurement of particles <2.5 μm ($PM_{2.5}$) may be more relevant for the health effects of air pollutants. There is even a suggestion that the measurement of ultrafine particles <0.1 μm (100 nm) in diameter may be most relevant to assess the toxic effects of air pollutants. This concept has not yet received wide acceptance.

PM_{10} particles will enter the bronchial tree, whereas $PM_{2.5}$ reaches the nonciliated distal airspaces. Ambient particles have been shown to have a wide size range and contain vast numbers of particles that are smaller than 1 μg in diameter.[11] Atmospheric particles have also been shown to be very acidic and often reach a pH as low as 2.

In cities, the sources of particles are from combustion, either from vehicle engines or from houses and factories. Most of the particulate matter (PM) from road transport comes from diesel vehicles. In winter, elevated PM_{10} concentrations are largely due to vehicle exhaust emissions, whereas a higher proportion of PM in summer is due to secondary particles.

Studies Linking Air Pollutants and COPD

The health effects of air pollutants on humans can be assessed in a number of different ways, including chamber studies, epidemiologic studies in panels of subjects at risk, and studies of hospital admissions or studies of mortality from records.[12] Chamber studies enable very accurately controlled doses of

pollutant to be delivered to volunteers under well-controlled conditions. The disadvantage is that usually these volunteers have only mild disease, and unlike real-life exposures, there is no coexposure to other pollutants; children are generally not studied for ethical reasons.[12] Data have also been gathered from epidemiologic studies that are concerned with real-life exposures at a population level.

When assessing epidemiologic studies of the effects of air pollutants, it is important to bear several points in mind. First, it is important to differentiate those studies that demonstrate acute from those that show chronic effects. This relates to effects that exacerbate COPD and to studies that suggest that air pollution may be a causal factor in the development of COPD. Since most people spend more than 95% of their time indoors, the indoor levels of air pollutants are most relevant to causing adverse effects, whereas most studies use outdoor measurements of air pollutants. Outdoor pollution penetrates readily into the indoor environment. However, it has been suggested that personal monitoring reveals much higher levels than are measured at outdoor sampling sites.[13] *Most of the adverse health effects of air pollutants have been shown in susceptible individuals, such as patients with COPD*. In addition, pollution exposures never involve single pollutants, so interactions between pollutants are likely. This is a disadvantage of epidemiologic studies since it is difficult to discriminate which pollutant is responsible for the effect.

The general effects of air pollution, excluding effects in COPD, are outlined in Table 2. They are an amalgam of chamber studies and acute and chronic epidemiologic studies of various end points in various countries and refer to exposures to plausible environmental levels.

Adverse Effects of Air Pollutants in COPD
Chamber Studies

Chamber exposure studies allow the effects of the delivery of usually single air pollutants to the lungs of normal subjects or those with mild airways disease to be studied. Often the concentrations of air pollutants used are higher than the average environmental concentrations.

Exposure studies in patients with COPD are relatively few for the major air pollutants. Exposure of normal healthy individuals to SO_2 at concentrations of ≤ 13.1 mg/m^3 (5 ppm) for periods of up to 4 hours produced only minimal changes in pulmonary function and mild upper respiratory tract symptoms. In comparison, in asthmatics, concentrations of 0.66 to 1.3 mg/m^3 (0.25–0.5 ppm) SO_2 produced bronchoconstriction, associated with increased airway resistance and clinical symptoms of wheezing.[14] The magnitude of the response is, however, very variable among asthmatics, implying different susceptibilities to the effect. There have been no comparable studies of exposure to SO_2 in COPD patients. Changes in pulmonary defenses relevant to COPD, such as a decrease in tracheobronchial mucocilliary clearance, have been shown

Pollutant	Population	Adverse Effect
SO$_2$	Normal	None or very little
	Asthmatic	Increased airway resistance
		Increased bronchial hyperreactivity
		Reduced peak flow
		Increased hospital admissions
	Other susceptible, eg, cardiovascular disease	Increased mortality
NO$_2$	Normal	None or very little
	Asthmatic	Small effect on bronchial responsiveness
		Enhancement of response to antigen
	Other susceptible, eg, cardiovascular disease	Possible increased mortality
Ozone	Normal	Small increases in airway resistance and bronchial hyperreactivity at high exposure
		Lung function change (FEV, FVC)
		Increased symptoms of cough and chest discomfort
		Inflammation caused by high exposures
	Asthmatic	Enhancement of response to antigen
		Small increases in airway resistance
	Other susceptible, eg, cardiovascular disease	Increased mortality
Particles (PM$_{10}$/PM$_{2.5}$)	Normal	Slight lung function decrease at very high exposure
	Asthmatic	Increased symptoms
		Increased hospitalizations
	Other susceptible, eg, cardiovascular disease	Increased mortality

Table 2 Effects of Air Pollutants

EPAQS report on SO$_2$; EPAQS report on NO$_2$; EPAQS report on ozone; EPAQS report on particles.

Adapted from Ayres JG[12] and Pope AC, Dockery DW.[167]

FEV = forced expiratory volume; FVC = forced vital capacity.

to occur following exposure to SO$_2$ in concentrations of 13.1 mg/m^3 (5 ppm).[15,16]

In the study of von Nieding and colleagues, COPD patients were exposed to very high levels (1.5 ppm) of NO$_2$.[17] This produced a small but detectable increase in airway resistance. Vagaggini and colleagues exposed seven COPD subjects to 0.3 ppm NO$_2$ for 1 hour with moderate intermittent exercise; there were no changes in the nasal lavage or induced sputum inflammatory profile of the COPD subjects following NO$_2$ exposure, but there was a mild decrease in forced expiratory volume in 1 second (FEV$_1$) 2 hours after NO$_2$ exposure in these patients, and the symptom score showed a mild increase.[18] To assess the expression of nuclear factor κB (NF-κB), cytokines, and

intercellular adhesion molecule 1 (ICAM-1) in the bronchial epithelium following NO$_2$ exposure, 12 healthy, young, non-smoking volunteers were exposed to 2 ppm of NO$_2$/filtered air (4 h/d) for 4 successive days. Fiberoptic bronchoscopy was performed 1 hour after air and final NO$_2$ exposures. Bronchial biopsy specimens were immunostained. Expression of interleukin (IL)-5, IL-10, IL-13, and ICAM-1 were all increased following NO$_2$ exposure, and there was a trend, not quite significant, for activation of NF-κB.

Solic and colleagues examined the effect of exposure to ozone at 0.2 ppm in COPD patients using a single crossover design with air as the control exposure.[19] During exposure to either air or ozone, the subjects exercised for 7.5 minutes every 30 minutes. There were no significant effects on respiratory mechanics following exposure to ozone, and, similarly, there was no change in ventilation or gas exchange. The only significant effect was that arterial oxygen saturation (SAO$_2$), measured by ear oximetry, was significantly lower at the end of ozone exposure than at the end of air exposure. This small but consistent decrease in oxygen saturation was suggested, by the authors, to demonstrate that indices of ventilation-perfusion distribution may be sensitive measures of ozone effects in COPD.

The development of particle concentrator technology has allowed exposure of humans to concentrated ambient particles (CAPs) and monitoring of the response. In such studies, normal subjects exposed to CAPs, up to about 300 μg/m^3, showed mild neutrophil inflammation in the bronchoalveolar lavage.[20] Gong and colleagues carried out a study of elderly individuals with and without COPD exposed to CAPS around 200 μg/m^3.[21] Maximal mid–expiratory flow and arterial oxygen saturation (measured by pulse oximetry) showed small but statistically significant decrements associated with CAPs that were more marked in healthy than in COPD subjects. The fact that healthy subjects showed a more adverse effect may be related to more efficient penetration and deposition of inhaled toxic particles in distal small airways.

Epidemiologic Studies

Several studies support the contention that COPD confers susceptibility to the effects of air pollution.

Mortality

To assess the risk of death, 1,845 men and 460 women who had visited emergency rooms because of COPD exacerbations during the period 1985 to 1989 were followed until death. The authors then assessed the acute association between levels of particulate air pollution and death. Particle levels, measured as black smoke, were associated with mortality for all causes but were stronger for respiratory causes (odds ratio 1.182; 95% confidence interval [CI] 1.025–1.365). In the large-scale APHEA study in Europe (Air Pollution and Health: a European Approach), the four main pollutants (NO, ozone, SO$_2$, and particles) were studied for their short-term association with adverse health effects, including mortality.[22] The daily number of deaths was associated with increases in the levels of particles, SO$_2$, ozone, and NO$_2$, and cardiovascular and respiratory deaths were associated with increases in particles, SO$_2$, and ozone.

Pathology Studies

In a unique study, Churg and colleagues examined at autopsy lungs from a group of never-smoking women from a high PM region, Mexico City, and compared them with the lungs of subjects from Vancouver, British Columbia, a city with low PM and air pollution generally.[23] The subjects had no history of smoking, occupational dust exposure, or exposure to bio-mass fuels during cooking. The lungs from Mexico City had more fibrosis and muscle assessed morphometrically in both the membranous and respiratory bronchioles and more luminal distortion. Evaluation of the particulate content of the airway walls by analytic electron microscopy showed chains and aggregates of carbonaceous spheres with the morphology of diesel exhaust particles in the Mexico City lungs. Therefore, even in the absence of smoking and occupational dust exposure, the high levels of PM and other pollutants had caused remodeling of the small airways. The lesions seen were described as essentially identical to the small airway lesions found in workers occupationally exposed to mineral dusts in the absence of other pollutants and therefore likely to be due to the PM exposure rather than other pollutants.

Studies assessing short-term effects of NO$_2$ levels on daily mortality or hospital admission rates related to obstructive airways disease are confounded by a strong correlation between daily PM$_{10}$ levels and NO$_2$ levels. Thus, it is difficult to differentiate the effects of NO$_2$ from those of PM$_{10}$. The APHEA study, which reported mortality and hospital admissions in 15 cities, found significant associations between NO$_2$ levels and daily death.[22] An increase in peak hourly levels of 50 μg/m^3 NO$_2$ produced an increase in the daily number of deaths of 1.3%. Although the effect diminished when other pollutants were taken into account, the association with NO$_2$ remained significant. In the same study in Spain, an increase in the daily NO$_2$ mean levels of 100 μg/m^3 NO$_2$ was associated with an increase of 3.4% in total mortality, largely from cardiovascular causes, with no effect on respiratory mortality.[24] However, a significant effect of NO$_2$ levels on respiratory mortality has been shown in studies in other European cities.[25]

Rossi and colleagues reported an association between a 12% increase in deaths from COPD and the mean level of airborne particulate 3 and 4 days prior to death.[26] In a study in Birmingham, England, Wordley and colleagues reported that deaths from COPD were significantly associated with the levels of PM$_{10}$ both 24 hours previously and on the same day.[27] A 10 μg/m^3 rise in PM$_{10}$ was also estimated to produce a 1.1% increase in all-cause mortality. In the well-documented "six cities" study, Schwartz and colleagues reported that a 10 μg/m^3 increase in 2-day mean PM$_{2.5}$ was associated with a 3.3% increase in deaths from COPD.[28] The relationship with PM$_{2.5}$ suggested that finer combustion-related particles may be important. In a study by Xu and colleagues, the heavily polluted areas of Beijing, which had maxima of 630 μg/m^3 of SO$_2$ and 1,003 μg/m^3 of TSP, were studied.[29] Regressions were carried out on SO$_2$ and TSP levels against deaths, controlling for the effects of temperature, humidity, and day of the week. Significant associations were seen between mortality from COPD and a doubling of SO$_2$ and a doubling of TSP. In their study of mortality in Philadelphia, Schwartz and Dockery reported that, for a 100 μg/m^3 increase in TSP, COPD deaths increased by 19% (95% CI 0.42%).[30]

Exacerbations

In the APHEA study, hospital emergency room visits for COPD in Barcelona were studied in relation to temporal trends in air pollution.[31] The results showed that a reduction of around 50 $\mu g/m^3$ in particles was accompanied by a reduction of about 6% in emergency room visits for COPD. Ozone levels were also associated with emergency room visits for COPD. Morgan and colleagues studied hospital admissions in Sydney, Australia, between 1990 and 1994.[32] An increase in daily maximum concentration of NO_2 from the 10th to the 90th percentile was associated with an increase of 4.6% (95% CI −0.17–9.61) in COPD admissions. A similar increase in daily maximum 1-hour particulate concentration was associated with an increase of 3.01% (95% CI 0.38–6.52) in COPD admissions. In a prospective study, Harre and colleagues followed 40 subjects with COPD who completed symptom diaries twice daily for 3 months during the winter of 1994.[33] All of the subjects lived within a 5 km radius of the regional council's air pollution monitoring site, and the daily and hourly mean pollutant levels (PM_{10}, NO_2, SO_2, and CO) were measured at the monitoring site. The pollution levels were low in that year, and the only significant association seen was between a rise in the PM_{10} concentration equivalent to the interquartile range and an increase in nighttime chest symptoms. A same-day rise in NO_2 concentration equivalent to the interquartile range was associated with increased inhaler use and 24-hour lag NO_2 concentrations with increased nebulizer use. Moolgavkar and colleagues investigated the association between air pollution and hospital admissions for COPD in Minneapolis–St. Paul and Birmingham, Alabama, over the period January 1, 1986, to December 31, 1991.[34] After adjustment for temperature, day of the week, season, and temporal trends, associations between air pollution and hospital admissions for respiratory causes were seen in Minneapolis–St. Paul but not in Birmingham. A 15 ppb increase in ozone on the previous day was associated with a 5.15% (95% CI 2.36–7.94%) increase in admissions. PM_{10}, SO_2, and NO_2 were also associated with hospital admissions, although none could be singled out as being more important than the others.

Studies linking NO_2 levels and hospital admission for respiratory diseases have produced inconsistent findings.[35] Analysis of data on hospitalizations specifically for exacerbations of COPD from the APHEA study in six European cities found an estimated relative risk (RR) of admission of 1.02, associated with a previous daily increase in NO_2 of 50 $\mu g/m^3$, which did not reach statistical significance.[36] In a study of hospital admissions in Sydney, Australia, between 1990 and 1994, an increase in daily maximum concentrations of NO_2 from the 10th to the 90th percentile was associated with an increase of 4.6% (95% CI −0.17–9.61) in COPD admissions.[32] However, other studies have not shown this association.[33]

In the APHEA study, Anderson and colleagues examined admissions for COPD in six European cities.[36] For all ages,

the RRs (95% CIs) of admission to hospital for COPD for a 50 $\mu g/m^3$ increase in the daily level of any pollutant were as follows: SO_2, 1.02 (0.08–1.06); black smoke, 1.04 (1.01–1.06); TSP, 1.02 (1.00–1.05); NO_2, 1.02 (1.00–1.05); and ozone, 1.04 (1.02–1.07). Wordley and colleagues reported on hospital admissions in Birmingham, England, in relation to particulate air pollution. The effect of a 10 $\mu g/m^3$ rise in PM_{10} was associated with a 2.4% increase in respiratory admissions, and this risk, although low, was linear, without evidence of a threshold. Dab and colleagues reported for the APHEA study on the relationship between air pollution and hospital admissions in Paris between 1987 and 1992.[37] PM_{10} and black smoke were associated with hospital admissions owing to all respiratory causes when the black smoke level exceeded its 5th percentile value by 100 $\mu g/m^3$. SO_2 levels consistently influenced hospital admissions for all respiratory causes, including COPD. Reporting for the APHEA study in the Netherlands, Schouten and colleagues showed that ozone had a significant effect on respiratory emergency admissions in Rotterdam but not in Amsterdam; although other trends were found, none were significant.[38] In the study of Higgins and colleagues, 75 patients with either asthma or COPD recorded their peak expiratory flow (PEF) rates and symptoms, such as wheeze, dyspnea, cough, and throat and eye irritation, and their bronchodilator use.[39] These were then related to pollution levels. On the basis of methacholine sensitivity, 36 patients were classified as "reactors." There were small but significant increases in PEF variability, bronchodilator use, and wheeze with increasing SO_2 level, whereas increased bronchodilator use, dyspnea, eye irritation, and minimum PEF recordings were related to ozone levels. In the subgroup of reactors, variability in peak flow and increase in wheeze and dyspnea and bronchodilator use were associated with increased levels of both SO_2 and ozone. These associations were seen with pollution levels on the same day, as well as those levels delayed by 24 or 48 hours. The RR of an increase of 100 $\mu g/m^3$ in daily PM_{10} for hospital admissions was 1.57 (95% CI 2.06–1.20). Notably, when days exceeding the national ambient air quality standard for PM_{10} were excluded, the association remained for COPD admissions (RR 1.54, 95% CI 2.06–1.16). Schwartz analyzed hospital admissions for the elderly in Birmingham, Alabama, in relation to air pollution levels.[40] Inhalable particles were a risk factor for admission for COPD (RR 1.27, 95% CI 1.08–1.50). An increase in ozone exposure of 50 ppb was more weakly associated with admissions for COPD with a 1-day lag (RR 1.17, 95% CI 0.86–1.60). Sunyer and colleagues studied the relationship between air pollution and emergency room admissions for COPD over 5 years in Barcelona, Spain.[41] An increase of 25 $\mu g/m^3$ of SO_2 produced adjusted changes of 6% and 9% in emergency room admissions for COPD during winter and summer, respectively. For particulate, expressed as black smoke, a similar change was found during winter, although the change was smaller in the summer. This association of each pollutant with COPD admissions remained significant after controlling for the other pollutant.

Several studies in Europe and the United States have shown increased RR of admission with an exacerbation of COPD associated with the levels of ozone,[42–45] although not all studies have supported this association.[46]

Numerous studies have shown an association between the levels of ozone and hospital admissions, particularly respiratory admissions, and some of these studies have specifically studied exacerbations of COPD.[47] In the APHEA study, a 50 µg/m³ decrease in ozone levels was associated with a 4% decrease in emergency room visits for COPD.[48] Moolgavkar and colleagues, in studies of hospital admissions in three US cities, found that a 15 ppb increase in oxygen on the previous day was associated with a 5.15% (95% CI 2.67–7.94) increase in admissions in at least one of the cities.[34] In several studies, Schwartz used Medicare data to assess the associations between air pollution and respiratory admissions in several US cities, including Birmingham, Alabama,[40] Detroit, Michigan,[49] Minneapolis–St. Paul, Minnesota,[50] Spokane, Washington,[51] Newhaven, Connecticut,[52] and Acoma, Washington.[52] Studies from these cities, excluding Birmingham, showed a significant association between ozone levels and hospital admissions for exacerbations of COPD. These associations were stronger than those found between ozone and asthma admissions.

Pulmonary Function

Jammes and colleagues studied the association between long-term exposure to outdoor air pollution and the severity of COPD and the prevalence of bronchial hyperreactivity.[53] Two groups of adult patients were chosen with similar ages and similar smoking habits who lived in a downtown district or in the outer, less polluted suburbs of Marseilles. The regions were similar with respect to SO_2 levels, but levels of NO and PM_{10} were higher in the downtown area than in the suburbs. Airway obstruction, as determined by a decrease in FEV_1, mean forced expiratory flow, and central airway resistance, was measured. Baseline lung function was altered more significantly in both male and female patients who lived in downtown Marseilles than in those who resided in the suburbs. The differences persisted regardless of the season during which the study occurred. Pope and Kanner assessed the association between PM_{10} and changes in FEV_1, FEV_1/forced vital capacity (FVC), and FVC in smokers with mild to moderate airflow limitation.[54] These spirometric data were obtained from Salt Lake City inhabitants from the Lung Health Study at two screening visits 10 to 90 days apart following an initial screening visit. Differences in pulmonary function were analyzed, and significant associations between changes in pulmonary function and PM_{10} were observed. The changes in FEV_1 and FEV_1/FVC were inversely associated with changes in PM_{10}. On average, an increase in PM_{10} equal to 100 µg/m³ was associated with a decline in FEV_1 equal to approximately 2%. The authors concluded that in current smokers, PM_{10} possibly had a small transient negative effect on lung function, not entirely obscured by their smoking habit.

There are relatively few studies of the long-term respiratory effects of NO_2 relevant to COPD. The only prospective cohort study was in over 6,000 Seventh Day Adventists in California, whose personal indoor NO_2 exposures were estimated, and NO_2 measurements were taken from the nearest outdoor monitor to an individual's home. This study showed no significant association between personal exposure to NO_2 and risk of chronic obstructive bronchitis, although statistical significance was reached when only the average outdoor NO_2 exposure was used in the analysis.[55] However, a cross-sectional study in over 9,000 Swiss adults showed an association between respiratory symptoms and decreasing lung function and the annual mean NO_2 levels.[56] Thus, there are therefore still insufficient data from epidemiologic studies to demonstrate a causal link between NO_2 levels and deterioration in lung function or exacerbations in COPD patients.

The toxic effects of carbon monoxide relate to interference with intracellular respiration by its binding to cytochrome oxidase and myoglobin and by the formation of carboxyhemoglobin, which interferes with the transport of oxygen. Accidental or deliberate exposure to carbon monoxide poisoning results in many deaths. Epidemiologic studies have shown associations between levels of ambient carbon monoxide concentrations and mortality and hospital admission in susceptible individuals with ischemic heart disease.[57] There have been no associations published between respiratory mortality and/or respiratory admissions and ambient carbon monoxide levels.

The chronic effects of ozone have been studied in Seventh Day Adventists in California and suggest that long-term exposure to ozone may induce new cases of asthma.[58] In addition, studies of students at the University of California at Berkley, who were lifelong residents in California, have shown that exposure to ozone was associated with a decline in respiratory function.[59] No studies have examined exposure to ozone and the risk of developing COPD.

Studies have also shown associations between the levels of particulate air pollution and both lung function and symptoms, particularly in children.[60–63] In a cohort of adults with COPD participating in the Lung Health Study, there was an association between the level of FEV_1 and PM_{10} concentrations.[64] At least 15 studies have shown associations between particulate air pollution levels and daily respiratory symptoms, particularly in asthmatics.[54]

The longer-term effects of chronic exposure to particulate air pollution have also been studied. Cohort-based studies have also shown associations between respiratory symptoms and long-term PM exposure in nonsmoking adults.[65,66] The results of several studies typically show that a 10 µg/m³ increase in PM_{10} is associated with a 5 to 20% increase in symptoms of bronchitis or chronic cough.[67,68] Analysis of data from the first and second National Health and Nutrition Examination Surveys (NHANES II and III)[66] and from studies in different areas in Switzerland[56] show a small but statistically significant association in most studies between lung function and long-term particulate air pollution exposure.

The results typically show that a 10 µg/m³ increase in PM₁₀ is associated with a decline in lung function of around 1 to 3%.

A summary of the percent change in health end points in chronic respiratory studies is shown in Figure 2.

Mechanisms of the Harmful Effects of Air Pollutants on the Lungs

Sulfur Dioxide

SO_2 interacts with water in the lung-lining fluid to form SO_3^{2-} and HSO_3^- ions, together with other compounds. Both SO_3^{2-} and HSO_3^- are readily oxidized by biologic molecules, and this can result in the formation of free radicals, such as superoxide anion and the hydroxyl and sulfoxyl radicals. It is thought that the oxidative stress so produced results in the injurious and inflammatory effects of SO_2 in the lungs.[9] Sulfate can also potentiate the inactivation of α_1-antitrypsin by peroxynitrite, so contributing to the protease/antiprotease imbalance, which is thought to be important in the pathogenesis of COPD. SO_2 can also lower the lung's antioxidant defenses by depleting the thiol antioxidant glutathione (GSH), by inhibition of GSH redox enzymes.[69] SO_2 has also been shown in a number of animal studies and *in-vitro* studies to reduce ciliary beat frequency[70–73] and to increase the expression of genes coding for mucus proteins.[74,75]

Nitrogen Dioxide

In the lung-lining fluid, NO and NO_2 dissolve to form nitrate, nitrite, and nitrous acid. Co-exposure to cigarette smoke or smog, which both contain hydrogen peroxide, results in the formation of the hydroxyl radical, which is extremely reactive and damaging to cells and results in the generation of oxidative stress in the lungs.

Ozone

Ozone is one of the most potent oxidizing compounds. When ozone dissolves in the lung-lining fluid, it forms hydrogen peroxide, hydroperoxides, and reactive aldehydes by a process known as ozonolysis, which can produce oxidative stress in the lungs and deplete antioxidant defenses.[76,77]

Particles

The mechanisms of the harmful effects of particulate air pollution in the lungs have been studied in some detail in recent years since particles are the most potent of the pollution components in ambient air. The reason why PM₁₀ is so toxic in such low concentrations remains a puzzle but may well be related to the inability of the lungs of susceptible individuals to protect themselves against inhaled particles. PM₁₀ has well-documented free radical activity and the potential to produce oxidative stress and inflammation.[78]

The components of the coarse and fine fraction of environmental particles have been described in this chapter.

From a toxicologic viewpoint, the question is: which of these components is (are) likely to drive the exacerbations of COPD? This is an important question from the viewpoint of the source apportionment of particles and their components, in focusing attempts to reduce the most harmful size fraction and components in designing exhaust emission-reduction systems. Knowledge of the most harmful component of the particle mix will result in targeting car exhaust systems and particle trap design to attain optimal effectiveness of emission reduction measures. The ability of the various components to produce oxidative stress and thereby initiate or prolong inflammation is a likely route whereby any particulate fraction might have an effect in COPD. Oxidative stress of environmental particle samples has been identified extensively as a mechanism for the adverse cellular effects of particles and

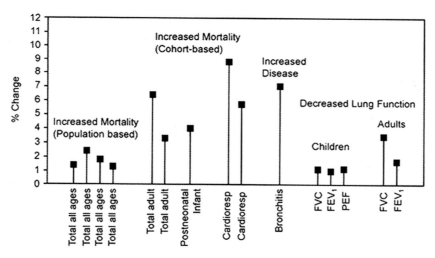

FIGURE 2. Summary of chronic exposure studies shown by the percent change in health end point for a 5 µg/m³ change in PM₂.₅. FEV₁ = forced expiratory volume in 1 second; FVC = forced vital capacity; PEF = peak expiratory flow.

pathogenesis generally (see elsewhere in this volume). However, it was recently suggested that sampling of particles to measure redox activity and spatial variation of PM redox activity could yield important information.[79] The long-term aim is therefore to build on the few studies that have used the oxidative stress potential of the particles sampled in epidemiologic studies[80] to link oxidative activity of PM to health end points in large population studies, with a view toward its adoption as a standard exposure metric. This is not suggested as a measure to replace the PM_{10} or $PM_{2.5}$ metrics at present but represents a complementary metric that more closely approaches the "biologically effective dose" that drives the toxic response to any substance.

There is little within the coarse fraction that is likely to have this effect composed, as it is, principally of salts and crustal components. However, in the fine and ultrafine fractions, there are components with the potential to cause oxidative stress when particles deposit in lung-lining fluid and interact with cells. Oxidative stress can arise directly from the particles themselves through the localized release of transition metals. For instance, in cell-free systems, we have shown that both Edinburgh PM_{10} and London PM_{10} have the ability to generate hydroxyl radical activity that is blockable by transition metal chelators.[81] Similar transition metal-mediated free radical generation has been demonstrated in particulate matter from Utah Valley[82] and for residual oil fly ash (ROFA).[83] This is further supported by studies in which the addition of particulates such as ROFA and PM_{10} to cells in culture cause metal-dependent oxidative stress and gene expression of proinflammatory mediators.[83,84] When the same types of particles are instilled into the lungs of animals, again, the subsequent inflammation that arises is driven by transition metals.[85–88]

Combustion-Derived Nanoparticles as the Most Toxicologically Potent Particle Type in PM

Ultrafine particles or nanoparticles (NPs) <100 nm are very readily measurable in urban air and comprise the greatest fraction by number of all of the size fractions. In conurbations, the NPs arise predominantly from combustion sources, are carbon-centered "soots" and combustion-derived nanoparticles (CDNPs), and have been identified as part of a group of highly potent particles with common oxidative stressing and proinflammatory properties.[89]

NP number concentrations across three European cities range from 15,000 to 18,000 particles/cm³,[90] compared with 10,000 to 50,000 particles/cm³ in a busy London street.[91] In a vehicle traveling in busy traffic in a study on US highways, exposure was 200 to 560×10^3 particles/cm³, predominantly NPs.[92,93] Indoor cooking, vacuuming, and burning wax candles all produce NPs.[94] CDNPs also arise from combustion of domestic gas, and in one study, three gas rings produced around 50,000 particles/cm³, which underwent rapid aggregation, with increases in particle size and a decrease in apparent number within a few minutes.[95] Secondary NPs may also

arise from environmental chemistry, for example, nitrates, but these are unlikely to be as toxicologically potent as CDNPs (see below). The mechanisms of the adverse effects of CDNPs have been extensively reviewed by the authors.[89,96] Direct epidemiologic evidence of their role in the adverse effects of PM_{10} is scanty because ultrafine particles are not routinely measured in urban air sampling programs. However, several epidemiologic studies have been able to identify traffic- and combustion-derived NPs as an important component in driving the adverse effects of PM.[97–105]

Toxicologic evidence supports the contention that CDNPs may be important mediators of adverse effects.[89,106,107] Ultrafine particles may also be found in the fine fraction since ultrafine particles aggregate, if they are in high enough concentration, to form secondary particles that have a larger aerodynamic diameter but are, in fact, composed of multiple ultrafine particles; these may then disaggregate in the lungs.

NPs in general deposit readily in the lungs, but in COPD, ultrafine particles were found to deposit in greater quantity than in normal lung, presumably owing to turbulence in the flow of air or the speed of airflow through inflamed or partially blocked airways.[108] Peters and colleagues reported that decrements in evening peak flow in a group of asthmatics were best associated with the ultrafine component of the airborne particles during a severe pollution episode[109]; COPD patients might also be at risk from ultrafine particles.

Animal studies have been used extensively to demonstrate that NPs have enhanced pathogenic potential compared with larger respirable particles of the same material.[89] Following instillation of ultrafine carbon black and fine carbon black at the same mass, there was substantially more inflammation with the NP carbon black and titanium dioxide (TiO_2) than the fine carbon black and TiO_2, respectively. Similar results have been shown for other ultrafine materials that are insoluble and nontoxic, including latex and TiO_2.[110,111] NPs have a relatively huge surface area compared with the same mass of larger particles, so it is important to discriminate whether the ability of NPs to cause inflammation is merely an ability to release from their large surface area high local concentrations of transition metals. Diesel exhaust and other combustion-derived, carbon-centered particles such as ROFA often have high levels of transition metals and organic molecules associated with them,[89] and the generation of free radicals by surfaces, metals, and organics underlies the oxidative and proinflammatory effects of CDNPs.[89] We have demonstrated that, at least in the case of ultrafine carbon black, the inflammation is not mediated by transition metals since treating the ultrafine particles with a transition metal chelator had no effect on the ability of the ultrafine carbon black to cause inflammation.[112] Additionally, a soluble extract of the ultrafine carbon black that would contain any transition metals was not inflammogenic. It is therefore necessary to consider the surface area of ultrafine particles an additional risk factor in addition to the transition metal content of any airborne PM$_{10}$ sample.[89] Marano and colleagues extensively studied the role of organics in generating proinflammatory effects and oxidative stress.[113]

Transition Metals, Organics, Free Radicals, and NP Toxicity

The production of free radicals in the lungs is being seen as a general mechanism mediating the biologic activity of a number of different pathogenic particles.[114,115] In the case of the environment particle cloud, which is highly heterogeneous, the CDNPs stand out as especially potent. The oxidative stress so produced is thought to arise first from the particles themselves and by the localized release from the particles of transition metals and organics.[89] This oxidative stress may be subsequently supplemented by the release of reactive oxygen species from inflammatory leukocytes that migrate into the airspaces as a result of the primary interaction between lung cells and particles (Figure 3). Oxidative stress is a general signaling mechanism within cells that produces the transcription of a number of proinflammatory genes for cytokines and adhesion molecules but also for protective antioxidant enzymes.[116] Under the influence of oxidative stress, the transcription factor NF-κB separates from its inhibitor, IκB, and translocates to the nucleus to bind to the promoter region of key genes for inflammatory mediators, allowing their transcription.[116] CDNPs can generate free radicals that would be a substantial stimulus to transcription.[89]

Recent data also suggest that PM$_{2.5}$ (PM < 2.5 μ in aerodynamic diameter) causes c-jun-dependent activator protein-1 (AP-1) activation.[117] The signal transduction pathway for these events may be through oxidant-mediated activation of

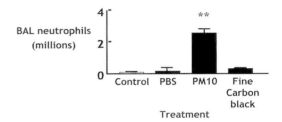

FIGURE 4. Influx of neutrophils into bronchoalveolar lavage (BAL) in rats following instillation of 125 μg of PM$_{10}$ and fine (260 nm diameter) carbon particles. Comparison data for animals that received no instillation (control) and instillation with phosphate-buffered saline (PBS) are shown. **$p < .01$ compared with PBS or fine carbon black.

Ras/mitogen-activated protein kinases.[118] As described above, the instillation of PM$_{10}$ into the lungs of rats produced neutrophil influx into the airspaces (Figure 4) and oxidative stress as shown by depletion of GSH in lung-lining fluid.[88] Importantly, PM$_{10}$ caused significantly more inflammation than a similar mass (125 μg) of carbon black that was 260 nm in diameter (ie, not in the ultrafine size range). Similar effects have been shown following inhalation of ultrafine but not fine carbon black.[119] These studies support the concept that the NP component of PM$_{10}$ is responsible for its toxic effects, through an oxidant-mediated mechanism.

ROFA has been used as a surrogate for PM$_{10}$, although it is very different in many respects from PM$_{10}$. ROFA causes pulmonary inflammation after instillation via a transition metal-mediated mechanism.[120] Furthermore, in rats instilled with ROFA, an intraperitoneal injection of the free radical scavenger dimethylthiourea (DMTU) decreased the extent of polymorphonuclear leukocyte influx to the lungs.[121] ROFA particles also caused increased transcription of cytokine genes by human bronchial epithelial cells *in vitro* via a transition metal-mediated mechanism,[122] as shown by the fact that the effect could be blocked with the metal chelator desferoxamine. Interestingly, the stimulation of cytokine production could be mimicked by vanadium salts in solution but not by iron or nickel sulfate, suggesting a possible important role for vanadium that affects protein kinase(s) activity.

Similarly, diesel oil particles and PM$_{10}$ were recently shown to enhance gene expression and the release of cytokines from primary cultures of airway epithelial cells *in vitro* by a metal-dependent oxidative stress mechanism.[83,84,123]

Activation of NF-κB in the Lungs by Particles

The transcriptional activator NF-κB is a nuclear factor of the Rel family that is translocated to the nucleus to permit expression of a wide range of proinflammatory genes.[116] The NF-κB heterodimer, comprising p65 and p50 proteins, is found in resting cells bound to its inhibitor, IκB, which masks the nuclear translocation signal and so prevents its translocation to the nucleus. Under oxidative stress or a range of other

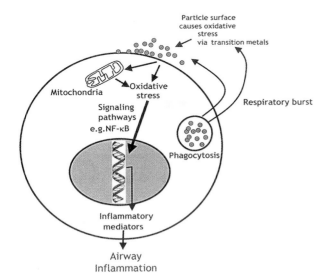

FIGURE 3. Hypothetical pathway for generation of oxidative stress and hence airway inflammation after exposure of airspace leukocytes to environmental particles. NF-κB = nuclear factor κB.

stimuli, such as tumor necrosis factor (TNF), the IκB is phosphorylated and then degraded via the ubiquitin proteosome system, allowing the NF-κB to relocate to the nucleus. Genes that have a κB binding site in their promoter include cytokines, growth factors, chemokines, and adhesion molecules and receptors.[116] We have demonstrated translocation of NF-κB from the cytoplasm to the nucleus by PM$_{10}$ in lung epithelial cells (Figure 5).[84] There is also evidence that increased intracellular calcium may be involved in the signaling pathways in cells in response to PM$_{10}$ and ultrafine particles in lung cells.[124] Brief inhalation of PM$_{2.5}$ CAPs (300 μg/m^3) for 6 hours in mice caused significant increases in steady-state messenger ribonucleic acid (mRNA) levels of a number of NF-κB- regulated genes, including TNF-α and -β, IL-6, interferon-γ, and transforming growth factor -β.[125]

PM$_{10}$ has also been shown to affect chromatin remodeling, which will enhance gene expression for proinflammatory cytokins. *In-vitro* studies indicate that histone deacetylase expression is reduced in epithelial cells exposed to PM$_{10}$, which would result in increased histone acetylation and unwinding of deoxyribonucleic acid (DNA) around the histone residues, so allowing access for transcription factors to DNA, causing enhanced gene transcription.[126]

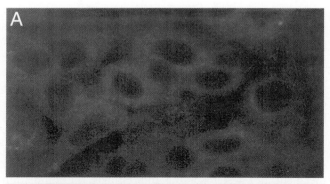
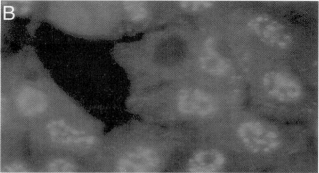

FIGURE 5. Type II alveolar epithelial cells were treated with a green fluorescently labeled antibody to the p50 component of nuclear factor κB (NF-κB). (*A*) In untreated cells, most of the fluorescently labeled NF-κB is in the cytosol. (*B*) Following treatment with 125 μg of PM$_{10}$, the fluorescently labeled NF-κB has now translocated to the nucleus. Reproduced with permission from Jimenez LA et al.[84]

The presence of the adenovirus regulatory gene *E1A* has been suggested to be a possible factor in susceptibility to inflammation caused by cigarette smoke. The *E1A* gene has been found to be present at a higher frequency in the lungs of COPD patients than in those of similar smokers without COPD.[127] The presence of *E1A* also enhances the inflammatory response of cells to endotoxin and oxidative stress.[128] Gilmour and colleagues measured IL-8 mRNA expression and protein release in response to PM$_{10}$ in human alveolar epithelial cells (A549) transfected with the *E1A* gene (E1A+ve).[126] The activation of the AP-1 and NF-κB was also assessed. E1A+ve cells showed an enhanced IL-8 mRNA and protein response following treatment with H$_2$O$_2$ and PM$_{10}$ compared with E1A−ve cells. Enhanced induction of IL-8 in E1A+ve cells was accompanied by increases in AP-1 and NF-κB nuclear binding and higher basal nuclear binding of these transcription factors. These data suggest that the presence of *E1A* primes the transcriptional machinery for oxidative stress signaling and therefore facilitates amplification of proinflammatory responses. Susceptibility to exacerbation of COPD in response to particulate air pollution may be conferred by this mechanism in COPD patients harboring *E1A* following adenoviral infection.

Implications of an Oxidative Stress-mediated Mechanism of Action of PM$_{10}$ for Susceptible Patients with Airways Disease

Since particles deposit on the epithelium, prior to phagocytosis, it seems likely that the airway epithelium is a target for PM$_{10}$ that may have a role in the observed increase in exacerbations of COPD. Within PM, the CDNP fraction seems to be especially important in driving inflammatory effects. The CDNPs in the PM$_{10}$ can compromise the epithelium by causing oxidative stress injury and inflammation. In addition, the underlying chronic inflammation in the airways of patients with COPD means that the airway cells are in a "primed" state for the further oxidative stress caused by depositing CDNPs.

The principal pulmonary effects of PM$_{10}$ are seen in susceptible populations, such as those with airways disease, including patients with COPD. If, as hypothesized here, PM$_{10}$ has its effect mainly via the CDNPs acting by a mechanism that involves oxidative stress, then these susceptible populations might be susceptible because of preexisting oxidative stress. The adenoviral *E1A* genes may be a mechanism whereby the COPD lung is primed for oxidative stress-induced inflammation from particles. We have demonstrated depleted antioxidant defenses in patients with airways disease.[129] Plasma from patients with COPD was found to have significantly lower antioxidant capacity than that from normal subjects, and a further decrease occurred during exacerbations of the disease. Clearly, these patients would be susceptible to an oxidative insult such as that hypothesized here to emanate from PM$_{10}$. Furthermore, only 15% of smokers develop COPD, and at least part of this susceptibility to the effects of COPD may be genetic,[130] relating to the ability of the subject to detoxify injurious components of cigarette smoke, including oxidants. Such genetic polymorphisms may also be associated with the susceptibility of patients with COPD to the effects of air pollutants.

Endotoxin

The ubiquitous gram-negative bacterial product endotoxin (lipopolysaccharide) is found in many PM_{10} samples. In some in-vitro studies, the endotoxin has been found to explain the biologic activity.[131–133] However, many studies show that the major biologic activity in a PM sample is not endotoxin but is, in fact, transition metal.[84] However, the multicomponent nature of PM_{10} does not preclude "networking" between cells in orchestrating an inflammatory response, for example, stimulation of macrophages by lipopolysaccharide and epithelial cells by metals or ultrafine particles.

Effects of Pollutants on the Airways

Any effects that pollutants have in promoting airway obstruction would very likely contribute to the worsening of COPD. Several studies demonstrate direct effects of pollutants on the mucociliary clearance system and mucus production by airway cells, and these are reviewed in the following section.

The mucociliary escalator is an important defense mechanism in the airways against inhaled particles. In the large proximal airways, goblet cells secrete mucus, which traps deposited particles. The mucus, with its trapped particles, is then propelled upward by ciliated cells to be either expectorated or swallowed. Mucus secretion is controlled by several genes,[134] whose expression may be induced by particles and other air pollutants.[74,135] Mucus has a major role in protecting the airways, particularly as it is a rich source of antioxidants.[136] However, mucus hypersecretion is the defining feature of chronic bronchitis.[137] Although mucus may, in some circumstances, have a protective role, induction of increased mucus secretion by particles may contribute to the development of exacerbations of COPD by increasing airway resistance by the development of mucus plugging in the smaller peripheral airways, a feature that is commonly present in patients dying of COPD.[138] In cigarette smokers and COPD patients, there is damage to the cilia, which, together with the excess amounts of mucus that is produced, overwhelms the mucociliary escalator and will reduce the ability of the lungs to deal adequately with inhaled particles.

Effects of Pollutants on the Airway Epithelium

Any effects that pollutants have in promoting airway obstruction would very likely contribute to the worsening of COPD. Several studies demonstrate the direct effects of pollutants on the mucociliary clearance system and mucus production by airway cells, and these are reviewed in the following section.

Effects on Ciliated Epithelial Cells

Kienast and colleagues investigated the influence of SO_2 on epithelial cells from nasal brushings from 12 healthy volunteers.[70] Nasal ciliated cells were exposed to SO_2, and ciliary beat frequency was measured. SO_2 exposure caused a dose-dependent decrease in ciliary beat frequency that ranged from 42.8% with 2.5 ppm SO_2 to 100% inhibition with 12.5 ppm SO_2. Majima and colleagues also demonstrated slowing of mucociliary transport in chickens exposed to 6 ppm SO_2.[71] This appeared to be a result of a change in the recoil distance of mucus caused by SO_2 exposure in vivo, and the authors proposed that SO_2 causes the formation of multiple points of adhesion of transit mucus between acinar gland cells and the emergent extracellular mucus; the net effect of this is for mucociliary transport to be retarded. Min and colleagues studied olfactory epithelium of mice exposed for up to 120 minutes to 20 ppm SO_2.[72] Exposure time, a surrogate for dose, was related to changes in ciliary loss, epithelial thinning, and desquamation; the changes were most pronounced 24 hours after exposure. Nikula and Wilson used rat tracheal organ cultures exposed to 1 ppm ozone and reported loss of ciliated cells and ciliated cell damage.[139] Kienast and colleagues used human respiratory epithelial cells from healthy volunteers.[70] The cells were grown on membranes at air-fluid interfaces and exposed to gaseous SO_2 for 30 minutes at 2 hours. Under these conditions, the cells exposed to air showed a 20% reduction in ciliary beat frequency but exposed to SO_2 (2.5–12.5 ppm) caused a concentration-dependent further decrease in ciliary frequency. In a related study, Riechelmann and colleagues described morphologic changes in guinea pig trachea exposed to SO_2 for 30 minutes.[73] Mucociliary activity was halved on exposure to SO_2, but, despite this, only minor morphologic alterations were observed. At high exposures, there was further slowing of ciliary activity, with widespread structural alterations such as sloughing, edema, and mitochondrial swelling. Tamaoki and colleagues exposed human bronchial epithelial cells to 3 ppm SO_2.[140] This rapidly decreased the ciliary beat frequency by 59% and was accompanied by a reduction in intracellular cyclic adenosine monophosphate levels to a quarter. Interestingly, this effect was prevented by pretreatment of cells with an antihistamine, azelastine. Carson and colleagues exposed human nasal epithelial cells to 2 ppm NO_2 for 4 hours.[141] The authors reported a trend toward structural alterations in six of seven nasal epithelial samples, characterized by excess matrix in the cilia, multiple ciliary axonemes, and vesiculations of the luminal border of the ciliary membranes. Chitano and colleagues exposed rats to 10 ppm NO_2 and ozone for 7 days and assessed lung inflammation and morphology, airway microvascular leakage, and in-vitro contractile responses of the main bronchi.[142] Histologic signs of increased inflammation were evident in the respiratory bronchioles and alveoli, and there was loss of cilia from the epithelium of the small airways. No alterations in microvascular permeability or smooth muscle responsiveness were found. Kakinoki and colleagues exposed rabbits for 24 hours to 3 ppm NO_2 and then assessed ciliary activity, mucociliary transport velocity in the trachea, and tracheal permeability.[143] In rabbits exposed to NO_2, ciliary activity was decreased, as was mucociliary transport velocity, whereas epithelial permeability was increased.

Effects on Mucus-Secreting Cells

Saldiva and colleagues took an interesting approach and housed rats either in the center of Sao Paulo, the largest city in South America, or in a nonpolluted area.[144] The rats housed in the polluted area developed secretory cell hyperplasia in their airways and alterations in cilia at the ultrastructural level and had more rigid mucus; all of these changes contributed to impairment of mucociliary clearance. Additionally, the number of inflammatory cells in the bronchoalveolar lavage was higher in the air pollution-exposed group than in the group kept in a nonpolluted area. Harkema and colleagues exposed Bonnet monkeys to 0.15 or 3 ppm ozone for 6 to 90 days for 8 hours per day.[145] The end points selected were quantitative morphologic changes as assessed by light and electron microscopy. Lesions consisting of necrotic ciliated cells, shortened cilia, and secretory cell hyperplasia were seen after 6- and 90-day exposure to both levels of ozone. Some adaptation was present, with inflammatory cell influx being present only at 6 days and not at 90 days.

Basbaum and colleagues measured steady-state levels of mucin mRNA following exposure to SO_2 in rats.[74] There was an increase in goblet cells from 0 to 4.5/mm in the trachea, from 0.2 to 6.2/mm in the mainstem bronchus, and from 0.2 to 22.7/mm in the distal airways. Concomitantly, mucin mRNA was increased up to ninefold in response to SO_2 exposure. Jany and colleagues measured mucin gene expression in rat airways following exposure to SO_2 and reported qualitative increases in mucin mRNA in Northern blots.[75] In an attempt to more closely mimic realistic exposure to mixtures of pollutants, Abraham and colleagues exposed sheep to a combined ozone and SO_2 cloud and measured tracheal mucus velocity and ciliary beat frequency.[146] On two separate occasions, sheep were exposed to either 0.3 ppm ozone and 3 ppm SO_2 or air. The combination of ozone and SO_2 depressed tracheal mucus velocity by 40% compared with the air exposure, with no corresponding change in ciliary beat frequency. Since the ciliary beat frequency was conserved, it must be assumed that either the contact between the cilia and the mucus or the mechanical properties of the mucus were changed by the exposure to ozone and SO_2.

In a potentially important study, guinea pigs were either exposed to ambient polluted air in Mexico City or were kept in filtered clean air. The guinea pigs exposed to the ambient air showed extreme damage to the epithelium. This included loss of cilia, detachment of epithelial cells, and eosinophil and macrophage migration toward alveolar spaces through type I pneumocytes with destruction of their basal membranes. In six guinea pigs in the exposed group, bacteria were seen along the airways, with an associated inflammatory response. This was interepreted as colonization of the respiratory epithelium by bacteria as the result of the impairment on the defense mechanism caused by the exposure to environmental ozone and PM_{10}.[147]

Jiang and colleagues used a panel of particulate samples that included ROFA; fly ash from a domestic oil burning furnace; ambient PM from St. Louis, Ottawa, and Washington, DC; and volcanic ash from Mount St. Helen's. All of these were tested for their effects on mucus secretion in guinea pig tracheal epithelial cells. Only ROFA produced significant stimulation of mucus secretion, and studies with antioxidants showed the mechanism to be an oxidant-mediated one. Furthermore, ROFA caused dramatic reductions in GSH by a transition metal-mediated mechanism. mRNA for the mucus gene *MUC2* was increased following ROFA treatment concomitantly with the increased secretion of mucus. A similar study was carried out by Longphre and colleagues, who measured the effect of ROFA on the mucin gene *MUC5ac* and lysozyme mRNA.[135] There was marked upregulation of the *MUC5ac* and lysozyme genes on exposure to ROFA and vanadium, which comprised 18.8% by weight of the ROFA and mediated the oxidative stress that caused the gene expression. The authors suggested that vanadium acts as a tyrosine phosphatase inhibitor favoring phosphorylation-dependent signaling pathways that lead to mucin and lysozyme secretion.

Interstitialization of Particles

Inhaled particles deposit in large numbers beyond the ciliated airways, in the terminal airways and proximal alveoli,[148] where the net flow of air is zero and where, for very small particles, deposition efficiency increases because of the high efficiency of deposition by diffusion.[149]

Interference with the normal process of phagocytosis and macrophage migration to the mucociliary escalator can lead to the adverse outcome of interstitialization.[150,151] Interstitialization results from the failure of the particles to be cleared by the normal pathways so that they will either remain in the interstitium, where they can chronically stimulate interstitial cells or will transfer to the lymph nodes. Interstitialization of particles was a prominent correlate of the onset of inflammation for ultrafine TiO_2 in the study of Ferin and colleagues.[152] In experimental studies, Churg and colleagues demonstrated that PM and NPs can cross the epithelium of organ cultures of airway[153] and can stimulate fibrogenic responses.[154–156]

In vivo, interstitialization is likely to occur when there is impaired clearance, which could result from (a) particle-mediated macrophage toxicity or impairment of macrophage motility[157,158] or (b) overload in the case of rats. Both of these events would allow increased interaction between particles and epithelium that would favor interstitialization. In studies with rats, ultrafine particles and PM_{10} cause increased epithelial permeability, which would also enhance interstitialization of particles.[88]

COPD and Exposure to Particles from Biomass Burning during Cooking

Almost 2.5 billion people across the world rely on burning of biomass for their cooking and heating needs, where the sources of biomass include coal, charcoal, wood, crops or other agricultural waste, dung, shrubs, grass, and straw, among others.[159] The global annual mortality of children alone from indoor air pollution has been calculated at 950,000.[159] Women and girls are also at high risk owing to their intimate daily involvement in domestic work, and cooking produces high, sustained exposure. World Health Organization figures suggest that in excess of 530,000 COPD deaths in women are attributable to indoor air pollution.[160] Men are not spared, however, and about 180,000 male COPD deaths can be attributed to indoor air pollution,[160] although there is clearly an important gender inequality in risk.

COPD results from this massive smoke exposure, which is also referred to as "hut lung" or "domestically acquired particulate lung disease."[161] Thus, environmental exposure in homes in developing countries is producing a disease that is also produced by workplace exposures in the developed world. The reason for this becomes clear when the airborne mass concentrations of particles are examined. In a home where there is unflued burning of biomass, airborne mass concentrations in the order of 1,000 to 13,000 $\mu g/m^3$ are reported,[161] compared with typical average outdoor levels in a busy conurbation such as London, which seldom exceed 50 $\mu g/m^3$.

Put into the context of this massive exposure, it is not surprising that studies have reported impaired lung function, increasing respiratory symptoms and incidence of lung infection, and even fibrosis, all typical of COPD in women working in unflued homes in Bangladesh,[161] Turkey,[162] Nepal,[163] Mexico,[164] and across Africa and Asia generally.[165]

Although the mechanisms of the effects of indoor burning of biomass are not understood at present, the CDNP model seems likely to be applicable.[89] In that regard, it has been noted that burning of dung, a common biomass fuel, produces a soot that is very rich in transition metals and oxidative stress potential.[166]

A research program is urgently needed to address and ameliorate this vast problem.

References

1. Evelyn J. Fumifugium or, the inconvenience of the aer. and smoke of London dissipated. J Chronic Dis 1965;12:1235–58.
2. Brimblecombe P. Air pollution and health history. In: Holgate ST, Samet JM, Koren HS, Maynard RL, editors. Air pollution and health. London: Academic Press; 1999. p. 5–18.
3. Russell R. Smoke in relation to fogs in London. London: National Smoke Abatement Institute; 1887.
4. Galton D. Preventable causes of impurity in London air. London: Sanitary Institute of Great Britain; 1880.
5. Russell WT. The influence of fog on mortality from respiratory diseases. Lancet 1924;II:335–9.
6. Ministry of Health. Mortality and morbidity during the London fog of December 2952. London: HMSO; 1954. Reports on Public Health and Medical Subjects No.: 95.
7. Logan WPD. Mortality in the London fog incident, 1952. Lancet 1953;1:336.
8. Bates DV. Setting the stage: critical risks. In: Environmental health risks and public policy. Decision making in free societies. Jessie and John Danz Lecture Series. Seattle: University of Washington Press; 1994. p. 6–56.
9. Wellburn A. Air pollution and climate change: the biological impact. New York: Longman; 1994.
10. Pryor WA, Church DF. Aldehydes, hydrogen peroxide, and organic radicals as mediators of ozone toxicity. Free Radic Biol Med 1991;11:41–6.
11. Expert Panel on Air Quality. Particles. London: HSO; 1995.
12. Ayres JG. Health effects of gaseous air pollutants. In: Hester RE, Harrison RM, editors. Issues in environmental science and technology 10. Air pollution and health. Cambridge, The Royal Society of Chemistry, 1998. p. 1–20.
13. Watt M, Godden D, Cherrie J, Seaton A. Individual exposure to particulate air pollution and its relevance to thresholds for health effects: a study of traffic wardens. Occup Environ Med 1995;52:790–2.
14. Sheppard D. Sulfur dioxide and asthma—a double-edged sword? J Allergy Clin Immunol 1988;82:961–4.
15. Newhouse MT, Wolff RK, Dolovich M, Obminski G. Effect of TLV levels of SO₂ and H₂ SO₄ on bronchial clearance in exercising man. Arch Environ Health 1978;33:24–32.
16. Wolff RK, Dolovich M, Rossman CM, Newhouse MT. Sulfur dioxide and tracheobronchial clearance in man. Arch Environ Health 1975;30:521–7.
17. von Nieding G, Wagner M, Krekeler H, et al. Minimum concentrations of NO₂ causing acute effects on the respiratory gas exchange and airway-resistance in patients with chronic bronchitis. Int Arch Arbeitsmed 1971;27:338–48.
18. Vagaggini B, Paggiaro PL, Giannini D, et al. Effect of short-term NO₂ exposure on induced sputum in normal, asthmatic and COPD subjects. Eur Respir J 1996;9:1852–7.
19. Solic JJ, Hazucha MJ, Bromberg PA. The acute effects of 0.2 ppm ozone in patients with chronic obstructive pulmonary disease. Am Rev Respir Dis 1982;125:664–9.
20. Ghio AJ, Kim C, Devlin RB. Concentrated ambient air particles induce mild pulmonary inflammation in healthy human volunteers. Am J Respir Crit Care Med 2000;162:981–8.
21. Gong H, Linn WS, Terrell SL, et al. Exposures of elderly volunteers with and without chronic obstructive pulmonary disease (COPD) to concentrated ambient fine particulate pollution. Inhal Toxicol 2004;16:731–44.
22. Touloumi G, Katsouyanni K, Zmirou D, et al. Short-term effects of ambient oxidant exposure on mortality: a combined analysis within the APHEA project. Air Pollution and Health: a European Approach. Am J Epidemiol 1997;146:177–85.
23. Churg A, Brauer M, Carmen Avila-Casado M, et al. Chronic exposure to high levels of particulate air pollution and small airway remodeling. Environ Health Perspect 2003;111:714–8.
24. Sunyer J, Castellsague J, Saez M, et al. Air pollution and mortality in Barcelona. J Epidemiol Community Health 1996;50 Suppl 1:s76–80.

25. Wietlisbach V, Pope CA, Ackermann-Liebrich U. Air pollution and daily mortality in three Swiss urban areas. Soz Praventivmed 1996;41:107–15.

26. Rossi G, Vigotti MA, Zanobetti A, et al. Air pollution and cause-specific mortality in Milan, Italy, 1980–1989. Arch Environ Health 1999;54:158–64.

27. Wordley J, Walters S, Ayres JG. Short term variations in hospital admissions and mortality and particulate air pollution. Occup Environ Med 1997;54:108–16.

28. Schwartz J, Dockery DW, Neas LM. Is daily mortality associated specifically with fine particles? J Air Waste Manage Assoc 1996;46:927–39.

29. Xu X, Gao J, Dockery DW, Chen Y. Air pollution and daily mortality in residential areas of Beijing, China. Arch Environ Health 1994;49:216–22.

30. Schwartz J, Dockery DW. Increased mortality in Philadelphia associated with daily air pollution concentrations. Am Rev Respir Dis 1992;145:600–4.

31. Tobias A, Campbell MJ, Saez M. Modelling asthma epidemics on the relationship between air pollution and asthma emergency visits in Barcelona, Spain. Eur J Epidemiol 1999; 15:799–803.

32. Morgan G, Corbett S, Wlodarczyk J. Air pollution and hospital admissions in Sydney, Australia, 1990 to 1994. Am J Public Health 1998;88:1761–6.

33. Harre ES, Price PD, Ayrey RB, et al. Respiratory effects of air pollution in chronic obstructive pulmonary disease: a three month prospective study. Thorax 1997;52:1040–4.

34. Moolgavkar SH, Luebeck EG, Anderson EL. Air pollution and hospital admissions for respiratory causes in Minneapolis-St. Paul and Birmingham. Epidemiology 1997;8:364–70.

35. Ackermann-Liebrich U, Rapp R. Epidemiological effects of oxides of nitrogen, especially NO_2. In: Holgate ST, Samet JM, Koren HS, Maynard RL, editors. Air pollution and health. London: Academic Press; 1999. p. 561–84.

36. Anderson HR, Spix C, Medina S, et al. Air pollution and daily admissions for chronic obstructive pulmonary disease in 6 European cities: results from the APHEA project. Eur Respir J 1997;10:1064–71.

37. Dab W, Medina S, Quenel P, et al. Short term respiratory health effects of ambient air pollution: results of the APHEA project in Paris. J Epidemiol Community Health 1996;50 Suppl 1:s42–6.

38. Schouten JP, Vonk JM, de Graaf A. Short term effects of air pollution on emergency hospital admissions for respiratory disease: results of the APHEA project in two major cities in the Netherlands, 1977–89. J Epidemiol Community Health 1996;50 Suppl 1:s22–9.

39. Higgins BG, Francis HC, Yates CJ, et al. Effects of air pollution on symptoms and peak expiratory flow measurements in subjects with obstructive airways disease. Thorax 1995;50:149–55.

40. Schwartz J. Air pollution and hospital admissions for the elderly in Birmingham, Alabama. Am J Epidemiol 1994; 139:589–98.

41. Sunyer J, Saez M, Murillo C, et al. Air pollution and emergency room admissions for chronic obstructive pulmonary disease: a 5-year study. Am J Epidemiol 1993;137:701–5.

42. Medina-Ramon M, Zanobetti A, Schwartz J. The effect of ozone and PM10 on hospital admissions for pneumonia and chronic obstructive pulmonary disease: a national multicity study. Am J Epidemiol 2006;163:579–88.

43. Delfino RJ, Becklake MR, Hanley JA. The relationship of urgent hospital admissions for respiratory illnesses to photochemical air pollution levels in Montreal. Environ Res 1994;67:1–19.

44. Dockery DW, Pope CA, Xu XP, et al. An association between air-pollution and mortality in 6 United States cities. N Engl J Med 1993;329:1753–9.

45. Higgins IT, D'Arcy JB, Gibbons DI, et al. Effect of exposures to ambient ozone on ventilatory lung function in children. Am Rev Respir Dis 1990;141:1136–46.

46. DerSimonian R, Laird N. Meta-analysis in clinical trials. Control Clin Trials 1986;7:177–88.

47. Thurston GD, Ito K. Epidemiological studies of ozone exposure effects. In: Holgate ST, Samet JM, Koren HS, Maynard RL, editors. Air pollution and health. London: Academic Press; 1999. p. 485–520.

48. Tobias GA, Sunyer DJ, Castellsague PJ, et al. Impact of air pollution on the mortality and emergencies of chronic obstructive pulmonary disease and asthma in Barcelona. Gaceta Sanitaria 1998;12:223–30.

49. Schwartz J. Air-pollution and hospital admissions for the elderly in Detroit, Michigan. Am J Respir Crit Care Med 1994;150:648–55.

50. Schwartz J. PM_{10}, ozone, and hospital admissions for the elderly in Minneapolis-St. Paul, Minnesota. Arch Environ Health 1994;49:366–74.

51. Schwartz J. Short term fluctuations in air pollution and hospital admissions of the elderly for respiratory disease. Thorax 1995;50:531–8.

52. Schwartz J. Air pollution and hospital admissions for respiratory disease. Epidemiology 1996;7:20–8.

53. Jammes Y, Delpierre S, Delvolgo MJ, et al. Long-term exposure of adults to outdoor air pollution is associated with increased airway obstruction and higher prevalence of bronchial hyperresponsiveness. Arch Environ Health 1998;53:372–7.

54. Pope CA III, Kanner RE. Acute effects of PM10 pollution on pulmonary function of smokers with mild to moderate chronic obstructive pulmonary disease. Am Rev Respir Dis 1993;147:1336–40.

55. Abbey DE, Colome SD, Mills PK, et al. Chronic disease associated with long-term concentrations of nitrogen dioxide. J Expo Anal Environ Epidemiol 1993;3:181–202.

56. Ackermann-Liebrich U, Leuenberger P, et al. Lung function and long term exposure to air pollutants in Switzerland. Study on Air Pollution and Lung Diseases in Adults (SAPALDIA) Team. Am J Respir Crit Care Med 1997;155:122–9.

57. Poloniecki JD, Atkinson RW, de Leon AP, Anderson HR. Daily time series for cardiovascular hospital admissions and previous day's air pollution in London, UK. Occup Environ Med 1997;54:535–40.

58. Nishino N, Abbey DE, McDonnell WF. Long term ambient concentrations of ozone and development of asthma: the ASHMOB study. Epidemiology 1996;7 (Suppl4):S31.

59. Kunzli N, Lurmann F, Segal M, et al. Association between lifetime ambient ozone exposure and pulmonary function in college freshmen—results of a pilot study. Environ Res 1997;72:8–23.

60. Dockery DW, Ware JH, Ferris BG Jr, et al. Change in pulmonary function in children associated with air pollution episodes. J Air Pollut Control Assoc 1982;32:937–42.

61. Brunekreef B, Kinney PL, Ware JH, et al. Sensitive subgroups and normal variation in pulmonary function response to air pollution episodes. Environ Health Perspect 1991; 90:189–93.

62. Hoek G, Brunekreef B. Acute effects of a winter air pollution episode on pulmonary function and respiratory symptoms of children. Arch Environ Health 1993;48:328–35.

63. Hoek G, Brunekreef B. Effects of low-level winter air pollution concentrations on respiratory health of Dutch children. Environ Res 1994;64:136–50.

64. Pope CA, Bates DV, Raizenne ME. Health effects of particulate air pollution: time for reassessment? Environ Health Perspect 1995;103:472–80.

65. Abbey DE, Hwang BL, Burchette RJ, et al. Estimated long-term ambient concentrations of PM10 and development of respiratory symptoms in a nonsmoking population. Arch Environ Health 1995;50:139–52.

66. Schwartz J. Lung function and chronic exposure to air pollution: a cross-sectional analysis of NHANES II. Environ Res 1989;50:309–21.

67. Schwartz J. Particulate air-pollution and chronic respiratory-disease. Environ Res 1993;62:7–13.

68. Dockery D, Pope CA. Epidemiology of acute health effects: summary of time-series studies. In: Wilson R, Spengler JD, editors. Particles in our air. Cambridge (MA): Harward University Press; 1996. p. 123–47.

69. Langley-Evans SC, Phillips GJ, Jackson AA. Sulphur dioxide: a potent glutathione depleting agent. Comp Biochem Physiol C Pharmacol Toxicol Endocrinol 1996;114:89–98.

70. Kienast K, Riechelmann H, Knorst M, et al. Combined exposures of human ciliated cells to different concentrations of sulfur dioxide and nitrogen dioxide. Eur J Med Res 1996;1:533–6.

71. Majima Y, Swift DL, Bang BG, Bang FB. Mechanism of slowing of mucociliary transport induced by SO_2 exposure. Ann Biomed Eng 1985;13:515–30.

72. Min YG, Rhee CS, Choo MJ, et al. Histopathologic changes in the olfactory epithelium in mice after exposure to sulfur dioxide. Acta Otolaryngol (Stockh) 1994;114:447–52.

73. Riechelmann H, Maurer J, Kienast K, et al. Respiratory epithelium exposed to sulfur dioxide-functional and ultrastructural alterations. Laryngoscope 1995;105:295–9.

74. Basbaum C, Gallup M, Gum J, et al. Modification of mucin gene expression in the airways of rats exposed to sulfur dioxide. Biorheology 1990;27:485–9.

75. Jany B, Gallup M, Tsuda T, Basbaum C. Mucin gene expression in rat airways following infection and irritation. Biochem Biophys Res Commun 1991;181:1–8.

76. Menzel DB. Antioxidant vitamins and prevention of lung disease. Ann N Y Acad Sci 1992;669:141–55.

77. Mudway IS, Kelly FJ. Ozone and the lung: a sensitive issue. Mol Aspects Med 2000;21:1–48.

78. MacNee W, Donaldson K. Mechanism of lung injury caused by PM_{10} and ultrafine particles with special reference to COPD. Eur Respir J Suppl 2003;40:47s–51s.

79. Borm PJ, Kelly F, Kunzli N, et al. Oxidant generation by particulate matter: from biologically effective dose to a promising, novel metric. Occup Environ Med 2007;64:73–4.

80. Kunzli N, Mudway IS, Gotschi T, et al. Comparison of oxidative properties, light absorbance, total and elemental mass concentration of ambient $PM_{2.5}$ collected at 20 European sites. Environ Health Perspect 2006;114:684–90.

81. Gilmour PS, Brown DM, Lindsay TG, et al. Adverse health effects of PM_{10} particles: involvement of iron in generation of hydroxyl radical. Occup Environ Med 1996;53:817–22.

82. Frampton MW, Ghio AJ, Samet JM, et al. Effects of aqueous extracts of PM(10) filters from the Utah valley on human airway epithelial cells. Am J Physiol 1999;277:L960–7.

83. Jiang N, Dreher KL, Dye JA, et al. Residual oil fly ash induces cytotoxicity and mucin secretion by guinea pig tracheal epithelial cells via an oxidant-mediated mechanism. Toxicol Appl Pharmacol 2000;163:221–30.

84. Jimenez LA, Thompson J, Brown DA, et al. Activation of NF-kappaB by PM(10) occurs via an iron-mediated mechanism in the absence of IkappaB degradation. Toxicol Appl Pharmacol 2000;166:101–10.

85. Costa DL, Dreher KL. Bioavailable transition metals in particulate matter mediate cardiopulmonary injury in healthy and compromised animal models. Environ Health Perspect 1997;105 Suppl 5:1053–60.

86. Dreher K, Jaskot R, Kodavanti U, et al. Soluble transition-metals mediate the acute pulmonary injury and airway hyperreactivity induced by residual oil fly-ash articles. Chest 1996;109:33S–34S.

87. Ghio AJ, Kadiiska MB, Xiang QH, Mason RP. In vivo evidence of free radical formation after asbestos instillation: an ESR spin trapping investigation. Free Radic Biol Med 1998;24:11–7.

88. Li XY, Gilmour PS, Donaldson K, MacNee W. Free radical activity and pro-inflammatory effects of particulate air pollution (PM_{10}) in vivo and in vitro. Thorax 1996; 51:1216–22.

89. Donaldson K, Tran L, Jimenez LA, et al. Combustion-derived nanoparticles: a review of their toxicology following inhalation exposure. Part Fibre Toxicol 2005;21:2–10.

90. de Hartog JJ, Hoek G, Mirme A, et al. Relationship between different size classes of particulate matter and meteorology in three European cities. J Environ Monit 2005;7:302–10.

91. Air Quality Expert Group. Patriculate matter in the United Kingdom. London: Department of Environment, Food and Rural Affairs; 2005.

92. Elder A, Gelein R, Finkelstein J, et al. On-road exposure to highway aerosols. 2. Exposures of aged, compromised rats. Inhal Toxicol 2004;16 Suppl 1:41–53.

93. Kittelson DB, Watts WF, Johnson JP, et al. On-road exposure to highway aerosols. 1. Aerosol and gas measurements. Inhal Toxicol 2004;16 Suppl 1:31–9.

94. Afshari A, Matson U, Ekberg LE. Characterization of indoor sources of fine and ultrafine particles: a study conducted in a full-scale chamber. Indoor Air 2005;15:141–50.

95. Dennekamp M, Howarth S, Dick CA, et al. Ultrafine particles and nitrogen oxides generated by gas and electric cooking. Occup Environ Med 2001;58:511–6.

96. Donaldson K, Jimenez LA, Rahman I, et al. Respiratory health effects of ambient air pollution particles: role of reactive species. In: Vallyathan V, Shi X, Castranova V, editors. Oxygen/nitrogen radicals: lung injury and disease. Lung biology in health and disease. Vol 187. New York: Marcel Dekker; 2004. p. 257–88.

97. Pope CA III, Hill RW, Villegas GM. Particulate air pollution and daily mortality on Utah's Wasatch Front 2. Environ Health Perspect 1999;107:567–73.

98. Laden F, Neas LM, Dockery DW, Schwartz J. Association of fine particulate matter from different sources with daily mortality in six U.S. cities. Environ Health Perspect 2000;108:941–7.

99. Schwartz J. What are people dying of on high air-pollution days? Environ Res 1994;64:26–35.

100. Ibald-Mulli A, Wichmann HE, Kreyling W, Peters A. Epidemiological evidence on health effects of ultrafine particles. J Aerosol Med 2002;15:189–201.

101. Peters A, von Klot S, Heier M, et al. Exposure to traffic and the onset of myocardial infarction. N Engl J Med 2004; 351:1721–30.

102. Dockery DW, Luttmann-Gibson H, Rich DQ, et al. Association of air pollution with increased incidence of ventricular tachyarrhythmias recorded by implanted cardioverter defibrillators. Environ Health Perspect 2005;113:670–4.

103. Schwartz J. Daily deaths are associated with combustion particles rather than SO(2) in Philadelphia. Occup Environ Med 2000;57:692–7.

104. Norris G, Larson T, Koenig J, et al. Asthma aggravation, combustion, and stagnant air. Thorax 2000;55:466–70.

105. Brunekreef B, Janssen NH, deHartog J, et al. Air pollution from truck traffic and lung function in children living near motorways. Epidemiology 1997;8:298–303.

106. Brown DM, Donaldson K, Borm PJ, et al. Calcium and ROS-mediated activation of transcription factors and TNF-alpha cytokine gene expression in macrophages exposed to ultrafine particles. Am J Physiol Lung Cell Mol Physiol 2004;286:L344–53.

107. Donaldson K, Stone V, Borm PJ, et al. Oxidative stress and calcium signaling in the adverse effects of environmental particles (PM$_{10}$). Free Radic Biol Med 2003;34:1369–82.

108. Bennett WD, Zeman KL, Kim C, Mascarella J. Enhanced deposition of fine particles in COPD patients spontaneously breathing at rest. Inhal Toxicol 1997;9:1–14.

109. Peters A, Wichmann HE, Tuch T, et al. Respiratory effects are associated with the number of ultrafine particles. Am J Respir Crit Care Med 1997;155:1376–83.

110. Brown DM, Wilson MR, MacNee W, et al. Size-dependent proinflammatory effects of ultrafine polystyrene particles: a role for surface area and oxidative stress in the enhanced activity of ultrafines. Toxicol Appl Pharmacol 2001;175:191–9.

111. Dick CA, Brown DM, Donaldson K, Stone V. The role of free radicals in the toxic and inflammatory effects of four different ultrafine particle types. Inhal Toxicol 2003; 15:39–52.

112. Brown DM, Stone V, Findlay P, et al. Increased inflammation and intracellular calcium caused by ultrafine carbon black is independent of transition metals or other soluble components. Occup Environ Med 2000;57:685–91.

113. Marano F, Boland S, Baeza-Squiban A. Particle-associated organics and proinflammatory signalling. In: Donaldson K, Borm PJA, editors. Particle toxicology. Boca Raton (FL): CRC Press; 2007. p. 211–26.

114. Kennedy TP, Dodson R, Rao NV, et al. Dusts causing pneumoconiosis generate .OH and produce hemolysis by acting as fenton catalysts. Arch Biochem Biophys 1989;269:359–64.

115. Donaldson K, Beswick PH, Gilmour PS. Free radical activity associated with the surface of particles: a unifying factor in determining biological activity? Toxicol Lett 1996;88:293–8.

116. Rahman I, MacNee W. Role of transcription factors in inflammatory lung diseases. Thorax 1998;53:601–12.

117. Timblin C, Berube KA, Churg A, et al. Ambient particulate matter causes activation of the c-jun kinase/stress activated protein kinase cascade and DNA synthesis in lung epithelial cells. Cancer Res 1998;58:4543–7.

118. Janssen YMW, Macara I, Mossman BT. Activation of NF-kappa B by reactive oxygen and nitrogen species in lung epithelial cells requires RAS/mitogen activated kinases. Am J Respir Crit Care Med 1998;157:A743.

119. Li XY, Donaldson K, MacNee W. Pro-inflammatory and oxidative activity of fine and ultrafine carbon black in rat lungs following instillation and inhalation. Am J Resp Crit Care Med 1998;157:A153.

120. Dreher KL, Jaskot RH, Lehmann JR, et al. Soluble transition metals mediate residual oil fly ash induced acute lung injury. J Toxicol Environ Health 1997;50:285–305.

121. Dye JA, Adler KB, Richards JH, Dreher KL. Epithelial injury induced by exposure to residual oil fly-ash particles: role of reactive oxygen species? Am J Respir Cell Mol Biol 1997;17:625–33.

122. Carter JD, Ghio AJ, Samet JM, Devlin RB. Cytokine production by human airway epithelial cells after exposure to an air pollution particle is metal-dependent. Toxicol Appl Pharmacol 1997;146:180–8.

123. Davis RJ, Bayram H, Abdelaziz MA. Effect of diesel exhaust particles on the release of inflammatory mediators from bronchial epithelial cells of atopic asthmatic patients and non-atopic asthmatic subjects. Am J Respir Crit Care Med 1998;157:A743.

124. Stone V, Tuinman M, Vamvakopoulos JE. 'Priming' of the calcium second messenger system in macrophages by ultrafine carbon black particles. Am J Respir Crit Care Med 1999;159:A27.

125. Shukla A, Timblin C, BeruBe K, et al. Inhaled particulate matter causes expression of nuclear factor (NF)-kappaB-related genes and oxidant-dependent NF-kappaB activation in vitro. Am J Respir Cell Mol Biol 2000;23:182–7.

126. Gilmour PS, Rahman I, Hayashi S, et al. Adenoviral E1A primes alveolar epithelial cells to PM(10)-induced transcription of interleukin-8. Am J Physiol Lung Cell Mol Physiol 2001;281:L598–606.

127. Hogg JC. Childhood viral infection and the pathogenesis of asthma and chronic obstructive lung disease. Am J Respir Crit Care Med 1999;160 (5 Pt 2):S26–8.

128. Keicho N, Higashimoto Y, Bondy GP, et al. Endotoxin-specific NF-kappaB activation in pulmonary epithelial cells harboring adenovirus E1A. Am J Physiol 1999;277:L523–32.

129. Rahman I, Morrison D, Donaldson K, MacNee W. Systemic oxidative stress in asthma, COPD, and smokers. Am J Respir Crit Care Med 1996;154:1055–60.

130. Sandford AJ, Weir TD, Pare PD. Genetic risk factors for chronic obstructive pulmonary disease. Eur Respir J 1997;10:1380–91.

131. Becker S, Soukup JM, Gilmour MI, Devlin RB. Stimulation of human and rat alveolar macrophages by urban air particulates: effects on oxidant radical generation and cytokine production. Toxicol Appl Pharmacol 1996;141:637–48.

132. Dreher K, Jaskot R. Role of particle-associated endotoxin in ambient air particulate matter induced pulmonary inflammation. FASEB J 1997;11:721.

133. Dong WM, Lewtas J, Luster MI. Role of endotoxin in tumor-necrosis-factor-alpha expression from alveolar macrophages treated with urban air particles. Exp Lung Res 1996; 22:577–92.

134. Jeffery PK, Li D. Airway mucosa: secretory cells, mucus and mucin genes. Eur Respir J 1997;10:1655–62.

135. Longphre M, Li D, Li J, et al. Lung mucin production is stimulated by the air pollutant residual oil fly ash. Toxicol Appl Pharmacol 2000;162:86–92.

136. Cross CE, van der Vliet A, O'Neill CA, et al. Oxidants, antioxidants, and respiratory tract lining fluids. Environ Health Perspect 1994;102 Suppl 10:185–91.

137. Definition and classification of chronic bronchitis for clinical and epidemiological purposes. A report to the Medical Research Council by their Committee on the Aetiology of Chronic Bronchitis. Lancet 1965;1:775–9.

138. Lamb D. Pathology. In: Calverley PMA, Pride NB, editors. Chronic obstructive pulmonary disease. London: Chapman & Hall; 1995. p. 9–34.

139. Nikula KJ, Wilson DW. Response of rat tracheal epithelium to ozone and oxygen exposure in vitro. Fundam Appl Toxicol 1990;15:121–31.

140. Tamaoki J, Chiyotani A, Sakai N, et al. Effect of azelastine on sulphur dioxide induced impairment of ciliary motility in airway epithelium. Thorax 1993;48:542–6.

141. Carson JL, Collier AM, Hu SC, Delvin RB. Effect of nitrogen dioxide on human nasal epithelium. Am J Respir Cell Mol Biol 1993;9:264–70.

142. Chitano P, Rado V, Di Stefano A, et al. Effect of subchronic in vivo exposure to nitrogen dioxide on lung tissue inflammation, airway microvascular leakage, and in vitro bronchial muscle responsiveness in rats. Occup Environ Med 1996;53:379–86.

143. Kakinoki Y, Ohashi Y, Tanaka A, et al. Nitrogen dioxide compromises defence functions of the airway epithelium. Acta Otolaryngol Suppl (Stockh) 1998;538:221–6.

144. Saldiva PH, King M, Delmonte VL, et al. Respiratory alterations due to urban air pollution: an experimental study in rats. Environ Res 1992;57:19–33.

145. Harkema JR, Plopper CG, Hyde DM, et al. Response of the macaque nasal epithelium to ambient levels of ozone. A morphologic and morphometric study of the transitional and respiratory epithelium. Am J Pathol 1987;128:29–44.

146. Abraham WM, Sielczak MW, Delehunt JC, et al. Impairment of tracheal mucociliary clearance but not ciliary beat frequency by a combination of low level ozone and sulfur dioxide in sheep. Eur J Respir Dis 1986;68:114–20.

147. Villegas-Castrejon H, Villalba-Caloca J, Meneses-Flores M, et al. Transmission electron microscopy findings in the respiratory epithelium of guinea pigs exposed to the polluted air of southwest Mexico City. J Environ Pathol Toxicol Oncol 1999;18:323–34.

148. Brody AR, Warheit DB, Chang LY, et al. Initial deposition pattern of inhaled minerals and consequent patho-genic events at the alveolar level. Ann N Y Acad Sci 1984; 428:108–20.

149. Anderson PJ, Wilson JD, Hiller FC. Respiratory tract deposition of ultrafine particles in subjects with obstructive or restrictive lung disease. Chest 1990;97:1115–20.

150. Morrow PE. Possible mechanisms to explain dust overloading of the lungs. Fundam Appl Toxicol 1988;10:369–84.

151. Churg A, Brauer M. Human lung parenchyma retains $PM_{2.5}$. Am J Respir Crit Care Med 1997;155:2109–11.

152. Ferin J, Oberdoerster G, Penney DP. Pulmonary retention of fine and ultrafine particles. Am J Respir Cell Mol Biol 1992;6:535–42.

153. Churg A, Stevens B, Wright JL. Comparison of the uptake of fine and ultrafine TiO_2 in a tracheal explant system. Am J Physiol 1998;274:L81–6.

154. Dai J, Xie C, Vincent R, Churg A. Air pollution particles produce airway wall remodeling in rat tracheal explants. Am J Respir Cell Mol Biol 2003;29:352–8.

155. Timblin CR, Shukla A, Berlanger I, et al. Ultrafine airborne particles cause increases in protooncogene expression and proliferation in alveolar epithelial cells. Toxicol Appl Pharmacol 2002;179:98–104.

156. Churg A, Gilks B, Dai J. Induction of fibrogenic mediators by fine and ultrafine titanium dioxide in rat tracheal explants. Am J Physiol 1999;277:L975–82.

157. Renwick LC, Brown D, Clouter A, Donaldson K. Increased inflammation and altered macrophage chemotactic responses caused by two ultrafine particle types. Occup Environ Med 2004;61:442–7.

158. Renwick LC, Donaldson K, Clouter A. Impairment of alveolar macrophage phagocytosis by ultrafine particles. Toxicol Appl Pharmacol. 2001;172:119–27.

159. Rehfuess E, Mehta S, Pruss-Ustun A. Assessing household solid fuel use: multiple implications for the Millennium Development Goals. Environ Health Perspect 2006;114:373–8.

160. Smith K, Maeusezahl-Feuz M. Indoor air pollution from household use of solid fuels. In: Ezzati M, Lopez AD, Rodgers A, Murray CJL, editors. Comparative quantification of health risks: global and regional burden of disease attributable to selected major risk factors. Geneva: World Health Organization; 2004. p. 1435–93.

161. Gold JA, Jagirdar J, Hay JG, et al. Hut lung. A domestically acquired particulate lung disease. Medicine (Baltimore) 2000;79:310–7.

162. Ozbay B, Uzun K, Arslan H, Zehir I. Functional and radiological impairment in women highly exposed to indoor biomass fuels. Respirology 2001;6:255–8.

163. Shrestha IL, Shrestha SL. Indoor air pollution from biomass fuels and respiratory health of the exposed population in Nepalese households. Int J Occup Environ Health 2005;11:150–60.

164. Diaz JV, Koff J, Gotway MB, et al. Case report: a case of wood-smoke-related pulmonary disease. Environ Health Perspect 2006;114:759–62.

165. Chan-Yeung M, Ait-Khaled N, White N, et al. The burden and impact of COPD in Asia and Africa. Int J Tuberc Lung Dis 2004;8:2–14.

166. Mudway IS, Duggan ST, Venkataraman C, et al. Combustion of dried animal dung as biofuel results in the generation of highly redox active fine particulates. Part Fibre Toxicol 2005;2:6.

167. Pope AC, Dockery DW. Epidemiology of particle effects. In: Holgate ST, Samet JM, Koren HS, Maynard RL, editors. Air pollution and health. San Diego (CA): Academic Press; 1999. p. 673–705.

CHAPTER 11

Mucus and Mucus-Secreting Cells in Chronic Obstructive Pulmonary Disease

Jin-Ah Park, PhD, Anne L. Crews, MS, Kimberly L. Raiford, PhD, and Kenneth B. Adler, PhD

Mucus overproduction and hypersecretion, with resulting airway obstruction and enhanced susceptibility to microbial infection and inflammation, are the major pathophysiologic lesions characterizing chronic bronchitis and also occur in other airway inflammatory diseases, such as asthma and cystic fibrosis. Under normal conditions, a thin layer of mucus lining the airways serves as a primary defense mechanism in the respiratory tract, protecting against impingement of inhaled particles and microbes and endogenously produced substances that could be detrimental (eg, cytokines, mediators of inflammation). The mucociliary escalator, in which the mucus interacts with cilia that line the airways to move these materials out of the lungs, is the primary defense mechanism that clears the airways of these substances that are trapped in the mucus. Mucus itself also contains additional components that can abet its defensive function, such as antioxidants and antimicrobial substances (eg, lysozyme and defensins). However, mucus hypersecretion as occurs in bronchitis and other diseases compromises the protective function of mucus as a physical barrier and mucociliary facilitator and may result in enhanced airway obstruction, microbial infection, and additional inflammatory responses.

Presently, there is no effective therapy that can affect mucus hypersecretion in the airways. Anti-inflammatory therapy, such as administration of inhaled corticosteroids and/or bronchodilatory agents, can be somewhat beneficial to patients with bronchitis, but there is no treatment that specifically can reduce mucus secretion. In this chapter, we review the structure and function of the mucus-secreting elements in the mammalian airways and present some of the newer findings related to intracellular mechanisms and signaling molecules that regulate the mucus secretory process. It is possible that some of these molecules and pathways can represent new therapeutic targets for which drugs can be developed that can reduce or control excess mucus secretion in airway inflammatory diseases.

Airway Epithelium

The mammalian airway is continuously exposed to the external environment. As the first point of contact, the airway epithelium acts as both a physical barrier and a mediator of airway homeostasis. Some of the specific functions of airway epithelium include lung fluid balance, metabolism of exogenous materials, mediation of inflammatory responses, regulation of smooth muscle tone, and secretion of mucins and surfactants.[1–3]

The airway epithelium is an integrated structure of pseudostratified columnar cells attached to a basement membrane, consisting of basal, ciliated, Clara, and goblet cells.[3] Basal cells have a high capacity for proliferation and regeneration[4] and are thought to be progenitors of goblet and ciliated cells.[5] In the distal conducting airways, Clara cells may act as progenitors in lieu of basal cells.[6] In addition to a role as progenitor cells, basal cells mediate inflammatory responses and transepithelial water movement and neutralize reactive oxygen species (ROS).[7] Ciliated epithelial cells, which make up over 50% of all epithelial cells in the human airway, have a primary role in mucociliary clearance.[8] Ciliated cells are believed to be terminally differentiated cell types arising from either basal or Clara cells, although there is some evidence of transdifferentiation of squamous or goblet cells into ciliated cells.[9,10] Clara cells are located in the bronchi and bronchioles and express Clara cell secretory protein (CCSP) and bronchiolar surfactant. In addition, Clara cells play a role in detoxification via their content of cytochrome P-450 and various antiproteases.[3,9] Goblet cells are filled with membrane-bound mucin granules and are mainly found in the bronchi and regular bronchioles. They are sparse in the terminal bronchioles and absent in the respiratory bronchioles under normal conditions.[6] The major function of goblet cells is production and secretion of mucin, the glycoprotein component of mucus that confers its physical and rheologic properties. However, in some disease states, goblet cell hyperplasia and metaplasia in both proximal and distal airways lead to mucus hypersecretion that is associated with failure of normal airway function as excess mucus causes increased pulmonary infection, impaired ciliary beating, and airway obstruction.[11,12]

Airway Mucus and Mucin Genes

Mucus produced by the epithelium of respiratory, gastrointestinal, and reproductive tracts provides a physical barrier between the external environment and the cellular components of the epithelial layer.[13] Airway mucus is a heterogeneous mixture of different secretions, including water, electrolytes, and organic compounds, such as mucin glycoproteins, proteoglycans, carbohydrates, peptides, serum proteins, soluble proteins, and lipids.[14] Hydrated gel-forming mucus humidifies the airways and serves to "trap" inhaled deleterious substances as part of the mucociliary clearance apparatus.[8]

The gel-forming properties of mucus are due to the major structural component of mucus, which is termed "mucin." Mucins, highly glycosylated oligomeric glycoproteins, are predominantly secreted from goblet cells of the airway epithelium and mucous cells of submucosal glands.[13,15] To date, 21 mucins have been identified in the human genome. They are categorized as secreted gel-forming mucins (*MUC2, MUC5AC, MUC5B, MUC6,* and *MUC19*), secreted non-gel-forming mucins (*MUC7, MUC8,* and *MUC9*), and membrane-associated mucins (*MUC1, MUC3A, MUC3B, MUC4, MUC11, MUC12, MUC13, MUC14, MUC15, MUC16, MUC17, MUC18,* and *MUC20*).[16,17]

The structure of mucin glycoproteins is based on the protein backbone encoded by each mucin gene, along with the heavily glycosylated side chains added via posttranslational glycosylation in the endoplasmic reticulum and Golgi apparatus.[13,18] The protein backbone contains an extensive number of tandem repeats (TRs) consisting of unique repeating amino acid sequences, including a high number of serine and threonine residues and at least one proline residue (with the exception of MUC14, -15, and -18). Amino and carboxyl terminal cysteine-rich domains are required for oligomerization of secreted mucins.[19,20]

Distinct from secreted mucins, transmembrane domains are included in the carboxyl termini of membrane-associated mucins.[17,21] Glycosylated side chains occupying about 50 to 90% of the mass of mucin are bound to the TR domains via N- or O-glycosidic linkages.[13,17] Highly diverse glycosylated side chains can serve as signaling receptors for incoming bacterial pathogens and environmental particles in the airway.[22]

Twelve mucins are known to be expressed in the airway, and the large number of publications related to gel-forming mucins reflects their significance.[17] The four gel-forming mucins (*MUC2, MUC5AC, MUC5B,* and *MUC19*) are expressed in the airway and contribute to the viscoelastic properties of airway mucus.[22–25] Disulfide bonds present in the cysteine-rich motifs are unique to gel-forming mucins.[19,20] *MUC5AC* and *MUC5B* are the predominant mucins in the airways, and their expression has been correlated with chronic airway diseases.[17,26] Two different populations of *MUC5B* (high- or low-charged forms owing to glycosylation differences) are present in the normal human airway.[27] *MUC2* mucin is a minor component of mucus as demonstrated by analysis of sputum collected from patients with chronic obstructive pulmonary disease (COPD) and measurement of mucin secretion in cultured differentiated epithelial cells.[23,28] *MUC19* was recently identified as a gel-forming mucin; however, its expression in airway disease has not yet been demonstrated.[24] With the exception of MUC19, all gel-forming mucin genes in the human are clustered on chromosome 11p15.5.[29,30]

COPD and Airway Mucin

COPD is characterized by slowly progressive and irreversible airway obstruction associated with long-term exposure to toxic gases or particulates, including cigarette smoke and coal dust.[31,32] Although the American Thoracic Society defined COPD as "airflow limitation due to chronic bronchitis or emphysema," it can often be caused by cystic fibrosis and chronic asthma.[33] The heterogeneity of the disease makes treatment difficult, and patients often suffer high morbidity or even mortality. In COPD, CD8[+] T-cells and macrophage recruitment are predominantly augmented with neutrophilic infiltration via increased neutrophilic chemokine (epithelium-derived neutrophil attractant 78, interleukin [IL]-8) expression during acute exacerbation.[34] Proteases released from neutrophils and macrophages are beneficial in host defense; however, protease overproduction owing to chronic inflammation can cause alveolar breakdown, resulting in emphysema.[35,36] A genetic deficiency in α_1-antitrypsin often results in the same pathology. An imbalance of oxidants and antioxidants is another factor contributing to COPD development. ROS are generated by inhalation of cigarette smoke, activation of macrophages or neutrophils, and inhalation of environmental pollutants such as ozone, nitrogen dioxide, or sulfur oxide.[32] Bacterial pathogens such as *Staphylococcus aureus* and *Haemophilus influenzae* can also commonly exacerbate bronchitis. In addition, bacterial products, including lipopolysaccharide and endotoxin, can cause goblet cell hyperplasia and potentiate ozone-induced goblet cell metaplasia in rodent models.[37,38]

In COPD, mucin hypersecretion results from mucous gland hyperplasia in the large airways and goblet cell metaplasia in the small airways.[16,39] Similar to asthma and cystic fibrosis, increased MUC5AC and MUC5B expression has also been demonstrated in COPD.[23] MUC5AC expression is increased in the bronchiolar epithelium, whereas increased MUC5B is found in the bronchiolar lumen compared with normal subjects.[40] The ratio of MUC5B to MUC5AC is increased, and there is an increase in the low-charged form of MUC5B in chronic bronchitis sputum compared with normal subjects.[23]

Mucin Gene Expression

The mechanisms involved in mucin gene expression have been thoroughly studied using both *in-vitro* and *in-vivo* models.[41] Specifically, augmented expression of *MUC5AC* and *MUC5B* is well characterized in disease states, including COPD and asthma.[23,42] Regulation of *MUC5AC* expression has been widely studied using a variety of cell culture systems, including lung carcinoma cell lines (NC1-H292, A549), primary normal human bronchial epithelial (NHBE) cells, and transfected human bronchial cell lines (HBE-1).[43–46]

The most extensively studied pathway of transcriptional regulation of mucin gene expression is the epidermal growth factor receptor (EGFR)-mediated pathway.[47] The EGFR expressed in epithelial cells is a transmembrane protein with tyrosine kinase activity, and it appears to have an important functional role in epithelial repair and differentiation.[48] Booth and colleagues demonstrated that airway remodeling is associated with EGFR activation induced in response to the T-helper 2 cytokine IL-13.[49] In their report, they showed that proliferative responses of airway epithelium are initiated by IL-13 in the absence of any inflammatory cells and based on release of the EGFR ligand transforming growth factor α, by the epithelial cells and an autocrine/paracrine-type response. Shao and colleagues showed that *MUC5AC* gene expression is regulated by an EGFR-mediated mechanism involving tumor necrosis factor (TNF-α)-converting enzyme (TACE) in NCI-H292 cells.[45] In addition, they reported that the TACE-EGFR signaling pathway is implicated in cigarette smoke–induced *MUC5AC* expression, a major pathogenic feature of COPD.[50] Despite the fact that the EGFR appears to be involved in goblet cell hyperplasia and metaplasia in COPD and other diseases, its value as a potential therapeutic target for treating COPD or other airway inflammatory diseases has yet to be demonstrated.

Along with the role of the EGFR, involvement of protein kinase C (PKC) has been suggested as a regulator of mucin gene expression associated with chronic airway diseases. PKC is a serine/threonine kinase involved in various cellular events such as proliferation, differentiation, gene expression, apoptosis, tumorigenesis, muscle contraction, and exocytosis.[51] Mucin gene expression is upregulated in a PKC-dependent manner in response to various stimuli, such as purinergic agonists,[52] ROS,[53] and inflammatory mediators,[54,55] but the specific PKC isoform and downstream pathways involved have not been elucidated.

Mucin Secretion and Mucin Granule Exocytosis

Increased amounts of mucin in the airway can result from both upregulated mucin gene expression and stimulated mucin granule exocytosis. Gel-forming mucins are secreted from goblet cells or glandular mucous cells into the airway lumen by a regulated event termed exocytosis.[16,56] Mucins are synthesized and stored within membrane-bound granules in the cytoplasm of these cells.[57] Excess mucin secretion as occurs in chronic bronchitis and other inflammatory airway diseases is the consequence of exposure to various secretory agonists, including pathophysiologic mediators, such as adrenergic, cholinergic, and purinergic agonists; bacterial products; cytokines; proteases; inflammatory mediators; and eicosanoids.[57,58] Intracellular signaling pathways of mucin secretion following secretagogue exposure have been studied for several years, but still relatively little is known about the mechanisms involved.

In contrast to constitutive exocytosis of integral proteins, regulated exocytosis is triggered by intracellular signals that are induced when the cell is stimulated. Regulated exocytosis involves the movement of secretory granules to the inner cell surface, docking, and then fusion of the lipid bilayer of the secretory granule to the plasma membrane.[16,56] These processes require well-regulated signaling pathways and coordination of the surrounding proteins. There is good evidence that the binding affinity between proteins involved in exocytosis is modulated by their phosphorylation. Using *in-vitro* phosphorylation of recombinant proteins, Evans and colleagues demonstrated that proteins associated with granules are phosphorylated by protein kinase A (PKA; cyclic adenosine monophosphate [cAMP]-dependent kinase) or PKC.[59]

As mentioned above, exocytosis involves fusion of secretory granule membranes with the plasma membrane following trafficking and docking of the granule (diagrammed in Figure 2 in Burgoyne and Morgan[56]). Recent studies have focused on the role of granule-associated proteins facilitating fusion of granules to the plasma membrane. Those granule-associated proteins include cysteine string protein (CSP), soluble N-ethylmaleimide-sensitive factor attachment protein (SNAP), Munc18/nSec1, and SNAP receptor (SNARE), including a complex of vesicle-associated membrane proteins (VAMPs), synaptosome-associated proteins (SNAP-23 and -25), and syntaxin.[56] The isoform expression of VAMP, SNAP, and syntaxin is cell specific.

The role of SNARE assembly in exocytosis has been studied extensively. The SNARE complex is composed of two helices of SNAP-25, a helix of syntaxin, and a helix of VAMPs. After the granule moves close to the plasma membrane, it binds to the lipid bilayer via a fully assembled SNARE complex (diagramed in Figure 6 in Burgoyne and Morgan[56]). Before the SNARE complex is completely assembled, one of the SNARE members, syntaxin, is not free to bind to other SNARE proteins owing to its association with Munc18. Following dissociation from Munc18, syntaxin is able to associate with other SNARE components. Dissociation of Munc18 from syntaxin may be mediated by its phosphorylation. Interactions between the SNARE proteins are demonstrated by *in-vitro* binding assays and coimmunoprecipitation.[60] Foster and colleagues demonstrated three different interactions: SNAP-23 and syntaxin-4, VAMP-2 and syntaxin-4, and VAMP-2 and SNAP-23.[60] Granule fusion is the important step in exocytosis, and regulating the interaction of each of the proteins with each other and the membrane may represent a potential target to modulate mucin secretion.

There also is good evidence that the binding affinity between proteins involved in exocytosis is modulated by their phosphorylation. Using *in-vitro* phosphorylation of recombinant proteins, Evans and colleagues demonstrated that proteins associated with granules are phosphorylated by PKA (cAMP-dependent kinase) or PKC.[59] Munc18, SNAP-25, and Rab3A are phosphorylated by PKC, and CSP is phosphorylated by PKA. They have also demonstrated that phosphorylation of CSP at the serine 10 residue inhibits its interaction with syntaxin *in vitro*, whereas it does not affect its interaction with heat shock protein 70. In addition, phosphorylation of CSP results in marked reduction in chromaffin cell secretion, suggesting that phosphorylation of CSP and CSP interactions with syntaxin have a role in exocytosis. Phosphorylation of Munc18 at the serine 313 residue inhibits interaction with syntaxin *in vitro*.[61,62] Interaction of SNAP-23 with syntaxin-4 is inhibited by either phosphorylation of syntaxin-4[63] or SNAP-23.[64] Chung and colleagues demonstrated that syntaxin is phosphorylated in human platelets treated with thrombin, and inhibition of syntaxin phosphorylation by PKC inhibitors reduces thrombin-mediated dense granule release from platelets.[63] They also showed that recombinant syntaxin is phosphorylated by various PKC isoforms *in vitro*, including PKCα, -β, -γ, -δ, -ε, and -ξ. They suggested that among the PKC isoforms, a novel-type PKC is a probable regulator of thrombin-mediated platelet secretion. Thus, either the δ or the ε isoform of PKC can be the target kinase regulating SNARE assembly. In studies from our laboratory, a number of fusion and docking proteins, especially CSP, have been implicated in mucin secretion by airway epithelial cells, as has the δ isoform of PKC. These are discussed below.

Neutrophils and Human Neutrophil Elastase

Neutrophil-predominant inflammation is a well-characterized aspect of chronic bronchitis.[65–67] In the airways, the presence of neutrophils is associated not only with declining airway function but also increased mucin production.[68,69] Neutrophils contain three distinct enzyme-containing granules within their cytoplasm, which are involved in innate immunity. Within azurophilic granules, three serine proteases (elastase, cathepsin, and protease-3) are known to mediate mucin overproduction.[70–75] Specific granules and storage granules contain collagenase (matrix metalloproteinase 8) and gelatinase (matrix metalloproteinase 9), respectively. These enzymes mediate cell migration and host defense against bacterial infection. However, persistent or excessive enzymatic activity, as seen in airway diseases such as COPD, can result in detrimental effects (even in the absence of α1-antitrypsin deficiency) central to the pathogenic processes. For example, it can lead to connective tissue degradation, secretory cell metaplasia, reduced ciliary beating, excess mucus secretion, bacterial proliferation, and recurrent infections.[35,76,77] In addition, all three serine proteases present in azurophilic granules can induce secretory cell metaplasia and emphysema in a hamster model.[78,79]

Among neutrophil proteases, human neutrophil elastase (HNE) has been of particular focus owing to its strong association with airway disease.[80] HNE is a serine protease (EC: 3.4.21.37) composed of 218-amino acid residues with two asparaginyl N-linked side chains and four intramolecular disulfide bridges. HNE functions as a potent hydrolyzer of most protein components of the extracellular matrix.[81] This 24 kDa protease contains a conserved triad of catalytic residues including Ser[195], His[57], and Asp[102]. The active-site serine is very nucleophilic, and it is inactivated by specific proteases, such as diisopropyl phosphofluoridate, phenylmethanesulfonyl fluoride, and 3,4-dichromisocoumarin.[82] In addition, when elastase is released from a neutrophil, it is quickly complexed to natural inhibitors such as α1-antitrypsin or α2-macroglobulin. These complexes are cleared by the liver or by macrophage phagocytosis. However, an imbalance in levels of HNE and protease inhibitors results in chronic disease states, which can lead to the destruction of alveolar walls.[36,83] HNE has been associated with many inflammatory disorders, such as emphysema, acute respiratory distress syndrome, shocked lung, rheumatoid arthritis, and glomerulonephritis.[80] Conversely, an HNE-deficient mouse study showed that HNE is critical to host defense against gram-negative bacteria, including *Klebsiella pneumoniae* and *Escherichia coli*.[84] Extensive research to develop potent HNE inhibitors that target its destructive and proinflammatory action has been ongoing for years.

HNE is found in high concentration (about 3.3 μm) in the sputum of patients with cystic fibrosis and chronic bronchitis.[85–88] HNE can degrade a variety of extracellular matrix proteins, including elastin, collagen, fibronectin, laminin, and proteoglycan, with a broad spectrum of substrates.[82] Under normal conditions, the proteolytic action of elastase is controlled by endogenous inhibitors such as α1-antitrypsin, α2-macroglobulin, and the secretory leukocyte protease inhibitor elafin.[82,89] In addition, persistent exposure to HNE leads to impaired ciliary motility, goblet cell metaplasia or hyperplasia, increased mucin production and secretion, and enhanced mucin gene expression.[70,86,88,90,91]

Several mechanisms have been proposed regarding HNE effects on mucin gene expression. Fischer and Voynow, and Voynow and colleagues, demonstrated that HNE induced MUC5AC expression by enhancing messenger ribonucleic acid stability via an oxidant-dependent mechanism in a lung adenocarcinoma cell line and NHBE cells.[43,92] In addition, they demonstrated that upregulated *MUC4* expression and activation of the ErbB2 receptor are involved in epithelial recovery following HNE exposure.[93] Shao and Nadel showed that upregulated *MUC5AC* expression is the result of the sequential activation of PKC, ROS, and TNF-α-converting enzyme in human pulmonary mucoepidermoid carcinoma cell lines and NHBE cells.[53,94] Goblet cell metaplasia was demonstrated in animal models after HNE exposure, resulting in mucin hypersecretion similar to what is seen in the small airways of patients suffering from chronic airway diseases.[70,91] Voynow and colleagues suggested that the proteolytic activity of HNE initiates an inflammatory process leading to goblet cell metaplasia by assessing keratinocyte-derived chemokine and IL-5 expression following HNE exposure with and without an HNE inhibitor (methoxysuccinyl Ala-Ala-Pro-Val chloromethylketone [AAPV-CMK]) in mouse lung.[82,91] *In-vitro* investigation of the role of HNE in mucin secretion is difficult owing to limited appropriate culture systems. Kim and colleagues showed that HNE mediated mucin release from primary hamster tracheal epithelial cell cultures *in vitro* and that an active catalytic site of HNE is required for both release and degradation of mucin.[71] Studies from our laboratory demonstrated that HNE provokes mucin secretion in well-differentiated NHBE cells and that the intracellular signaling pathway regulating HNE-induced mucin hypersecretion involved PKC, specifically the δ isoform.[95] In fact, PKC could be a "universal" mediator of mucin secretion in response to most if not all secretory stimuli.

Protein Kinase C

PKC is a serine/threonine kinase involved in various cellular events, such as proliferation, differentiation, gene expression, apoptosis, tumorigenesis, muscle contraction, and exocytosis.[51] PKC isoforms have been classified into three subfamilies depending on their mode of activation: 1) conventional (α, β, γ) PKCs, which are activated by phosphatidylserine (PS), diacylglycerol (DAG), phorbol ester (12-O-tetradecanoyl-phorbol-13-acetate [TPA] or phorbol 12-myristate 13-acetate [PMA]); 2) novel (δ, ε, η, θ, μ) PKCs, which are PS, DAG, or TPA dependent but Ca^{2+} independent; and 3) atypical (ξ, ι/λ) PKCs, which are either Ca^{2+} or PS, DAG, or TPA independent for their activation.[51,96] In addition, a newly discovered member of the PKC family, called the protein kinase C—related kinase (PRK; PRK1,2,3), has sequence homology to PKC.[97] The PRK family does not require DAG or PMA for its activation.[98] Newly found novel-type PKCs are termed protein kinase D (PKD).[99,100] Initially, PKDs were designated as novel-type isoforms owing to their requirement for DAG or PS for activation; these include PKCμ and PKCν.[101]

Traditionally, PKC activation is accomplished in a stepwise manner that involves the translocation of inactive PKC localized within the cytosol to the cellular membrane.[51] PKC in the cytosol remains inactive by binding of a pseudosubstrate domain to C4 regions in its catalytic domain. Conversion of PKC into the active form occurs when the affinity of the pseudosubstrate domain for the C4 domain decreases following the binding of DAG to the C1 domain. Additional interaction with the anionic phospholipids on the membrane is followed by a critical conformational change, which allows PKC to bind to the substrate as well as adenosine triphosphate (ATP). Then active PKC mediates the phosphorylation of the substrate at the serine and threonine residues. Sustained PKC activation is followed by degradation of PKC by a protease (calpain) or by the ubiquitin-proteasome pathway.[102–104]

The distribution of PKCs shows tissue-specific patterns. PKCα expression is ubiquitous, PKCγ is expressed exclusively in the central nervous system, and PKCβ, -δ, and -ε are widely expressed in most tissues.[105] All isoforms (except PKCγ) are expressed in mammalian lung tissue.[106] We have found that primary NHBE cells in culture contain all except θ and γ. PKC isoforms expressed in the lung have been implicated in a number of cellular responses, including permeability, smooth muscle contraction, inflammatory cell migration, proliferation, differentiation, hypertrophy, apoptosis, and secretion.[106–109]

As mentioned above, the PKC isoform that appears to be related to mucin secretion is PKCδ. PKCδ is the most widely studied member of the novel PKC family owing to its extensive roles in a variety of cellular signaling pathways, including

cell growth, differentiation, proliferation, apoptosis, tumor promotion, and carcinogenesis.[110,111] PKCδ protein is expressed in brain, heart, spleen, lung, liver, ovary, pancreas, and adrenal tissues and a variety of inflammatory cells.[105,107]

PKCδ was cloned from a rat brain complementary deoxyribonucleic acid (cDNA) library by Ono and colleagues in 1987.[112] The amino acid sequence of PKCδ shows 58% homology to PKCα. The *PKCδ* gene is clustered at human chromosome 3p21, rat chromosome 19p14, and mouse chromosome 14.[113,114] *PKCδ* comprises 18 exons in humans and mice and 19 exons in rats. It is composed of 676 amino acids in human and 673 amino acids in rats, and its genomic structure is highly conserved in mammals.

PKCδ has been shown to play multiple roles in cell growth, proliferation and differentiation,[115–121] apoptosis,[122–133] and inflammation.[134–140] Relevant to mucin secretion, a large body of evidence suggests that PKCδ controls various exocytotic events, including the secretion of insulin,[115,116,141] gastric peptides,[116] enzymes,[117] platelet-dense granules,[118] and inflammatory cell degranulation.[119–121] In human platelets, PKCδ is activated in response to protease-activated receptor agonist peptides (SFLLRN and AYPGKF), leading to dense granule release.[118] In addition, the protease-activated receptor (PAR) agonist peptide-induced dense granule release is blocked by rottlerin (a specific PKCδ inhibitor) but not by Go6976 (a conventional PKC inhibitor). Ishikawa and colleagues demonstrated that carbachol-stimulated insulin secretion is associated with translocation of PKCδ in rat pancreatic islets.[115] Carbachol-stimulated insulin secretion is not reduced by Go6976 but is significantly suppressed by an ambiguous PKC inhibitor, chelerythrine. Ishikawa and colleagues' report suggested that one of the novel PKC isoforms, δ or ε, might play a regulatory role in carbachol-stimulated insulin secretion. Cho and colleagues demonstrated that PKCδ activation is involved in antigen-induced mast cell degranulation, which is subsequently inhibited by rottlerin or transfection of a dominant negative mutant of PKCδ.[120] These results were in contrast to those of Leitges and colleagues, who suggested that PKCδ is a negative regulator of antigen-induced mast cell degranulation.[121] Despite the controversy, PKCδ appears to be a key molecule in antigen-induced mast cell degranulation *in vivo* and *in vitro*.

Recent studies have shown that PKCδ also is an integral component of airway mucin secretion. Abdullah and colleagues showed that the PKCδ isoform plays a role in the mucin secretion pathway in response to purinergic agonists (ATPγS) and PMA in mouse goblet cells.[122] Park and colleagues recently demonstrated that the PKCδ isoform modulates mucin secretion in response to HNE in well-differentiated NHBE cells.[123] Transfection of a dominant-negative PKCδ construct into HBE-1 cells resulted in decreased mucin secretion in response to PMA stimulation, whereas overexpression of PKCδ enhanced secretion.[123] It is of particular interest that this isoform appears to be the PKC subtype that is most effective in phosphorylating MARCKS protein as a key step in the mucin secretion pathway.

MARCKS (Myristoylated Alanine-Rich C Kinase Substrate)

MARCKS, widely distributed in many cell types (including epithelial cells), is a well-known PKC substrate. MARCKS has been implicated in many cellular functions, such as cell motility, phagocyte activation, exocytosis, membrane trafficking, and mitogenesis, through regulation of cytoskeletal structures.[124–126] In humans, MARCKS consists of 323 amino acids. Its expected molecular weight based on the number of amino acids is 40 kDa, but it is detected near 85 kDa by Western blot analysis owing to its rod-like shape. MARCKS has three conserved domains: the amino-terminus myristoylated domain, the multiple homology 2 (MH2) domain, and the phosphorylation site domain (PSD).[128] The N-terminal glycine is the site of myristoylation, which allows for effective binding of MARCKS protein to the plasma membrane.[128,129] The function of the MH2 domain has not been elucidated. The phosphorylation target of PKC, the PSD site, has the ability to bind to membranes with a highly basic region containing 12 to 13 positively charged Lys/Arg residues and to actin, where it crosslinks actin filaments together. These functions can be disrupted by Ca^{2+}/calmodulin or phosphorylation of MARCKS by PKC.[130,131]

MARCKS is phosphorylated by PKC at serine residues 152, 156, and 163, which are located in its PSD.[132] Phosphorylation of MARCKS in the PSD has been shown to be central to the function of MARCKS protein.[124,130,133,134] MARCKS is a prominent PKC substrate, and its phosphorylation is differentially regulated depending on the specificity of each PKC isoform. Herget and colleagues performed PKC phosphorylation assays in vitro to demonstrate the differential efficiency of each PKC isoform in phosphorylation of MARCKS.[132] MARCKS is phosphorylated by PKCα, β₁, β₂, γ, δ, and ε but not by ξ. Additionally, it has been suggested that the intact MARCKS protein is an excellent substrate for PKCβ₁, δ, and ε. However, it is PKCδ that appears to be the most potent isoform responsible for the phosphorylation of MARCKS, followed by the ε and β₁ isoforms, as determined by Vmax to Km catalytic efficiency ratios. This finding was supported by a study conducted by Fujise and colleagues, which also demonstrated that PKCδ has a high affinity for MARCKS.[135]

Involvement of MARCKS in exocytosis in conjunction with PKC activation has been reported. Transfection of deletion mutation constructs lacking the PSD results in attenuation of mucin secretion in response to PMA in HBE-1 cells.[126] Glutamate exocytosis from synaptosome is increased by PKC in cooperation with phosphorylation of MARCKS and increased intracellular calcium concentrations.[136] MARCKS protein is involved in chromaffin cell secretion.[137] Trifaro and colleagues suggested that chromaffin cell secretion is the result of two cooperating pathways: calcium influx into cells with scinderin activation and phosphorylation of MARCKS by PKC. They also suggested that those two separate steps lead to control of actin filaments, which serve as a barrier under the membrane. Association of actin with MARCKS during exocytosis has been demonstrated in oxytocin exocytosis from bovine luteal cells in response to prostaglandin F$_{2-\alpha}$.[125]

In a series of studies from the Adler laboratory in North Carolina, MARCKS was shown to be a key molecule regulating mucin secretion by airway goblet cells. Stimulation of mucin secretion by a variety of secretagogues results in phosphorylation of MARCKS in human airway epithelial cells in vitro; a peptide identical to the MARCKS N-terminus attenuates mucin hypersecretion induced by PKC-activating agents in a concentration-dependent manner in well-differentiated NHBE cells in vitro, and in response to cholinergically stimulated mucin secretion in ovalbumin-sensitized mice[138] when administered intratracheally. Instillation of this peptide also inhibited airway obstruction in these mice.[139] Additional chaperones associated with MARCKS-related mucin secretion include CSP and heat shock protein 70.[140] The results of these studies support a hypothetical mechanism whereby PKC-dependent phosphorylation of MARCKS results in release of MARCKS from the plasma membrane into the cytoplasm. In the cytoplasm, in conjunction with the chaperone CSP, MARCKS appears to associate with membranes of intracellular mucin granules as a key step in the mucin secretory process. As MARCKS has been shown to bind to both actin and myosin in the cytoplasm of airway epithelial cells,[126] it is possible that MARCKS can serve to tether mucin granules to the cellular contractile apparatus, mediating subsequent granule movement and exocytosis. The hypothetical mechanism of mucin secretion involving MARCKS and related chaperone and fusion, scaffolding, and docking proteins is illustrated in Figure 1.

Conclusion

Constitutive and low-level mucin secretion from healthy airway epithelium protects upper and lower airways by capturing and expelling inhaled exogenous substances and endogenous materials, which could be deleterious. However, persistent mucus hypersecretion as commonly observed in patients with chronic bronchitis can lead to airway obstruction, enhanced microbial infection, and inflammation. Excess mucus can result from increased production of mucus, hyperplastic and metaplastic changes in the mucin-secreting cellular apparatus, and enhanced secretion of stored mucus via an exocytotic mechanism. Mucin secretion has been shown to involve signaling molecules such as MARCKS protein, PKC, especially the δ isoform, and numerous other fusion and docking proteins that regulate the actual release of mucin from the secretory cells to the airway lumen. Excess mucus is the primary lesion of chronic bronchitis, yet, presently, there is no effective therapy targeted to the secretory process. Clearly, controlling excessive mucus in the airway, via regulating mucus production and/or secretion, is a major goal for better treatment of COPD patients.

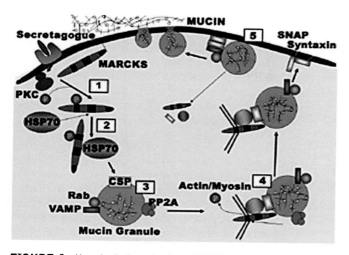

FIGURE 1. Hypothetical mechanism of MARCKS-related mucin hypersecretion by airway goblet cells. When a secretagogue binds to a surface receptor, as illustrated in the upper left corner (or if the cell is stimulated by a non-receptor-mediated signal), it sets into motion the following sequence of events: (1) protein kinase C (PKC) is activated (most likely the δ isoform) and moves from cytoplasm to membrane. On the plasma membrane, PKC phosphorylates MARCKS, which is found attached to the inner face of the membrane. After being phosphorylated, MARCKS detaches from the plasma membrane and translocates to the cytoplasm. (2) In the cytoplasm, MARCKS binds to heat shock protein 70 (HSP70) via the MARCKS MH2 domain. (3) The MARCKS-HSP70 complex then gets targeted to mucin granule membranes owing to interactions between HSP70 and cysteine string protein (CSP) bound to the mucin granule membrane. The MARCKS-HSP70 complex then binds to the mucin granule via CSP, forming a trimeric MARCKS-HSP70-CSP complex on the granule membrane, with the N-terminus of MARCKS inserting into the membrane. (4) MARCKS is then dephosphorylated by a protein phosphatase type 2 that is localized to the granule membrane. Dephosphorylation of MARCKS allows MARCKS to bind to actin via the MARCKS phosphorylation site domain. Contraction of the actin-myosin cytoskeleton then allows for the entire complex to translocate to the plasma membrane, where, (5) in conjunction with a variety of fusion, scaffolding, and docking proteins (SNAPs, syntaxins, SNAREs, Muncs), the granule membrane fuses with the plasma membrane and the contents of the granule (mucins) are released into the airway lumen via an exocytotic process.

Acknowledgment

This work was supported by Grant R37 HL36982 from the National Institutes of Health.

References

1. Holgate ST, Lackie P, Wilson S, et al. Bronchial epithelium as a key regulator of airway allergen sensitization and remodeling in asthma. Am J Respir Crit Care Med 2000;162(3 Pt 2):S113–7.
2. Knight D. Epithelium-fibroblast interactions in response to airway inflammation. Immunol Cell Biol 2001;79:160–4.
3. Knight DA, Holgate ST. The airway epithelium: structural and functional properties in health and disease. Respirology 2003;8:432–46.
4. Hong KU, Reynolds SD, Watkins S, et al. Basal cells are a multipotent progenitor capable of renewing the bronchial epithelium. Am J Pathol 2004;164:577–88.
5. Boers JE, Ambergen AW, Thunnissen FB. Number and proliferation of basal and parabasal cells in normal human airway epithelium. Am J Respir Crit Care Med 1998;157(6 Pt 1):2000–6.
6. Boers JE, Ambergen AW, Thunnissen FB. Number and proliferation of Clara cells in normal human airway epithelium. Am J Respir Crit Care Med 1999;159(5 Pt 1):1585–91.
7. Evans MJ, Van Winkle LS, Fanucchi MV, Plopper CG. Cellular and molecular characteristics of basal cells in airway epithelium. Exp Lung Res 2001;27:401–15.
8. Chilvers MA, O'Callaghan C. Local mucociliary defence mechanisms. Paediatr Respir Rev 2000;1:27–34.
9. Park KS, Wells JM, Zorn AM, et al. Transdifferentiation of ciliated cells during repair of the respiratory epithelium. Am J Respir Cell Mol Biol 2006;34:151–7.
10. Tyner JW, Kim EY, Ide K, et al. Blocking airway mucous cell metaplasia by inhibiting EGFR antiapoptosis and IL-13 transdifferentiation signals. J Clin Invest 2006;116:309–21.
11. Boucher RC. Relationship of airway epithelial ion transport to chronic bronchitis. Proc Am Thorac Soc 2004;1:66–70.
12. Gilligan PH. Microbiology of airway disease in patients with cystic fibrosis. Clin Microbiol Rev 1991;4:35–51.
13. Rose MC. Mucins: structure, function, and role in pulmonary diseases. Am J Physiol 1992;263(4 Pt 1):L413–29.
14. Verdugo P. Goblet cells secretion and mucogenesis. Annu Rev Physiol 1990;52:157–76.
15. Rogers DF. The airway goblet cell. Int J Biochem Cell Biol 2003;35:1–6.
16. Williams OW, Sharafkhaneh A, Kim V, et al. Airway mucus: from production to secretion. Am J Respir Cell Mol Biol 2006;34:527–36.
17. Rose MC, Voynow JA. Respiratory tract mucin genes and mucin glycoproteins in health and disease. Physiol Rev 2006;86:245–78.
18. Perez-Vilar J. Mucin granule intraluminal organization. Am J Respir Cell Mol Biol 2007;36:183–90.
19. van de Bovenkamp JH, Hau CM, Strous GJ, et al. Molecular cloning of human gastric mucin MUC5AC reveals conserved cysteine-rich D-domains and a putative leucine zipper motif. Biochem Biophys Res Commun 1998;245:853–9.
20. Desseyn JL, Buisine MP, Porchet N, et al. Genomic organization of the human mucin gene MUC5B. cDNA and genomic sequences upstream of the large central exon. J Biol Chem 1998;273:30157–64.
21. Moniaux N, Escande F, Porchet N, et al. Structural organization and classification of the human mucin genes. Front Biosci 2001;6:D1192–206.
22. Thornton DJ, Sheehan JK. From mucins to mucus: toward a more coherent understanding of this essential barrier. Proc Am Thorac Soc 2004;1:54–61.
23. Kirkham S, Sheehan JK, Knight D, et al. Heterogeneity of airways mucus: variations in the amounts and glycoforms of the major oligomeric mucins MUC5AC and MUC5B. Biochem J 2002;361(Pt 3):537–46.
24. Chen Y, Zhao YH, Kalaslavadi TB, et al. Genome-wide search and identification of a novel gel-forming mucin MUC19/Muc19 in glandular tissues. Am J Respir Cell Mol Biol 2004;30:155–65.

25. Copin MC, Devisme L, Buisine MP, et al. From normal respiratory mucosa to epidermoid carcinoma: expression of human mucin genes. Int J Cancer 2000;86:162–8.

26. Rogers DF, Barnes PJ. Treatment of airway mucus hypersecretion. Ann Med 2006;38:116–25.

27. Wickstrom C, Davies JR, Eriksen GV, et al. MUC5B is a major gel-forming, oligomeric mucin from human salivary gland, respiratory tract and endocervix: identification of glycoforms and C-terminal cleavage. Biochem J 1998;334(Pt 3):685–93.

28. Gray T, Koo JS, Nettesheim P. Regulation of mucous differentiation and mucin gene expression in the tracheobronchial epithelium. Toxicology 2001;160:35–46.

29. Pigny P, Guyonnet-Duperat V, Hill AS, et al. Human mucin genes assigned to 11p15.5: identification and organization of a cluster of genes. Genomics 1996;38:340–52.

30. Desseyn JL, Aubert JP, Porchet N, Laine A. Evolution of the large secreted gel-forming mucins. Mol Biol Evol 2000;17:1175–84.

31. MacNee W. Oxidants/antioxidants and COPD. Chest 2000;117(5 Suppl 1):303S–17S.

32. Rahman I, MacNee W. Role of oxidants/antioxidants in smoking–induced lung diseases. Free Radic Biol Med 1996;21:669–81.

33. Mannino DM. Chronic obstructive pulmonary disease: definition and epidemiology. Respir Care 2003;48:1185–91; discussion 1191–3.

34. Qiu Y, Zhu J, Bandi V, et al. Biopsy neutrophilia, neutrophil chemokine and receptor gene expression in severe exacerbations of chronic obstructive pulmonary disease. Am J Respir Crit Care Med 2003;168:968–75.

35. Stockley RA. Neutrophils and protease/antiprotease imbalance. Am J Respir Crit Care Med 1999;160(5 Pt 2):S49–52.

36. Cantin A, Crystal RG. Oxidants, antioxidants and the pathogenesis of emphysema. Eur J Respir Dis Suppl 1985;139:7–17.

37. Wagner JG, Van Dyken SJ, Hotchkiss JA, Harkema JR. Endotoxin enhancement of ozone-induced mucous cell metaplasia is neutrophil-dependent in rat nasal epithelium. Toxicol Sci 2001;60:338–47.

38. Wagner JG, Hotchkiss JA, Harkema JR. Effects of ozone and endotoxin coexposure on rat airway epithelium: potentiation of toxicant-induced alterations. Environ Health Perspect 2001;109 Suppl 4:591–8.

39. Saetta M, Turato G, Baraldo S, et al. Goblet cell hyperplasia and epithelial inflammation in peripheral airways of smokers with both symptoms of chronic bronchitis and chronic airflow limitation. Am J Respir Crit Care Med 2000;161 (3 Pt 1):1016–21.

40. Caramori G, Di Gregorio C, Carlstedt I, et al. Mucin expression in peripheral airways of patients with chronic obstructive pulmonary disease. Histopathology 2004;45:477–84.

41. Voynow JA, Gendler SJ, Rose MC. Regulation of mucin genes in chronic inflammatory airway diseases. Am J Respir Cell Mol Biol 2006;34:661–5.

42. Groneberg DA, Eynott PR, Oates T, et al. Expression of MUC5AC and MUC5B mucins in normal and cystic fibrosis lung. Respir Med 2002;96:81–6.

43. Fischer B, Voynow J. Neutrophil elastase induces MUC5AC messenger RNA expression by an oxidant-dependent mechanism. Chest 2000;117(5 Suppl 1):317S–20S.

44. Fischer BM, Voynow JA. Neutrophil elastase induces MUC5AC gene expression in airway epithelium via a pathway involving reactive oxygen species. Am J Respir Cell Mol Biol 2002;26:447–52.

45. Shao MX, Ueki IF, Nadel JA. Tumor necrosis factor alpha-converting enzyme mediates MUC5AC mucin expression in cultured human airway epithelial cells. Proc Natl Acad Sci U S A 2003;100:11618–23.

46. Yuan-Chen Wu D, Wu R, Reddy SP, et al. Distinctive epidermal growth factor receptor/extracellular regulated kinase-independent and -dependent signaling pathways in the induction of airway mucin 5B and mucin 5AC expression by phorbol 12-myristate 13-acetate. Am J Pathol 2007;170:20–32.

47. Nadel JA. Role of epidermal growth factor receptor activation in regulating mucin synthesis. Respir Res 2001;2:85–9.

48. Ingram JL, Bonner JC. EGF and PDGF receptor tyrosine kinases as therapeutic targets for chronic lung diseases. Curr Mol Med 2006;6:409–21.

49. Booth BW, Adler KB, Bonner JC, et al. Interleukin-13 induces proliferation of human airway epithelial cells in vitro via a mechanism mediated by transforming growth factor-alpha. Am J Respir Cell Mol Biol 2001;25:739–43.

50. Shao MX, Nakanaga T, Nadel JA. Cigarette smoke induces MUC5AC mucin overproduction via tumor necrosis factor-alpha-converting enzyme in human airway epithelial (NCI-H292) cells. Am J Physiol Lung Cell Mol Physiol 2004; 287:L420–7.

51. da Rocha AB, Mans DR, Regner A, Schwartsmann G. Targeting protein kinase C: new therapeutic opportunities against high-grade malignant gliomas? Oncologist 2002;7:17–33.

52. Chen Y, Zhao YH, Wu R. Differential regulation of airway mucin gene expression and mucin secretion by extracellular nucleotide triphosphates. Am J Respir Cell Mol Biol 2001;25:409–17.

53. Shao MX, Nadel JA. Dual oxidase 1-dependent MUC5AC mucin expression in cultured human airway epithelial cells. Proc Natl Acad Sci U S A 2005;102:767–72.

54. Kim YD, Jeon JY, Woo HJ, et al. Interleukin-1beta induces MUC2 gene expression and mucin secretion via activation of PKC-MEK/ERK, and PI3K in human airway epithelial cells. J Korean Med Sci 2002;17:765–71.

55. Song JS, Kang CM, Yoo MB, et al. Nitric oxide induces MUC5AC mucin in respiratory epithelial cells through PKC and ERK dependent pathways. Respir Res 2007;8:28.

56. Burgoyne RD, Morgan A. Secretory granule exocytosis. Physiol Rev 2003;83:581–632.

57. Jackson AD. Airway goblet-cell mucus secretion. Trends Pharmacol Sci 2001;22:39–45.

58. Adler KB, Li Y. Airway epithelium and mucus: intracellular signaling pathways for gene expression and secretion. Am J Respir Cell Mol Biol 2001;25:397–400.

59. Evans GJ, Wilkinson MC, Graham ME, et al. Phosphorylation of cysteine string protein by protein kinase A. Implications for the modulation of exocytosis. J Biol Chem 2001;276: 47877–85.

60. Foster LJ, Yeung B, Mohtashami M, et al. Binary interactions of the SNARE proteins syntaxin-4, SNAP23, and VAMP-2 and their regulation by phosphorylation. Biochemistry 1998;37:11089–96.

61. Fujita Y, Sasaki T, Fukui K, et al. Phosphorylation of Munc-18/n-Sec1/rbSec1 by protein kinase C: its implication in regulating the interaction of Munc-18/n-Sec1/rbSec1 with syntaxin. J Biol Chem 1996;271:7265–8.

62. Barclay JW, Craig TJ, Fisher RJ, et al. Phosphorylation of Munc18 by protein kinase C regulates the kinetics of exocytosis. J Biol Chem 2003;278:10538–45.

63. Chung SH, Polgar J, Reed GL. Protein kinase C phosphorylation of syntaxin 4 in thrombin-activated human platelets. J Biol Chem 2000;275:25286–91.

64. Polgar J, Lane WS, Chung SH, et al. Phosphorylation of SNAP-23 in activated human platelets. J Biol Chem 2003;278:44369–76.

65. Jeffery PK. Differences and similarities between chronic obstructive pulmonary disease and asthma. Clin Exp Allergy 1999;29 Suppl 2:14–26.

66. Fahy JV, Kim KW, Liu J, Boushey HA. Prominent neutrophilic inflammation in sputum from subjects with asthma exacerbation. J Allergy Clin Immunol 1995;95:843–52.

67. Stockley RA. Role of inflammation in respiratory tract infections. Am J Med 1995;99(6B):8S–13S.

68. Stanescu D, Sanna A, Veriter C, et al. Airways obstruction, chronic expectoration, and rapid decline of FEV_1 in smokers are associated with increased levels of sputum neutrophils. Thorax 1996;51:267–71.

69. Fahy JV, Schuster A, Ueki I, et al. Mucus hypersecretion in bronchiectasis. The role of neutrophil proteases. Am Rev Respir Dis 1992;146:1430–3.

70. Breuer R, Christensen TG, Lucey EC, et al. An ultrastructural morphometric analysis of elastase-treated hamster bronchi shows discharge followed by progressive accumulation of secretory granules. Am Rev Respir Dis 1987;136:698–703.

71. Kim KC, Wasano K, Niles RM, et al. Human neutrophil elastase releases cell surface mucins from primary cultures of hamster tracheal epithelial cells. Proc Natl Acad Sci USA 1987;84:9304–8.

72. Nadel JA. Protease actions on airway secretions. Relevance to cystic fibrosis. Ann N Y Acad Sci 1991;624:286–96.

73. Sommerhoff CP, Nadel JA, Basbaum CB, Caughey GH. Neutrophil elastase and cathepsin G stimulate secretion from cultured bovine airway gland serous cells. J Clin Invest 1990;85:682–9.

74. Rao NV, Marshall BC, Gray BH, Hoidal JR. Interaction of secretory leukocyte protease inhibitor with proteinase-3. Am J Respir Cell Mol Biol 1993;8:612–6.

75. Renesto P, Halbwachs-Mecarelli L, Nusbaum P, et al. Proteinase 3. A neutrophil proteinase with activity on platelets. J Immunol 1994;152:4612–7.

76. Stockley RA, Burnett D. Alpha,-antitrypsin and leukocyte elastase in infected and noninfected sputum. Am Rev Respir Dis 1979;120:1081–6.

77. Gadek JE. Adverse effects of neutrophils on the lung. Am J Med 1992;92(6A):27S–31S.

78. Lucey EC, Stone PJ, Breuer R, et al. Effect of combined human neutrophil cathepsin G and elastase on induction of secretory cell metaplasia and emphysema in hamsters, with in vitro observations on elastolysis by these enzymes. Am Rev Respir Dis 1985;132:362–6.

79. Kao RC, Wehner NG, Skubitz KM, et al. Proteinase 3. A distinct human polymorphonuclear leukocyte proteinase that produces emphysema in hamsters. J Clin Invest 1988; 82:1963–73.

80. Tremblay GM, Janelle MF, Bourbonnais Y. Anti-inflammatory activity of neutrophil elastase inhibitors. Curr Opin Investig Drugs 2003;4:556–65.

81. Takahashi H, Nukiwa T, Yoshimura K, et al. Structure of the human neutrophil elastase gene. J Biol Chem 1988;263:14739–47.

82. Bode W, Meyer E Jr, Powers JC. Human leukocyte and porcine pancreatic elastase: x-ray crystal structures, mechanism, substrate specificity, and mechanism-based inhibitors. Biochemistry 1989;28:1951–63.

83. Gadek JE, Fells GA, Zimmerman RL, et al. Antielastases of the human alveolar structures. Implications for the protease-antiprotease theory of emphysema. J Clin Invest 1981;68:889–98.

84. Belaaouaj A, McCarthy R, Baumann M, et al. Mice lacking neutrophil elastase reveal impaired host defense against gram negative bacterial sepsis. Nat Med 1998;4:615–8.

85. Fick RB Jr, Naegel GP, Squier SU, et al. Proteins of the cystic fibrosis respiratory tract. Fragmented immunoglobulin G opsonic antibody causing defective opsonophagocytosis. J Clin Invest 1984;74:236–48.

86. Suter S, Schaad UB, Tegner H, et al. Levels of free granulocyte elastase in bronchial secretions from patients with cystic fibrosis: effect of antimicrobial treatment against Pseudomonas aeruginosa. J Infect Dis 1986;153:902–9.

87. Doring G, Goldstein W, Botzenhart K, et al. Elastase from polymorphonuclear leucocytes: a regulatory enzyme in immune complex disease. Clin Exp Immunol 1986;64:597–605.

88. Goldstein W, Doring G. Lysosomal enzymes from polymorphonuclear leukocytes and proteinase inhibitors in patients with cystic fibrosis. Am Rev Respir Dis 1986;134:49–56.

89. Bainton DF, Ullyot JL, Farquhar MG. The development of neutrophilic polymorphonuclear leukocytes in human bone marrow. J Exp Med 1971;134:907–34.

90. Vignola AM, Bonanno A, Mirabella A, et al. Increased levels of elastase and alpha1-antitrypsin in sputum of asthmatic patients. Am J Respir Crit Care Med 1998;157:505–11.

91. Voynow JA, Fischer BM, Malarkey DE, et al. Neutrophil elastase induces mucus cell metaplasia in mouse lung. Am J Physiol Lung Cell Mol Physiol 2004;287:L1293–302.

92. Voynow JA, Young LR, Wang Y, et al. Neutrophil elastase increases MUC5AC mRNA and protein expression in respiratory epithelial cells. Am J Physiol 1999;276(5 Pt 1):L835–43.

93. Fischer BM, Cuellar JG, Byrd AS, et al. ErbB2 activity is required for airway epithelial repair following neutrophil elastase exposure. FASEB J 2005;19:1374–6.

94. Shao MX, Nadel JA. Neutrophil elastase induces MUC5AC mucin production in human airway epithelial cells via a cascade involving protein kinase C, reactive oxygen species, and TNF-alpha-converting enzyme. J Immunol 2005; 175:4009–16.

95. Park JA, He F, Martin LD, et al. Human neutrophil elastase induces hypersecretion of mucin from well-differentiated human bronchial epithelial cells in vitro via a protein kinase CΔ-mediated mechanism. Am J Pathol 2005;167:651–61.

96. Nishizuka Y. Intracellular signaling by hydrolysis of phospholipids and activation of protein kinase C. Science 1992;258:607–14.

97. Kitagawa M, Mukai H, Shibata H, Ono Y. Purification and characterization of a fatty acid-activated protein kinase (PKN) from rat testis. Biochem J 1995;310(Pt 2):657–64.

98. Palmer RH, Ridden J, Parker PJ. Cloning and expression patterns of two members of a novel protein-kinase-C-related kinase family. Eur J Biochem 1995;227:344–51.

99. Johannes FJ, Prestle J, Eis S, et al. PKCu is a novel, atypical member of the protein kinase C family. J Biol Chem 1994;269:6140–8.

100. Rozengurt E, Rey O, Waldron RT. Protein kinase D signaling. J Biol Chem 2005;280:13205–8.

101. Hayashi A, Seki N, Hattori A, et al. PKCnu, a new member of the protein kinase C family, composes a fourth subfamily with PKCmu. Biochim Biophys Acta 1999;1450:99–106.

102. Kishimoto A, Mikawa K, Hashimoto K, et al. Limited proteolysis of protein kinase C subspecies by calcium-dependent neutral protease (calpain). J Biol Chem 1989;264:4088–92.

103. Lee MW, Severson DL. Signal transduction in vascular smooth muscle: diacylglycerol second messengers and PKC action. Am J Physiol 1994;267(3 Pt 1):C659–78.

104. Lu Z, Liu D, Hornia A, et al. Activation of protein kinase C triggers its ubiquitination and degradation. Mol Cell Biol 1998;18:839–45.

105. Wetsel WC, Khan WA, Merchenthaler I, et al. Tissue and cellular distribution of the extended family of protein kinase C isoenzymes. J Cell Biol 1992;117:121–33.

106. Webb BL, Hirst SJ, Giembycz MA. Protein kinase C isoenzymes: a review of their structure, regulation and role in regulating airways smooth muscle tone and mitogenesis. Br J Pharmacol 2000;130:1433–52.

107. Harrington EO, Loffler J, Nelson PR, et al. Enhancement of migration by protein kinase Calpha and inhibition of proliferation and cell cycle progression by protein kinase Cdelta in capillary endothelial cells. J Biol Chem 1997;272:7390–7.

108. Abe MK, Kartha S, Karpova AY, et al. Hydrogen peroxide activates extracellular signal-regulated kinase via protein kinase C, Raf-1, and MEK1. Am J Respir Cell Mol Biol 1998;18:562–9.

109. Lucas M, Sanchez-Margalet V. Protein kinase C involvement in apoptosis. Gen Pharmacol 1995;26:881–7.

110. Gschwendt M. Protein kinase C delta. Eur J Biochem 1999;259:555–64.

111. Steinberg SF. Distinctive activation mechanisms and functions for protein kinase Cdelta. Biochem J 2004;384(Pt 3):449–59.

112. Ono Y, Fujii T, Ogita K, et al. Identification of three additional members of rat protein kinase C family: delta-, epsilon- and zeta-subspecies. FEBS Lett 1987;226:125–8.

113. Huppi K, Siwarski D, Goodnight J, Mischak H. Assignment of the protein kinase C delta polypeptide gene (PRKCD) to human chromosome 3 and mouse chromosome 14. Genomics 1994;19:161–2.

114. Kofler K, Erdel M, Utermann G, Baier G. Molecular genetics and structural genomics of the human protein kinase C gene module. Genome Biol 2002;3: research0014.1–research0014.10.

115. Ishikawa T, Iwasaki E, Kanatani K, et al. Involvement of novel protein kinase C isoforms in carbachol-stimulated insulin secretion from rat pancreatic islets. Life Sci 2005;77:462–9.

116. Li J, Hellmich MR, Greeley GH Jr, et al. Phorbol ester-mediated neurotensin secretion is dependent on the PKC-alpha and -delta isoforms. Am J Physiol Gastrointest Liver Physiol 2002;283:G1197–206.

117. Ridge KM, Dada L, Lecuona E, et al. Dopamine-induced exocytosis of Na,K-ATPase is dependent on activation of protein kinase C-epsilon and -delta. Mol Biol Cell 2002;13:1381–9.

118. Murugappan S, Tuluc F, Dorsam RT, et al. Differential role of protein kinase C delta isoform in agonist-induced dense granule secretion in human platelets. J Biol Chem 2004;279:2360–7.

119. Ozawa K, Szallasi Z, Kazanietz MG, et al. Ca(2+)-dependent and Ca(2+)-independent isozymes of protein kinase C mediate exocytosis in antigen-stimulated rat basophilic RBL-2H3 cells. Reconstitution of secretory responses with Ca2+ and purified isozymes in washed permeabilized cells. J Biol Chem 1993;268:1749–56.

120. Cho SH, Woo CH, Yoon SB, Kim JH. Protein kinase Cdelta functions downstream of Ca2+ mobilization in FcepsilonRI signaling to degranulation in mast cells. J Allergy Clin Immunol 2004;114:1085–92.

121. Leitges M, Gimborn K, Elis W, et al. Protein kinase C-delta is a negative regulator of antigen-induced mast cell degranulation. Mol Cell Biol 2002;22:3970–80.

122. Abdullah LH, Bundy JT, Ehre C, Davis CW. Mucin secretion and PKC isoforms in SPOC1 goblet cells: differential activation by purinergic agonist and PMA. Am J Physiol Lung Cell Mol Physiol 2003;285:L149–60.

123. Park JA, Crews AL, Adler KB. Protein kinase C delta regulates airway mucin secretion via phosphorylation of MARCKS protein. Proc Am Thorac Soc 2007;175:A752.

124. Glaser M, Wanaski S, Buser CA, et al. Myristoylated alanine-rich C kinase substrate (MARCKS) produces reversible inhibition of phospholipase C by sequestering phosphatidylinositol 4,5-bisphosphate in lateral domains. J Biol Chem 1996;271:26187–93.

125. Salli U, Supancic S, Stormshak F. Phosphorylation of myristoylated alanine-rich C kinase substrate (MARCKS) protein is associated with bovine luteal oxytocin exocytosis. Biol Reprod 2000;63:12–20.

126. Li Y, Martin LD, Spizz G, Adler KB. MARCKS protein is a key molecule regulating mucin secretion by human airway epithelial cells in vitro. J Biol Chem 2001;276:40982–90.

127. Blackshear PJ. The MARCKS family of cellular protein kinase C substrates. J Biol Chem 1993;268:1501–4.

128. Seykora JT, Myat MM, Allen LA, et al. Molecular determinants of the myristoyl-electrostatic switch of MARCKS. J Biol Chem 1996;271:18797–802.

129. Boutin JA. Myristoylation. Cell Signal 1997;9:15–35.

130. McIlroy BK, Walters JD, Blackshear PJ, Johnson JD. Phosphorylation-dependent binding of a synthetic MARCKS peptide to calmodulin. J Biol Chem 1991;266: 4959–64.

131. McLaughlin S, Aderem A. The myristoyl-electrostatic switch: a modulator of reversible protein-membrane interactions. Trends Biochem Sci 1995;20:272–6.

132. Herget T, Oehrlein SA, Pappin DJ, et al. The myristoylated alanine-rich C-kinase substrate (MARCKS) is sequentially phosphorylated by conventional, novel and atypical isotypes of protein kinase C. Eur J Biochem 1995;233:448–57.

133. Song JC, Hrnjez BJ, Farokhzad OC, Matthews JB. PKC-epsilon regulates basolateral endocytosis in human T84 intestinal epithelia: role of F-actin and MARCKS. Am J Physiol 1999;277(6 Pt 1):C1239–49.

134. Elzagallaai A, Rose SD, Trifaro JM. Platelet secretion induced by phorbol esters stimulation is mediated through phosphorylation of MARCKS: a MARCKS-derived peptide blocks MARCKS phosphorylation and serotonin release without affecting pleckstrin phosphorylation. Blood 2000;95:894–902.

135. Fujise A, Mizuno K, Ueda Y, et al. Specificity of the high affinity interaction of protein kinase C with a physiological substrate, myristoylated alanine-rich protein kinase C substrate. J Biol Chem 1994;269:31642–8.

136. Coffey ET, Herrero I, Sihra TS, et al. Glutamate exocytosis and MARCKS phosphorylation are enhanced by a metabotropic glutamate receptor coupled to a protein kinase C synergistically activated by diacylglycerol and arachidonic acid. J Neurochem 1994;63:1303–10.

137. Trifaro J, Rose SD, Lejen T, Elzagallaai A. Two pathways control chromaffin cell cortical F-actin dynamics during exocytosis. Biochimie 2000;82:339–52.

138. Singer M, Martin LD, Vargaftig BB, et al. A MARCKS-related peptide blocks mucus hypersecretion in a mouse model of asthma. Nat Med 2004;10:193–6.

139. Agrawal A, Rengarajan S, Adler KB, et al. Inhibition of mucin secretion with MARCKS-related peptide improves airway obstruction in a mouse model of asthma. J Appl Physiol 2007;102:399–405.

140. Park J, Fang S, Adler KB. Regulation of airway mucin secretion by MARCKS protein involves the chaperones heat shock protein 70 and cysteine string protein. Proc Am Thorac Soc 2006;3:493.

141. Yaney GC, Fairbanks JM, Deeney JT, et al. Potentiation of insulin secretion by phorbol esters is mediated by PKC-alpha and nPKC isoforms. Am J Physiol Endocrinol Metab 2002;283:E880–8.

CHAPTER 12

OTHER LARGE-AIRWAY DISEASES THAT LIMIT AIRFLOW

CARLOS E. GIROD, MD, AND MARVIN I. SCHWARZ, MD

THE TERM *CHRONIC OBSTRUCTIVE PULMONARY DISEASES* (COPD) defines the pulmonary disorders that cause progressive airflow obstruction and have minimal reversibility. The diseases that define COPD are chronic bronchitis and emphysema.[1,2] The main focus of this chapter is to describe other airway diseases that result in airflow limitation. By mimicking chronic bronchitis, emphysema, and asthma, these less common diseases present diagnostic and therapeutic challenges. They are often misdiagnosed, leading to either incorrect or inadequate treatment.[1,3,4]

Airflow obstruction can occur at any generation of airway branching. Airflow limitation depends on the number of involved airways and the degree of obstruction. There are three primary sites of airway obstruction: the upper airway, large (central) airways, and small (peripheral) airways. The classification of obstructive pulmonary diseases other than emphysema and chronic bronchitis is shown in Figure 1 and is based on the anatomic site of airflow obstruction.

In the normal lung, the greatest contribution to airway resistance (60–70%) is made by the large (central) airways. This is due to reduced total cross-sectional area and resultant turbulent airflow.[5] Therefore, a small decrease in luminal diameter can account for significant airflow limitation. This chapter focuses on diseases of the upper airway, trachea, and large (central) airways. Chapter 13, "Diffuse Interstitial Lung Diseases Resulting in Airflow Limitation," discusses the interstitial and parenchymal lung diseases that involve the small (peripheral) airways.

Diseases of the Upper Airway: Larynx and Trachea

The upper airway includes the airways that extend from the nose to the carina. These are divided into extrathoracic or intrathoracic components, depending on whether the obstruction is located above or below the thoracic inlet. The larynx is extrathoracic and is divided into the supraglottis, glottis, and subglottis. It normally accounts for 40% of the airflow resistance during quiet breathing. During increasing respiratory demands, the resistance is reduced by reflex dilatation of the laryngeal lumen.[5] The trachea is approximately 10 to 13 cm in length and is divided into extra- and intrathoracic components.[6] Significant airflow limitation can occur when it is compressed, narrowed, or stenosed. The diseases leading to obstruction of the upper airway are extensive;

a recent review listed more than 50 disorders.[7] This discussion focuses on upper airway lesions that present with chronic airflow limitation and can be confused with COPD.[3]

Chronic upper airway obstruction presents with cough (sometimes "barking"), recurrent infection, stridor, dyspnea, and hoarseness. It is important to determine whether the patient has a previous history of endotracheal intubation or tracheostomy. Dyspnea with exertion and stridor is usually associated with critical airway narrowing to a diameter of 5 to 8 mm. At this diameter, reduced inspiratory or expiratory flow rates are easily detected.[3,7] Intrathoracic airway obstruction (predominantly from tracheal lesions) is characterized by abnormalities in the expiratory portion of the flow-volume loop. During forced exhalation, the pleural pressure becomes greater than the intraluminal tracheal pressure, leading to further collapse of the airway and accentuation of the tracheal stenosis (Figure 2A). If the lesion is extrathoracic, a flattening or "serration" of the inspiratory flow-volume loop is seen. This is due to worsening of the stenosis caused by collapse during inspiration at a time when the intraluminal tracheal pressures fall below atmospheric pressure (Figure 2B). If the lesion is fixed in the trachea, a fixed intrathoracic obstruction develops, affecting both the inspiratory and expiratory flow-volume loops (Figure 3).[3,7]

Several upper airway diseases present with subacute or chronic symptoms that may be confused with emphysema and chronic bronchitis (Table 1).[3,8] The most common of these are vocal cord paralysis or tumors, tracheal stenosis or tumors, and tracheobronchomalacia.

Vocal Cord Paralysis or Tumors

Vocal cord paralysis represents the most frequent cause of a variable extrathoracic airway obstruction.[8] This may result from trauma, iatrogenic injury (intubation, endoscopy, damage to recurrent laryngeal nerve), or laryngeal or intrathoracic tumors. Vocal cord paralysis causes dyspnea, hoarseness, wheezing, and stridor. Of interest, voice may be preserved with bilateral vocal cord paralysis or with gradual unilateral paralysis. This is related to equal bilateral vibration of the vocal cords, allowing the preservation of speech.[7] Vocal cord tumors can be supraglottic or glottic and can demonstrate a flow-volume loop with variable extrathoracic airway obstruction (see Figure 2B). The presence of a vocal

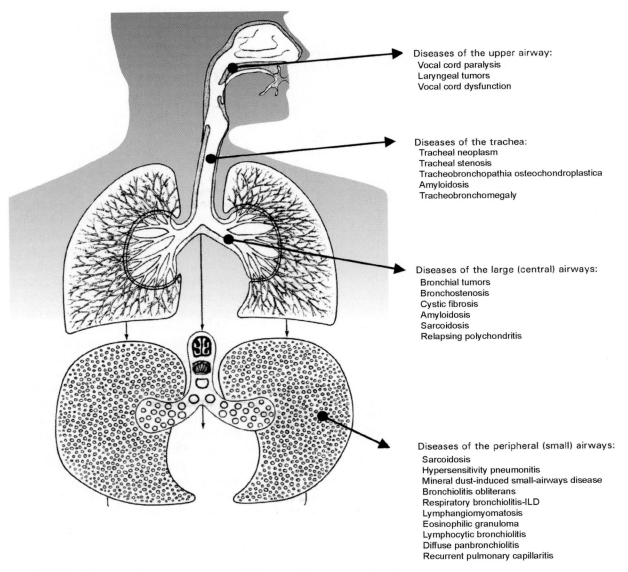

Diseases of the upper airway:
  Vocal cord paralysis
  Laryngeal tumors
  Vocal cord dysfunction

Diseases of the trachea:
  Tracheal neoplasm
  Tracheal stenosis
  Tracheobronchopathia osteochondroplastica
  Amyloidosis
  Tracheobronchomegaly

Diseases of the large (central) airways:
  Bronchial tumors
  Bronchostenosis
  Cystic fibrosis
  Amyloidosis
  Sarcoidosis
  Relapsing polychondritis

Diseases of the peripheral (small) airways:
  Sarcoidosis
  Hypersensitivity pneumonitis
  Mineral dust-induced small-airways disease
  Bronchiolitis obliterans
  Respiratory bronchiolitis-ILD
  Lymphangiomyomatosis
  Eosinophilic granuloma
  Lymphocytic bronchiolitis
  Diffuse panbronchiolitis
  Recurrent pulmonary capillaritis

FIGURE 1. Classification of obstructive pulmonary diseases other than emphysema or chronic bronchitis by anatomic site of airflow obstruction. Reproduced with permission from Netter FH. The respiratory system. In: Divertie MB, Brass A, eds. The CIBA collection of medical illustration. Vol 7. 2nd ed. Summit [NJ]: CIBA; 1980. p. 55. Copyright 1997. Icon Learning Systems, LLC, a subsidiary of Medi Media USA Inc. Reprinted with permission from ICON Learning Systems, LLC, illustrated by Frank H. Netter, MD. All rights reserved. Classification scheme designed by authors CE Girod and MI Schwarz. ILD = interstitial lung disease.

cord lesion is confirmed by direct laryngoscopy. Urgent treatment requires the administration of helium-oxygen mixtures that decrease inhaled gas viscosity and prompt evaluation for tracheostomy.

Vocal Cord Dysfunction

In 1983, Christopher and colleagues described vocal cord dysfunction in five patients whose clinical course mimicked asthma.[9] This condition is also called "paradoxical laryngeal dysfunction"[10] and is believed to represent a conversion disorder in which patients demonstrate paradoxical and involuntary closure of the true and false vocal cords during

inspiration and, sometimes, expiration. It can be severe, necessitating emergency room visits, hospitalization, and urgent endotracheal intubation.[11] Vocal cord dysfunction is more common in women and is associated with a high incidence of psychiatric disorders and previous physical or sexual abuse. Physical examination reveals inspiratory and expiratory wheezing that is more prominent in the neck. The flow-volume loop will reveal blunting or truncation of the inspiratory limb of the flow-volume loop consistent with a classic variable extrathoracic airflow obstruction (see Figure 2B). A diagnosis of vocal cord dysfunction is confirmed by direct laryngoscopy during an attack or

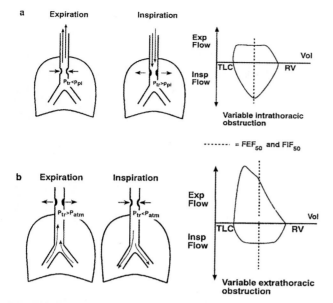

FIGURE 2. Diagram of flow-volume loops demonstrating intra- and extrathoracic airway obstruction. Reproduced with permission from St John RC et al.[3] Exp = expiratory; FEF = forced expiratory flow; FIF = forced inspiratory flow; Insp = inspiratory; Ppl = pleural pressure; Ptm = atmospheric pressure; Ptr = tracheal pressure; RV = residual volume; TLC = total lung capacity.

Table 1   Causes of Upper Airway Obstruction Mimicking Chronic Obstructive Pulmonary Disease

Variable intrathoracic obstruction
  Tracheal tumors
  Tracheobronchomalacia
  Tracheobronchomegaly (Mounier-Kuhn syndrome)

Variable extrathoracic obstruction
  Vocal cord dysfunction
  Glottic stricture
  Laryngeal tumor
  Wegener granulomatosis

Fixed obstruction
  Bilateral vocal cord paralysis
  Tracheal stenosis
  Tracheal tumors
  Extrinsic compression from goiter, lymphoadenopathy, or tumor
  Fibrosing mediastinitis
  Tracheobronchopathia osteochondroplastica
  Tracheobronchial amyloidosis

Adapted from St John RC et al.[3]

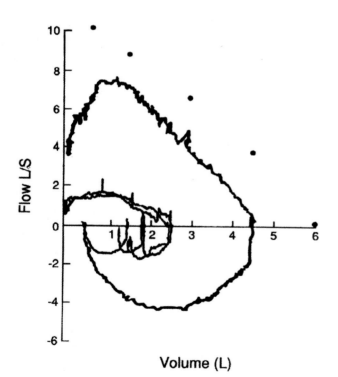

FIGURE 3. Flow-volume loop demonstrating a fixed intrathoracic airway obstruction (smaller loop) relieved with stenting (larger loop). Reproduced with permission from Mehta AC et al.[17] L/S = liters per second.

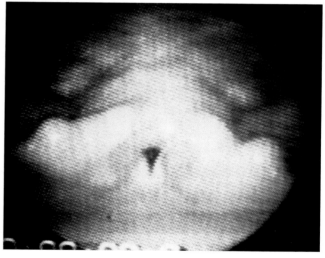

FIGURE 4. Laryngeal narrowing during inspiration, demonstrating a posterior "chink" in a patient with vocal cord dysfunction.

when induced with a methacholine inhalational challenge (Figure 4).[11–13] Laryngeal function is normal between attacks. Treatment is problematic and requires the patient's acceptance of the diagnosis. Speech therapy and psychotherapy can be helpful in teaching relaxed throat breathing and relaxation techniques. Injection with botulinum toxin has been reported but remains controversial and experimental.[14] The use of inhaled helium-oxygen mixtures may abort an acute attack.[14]

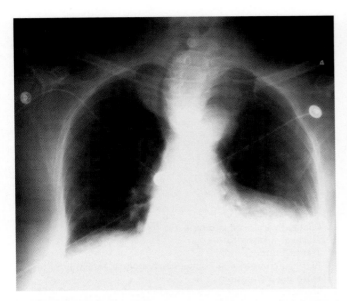

FIGURE 5. Chest radiograph showing tracheal narrowing and displacement owing to a goiter of the thyroid, causing stridor and respiratory failure.

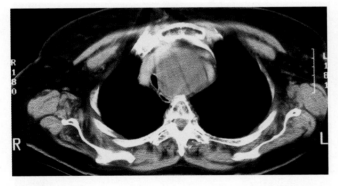

FIGURE 6. Computed tomographic scan demonstrating tracheal narrowing and displacement owing to a goiter, causing stridor and respiratory failure.

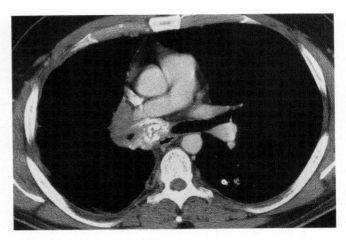

FIGURE 7. Marked narrowing of the right mainstem bronchus owing to fibrosing mediastinitis, as shown by computed tomography.

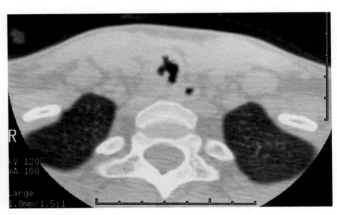

FIGURE 8. Tracheal stenosis in a patient with previous prolonged endotracheal intubation.

Tracheal Compression, Strictures, and Tumors

Tracheal narrowing from extrinsic compression, postintubation stenosis, or tumors can gradually progress, with the development of symptoms that suggest COPD.[3,7,8] The tracheal lumen has to be narrowed from its normal diameter of 13 to 25 mm to approximately 6 to 8 mm before symptoms or spirometric abnormalities develop. At that point, the flow-volume loops will demonstrate an inspiratory or expiratory cutoff, depending on the location of the lesion in the intra- or extrathoracic trachea.[7]

Mediastinal or esophageal tumors, lymphadenopathy, fibrosing mediastinitis, vascular anomalies, and goiters can cause extrinsic compression of the trachea (Figures 5, 6, and 7). A tracheal stricture is either congenital or occurs after

intubation or tracheostomy (Figure 8). Patients can present with a fixed intrathoracic airway obstruction months to years after the endotracheal intubation or tracheostomy.[8] Its pathogenesis is related to the necrosis of the tracheal mucosa caused by the inflated balloon cuff of the endotracheal or tracheostomy tube. Prospective studies demonstrate a 10 to 19% incidence of tracheal stenosis after endotracheal intubation, but most tracheal stenoses were clinically "silent." Risk factors for the development of this complication include diabetes, severe underlying respiratory failure, prolonged intubation, female gender, larger endotracheal tubes, and overinflation of the balloon cuff.[7,8] Percutaneous dilation tracheostomy may be a risk factor for development of suprastomal tracheal stenosis.[15] The diagnosis is suggested by a fixed intrathoracic airway obstruction on the flow-volume loop (see Figure 3) and is confirmed by either flexible laryngoscopy or ultrafast cine–computed tomography (CT) with image reconstruction of the trachea and

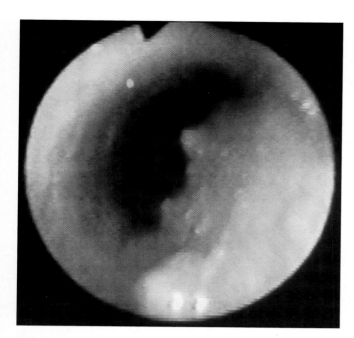

FIGURE 9. Marked narrowing of the trachea owing to directed extension of a papillary thyroid carcinoma.

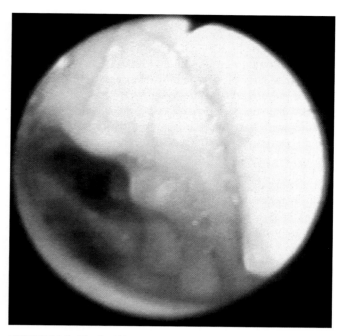

FIGURE 10. The "cobblestone" appearance of the trachea in a patient with tracheobronchopathia osteochondroplastica.

subglottic regions. Virtual bronchoscopy also allows for detection and measurement of central airway stenotic lesions by digitally reconstructing the trachea and airways with images acquired with multirow detector CT.[16] Treatment of benign tracheal stenosis or stricture requires airway stenting, laser therapy, or surgical resection.[7,17,18]

Other causes of tracheal obstruction that present with chronic airflow obstruction include benign and malignant tracheal tumors (Figure 9). These lesions can present with fixed or variable intra- and extrathoracic airway obstruction. The most common tumors are squamous cell carcinoma, adenoid cystic carcinoma, Hodgkin disease, Kaposi sarcoma, and chondrosarcoma.[7,19]

Tracheobronchopathia Osteochondroplastica

TO is a rare benign disorder that affects the larynx, trachea, and major bronchi. The original description was made by Wilks in the 1800s.[20] This disease is usually asymptomatic and is found incidentally by CT or during postmortem examination.[21,22] The striking feature of TO is the endoscopic appearance of a deformed trachea with a beaded, nodular, and "cobblestone" appearance (Figure 10). This appearance is due to submucosal nodules that contain cartilage, bone, acellular proteinaceous material, calcifications, and hematopoietic cells. The nodules usually involve the cartilaginous trachea, sparing the membranous trachea.[23] The pathogenesis is unknown; various possibilities include a congenital anomaly or a sequela of chronic infection, environmental exposure, metabolic abnormality, or a variant of TBA. Virchow postulated that TO nodules develop from echondrosis and exostosis of tracheal cartilage. The currently accepted hypothesis is that TO originates from elastic connective tissue that undergoes cartilaginous and bony metaplasia.[21–25]

The incidence of TO is unknown and is likely underestimated owing to the lack of radiographic abnormalities.[21] There is no sex predilection, and TO is usually discovered in patients aged 50 years or older. Patients can be symptomatic or can exhibit a nonproductive or productive cough, recurrent episodes of bronchitis, dyspnea, and hemoptysis. Clinically, it is difficult to distinguish from COPD.[21,22] Spirometry may be normal or may demonstrate an obstructive pattern.[22] During bronchoscopy, nodules with hard consistency are detected on the anterolateral walls of the trachea, producing a "grinding" sensation when the bronchoscope is advanced over them.[22] Despite the fact that endobronchial biopsies are problematic owing to forceps slippage, a diagnosis is achieved in approximately 70% of cases. The presence of submucosal cartilage, bone, or calcification is diagnostic.[22] On follow-up, most patients demonstrate preserved lung function, suggesting a benign course. Nevertheless, there are reports of accelerated or progressive TO with tracheal stenosis and respiratory compromise.[22,26,27] Treatment is primarily supportive, with antibiotics for bronchitis or infections. Laser ablative therapy or surgical resection may be required.

Tracheobronchial Amyloidosis

Amyloidosis involves the respiratory system in several patterns: the alveolar septal form (which mimics interstitial lung disease or pulmonary hypertension), pulmonary nodules or masses, and tracheobronchial deposition. TBA is rare; fewer than 100 cases have been reported in the literature. It represents a localized form of primary amyloidosis characterized by local clonal expansion of plasma cells producing light-chain immunoglobulin fractions that accumulate in these large airways.[28–30] It represents 10 to 25% of all cases of pulmonary amyloidosis.[28,31–33]

TBA has no sex predilection and usually occurs in middle-aged patients. The symptoms reported include cough, hoarseness, hemoptysis, and dyspnea. A delay in diagnosis of 1 to 2 years is common as patients are misdiagnosed as having pneumonia, chronic bronchitis, and asthma. Unless atelectasis or lobar collapse develops, airway involvement is not identifiable by chest radiography. Negative results of fat pad biopsy, protein electrophoresis, and bone marrow biopsy exclude systemic amyloidosis in these patients.[28,31] Pulmonary function studies demonstrate an obstructive pattern, with air trapping in most cases. Depending on the degree and location of the luminal obstruction, a fixed airway obstruction may be seen on the flow-volume loop. TBA involves the distal trachea, the carina, and mainstem bronchi. The gross appearance of TBA ranges from round yellowish lesions to "cobblestoning," with diffuse inflammation of the tracheal mucosa. In some cases, the gross appearance of the airways is normal, even though calcifications and thickening of the tracheal and bronchial walls are detected by CT.[28]

O'Regan and colleagues reported that TBA was usually stable 12 to 24 months from diagnosis.[28] But with follow-up (average of 8 years), a slowly progressive pattern of infiltration with airway narrowing and obstruction develops. Severe obstruction requires laser débridement with a rigid bronchoscope. The lesions can recur after treatment.[28,30–32] Patients with upper airway disease may require tracheostomy. Progression of TBA to diffuse systemic amyloidosis has not been described. Treatment with colchicine, melphalan, and prednisone has been attempted, but efficacy has not been confirmed. Low-dose radiation therapy for TBA has been proposed and is supported by the well-known radiosensitivity of plasma cells.[28,30,32] Up to 25% of patients with TBA die from respiratory failure, pneumonia, or post-tracheostomy bleeding.[34]

Tracheobronchomegaly: Mounier-Kuhn Syndrome

Mounier-Kuhn syndrome (MKS) was first described in 1932. It is characterized by flaccid dilatation and malacia of the trachea and major bronchi.[35] This syndrome is rare, with approximately 80 cases reported in the literature.[36] It mimics chronic bronchitis and emphysema. The diagnosis can be elusive and is usually discovered after the patient undergoes chest CT. It usually presents in the third or fourth decade of life. Males with a smoking history are more commonly affected. It is unclear if MKS is an acquired or congenital disease, although it is suspected to be a congenital disorder.[35] Familial cases have been described.[36] Secondary tracheobronchomegaly can occur with prolonged intubation, tracheostomy, chronic bronchiectasis, relapsing polychondritis (RP), tracheal tumors, Ehlers-Danlos syndrome, and congenital cutis laxa.[36,37]

The symptoms of MKS mimic those of chronic bronchitis and bronchiectasis. A deep "barking" cough and dyspnea are common, although some patients remain asymptomatic. Complications include pneumonia, bronchiectasis, emphysema, respiratory failure, and even death. These complications are due to distal pooling of secretions caused by dynamic collapse of the trachea and mainstem bronchi during forceful coughing. Pulmonary function tests reveal decreased flow rates and air trapping. The diagnosis relies on CT-guided measurement of the trachea, right mainstem bronchus, and left mainstem bronchus diameters larger than 3.0, 2.4, and 2.3 cm, respectively (Figures 11, 12, and 13).[38,39] Bronchoscopy demonstrates enlargement and dynamic collapse of the trachea and mainstem bronchi, with saccular dilatation, redundant folds, and pseudodiverticula. Histologically, the trachea and mainstem bronchi demonstrate decreased and atrophic longitudinal elastic fibers, enlarged cartilaginous rings, and thinning of the muscularis layer.[36] Treatment is supportive and is focused on improving secretion clearance, with rotating antibiotics to treat the associated bronchiectasis, chest percussion, and the use of nocturnal continuous positive airway pressure to prevent expiratory airway collapse.[36,40] Bilateral lung transplantation has been attempted with poor outcomes owing to anastomosis problems and persistent bacterial colonization and infection.[38,41]

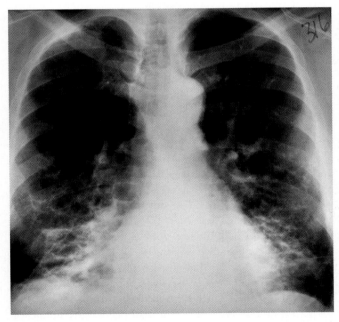

FIGURE 11. Chest radiograph of a patient with Mounier-Kuhn syndrome demonstrates diffuse bronchiectasis and marked dilatation of the trachea and bronchi.

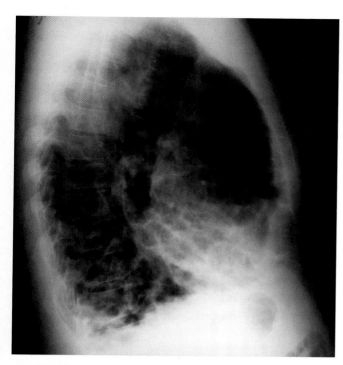

FIGURE 12. Chest radiograph of the same patient shown in Figure 11 demonstrates diffuse bronchiectasis and marked dilatation of the trachea and bronchi.

Diseases of the Large (Central) Airways

The large (central) airways are bronchi with luminal diameters >3 mm. The most prevalent diseases are asthma and chronic bronchitis. However, other entities should be considered (Table 2).

Anatomic obstruction of the large (central) airways is a complication of bronchial tumors and bronchostenosis.

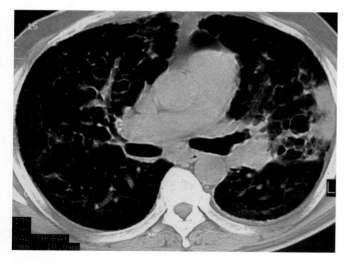

FIGURE 13. Computed tomographic features of Mounier-Kuhn syndrome, with diffuse bronchiectasis and dilatation of the mainstem bronchi.

Table 2 Important Causes of Large (Central) Airway Obstruction Mimicking Chronic Obstructive Pulmonary Disease
Bronchial tumors
Bronchostenosis
Bronchomalacia
Bronchiectasis
Cystic fibrosis
Sarcoidosis
Relapsing polychondritis

Bronchial tumors can present with slow onset of airflow obstruction. The most common benign bronchial tumors are adenomas, papillomas, hamartomas, and angiomas.[42] Malignant tumors include bronchogenic carcinoma, metastatic tumors, carcinoid tumors, and cylindromas.[43] Bronchostenosis is a benign stricture with stenosis of a major bronchus and is usually a sequela of endobronchial or lower lung field tuberculosis.[44] Van den Brande and colleagues observed 11 elderly patients with endobronchial tuberculosis and found that 6 of these patients developed bronchostenosis despite antituberculous treatment.[45] Bronchostenosis patients can present with chronic cough, wheezing (sometimes focal), and dyspnea.[45] The stenosis is treated with endoscopic dilatation and/or endobronchial stenting.[45,46]

Bronchiectasis

Bronchiectasis is a disorder characterized by irreversible bronchial wall destruction and dilatation. It is caused by several congenital, inflammatory, acquired, and obstructive disorders.[47–51] It has been referred to as the "other" obstructive lung disease.[47,49] In fact, 29% of patients diagnosed by their primary care physicians with COPD have bronchiectasis by CT criteria.[52] Bronchiectasis involves medium-sized airways, causing bronchial distortion and dilatation. The mechanism causing airflow limitation in bronchiectasis is unclear.[47] Possible explanations include the presence of dynamic airway collapse and associated small airways disease. Using high-resolution computed tomography (HRCT), Kang and colleagues demonstrated changes consistent with involvement of the small airways in over 50% of patients undergoing resection for bronchiectasis.[53] Of the resected lobes, 85% demonstrated bronchiolitis obliterans.[47,53] The development of bronchiectasis requires the presence of infection, obstruction, traction, and abnormal host inflammatory, cellular, and cytokine responses.[51,54] This process is sustained by either a congenital or an acquired defect in mucociliary clearance that leads to chronic infection and subsequent inflammation of the bronchial mucosa and lumen.

CLASSIFICATION AND ASSOCIATED DISORDERS

Reid classified bronchiectasis into three forms on the basis of their morphologic patterns: cylindrical, varicose, and saccular (cystic) bronchiectasis.[55] Reid's classification lacks clinical utility since no correlation exists between the pattern of bronchiectasis and the underlying pathogenesis or physiologic impairment. Nonetheless, the presence of saccular (cystic) bronchiectasis suggests severe and advanced disease.[47,49] Bronchiectasis is best classified by its predisposing conditions, as illustrated in Table 3. In approximately 40% of patients, the predisposing disorder is unknown.[47,56]

Postinfectious and infectious diseases are the most common causes of bronchiectasis. The incidence of infection-related bronchiectasis has declined with the introduction of mass vaccination and antibiotics. Measles, pertussis, adenovirus, tuberculosis, and *Mycobacterium avium-intracellulare* are important pathogens.[56] *Mycobacterium avium-intracellulare* causes a syndrome of chronic bronchitis in immunocompetent, nonsmoking, elderly women.[51,57] This disease is characterized by productive cough, night sweats, low-grade fever, malaise, weight loss, and airflow limitation. The chest radiograph can be rather unimpressive. HRCT demonstrates nodular bronchiectasis, with predominant involvement of the middle lobe and lingula (Figures 14 and 15). Treatment with rifabutin, ethambutol, and clarithromycin is successful in most patients.[57]

In adults, common variable hypogammaglobulinemia is an important cause of bronchiectasis. Immunoglobulin (Ig)A, IgM, IgG, and IgG subclass deficiencies have been associated with the development of bronchiectasis.[50,51]

Allergic bronchopulmonary aspergillosis usually presents with upper lobe and central (proximal) bronchiectasis and a clinical picture of chronic refractory asthma (Figure 16). It is characterized by intermittent wheezing, fever, cough, peripheral eosinophilia, transient pulmonary infiltrates, and bronchial plug expectoration. Patients usually have elevated IgE levels, *Aspergillus* serum precipitins, and immediate hypersensitivity to *Aspergillus* antigens by skin testing. Treatment consists of environmental control, oral corticosteroids, and, in some cases, antifungal therapy.[58,59]

Table 3 Conditions and Disorders Associated with Bronchiectasis

Severe inflammation
  Infection
    Mycobacterium (tuberculosis, MAI)
    Bacterial (*Staphylococcus aureus, Pseudomonas, Bordetella pertussis*)
    Viral (measles, influenza, rubeola, adenovirus, HIV)
    Fungal (histoplasmosis, coccidiomycosis)
  Hypersensitivity
    Allergic bronchopulmonary aspergillosis
  Inhalational injury
    Smoke
    Sulfur dioxide
    Ammonia
  Other
    Gastric aspiration
    Diffuse panbronchiolitis
	Airway obstruction
	  Foreign body
	  Bronchial stricture
	  Bronchial tumor
	
	Bronchial nodule
	  Sarcoidosis
	  Amyloidosis
	  Broncholithiasis
	Extrinsic bronchial compression
	  Mediastinal mass or lymph node
	  Lung cancer
	  Vascular aneurysm
	  Mediastinal fibrosis

Autoimmune disorders
  Relapsing polychondritis
  Behçet syndrome
  Sjögren syndrome
  Rheumatoid arthritis
  Ulcerative colitis
	Immunodeficiency
	  Hypogammaglobulinemia
	  Caused by cancer (chronic lymphocytic leukemia)
	    or chemotherapy
	Traction
	  Pulmonary fibrosis
	  Radiation
	  Sarcoidosis

Congenital syndromes
  Cystic fibrosis
  α_1-Antitrypsin
  Primary ciliary dyskinesia
    Kartagener syndrome (situs inversus, sinusitis, bronchiectasis)
  Chronic granulomatous disease
  Young syndrome (azoospermia and sinopulmonary syndrome)
  Yellow nail syndrome (lymphedema and pleural effusions)
	Anatomic malformations or variants
	  Bronchomalacia
	  Williams-Campbell syndrome (cartilage deficiency)
	  Mounier-Kuhn syndrome (tracheobronchomegaly)
	  Swyer-James syndrome
	  Right middle lobe syndrome
	  Pulmonary sequestration

Adapted with permission from Mysliwiec V and Pina JS[47] and Schwartz MN.[54]
HIV = human immunodeficiency virus; MAI = *Myobacterium avium-intracellulare*

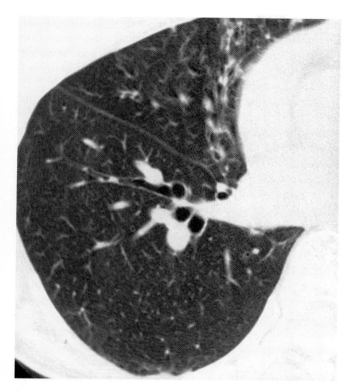

FIGURE 14. Middle lobe bronchiectasis in a woman with *Mycobacterium avium-intracellulare* infection.

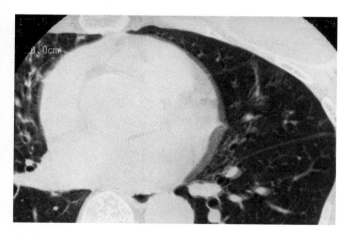

FIGURE 15. Computed tomographic scan showing lingular bronchiectasis in a woman with *Mycobacterium avium-intracellulare* infection (same patient as shown in Figure 14).

Yellow nail syndrome is a rare syndrome characterized by bronchiectasis, slow-growing yellow nails, lymphedema, and chylothorax associated with hypoplasia of the lymphatic system.[60,61]

Primary ciliary dyskinesia and Kartagener syndrome are congenital abnormalities characterized by defective ciliary

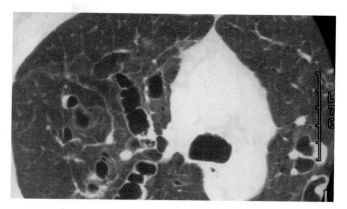

FIGURE 16. Computed tomographic scan demonstrating central bronchiectasis in a patient with allergic bronchopulmonary aspergillosis.

function owing to deficiencies in the components of the microtubular system. *DNAH5*, a gene located in chromosome 5p15-p14, encodes for the heavy chain of the dyenin arm and is associated with primary ciliary diskinesia.[51] Patients with these syndromes experience chronic rhinosinusitis, otitis, bronchiectasis (30%), sterility, olfactory defects, and corneal malformations. The diagnosis requires electron microscopic examination of a sinus or bronchial mucosal biopsy specimen. Kartagener syndrome accounts for 50% of the primary ciliary dyskinesia syndromes and is an autosomal recessive trait characterized by the clinical triad of sinusitis, situs inversus, and bronchiectasis (Figures 17 and 18).[51,56]

Young syndrome mimics the primary ciliary dyskinesia syndromes, except for the absence of microtubular abnormalities. It is characterized by the presence of obstructive azoospermia, chronic sinusitis, and bronchiectasis (seen in 30 to 70% of cases). The pulmonary presentation is as a mild form of bronchiectasis, with cough, sputum, and airflow limitation. It can be differentiated from cystic fibrosis (CF) by normal pancreatic function, normal sweat chloride levels, and the absence of a family history.[56] Young syndrome may be a milder clinical phenotype of CF presenting with normal sweat chloride and pancreatic function. Mutations in the CF *CFTR* gene, such as the Q1291H mutation, have been identified in patients with Young syndrome.[62,63]

CLINICAL AND RADIOGRAPHIC PRESENTATION

Despite the variety of disorders predisposing individuals to bronchiectasis, their clinical and radiographic presentations are similar. In the past, bronchiectasis was primarily a sequela of severe viral, mycobacterial, or bacterial infection. It was characterized by severe bronchorrhea, hemoptysis, respiratory failure, and death. Since the advent of immunization and antibiotics, bronchiectasis now occurs with a more subtle clinical presentation and is often confused with chronic bronchitis or COPD. Symptoms include chronic

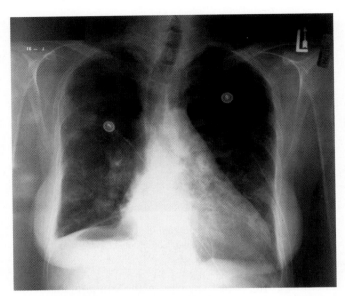

FIGURE 17. Radiograph from a patient with Kartagener syndrome (primary ciliary dyskinesia), demonstrating partial situs inversus (note the stomach gas pattern under the right diaphragm) and diffuse bronchiectasis.

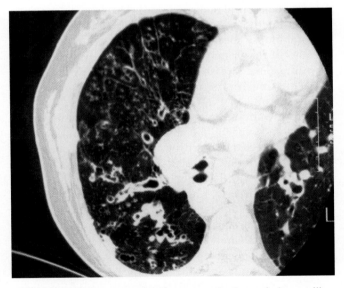

FIGURE 18. A patient with Kartagener syndrome (primary ciliary dyskinesia) shows diffuse bronchiectasis.

cough and sputum production that are usually worse in the morning or after the patient assumes a supine position. Daily sputum production of as much as 600 cc has been quantified. A dry cough with intermittent exacerbations suggests "dry" bronchiectasis. As exacerbations increase, fever, dyspnea, wheezing, chest pain, hemoptysis, anorexia, and weight loss develop. The evaluation of bronchiectasis should include a full history with a focus on childhood illnesses and any previous history of pneumonia. Careful

investigation for sinus disease and infertility is also important. Physical examination can reveal inspiratory coarse or "moist" crackles, rhonchi, and airway "popping" noises. Clubbing is seen in 3% of cases. Cor pulmonale is rare and accompanies advanced bronchiectasis.[51,52,54,56]

One reason bronchiectasis is confused with COPD is that 50% of patients lack chest radiographic abnormalities.[47,51,64] Radiographic findings that suggest bronchiectasis include thickening of the bronchial walls, volume loss at the lung bases, and parallel lines ("tram tracks") that correlate with bronchial wall thickening and dilatation. Severe bronchiectasis can present with cystic or "ring" shadows and/or dilated bronchi with mucous plugging ("gloved finger" sign).

DIAGNOSIS

The diagnosis of bronchiectasis has improved with the use of HRCT. This technique allows for 1 to 1.5 mm sections every 10 mm from the apex to the base of the lung and has made previous diagnostic technology obsolete. It is very sensitive for diagnosing early bronchiectasis and even for suggesting a specific underlying disease.[48,51,65] Widespread bronchiectasis with symmetric upper lobe predominance is associated with CF. Unilateral mild upper lobe involvement is seen with tuberculosis. Central bronchiectasis characterizes allergic bronchopulmonary aspergillosis. Hypogammaglobulinemia and immotile cilia syndrome typically involve the middle lobe.[63] *Mycobacterium avium-intracellulare*–associated bronchiectasis is characterized by nodular bronchiectasis of the middle lobe and lingula.[51,57]

Pulmonary function tests usually reveal airflow limitation and air trapping.[66] In 40% of patients, a bronchodilator response with greater than 15% increase in forced expiratory volume in 1 second (FEV$_1$) is observed.[51,54] Bronchoscopy is performed when an obstructive cause is suspected in cases of focal bronchiectasis. Depending on the clinical suspicion, measurement of sweat chloride, immunoglobulins, IgE, α_1-antitrypsin levels, and *Aspergillus* precipitins and skin testing are indicated.[51,54] Mucosal biopsy for ciliary abnormalities may also be indicated.[56]

TREATMENT

Treatment should focus on the predisposing condition. Adequate bronchial hygiene and secretion clearance can be achieved with chest percussion, postural drainage, mucolytics, and bronchodilators. Recent studies suggest that inhaled steroids reduce sputum production and improve FEV$_1$.[51,54] Acute exacerbations of bronchiectasis require specific antibiotic therapy directed to the predominant organism isolated in sputum. Empiric therapy with ampicillin, amoxicillin, doxycycline, trimethoprim-sulfamethoxazole, or amoxicillin-clavulanate is usually adequate for mild bronchiectasis. Severe bronchiectasis with suspected *Pseudomonas aeruginosa* requires double antipseudomonal coverage. Inhaled tobramycin or gentamycin may be used to treat exacerbations.[54] In cases of bronchiectasis with frequent exacerbations, chronic rotating antibiotic therapy is used. Surgery is reserved for localized bronchiectasis refractory to therapy or for patients with recurrent hemoptysis.[49,56,67]

Cystic Fibrosis

CF is the most prevalent lethal genetic disorder in the United States. It primarily affects Caucasians, with an incidence of 1 in 2,500 live births. CF is an autosomal recessive disorder, and 1 in 25 Caucasians in the United States are asymptomatic carriers of the disease. The disease is also seen in African Americans, with a much lower incidence of 1 in 17,000 births.[68–70] The CF gene has been mapped to chromosome 7. The gene product is the cystic fibrosis transmembrane conductance regulator (CFTR), a protein essential to chloride epithelial transport.[70] The most common genetic mutation, seen in approximately 70% of patients, is the deletion of three base pairs at codon 508 (F508) coding for phenylalanine. The defect in airway chloride transport is associated with increased sodium absorption with desiccation of mucus, bronchial obliteration, infection, and bronchiectasis.[70,71]

CF is characterized by the development of chronic airflow obstruction, bronchiectasis, recurrent pulmonary infections, pancreatic insufficiency, diabetes, and dysfunction of the liver and the gastrointestinal and reproductive systems.[70,72] Diagnosis involves recognition of characteristic clinical features, determination of an elevated sweat chloride level (>60 mEq/L), detection of a CFTR gene mutation by polymerase chain reaction (PCR), and measurement of abnormal nasal epithelial electrolyte ion transport.[72,73]

CF is usually diagnosed in early childhood (95% of patients are diagnosed by the age of 8 years) and is therefore treated by pediatricians and pediatric pulmonologists.[70,73,74] Recent developments in the treatment of CF have increased the mean life span of CF patients to 30 years of age.[72] Therefore, an increasing number of adult CF patients are currently under the care of internists and adult pulmonary specialists.[75,76]

Increasing attention is now given to reports of adults with milder forms of CF that elude diagnosis until adulthood.[45,70,74] These older patients present with a clinical picture that suggests chronic asthma, chronic bronchitis, bronchiectasis, or nontuberculous mycobacterial infection.[77] The diagnosis is elusive since these patients may present with subtle clinical findings or may have borderline or normal sweat chloride values.[78] The diagnosis of CF in adults is usually suspected when diffuse bronchiectasis is detected by HRCT or a mucoid Pseudomonas strain is isolated in a routine sputum culture.[74] Older CF patients have less pancreatic insufficiency, milder lung disease, atypical mutations of the CFTR gene, and an improved clinical course.[70,79] The current explanation for the late appearance of CF is the presence of residual chloride airway secretion and protection by other genetic and environmental influences.[77,80] A recent study by Ziedalski and colleagues reported a 20% incidence of CFTR mutations or an abnormal sweat chloride concentration in adult patients referred for evaluation of bronchiectasis and/or nontuberculous mycobacterial infection.[77] This finding suggests that mutations of the CFTR gene may lead to a wide spectrum of diseases from mild bronchiectasis to the extreme presentation of "classic" CF.

Over 90% of deaths from "classic" CF are due to lung disease. CF is characterized by a progressive deterioration in lung function and an increase in the frequency of acute exacerbations. The deterioration of lung function is associated with early colonization with Staphylococcus aureus and Haemophilus influenzae and later with mucoid and nonmucoid strains of Pseudomonas.[71,73]

Pulmonary function tests demonstrate a predominant obstructive pattern with decreased expiratory flows and air trapping (increased residual volume to total lung capacity ratio).[81] The diffusion capacity for carbon monoxide (DL_{CO}), a marker of pulmonary alveolocapillary surface area, is usually preserved until late in the disease.[75] Radiographs in CF patients may be normal at initial presentation but later demonstrate hyperinflation, lobar collapse, peribronchial "cuffing," and progressive bronchiectasis. In adult CF, chest radiography demonstrates features of bronchiectasis, such as "tram tracks," ring shadows, nodular opacities, and cysts with air-fluid levels. HRCT is very sensitive for the detection of bronchial wall thickening and cylindrical, varicose, and cystic bronchiectasis.[69]

The diagnosis of CF in adults should be suspected in cases of unexplained diffuse bronchiectasis, recurrent pulmonary infections, atypical nontuberculous mycobaterial infection, or unexplained COPD. PCR analysis for CFTR mutations may be necessary in patients with normal or borderline sweat chloride values.[71,74,80,82] The treatment of CF patients requires referral to a center of specialized care focusing on pulmonary, gastrointestinal, mineral metabolism, and dietary issues. Treatment is geared to the clearance and lysis of mucous secretions,[83] bronchodilatation, antibiotics, anti-inflammatory therapy (corticosteroids and nonsteroidal anti-inflammatory drugs), and the management of secondary complications such as hypoxemia, hemoptysis, and pneumothorax.[70–72] A recent study demonstrated the effectiveness of nebulized hypertonic 7% saline in aiding mucus clearance and improving FEV_1 and forced vital capacity (FVC).[84]

Sarcoidosis

Sarcoidosis is a common disorder that is usually associated with mediastinal or hilar lymphadenopathy and pulmonary parenchymal nodular or interstitial disease. Although sarcoidosis is considered an interstitial lung disease, 4 to 67% of patients demonstrate airflow obstruction during pulmonary function testing.[85–87] The anatomic site of airflow obstruction in sarcoidosis appears to be the small (peripheral) airways (see Chapter 13). Approximately 2 to 26% of patients with sarcoidosis present with chronic airflow limitation owing to granulomatous inflammation and nodules of the large

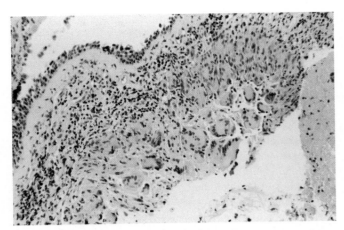

FIGURE 19. Photomicrograph of an endobronchial biopsy confirming granulomatous inflammation (sarcoidosis) involving the large (central) airways in a patient with cough and chronic airflow limitation.

(central) airways and bronchostenosis (Figure 19).[86,88–91] Of note, endobronchial sarcoid may be present in the absence of pulmonary parenchymal involvement.[92]

Patients with bronchostenosis of the large (central) airways owing to sarcoidosis present with cough, focal wheezing, and stridor. Pulmonary function tests reveal moderate to severe airflow limitation. Bronchoscopy usually reveals multiple sites of segmental narrowing.[91] Balloon dilatation of the stenotic airways is occasionally successful.[93,94] Early treatment with corticosteroids or methotrexate may prevent progression to fixed bronchostenosis.[88]

Relapsing Polychondritis

RP presents with airflow limitation in the large (central) airway. Originally described by Jaksch-Watenhorst in 1923,[95] RP is an unusual disease (approximately 600 cases have been reported). It is characterized by severe "relapsing" inflammation and destruction of cartilage and proteoglycan-rich tissues.[96] RP involves the external ear, vestibular system, eyes, nose, large joints, aortic root, chest wall, larynx, and major airways. The clinical presentation can mimic that of either rheumatoid arthritis or Wegener granulomatosis.[97] An autoimmune etiology for RP is suspected on the basis of its frequent association with other connective tissue diseases and immunohistochemical demonstration of immunoglobulin and complement deposition in cartilage. Serum antibodies to type II collagen are present in up to 20% of patients.[97–99] Recent reports suggest a primary T-helper-1-mediated immune response in RP as evident by high levels of interferon-γ, interleukin (IL)-12, and IL-2.[100]

Respiratory tract involvement is the presenting manifestation in up to 66% of patients, and such involvement portends a poor prognosis.[96,101] The leading cause of death in RP patients is involvement of the respiratory system, causing recurrent pneumonias and respiratory failure owing to loss of airway stability. The central airways (glottis, trachea, and mainstem bronchi) are preferentially involved. Women are predominantly affected. These patients present with hoarseness, cough, pain over the anterior trachea, dyspnea, hemoptysis, wheezing, and (sometimes) respiratory distress requiring intubation or emergent tracheostomy.[96,98,101] As reported by Tillie-Leblond and colleagues, pulmonary function tests reveal moderate to severe airflow limitation, with reduced FEV_1 to FVC ratios.[96] Some patients may present with primary tracheal involvement with either a variable extrathoracic or fixed intrathoracic airflow obstruction by flow-volume loops. All patients had normal DL_{CO}, suggesting the preservation of lung parenchyma.[95,98]

Bronchoscopic examination of patients with airway obstruction reveals laryngeal and upper tracheal involvement. Rarely, patients present with isolated mainstem bronchi involvement. The airways show inflammation, dynamic collapse, and stenosis. Imaging with multirow detector chest CT scans allows for airway reconstruction that provide a clear determination of the severity of airway involvement.[96,98]

Bronchoscopy-directed biopsy of the RP lesion is usually nondiagnostic unless deep cartilage is sampled. Since there is no reliable serologic test for RP, the diagnosis is usually delayed an average of 2 to 3 years from the onset of symptoms. Patients may present with an elevated sedimentation rate, anemia, leukocytosis, eosinophilia, and hypergammaglobulinemia.[97] The clinical criteria for diagnosing RP include (1) bilateral auricular cartilage involvement, (2) nonerosive polyarthritis, (3) nasal cartilage chondritis, (4) eye inflammation (episcleritis, scleritis), (5) airway involvement, and (6) cochlear or vestibular involvement.[102] A diagnosis of RP is made (a) when three or more of these clinical features are present or (b) when two or more sites are involved and the response to corticosteroids or analysis of biopsy specimens demonstrates chondritis at one or more sites.[98]

The treatment of airway involvement with RP requires a multidisciplinary approach. For acute exacerbations of laryngeal or airways disease, high-dose prednisone at 0.75 to 1 mg/kg/d is recommended. Steroids should be tapered slowly, with maintenance therapy continued during remissions. Cytotoxic therapy with azathioprine, cyclophosphamide, dapsone, penicillamine, and cyclosporine has been reported. Oral methotrexate at a dose of 17.5 mg/wk remains an important steroid-sparing therapy.[97] Infliximab, a monoclonal antibody against tumor necrosis factor-α, has achieved disease remission in cases of refractory RP.[103] Tracheostomy is necessary in cases with upper airway compromise. Surgical resection, airway stenting (with a Montgomery tube or collapsible silicone or metallic stents), and balloon dilatation have been successful for severe tracheobronchostenosis.[98] Aggressive treatment in patients with airway strictures has led to an improved survival rate of 94% at 8 years.[97,104]

Summary

This chapter reviewed other diseases of the large (central) airways that are often misdiagnosed as COPD. The patients may be smokers or ex-smokers, with dyspnea, cough, sputum production, and wheezing consistent with either emphysema or chronic bronchitis. The clinician may find the results of physical examination, chest radiography, and pulmonary function tests to be compatible with a diagnosis of COPD. Correct diagnosis and treatment of these less common large (central) airways diseases may thus be delayed.[3] Therefore, it is imperative to have a measure of healthy skepticism when examining a patient with airflow obstruction that does not fit the usual COPD pattern or fails to respond to therapy as expected.

The clinician should suspect one of these other obstructive pulmonary diseases when dealing with a patient with chronic airflow obstruction and the following conditions:

- Little or no smoking history (< 20 packs per year)[1,3]
- Onset of disease before the fourth decade or after the seventh decade of life
- Rapid fall in FEV_1 (>75 cc/yr)[1,3,105]
- Presence of connective tissue disease[106]
- Exposure to occupational or environmental factors[107]
- Unexplained systemic illness
- Multisystem organ dysfunction

References

1. GOLD Executive Committee. Global strategy for the diagnosis, management, and prevention of chronic obstructive pulmonary disease. Available at: http://www.goldcopd.com. (Accessed February 17, 2008.)
2. Pauwels RA, Buist AS, Calverley PMA, et al. Global strategy for the diagnosis, management, and prevention of chronic obstructive pulmonary disease. NHLBI/WHO Global Initiative for Chronic Obstructive Lung Disease (GOLD) workshop summary. Am J Respir Crit Care Med 2001;163:1256–76.
3. St John RC, Gadek JE, Pacht ER. Chronic obstructive disease: less common causes—an algorithm for the primary care physician. J Gen Intern Med 1993;8:564–72.
4. Murin S, Bilello KS, Matthay R. Other smoking-affected pulmonary diseases. Clin Chest Med 2000;21:121–37, ix.
5. Murray JF. Ventilation. In: Murray JF, editor. The normal lung. 2nd ed. Philadelphia: W.B. Saunders; 1986. p. 83–119.
6. Gamsu G, Webb WR. Computed tomography of the trachea and mainstem bronchi. Semin Roentgenol 1983;18:51–60.
7. Aboussouan LS, Stoller JK. Diagnosis and management of upper airway obstruction. Clin Chest Med 1994;15:35–53.
8. Braman SS, Gaiser HA. Upper airway obstruction. In: Fishman AP, editor. Pulmonary diseases and disorders. 3rd ed. New York: McGraw-Hill; 1998. p. 783–801.
9. Christopher KL, Wood RP 2nd, Eckert RC, et al. Vocal-cord dysfunction presenting as asthma. N Engl J Med 1983;308:1566–70.
10. Tilles SA, Nelson HS. Differential diagnosis of adult asthma. Med Clin North Am 2006;90:61–76.
11. Newman KB, Mason UG 3rd, Schmaling KB. Clinical features of vocal cord dysfunction. Am J Respir Crit Care Med 1995;152(4 Pt 1):1382–6.
12. Guss JMD, Mirza NMD. Methacholine challenge testing in the diagnosis of paradoxical vocal fold motion. Laryngoscope 2006;116:1558–61.
13. Perkins PJ, Morris MJ. Vocal cord dysfunction induced by methacholine challenge testing. Chest 2002;122:1988–93.
14. Bahrainwala AH, Simon MR. Wheezing and vocal cord dysfunction mimicking asthma. Curr Opin Pulm Med 2001;7:8–13.
15. Koitschev A, Simon C, Blumenstock G, et al. Suprastomal tracheal stenosis after dilational and surgical tracheostomy in critically ill patients. Anaesthesia 2006;61:832–7.
16. Hoppe H, Dinkel HP, Walder B, et al. Grading airway stenosis down to the segmental level using virtual bronchoscopy. Chest 2004;125:704–11.
17. Mehta AC, Harris RJ, De Boer GE. Endoscopic management of benign airway stenosis. Clin Chest Med 1995;16:401–13.
18. Rafanan AL, Mehta AC. Stenting of the tracheobronchial tree. Radiol Clin North Am 2000;38:395–408.
19. Maish M, Vaporciyan AA. Chondrosarcoma arising in the trachea: a case report and review of the literature. J Thorac Cardiovasc Surg 2003;126:2077–80.
20. Wilks, S. Ossific deposits on the larynx, trachea, and bronchi. Trans Pathol Soc Land 1857;8: 88.
21. Meyer CN, Dossing M, Broholm H. Tracheobronchopathia osteochondroplastica. Respir Med 1997;91:499–502.
22. Leske V, Lazor R, Coetmeur D, et al. Tracheobronchopathia osteochondroplastica: a study of 41 patients. Medicine (Baltimore) 2001;80:378–90.
23. Akyol MU, Martin AA, Dhurandhar N, Miller RH. Tracheobronchopathia osteochondroplastica: a case report and a review of the literature. Ear Nose Throat J 1993;72:347–50.
24. Mariotta S, Pallone G, Pedicelli G, Bisetti A. Spiral CT and endoscopic findings in a case of tracheobronchopathia osteochondroplastica. J Comput Assist Tomogr 1997;21:418–20.
25. Spencer H. Pathology of the Lung. Volume 2, 3rd. ed. Oxford: Pergamon Press, 1977. p. 688.
26. Lundgren R, Stjernberg NL. Tracheobronchopathia osteochondroplastica. A clinical bronchoscopic and spirometric study. Chest 1981;80:706–9.
27. Tukiainen H, Torkko M, Terho EO. Lung function in patients with tracheobronchopathia osteochondroplastica. Eur Respir J 1988;1:632–5.
28. O'Regan A, Fenlon HM, Beamis JF Jr, et al. Tracheobronchial amyloidosis. The Boston University experience from 1984 to 1999. Medicine (Baltimore) 2000;79:69–79.
29. Toyoda M, Ebihara Y, Kato H, Kita S. Tracheobronchial AL amyloidosis: histologic, immunohistochemical, ultrastructural, and immunoelectron microscopic observations. Hum Pathol 1993;24:970–6.
30. Monroe AT, Walia R, Zlotecki RA, Jantz MA. Tracheobronchial amyloidosis: a case report of successful treatment with external beam radiation therapy. Chest 2004;125:784–9.
31. Utz JP, Swensen SJ, Gertz MA. Pulmonary amyloidosis. The Mayo Clinic experience from 1980 to 1993. Ann Intern Med 1996;124:407–13.

32. Kurrus JA, Hayes JK, Hoidal JR, et al. Radiation therapy for tracheobronchial amyloidosis. Chest 1998;114:1489–92.

33. Cordier JF, Loire R, Brune J. Amyloidosis of the lower respiratory tract. Clinical and pathologic features in a series of 21 patients. Chest 1986;90:827–31.

34. Rubinow A, Celli BR, Cohen AS, et al. Localized amyloidosis of the lower respiratory tract. Am Rev Respir Dis 1978;118:603–11.

35. Woodring JH, Howard RS 2nd, Rehm SR. Congenital tracheobronchomegaly (Mounier-Kuhn syndrome): a report of 10 cases and review of the literature. J Thorac Imaging 1991;6(2):1–10.

36. Johnston RF, Green RA. Tracheobronchiomegaly. Report of five cases and demonstration of familial occurrence. Am Rev Respir Dis 1965;91:35–50.

37. Feist JH, Johnson TH, Wilson RJ. Acquired tracheomalacia: etiology and differential diagnosis. Chest 1975;68:340–5.

38. Shah SS, Karnak D, Mason D, et al. Pulmonary transplantation in Mounier-Kuhn syndrome: a case report. J Thorac Cardiovasc Surg 2006;131:757–8.

39. Shin MS, Jackson RM, Ho KJ. Tracheobronchomegaly (Mounier-Kuhn syndrome): CT diagnosis. AJR Am J Roentgenol 1988;150:777–9.

40. Kanter RK, Pollack MM, Wright WW, Grundfast KM. Treatment of severe tracheobronchomalacia with continuous positive airway pressure (CPAP). Anesthesiology 1982;57:54–6.

41. Minai OA, Mehta AC, Pettersson G, Demet K. Lung transplantation in a patient with Mounier-Kuhn syndrome. J Thorac Cardiovasc Surg 2006;132:737–8.

42. Shah H, Garbe L, Nussbaum E, et al. Benign tumors of the tracheobronchial tree. Endoscopic characteristics and role of laser resection. Chest 1995;107:1744–51.

43. Keller SM, Katariya K. Primary lung tumors other than bronchogenic carcinoma: benign and malignant. In: Fishman AP, editor. Pulmonary diseases and disorders. 3rd ed. New York: McGraw-Hill; 1998. p. 1833–40.

44. Smith LS, Schillaci RF, Sarlin RF. Endobronchial tuberculosis. Serial fiberoptic bronchoscopy and natural history. Chest 1987;91:644–7.

45. Van den Brande PM, Van de Mierop F, Verbeken EK, Demedts M. Clinical spectrum of endobronchial tuberculosis in elderly patients. Arch Intern Med 1990;150:2105–8.

46. Satoh S, Mori M, Inoue Y. Expandable metallic stents applied to benign bronchostenosis. Chest 1993;103:1302–3.

47. Hansell DM. Bronchiectasis. Radiol Clin North Am 1998;36:107–28.

48. Westcott JL. Bronchiectasis. Radiol Clin North Am 1991;29:1031–42.

49. Mysliwiec V, Pina JS. Bronchiectasis: the 'other' obstructive lung disease. Postgrad Med 1999;106:123–6, 128–31.

50. Barker AF, Bardana EJ Jr. Bronchiectasis: update of an orphan disease. Am Rev Respir Dis 1988;137:969–78.

51. Barker AF. Bronchiectasis. N Engl J Med 2002;346:1383–93.

52. King PT, Holdsworth SR, Freezer NJ, et al. Characterisation of the onset and presenting clinical features of adult bronchiectasis. Respir Med 2006;100:2183–9.

53. Kang EY, Miller RR, Muller NL. Bronchiectasis: comparison of preoperative thin-section CT and pathologic findings in resected specimens. Radiology 1995;195:649–54.

54. King P, Holdsworth S, Freezer N, Holmes P. Bronchiectasis. Intern Med J 2006;36:729–37.

55. Reid LM. Reduction in bronchial subdivision in bronchiectasis. Thorax 1950;5:233–47.

56. Schwartz MN. Bronchiectasis. In: Fishman AP, editor. Pulmonary diseases and disorders. 3rd ed. New York: McGraw-Hill; 1998. p. 2045–70.

57. Griffith DE, Aksamit T, Brown-Elliott BA, et al. An official ATS/IDSA statement: diagnosis, treatment, and prevention of nontuberculous mycobacterial diseases. Am J Respir Crit Care Med 2007;175:367–416.

58. Virnig C, Bush RK. Allergic bronchopulmonary aspergillosis: a US perspective. Curr Opin Pulm Med 2007;13:67–71.

59. Greenberger PA. Allergic bronchopulmonary aspergillosis, allergic fungal sinusitis, and hypersensitivity pneumonitis. Clin Allergy Immunol 2002;16:449–68.

60. Hiller E, Rosenow EC 3rd, Olsen AM. Pulmonary manifestations of the yellow nail syndrome. Chest 1972;61:452–8.

61. Alkadhi H, Wildermuth S, Russi EW, Boehm T. Yellow nail syndrome. Respiration 2005;72:197.

62. Wellesley D, Schwarz M. Cystic fibrosis, Young's syndrome, and normal sweat chloride. Lancet 1998;352(9121):38.

63. Hirsh A, Williams C, Williamson B. Young's syndrome and cystic fibrosis mutation delta F508. Lancet 1993;342(8863):118.

64. Currie DC, Cooke JC, Morgan AD, et al. Interpretation of bronchograms and chest radiographs in patients with chronic sputum production. Thorax 1987;42:278–84.

65. Cartier Y, Kavanagh PV, Johkoh T, et al. Bronchiectasis: accuracy of high-resolution CT in the differentiation of specific diseases. AJR Am J Roentgenol 1999;173:47–52.

66. Nicotra MB, Rivera M, Dale AM, et al. Clinical, pathophysiologic, and microbiologic characterization of bronchiectasis in an aging cohort. Chest 1995;108:955–61.

67. Marwah OS, Sharma OP. Bronchiectasis. How to identify, treat, and prevent. Postgrad Med 1995;97:149–50, 153–6, 159.

68. Bye MR, Ewig JM, Quittell LM. Cystic fibrosis. Lung 1994;172:251–70.

69. Ruzal-Shapiro C. Cystic fibrosis. An overview. Radiol Clin North Am 1998;36:143–61.

70. Accurso FJ. Update in cystic fibrosis 2005. Am J Respir Crit Care Med 2006;173:944–7.

71. Davis PB, Drumm M, Konstan MW. Cystic fibrosis. Am J Respir Crit Care Med 1996;154:1229–56.

72. Davis PB. Cystic fibrosis since 1938. Am J Respir Crit Care Med 2006;173:475–82.

73. Rosenstein BJ, Cutting GR. The diagnosis of cystic fibrosis: a consensus statement. Cystic Fibrosis Foundation Consensus Panel. J Pediatr 1998;132:589–95.

74. Rosenbluth D, Goodenberger D. Cystic fibrosis in an elderly woman. Chest 1997;112:1124–6.

75. di Sant'agnese PA, Davis PB. Cystic fibrosis in adults. 75 cases and a review of 232 cases in the literature. Am J Med 1979;66:121–32.

76. Shwachman H, Kowalski M, Khaw KT. Cystic fibrosis: a new outlook. 70 patients above 25 years of age. Medicine (Baltimore) 1977;56:129–49.

77. Ziedalski TM, Kao PN, Henig NR, et al. Prospective analysis of cystic fibrosis transmembrane regulator mutations in adults with bronchiectasis or pulmonary nontuberculous mycobacterial infection. Chest 2006;130:995–1002.

78. Stewart B, Zabner J, Shuber AP, et al. Normal sweat chloride values do not exclude the diagnosis of cystic fibrosis. Am J Respir Crit Care Med 1995;151(3 Pt 1):899–903.

79. Gan KH, Geus WP, Bakker W, et al. Genetic and clinical features of patients with cystic fibrosis diagnosed after the age of 16 years. Thorax 1995;50:1301–4.

80. Thomas SR, Jaffe A, Geddes DM, et al. Pulmonary disease severity in men with deltaF508 cystic fibrosis and residual chloride secretion. Lancet 1999;353(9157):984–5.

81. Schluchter MD, Konstan MW, Drumm ML, et al. Classifying severity of cystic fibrosis lung disease using longitudinal pulmonary function data. Am J Respir Crit Care Med 2006;174:780–6.

82. Augarten A, Kerem BS, Yahav Y, et al. Mild cystic fibrosis and normal or borderline sweat test in patients with the 3849 + 10 kb C->T mutation. Lancet 1993;342(8862):25–6.

83. Kendrick AH. Airway clearance techniques in cystic fibrosis. Eur Respir J 2006;27:1082–3.

84. Donaldson SH, Bennett WD, Zeman KL, et al. Mucus clearance and lung function in cystic fibrosis with hypertonic saline. N Engl J Med 2006;354:241–50.

85. Newman LS, Rose CS, Maier LA. Sarcoidosis. N Engl J Med 1997;336:1224–34.

86. Harrison BD, Shaylor JM, Stokes TC, Wilkes AR. Airflow limitation in sarcoidosis—a study of pulmonary function in 107 patients with newly diagnosed disease. Respir Med 1991;85:59–64.

87. Handa T, Nagai S, Fushimi Y, et al. Clinical and radiographic indices associated with airflow limitation in patients with sarcoidosis. Chest 2006;130:1851–6.

88. Chambellan A, Turbie P, Nunes H, et al. Endoluminal stenosis of proximal bronchi in sarcoidosis: bronchoscopy, function, and evolution. Chest 2005;127:472–81.

89. Udwadia ZF, Pilling JR, Jenkins PF, Harrison BD. Bronchoscopic and bronchographic findings in 12 patients with sarcoidosis and severe or progressive airways obstruction. Thorax 1990;45:272–5.

90. Armstrong JR, Radke JR, Kvale PA, et al. Endoscopic findings in sarcoidosis. Characteristics and correlations with radiographic staging and bronchial mucosal biopsy yield. Ann Otol Rhinol Laryngol 1981;90(4 Pt 1):339–43.

91. Stjernberg N, Thunell M. Pulmonary function in patients with endobronchial sarcoidosis. Acta Med Scand 1984;215:121–6.

92. Sheffield EA. Pathology of sarcoidosis. Clin Chest Med 1997;18:741–54.

93. Brown KT, Yeoh CB, Saddekni S. Balloon dilatation of the left main bronchus in sarcoidosis. AJR Am J Roentgenol 1988;150:553–4.

94. Fouty BW, Pomeranz M, Thigpen TP, Martin RJ. Dilatation of bronchial stenoses due to sarcoidosis using a flexible fiberoptic bronchoscope. Chest 1994;106:677–80.

95. Jaksch-Watenhorst R. Polychondropathia. Wien Arch Inn Med 1923;6:93–100.

96. Tillie-Leblond I, Wallaert B, Leblond D, et al. Respiratory involvement in relapsing polychondritis. Clinical, functional, endoscopic, and radiographic evaluations. Medicine (Baltimore) 1998;77:168–76.

97. Trentham DE, Le CH. Relapsing polychondritis. Ann Intern Med 1998;129:114–22.

98. Lee-Chiong TL Jr. Pulmonary manifestations of ankylosing spondylitis and relapsing polychondritis. Clin Chest Med 1998;19:747–7, ix.

99. Terato K, Shimozuru Y, Katayama K, et al. Specificity of antibodies to type II collagen in rheumatoid arthritis. Arthritis Rheum 1990;33:1493–500.

100. Kraus VB, Stabler T, Le ET, et al. Urinary type II collagen neoepitope as an outcome measure for relapsing polychondritis. Arthritis Rheum 2003;48:2942–8.

101. Eng J, Sabanathan S. Airway complications in relapsing polychondritis. Ann Thorac Surg 1991;51:686–92.

102. McAdam LP, O'Hanlan MA, Bluestone R, Pearson CM. Relapsing polychondritis: prospective study of 23 patients and a review of the literature. Medicine (Baltimore) 1976;55:193–215.

103. Mpofu S, Estrach C, Curtis J, Moots RJ. Treatment of respiratory complications in recalcitrant relapsing polychondritis with infliximab. Rheumatology (Oxford) 2003;42:1117–8.

104. Segel MJ, Godfrey S, Berkman N. Relapsing polychondritis: reversible airway obstruction is not always asthma. Mayo Clin Proc 2004;79:407–9.

105. Brandstetter RD, Kazemi H. Aging and the respiratory system. Med Clin North Am 1983;67:419–31.

106. Wells AU, du Bois RM. Bronchiolitis in association with connective tissue disorders. Clin Chest Med 1993;14:655–66.

107. Wright JL, Cagle P, Churg A, et al. Diseases of the small airways. Am Rev Respir Dis 1992;146:240–62.

CHAPTER 13

Diffuse Interstitial Lung Diseases Resulting in Airflow Limitation

Carlos E. Girod, MD, and Marvin I. Schwarz, MD

Interstitial lung diseases are considered to be restrictive lung diseases; however, there are those that also involve small airways, leading to airflow limitation. The term *small airways* refers to peripheral airways with a luminal diameter less than 3 mm.[1] These airways consist of small bronchi and bronchioles (≤2 mm in diameter).[2,3] The bronchioles are differentiated from bronchi by their lack of cartilaginous support. There are 8 to 14 branching airways before the lobular bronchioles, the small airways that feed the secondary pulmonary lobule (also known as the lobule of Miller). This lobule represents the smallest discrete unit of lung surrounded by interlobular septa. The lobular bronchiole then forms the acinus by dividing into various terminal bronchioles, which, in turn, branch into the respiratory bronchioles. The respiratory bronchiole divides into three subsequent generations that have increasing numbers of alveoli in their walls and that end in the alveolar ducts and alveolar sacs (Figure 1).[4]

The total cross-sectional areas of the membranous bronchioles and respiratory bronchioles are 53 cm^2 and 186 cm^2, respectively. This represents a larger surface area than that of the major bronchi. It was once thought that the small airways contributed little (10–20%) to the overall airway resistance; therefore, these airways were referred to as "silent airways."[3,5,6] This suggested that significant small airway destruction or narrowing had to occur before airflow limitation could be detected by conventional pulmonary function testing or became clinically significant. Current data suggest that the contribution of the small airways to airflow resistance is as high as 30 to 40%.[7–10] Therefore, it is now recognized that diseases that primarily affect the small airways can lead to significant airflow limitation with symptoms and signs consistent with chronic obstructive pulmonary disease (COPD).[3]

The study of the small (peripheral) airways was previously hampered by the lack of reproducible pulmonary function tests,[11] sensitive radiographic imaging, or adequate lung biopsy specimens. The introduction of high-resolution computed tomography (HRCT) of the chest has revolutionized the study of small airways diseases (see Figure 1).[3,9,12,13] Some of the abnormalities found by HRCT that correlate with histologic small airways disease are summarized in Table 1. Other abnormalities associated with bronchiolar obstruction include parenchymal cyst formation, secondary emphysema (airspace dilatation), and bronchiolectasis with luminal impaction

("tree-in-bud" pattern).[3] For unexplained cases of chronic airflow limitation, HRCT will not only suggest the presence of small airways disease but will also exclude bronchiectasis and emphysema.

Interstitial Lung Diseases Involving the Small (Peripheral) Airways

Several interstitial lung diseases involving the small airways present with the symptoms, signs, and physiology of chronic airflow obstruction (Table 2).

Sarcoidosis

Sarcoidosis is an interstitial lung disease with restrictive lung function. Nevertheless, up to 67% of patients present with

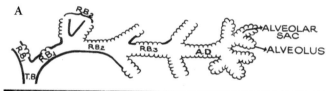

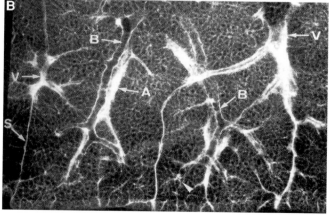

FIGURE 1. (*A*) Illustration of small airways leading to the acinar structure, the gas exchange unit of the lung. Reproduced with permission from Thurlbeck WM.[7] (*B*) High-resolution computed tomography of a resected lung specimen, demonstrating the anatomy of the secondary pulmonary lobule or lobule of Miller. The lobule is demarcated by the interlobular septa (S). The lobular bronchiole (B) and artery (A) feed the pulmonary lobule. Reproduced with permission from Itoh H, Murata K, Konishi J, et al. Diffuse lung disease: pathologic basis for the high-resolution computed tomography findings. J Thorac Imaging 1993;8:176–88.

Table 1 Histologic and Computed Tomographic Features and Correlations of Small-Airway Diseases that Present with Chronic Airflow Limitation

Histologic Feature	HRCT Correlation
Bronchiolar wall thickening and inflammation	Centrilobular nodules
Bronchiolar dilatation and luminal impaction	Branching centrilobular opacities or "tree-in-bud"
Partial or complete bronchiolar obstruction	Air trapping with "mosaic" pattern Parenchymal cysts Areas of low attenuation

Adapted from Worthy SA and Muller NL[13] and Chabat F, Yang G-Z, Hansell DM. Obstructive lung diseases: texture classification for differentiation at CT. Radiology 2003;228:871–7.

HRCT = high-resolution computed tomography.

airflow limitation owing to either a large airway lesion (leading to stenosis) or small airway inflammation (bronchiolitis).[14,15] In one study of sarcoidosis patients undergoing open lung biopsy, 57% demonstrated granulomatous inflammation of the small airways (Figure 2).[16] The mechanisms for bronchiolar obstruction in sarcoidosis include direct granulomatous inflammation of the bronchiolar wall, extrusion of granulomas into the bronchiolar lumen, and proximal extension of alveolar fibrosis, leading to concentric bronchiolar narrowing.[11,16] Clinical features that correlate with airflow obstruction include stage IV classification, older age, smoking history, and HRCT finding of bronchovascular bundle involvement.[14]

Rarely, patients with sarcoidosis present with chest radiographs, HRCT scans, and pulmonary function tests that suggest advanced emphysema. Zar and Cole reported a 39-year-old man with a brief smoking history of 9 pack-years and symptoms of COPD, along with a chest CT scan showing mediastinal adenopathy and changes consistent with emphysema.[17] Transbronchial biopsy specimens revealed noncaseating granulomas consistent with sarcoidosis. Judson and Strange reported on three patients (two smokers and one nonsmoker) with a diagnosis of bullous sarcoidosis with severe airflow limitation.[18] Sarcoidosis was suspected in all three after CT scans revealed mediastinal lymphadenopathy. Open lung or thoracoscopic lung biopsy specimens confirmed a diagnosis of sarcoidosis in all three patients. One patient required lung transplantation, and another improved with corticosteroid therapy. Although it is possible that these patients had both smoking-related emphysema and sarcoidosis, the pathology specimens revealed significant bronchiolar involvement, with granulomatous inflammation and fibrosis. Of interest, Keller and colleagues reported a 9% incidence of occult sarcoidosis in patients undergoing lung volume reduction surgery for the treatment of emphysema.[19]

Table 2 Interstitial Lung Diseases Involving the Small (Peripheral) Airways and Mimicking Chronic Obstructive Pulmonary Disease

Sarcoidosis

Hypersensitivity pneumonitis

Primary bronchiolar disorders
  Constrictive bronchiolitis
  Proliferative bronchiolitis
  Respiratory bronchiolitis
  Diffuse panbronchiolitis
  Follicular bronchiolitis
  Mineral dust-induced airway disease

Lymphangioleiomyomatosis

Pulmonary Langerhans cell histiocytosis

Recurrent diffuse alveolar hemorrhage and vasculitis

Adapted from King TE[30] and Ryu JH et al.[3]

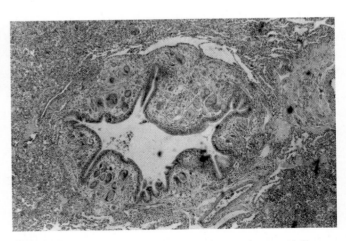

FIGURE 2. Photomicrograph demonstrating granulomatous inflammation in the wall of a terminal bronchiole owing to sarcoidosis.

Hypersensitivity Pneumonitis

Hypersensitivity pneumonitis (HP) is a disorder characterized by the development of a local pulmonary immunologic reaction in response to repeated inhalation of organic and inorganic antigens.[20–22] This section focuses on the involvement of the small airways. In HP, the inflammatory reaction primarily occurs in the distal lung parenchyma, including the bronchioles and the interstitium. The clinical presentation can be consistent with either acute pneumonia or a more indolent interstitial lung disease. Nevertheless, small airways disease owing to bronchiolocentric granulomatous inflammation with symptoms of airflow limitation is seen in the acute, subacute, and chronic forms of HP.[23]

More than 200 different inorganic and organic antigens are associated with the development of HP.[21,24] The most common include bird fancier's lung and farmer's lung. The inhaled antigens that cause bird fancier's lung originate from avian droppings, serum, feathers, and eggs. In farmer's lung, thermophilic actinomycetes or saprophytic fungi are the presumed inhaled antigen.[22] The organic antigen must be an average of 0.3 to 5 microns in size to reach the terminal airways and alveolar structures. On repeated inhalation, the patient becomes sensitized and develops a type III immune response with antibody-antigen complex deposition in the early phases. This leads to an alveolitis characterized by lymphocytic and mononuclear cell infiltration. On persistent inhalation of the antigen, a T cell–mediated type IV delayed hypersensitivity develops with CD8+ cytotoxic lymphocyte and macrophage activation, granuloma formation, and development of fibrosis.[3,20–23,25–27]

Acute HP develops after a short-term, high-level antigen exposure in a previously primed host and usually presents with a syndrome that mimics acute pneumonia. Subacute HP is considered to be a more lengthy form of acute HP and has a more indolent course, characterized by chronic respiratory complaints and interstitial opacities and nodules on chest radiography or HRCT. Chronic HP accounts for approximately 5% of HP patients. It is characterized by repeated exposure to low levels of inhaled antigen and presents with a clinical picture consistent with chronic interstitial lung disease.[21] Some chronic HP patients may also develop progressive respiratory failure and hypoxemia owing to the obliteration of bronchioles and the development of obstructive lung disease (Figures 3 and 4).[20,22,23,28]

An obstructive pattern owing to small airways disease is seen in 10 to 42% of patients with HP.[21,24] Fifty-four to 86% of patients with HP demonstrate evidence of small airways disease on HRCT, with air trapping ("mosaic" pattern) or centrilobular nodules (Figure 5).[13,29] In up to 60% of biopsy specimens from patients with either acute or chronic HP, mononuclear cell and granulomatous inflammation of the bronchioles is present (Figure 6).[23] The term *cellular bronchiolitis* has been applied to this type of small airway inflammation.[13,30] Despite these findings, most patients with HP present with a restrictive lung disease rather than an obstruc

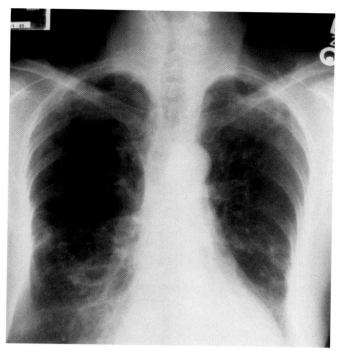

FIGURE 3. Chest radiograph of a patient with proven chronic hypersensitivity pneumonitis, demonstrating overdistention. Physiology studies indicated an obstructive pattern.

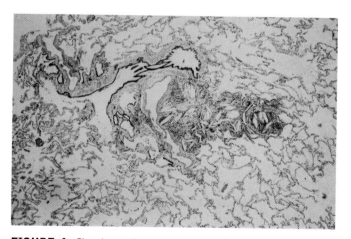

FIGURE 4. Chronic scarring and narrowing of a respiratory bronchiole in a patient with chronic hypersensitivity pneumonitis.

tive pattern.[23] Perez-Padilla and colleagues reviewed 36 open lung biopsy specimens of patients with chronic pigeon breeder's lung disease, focusing on the bronchiolar lesions.[31] The severity of the bronchiolitis equaled and paralleled the degree of inflammation and fibrosis seen in the lung parenchyma and interstitium. Thus, the contribution of the small airways disease in HP is overshadowed by the widespread alveolar and interstitial inflammation.

Despite the fact that > 95% of patients with HP are nonsmokers,[21] a clinical syndrome consistent with a diagnosis of chronic bronchitis is seen in approximately 20 to 50% of

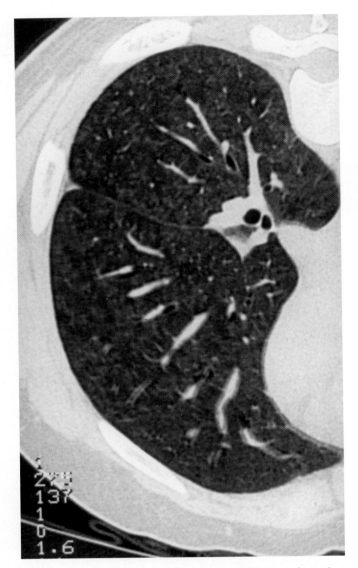

FIGURE 5. High-resolution computed tomographic scan of a patient with subacute hypersensitivity pneumonitis, demonstrating diffuse centrilobular nodules indicating peribronchiolar inflammation.

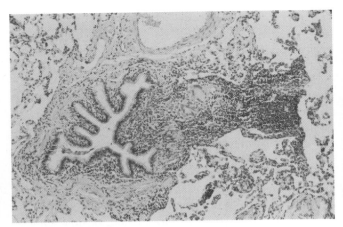

FIGURE 6. Photomicrograph of a patient with subacute hypersensitivity pneumonitis, showing bronchiolocentric granulomatous inflammation.

Primary Bronchiolar Disorders

The primary bronchiolar disorders (PBDs) should always be considered in patients presenting with unexplained chronic airflow limitation. Patients with PBDs have progressive airflow limitation that leads to significant exercise limitation and respiratory failure. The first description of a bronchiolitis was made by Lange in 1901 in two patients who died with advanced lung disease and who demonstrated histologic features of bronchiolitis obliterans, now termed cryptogenic organizing pneumonia (COP).[3,30] It was not until the 1970s that the clinical, radiographic, and histologic manifestations of these diseases were described and recognized. In a recent review by Ryu and colleagues, the PBDs were classified into distinct types (Table 3).[3]

The PBDs cause progressive dyspnea, airflow limitation, and hypoxemia, sometimes in the absence of radiographic parenchymal consolidation or significant parenchymal lung disease.[9] Pulmonary function testing usually reveals a reduced forced expiratory volume in 1 second (FEV_1), forced vital capacity (FVC), FEV_1 to FVC ratio, and diffusion capacity for carbon monoxide (DL_{CO}).[11] The emergence of HRCT and lung biopsy by video-assisted thoracoscopy has led to an increased recognition of this entity. A PBD or bronchiolitis obliterans has been identified as the cause of chronic airflow obstruction in 5 to 7% of patients being evaluated for COPD.[34]

CONSTRICTIVE BRONCHIOLITIS

Constrictive bronchiolitis, also called "obliterative bronchiolitis" or "bronchiolitis obliterans," causes progressive and irreversible airflow obstruction. These patients have dyspnea, cough, and either normal or hyperinflated lungs on chest radiography (Figure 7). A diagnosis of constrictive bronchiolitis should be suspected in patients with low FEV_1 and unexplained airflow limitation regardless of smoking history. The history may identify the predisposing conditions or

patients with serum precipitins to bird fancier's or farmer's lung antigens. In these patients, HRCT imaging has demonstrated emphysema in up to 50% of cases.[22] Many of these patients with documented emphysema were nonsmokers.[24,32,33] This presentation can mimic COPD with cough, sputum production, and dyspnea and may be the sole presentation of exposure to the antigen in the absence of typical physiologic and radiographic features of HP.[23]

The clinician must be aware that some patients with HP can present with severe airflow limitation, with symptoms indistinguishable from those of COPD. Some of these patients may demonstrate emphysematous changes by CT or lung biopsy.[22,23] A careful history for occupational and environmental exposures should be obtained from all patients evaluated for chronic airflow limitation.

Table 3   Classification of Bronchiolar Disorders

Primary Bronchiolar Disorders	Interstitial Lung Diseases with a Prominent Bronchiolar Involvement	Large-Airway Diseases with Bronchiolar Involvement
Constrictive bronchiolitis (bronchiolitis obliterans)	Hypersensitivity pneumonitis	Chronic bronchitis
Acute bronchiolitis	Respiratory bronchiolitis-interstitial lung disease	Bronchiectasis
Respiratory bronchiolitis	Cryptogenic organizing pneumonia (idiopathic bronchiolitis obliterans organizing pneumonia or proliferative bronchiolitis)	Asthma
Diffuse panbronchiolitis	Miscellaneous disorders	
Follicular bronchiolitis	Pulmonary Langerhans cell histiocytosis	
Mineral dust-induced airway disease	Sarcoidosis	
	Bronchiolocentric interstitial pneumonia	

Adapted from Ryu JH et al.[3]

exposures listed in Table 4. In constrictive bronchiolitis, the physical examination can be normal, or it may reveal wheezing, inspiratory "squeaks," or crackles. Pulmonary function tests demonstrate varying degrees of airflow limitation without a bronchodilator response.[3] Of note, the DL$_{CO}$ may be normal or relatively preserved for the degree of expiratory flow impairment.

Expiratory HRCT shows air trapping and a "mosaic" pattern in the majority of patients (Figure 8). The mosaic pattern represents patchy areas of decreased lung attenuation owing to hyperinflated lung lobules, with associated reflex vasoconstriction interposed with uninvolved lung. Of note, a normal HRCT scan does not exclude constrictive bronchiolitis.[3,12,13,35]

Histologic evaluation of the lung in constrictive bronchiolitis reveals a patchy and nodular inflammation of the membranous and respiratory bronchioles, with submucosal scarring and fibrosis, leading to gradual luminal obliteration (Figures 9 to 11).[35] Smooth muscle hypertrophy and bronchiolectasis may be present.[9,30,36,37] The histologic pattern suggests a bronchiolar repair process after an inhalational or bloodborne injury. The repair is similar to that seen in idiopathic pulmonary fibrosis. Airway epithelial injury leads to fibroproliferation and exudation of mesenchymal cells into the bronchial wall, airway lumen, and surrounding interstitium, leading to constriction and obliteration of the small airways.[3,36,38,39]

Although the chest HRCT scan may be very suggestive of constrictive bronchiolitis, surgical lung biopsy is often required for definitive confirmation. Based on the patchy nature of the bronchiolitis, transbronchial lung biopsies will not provide sufficient tissue for diagnosis.[3] Some authors have suggested that a combination of clinical and radiographic features and the results of bronchoalveolar lavage (BAL) can establish a noninvasive diagnosis of constrictive bronchiolitis. This combination, which included (a) lack of smoking history, (b) dry cough and dyspnea, (c) severe airflow limitation without response to bronchodilators, (d) suggestive HRCT, and (e) greater than 25% neutrophils in BAL, was highly predictive of constrictive bronchiolitis.[39,40]

The clinical course is one of progressive airflow limitation despite anti-inflammatory and immunosuppressive therapy. Postviral or cryptogenic bronchiolitis has a better prognosis, with patients surviving from 5 to 10 years. Constrictive bronchiolitis in posttransplant patients, called bronchiolitis obliterans syndrome (BOS), is more rapidly progressive, with survival often measured in months.[3,12] BOS is usually treated

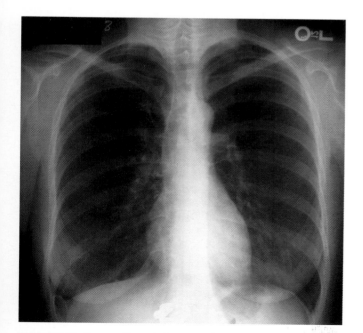

FIGURE 7. Chest radiograph demonstrating lung overdistention as the sole finding in a patient with constrictive bronchiolitis complicating rheumatoid arthritis.

Table 4   Conditions or Exposures Associated with Constrictive Bronchiolitis
Idiopathic (4%); called "cryptogenic" BO
Postinfectious (*Mycoplasma*, HIV, viral)
Chronic asthma, bronchiectasis, cystic fibrosis
Toxic agent or fume inhalation (nitrogen dioxide, sulfur dioxide, ammonia, chlorine)
Connective tissue disease (rheumatoid arthritis, SLE, secondary Sjögren syndrome)
Bone marrow, heart/lung, and lung transplantation (may occur in 35–60% of patients and is also called "bronchiolitis obliterans syndrome")
Drug reactions (penicillamine, gold, amiodarone, cocaine)
Healed ARDS or diffuse alveolar damage
Hypersensitivity pneumonitis
Inflammatory bowel disease
Paraneoplastic pemphigus
Neuroendocrine cell hyperplasia
IgA nephropathy
Popcorn worker's lung (diacetyl)
World Trade Center lung
Chronic aspiration

Adapted with permission from Ryu JH et al,[3] Couture C and Colby TV,[1] and Ryu JH.[38]

ARDS = acute respiratory diseases; BO = bronchiolitis obliterans; HIV = human immunodeficiency virus; IgA = immunoglobin A; SLE = systemic lupus erythematosus.

with accentuation of immunosuppressive therapy.[30,41] A recent case series demonstrated the potential benefit of chronic macrolide therapy (ie, azithromycin) in patients with established BOS.[38,42]

In patients with constrictive bronchiolitis from causes other than posttransplantation, a suggested regimen is prednisone at 1 mg/kg/d for 12 weeks, followed by a tapering to 20 mg/d continued for several months. Alternate-day maintenance dosing should then be continued for 2 years.[39] Evaluation for lung transplantation should be considered early in the disease course.

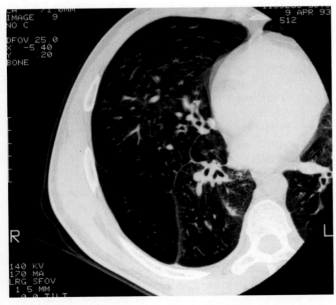

FIGURE 8. High-resolution computed tomographic scan demonstrating a "mosaic" pattern (owing to air trapping causing decreased attenuation) interposed with uninvolved lungs.

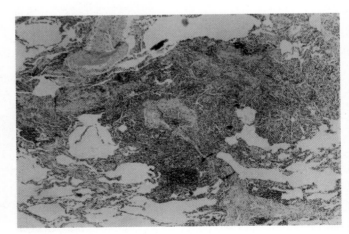

FIGURE 9. Constrictive bronchiolitis in a patient with rheumatoid arthritis. Note the peripheral lymphocytic infiltration and the central concentric fibrosis and obliteration of the bronchiolar lumen.

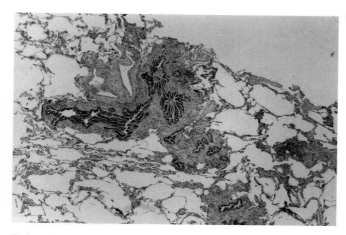

FIGURE 10. An example of concentric fibrous obliteration of the bronchiolar lumens in an autologous bone marrow transplantation patient.

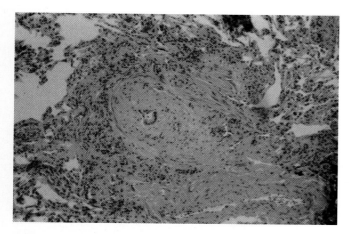

FIGURE 11. An example of concentric fibrous obliteration of bronchiolar lumens in a patient with constrictive bronchiolitis.

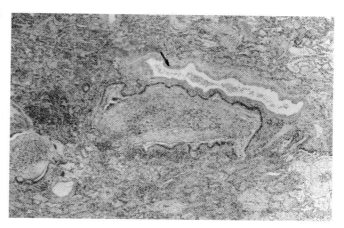

FIGURE 12. Proliferative bronchiolitis in a patient with cryptogenic organizing pneumonia (bronchiolitis obliterans organizing pneumonia) demonstrating an inflammatory polyp consisting of proliferating fibroblasts, mucopolysaccharide, and inflammatory cells obliterating the bronchiolar lumen.

PROLIFERATIVE BRONCHIOLITIS

Proliferative bronchiolitis is another clinical and histologic form of a PBD that is usually associated with organizing pneumonia. It is also referred to as bronchiolitis obliterans organizing pneumonia (BOOP) or COP.[3,30,38] Proliferative bronchiolitis is primarily a luminal disease in which the structures and the membranous bronchioles become filled with inflammatory polyps (Figure 12).[3] Its clinical presentation differs significantly from that of constrictive bronchiolitis, and it causes restrictive (as opposed to obstructive) pulmonary dysfunction. In 11 to 28% of patients with BOOP or COP, an obstructive or mixed restrictive/obstructive ventilatory pattern is seen.[3,43] There is parenchymal consolidation on radiographic studies. Proliferative bronchiolitis is associated with the conditions listed in Table 5. As is the case for constrictive bronchiolitis, proliferative bronchiolitis represents an exuberant inflammatory response and repair as a result of injury. Most cases are idiopathic (70–90%) and are associated with an organizing pneumonia.[3,36,38,44,45] In contrast to constrictive bronchiolitis, proliferative bronchiolitis responds to corticosteroid treatment.[36] In unresponsive cases, progression to pulmonary fibrosis occurs.

RESPIRATORY BRONCHIOLITIS

Respiratory bronchiolitis is a common bronchiolitis predominantly seen in smokers[46] and may be the precursor lesion of emphysema.[47] This bronchiolitis is characterized by pigmented, "dust-laden" macrophages at the center of the pulmonary lobules, development of squamous metaplasia, and accumulation of connective tissue.[46,48–51] Smokers with this lesion are usually asymptomatic but have observable HRCT abnormalities that include parenchymal nodules, bronchial wall thickening, and ground-glass opacities.[52,53] Radiologic and histologic correlations have demonstrated that the HRCT abnormalities seen in smokers represent accumulation of pigmented macrophages, bronchiolectasis, and peribronchiolar fibrosis.[54] This inflammatory bronchiolitis may provide the inflammatory milieu for elastin degradation and bronchiolar obstruction associated with early emphysema.[47] Previous work by Brody and Craighead suggested that the pigmented macrophages of respiratory bronchiolitis contain kaolinite (aluminum silicate), a common component of clay soils that has also been identified in commercial cigarette brands.[55] This form of bronchiolitis may be a form of chronic dust-induced disease induced by inhalation of kaolinite or aluminum silicate contained in cigarettes.[47]

A small percentage of smokers develop an idiopathic interstitial pneumonia in association with respiratory bronchiolitis called respiratory bronchiolitis–associated interstitial lung disease (RB-ILD).[46] In contrast with the typical respiratory bronchiolitis seen in virtually all smokers, this unique entity affects not only the respiratory bronchioles but also the surrounding lung parenchyma, with clinical features suggesting

Table 5 Conditions and Exposures Associated with Proliferative Bronchiolitis
Proliferative BOOP
Idiopathic PB or BOOP (70–90%), called cryptogenic organizing pneumonia
Collagen vascular disease (rheumatoid arthritis, SLE, polymyositis, dermatomyositis, progressive systemic sclerosis, Behçet disease, Sjögren syndrome)
Organizing acute infection (bacteria, *Mycoplasma, Cryptococcus, Nocardia,* viruses)
Inhalational injury (silo filler's, paraquat, paint aerosols)
Organ transplantation
Radiation therapy
Drug induced
Organizing diffuse alveolar damage or ARDS
Chronic eosinophilic pneumonia
Vasculitis (especially Wegener granulomatosis)
Hypersensitivity pneumonitis
Eosinophilic pneumonias
Aspiration
Hematologic malignancies
Wegener granulomatosis
Miscellaneous
IgA nephropathy
Sweet's syndrome
Hepatitis C
Common variable hypogammaglobulinemia
Thyroiditis

Adapted with permission from King TE[30] and Ryu JH et al.[3]

ARDS = acute respiratory diseases; BOOP = bronchiolitis obliterans organizing pneumonia; IgA = immunoglobulin A; PB = proliferative bronchiolitis; SLE = systemic lupus erythematosus.

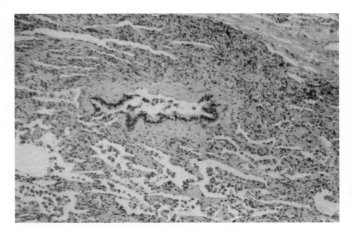

FIGURE 13. Respiratory bronchiolitis-associated interstitial lung disease. Note the increase in connective tissue surrounding the respiratory bronchiole and the pigmented (smoker's) macrophages in the adjacent alveoli.

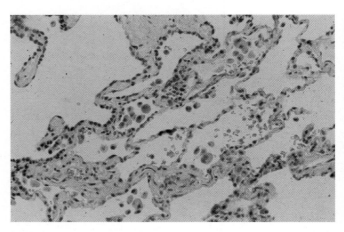

FIGURE 14. Respiratory bronchiolitis-associated interstitial lung disease. There is broadening of the alveolar walls owing to increased collagen in the alveolar walls adjacent to the affected bronchioles.

an interstitial lung disease.[56–59] Patients with RB-ILD are almost always smokers and present with dyspnea and cough, mixed restrictive/obstructive pulmonary function, a low diffusing capacity (ie, DL_{CO}), and hypoxemia. Lung biopsy specimens demonstrate the accumulation of brown-pigmented macrophages (smoker's macrophages) within respiratory bronchioles and adjacent alveoli (Figure 13). The respiratory bronchioles demonstrate increased connective tissue in their walls but no luminal obliteration. In contrast with respiratory bronchiolitis, RB-ILD demonstrates significant interstitial fibrosis in a bronchiolocentric pattern (Figure 14). Approximately 57% of patients with RB-ILD also manifest premature centrilobular emphysema.[46] In 1987,

Myers and colleagues first described RB-ILD in six young smokers with progressive respiratory deterioration accompanied by restrictive pulmonary function, decreased DL_{CO}, and hypoxemia.[56,57,60]

The age of RB-ILD patients ranges from 22 to 53 years. It is more common in men, and there is no ethnic predilection.[46] Affected individuals have smoked from 7 to 75 pack-years. Chronic symptoms consist of dyspnea (70%), sputum production (44%), cough (58%), and chest pain persistent for up to 5 years prior to diagnosis.[46] Rare asymptomatic patients have been reported in each series.

The physical examination may reveal inspiratory bibasilar crackles that are coarser than the "Velcro-like" crackles of idiopathic pulmonary fibrosis.[46] Laboratory data are unremarkable except for hypoxemia at rest or with exercise. Although pulmonary function tests are primarily restrictive,

30% of patients may present with an obstructive process. Most patients demonstrate a mixed obstructive/restrictive pattern with a characteristically low DL_{CO}.[60] An interesting feature seen in a few cases is a dramatic reversal of the restrictive/obstructive pattern after bronchodilator administration. This phenomenon, called "reversible restriction," is believed to be secondary to bronchodilation of small airways and alveolar ducts.[61] The chest radiographs may be normal in up to 28% of patients or show bronchial wall thickening and diffuse, ill-defined reticulonodular infiltrates (Figure 15).[46] Findings on HRCT range from normal to ground-glass opacification, centrilobular nodules, linear opacities, atelectasis, and emphysema (Figure 16).[3,53,59,62]

RB-ILD should be suspected in a young smoker who has unexplained dyspnea, cough, significant restrictive or mixed physiology, and a low DL_{CO}. Open lung biopsy specimens reveal an inflammatory lesion composed of mononuclear cells in the submucosa of membranous and respiratory bronchioles. The key feature is the predominance of associated fibrosis extending in stellate fashion from the respiratory

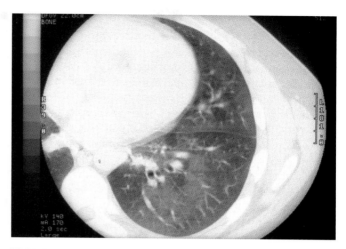

FIGURE 16. Respiratory bronchiolitis-associated interstitial lung disease. High-resolution computed tomography demonstrates a nonspecific ground-glass pattern.

bronchioles to the surrounding alveolar walls.[58] Smoking cessation is the key component of treatment.[57] In a recent series by Ryu and colleagues, corticosteroids led to improvement in pulmonary function tests and HRCT scan abnormalities in up to 64% of patients.[60] Nevertheless, recurrence of symptoms and abnormal physiology may occur after discontinuation of oral prednisone therapy.[60]

DIFFUSE PANBRONCHIOLITIS

Diffuse panbronchiolitis (DPB) is an inflammatory small airways disease involving respiratory bronchioles. Because of productive cough and airflow obstruction, this condition is often confused with COPD or bronchiectasis.[2,63]

Found primarily in Japanese and Korean adults,[64] DPB is a disease of unknown etiology. The increased incidence of DPB in these populations is associated with a high incidence (11–14%) of human leukocyte antigen B54 (HLA-B54), which is seen in 63% of DPB patients, with a reported relative risk of 13.30.[30,63,64] Keicho and colleagues mapped the human leukocyte antigen (HLA)-associated major susceptibility gene to the 200 kb class I telomeric region of the HLA-B locus on chromosome 6p21.3.[65] Recently, Kamio and colleagues demonstrated increased frequency of polymorphism of the mucin gene *MUC5B* in patients with DPB. An increase in the expression of *MUC5B* is associated with mucus hypersecretion, which may explain the development of DPB.[66] Cases have also been reported in China, Latin America, and the United States.[67–69] Fitzgerald and colleagues reported on five US citizens with progressive obstructive pulmonary disease and biopsy-proven DPB.[69] It is likely that DPB is underdiagnosed since it is easily confused with chronic bronchitis. It should be suspected in patients with unexplained COPD or bronchiolitis, especially if sinusitis is present.[69]

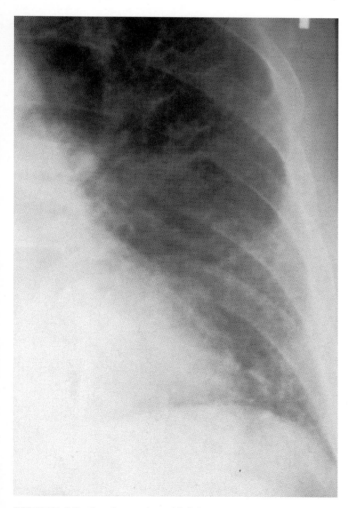

FIGURE 15. Respiratory bronchiolitis-associated interstitial lung disease. Chest radiograph demonstrating ill-defined infiltrates.

DPB usually affects males in their fourth and fifth decades of life. Its symptoms are similar to those of chronic bronchitis, sinusitis, and bronchiectasis. All patients report a history of paranasal sinusitis in their second and third decades of life. In the Japanese DPB patients, approximately 66% smoked.[64,69] Initially, there is isolation of *Haemophilus influenzae* from the sputum, and this is followed by *Pseudomonas* species. Of note, these patients have normal immunoglobulin levels, have no connective tissue disease, and are not immunosuppressed.

The chest radiography reveals hyperinflation and may demonstrate ill-defined nodules of <2 mm in the lung bases. In advanced disease, "tram lines" suggestive of bronchiectasis are seen (Figure 17). HRCT demonstrates peripheral centrilobular nodules or branching structures ("tree-in-bud"), consistent with bronchiolectasis (Figures 18 and 19). Bronchial wall thickening, diffuse bronchiectasis, and air trapping are also observed.[3,30,64,69] Pulmonary function tests reveal an obstructive pattern, air trapping (increased residual volume to total lung capacity ratio), reduced diffusion capacity, and hypoxemia.[64,69]

The confirmation of DPB usually requires a lung biopsy. The histology is characteristic, with the gross pathology revealing inflammatory nodules (gray-white to yellow) with centrilobular distribution. There is inflammation centered at the terminal and respiratory bronchioles, with dense peribronchiolar and luminal accumulation of neutrophils, lymphocytes, plasma cells, and histiocytes. There is associated proliferation of bronchial-associated lymphoid follicles and a characteristic accumulation of interstitial foamy macrophages (Figures 20 and 21).[3,37,64,69,70] Of note, these histologic features are also seen in bronchiolitis associated with bronchiectasis and rheumatoid arthritis.[3]

This disease is progressive, and if untreated, the 5-year and 10-year survival rates are 42% and 25%, respectively. DPB has a high incidence of elevated cold agglutinin titers despite absent *Mycoplasma* antibodies.[3] This finding has led to empiric therapy with macrolides, with an improvement in the 5-year survival to 91%. Patients are usually treated with low-dose erythromycin at 400 to 600 mg/d for an average of 20 months.

DPB is an example of how the study of a rare disease can yield insight into the treatment of common disorders. The

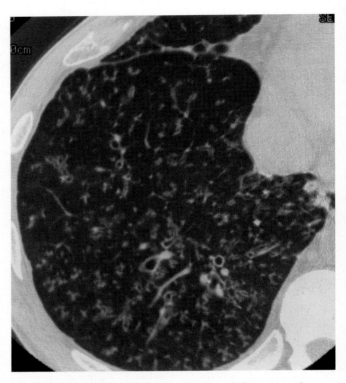

FIGURE 18. Diffuse panbronchiolitis. High-resolution computed tomography demonstrates bronchiectasis and a peripheral "tree-in-bud" pattern, indicating bronchiolectasis.

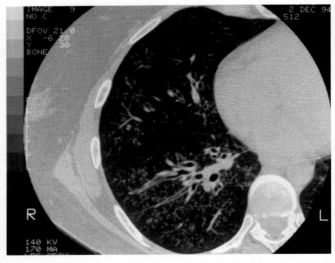

FIGURE 19. Diffuse panbronchiolitis. In addition to the bronchiectasis and bronchiolectasis, high-resolution computed tomography demonstrates centrilobular nodules.

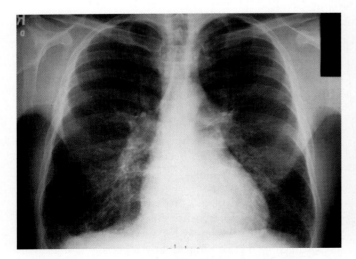

FIGURE 17. Diffuse panbronchiolitis. Chest radiograph demonstrating interstitial nodules with "tram lines."

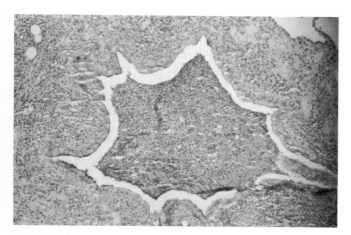

FIGURE 20. Respiratory bronchiole in a patient with diffuse panbronchiolitis, showing intraluminal mucus with inflammatory cells and diffuse inflammation of the entire bronchiolar wall.

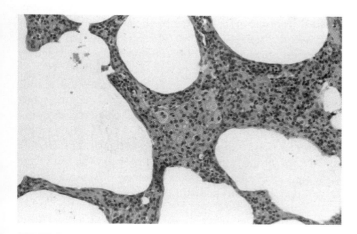

FIGURE 21. Photomicrograph demonstrating the characteristic interstitial collection of foamy macrophages in a case of diffuse panbronchiolitis.

impact of chronic macrolide therapy for DPB has initiated studies into the anti-inflammatory effects of macrolides on the bronchial and bronchiolar mucosa. These anti-inflammatory effects are not related to the antimicrobial properties of these agents and are likely due to the inhibition of local proinflammatory cytokine and chemokine production.[71] Abe and colleagues recently demonstrated that clarithromycin inhibited interleukin-8 and interleukin-1β secretion in human bronchial epithelial cell lines.[3,72] The effects of macrolides on other large and small airways diseases, such as bronchiectasis, cystic fibrosis, chronic bronchitis, and bronchiolitis obliterans, are under active investigation.[42,73]

FOLLICULAR BRONCHIOLITIS

Follicular bronchiolitis may present with airflow limitation and symptoms of dyspnea that may mimic COPD. This disease is associated with cystic fibrosis, chronic bronchiectasis, chronic aspiration syndromes, connective tissue disease,

acquired immune deficiency syndrome (AIDS), acquired hypogammaglobulinemia, chronic pulmonary infections, and hypersensitivity reactions.[30,38] It may also be a manifestation or association of a primary lymphoid hyperplasia and lymphocytic interstitial pneumonitis.[3,74] The small airways are affected via direct compression by proliferating and enlarged peribronchiolar lymphoid follicles.[38] The patient presents with dyspnea, cough, occasional fever, and obstructive or mixed pulmonary function studies.[30] The radiographs may be normal or demonstrate nodular or reticulonodular infiltrates with associated mediastinal adenopathy. Common HRCT scan findings include bilateral centrilobular nodules and ground-glass opacities.[3,75] Thin-walled cysts, which should be easily distinguishable from emphysema, have been reported.[74] Treatment is directed at the predisposing condition. Systemic corticosteroids and inhaled bronchodilators are often used, with conflicting results.[3,30]

MINERAL DUST-INDUCED AIRWAY DISEASE

Mineral dusts, such as silica and asbestos, are well-known causes of pulmonary fibrosis with associated restrictive physiology. Nevertheless, small airways disease is a more frequent and early complication of mineral dust inhalation. Various reviews and case series of miners and workers have revealed a high incidence of obstructive pulmonary function tests compatible with COPD.[3,9,30,38] This observation is confounded by concomitant cigarette smoking, but epidemiologic studies suggest an additive effect of mineral dust inhalation.[76] Histologic studies of chronic inorganic dust inhalation demonstrate preferential accumulation in the membranous, respiratory bronchioles and alveolar ducts, leading to inflammation, fibrosis, and luminal distortion.[3,30,77] Typically, these small airways demonstrate an accumulation of pigmented and anthracotic dust material with increased macrophage accumulation.[1,9,77] This bronchiolitis has been reported in subjects with chronic exposure to a variety of inorganic dusts, such as asbestos, talc, mica, kaolin, silicates, aluminum oxide, iron oxide, talc, and coal.[3,30,47] Therefore, it is important to obtain a full environmental and occupational history in patients with unexplained or premature COPD.

Lymphangioleiomyomatosis

Lymphangioleiomyomatosis (LAM) is a rare disease that affects nonsmoking women, usually in their childbearing years. It may occur as a sporadic disease or in 33% of women with a diagnosis of tuberous sclerosis (TS).[78–80] The reported incidence of sporadic disease is approximately one per million persons.[81] It is characterized by progressive airflow limitation that leads to respiratory failure and, ultimately, to death. LAM is associated with hamartomatous smooth muscle proliferation involving the small airways, interstitium, blood vessels, and lymphatics of the lungs (Figure 22). The involvement of the interstitium and small airways leads to obstruction and to the formation of thin-walled cysts.[80–84] Although classified as an interstitial lung disease, it primarily

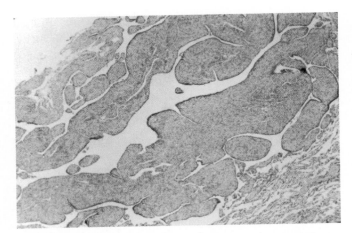

FIGURE 22. Lymphangioleiomyomatosis. Smooth muscle proliferation in the wall of a respiratory bronchiole.

affects the small (peripheral) airways, leading to severe airflow limitation and hyperinflation.

LAM is often confused with asthma, COPD, idiopathic pulmonary fibrosis, sarcoidosis, and tuberculosis. The diagnosis is usually delayed for 3 to 4 years after the onset of symptoms.[81,84] The mean age at presentation is 34 years of age (range 18–76 years old), and the disease affects primarily Caucasian women.[84,85] Rarely, it can present in postmenopausal women. One series reported eight postmenopausal patients; six of them were receiving estrogen replacement therapy.[86] Patients present with dyspnea or spontaneous pneumothorax (55% of patients).[85,87] Other symptoms include a nonproductive cough, hemoptysis, and fatigue.[88] Involvement of lymph nodes or obstruction of lymph flow in the chest and abdomen leads to chylothorax or chylous ascites. Hemoptysis is likely due to involvement and rupture of the pulmonary veins.

The physical examination is usually normal or detects crackles and/or rhonchi. Clubbing is rarely seen.[84] Approximately 33 to 60% of LAM patients have renal angiomyolipomas and have a picture suggestive of TS.[89] Nevertheless, LAM patients do not have the mental retardation, seizure disorder, or facial angiofibromas seen in TS. LAM has been referred to as a *forme fruste* or part of the clinical spectrum of TS since 26 to 39% of women with TS have chest CT features consistent with LAM.[81,84,89,90]

The association between TS and LAM is explained by a common genetic mutation. The genetic mutation in TS has been characterized as a germ cell mutation in either the *TSC1* or *TSC2* tumor suppressor gene (mapped to chromosome 9q34 and 16p13, respectively).[89] The *TSC1* gene codes for hamartin, a protein with tumor suppressor activity. The *TSC2* gene product is tuberin, a 200 kDa protein that, when inactivated, leads to cell growth and protein translation conducive to hamartomatous growth.[80,89] In LAM, a germ cell mutation is not seen, but it is suspected that a spontaneous somatic cell mutation in combination with a loss of heterozygosity leads

to absent TSC2 protein.[81,91] The *TSC2* gene mutation has been identified in both angiomyolipoma and LAM cells, suggesting that the LAM cells may be "metastatic" from the renal angiomyolipoma lesion.[89] In the lung, these "benign metastatic" cells proliferate with a hamartomatous smooth muscle proliferation, leading to the bronchiolar obstruction, cyst formation, and airflow limitation.[89,91]

The diagnosis of LAM is suspected in women of childbearing age with dyspnea, spontaneous pneumothorax, hemoptysis, chylothorax, or unexplained airflow limitation.[80] Chest radiography may demonstrate a reticular or reticulonodular pattern with hyperinflation, pneumothorax, or pleural effusion (Figure 23). Pulmonary function tests range from normal early on to severe airflow obstruction, decreased DL_{CO}, and hypoxemia.[80,85] The HRCT scan of the chest is often diagnostic, revealing the presence of diffuse thin-walled (2–5 mm) cysts in the lung parenchyma (Figure 24). With disease progression, the cysts become more numerous and enlarged. Emphysematous cysts are distinguished from the cysts of LAM by their lack of walls and by their apical distribution.[78,82,84] The cyst formation in LAM may be due to the action of metalloproteinases secreted by LAM cells on the lung collagen and elastic structure.[78,92]

The diagnosis of LAM is confirmed after a surgical lung biopsy, although the clinical and radiographic picture is adequate for the majority of cases.[80] The histology reveals nodular proliferation of smooth muscle cells ("LAM cells") within the alveolar walls, lymphatics, and blood vessels. This smooth muscle cell proliferation obliterates bronchioles, leading to distal cyst formation. LAM cells are likely of smooth muscle origin; they have estrogen and progesterone receptors (50%

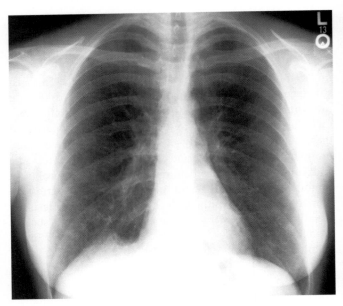

FIGURE 23. Chest radiograph of lymphangioleiomyomatosis in a 34-year-old nonsmoking woman, showing hyperinflation and ill-defined infiltrates.

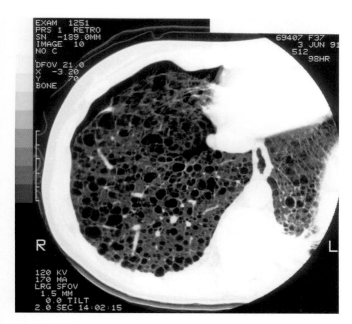

FIGURE 24. Lymphangioleiomyomatosis. High-resolution computed tomography demonstrates multiple thin-walled cysts and spontaneous pneumothorax.

of cases) and stain positively with the melanoma HMB45 antibody.[80,81] There are reports of establishing a diagnosis of LAM with the combination of a highly suggestive HRCT scan and positive staining of transbronchial lung biopsy specimens for the HMB45 melanoma antigen.[81,84,93]

The treatment is largely derived from results of small series or case reports. Patients may have variable courses with a prolonged life expectancy to a more rapid deterioration with onset of respiratory failure and death within 10 years.[80,92] Survival data indicate that 78% of patients are alive at 8.5 years from the onset of disease.[94] Progesterone treatment slows the progression of the disease. Pregnancy and estrogen therapy are associated with either the onset of LAM or a worsening of clinical manifestations, suggesting the importance of hormonal influences in this disease. Estrogen is believed to potentiate smooth muscle proliferation by downregulating tuberin, the *TSC2* gene product. Estrogen may also indirectly inhibit apoptosis of LAM cells.[84,85]

Ten percent of patients demonstrate a bronchodilator response and should be treated with inhaled β2-agonists.[81] Corticosteroids are not effective. The treatment is primarily focused on hormonal manipulation. The literature reports variable results with progesterone therapy, oophorectomy, and tamoxifen administration; the data are most convincing for progesterone therapy. Recently, a retrospective evaluation of the National Institutes of Health registry revealed that progesterone therapy did not appear to alter the decline in lung function in LAM.[79] In a recent case report, the prolonged administration of doxycycline, a potent inhibitor of matrix metalloproteinase, led to dramatic improvement in lung function and oxygenation in a patient with advanced LAM.[92]

Pulmonary Langerhans Cell Histiocytosis

Pulmonary Langerhans cell histiocytosis (PLCH) occurs almost exclusively in cigarette smokers. Other names for this disease are histiocytosis X and eosinophilic granuloma.[95,96] The first cases of "eosinophilic granuloma of the lung" were reported in 1951 by Farinacci.[97,98] This disease involves the small (peripheral) airways and is characterized by bronchiolocentric granulomatous inflammation containing proliferating Langerhans cells (LCs).[34,97,99]

The incidence is unknown.[96] One review mentions a total of 200 cases reported in the literature in a 30-year period.[100] The patients are almost exclusively current or former smokers (> 95%) and present in the third to fifth decades of life.[96] Cough and dyspnea are present in 70% of cases. About one-third of the cases present with systemic symptoms, including fever, weight loss, fatigue, and generalized malaise.[98] Spontaneous pneumothorax is seen in about 25% of cases and may be the initial manifestation. In 15% of cases, there is involvement of the bones, pituitary gland, skin, lymph nodes, liver, and spleen[95,99]; in the remainder of cases, the disease is found only in the lungs. The physical examination is normal in 62% of patients. Decreased breath sounds, rales, and wheezes are less common findings. Peripheral blood eosinophilia is not seen.[100]

LCs are dendritic cells of monocyte-macrophage lineage, with antigen-presenting capacity and expression of CD1a surface glycoprotein and cytoplasmic S-100 protein. These cells are identified by the presence of Birbeck granules, which are rod-shaped pentalaminar intracellular cytoplasmic inclusions detected by electron microscopy.[96,98,101] The strong association between smoking and PLCH suggests the direct effects of cigarette smoke on LC proliferation in the lung. Smoking leads to increased secretion of bombesin-like peptides that stimulate macrophage cytokine secretion and recruitment of LCs, with resultant fibroblast proliferation.[96,98] One hypothesis suggested that PLCH represents a local "malignant" proliferation of LCs; however, recent data do not support this pathogenic mechanism.[95–98]

The pulmonary function tests of patients with PLCH can range from normal to obstructive or a mixed restrictive/obstructive pattern. A low DL_{CO} is present in 60 to 90% of patients. The degree of airflow obstruction correlates with the histology, which demonstrates peribronchiolar inflammation and fibrosis.[95,100] The chest radiographs are usually abnormal, revealing bilateral upper and middle lobe nodular or reticulonodular infiltrates in association with cysts (Figure 25).[95,97] Lung volumes are often preserved or increased, differentiating PLCH from other interstitial lung diseases. HRCT may be diagnostic.[82,95,98,102,103] Early on, HRCT demonstrates nodular lesions and cysts. In combination with the right clinical presentation, the presence of

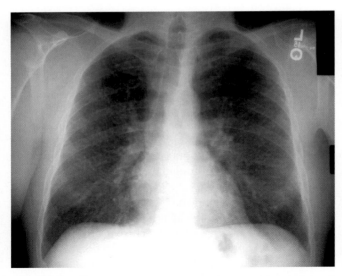

FIGURE 25. Pulmonary Langerhans cell histiocytosis. Chest radiograph demonstrating multiple diffuse nodules with upper zone predilection. Small cystic structures can also be appreciated.

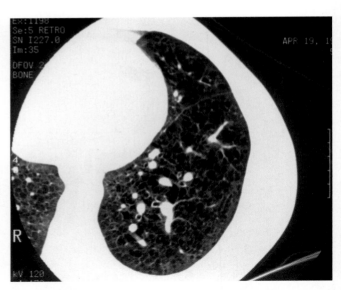

FIGURE 27. Pulmonary Langerhans cell histiocytosis. High-resolution computed tomography shows diffuse cystic change in a man with moderately severe airflow limitation.

upper lobe cysts and peribronchiolar nodules is highly suggestive of PLCH (Figures 26 and 27).[101] The diagnosis is confirmed after open lung biopsy. Recent reports demonstrated that a BAL demonstrating ≥5% LCs (CD1a-positive cells) is highly suggestive of PLCH and may eliminate the need for tissue diagnosis in a patient with a compatible clinical picture and HRCT scan.[95,96]

The histologic abnormalities follow a peribronchiolar distribution. Early on, there is bronchiolocentric proliferation of

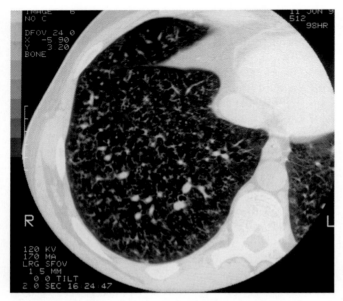

FIGURE 26. Pulmonary Langerhans cell histiocytosis. High-resolution computed tomography demonstrates scattered cysts and centrilobular nodules.

LCs (Figures 28 and 29). These proliferating cells form characteristic stellate nodules measuring 0.4 to 1.3 cm in size and containing LCs, eosinophils, histiocytes, lymphocytes, plasma cells, and pigmented macrophages. Eosinophils are often admixed with the LCs or are at the periphery of the histiocytic inflammation. With progression, the stellate nodules coalesce, cavitate, and undergo fibrotic transformation, resulting in bronchiolar obliteration. The obliteration of the terminal and respiratory bronchioles results in airflow limitation and cyst formation.[95,96,100,104]

The natural history of PLCH is variable, and approximately 75% of patients improve or stabilize following smoking cessation.[98] Less than 10% of cases progress to respiratory failure and death.[105] Predictors of decreased survival include an obstructive pulmonary function test pattern, reduced DL_{CO}, advanced age, systemic involvement, honeycomb lung, and a large number of lung cysts.[96,105] Steroid treatment results in disease stabilization in some cases. Current recommendations reserve corticosteroid use for patients with progressive disease despite smoking cessation.[95,96] Rapidly progressive or systemic disease has been treated with chemotherapy and cytotoxic agents without success.[96,98] Transplantation has been performed, and recurrences of PLCH in the transplanted lung have been reported.

Recurrent Diffuse Alveolar Hemorrhage and Vasculitis

Recurring episodes of diffuse alveolar hemorrhage secondary to pulmonary capillaritis, a small vessel vasculitis characterized by recurrent interstitial neutrophilic infiltration with fragmentation, have resulted in a progressive obstructive lung disease indistinguishable from emphysema.

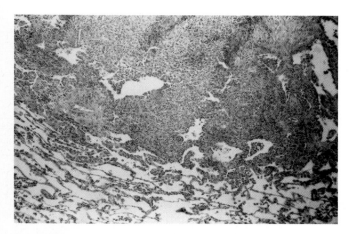

FIGURE 28. Pulmonary Langerhans cell histiocytosis. Photomicrograph of bronchiolocentric inflammation.

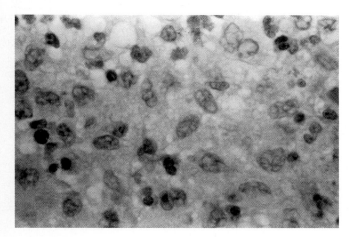

FIGURE 29. Pulmonary Langerhans cell histiocytosis. High-power photomicrograph of same patient seen in Figure 28, demonstrating characteristic Langerhans cells.

Microscopic polyangiitis, a systemic vasculitis, was reported to develop a severe irreversible airflow limitation and hyperinflation in three cases.[106,107] Ten years following the initial episode of diffuse alveolar hemorrhage, the physiologic testing and HRCT indicated the development of emphysema after recurrent episodes of diffuse alveolar hemorrhage. Whether the mechanism is due to the repeated neutrophilic infiltration and their eventual death occasioning the release of oxygen radicals and proteolytic enzymes, leading to alveolar destruction and emphysema, still remains unclear.

Hypocomplementemic urticarial vasculitis syndrome (HUVS) is an uncommon disorder characterized by complement accumulation, and with precipitation of serum $C1_q$, a syndrome results, consisting of urticarial vasculitis, angioedema, arthralgia, ocular inflammation, glomerulonephritis, and an obstructive lung disease.[108,109] A recent report indicated that in one case of HUVS during the course of the disease, a biopsy showed pulmonary capillaritis, and despite treatment with corticosteroids, the obstructive lung disease progressed. Eventually, the patient underwent successful double lung transplantation.[109] The explanted lung showed evidence of active pulmonary capillaritis and severe panacinar emphysema. The occurrence of obstructive lung disease in association with HUVS is fairly common, developing in as many as 50% of the patients. In these patients, there is no association with cigarette smoking.

Significant airflow limitation has also been reported after recurrent diffuse alveolar hemorrhage from idiopathic pulmonary hemosiderosis (IPH).[110] In IPH, the hemorrhagic episodes are bland and not associated with pulmonary capillaritis. The question remains in some of these patients with IPH whether pulmonary capillaritis was present as many of them did not undergo surgical biopsy.

Summary

This chapter has described diffuse interstitial lung diseases that result in airflow limitation owing to small airway involvement. These disorders should be considered in patients with chronic airflow obstruction who have too rapid a fall in spirometric values, have minimal or no smoking history, or who are young. A systematic approach to the diagnosis of these diseases should include the use of chest radiography and complete pulmonary function testing, including examination of flow-volume loops, spirometric values, lung volumes, and DL_{CO}. In patients with atypical presentations and unrevealing radiographs, HRCT of the chest with inspiratory and expiratory cuts may provide evidence of small airways disease. When suspected, these patients should be referred to a pulmonary disease specialist for further evaluation and possible lung biopsy.

References

1. Couture C, Colby TV. Histopathology of bronchiolar disorders. Semin Respir Crit Care Med 2003;24:489–98.
2. Colby TV. Bronchiolitis. Pathologic considerations. Am J Clin Pathol 1998;109:101–9.
3. Ryu JH, Myers JL, Swensen SJ. Bronchiolar disorders. Am J Respir Crit Care Med 2003;168:1277–92.
4. Muller NL, Miller RR. Diseases of the bronchioles: CT and histopathologic findings. Radiology 1995;196:3–12.
5. Mead J. The lung's "quiet zone." N Engl J Med 1970;282:1318–9.
6. Hogg JC, Macklem PT, Thurlbeck WM. Site and nature of airway obstruction in chronic obstructive lung disease. N Engl J Med 1968;278:1355–60.
7. Thurlbeck WM. Pathology of chronic airflow obstruction. In: Cherniack NS, editor. Chronic obstructive pulmonary disease. 1st ed. Philadelphia: W.B. Saunders; 1991. p. 3–20.
8. Thurlbeck WM, Wright JL. Airflow obstruction due to disease in the small airways. In: Thurlbeck WM, Wright JL, editors. Thurlbeck's chronic airflow obstruction. 2nd ed. Hamilton (ON): BC Decker; 1999. p. 223–54.

9. Wright JL, Cagle P, Churg A, et al. Diseases of the small airways. Am Rev Respir Dis 1992;146:240–62.

10. Niewoehner DE, Knoke JD, Kleinerman J. Peripheral airways as a determinant of ventilatory function in the human lung. J Clin Invest 1977;60:139–51.

11. Shaw RJ, Djukanovic R, Tashkin DP, et al. The role of small airways in lung disease. Respir Med 2002;96:67–80.

12. Desai SR, Hansell DM. Small airways disease: expiratory computed tomography comes of age. Clin Radiol 1997;52:332–7.

13. Worthy SA, Muller NL. Small airway diseases. Radiol Clin North Am 1998;36:163–73.

14. Handa T, Nagai S, Fushimi Y, et al. Clinical and radiographic indices associated with airflow limitation in patients with sarcoidosis. Chest 2006;130:1851–6.

15. Westall GP, Stirling RG, Cullinan P, Dubois RM. Sarcoidosis. In: Schwarz MI, King TE, editors. Interstitial lung disease. 4th ed. Hamilton (ON): BC Decker; 2003. p. 332–86.

16. Sheffield EA. Pathology of sarcoidosis. Clin Chest Med 1997;18:741–54.

17. Zar HJ, Cole RP. Bullous emphysema occurring in pulmonary sarcoidosis. Respiration 1995;62:290–3.

18. Judson MA, Strange C. Bullous sarcoidosis: a report of three cases. Chest 1998;114:1474–8.

19. Keller CA, Naunheim KS, Osterloh J, et al. Histopathologic diagnosis made in lung tissue resected from patients with severe emphysema undergoing lung volume reduction surgery. Chest 1997;111:941–7.

20. Fink JN. Hypersensitivity pneumonitis. Clin Chest Med 1992;13:303–9.

21. Mohr LC. Hypersensitivity pneumonitis. Curr Opin Pulm Med 2004;10:401–11.

22. Sélman M. Hypersensitivity Pneumonitis. In: Schwarz MI, King TE, editors. Interstitial lung disease. 4th ed. Hamilton (ON): BC Decker; 2003. p. 452–84.

23. Selman-Lama M, Perez-Padilla R. Airflow obstruction and airway lesions in hypersensitivity pneumonitis. Clin Chest Med 1993;14:699–714.

24. Glazer CS, Rose CS, Lynch DA. Clinical and radiologic manifestations of hypersensitivity pneumonitis. Thorac Imaging 2002;17:261–72.

25. Salvaggio JE. Extrinsic allergic alveolitis (hypersensitivity pneumonitis): past, present and future. Clin Exp Allergy 1997;27 Suppl 1:18–25.

26. Craig TJ, Richerson HB. Update on hypersensitivity pneumonitis. Compr Ther 1996;22:559–64.

27. Ismail T, McSharry C, Boyd G. Extrinsic allergic alveolitis. Respirology 2006;11:262–8.

28. Reynolds HY. Hypersensitivity pneumonitis. Clin Chest Med 1982;3:503–19.

29. Hansell DM, Wells AU, Padley SP, Muller NL. Hypersensitivity pneumonitis: correlation of individual CT patterns with functional abnormalities. Radiology 1996;199:123–8.

30. King TE. Bronchiolitis. In: Schwarz MI, King TE, editors. Interstitial lung disease. 4th ed. Hamilton (ON): BC Decker; 2003. p. 787–837.

31. Perez-Padilla R, Gaxiola M, Salas J, et al. Bronchiolitis in chronic pigeon breeder's disease. Morphologic evidence of a spectrum of small airway lesions in hypersensitivity pneumonitis induced by avian antigens. Chest 1996;110:371–7.

32. Erkinjuntti-Pekkanen R, Rytkonen H, Kokkarinen JI, et al. Long-term risk of emphysema in patients with farmer's lung and matched control farmers. Am J Respir Crit Care Med 1998;158:662–5.

33. Remy-Jardin M, Remy J, Wallaert B, Muller NL. Subacute and chronic bird breeder hypersensitivity pneumonitis: sequential evaluation with CT and correlation with lung function tests and bronchoalveolar lavage. Radiology 1993;189:111–8.

34. St John RC, Gadek JE, Pacht ER. Chronic obstructive pulmonary disease: less common causes—an algorithm for the primary care physician. J Gen Intern Med 1993;8:564–72.

35. Chan A, Allen R. Bronchiolitis obliterans: an update. Curr Opin Pulm Med 2004;10:133–41.

36. King TE. Bronchiolitis. In: Schwarz MI, King TE, editors. Interstitial lung disease. 3rd ed. Hamilton (ON): BC Decker; 1998. p. 645–84.

37. Myers JL, Colby TV. Pathologic manifestations of bronchiolitis, constrictive bronchiolitis, cryptogenic organizing pneumonia, and diffuse panbronchiolitis. Clin Chest Med 1993;14:611–22.

38. Ryu JH. Classification and approach to bronchiolar diseases. Curr Opin Pulm Med 2006;12:145–51.

39. St John RC, Dorinsky PM. Cryptogenic bronchiolitis. Clin Chest Med 1993;14:667–75.

40. Kindt GC, Weiland JE, Davis WB, et al. Bronchiolitis in adults. A reversible cause of airway obstruction associated with airway neutrophils and neutrophil products. Am Rev Respir Dis 1989;140:483–92.

41. Dudek AZ, Mahaseth H. Hematopoietic stem cell transplant-related airflow obstruction. Curr Opin Oncol 2006;18:115–9.

42. Yates B, Murphy DM, Forrest IA, et al. Azithromycin reverses airflow obstruction in established bronchiolitis obliterans syndrome. Am J Respir Crit Care Med 2005;172:772–5.

43. Cordier JF. Cryptogenic organizing pneumonitis. Bronchiolitis obliterans organizing pneumonia. Clin Chest Med 1993;14:677–92.

44. Epler GR, Colby TV, McLoud TC, et al. Bronchiolitis obliterans organizing pneumonia. N Engl J Med 1985;312:152–8.

45. Alasaly K, Muller N, Ostrow DN, et al. Cryptogenic organizing pneumonia. A report of 25 cases and a review of the literature. Medicine 1995;74:201–11.

46. King TE. Idiopathic interstitial pneumonias. In: Schwarz MI, King TE, editors. Interstitial lung disease. 4th ed. Hamilton (ON): BC Decker; 2003. p. 701–86.

47. Girod CE, King TE Jr. COPD: a dust-induced disease? Chest 2005;128:3055–64.

48. Fraig M, Shreesha U, Savici D, Katzenstein AL. Respiratory bronchiolitis: a clinicopathologic study in current smokers, ex-smokers, and never-smokers. Am J Surg Pathol 2002;26:647–53.

49. Adesina AM, Vallyathan V, McQuillen EN, et al. Bronchiolar inflammation and fibrosis associated with smoking. A morphologic cross-sectional population analysis. Am Rev Respir Dis 1991;143:144–9.

50. Niewoehner DE, Kleinerman J, Rice DB. Pathologic changes in the peripheral airways of young cigarette smokers. N Engl J Med 1974;291:755–8.

51. Allan PF, Perkins P. A review of respiratory bronchiolitis and respiratory bronchiolitis-associated interstitial lung disease. Clin Pulm Med 2004;11:219–27.

52. Remy-Jardin M, Remy J, Boulenguez C, et al. Morphologic effects of cigarette smoking on airways and pulmonary parenchyma in healthy adult volunteers: CT evaluation and correlation with pulmonary function tests. Radiology 1993;186:107–15.

53. Lynch DA, Travis WD, Muller NL, et al. Idiopathic interstitial pneumonias: CT features. Radiology 2005;236:10–21.

54. Remy-Jardin M, Remy J, Gosselin B, et al. Lung parenchymal changes secondary to cigarette smoking: pathologic-CT correlations. Radiology 1993;186:643–51.

55. Brody AR, Craighead JE. Cytoplasmic inclusions in pulmonary macrophages of cigarette smokers. Lab Invest 1975;32:125–32.

56. Myers JL, Veal CF Jr, Shin MS, Katzenstein AL. Respiratory bronchiolitis causing interstitial lung disease. A clinicopathologic study of six cases. Am Rev Respir Dis 1987;135:880–4.

57. Yousem SA, Colby TV, Gaensler EA. Respiratory bronchiolitis-associated interstitial lung disease and its relationship to desquamative interstitial pneumonia. Mayo Clin Proc 1989;64:1373–80.

58. King TE Jr. Respiratory bronchiolitis-associated interstitial lung disease. Clin Chest Med 1993;14:693–8.

59. Holt RM, Schmidt RA, Godwin JD, Raghu G. High resolution CT in respiratory bronchiolitis-associated interstitial lung disease. J Comput Assist Tomogr 1993;17:46–50.

60. Ryu JH, Myers JL, Capizzi SA, et al. Desquamative interstitial pneumonia and respiratory bronchiolitis-associated interstitial lung disease. Chest 2005;127:178–84.

61. Kaminsky DA, Irvin CG. Anatomic correlates of reversible restrictive lung disease. Chest 1993;103:928–31.

62. Gruden JF, Webb WR. CT findings in a proved case of respiratory bronchiolitis. AJR Am J Roentgenol 1993;161:44–6.

63. Homma S, Kawabata M, Kishi K, et al. Diffuse panbronchiolitis in rheumatoid arthritis. Eur Respir J 1998;12:444–52.

64. Sugiyama Y. Diffuse panbronchiolitis. Clin Chest Med 1993;14:765–72.

65. Keicho N, Ohashi J, Tamiya G, et al. Fine localization of a major disease-susceptibility locus for diffuse panbronchiolitis. Am J Hum Genet 2000;66:501–7.

66. Kamio K, Matsushita I, Hijikata M, et al. Promoter analysis and aberrant expression of the MUC5B gene in diffuse panbronchiolitis. Am J Respir Crit Care Med 2005;171:949–57.

67. Tsang KW, Ooi CG, Ip MS, et al. Clinical profiles of Chinese patients with diffuse panbronchiolitis. Thorax 1998;53:274–80.

68. Martinez JA, Guimaraes SM, Ferreira RG, Pereira CA. Diffuse panbronchiolitis in Latin America. Am J Med Sci 2000;319:183–5.

69. Fitzgerald JE, King TE Jr, Lynch DA, et al. Diffuse panbronchiolitis in the United States. Am J Respir Crit Care Med 1996;154(2 Pt 1):497–503.

70. Fisher MS Jr, Rush WL, Rosado-de-Christenson ML, et al. Diffuse panbronchiolitis: histologic diagnosis in unsuspected cases involving North American residents of Asian descent. Arch Pathol Lab Med 1998;122:156–60.

71. Rubin BK, Henke MO. Immunomodulatory activity and effectiveness of macrolides in chronic airway disease. Chest 2004;125:70S–8S.

72. Abe S, Nakamura H, Inoue S, et al. Interleukin-8 gene repression by clarithromycin is mediated by the activator protein-1 binding site in human bronchial epithelial cells. Am J Respir Cell Mol Biol 2000;22:51–60.

73. Stover DE, Mangino D. Macrolides: a treatment alternative for bronchiolitis obliterans organizing pneumonia? Chest 2005;128:3611–7.

74. Silva CI, Flint JD, Levy RD, Muller NL. Diffuse lung cysts in lymphoid interstitial pneumonia: high-resolution CT and pathologic findings. J Thorac Imaging 2006;21:241–4.

75. Howling SJ, Hansell DM, Wells AU, et al. Follicular bronchiolitis: thin-section CT and histologic findings. Radiology 1999;212:637–42.

76. Garshick E, Schenker MB, Dosman JA. Occupationally induced airways obstruction. Med Clin North Am 1996;80:851–78.

77. Churg A, Wright JL. Airway wall remodeling induced by occupational mineral dusts and air pollutant particles. Chest 2002;122:306S–9S.

78. Niku S, Stark P, Levin DL, Friedman PJ. Lymphangioleiomyomatosis: clinical, pathologic, and radiologic manifestations. J Thorac Imaging 2005;20:98–102.

79. Taveira-DaSilva AM, Stylianou MP, Hedin CJ, et al. Decline in lung function in patients with lymphangioleiomyomatosis treated with or without progesterone. Chest 2004;126:1867–74.

80. Kristoff AS, Moss J. Lymphangioleiomyomatosis. In: Schwarz MI, King TE, editors. Interstitial lung disease. 4th ed. Hamilton (ON): BC Decker; 2003. p. 851–64.

81. Johnson S. Rare diseases 1: lymphangioleiomyomatosis: clinical features, management and basic mechanisms. Thorax 1999;54:254–64.

82. Webb WR. High-resolution computed tomography of obstructive lung disease. Radiol Clin North Am 1994;32:745–57.

83. Oh YM, Mo EK, Jang SH, et al. Pulmonary lymphangioleiomyomatosis in Korea. Thorax 1999;54:618–21.

84. Sullivan EJ. Lymphangioleiomyomatosis: a review. Chest 1998;114:1689–703.

85. Ryu JH, Moss J, Beck GJ, et al. The NHLBI Lymphangioleiomyomatosis Registry: characteristics of 230 patients at enrollment. Am J Respir Crit Care Med 2006;173:105–11.

86. Baldi S, Papotti M, Valente ML, et al. Pulmonary lymphangioleiomyomatosis in postmenopausal women: report of two cases and review of the literature. Eur Respir J 1994;7:1013–6.

87. Almoosa KF, Ryu JH, Mendez J, et al. Management of pneumothorax in lymphangioleiomyomatosis: effects on recurrence and lung transplantation complications. Chest 2006;129:1274–81.

88. Cohen MM, Pollock-BarZiv S, Johnson SR. Emerging clinical picture of lymphangioleiomyomatosis. Thorax 2005;60:875–9.

89. Crino PB, Nathanson KL, Henske EP. The tuberous sclerosis complex. N Engl J Med 2006;355:1345–56.

90. Bonetti F, Chiodera P. Lymphangioleiomyomatosis and tuberous sclerosis: where is the border? Eur Respir J 1996;9:399–401.

91. Smolarek TA, Wessner LL, McCormack FX, et al. Evidence that lymphangiomyomatosis is caused by TSC2 mutations: chromosome 16p13 loss of heterozygosity in angiomyolipomas and lymph nodes from women with lymphangiomyomatosis. Am J Hum Genet 1998;62:810–5.

92. Moses MA, Harper J, Folkman J. Doxycycline treatment for lymphangioleiomyomatosis with urinary monitoring for MMPs. N Engl J Med 2006;354:2621–2.

93. Guinee DG Jr, Feuerstein I, Koss MN, Travis WD. Pulmonary lymphangioleiomyomatosis. Diagnosis based on results of transbronchial biopsy and immunohistochemical studies and correlation with high-resolution computed tomography findings. Arch Pathol Lab Med 1994;118:846–9.

94. Taylor JR, Ryu J, Colby TV, Raffin TA. Lymphangioleiomyomatosis. Clinical course in 32 patients. N Engl J Med 1990;323:1254–60.

95. Vassallo R, Ryu JH, Colby TV, et al. Pulmonary Langerhans'-cell histiocytosis. N Engl J Med 2000;342:1969–78.

96. Vassallo R, Limper AH. Pulmonary Langerhans cell histiocytosis. In: Schwarz MI, King TE, editors. Interstitial lung disease. 4th ed. Hamilton (ON): BC Decker; 2003. p. 838–50.

97. Aubry MC, Wright JL, Myers JL. The pathology of smoking-related lung diseases. Clin Chest Med 2000;21:11–35, vii.

98. Abbott GF, Rosado-de-Christenson ML, Franks TJ, et al. From the archives of the AFIP: pulmonary Langerhans cell histiocytosis. Radiographics 2004;24:821–41.

99. Murin S, Bilello KS, Matthay R. Other smoking-affected pulmonary diseases. Clin Chest Med 2000;21:121–37, ix.

100. Friedman PJ, Liebow AA, Sokoloff J. Eosinophilic granuloma of lung. Clinical aspects of primary histiocytosis in the adult. Medicine 1981;60:385–96.

101. Sundar KM, Gosselin MV, Chung HL, Cahill BC. Pulmonary Langerhans cell histiocytosis: emerging concepts in pathobiology, radiology, and clinical evolution of disease. Chest 2003;123:1673–83.

102. Muller NL. Computed tomography in chronic interstitial lung disease. Radiol Clin North Am 1991;29:1085–93.

103. Brauner MW, Grenier P, Tijani K, et al. Pulmonary Langerhans cell histiocytosis: evolution of lesions on CT scans. Radiology 1997;204:497–502.

104. Housini I, Tomashefski JF Jr, Cohen A, et al. Transbronchial biopsy in patients with pulmonary eosinophilic granuloma. Comparison with findings on open lung biopsy. Arch Pathol Lab Med 1994;118:523–30.

105. Vassallo R, Ryu JH, Schroeder DR, et al. Clinical outcomes of pulmonary Langerhans'-cell histiocytosis in adults. N Engl J Med 2002;346:484–90.

106. Schwarz MI, Mortenson RL, Colby TV, et al. Pulmonary capillaritis. The association with progressive irreversible airflow limitation and hyperinflation. Am Rev Respir Dis 1993;148:507–11.

107. Brugiere O, Raffy O, Sleiman C, et al. Progressive obstructive lung disease associated with microscopic polyangiitis. Am J Respir Crit Care Med 1997;155:739–42.

108. Wisnieski JJ, Baer AN, Christensen J, et al. Hypocomplementemic urticarial vasculitis syndrome. Clinical and serologic findings in 18 patients. Medicine 1995;74:24–41.

109. Hunt DP, Weil R, Nicholson AG, et al. Pulmonary capillaritis and its relationship to development of emphysema in hypocomplementaemic urticarial vasculitis syndrome. Sarcoidosis Vasc Diffuse Lung Dis 2006;23:70–2.

110. Wright PH, Buxton-Thomas M, Keeling PW, Kreel L. Adult idiopathic pulmonary haemosiderosis: a comparison of lung function changes and the distribution of pulmonary disease in patients with and without coeliac disease. Br J Dis Chest 1983;77:282–92.

CHAPTER 14

Bacterial Infection in Chronic Obstructive Pulmonary Disease

Sanjay Sethi, MD

Several potential contributions of bacterial infection to the etiology, pathogenesis, and the clinical course of chronic obstructive pulmonary disease (COPD) can be identified.[1] However, the precise role of bacterial infection in COPD has been a source of controversy for several decades.[2–4] Opinion has ranged from a preeminent role (along with mucus hypersecretion) as embodied in the British hypothesis in the 1950s and 1960s to bacterial infection being regarded as a mere epiphenomenon in the 1970s and 1980s.[2–4] In the last two decades, modern research techniques have shed new light on the contribution of bacterial infection to this disease.

Five potential pathways by which bacteria could contribute to the etiopathogenesis of COPD can be identified as follows: (1) childhood lower respiratory tract infection impairs lung growth reflected in smaller lung volumes in adulthood; (2) bacteria cause a substantial proportion of acute exacerbations of COPD, with consequent morbidity and mortality; (3) chronic colonization of the lower respiratory tract by bacterial pathogens amplifies the chronic airway inflammation present in COPD and accelerates progressive airway obstruction (vicious circle hypothesis); (4) bacterial pathogens invade and persist in respiratory tissues, alter the host response to cigarette smoke, or induce a chronic inflammatory response and thus contribute to the pathogenesis of COPD; (5) bacterial antigens in the lower airway induce hypersensitivity that enhances airway hyperreactivity and induces eosinophilic inflammation. These pathways are used as a framework to discuss the potential roles of bacterial infection in this chapter, with an emphasis on information gained from newer research techniques in the last two decades.

Childhood Lower Respiratory Tract Infection and Adult Lung Function

Four cross-sectional studies have reported lung function (measured by spirometry) in cohorts of adult patients for whom reliable information was available regarding the incidence of lower respiratory tract infection (bronchitis, pneumonia, whooping cough) in childhood (<14 years of age) (Table 1).[5–8] These studies have consistently shown a lower forced expiratory volume in 1 second (FEV_1) and often a lower forced vital capacity (FVC) in association with a history of childhood lower respiratory tract infection, after controlling for confounding factors such as tobacco exposure.[5–8] The magnitude of this defect in FEV_1 tends to be greater in older cohorts but is not large enough to cause symptomatic pulmonary disease by itself. However, this defect in FEV_1 could make the individual susceptible to the effects of additional injurious agents such as tobacco smoke and environmental or occupational exposure to airborne pollutants. The defect in lung function is not obstructive as the FEV_1 to FVC ratio is preserved. Instead, it is consistent with "smaller lungs," suggesting impaired lung growth. This is supported by recent observations by Marossy and colleagues that the decline in FEV_1 between the ages of 35 and 45 years in the British birth cohort was not faster in those with a history of childhood lower respiratory tract illness.[9]

Although the association between childhood lower respiratory tract infection and impaired lung function in adulthood is now well established, there is ongoing debate as to whether a cause-and-effect relationship exists. Such a relationship could be due to damage to a vulnerable lung undergoing rapid postnatal growth and maturation by the infectious process. If this was the case, then the effect of infection on lung function should be seen only in the first 2 years of life, the major period of postnatal lung growth, and not in later childhood (3–14 years). However, this has not been a consistent observation in the studies to date.[5–8] An alternative explanation for the observed association is that an undetermined genetic factor predisposes these individuals to lower respiratory tract infections in childhood and a lower FEV_1 in adulthood. This explanation implies that impaired lung growth antedates the respiratory tract infection, with the infectious episode being a marker of the vulnerability of smaller lungs to infection in childhood.

The etiology of childhood lower respiratory tract infection was not established in these studies; therefore, whether the impact of viral infection differs from bacterial infection is not known. Although a substantial proportion of childhood respiratory infections are viral, bacterial infections, especially with *Streptococcus pneumoniae* and *Haemophilus influenzae*, are common causes of severe pneumonia in children.[10] The impact of childhood bacterial lower respiratory tract infection on lung growth and therefore the prevalence of COPD is likely to be greater in developing countries, where such infections are common and often inadequately treated.

Table 1 Association of Childhood Lower Respiratory Tract Infection with Lung Function in Adults				
Study	n	Childhood Lower Respiratory Tract Infection	Age at Follow-up (yr)	Effect on Forced Expiratory Volume in 1 s
Barker et al, 1991[5]	639 (all male)	Bronchitis or pneumonia in first yr	59–67	↓ 200 mL
Shaheen et al, 1995[7]	618	Pneumonia in first 2 yr Bronchitis in first 2 yr	67–74	↓ 650 mL (in males with pneumonia)
Johnston et al, 1998[6]	1,392	Pneumonia in first 7 yr Whooping cough in first 7 yr	34–35yr	↓ 102 mL (with pneumonia)
Shaheen et al, 1998[8]	239	Pneumonia in first 14 yr Bronchitis in first 14 yr	57.6 ± 4.3yr	↓ 390 mL (with pneumonia in first 2 yr) ↓ 130 mL (with bronchitis in first 2 yr)

Bacterial Pathogens as a Cause of Acute Exacerbations of COPD

Bacteria are isolated from sputum in 40 to 60% of acute exacerbations of COPD.[11] Table 2 summarizes the sputum bacteriology obtained in 14 clinical trials of antibiotics in acute exacerbations.[12–25] These studies enrolled 9,614 patients. Variation in the relative incidence of specific pathogens may relate to patient inclusion criteria and sputum culture techniques. The three predominant bacterial species isolated are nontypeable *H. influenzae*, *Moraxella catarrhalis*, and *S. pneumoniae* (Figure 1). Other less frequently isolated potential pathogens are *Haemophilus parainfluenzae*, *Staphylococcus aureus*, *Pseudomonas aeruginosa*, and gram-negative enterobacteria. More recent trials than those included in the table demonstrate a similar incidence and pattern of sputum bacteriology in exacerbations.[26–32]

Whether isolation from sputum of a potential pathogen represents infection of the lower airway causing the exacerbation has been a controversial issue for several decades. In the 1950s and 1960s, the British hypothesis of the pathogenesis of COPD included as major contributors recurrent bacterial infection and mucus hypersecretion.[33] Several longitudinal cohort studies in the 1960s and 1970s demonstrated that the incidence of bacterial isolation from sputum was not greater during exacerbations of COPD than during stable

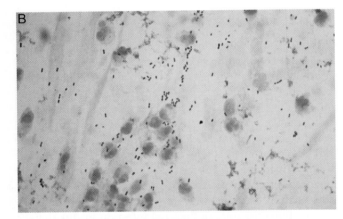

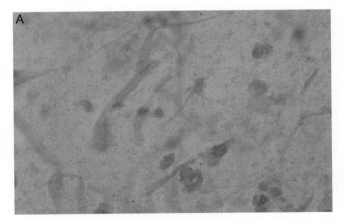

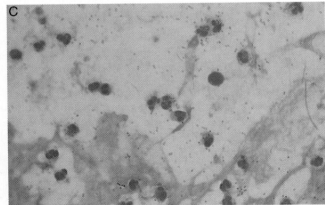

FIGURE 1. Gram-stained smears of sputum specimens obtained during acute exacerbations of chronic obstructive pulmonary disease demonstrating the three predominant bacterial pathogens: *A*, nontypeable *Haemophilus influenzae*; *B*, *Streptococcus pneumoniae*; *C*, *Moraxella (Branhamella) catarrhalis*.

Table 2 Bacterial Pathogens Isolated from Sputum in Recent Studies of Acute Exacerbation of Chronic Bronchitis

	No. of Patients	% Sputum Culture + for PPB*	Total Bacterial Isolates (%)						
			Nontypeable *Haemophilus influenzae*	*Streptococcus pneumoniae*	*Moraxella catarrhalis*	Entero-bacteria	*Haemophilus parainfluenzae*	*Staphylococcus aureus*	*Pseudomonas aeruginosa*
Mean	687	53.7	31.2	14.2	14	11.4	9.4	6.4	5.8
Range	140–2,180	28.1–88.6	13–50	7–26	4–21	3–19	0–32	1–20	1–13

Adapted from references 12 to 25.
*Potentially pathogenic bacteria.

disease.[34,35] These studies also failed to demonstrate an increase in bacterial titers in sputum during acute exacerbations.[34] Serologic studies conducted in the same time period of serum antibody titers to bacterial pathogens such as nontypeable *H. influenzae* in patients with COPD compared with controls arrived at contradictory conclusions.[1] The results of placebo-controlled antibiotic trials in acute exacerbations have also been inconsistent, demonstrating either a small or no benefit with antibiotic therapy.[36,37]

One interpretation of these observations has been that isolation of bacteria from sputum during exacerbations represents chronic colonization, an "innocent bystander" role.[3,4,38,39] Alternative explanations for the contradictory observations from serologic studies and antibiotic therapy should be considered.[1,40] In the last decade, several investigators have reexamined the issue of whether bacteria cause acute exacerbations of COPD using either new diagnostic modalities or research techniques (Table 3). These methods provide a more rigorous evaluation of the etiology of exacerbations.

Bronchoscopic Sampling of the Lower Respiratory Tract in Exacerbations of COPD

An attractive approach to understanding the role of bacterial infection in exacerbations of COPD is to determine bacterial concentrations in the distal airways by quantitative culture of distal airway secretions obtained by protected specimen brush (PSB) or by bronchoalveolar lavage (BAL). Samples obtained from the distal airways with these techniques are

Table 3 New Approaches to Understanding the Role of Bacteria in Exacerbations of Chronic Obstructive Pulmonary Disease

Bronchoscopic sampling of the lower respiratory tract

Molecular epidemiology of bacterial pathogens

Immune response to bacterial pathogens in exacerbations

Airway inflammation measurement and correlation with bacteriology

Antibiotic trials with better design and unconventional end points

uncontaminated by upper respiratory tract secretions. Furthermore, bacterial concentrations above certain thresholds on quantitative culture of these samples correlate with tissue infection in patients with pneumonia.[41] Four studies that have used this methodology in acute exacerbations of COPD have consistently shown significant bacterial concentrations in the distal airways in approximately 50% of patients experiencing an exacerbation (Table 4).[38,42–44] Bacterial species isolated in these studies mirror those commonly isolated from sputum cultures.

Rosell and colleagues recently performed a pooled analysis of bronchoscopic PSB cultures in controls, stable COPD, and exacerbations of COPD performed in different studies published between 1993 and 2002.[45] The presence of potentially pathogenic microorganisms of at least 100 colony-forming units/mL was 4% in healthy controls, 29% in stable COPD, and 54% during exacerbation. Furthermore, high microbial load defined as at least 10,000 colony-forming units/mL was seen in 1% of healthy controls, 8% of stable patients, and 21% of patients with exacerbations (Figure 2).[45] The spectrum of pathogens isolated in stable disease and exacerbations was similar. In a more severely ill population of patients placed on

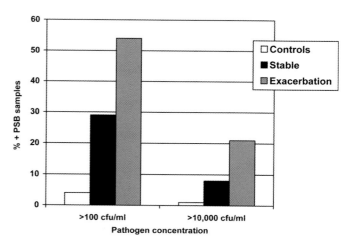

FIGURE 2. Culture results of bronchoscopic samples obtained from healthy controls, in stable chronic obstructive pulmonary disease (COPD), and during exacerbations of COPD. Adapted from Rosell and colleagues.[45] cfu/ml = colony-forming units of pathogenic bacteria per milliliter of PSB sample; PSB = protected specimen brush.

				Bacterial Pathogens Isolated						
Study	*Subjects*	*Diagnostic Methods*	*Bacterial Pathogen Present*	*H. influenzae*	*M. catarrhalis*	*S. pneumoniae*	*H. para influenzae*	*P. aeruginosa*	Other Gram Negative	Other Gram Positive
Fagon et al[38]	50 ICU Patients on ventilator	Protected specimen brush	50*	6	3	7	11	3	5	9
Monso et al[42]	29 outpatients	Protected specimen brush	51.7	10	2	3	—	2	—	—
Soler et al[44]	50 ICU Patients on ventilator	Protected specimen brush, BAL, endotracheal aspirate	56†	11	4	4	—	9	6	—
Pela et al[43]	40 outpatients	Protected specimen brush	52.5	1	2	10	1	—	1	7

Table 4 Bronchoscopic Studies in Acute Exacerbations of Chronic Obstructive Pulmonary Disease

BAL = bronchoalveolar lavage; ICU = intensive care unit.
*≥ 10^2 colony-forming units/mL was used to define a positive culture instead of the usual ι ^{103} colony-forming units/mL.
†21 patients had antimicrobial therapy in the 24 hours prior to admission to the ICU.

mechanical ventilation for an acute exacerbation, the distribution of specific bacterial pathogens isolated from the distal airways is remarkable for a large proportion of *P. aeruginosa* and other gram-negative bacilli (14 of 50; 28%).[44] Two studies using sputum cultures have also demonstrated an increasing frequency of isolation of these groups of pathogens in exacerbations of severe COPD.[46,47] Whether this is due to environmental factors (such as antibiotic selection pressure or exposure to hospital flora from frequent exacerbations) or is related to a greater degree of host immune compromise is not clear. Furthermore, among patients receiving noninvasive ventilation for severe exacerbations, Ferrer and colleagues found that the presence of nonfermenting gram-negative bacteria (predominantly *P. aeruginosa*) in sputum was clearly associated with clinical failure of noninvasive ventilation.[48]

In a recent interesting study, Soler and colleagues demonstrated a very close correlation between positive PSB cultures and sputum purulence by history at the time of exacerbation.[49] When sputum purulence was present, 77% of bronchoscopic cultures yielded significant bacterial growth, whereas in the absence of sputum purulence, the proportion of positive PSB cultures decreased to 6%. Such clinical correlation of the presence of bacteria in bronchoscopic cultures at exacerbation implies that such isolation represents true infection.

The consistent rate of isolation of pathogenic bacteria in the bronchoscopic studies at exacerbation, the increased rate of isolation of pathogenic bacteria during exacerbations compared to clinically stable periods, and the clinical correlation of positive bronchoscopic cultures with sputum purulence support the pathogenic role of bacteria in a proportion of exacerbations of COPD.

Bacterial Pathogenesis of Exacerbation: New Model

Changes in bacterial concentration (or load) in the airways have been proposed to explain how bacteria cause exacerbations in the face of chronic colonization.[50] In a recent study, we compared bacterial pathogen titers in sputum culture from a large number of sputum samples obtained in a prospective observational cohort study.[50] We were unable to find increased titers of bacteria at exacerbation compared to a stable state, especially in strains that were already present in sputum before the onset of the exacerbation. These data suggest that increased airway bacterial load alone is unlikely to represent the primary mechanism of bacterial exacerbation in COPD.

Advances in our understanding of bacterial pathogenesis have made it clear that previous studies in bacterial infection in exacerbations had used methods that would be considered inadequate by current standards.[51,52] Recent observations with newer molecular and immunologic techniques on the bacterial pathogenesis of exacerbations form the basis of a new model of bacterial exacerbation pathogenesis (Figure 3). Rather than an increase in airway bacterial load, the major initiating factor for exacerbations is acquisition of new strains from the environment of *H. influenzae*, *M. catarrhalis*, and *S. pneumoniae*. These three species of bacteria, which are predominant causes of most upper and lower respiratory infections, are exclusively human pathogens whose natural niche is colonization of the upper respiratory tract. They are readily exchanged among humans by aerosolization and fomite transfer. However, when acquired by patients with abnormalities in host defense in the respiratory tract, such as COPD, these bacteria cause mucosal and, occasionally, systemic infections. Evidence to support individual components of this pathogenetic model is presented below.

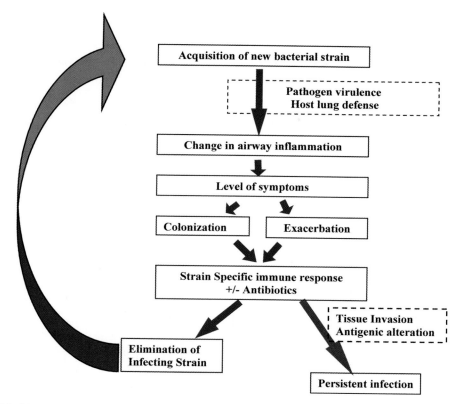

FIGURE 3. Proposed model of bacterial infection in chronic obstructive pulmonary diseaes. Reproduced with permission from Veeramachaneni SB and Sethi S.[119]

Acquisition of New Strains of Bacteria and Exacerbation

Variation in the antigenic structure among strains of a bacterial species is now understood to be a major mechanism for the evasion of the human immune response and causation of bacterial infection.[51,52] Therefore, simply culturing and enumerating colony counts of pathogens from bodily fluids are inadequate in understanding this infectious process, as was done in several older longitudinal cohort investigations conducted to elucidate the role of bacteria in exacerbations of COPD.[35,53] A recent longitudinal COPD cohort study has addressed the limitations of previous studies and better elucidated the dynamics of bacterial infection in this disease.[54] In this study, strains of potential respiratory pathogens isolated from sputum were characterized by molecular techniques, to identify when new strains were acquired by a patient and when those strains were cleared from the respiratory tract. Using this approach, acquisition of new strains of certain bacterial species was found to be clearly associated with a greater than twofold increased risk of exacerbation (Figure 4, Table 5).[54] The time frame of increased risk appears to be up to 4 to 8 weeks after acquisition of a new strain. By pathogen, increased risk of exacerbations with new strain acquisition was seen for *H. influenzae*, *M. catarrhalis*, and *S. pneumoniae* but not for *P. aeruginosa* (see Table 5). Strain

characterization for *H. parainfluenzae*, *S. aureus*, and Enterobacteriaceae was not performed in this study.

Pathogen Virulence as a Determinant of Exacerbation

As in most infectious diseases, a complex host-pathogen interaction likely determines the outcome of each new bacterial strain acquisition in COPD. Therefore, it is not surprising that not every new strain acquisition of bacterial pathogens is associated with exacerbation. Conceptually, the balance between host defense and pathogen virulence determines the level of airway inflammation induced by the pathogen, which, in turn, determines the level of symptoms in the patient (see Figure 3). To add to the complexity, patient perception and physician interpretation of symptoms are additional determinants of exacerbation.

Although *H. influenzae*, *M. catarrhalis*, and *S. pneumoniae* are well-recognized respiratory pathogens, their virulence determinants in airway mucosal infection are not well described. Putative pathogen virulence factors include adhesion to and invasion of airway epithelial cells, inactivation of host defense mechanisms, and elicitation of inflammatory mediators from airway cells. Chin and colleagues compared (using *in-vitro* and *in-vivo* models) the virulence of well-characterized *H. influenzae* strains that were isolated from the

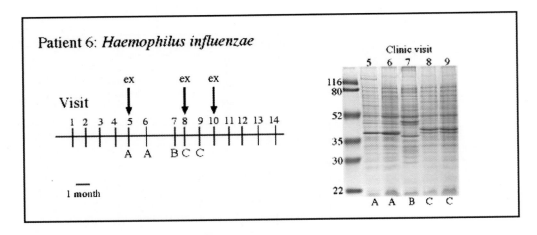

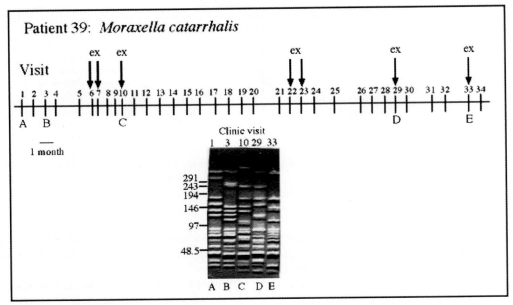

FIGURE 4. Timelines and molecular typing for patients with chronic obstructive pulmonary disease. The *horizontal line* is a timeline, with each number indicating a clinic visit The *arrows* indicate exacerbations. Isolates of H. *influenzae* and M. *catarrhalis* were assigned types based on sodium dodecyl sulfate–polyacrylamide gel and pulsed-field gel electrophoresis, respectively. The types are indicated by letters *A* to *E*. Molecular mass standards are noted on the left of the gels. Reproduced with permission from Sethi S et al.[54] Sethi S, Evans N, Grant BJB, Murphy TF. Acquisition of a new bacterial strain and occurrence of exacerbations of chronic obstructive pulmonary disease. N Engl J Med 2002;347:465–71. Copyright © Massachusetts Medical Society. All rights reserved.

Table 5 Isolation of a New Strain of a Bacterial Pathogen Increases the Risk of Exacerbation of Chronic Obstructive Pulmonary Disease

New Strain	Relative Risk of Exacerbation	95% Confidence Interval of Relative Risk
Any pathogen	2.15	1.83–2.53
H. influenzae	1.69	1.37–2.09
M. catarrhalis	2.96	2.39–3.67
S. pneumoniae	1.77	1.14–2.75
P. aeruginosa	0.61	0.21–1.82

Adapted from Sethi S et al.[54]

sputum of patients in the COPD cohort study discussed above.[55] Strains isolated during exacerbations were compared with colonizing strains. Exacerbation strains induced greater airway neutrophil recruitment in a mouse pulmonary clearance model than colonizing strains. Furthermore, exacerbation strains adhered in significantly higher numbers to and elicited more interleukin (IL)-8 from primary airway human airway epithelial cells in culture when compared with colonizing strains.

Strains of *H. influenzae* associated with symptomatic infection are more likely to produce immunoglobulin (Ig)A protease than strains that colonize the nasopharynx.[56] Exacerbation and colonizing strains of *H. influenzae* from the above-mentioned COPD cohort study were compared with a genomics approach to determine if genetic differences underlie the pathogenic potential of these strains. A specific combination of genes was found to be related to exacerbation.[57] One of these genes is a novel IgA protease, suggesting that inactivation of host defenses is an important determinant of disease expression among bacterial strains. These observations support pathogen virulence as an important determinant of clinical manifestations of new bacterial strain acquisition in COPD. However, our understanding of pathogen virulence with relevance to COPD is still in its infancy, and additional observations are needed.

Host Defense as a Determinant of Exacerbations

There appears to be a failure of innate lung defense mechanisms in COPD, allowing bacterial proliferation and persistence in the lower airways. This elicits adaptive immune responses to control and eradicate the infection. When immune responses to new strains of *M. catarrhalis* associated with COPD exacerbation and colonization were compared, a mucosal IgA response to the infecting strain was more common and vigorous with colonization, whereas a systemic IgG immune response was more common and vigorous with exacerbations.[58] Therefore, the pattern of host immune response could dictate the clinical expression of a bacterial strain acquisition in COPD. A vigorous mucosal IgA response could "exclude" the bacteria from interaction with the epithelial mucosa, resulting in less airway inflammation and therefore favoring colonization. An alternative explanation is that the clinical scenario determines the consequent immune response, with colonization resulting in more of a mucosal than a systemic antigen burden. Further studies to determine which of these mechanisms are operational in COPD are being performed.

Systemic cellular host defense and exacerbation occurrence in COPD also appear to be related when peripheral blood mononuclear cell proliferation on exposure to a conserved *H. influenzae* antigen, outer membrane protein P6, was examined. A history of exacerbation with *H. influenzae* in the preceding 12 months among patients with COPD was associated with a diminished response to P6.[59] COPD patients who had not experienced such *H. influenzae* exacerbations had proliferative responses to P6 that were comparable to those of healthy controls. One can speculate that a normal cellular response to *H. influenzae* antigens suppresses or even eradicates newly acquired strains of *H. influenzae* and therefore prevents infection. Enhanced understanding of the determinants of host immune response that influence the outcome of a bacterial acquisition in a patient with COPD is essential and could yield new and unique approaches to prevent and treat exacerbations.

Airway Inflammation as a Determinant of Exacerbation

Several studies now clearly support the concept that exacerbations of COPD are inflammatory events, with both airway and systemic inflammation seen. However, this inflammatory process is not uniform among exacerbations and is related to the etiology of the exacerbation. In most studies, exacerbations associated with bacterial pathogens exhibit significantly more neutrophilic inflammation than nonbacterial episodes.[60,61] Specifically, when compared with nonbacterial exacerbations, higher levels of IL-8, tumor necrosis factor α (TNF-α), and neutrophil elastase (NE) were seen in exacerbations associated with *H. influenzae*, whereas significantly higher TNF-α and NE were seen in exacerbations associated with *M. catarrhalis*.[60] Airway bacterial concentrations and intensity of neutrophilic inflammation are also related, suggesting a stimulus-response relationship.[60,61] Furthermore, a significant correlation between the clinical severity of an exacerbation and the level of sputum NE has been demonstrated.[61]

Resolution of symptoms of exacerbations associated with purulent sputum is associated with a consistent decrease in neutrophilic airway inflammation, as measured in levels of sputum IL-8, leukotriene B$_4$ (LTB$_4$), NE, and myeloperoxidase (MPO).[62] Furthermore, a more marked reduction in airway inflammation is seen when such clinical resolution is accompanied by bacteriologic eradication of the offending pathogen, compared with when bacterial pathogens persist in the airway in spite of clinical resolution.[62] Papi and colleagues, in a recent study, observed a relationship between eosinophilic inflammation and the presence of viral infection as a cause of COPD.[63] This observation may explain the efficacy of systemic steroids in the treatment of exacerbations.

Lower airway bacterial "colonization" in the absence of increased symptoms is also associated with airway inflammation (see below). The model in Figure 3 would suggest that this inflammatory response would be of a lesser magnitude than that elicited during exacerbations; however, direct evidence for this concept is not available.

Strain-Specific Immune Response

Development of an adaptive immune response is strong evidence of an infective process. However, to reliably study immune response to bacterial infection, several considerations in the experimental design have emerged. Infecting (homologous) strains responsible should be used as the antigen to account for antigenic diversity among strains. To account for baseline antibodies, samples (serum or mucosal secretions) obtained after infection should be compared with preinfection samples to clearly distinguish antibodies that develop following infection. The results can also be confounded by cross-reactive antibodies, which often bind to non-surface-exposed epitopes of bacteria. Therefore, the immunoassays used should be specific for antibodies that bind to surface antigens of the bacterial pathogen.[1,32]

Recent studies in which these design criteria were met have clearly demonstrated the development of antibodies that bind to the bacterial cell surface following exacerbations of COPD associated with *H. influenzae*, *M. catarrhalis*, and *S. pneumoniae*, as well as following colonization with *M. catarrhalis*.[58,64,65] Furthermore, for *H. influenzae*, these antibodies have been demonstrated to be bactericidal for the infecting strain but to have a strong degree of strain specificity (Figure 5). This strain specificity likely allows other strains of *H. influenzae* with antigenically diverse surface antigens to infect the same patient and cause exacerbations. Strain-specificity of the antibodies directed against *M. catarrhalis* and *S. pneumoniae* has not been directly demonstrated. However, it is likely present based on the susceptibility of these patients to recurrent infection with the same species.

Development of adaptive immune responses following exacerbation with these respiratory bacterial pathogens supports the pathogenic role of these organisms in the lower airway. The strain specificity of these immune responses accounts for the recurrent exacerbations seen in COPD.

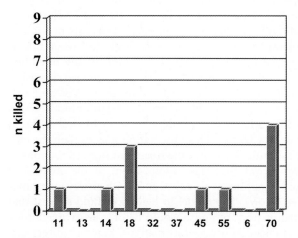

FIGURE 5. Sera obtained after exacerbation from 10 patients that were bactericidal for the infecting strain were tested in bactericidal assays with a panel of nine heterologous strains. The y axis shows the number of heterologous strains killed with each of the 10 sera. Adapted from Sethi S et al[65] and reproduced with permission from Sethi S: New developments in the pathogenesis of acute exacerbations of chronic obstructive pulmonary disease. Curr Opin Infect Dis 2004;17:113–9. © Lippincott, Williams and Wilkins.[120]

Other Potential Mechanisms of Bacterial Exacerbations

P. aeruginosa, a significant airway pathogen in bronchiectasis and cystic fibrosis, is regularly seen in sputum and bronchoscopic samples in COPD exacerbations, usually with underlying moderate or severe airflow obstruction. As discussed above, isolation of this pathogen in severe exacerbations is associated with worse outcomes.[48] However, an association between exacerbations and new strain isolation was not identified for *P. aeruginosa* in COPD and in cystic fibrosis.[54,66] This suggests alternative mechanisms underlying exacerbations owing to this pathogen. Biofilms are complex communities enclosed in matrix of extracellular polymeric substances. *P. aeruginosa* forms biofilms in the airways in cystic fibrosis, and a change from this biofilm state to a free-floating planktonic state has been associated with exacerbations of this disease.[67] *H. influenzae* can also form biofilms *in vitro* and in the airways of cystic fibrosis. It is possible that biofilm formation by these pathogens is prevalent in COPD airways and is a mechanism of persistence and exacerbations.

Other gram-negative enteric bacteria and *S. aureus* are often isolated from sputum during exacerbations. They also have been found in bronchoscopic samples obtained during exacerbations of severe COPD.[44] Data regarding strain changes and immune and inflammatory responses to these pathogens are unavailable. Therefore, whether these pathogens cause exacerbations and the mechanism of such exacerbations are unclear.

Vicious Circle Hypothesis

A small proportion (30–40%) of smokers develops COPD. Susceptibility to tobacco smoke could be due to one or more cofactors that contribute to the pathogenesis of COPD, which include genetic predisposition, nutritional factors, chronic infection, and autoimmunity. The healthy human tracheobronchial tree and lung parenchyma have a remarkable ability to maintain sterility, in spite of repetitive exposure to microbial inocula from microaspiration and inhalation. Maintenance of a sterile lung is dependent on a very efficient innate lung defense system, which is multifaceted and redundant. Disruption of this innate immunity would permit recurrent or chronic lung infections. COPD appears to be one such disease in which the innate lung defense appears to be disrupted because both recurrent acute and chronic infections are seen in almost all patients with this disease. Several years ago, we proposed a "vicious circle hypothesis" to explain how chronic bacterial "colonization" of the lower airways in patients with COPD can perpetuate inflammation and contribute to progression of the disease.[1,68] An updated version of this hypothesis is shown in Figure 6, and *in-vitro* and *in-vivo* evidence supporting this hypothesis are discussed. Several microbial pathogens, including typical bacteria, *Chlamydia*, *Pneumocystis*, and viruses, have been shown to colonize the lung in COPD and may contribute to COPD pathogenesis.[69–73] This discussion is confined to typical bacteria.

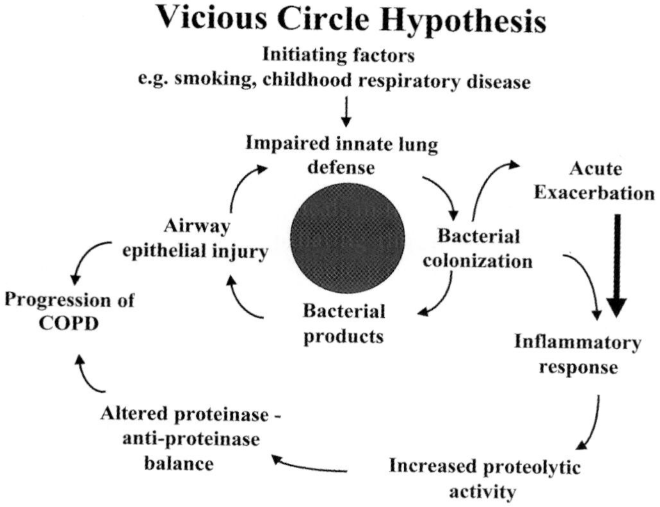

Vicious Circle Hypothesis

Initiating factors
e.g. smoking, childhood respiratory disease

FIGURE 6. Diagrammatic representation of the vicious circle hypothesis of how bacterial colonization and exacerbations contribute to the progression of chronic obstructive pulmonary disease (COPD). Reproduced with permission from Eldika N and Sethi S: Role of nontypeable haemophilus influenzae in exacerbations and progression of chronic obstructive pulmonary disease. Curr Opin Pulm Med 2006;12:118–24. © Lippincott, Williams and Wilkins.[121]

The presence of microbial pathogens in the lower airway in COPD when the patient is at his or her baseline level of symptoms (ie, stable) is usually referred to as colonization. This terminology implies that the presence of bacteria in the lower airway in stable COPD is innocuous and therefore does not require further investigation or treatment. As discussed below, based on growing evidence, this may not be the case; therefore, the term *colonization* is likely inappropriate. The presence of a microbial pathogen in a host is appropriately referred to as colonization when there is no host immune response to the pathogen and no evidence that the microbial pathogen is damaging the host. Therefore, the absence of increased symptoms of exacerbation does not satisfy the above criteria.

Mechanisms of Chronic Microbial Colonization in COPD

Several components of the lung defense appear to be compromised in COPD and could allow bacterial colonization. Bacterial colonization and its associated inflammation, in turn, could worsen lung defense mechanisms, thereby allowing bacterial persistence and setting up the vicious circle.

A major mechanism that maintains the sterility of the normal tracheobronchial tree is the mucociliary escalator, by effectively trapping and clearing particles.[74] Vastag and colleagues showed that abnormal mucociliary clearance was universal in moderate and heavy smokers, although there was large variability in the degree of impairment.[75] Bacteria, viruses, and particulate matter can enter the tracheobronchial tree by inhalation and by microaspiration of oropharyngeal contents during sleep.[76] Inadequate mucociliary clearance would allow these agents to persist in the respiratory tract and interact with airway epithelial cells and macrophages, leading to an inflammatory response.

Impairment of mucociliary clearance can be due to enhanced mucus secretion, disruption of normal ciliary activity, and airway epithelial injury. Experimental evidence demonstrates that respiratory tract pathogens and their products can cause all of these effects *in vitro*. Cell-free filtrates of broth cultures of some strains of nontypeable *H. influenzae*, *S. pneumoniae*, and *P. aeruginosa* stimulate secretion of mucous glycoproteins by explanted guinea pig airway tissue.[77] This stimulation is a true secretory effect and not passive release of preformed intracellular macromolecules owing to cellular damage. The *Pseudomonas* stimulatory products are 60 to 100 kDa proteases. The *Haemophilus* and pneumococcal stimulatory exoproducts are 50 to 300 kDa in size and do not possess proteolytic activity. Cell-free supernatants of nontypeable *H. influenzae* and *P. aeruginosa* rapidly inhibit ciliary beat frequency of strips of human nasal ciliary epithelium by inducing ciliary dyskinesia and ciliostasis.[78] Human NE inhibits ciliary activity and damages respiratory epithelium.[79,80] Bacterial products in the airways may be a potent stimulus for neutrophil migration into the airways, and elastase released from these neutrophils can act synergistically with bacterial products and cause further inhibition of tracheobronchial ciliary function.

An increasing number of polypeptides with antimicrobial activity have been identified in the airway surface fluid that may play an important role in host defense in the respiratory tract.[81–83] Although several alterations in the levels of these airway antimicrobial peptides in COPD have been described, how this relates to bacterial colonization and whether colonizing bacteria can, in turn, modify these peptides have not been systematically investigated.

Compromised mucociliary clearance and antimicrobial defenses on the airway surface could allow bacteria to interact with the airway epithelium. Subsequent interaction of the microbial pathogen and epithelial cells could be significant determinants of colonization and airway inflammation. Nontypeable *H. influenzae* caused airway epithelial injury in an *in-vitro* tissue culture model of nasal turbinate epithelium.[84] At 14 hours, patchy injury developed to the airway epithelium, with bacterial cells now associating with these damaged epithelial cells but not with intact epithelium. At 24 hours, detached epithelial cells with adherent bacteria were seen.

Increased adherence of bacterial pathogens to oropharyngeal cells has been described in smokers, in persons prone to respiratory infections, and in exacerbation-prone COPD patients.[85–89] Increased adherence also has been associated with more frequent bacterial colonization of the upper respiratory tract in COPD.[86] Whether such a propensity extends to the lower respiratory tract is not known.

The airway epithelium recognizes microbial agents through pattern recognition receptors such as Toll-like receptors. This results in the production of inflammatory and chemotactic mediators, as well as antimicrobial substances.[81,90] An inflammatory response appropriate to the stimulus should result in efficient clearance of the stimulus.

However, a dysregulated inflammatory response could be disadvantageous to the host. Whether such dysregulation exists in COPD is under active investigation.

The alveolar macrophage is the resident mononuclear phagocyte of the lung and functions as a key defense against inhaled particulate matter and pathogens.[91,92] We recently showed that alveolar macrophages in COPD are hyporesponsive to *H. influenzae* antigens and demonstrate impaired phagocytosis for *H. influenzae*.[93] This suggests that immunologically impaired macrophages in COPD promote increased bacterial colonization.[94]

Inflammation Related to Microbial Colonization in COPD

Demonstration of an inflammatory response to "colonization" would add credence to the potential pathogenic role of the specific microbial pathogen. Recent studies have demonstrated such an association, with the best data for typical bacterial pathogens, including nontypeable *H. influenzae*.

Exposure of explant cultures of human bronchial epithelium to lipo-oligosaccharide (endotoxin) from nontypeable *H. influenzae* significantly increases IL-6, IL-8, and TNF-α secretion and intercellular adhesion molecule 1 expression in the explanted tissue.[95] The levels of inflammatory mediators attained in the culture medium are adequate to increase neutrophil chemotaxis and adherence *in vitro*. We recently showed that components of *H. influenzae*, especially an outer membrane lipoprotein, P6, are potent inducers of IL-8 and TNF-α from alveolar and blood macrophages obtained from healthy controls and COPD.[96]

Bresser and colleagues identified chronic bronchitis patients who were chronically infected with *H. influenzae*. Sputum levels of inflammatory mediators, specifically MPO, TNF-α, and IL-8, as well as the degree of plasma protein leakage into the sputum, were significantly higher in the *H. influenzae*-infected group compared with noninfected patients.[97] In a recent study, Banerjee and colleagues showed that patients with moderate to severe stable COPD who were "colonized" with bacterial pathogens, including *H. influenzae*, had a worse health status and more airway inflammation, as reflected in higher levels of IL-8, LTB4, TNF-α, NE, and increased neutrophil chemotaxis, in comparison with COPD patients who were not colonized with such bacteria.[98]

The above studies are very interesting and provocative; however, sputum mainly reflects the inflammatory process in the larger airways and not the major site of airway obstruction in COPD, which is the peripheral tracheobronchial tree. Bronchoscopically obtained samples, specifically protected specimen brushings and BAL, sample the peripheral airways and the alveolar space. Such samples therefore are more informative; however, they are difficult to obtain. Two studies have used bronchoscopic sampling to examine the impact of airway bacterial colonization on inflammation in COPD. Soler and colleagues examined inflammation and colonization in BAL samples in stable COPD, smokers without

COPD, and nonsmokers.[99] Bacterial colonization was seen in 32% of COPD subjects. None of the nonsmokers were colonized; however, surprisingly, 42% of "healthy smokers" also demonstrated bacterial colonization. Colonized subjects, with or without COPD had more bronchial neutrophilia and higher levels of TNF-α in the BAL compared with noncolonized subjects.

The findings of this study, although exciting, are limited because of the significant findings seen only when smokers with and without COPD were combined. Furthermore, smoking-induced inflammation shares the same characteristics as bacterial colonization-associated inflammation, making the findings difficult to interpret. An optimal study would be confined to ex-smokers to more reliably demonstrate the association between bacterial colonization and airway inflammation. We recently completed such a study in which 35% of ex-smokers with stable COPD were found to be "colonized" with bacterial pathogens, predominantly *Haemophilus* spp.[100] None of the ex-smokers without COPD were colonized, and 1 of 15 (7%) healthy nonsmokers demonstrated colonization. Colonization was associated with greater numbers of neutrophils and higher levels of IL-8, matrix metalloproteinase 9, and endotoxin in the lavage fluid (Figure 7).

These studies provide evidence that bacterial colonization of the central and peripheral airways is common in COPD and associated with neutrophilic inflammation. Furthermore, bacterial colonization and associated inflammation develop early in the disease, in healthy smokers with chronic bronchitis, and persist in ex-smokers who have developed COPD. Therefore, colonization-induced inflammation could contribute to the development of COPD at all stages of this disease.

Immune Response to Colonization in COPD

Failure of innate lung defense, leading to establishment of chronic infection in the airways, should lead to an adaptive immune response to the pathogen, in an attempt to eradicate or contain it. Therefore, another line of evidence that microbial presence in the lower airways is not mere "colonization" would be the development of specific immune responses to the pathogen following colonization. This question has not been adequately studied, but there is emerging evidence that such immune responses do develop in COPD. We have shown that following *M. catarrhalis* colonization, a substantial proportion of patients with COPD develop systemic (serum IgG) and mucosal (sputum IgA) antibodies to the infecting strain.[58] Similar observations of adaptive immune response following colonization with nontypeable *H. influenzae*, *Pseudomonas*, and *S. pneumoniae* have been made (unpublished data, 2007).

The observations of increased airway inflammation and development of specific immune response to "colonizing" bacteria in COPD support the paradigm that this "colonization" actually is a low-grade smoldering infection that

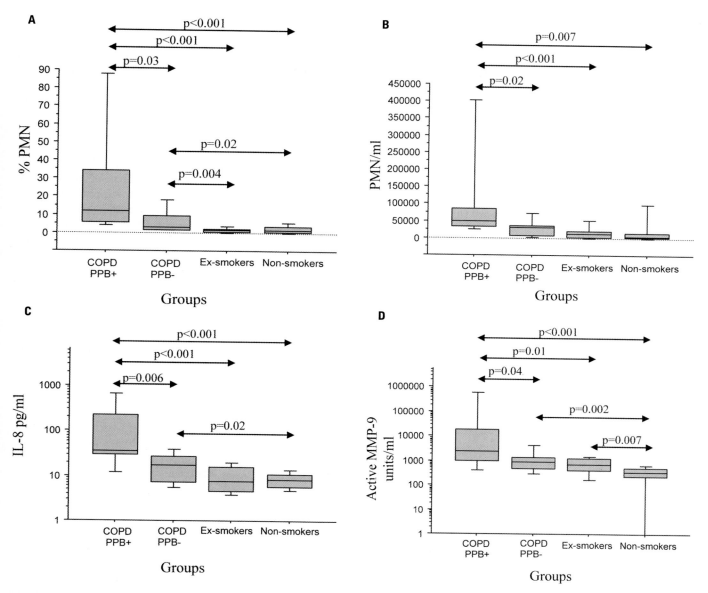

FIGURE 7. Comparison of bronchoalveolar lavage fluid measurements among patients with chronic obstructive pulmonary disease colonized (COPD, PPB+) and not colonized (COPD, PPB-) with potentially pathogenic bacteria, ex-smokers and nonsmokers. The *horizontal lines* represent median values, the *boxes* represent 25th to 75th quartiles, and the *vertical lines* represent 10th to 90th percentile values. Significant differences between groups are represented by *double-sided arrows* with associated p values by Mann-Whitney *U* rank test. Reproduced with permission from Sethi S et al.[100] *A*, Relative neutrophil count (PMN%); *B*, absolute neutrophil count (PMN); *C*, interleukin-8 level (IL-8, pg/mL); *D*, active matrix metalloproteinase 9 level (MMP-9, units/mL).

induces chronic airway inflammation. In the large airways, such inflammation would contribute to mucus production, and in the small airways, it could contribute to respiratory bronchiolitis and progressive airway obstruction.[101,102] Therefore, the vicious circle appears to exist; however, its importance in the natural history of COPD is as yet unknown. Studies to determine if development and progression of COPD are related to bacterial colonization are needed; however, they will be large, long, and expensive. Alternatively, attempts to interrupt the vicious circle in estab-

lished COPD with agents that decrease lower airway bacterial colonization could provide similar evidence.

Chronic Bacterial Infection of Respiratory Tissues

In the past, documentation of chronic infection in COPD has relied on culturing of respiratory secretions. These cultures, although specific and allowing recovery of the pathogen for further study, are insensitive and not able to detect fastidious strains of microbial pathogens. In the past few years, molecular and immunologic diagnostic techniques, including polymerase chain reaction (PCR), in situ hybridization, and fluorescent antibody staining, have been applied to respiratory secretions and lung tissue samples to better elucidate the presence of microbial pathogens in the lung in stable COPD.

Several studies have now shown that nontypeable *H. influenzae* is detected with much higher frequency in COPD by these new detection methods compared with culture. We showed by PCR detection that *H. influenzae* persists in sputum obtained from patients with COPD even when cultures are negative (Figure 8).[103] Bandi and colleagues demonstrated *H. influenzae* by fluorescent staining with a monoclonal antibody in a third of bronchial biopsies obtained from patients with stable COPD.[104] Moller and colleagues demonstrated that in lung explants obtained from patients undergoing lung transplantation, *H. influenzae* was diffusely present in lung tissue by in situ hybridization and PCR.[71]

Integration of the adenovirus *E1A* gene into the genome of lung cells has been shown to occur with increased frequency in smokers with COPD.[70] In animal models, this integration has been shown to enhance the inflammation engendered by smoke exposure.[105] Chronic *C. pneumoniae* infection has been detected by PCR and serology in 71% of patients with severe COPD and 46% of mild to moderate COPD compared with 0% in the control group.[69] Respiratory syncytial virus and *Pneumocystis jiroveci* are two additional pathogens detected in lung tissue or secretions in COPD, again based on molecular techniques.[72,73]

Although molecular techniques are undoubtedly more sensitive than culture, one has to be aware of their limitations. They are very prone to contamination and therefore false-positive results. They do not provide a microbial isolate for further study; therefore, one cannot confirm the significance of microbial presence by complementary techniques such as immunoassays. Because of their extreme sensitivity, one can question the pathogenetic significance of the presence of a microbial pathogen in very low concentrations and therefore the significance of a positive result with these techniques.

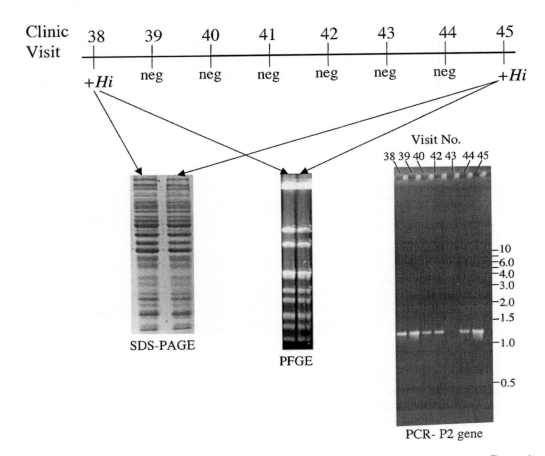

FIGURE 8. Timeline from a study clinic patient depicting clinic visits 38 through 45, which occurred about 1 month apart. The results of sputum culture are noted below each clinic visit. +Hi = positive culture for H. influenzae; neg = negative culture for H. influenzae. Identical results of typing by sodium dodecyl sulfate-polyacrylamide gel (SDS-PAGE) and pulsed-field gel electrophoresis (PFGE) are shown for the strains isolated at visits 38 and 45. An agarose gel at the right shows the results of polymerase chain reaction (PCR) of the P2 gene (about 1.2 kb) of the sputum pellets from clinic visits as noted at the top of the gel. Molecular mass markers are noted in kilobases on the right. Note that no sputum pellet was available at visit 31 and that visit 43 yielded a negative result on PCR. Sputum from all other visits yielded a PCR product of about 1.2 kb. Reproduced with permission from Murphy TF et al.[103]

Intracellular and Intercellular Invasion of Nontypeable *H. influenzae*

Nontypeable *H. influenzae* is present in the lumen of the respiratory tract, binds with specificity to mucin, and adheres to the surface of respiratory epithelial cells. More recently, research from several groups has shown that the organism's niche in the human respiratory tract is not limited to the surface of epithelial cells. Studies using cultures of human epithelial cells have revealed that a small percentage of adherent nontypeable *H. influenzae* enter epithelial cells in a process that involves actin filaments and microtubules.[106] Organ culture studies using lung epithelial cells on permeable supports revealed clusters of *H. influenzae* between cells, indicating that bacteria penetrated by paracytosis or passage between cells.[107] Nontypeable *H. influenzae* that penetrate the epithelial cell layer in this model system are protected from the bactericidal activity of several antibiotics and antibody-mediated bactericidal activity.[108] In assays employing primary human airway cultures, nontypeable *H. influenzae* adheres to and enters exclusively nonciliated cells in the population by the process of macropinocytosis.[109]

In addition to these elegant *in-vitro* studies, *in-vivo* studies confirm that nontypeable *H. influenzae* penetrate the mucosal surface during colonization of the human respiratory tract. In situ hybridization and selective cultures revealed that viable nontypeable *H. influenzae* are present in macrophage-like cells in adenoids of children.[110] The studies by Bandi and colleagues and Moller and colleagues referred to earlier demonstrate a similar presence of *H. influenzae* in the tissues of the lower respiratory tract.[71,104]

Bacteria in tissues are protected from antibiotics and bactericidal antibodies and may act as reservoirs of infection.[108] Tissue infection by nontypeable *H. influenzae* could also contribute to the pathogenesis of COPD directly or indirectly. Chronic low-grade infection could directly induce a chronic inflammatory response in the parenchyma and the airways of the lung that could be additive or synergistic to the inflammatory effects of tobacco smoke. Indirectly, such an infection could enhance the damaging effects of tobacco smoke on respiratory tissues. On the other hand, it is possible that this tissue infection is simply a marker of compromised local immunity. Whether tissue infection by nontypeable *H. influenzae* is seen in early COPD and the effect of this infection on airway inflammation need to be investigated.

Chronic *Chlamydia pneumoniae* Infection in COPD

Chlamydia pneumoniae is an obligate intracellular atypical bacterial pathogen. Acute *C. pneumoniae* infection can cause bronchitis, pneumonia, and acute exacerbations of COPD. Chronic infection with *C. pneumoniae* is being actively investigated as a cause of several systemic diseases, especially coronary artery disease.[111] In one study, the incidence of chronic *C. pneumoniae* infection (as defined below) was 71% in patients with severe COPD, 46% in mild to moderate COPD,

and 0% in the control group.[69] The presence of chronic *C. pneumoniae* infection was determined by three different methods: serum antibodies to *C. pneumoniae* (IgG and IgA and circulating immune complexes), sputum IgA antibodies to *C. pneumoniae*, and PCR of sputum for *C. pneumoniae* deoxyribonucleic acid (DNA). Infection was defined by positive results in two of the three methods in a patient.[69] Whether this chronic infection contributes to the pathogenesis of COPD as discussed above or is a reflection of compromised local immunity warrants further investigation.

Hypersensitivity to Bacterial Antigens in COPD

Allergic bronchopulmonary aspergillosis is a model of an infectious disease with predominantly allergic manifestations mediated by a T-helper 2 (Th2)-type immune response and characterized by IgE and eosinophil predominance.[112] Inefficient removal of bacteria from the lower respiratory tract is characteristic of chronic bronchitis, resulting in prolonged contact between the airway lymphoid tissue and bacterial antigens. This could lead to the emergence of IgE antibodies to bacterial antigens, which could induce eosinophil infiltration and mast cell degranulation on repeated exposures to the bacterial antigens. An increased number of eosinophils is a component of airway inflammation in patients with COPD, and tissue and airway lumen eosinophilia become more prominent during exacerbations.[113] Furthermore, a small subgroup of patients with COPD have an eosinophilic bronchitis that is responsive to steroids.[114]

The ability of bacterial pathogens to induce histamine release, hypersensitivity, and IgE-mediated inflammation has been sporadically investigated. Mast cells release histamine by non-IgE-mediated and IgE-mediated mechanisms. Formalin-killed suspensions of nontypeable *H. influenzae* and *S. aureus* induce non-IgE-mediated and enhanced IgE-mediated histamine release from human airway mast cells.[115] The enhancement of IgE-mediated histamine release appears to be mediated by the endotoxin (lipooligosaccharide) of nontypeable *H. influenzae*.[116] Histamine increases bronchial epithelial permeability, stimulates mucus secretion, and induces bronchoconstriction.

Patients with acute exacerbations of chronic bronchitis have basophil-bound IgE and serum IgE to homologous strains of nontypeable *H. influenzae* and *S. pneumoniae* isolated from sputum with the acute exacerbation.[119] In another study in asthmatics, 29% of patients had serum IgE antibodies to nontypeable *H. influenzae* and/or *S. pneumoniae*.[118] This sensitization to bacterial antigens may contribute to the bronchoconstriction and airway inflammation seen with acute exacerbations of COPD.

These observations regarding histamine release and IgE to bacterial antigens suggest that bacterial pathogens, either directly or indirectly via a Th2-type immune response, could contribute to the eosinophilia, airway hyperreactivity, and bronchoconstriction seen in patients with COPD. Further investigation in this area is warranted, especially in the group of COPD patients with eosinophilic bronchitis.[114]

Future Directions

Substantial new information has emerged regarding the contribution of bacterial infection to the course of COPD. However, several important questions remain to be answered to allow precise delineation of the role of bacterial infection in COPD. Longitudinal cohort studies in which the etiology of childhood lower respiratory tract infection is defined are needed to demonstrate if bacterial infection in childhood is associated with impaired lung function and a predisposition to COPD in adulthood. Mechanisms of infection and the human immune response to bacterial pathogens during exacerbations need further investigation to develop better preventive strategies. Although bacterial infection appears to be a stimulus for airway inflammation during exacerbations and in the stable phase of COPD, whether this leads to progression of airway obstruction or contributes to the symptoms of COPD has not been determined. Tissue infection by pathogens such as nontypeable *H. influenzae* of the airways has been shown in end-stage COPD. Whether such an infection is seen in the earlier stages of COPD is unknown. In addition, whether this tissue infection contributes to progression of disease or is simply a marker of compromised bacterial clearance and local immunity needs investigation.

Patients with COPD are a heterogeneous group, and the role of bacteria and the pathways by which infection contributes to its pathogenesis is likely to vary among subsets of patients with COPD. For example, hypersensitivity to bacterial antigens may play a role in COPD patients with eosinophilic bronchitis, or tissue invasion by bacteria may be important in patients with predominant chronic bronchitis. Regarding bacterial infection as the central mechanism of development of all COPD and dismissing it as an epiphenomenon are unlikely to be correct viewpoints. Most likely, in a subset of patients with COPD, bacterial infection contributes substantially to progression of their disease. Identification of this subset of patients could lead to therapeutic interventions to alter the natural history of their disease.

Acknowledgment

Adeline Thurston is thanked for her expertise in preparing the manuscript.

References

1. Murphy TF, Sethi S. Bacterial infection in chronic obstructive pulmonary disease. Am Rev Respir Dis 1992;146:1067–83.
2. Leeder SR. Role of infection in the cause and course of chronic bronchitis and emphysema. J Infect Dis 1975;131:731–42.
3. Speizer FE, Tager IB. Epidemiology of chronic mucus hypersecretion and obstructive airways disease. Epidemiol Rev 1979;1:124–42.
4. Tager I, Speizer FE. Role of infection in chronic bronchitis. N Engl J Med 1975;292:563–71.
5. Barker DJP, Godfrey KM, Fall C, et al. Relation of birth weight and childhood respiratory infection to adult lung function and death from chronic obstructive airways disease. BMJ 1991;303:671–5.
6. Johnston IDA, Strachan DP, Anderson HR. Effect of pneumonia and whooping cough in childhood on adult lung function. N Engl J Med 1998;338:581–7.
7. Shaheen SO, Barker DJP, Holgate ST. Do lower respiratory tract infections in early childhood cause chronic obstructive pulmonary disease? Am J Respir Crit Care Med 1995;151:1649–52.
8. Shaheen SO, Sterne JAC, Tucker JS, Florey CD. Birth weight, childhood lower respiratory tract infection, and adult lung function. Thorax 1998;53:549–53.
9. Marossy AE, Strachan DP, Rudnicka AR, Anderson HR. Childhood chest illness and the rate of decline of adult lung function between ages 35 and 45 years. Am J Respir Crit Care Med 2007;175:355–9.
10. Vuori E, Peltola H, Kallio MJT, et al. Etiology of pneumonia and other common childhood infections requiring hospitaliation and parenteral antimicrobial therapy. Clin Infect Dis 1998;27:566–72.
11. Sethi S. Etiology and management of infections in chronic obstructive pulmonary disease. Clin Pulm Med 1999;6:327–32.
12. Allegra L, Konietzko N, Leophonte P, et al. Comparative safety and efficacy of sparfloxacin in the treatment of acute exacerbations of chronic obstructive pulmonary disease: a double–blind, randomised, parallel, multicentre study. J Antimicrob Chemother 1996;37:93–104.
13. Anzueto A, Niederman MS, Tillotson GS, Bronchitis Study G. Etiology, susceptibility, and treatment of acute bacterial exacerbations of complicated chronic bronchitis in the primary care setting: ciprofloxacin 750 mg bid vs clarithromycin 500 mg bid. Clin Ther 1998;20:885–900.
14. Chodosh S, Lakshminarayan S, Swarz H, Breisch S. Efficacy and safety of a 10-day course of 400 or 600 milligrams of grepafloxacin once daily for treatment of acute bacterial exacerbations of chronic bronchitis: comparison with a 10–day course of 500 milligrams of ciprofloxacin twice daily. Antimicrob Agents Chemother 1998;42:114–20.
15. Chodosh S, McCarty J, Farkas S, et al, Bronchitis Study G. Randomized, double-blind study of ciprofloxacin and cefuroxime axetil for treatment of acute bacterial exacerbations of chronic bronchitis. Clin Infect Dis 1998;27:722–9.
16. Chodosh S, Schreurs JM, Siami G, et al, Bronchitis Study G. Efficacy of oral ciprolfoxacin vs clarithromycin for treatment of acute bacterial exacerbations of chronic bronchitis. Clin Infect Dis 1998;27:730–8.
17. Davies BI, Maesen FPV. Clinical effectiveness of levofloxacin in patients with acute purulent exacerbations of chronic bronchitis: the relationship with in-vitro activity. J Antimicrob Chemother 1999;43:83–90.
18. DeAbate CA, Henry D, Bensch G, et al, Sparfloxacin Multicenter ASG. Sparfloxacin vs. ofloxacin in the treatment of acute bacterial exacerbations of chronic bronchitis. Chest 1998;114:120–130.

19. Habib MP, Gentry LO, Rodriguez-Gomez G, et al. Multicenter, randomized study comparing efficacy and safety of oral levofloxacin and cefaclor in treatment of acute bacterial exacerbations of chronic bronchitis. Infect Dis Clin Pract 1998;7:101–9.

20. Langan C, Clecner B, Cazzola CM, et al. Short-course cefuroxime axetil therapy in the treatment of acute exacerbations of chronic bronchitis. Int J Clin Pract 1998;52:289–97.

21. Langan CE, Cranfield R, Breisch S, Pettit R. Randomized, double-blind study of grepafloxacin versus amoxicillin in patients with acute bacterial exacerbations of chronic bronchitis. J Antimicrob Chemother 1997;40:63–72.

22. Langan CE, Zuck P, Vogel F, et al. Randomized, double-blind study of short-course (5 day) grepafloxacin versus 10 day clarithromycin in patients with acute bacterial exacerbations of chronic bronchitis. J Antimicrob Chemother 1999; 44:515–23.

23. Read RC, Kuss A, Berrisoul F, et al. The efficacy and safety of a new ciprofloxacin suspension compared with co-amoxiclav tablets in the treatment of acute exacerbations of chronic bronchitis. Respir Med 1999;93:252–61.

24. Shah PM, Maesen FPV, Dolmann A, et al. Levofloxacin versus cefuroxime axetil in the treatment of acute exacerbation of chronic bronchitis: results of a randomized, double-blind study. J Antimicrob Chemother 1999;43:529–39.

25. Wilson R, Kubin R, Ballin I, et al. Five day moxifloxacin therapy compared with 7 day clarithromycin therapy for the treatment of acute exacerbations of chronic bronchitis. J Antimicrob Chemother 1999;44:501–13.

26. Aubier M, Aldons PM, Leak A, et al. Telithromycin is as effective as amoxicillin/clavulanate in acute exacerbations of chronic bronchitis. Respir Med 2002;96:862–71.

27. Wilson R, Allegra L, Huchon G, et al. Short-term and long-term outcomes of moxifloxacin compared to standard antibiotic treatment in acute exacerbations of chronic bronchitis. Chest 2004;125:953–64.

28. File T, Schlemmer B, Garau J, et al. Gemifloxacin versus amoxicillin/clavulanate in the treatment of acute exacerbations of chronic bronchitis. The 070 Clinical Study Group. J Chemother 2000;12:314–25.

29. Martinez FJ, Grossman RF, Zadeikis N, et al. Patient stratification in the management of acute bacterial exacerbation of chronic bronchitis: the role of levofloxacin 750 mg. Eur Respir J 2005;25:1001–10.

30. Sethi S, Breton J, Wynne B. Efficacy and safety of pharmacokinetically enhanced amoxicillin-clavulanate at 2,000/125 milligrams twice daily for 5 days versus amoxicillin-clavulanate at 875/125 milligrams twice daily for 7 days in the treatment of acute exacerbations of chronic bronchitis. Antimicrob Agents Chemother 2005;49:153–60.

31. Starakis I, Gogos CA, Bassaris H. Five-day moxifloxacin therapy compared with 7-day co-amoxiclav therapy for the treatment of acute exacerbation of chronic bronchitis. Int J Antimicrob Agents 2004;23:129–37.

32. Yi K, Sethi S, Murphy T. Human immune response to nontypeable *Haemophilus influenzae* in chronic bronchitis. J Infect Dis 1997;176:1247–52.

33. Medical Research Council. Definitions and classification of chronic bronchitis for clinical and epidemiological purposes. A report to the Medical Research Council by their committee on the aetiology of chronic bronchitis. Lancet 1965;1:775–9.

34. Gump DW, Phillips CA, Forsyth BR, et al. Role of infection in chronic bronchitis. Am Rev Respir Dis 1976;113:465–73.

35. McHardy VU, Inglis JM, Calder MA, Crofton JW. A study of infective and other factors in exacerbations of chronic bronchitis. Br J Dis Chest 1980;74:228–38.

36. Anthonisen NR, Manfreda J, Warren CPW, et al. Antibiotic therapy in exacerbations of chronic obstructive pulmonary disease. Ann Intern Med 1987;106:196–204.

37. Saint S, Bent S, Vittinghoff E, Grady D. Antibiotics in chronic obstructive pulmonary disease exacerbations. A meta-analysis. JAMA 1995;273:957–96.

38. Fagon JY, Chastre J, Trouillet JL, et al. Characterization of distal bronchial microflora during acute exacerbation of chronic bronchitis. Am Rev Respir Dis 1990;142:1004–8.

39. Nicotra MB, Kronenberg S. Con: antibiotic use in exacerbations of chronic bronchitis. Semin Respir Infect 1993;8:254–8.

40. Isada CM. Pro: antibiotics for chronic bronchitis with exacerbations. Semin Respir Infect 1993;8:243–53.

41. Chastre J, Fagon JY, Bornet-Lesco M, et al. Evaluation of bronchoscopic techniques for the diagnosis of nosocomial pneumonia. Am J Respir Crit Care Med 1995;152:231–40.

42. Monso E, Ruiz J, Rosell A, et al. Bacterial infection in chronic obstructive pulmonary disease. A study of stable and exacerbated outpatients using the protected specimen brush. Am J Respir Crit Care Med 1995;152:1316–20.

43. Pela R, Marchesani F, Agostinelli C, et al. Airways microbial flora in COPD patients in stable clinical conditions and during exacerbations: a bronchoscopic investigation. Monaldi Arch Chest Dis 1998;53:262–7.

44. Soler N, Torres A, Ewig S, et al. Bronchial microbial patterns in severe exacerbations of chronic obstructive pulmonary disease (COPD) requiring mechanical ventilation. Am J Respir Crit Care Med 1998;157:1498–505.

45. Rosell A, Monso E, Soler N, et al. Microbiologic determinants of exacerbation in chronic obstructive pulmonary disease. Arch Intern Med 2005;165:891–7.

46. Eller J, Ede A, Schaberg T, et al. Infective exacerbations of chronic bronchitis. Relation between bacteriologic etiology and lung function. Chest 1998;113:1542–8.

47. Miravitlles M, Espinosa C, Fernandez-Laso E, et al. Relationship between bacterial flora in sputum and functional impairment in patients with acute exacerbations of COPD. Study Group of Bacterial Infection in COPD. Chest 1999;116:40–6.

48. Ferrer M, Ioanas M, Arancibia F, et al. Microbial airway colonization is associated with noninvasive ventilation failure in exacerbation of chronic obstructive pulmonary disease. Crit Care Med 2005;33:2003–9.

49. Soler N, Agusti C, Angrill J, et al. Bronchoscopic validation of the significance of sputum purulence in severe exacerbations of chronic obstructive pulmonary disease. Thorax 2007;62:29–35.

50. Sethi S, Sethi R, Eschberger K, et al. Airway bacterial concentrations and exacerbations of chronic obstructive pulmonary disease. Am J Respir Crit Care Med 2007;76(4):356–61. Epub May 3, 2007.

51. Brunham RC, Plummer FA, Stephens RS. Bacterial antigenic variation, host immune response and pathogen-host coevolution. Infect Immun 1993;61:2273–6.

52. Maslow JN, Mulligan ME, Arbeit RD. Molecular epidemiology: application of contemporary techniques to the typing of microorganisms. Clin Infect Dis 1993;17:153–64.

53. Gump DW, Christmas WA, Forsyth BR, et al. Serum and secretory antibodies in patients with chronic bronchitis. Arch Intern Med 1973;132:847–51.

54. Sethi S, Evans N, Grant BJB, Murphy TF. Acquisition of a new bacterial strain and occurrence of exacerbations of chronic obstructive pulmonary disease. N Engl J Med 2002;347:465–71.

55. Chin CL, Manzel LJ, Lehman EE, et al. *Haemophilus influenzae* from patients with chronic obstructive pulmonary disease exacerbation induce more inflammation than colonizers. Am J Respir Crit Care Med 2005;172:85–91.

56. Vitovski S, Dunkin KT, Howard AJ, Sayers JR. Nontypeable *Haemophilus influenzae* in carriage and disease: a difference in IgA1 protease activity levels. JAMA 2002;287:1699–705.

57. Fernaays MM, Lesse AJ, Sethi S, et al. Differential genome contents of nontypeable *Haemophilus influenzae* strains from adults with chronic obstructive pulmonary disease. Infect Immun 2006;74:3366–74.

58. Murphy TF, Brauer AL, Grant BJ, Sethi S. *Moraxella catarrhalis* in chronic obstructive pulmonary disease: burden of disease and immune response. Am J Respir Crit Care Med 2005;172:195–9.

59. Abe Y, Murphy TF, Sethi S, et al. Lymphocyte proliferative response to p6 of *Haemophilus influenzae* is associated with relative protection from exacerbations of chronic obstructive pulmonary disease. Am J Respir Crit Care Med 2002;165:967–71.

60. Sethi S, Muscarella K, Evans N, et al. Airway inflammation and etiology of acute exacerbations of chronic bronchitis. Chest 2000;118:1557–65.

61. Gompertz S, Bayley DL, Hill SL, Stockley RA. Relationship between airway inflammation and the frequency of exacerbations in patients with smoking related COPD. Thorax 2001;56:36–41.

62. White AJ, Gompertz S, Bayley DL, et al. Resolution of bronchial inflammation is related to bacterial eradication following treatment of exacerbations of chronic bronchitis. Thorax 2003;58:680–5.

63. Papi A, Bellettato CM, Braccioni F, et al. Infections and airway inflammation in chronic obstructive pulmonary disease severe exacerbations. Am J Respir Crit Care Med 2006;173:1114–21.

64. Sethi S, Wrona C, Grant BJB, Murphy TF. Strain specific immune response to *Haemophilus influenzae* in chronic obstructive pulmonary disease. Am J Respir Crit Care Med 2004;169:448–53.

65. Bogaert D, van der Valk P, Ramdin R, et al. Host–pathogen interaction during pneumococcal infection in patients with chronic obstructive pulmonary disease. Infect Immun 2004;72:818–23.

66. Aaron SD, Ramotar K, Ferris W, et al. Adult cystic fibrosis exacerbations and new strains of *Pseudomonas aeruginosa*. Am J Respir Crit Care Med 2004;169:811–5.

67. Gibson RL, Burns JL, Ramsey BW. Pathophysiology and management of pulmonary infections in cystic fibrosis. Am J Respir Crit Care Med 2003;168:918–51.

68. Cole P. Host–microbe relationships in chronic respiratory infection. Respiration 1989;55:5–8.

69. von Hertzen L, Alakarppa H, Koskinen R, et al. *Chlamydia pneumoniae* infection in patients with chronic obstructive pulmonary disease. Epidemiol Infect 1997;118:155–64.

70. Matsuse T, Hayashi S, Kuwano K, et al. Latent adenoviral infection in the pathogenesis of chronic airways obstruction. Am Rev Respir Dis 1992;146:177–84.

71. Moller LVM, Timens W, van der Bij W, et al. *Haemophilus influenzae* in lung explants of patients with end-stage pulmonary disease. Am J Respir Crit Care Med 1998;157:950–6.

72. Seemungal T, Harper–Owen R, Bhowmik A, et al. Respiratory viruses, symptoms, and inflammatory markers in acute exacerbations and stable chronic obstructive pulmonary disease. Am J Respir Crit Care Med 2001;164:1618–23.

73. Morris A, Sciurba FC, Lebedeva IP, et al. Association of chronic obstructive pulmonary disease severity and pneumocystis colonization. Am J Respir Crit Care Med 2004; 170(4):408–13. Epub 2004 Apr 29.

74. Wanner A, Salathe M, O'Riordan TG. Mucociliary clearance in the airways. Am J Respir Crit Care Med 1996;154:1868–902.

75. Vastag E, Matthys H, Zsamboki G, et al. Mucociliary clearance in smokers. Eur J Respir Dis 1986;68:107–13.

76. Gleeson K, Eggli DF, Maxwell SL. Quantitative aspiration during sleep in normal subjects. Chest 1997;111:1266–72.

77. Adler KB, Hendley DD, Davis GS. Bacteria associated with obstructive pulmonary disease elaborate extracellular products that stimulate mucin secretion by explants of guinea pig airways. Am J Pathol 1986;125:514.

78. Wilson R, Roberts D, Cole P. Effect of bacterial products on human ciliary function in vitro. Thorax 1984;40:125–31.

79. Amitani R, Wilson R, Rutman A, et al. Effects of human neutrophil elastase and *Pseudomonas aeruginosa* proteinases on human respiratory epithelium. Am J Respir Cell Mol Biol 1991;4:26–32.

80. Hiemstra PS, van Wetering S, Stolk J. Neutrophil serine proteinases and defensins in chronic obstructive pulmonary disease: effects on pulmonary epithelium. Eur Respir J 1998;12:1200–8.

81. Bals R, Hiemstra PS. Innate immunity in the lung: how epithelial cells fight against respiratory pathogens. Eur Respir J 2004;23:327–33.

82. Ganz T. Antimicrobial polypeptides. J Leukoc Biol 2004;75:34–8.

83. Crouch EC. Collectins and pulmonary host defense. Am J Respir Cell Mol Biol 1998;19:177–201.

84. Read RC, Wilson R, Rutman A, et al. Interaction of nontypable Haemophilus influenzae with human respiratory mucosa in vitro. J Infect Dis. 1991 Mar;163(3):549–58.

85. El Ahmer OR, Essery SD, Saadi AT, et al. The effect of cigarette smoke on adherence of respiratory pathogens to buccal epithelial cells. FEMS Immunol Med Microbiol 1999;23:27–36.

86. Taylor D, Clancy R, Cripps A, et al. An alteration in the host–parasite relationship in subjects with chronic bronchitis prone to recurrent episodes of acute bronchitis. Immunol Cell Biol 1994;72:143–51.

87. Arcavi L, Benowitz NL. Cigarette smoking and infection. Arch Intern Med 2004;164:2206–16.

88. Mbaki N, Rikitomi N, Akiyama M, Matsumoto K. In vitro adherence of *Streptococcus pneumoniae* to oropharyngeal cells: enhanced activity and colonization of the upper respiratory tract in patients with recurrent respiratory infections. Tohoku J Exp Med 1989;157:345–54.

89. Fainstein V, Musher DM. Bacterial adherence to pharyngeal cells in smokers, nonsmokers, and chronic bronchitics. Infect Immun 1979;26:178–82.

90. Kadioglu A, Andrew PW. The innate immune response to pneumococcal lung infection: the untold story. Trends Immunol 2004;25:143–9.

91. Hocking WG, Golde DW. The pulmonary-alveolar macrophage (first of two parts). N Engl J Med 1979;301:580–7.

92. Fels AO, Cohn ZA. The alveolar macrophage. J Appl Physiol 1986;60:353–69.

93. Berenson C, Maloney J, Grove L, et al. Impaired alveolar macrophage response to *haemophilus* antigens in chronic obstructive lung disease. Am J Respir Crit Care Med 2006;174(1):31–40.

94. Barnes PJ. Mediators of chronic obstructive pulmonary disease. Pharmacol Rev 2004;56:515–48.

95. Khair OA, Devalia JL, Abdelaziz MM, et al. Effect of *Haemophilus influenzae* endotoxin on the synthesis of IL–6, IL-8, TNF–α and expression of ICAM-1. Eur Respir J 1994;7:2109–16.

96. Sha Q, Truong-Tran AQ, Plitt JR, et al. Activation of airway epithelial cells by Toll-like receptor agonists. Am J Respir Cell Mol Biol 2004;31:358-64.

97. Bresser P, Out TA, van Alphen L, et al. Airway inflammation in nonobstructive and obstructive chronic bronchitis with chronic haemophilus influenzae airway infection. Comparison with noninfected patients with chronic obstructive pulmonary disease. Am J Respir Crit Care Med 2000 Sep;162(3 Pt 1):947–52.

98. Banerjee D, Khair OA, Honeybourne D. Impact of sputum bacteria on airway inflammation and health status in clinical stable COPD. Eur Respir J 2004;23:685–91.

99. Soler N, Ewig S, Torres A, et al. Airway inflammation and bronchial microbial patterns in patients with stable chronic obstructive pulmonary disease. Eur Respir J 1999; 14:1015–22.

100. Sethi S, Maloney J, Grove L, et al. Airway inflammation and bronchial bacterial colonization in chronic obstructive pulmonary disease. Am J Respir Crit Care Med 2006;173:991–8.

101. Di Stefano A, Capelli A, Lusuardi M, et al. Severity of airflow limitation is associated with severity of airway inflammation in smokers. Am J Respir Crit Care Med 1998;158:1277–85.

102. Thompson AB, Daughton D, Robbins RA, et al. Intraluminal airway inflammation in chronic bronchitis. Characterization and correlation with clinical parameters. Am Rev Respir Dis 1989;140:1527–37.

103. Murphy TF, Brauer AL, Schiffmacher AT, Sethi S. Persistent colonization by *Haemophilus influenzae* in chronic obstructive pulmonary disease. Am J Respir Crit Care Med 2004;170:266–72.

104. Bandi V, Apicella MA, Mason E, et al. Nontypeable *Haemophilus influenzae* in the lower respiratory tract of patients with chronic bronchitis. Am J Respir Crit Care Med 2001;164:2114–9.

105. Keicho N, Elliott WM, Hogg JC, Hayashi S. Adenovirus E1A gene dysregulates ICAM–1 expression in transformed pulmonary epithelial cells. Am J Respir Cell Mol Biol 1997;16:23–30.

106. St. Geme JW III, Falkow S. *Haemophilus influenzae* adheres to and enters cultured human epithelial cells. Infect Immun 1990;58:4036–44.

107. van Schilfgaarde M, van Alphen L, Eijk PP, et al. Paracytosis of *Haemophilus influenzae* through cell layers of NCI-H292 lung epithelial cells. Infect Immun 1995;63:4729–37.

108. Murphy TF. Immunity to nontypeable *Haemophilus influenzae*: elucidating protective responses. Am J Respir Crit Care Med 2003;167:486–7.

109. Ketterer MR, Shao JQ, Hornick DB, et al. Infection of primary human bronchial epithelial cells by *Haemophilus influenzae*: macropinocytosis as a mechanism of airway epithelial cell entry. Infect Immun 1999;67:4161–70.

110. Forsgren J, Samuelson A, Ahlin A, et al. *Haemophilus influenzae* resides and multiplies intracellularly in human adenoid tissue as demonstrated by in situ hybridization and bacterial viability assay. Infect Immun 1994;62:673–9.

111. Linnanmaki E, Leinonen M, Mattila K, et al. *Chlamydia pneumoniae*-specific circulating immune complexes in patients with chronic coronary heart disease. Circulation 1993;87:1130–4.

112. Kauffman HF, Tomee JF, van der Werf TS, et al. Review of fungus–induced asthmatic reactions. Am J Respir Crit Care Med 1995;151:2109–16.

113. Saetta M, Di Stefano A, Maestrelli P, et al. Airway eosinophilia in chronic bronchitis during exacerbations. Am J Respir Crit Care Med 1994;150:1646–52.

114. Hargreave FE, Leigh R. Induced sputum, eosinophilic bronchitis, and chronic obstructive pulmonary disease. Am J Respir Crit Care Med 1999;160(5 Pt 2):S53–7.

115. Clementsen P, Larsen FO, Milman N, et al. *Haemophilus influenzae* release histamine and enhance histamine release from human bronchoalveolar cells. APMIS 1995;103:806–12.

116. Clementsen P, Milman N, Kilian M, et al. Endotoxin from *Haemophilus influenzae* enhances IgE-mediated and non-immunological histamine release. Allergy 1990;45:10–7.

117. Kjaergard LL, Larsen FO, Norn S, et al. Basophil-bound ige and serum IgE directed against *Haemophilus influenzae* and *Streptococcus pneumoniae* in patients with chronic bronchitis during acute exacerbations. APMIS 1996;104:61–7.

118. Pauwels R, Verschraegen G, van der Straeten M. IgE antibodies to bacteria in patients with bronchial asthma. Allergy 1980;157:665–9.

119. Veeramachaneni SB, Sethi S. Pathogenesis of bacterial exacerbations of COPD. COPD 2006;3:109–15.

120. Sethi S. New developments in the pathogenesis of acute exacerbations of chronic obstructive pulmonary disease. Curr Opin Infect Dis 2004;17:113–9.

121. Eldika N, Sethi S. Role of nontypeable *Haemophilus influenzae* in exacerbations and progression of chronic obstructive pulmonary disease. Curr Opin Pulm Med 2006;12(2):118–24.

CHAPTER 15

Viral Infections and Chronic Obstructive Pulmonary Disease

Patrick Mallia, MD, MRCP, PhD, and Sebastian L. Johnston, MBBS, PhD

Exacerbations of chronic obstructive pulmonary disease (COPD) account for many of the morbidity, mortality, and health care costs associated with COPD. Recent studies have implicated respiratory virus infections as a major cause of COPD exacerbations. There is also evidence that chronic virus infection occurs in COPD and may be one mechanism that enhances smoking–induced inflammation and contributes to the pathogenesis of COPD. Current treatments for COPD are not very effective at preventing or treating acute exacerbations, and new treatments specifically addressing prevention and treatment of exacerbations are urgently needed.

Viruses and COPD Exacerbations

Viral infections of the respiratory tract are the most common infectious syndromes in humans; therefore, respiratory virus infections in COPD patients are likely to occur commonly. For many years, there was little research into the potential role of respiratory viruses in COPD exacerbations. However, recently, the identification of viruses in clinical samples has been revolutionized with the development of new molecular techniques based on the amplification of nucleic acids. This has led to a major reappraisal of our knowledge concerning the role of respiratory viruses in a number of disease syndromes, including COPD exacerbations.

Clinical Syndromes Associated with Respiratory Viruses

A wide variety of viruses can infect the human respiratory tract and cause a spectrum of clinical syndromes ranging from self-limiting upper respiratory infection (the common cold) to life-threatening lower respiratory tract infections (pneumonia, bronchiolitis). The field of respiratory virology continues to evolve rapidly owing to the discovery of new pathogens (eg, human metapneumovirus [hMPV]), new understanding of the role of previously recognized viruses (eg, rhinoviruses), and the ability of viruses to mutate and cause new clinical syndromes (eg, severe acute respiratory syndrome [SARS], avian influenza). Polymerase chain reaction (PCR)-based methods have been shown to markedly improve the detection rate of respiratory viruses in clinical samples when compared with culture and antigen detection techniques.[1,2] This is especially true for viruses that are difficult to detect with standard techniques such as coronaviruses and rhinoviruses. Rhinoviruses are difficult to culture, and serology is impractical owing to the large number of serotypes (> 100) that exist. Rhinoviruses are the most common etiologic agent of the common cold, with peaks occurring in autumn and spring, when they account for up to 80% of upper respiratory tract infections.[3] Until relatively recently, rhinoviruses were considered to be trivial pathogens that infected the upper respiratory tract, causing mainly self-limiting upper respiratory tract illness. With the development of PCR, the diagnosis of rhinovirus infections has been transformed, and it has become clear that they are involved in a wider range of clinical syndromes than was previously recognized. In addition, there is now compelling evidence that rhinovirus infection is not confined to the upper respiratory tract but that rhinoviruses can infect the lower airways also.[4] Studies in asthma using PCR have revealed that viruses are the major cause of asthma exacerbations, responsible for 85% of exacerbations in children, and the most common viruses detected were rhinoviruses.[5] Subsequent studies in both children and adults have confirmed that respiratory viruses are associated with the majority of asthma exacerbations.[6] Rhinoviruses have also been implicated in other respiratory clinical syndromes, such as bronchiolitis[7] and pneumonia.[8] These data regarding the role of rhinoviruses in asthma and other lower respiratory tract disease have led investigators to examine a possible role for respiratory viruses in COPD.

Studies Linking Respiratory Virus Infection with COPD Exacerbations

An association between upper respiratory tract infection and COPD exacerbations has long been recognized, and in clinical practice, patients often report colds preceding exacerbations.[9,10] A number of studies in the 1960s and 1970s analyzed the role of respiratory viruses in patients with chronic bronchitis and symptoms of acute lower respiratory tract infection. Scott and colleagues detected a rhinovirus in 13 of 87 (14.9%) exacerbations of chronic bronchitis,[11] and Gregg and Inglis detected a number of different viruses in 30% of exacerbations.[12] A study of 25 patients followed over a 4-year period detected a respiratory virus or *Mycoplasma pneumoniae* in 33.6% of 116 exacerbations, but rhinovirus was detected in only 3.4%.[13] Buscho and colleagues studied 46 men with chronic bronchitis also over a 4-year period and detected a virus in 25% of 166 exacerbations and 14% of stable periods ($p = .02$).[14] Rhinoviruses were detected in only 2.7% of exacerbation samples and 0.55% of stable samples ($p > .05$). A study in patients with chronic bronchitis and airflow obstruction reported a virus detection rate of 18% in exacerbations and 6% in stable patients ($p < .01$). Therefore, these early studies using the virus detection methods available at the time implicated virus infection in at least 15 to 30% of exacerbations of chronic bronchitis. However, these initial results failed to stimulate further research into the role of viruses in COPD. In contrast, a large number of studies focused on the role of bacteria and antibiotic therapy in COPD exacerbations, and this remained the main focus of research into the etiology of COPD exacerbations up until relatively recently. The development of PCR led a number of investigators to reevaluate the role of viruses in COPD exacerbations using this new diagnostic technique. The first studies using PCR to detect respiratory viruses in COPD were carried out by the East London group in patients with mild exacerbations treated as outpatients. In a cohort of patients with moderate to severe COPD (mean forced expiratory volume in 1 second [FEV_1] 40% predicted), 43 exacerbations were examined for the presence of rhinovirus in sputum. Twenty-three percent of exacerbation samples were positive for rhinovirus ribonucleic acid (RNA) compared with zero number of samples collected from stable patients.[15] In a subsequent report from this group, respiratory samples from COPD patients were analyzed for a panel of common respiratory viruses. A respiratory virus was detected in 39% of exacerbations and in 16% of stable patients. The most common viruses detected were rhinoviruses, which accounted for 58%.[9] In this study, symptom data were also collected, and 64% of the exacerbations were preceded by symptoms of a cold. Therefore, this figure may be an underestimate of the true frequency of viral infection, which could be accounted for by a number of factors in the study:

1. Samples were taken within 48 hours of the onset of lower respiratory tract symptoms. Upper respiratory tract infection may precede the exacerbation by several days; therefore, the virus may no longer be detectable by the time of exacerbation of COPD.
2. Only nasal aspirate samples were taken, whereas in the previous study from this group, both sputum and nasal samples were taken. When both samples were collected, 40% more sputum samples were positive compared with nasal samples,[15] so samples collected from the upper respiratory tract only may give a low estimate of the contribution of viruses to COPD exacerbations.

COPD exacerbations are a major cause of hospitalization in COPD patients, and hospital admissions are the main driver of the health care costs associated with COPD. Hospital admissions owing to COPD exacerbations are more common in winter, when there is the greatest circulation of respiratory viruses in the community.[16] A study of the relationship between viral respiratory illnesses in children and hospital admissions of patients with COPD reported significant correlations between the frequency of childhood viral infections and the number of adult COPD hospitalizations.[17] Several studies have directly evaluated the frequency of viral infection in patients admitted to hospital with COPD exacerbations. A German study assessed the incidence of virus infection using PCR in 85 COPD patients (mean FEV_1 49% predicted) admitted to hospitals with an acute exacerbation and a group of patients with stable COPD. A respiratory virus was detected in 56% of exacerbated patients and 19% of controls ($p < .001$). Rhinoviruses were the most common viruses detected (36% of virus-associated exacerbations), and there was a higher detection rate in sputum, again indicating that this is superior to testing upper respiratory tract samples only. A study from the United States in a mixture of hospitalized and ambulatory patients reported that 41.8% of exacerbations were associated with a respiratory virus, with rhinoviruses accounting for half of these.[2] An Italian study detected a respiratory virus in 48.4% of exacerbations and 6.25% of stable COPD patients ($p < .001$), 54.8% of which were rhinoviruses.[18] The only study in which rhinoviruses were not the most common viruses detected was a study from Singapore of COPD patients hospitalized with an acute exacerbation of COPD.[19] In this study, 64% of exacerbations were positive for a virus, and influenza was the most common virus.

The most severe manifestation of COPD exacerbations is the development of respiratory failure and requirement for mechanical ventilation. Mortality in patients with exacerbations requiring assisted ventilation is high, as is the cost of treating such events, which often result in a prolonged stay in intensive care units. Two studies have assessed the role of virus infection in COPD patients with more severe exacerbations requiring either noninvasive ventilation or intubation and mechanical ventilation. A respiratory virus was identified in 47% of exacerbations requiring mechanical ventilation in the United Kingdom[20] and 43% of exacerbations in a study from Australia.[21] The Australian study provided data regarding virus types, and the most common virus detected was influenza A (26%), with rhinovirus detected in 13% of virus–associated episodes.[21]

Therefore, studies using PCR have implicated a respiratory virus in 40 to 60% of acute COPD exacerbations. These findings have been replicated in a range of geographic settings and exacerbation severity. Studies in the northern hemisphere have consistently identified rhinoviruses as the most common virus detected, whereas studies from Hong Kong and Australia have reported influenza to be more common. These studies suggest that respiratory virus infection is at least as common a cause of COPD exacerbations as bacterial infection.

Recently Discovered Viruses and COPD Exacerbations

In up to 10 to15% of patients with acute respiratory illnesses, no pathogen can be found even when PCR technology is used.[5] A number of previously unknown viruses have recently been identified, and these, together with as yet unidentified viruses, may account for these PCR-negative illnesses. One recently described virus is the human metapneumovirus (hMPV), a novel paramyxovirus that was first identified in children in Holland in 2001.[22] Since that initial report, hMPV has been identified globally and has been detected in both children and adults with various clinical syndromes, such as upper and lower respiratory tract infections and wheezing.[23,24] A number of studies have evaluated whether hMPV is involved in COPD exacerbations. Beckham and colleagues failed to detect any hMPV infections in patients with COPD exacerbations,[2] whereas Martinello and colleagues identified hMPV in 12% of patients admitted to hospital in the United States with an acute exacerbation of COPD.[25] Other studies have reported detection rates of 2.3%,[26] 4.1%,[27] and 4.7%[18] in studies from Germany, Canada, and Italy, respectively.

Other new viruses that infect the human respiratory tract have been described recently, including two new human parvoviruses termed the "human bocavirus" (HBoV) and PARV4.[28,29] Studies in children have implicated these viruses as common viral pathogens in respiratory syndromes.[30,31] No studies have yet reported on these viruses in COPD, so it is not known whether they play a role in exacerbations. However, the discovery of previously unidentified viruses that cause respiratory illness illustrates the continual new developments occurring in this field.

Do Viruses Cause Exacerbations?

The detection of a microorganism in the respiratory tract during an illness and a significantly lower incidence of infection among subjects without the disease syndrome shows an association between the two but does not definitively prove that the organism is causing the disease. The studies detecting viruses in COPD exacerbations do not definitively prove that viruses cause exacerbations. Definitive proof of causality is difficult and used to depend on fulfilling Koch's postulates. It is now recognized that microorganisms exist that do not fulfill all of the postulates but whose pathogenicity is not in doubt. Suitable animal models are often not available, and this is especially the case for rhinoviruses, for which no small animal model currently exists. Proof of causality often depends on the accumulation of a number of lines of evidence, including the presence of an organism in samples collected from patients with the disease and not in controls, the development of specific immune responses, and consistent association of an organism with a particular disease syndrome. For many respiratory viruses, further evidence of pathogenicity has come from experimental infection studies involving controlled inoculation of adult volunteers with the virus and the induction of clinical illness. Such infection studies have been carried out for rhinoviruses,[32–34] parvovirus,[35] respiratory syncytial virus (RSV),[32,36] coronaviruses,[32] and influenza.[37] Furthermore, experimental rhinovirus infection has been carried out in asthmatic volunteers and has induced many of the features of a mild asthma exacerbation, thus providing further evidence for a link between virus infection and asthma exacerbations.[38–40] Our group recently carried out a pilot study in which we inoculated COPD patients with a rhinovirus to determine whether it might be possible to establish a human model of virus-induced COPD exacerbation.[41] Successful infection with rhinovirus led to the typical symptoms of exacerbation, together with increased airflow obstruction, evidence of viral replication in the respiratory tract, and nasal inflammation;[41] these findings are currently being replicated in a larger number of COPD patients (unpublished data, 2008). Therefore, this study has provided further evidence that respiratory viruses can cause acute exacerbations of COPD. The prevention of exacerbations with antiviral treatments or vaccines will be another important step in proving causation.

Interactions between Viruses and Bacteria

The human respiratory tract is continually exposed to microorganisms, including both viruses and bacteria, and infection with more than one organism is likely to be a common event. It is widely stated that viral infection predisposes individuals to bacterial infection, but with the exception of influenza, there are surprisingly few published data to support this. There is epidemiologic evidence linking influenza and RSV with bacterial infections,[42,43] but for other viruses, such as the rhinoviruses, the effect on bacterial infection is less well established. Studies evaluating associations between respiratory viruses and bacterial infection have often had conflicting results. A number of studies have found no significant association between respiratory virus infections and bacterial infections in both children[44–46] and adults.[47] One study of viral and bacterial pathogens in the nasopharynx of otitis-prone children found a positive association between respiratory virus and *Moraxella catarrhalis* but not *Haemophilus influenzae* or *Streptococcus pneumoniae*.[48] There is *in-vitro* evidence that rhinoviruses can increase adherence of *S. pneumoniae* and *Staphylococcus aureus* to airway epithelial cells,[49,50] but it is not known whether this occurs *in vivo*. In addition, it has been shown that bacterial infection can increase the susceptibility of respiratory epithelial cells to rhinovirus infection; therefore, bacterial infection may predispose individuals to virus infection in the airways.[51]

Viruses and Bacteria in COPD Exacerbations

Bacterial colonization of the airways in COPD patients is common, being present in up to 25% of stable patients and 50% of exacerbations.[52] Therefore, it is likely that acute virus infections in patients colonized with bacteria and dual infection with viruses and bacteria occur. Few studies have been carried out evaluating whether dual infection with bacteria and viruses plays a role in COPD exacerbations. Two studies of viral and bacterial infections in patients with chronic bronchitis reported conflicting findings, with one reporting positive but nonsignificant relationships between viruses and bacteria[53] and another reporting no association.[13] A more recent study examined sputum for evidence of both bacterial and virus infection in 64 patients hospitalized with a COPD exacerbation and detected a respiratory pathogen in 78% of exacerbations.[18] Of these, 29.7% were bacterial and 23.4% were viral (55% rhinoviruses), and in 25% of exacerbations, both viral and bacterial infections were present. Exacerbations in which coinfection were present were associated with more marked lung function impairment and longer hospitalizations compared with those in which no organism was detected, but there were no differences between exacerbations with a single pathogen and those in which dual infection was present. A report from the East London COPD cohort examined the incidence of coinfection with rhinoviruses and bacteria in COPD exacerbations treated as outpatients; 69.6% of exacerbations were associated with a bacterial pathogen, most commonly *H. influenzae*, and rhinovirus was identified in 19.6% of exacerbations.[54] Exacerbations associated with both *H. influenzae* and rhinovirus exhibited a greater bacterial load and serum interleukin (IL)-6, but the frequency of coinfection was not reported. Another study from this group reported that in exacerbations in which a rhinovirus was detected, coinfection with a bacteria was present in 70%.[55] In severe COPD exacerbations requiring ventilation, mixed infection was present in 10%.[21] Bandi and colleagues studied the incidence of virus infection in acute COPD exacerbations in which nontypeable *H. influenzae* was isolated in sputum.[56] A virus was detected in 45.7% of exacerbations, and 31.4% were associated with the development of new serum immunoglobulin G (IgG) to *H. influenzae*, but only 8.6% of exacerbations were associated with both virus infection and a new serum IgG response to *H. influenzae*.

The relationships between viruses and bacteria in COPD are undoubtedly complex. All studies published to date examining the role of coinfection have sampled at single time points during an exacerbation. If viral infection predisposes individuals to bacterial infection, it is possible that viral infection may occur first and is then followed by a bacterial infection. There may be a period of time when only viruses or bacteria are detectable in the airways, and sampling at a single time point may fail to detect the relationship between the two. A proportion of exacerbations in which only bacteria are isolated may have been preceded by a viral infection that is no longer detectable but contributed to the pathogenesis of the exacerbation. Studies are needed in which longitudinal sampling is carried out in COPD patients for viruses and bacteria to determine the relationship between them and their effect on exacerbations.

Susceptibility to Viruses and COPD

Respiratory virus infections are common in COPD patients, but it is not known whether COPD patients are more susceptible to virus infection compared with individuals without COPD. Few studies have examined this topic, and those that are available have had conflicting results. A community study of rhinovirus illnesses in Michigan reported significantly more rhinovirus infections in males with chronic bronchitis.[57] However, in this study, the diagnosis of infection relied on serology alone, and only 5 (of > 100) respiratory virus serotypes were tested. A more recent study evaluating rates of respiratory virus respiratory tract illness in COPD patients and age-matched controls found that the rates of lower respiratory tract illnesses were more frequent in the COPD group and that there were significantly more hospitalizations in patients with moderate to severe COPD.[16] Respiratory virus infections were detected in 44% of episodes of acute respiratory illness in the controls and 27% of episodes in the COPD group, suggesting that COPD patients are, in fact, less susceptible to respiratory virus infection. However, this study did not use PCR, which is very much more sensitive than cell culture in detecting rhinovirus in airway samples.[58] Therefore, an alternative explanation of these results is that in COPD patients, lower levels of virus that were not able to be detected by culture can cause clinical illness. In an outbreak of rhinovirus illness among the residents of a long-term care facility, those infected were more likely to have COPD than those not infected, but this difference was not significant (52% compared with 36%; $p = .07$). No information was provided regarding smoking rates in the two groups, so it is not clear whether the higher infection rates in the COPD group were related to a higher frequency of smoking in the COPD patients. A study of 121 elderly adults with confirmed respiratory virus infection found that chronic lung disease and smoking were associated with a greater risk of lower respiratory tract complications.[59] Therefore, the results of the studies published to date regarding COPD and susceptibility to virus infection are equivocal. To address this question, studies are needed with control groups matched for age and smoking with the COPD patients and using PCR for virus detection. COPD is a heterogeneous disease, and the response to virus infection may well vary between patients. One study of the relationship between colds and exacerbations in COPD patients reported that those COPD patients with more frequent exacerbations suffered more frequent colds.[60] Therefore, it may be that there is a subset of COPD patients with increased susceptibility to respiratory virus infection and exacerbations. However, this study used a symptomatic definition of a cold and did not carry out virologic sampling, so its results are not conclusive.

Respiratory Viruses and Airway Inflammation in COPD Exacerbations

COPD is associated with pulmonary and systemic inflammation even in patients who are clinically stable. During exacerbations, inflammation is further increased above that present in stable patients. There are increased numbers of leukocytes in sputum during exacerbations,[61] although the results of different studies have not been consistent, with some studies reporting no increases in leukocytes in sputum in exacerbations.[62,63] Few studies have evaluated whether the inflammatory response differs according to the etiologic agent of exacerbation and whether viruses are associated with a specific inflammatory profile. Exacerbations of chronic bronchitis in which *H. influenzae* or *M. catarrhalis* had been identified were associated with higher levels of IL-8, tumor necrosis factor α (TNF-α), and neutrophil elastase (NE) in sputum than those in which no bacterial pathogen was isolated.[64] Exacerbations associated with purulent sputum (and a high incidence of bacterial infection) were associated with significantly higher levels of IL-8, TNF-α, leukotriene B4, and myeloperoxidase compared with those associated with mucoid sputum.[65] Presumably, many of the culture-negative and mucoid exacerbations were due to virus infection; therefore, these studies suggest that bacterial exacerbations are associated with more severe airway inflammation. However, a study of virus-associated exacerbations reported that they were associated with more symptoms and higher levels of sputum IL-6 compared with those in which no virus was detected, although this study did not investigate the role of bacterial infection.[15] Another study reported that endothelin-1 levels in sputum were higher in COPD patients with documented viral or chlamydial infection than those without, although the numbers were small and the difference did not reach statistical significance.[62]

Other studies have reported that the increases in airway inflammatory markers in the airways of patients with an acute exacerbation of COPD occur independently of a demonstrable viral or bacterial infection[66] and that neutrophil numbers are not related to the presence of viral infection.[20] One study of bacterial and virus infections in COPD exacerbations reported increased neutrophils and eosinophils in sputum.[18] When the cell types were related to the etiologic agent of the exacerbation, eosinophilia occurred in the virus-associated exacerbations only. Further studies are needed in which sampling is carried out for both bacteria and viruses to determine the effect of different etiologic agents on the specific cellular and molecular inflammatory profile in COPD exacerbations.

Markers of Virus Infection in COPD Exacerbations

Viruses have been implicated in at least 40 to 60% of exacerbations of COPD. Identifying exacerbations with a viral etiology is important as it could lead to more targeted therapy and reduce unnecessary antibiotic use. Antibiotics are of undoubted benefit in COPD exacerbations, but it is likely that this is due to a large effect in some patients, with less or no effect in others. This has been suggested since the classic study of Anthonisen and colleagues in 1978.[10] However, the reality of antibiotic use in COPD exacerbations is that the majority of patients receive antibiotics. Investigators have attempted to determine whether clinical characteristics can provide evidence regarding exacerbation etiology, but the results have been mixed. Anthonisen and colleagues stratified exacerbations into those in which the three symptoms of dyspnea, sputum volume, and sputum purulence were increased (type I), type II exacerbations (two symptoms), and type III (one symptom plus minor criteria). The greatest treatment benefits with antibiotics were seen in type I exacerbations, implying that bacteria played a significant role in exacerbations characterized by these symptoms. Some studies have reported that sputum purulence is associated with a higher incidence of bacterial infection than exacerbations associated with mucoid sputum,[67,68] whereas others have not found this association.[69,70]

As clinical factors may not be sensitive or specific enough to distinguish between bacterial and viral infection, the development of a marker that could do so would be a major clinical breakthrough. A recent approach that holds considerable promise is the measurement of serum procalcitonin. Procalcitonin is a protein that is normally undetectable but increases markedly in bacterial infections. In infections owing solely to viral infection, procalcitonin is not elevated, so it has potential as a specific marker of bacterial infection. Use of procalcitonin-guided treatment in adults with lower respiratory tract infections has shown that this is associated with a reduction in antibiotic use and no adverse clinical outcomes owing to undertreatment.[71] In a subgroup of patients in this study with COPD exacerbations, the use of antibiotics was reduced by 56% using procalcitonin-guided therapy. A study evaluating procalcitonin specifically in COPD exacerbations found that procalcitonin-guided therapy reduced antibiotic use without compromising clinical outcomes, including improvement in lung function, exacerbation rate, and time to the next exacerbation.[70] There was an absolute risk reduction of 31.5% in antibiotic exposure. Procalcitonin levels were similar in patients with and without sputum purulence and did not differ between patients with Anthonisen type I, II, or III exacerbations, further suggesting that these parameters alone do not distinguish exacerbation etiology. Therefore, procalcitonin holds promise as a marker of bacterial infection in respiratory infections, including COPD exacerbations.

The two studies published to date have been performed in a single center and therefore require replication in other centers to confirm the widespread applicability of these results.

Mechanisms Linking Virus Infection with COPD Exacerbations

It is well established that viruses are triggers of asthma and COPD exacerbations, but the mechanisms whereby viruses induce exacerbations are largely undetermined. Respiratory viruses infect the airway epithelium and generate local and systemic immune and inflammatory responses. Different viruses have diverse effects on the airways, with some viruses, such as influenza and adenovirus, having a marked cytopathic effect on the airway epithelium, whereas rhinoviruses appear to cause less cell death. As rhinoviruses are the most common viral cause of exacerbations and there are more data available on the pathogenesis of rhinovirus infections, we discuss current knowledge regarding the mechanisms of rhinovirus-induced airway pathology and its potential applicability to COPD exacerbations.

The number of epithelial cells infected by rhinoviruses is low, although this has been studied only in healthy subjects and may not be true in asthma or COPD. One current model of rhinovirus disease pathogenesis is that much of the pathology results from rhinovirus-infected epithelial cells producing proinflammatory cytokines.[72,73] The proinflammatory mediators induced by rhinovirus infection have been studied using both *in-vitro* models of virus infection of epithelial cell lines and *in-vivo* models in clinical samples. Some of the mediators and chemokines that are induced by rhinovirus and their main functions are listed in Table 1.[74–105]

These mediators function as chemoattractants, leading to the recruitment of inflammatory cells such as neutrophils, lymphocytes, and eosinophils to the airways. Inflammatory cells release a wide range of mediators, such as proteases, reactive oxygen species, cationic granule proteins, and lipid mediators. These cells are an essential component of the immune response to infection, but the products released can cause host tissue damage and contribute to the pathogenesis of respiratory virus infection. The severity of cold symptoms correlates with concentrations of IL-6,[98,106] IL-8,[87,106] granulocyte colony-stimulating factor,[40] and neutrophils[106] in nasal secretions, highlighting the importance of these in the pathogenesis of upper respiratory tract infections. In asthma exacerbation, severity correlates with markers of neutrophil necrosis lactate dehydrogenase (LDH) and degranulation (NE) and eosinophilic cationic protein (ECP) levels in sputum[6,107] and IL-8 in nasal washings.[108] It was recently shown that rhinoviruses can also infect and replicate within airway macrophages and this can induce high levels of proinflammatory cytokines; thus, this may also be an important source of inflammatory mediators involved in the pathogenesis of

respiratory virus-induced disease.[109] The vast majority of *in-vivo* studies have been carried out in normal volunteers or asthmatics. The only data regarding inflammatory mediators in virus-induced COPD exacerbations are the detection of IL-8 and IL-6 in nasal lavage in experimental rhinovirus infection in COPD[41] and IL-6 in sputum in rhinovirus-associated exacerbations.[15] Further studies are required to determine whether a similar profile of inflammatory mediators and cytokines drives the inflammatory process of exacerbation in COPD.

Rhinovirus infection has also been shown to stimulate mucus production. Rhinovirus increases expression of a number of mucin genes *in vitro* in primary human airway cells[110,111] and *in vivo*.[112] As increased sputum production is a common clinical feature of COPD exacerbations, this may be an important mechanism of virus-induced exacerbations.

Innate Immune Response and Respiratory Virus Infections

Rhinovirus infections are associated with increased lower respiratory tract symptom severity in asthmatics compared with nonasthmatics.[113] Although it is well established that virus infections induce proinflammatory cytokines, it has not been shown conclusively that the inflammatory response differs in asthmatics. Therefore, the mechanism of increased severity of virus infection in asthma remains undetermined. A novel potential mechanism that was recently identified is a deficiency in the innate immune response to rhinovirus infection in asthmatics. The type I ($\alpha\beta$) interferons (IFNs) are important components of the antiviral innate immune response that have a direct antiviral effect on infected and adjacent cells, while also promoting acquired antiviral immune responses. One important mechanism of action of $\alpha\beta$ IFNs is the induction of apoptosis in virus-infected cells, which prevents viral replication and promotes phagocytosis of infected cells.[114] Bronchial epithelial cells from asthma patients infected with rhinovirus support more virus replication and release compared with cells derived from subjects without asthma.[115] This is accompanied by a greater degree of cell necrosis rather than apoptosis and is due to a deficiency in IFN-β in cells from asthma patients. In addition to this, a deficiency in another IFN family, the IFN-λs, has also been reported in asthma patients and related to clinical outcomes after experimental rhinovirus infection.[116] Whether this mechanism plays a role in virus-induced exacerbations in COPD is as yet unknown. It has been shown *in vitro* that cigarette smoke impairs the ability of cell lines to produce IFN-α/β[117]; therefore, further research in this field is needed to elucidate the role of interferons in COPD exacerbations.

Another component of the innate immune response involved in antiviral defense is nitric oxide (NO). NO is produced from L-arginine by the enzyme nitric oxide synthase (NOS), which exists in three isoforms. Type I and III NOS are

Table 1   Cytokines and Inflammatory Mediators Induced by Rhinovirus Infection

Mediator	Principal Actions	In-Vitro Studies	In-Vivo Studies
Interleukin-8 (CXCL8/IL-8)	Neutrophil chemoattractant/activator Eosinophil chemoattractant Induces release of histamine from basophils	BEAS-2B cell line[74–80] A549 cell line[81] Primary human airway epithelial cells[4,80,82–85]	Nasal washings (normals)[83,86,87] Nasal washings (asthmatics)[86,88–90] Nasal washings (COPD)[41] Sputum (asthmatics)[91,92] Sputum (normals)[92]
Regulated on activation normal T-cell expressed and secreted (CCL5/RANTES)	Eosinophil chemoattractant T-cell chemoattractant Monocyte chemoattractant Basophil chemoattractant	A549[93,94] BEAS-2B[75,80] Primary human airway epithelial cells[4,80,82,93]	Nasal aspirates[95,96] Sputum (normals)[97] Sputum (asthmatics)[97]
Interleukin-6 (IL-6)	T-cell growth/activation B-cell differentiation/antibody production Acute-phase protein synthesis	BEAS-2B[74,76–79] A549[98] Primary human airway epithelial cells[4,84,85]	Nasal washings (normals)[86,98,99] Nasal washings (asthmatics)[86] Nasal washings (COPD)[41] Sputum (normals)[86] Sputum (asthmatics)[86,91]
Growth-regulated oncogene α (CXCL1/GRO-α)	Neutrophil chemoattractant/activator	A549[94] BEAS-2B[79]	
Tumor necrosis factor α (TNF-α)	Neutrophil chemoattractant/activator Induces airway hyperresponsiveness	Primary human airway epithelial cells[84,85]	BAL (allergic subjects)[100]
Interleukin-1β (IL-1β)	Upregulates adhesion molecules on endothelial cells	Primary human airway epithelial cells[84,85] BEAS-2B[79]	Nasal washings (normals)[99] Nasal washings (asthmatics)[88]
Interferon-γ-inducible protein 10 (CXCL10/IP10)	Activated T-cell chemoattractant Activated NK cell chemoattractant	Primary human airway epithelial cells[80,101]	Nasal washings (normals)[101]
Eotaxin-1/eotaxin-2	Eosinophil-specific chemoattractants	BEAS-2B[75]	Nasal washings (atopics)[102]
Epithelial-neutrophil activating peptide 78 (CXCL5/ENA-78)	Neutrophil chemoattractant Increases intracellular free calcium Increases elastase release	BEAS-2B[79,103] Primary human airway epithelial cells[80,103]	
Granulocyte-macrophage colony-stimulating factor (GM-CSF)	Primes neutrophils/eosinophils for enhanced activation Increases adhesion molecule expression Cofactor for eosinophil superoxide production	BEAS-2B[74,78,79,104] Primary human airway epithelial cells[82]	
Interleukin-11 (IL-11)	Activates B cells Induces AHR in mice	A549[105]	Nasal washings (normals)[105]
Macrophage inflammatory protein 1α MIP-1α/CCL3	Chemotactic for and activator of monocytes and T cells	BEAS-2B[75]	Sputum (normals and asthmatics)[97]
Interleukin-10 (IL-10)	Immunomodulatory functions		Sputum (asthmatics)[97]

AHR = airway hyperresponsiveness; BAL = bronchoalveolar lavage; COPD = chronic obstructive pulmonary disease; NK = natural killer.

constitutively expressed, whereas type II NOS (iNOS) is inducible by inflammatory cytokines and microbial products. Epithelial cells express all three isoforms of NOS, but iNOS is the predominant form. Rhinovirus infection increases epithelial iNOS expression both *in vitro* and *in vivo*,[118,119] and during experimental rhinovirus infections, levels of exhaled NO increase.[119,120] There is also evidence that NO has an inhibitory effect on rhinovirus as in cell lines it inhibits the replication of rhinoviruses and the rhinovirus-induced production of cytokines.[77,104] In clinical studies, an inverse correlation has been shown between NO levels and both severity of symptoms[119] and changes in airway hyperresponsiveness in asthma patients during rhinovirus infection,[120] suggesting that NO may play a protective role in the airways in respiratory virus infection. There is evidence that NO is reduced in smokers,[121] and this may be a mechanism whereby smoking increases susceptibility to respiratory virus infection.

Chronic Virus Infection and COPD

Although exposure to tobacco smoke is the main risk factor for COPD, only a proportion of smokers lose lung function at an accelerated rate and progress to develop airflow obstruction. Smokers who develop COPD have an enhanced inflammatory response to cigarette smoke, but the mechanisms underlying this remain undetermined. Acute respiratory tract infections likely contribute to disease progression in COPD as frequent exacerbations are associated with an accelerated decline in lung function.[122,123] In addition to acute infections, a possible role for chronic virus infection in COPD has been reported.

Latent Virus Infection in COPD

Some viruses are able to remain in host cells in a latent form in which viral genes are incorporated into the host genome and expressed, but active viral replication does not occur. One such virus type is the adenoviruses, double-stranded deoxyribonucleic acid (DNA) viruses that infect the human respiratory tract and cause acute respiratory illness in children and adults. Host airway epithelial cells infected with adenoviruses express the protein product of the early region 1A (*E1A*) viral gene. Human epithelial cell lines infected with adenovirus have increased production of inflammatory mediators such as intercellular adhesion molecule 1 and IL-8,[124–127] and growth factors such as connective tissue growth factor and transforming growth factor β_1.[128] In addition, *E1A* suppresses the production of the antiproteases elafin and secretory leukoprotease inhibitor.[129] Studies in animal models and in humans have also implicated chronic adenovirus infection in the pathogenesis of COPD. In the guinea pig, exposure to a single dose of cigarette smoke resulted in an increased inflammatory response in animals infected with adenovirus compared with uninfected controls.[130] Chronic cigarette exposure in infected animals resulted in increased inflammation and the development of lesions similar to human emphysema.[131] Exposure to

cigarette smoke alone led to an increase in the CD4+ subset of T cells, whereas the presence of adenoviral infection was associated with an increase in CD8+ lymphocytes.[131] Human studies have also provided evidence for a role of chronic adenovirus infection in COPD. Increased numbers of alveolar epithelial cells expressing *E1A* have been reported in COPD patients compared with smokers without airflow obstruction.[132] Severe emphysema is associated with increased numbers of alveolar epithelial cells expressing *E1A* compared with mild disease, and this increased *E1A* expression is also associated with increased numbers of inflammatory cells in the lung.[133] Therefore, latent adenovirus infection may be one mechanism that amplifies the inflammatory effect of cigarette smoke and contributes to the development of airflow obstruction in smokers.

Persistent Virus Infection in COPD

RSV is a single-stranded RNA virus that causes acute respiratory tract infections in children and is a significant pathogen in adults, especially in the elderly.[134] One study of virus infection in COPD found a higher frequency of RSV infection in airway samples taken from stable COPD than in samples collected during exacerbations. RSV was detected in 23.5% of stable COPD patients and in 14.2% of patients during exacerbations.[9] The presence of RSV in stable COPD was associated with a higher mean arterial partial pressure of carbon dioxide, higher serum IL-6 and plasma fibrinogen levels, and more frequent exacerbations, suggesting a link with disease severity and systemic inflammation. Another study from the same group detected RSV in 32.8% of sputum samples collected from COPD patients over a 2-year period.[135] Patients in whom RSV was more frequently detected (> 50% of samples were RSV PCR positive) had more airway inflammation and faster FEV_1 decline compared with those with less frequent detection of RSV (101.4 mL/yr (95% confidence interval [CI] 57.1–145.8) versus 51.2 mL/yr (95% CI 31.7–70.8); $p = .01$). The relationship between RSV detection and accelerated lung function decline was independent of smoking status, exacerbation frequency, and lower airway bacterial load. A study from Germany reported that RSV-A infection was present in 28% of nasal lavage and sputum samples taken from stable COPD patients.[136] Quantitative real-time PCR performed on these samples and on samples taken from children with acute respiratory tract infections found that the viral load in the infants with acute infection was almost 2,000-fold higher than in the COPD patients. This would suggest that in COPD, low-grade RSV infection is present. However, a study from the United States failed to detect a high prevalence of RSV infection in COPD patients.[137] In 112 COPD patients, RSV was detected by reverse transcriptase-PCR in 6.8% of nasal and sputum samples taken during exacerbations and only 0.3% of samples in stable patients. Therefore, the role of persistent RSV infection in COPD and its role in disease progression remain unclear.

Non-Respiratory Virus Infection and COPD

In addition to the role of respiratory virus infections—both acute and chronic—in COPD, associations have been reported between infection with viruses that do not infect the respiratory tract and COPD. Emphysema-like lesions have been described in individual patients with human immunodeficiency virus (HIV) infection,[138] and an association was confirmed in a case-control study in which HIV-positive patients were compared with a HIV-negative group matched for age and smoking history.[139] The presence of emphysema was assessed with high-resolution computed tomography and lung function tests, and the incidence of emphysema was 15% in the HIV-positive group compared with 2% in the control group. Among those with a smoking history of 12 pack-years or more, 37% of patients in the HIV-positive group had emphysema, whereas none of the controls did. Bronchoalveolar lavage in the HIV-positive patients found no differences in the numbers of neutrophils, macrophages, or total T cells between those with emphysema and those without, but there was a significantly higher number of CD8+ T cells in the emphysema group. A subsequent study examined the prevalence of COPD in HIV-positive patients receiving highly active antiretroviral therapy and reported a 50% increased risk of developing emphysema compared with HIV-negative individuals.[140]

An association between impaired lung function and chronic hepatitis C-infection has also been reported.[141] Kanazawa and colleagues assessed the effect of hepatitis C status on lung function in COPD by comparing the rate of annual decline in FEV_1 and diffusing capacity in COPD patients with and without concurrent hepatitis C infection. The combination of current smoking and positive hepatitis C status was associated with a faster decline in FEV_1 and diffusing capacity compared with current smokers who were hepatitis C-negative. Ex-smokers who were hepatitis C positive had a rate of decline in lung function equivalent to hepatitis C-negative current smokers.

The mechanisms by which HIV and hepatitis C infection contribute to the development of COPD are unknown but may be related to immune mechanisms or other infections. Both HIV and hepatitis C infection are associated with increased numbers of lymphocytes in the lung.[142,143] In HIV patients, these are predominantly CD8+ T cells, and CD8+ T cells are associated with airflow obstruction in COPD.[144] CD8+ lymphocytes also secrete large amounts of IFN-γ,[145] and overexpression of IFN-γ has been shown to cause emphysema in animal models.[146] Chronic viral infection may result in increased numbers of circulating cytotoxic T cells, and smoking may induce local chemotactic factors, leading to their localization in the lung, where they contribute to the development of parenchymal lung destruction. In HIV-positive patients, repeated episodes of infection may contribute to the development of airway obstruction. Both bacterial pneumonia and infection with *Pneumocystis jiroveci* are common infections in HIV patients and are associated with decline in lung function.[147] In addition, colonization with *P. jiroveci* has been associated with the presence and severity of COPD in patients who are not infected with HIV.[148]

Conclusions

COPD is a major public health problem that will continue to grow in importance in the next decades. A large part of the burden of COPD is due to the occurrence of acute exacerbations, which are common events in COPD and account for much of the morbidity, mortality, and health care costs associated with the disease. Recent studies using PCR have established an association between respiratory virus infection and at least 40 to 60% of COPD exacerbations, with the most common viruses being the rhinoviruses. These studies should provide the impetus for further research into the mechanisms linking viruses to COPD exacerbations and the use of antiviral agents in COPD. It is hoped that a better understanding of these mechanisms will lead to the development of novel therapeutic agents that can be used to prevent or treat virus-induced COPD exacerbations.

References

1. Xiang X, Qiu D, Chan KP, et al. Comparison of three methods for respiratory virus detection between induced sputum and nasopharyngeal aspirate specimens in acute asthma. J Virol Methods 2002;101:127–33.
2. Beckham JD, Cadena A, Lin J, et al. Respiratory viral infections in patients with chronic, obstructive pulmonary disease. J Infect 2005;50:322–30.
3. Arruda E, Pitkaranta A, Witek TJ Jr, et al. Frequency and natural history of rhinovirus infections in adults during autumn. J Clin Microbiol 1997;35:2864–8.
4. Papadopoulos NG, Bates PJ, Bardin PG, et al. Rhinoviruses infect the lower airways. J Infect Dis 2000;181:1875–84.
5. Johnston SL, Pattemore PK, Sanderson G, et al. Community study of role of viral infections in exacerbations of asthma in 9–11 year old children. BMJ 1995;310:1225–9.
6. Wark PA, Johnston SL, Moric I, et al. Neutrophil degranulation and cell lysis is associated with clinical severity in virus-induced asthma. Eur Respir J 2002;19:68–75.
7. Papadopoulos NG, Moustaki M, Tsolia M, et al. Association of rhinovirus infection with increased disease severity in acute bronchiolitis. Am J Respir Crit Care Med 2002;165:1285–9.
8. Hicks LA, Shepard CW, Britz PH, et al. Two outbreaks of severe respiratory disease in nursing homes associated with rhinovirus. J Am Geriatr Soc 2006;54:284–9.
9. Seemungal T, Harper-Owen R, Bhowmik A, et al. Respiratory viruses, symptoms, and inflammatory markers in acute exacerbations and stable chronic obstructive pulmonary disease. Am J Respir Crit Care Med 2001;164:1618–23.
10. Anthonisen NR, Manfreda J, Warren CP, et al. Antibiotic therapy in exacerbations of chronic obstructive pulmonary disease. Ann Intern Med 1987;106:196–204.
11. Scott EJ, Grist NR, Eadie MB. Rhinovirus infections in chronic bronchitis: isolation of eight possibly new rhinovirus serotypes. J Med Microbiol 1968;1:109–17.

12. Gregg I, Inglis JM. Exacerbations in chronic bronchitis. Br Med J 1969;4:807.

13. Gump DW, Phillips CA, Forsyth BR, et al. Role of infection in chronic bronchitis. Am Rev Respir Dis 1976;113:465–74.

14. Buscho RO, Saxtan D, Shultz PS, et al. Infections with viruses and *Mycoplasma pneumoniae* during exacerbations of chronic bronchitis. J Infect Dis 1978;137:377–83.

15. Seemungal TA, Harper-Owen R, Bhowmik A, et al. Detection of rhinovirus in induced sputum at exacerbation of chronic obstructive pulmonary disease. Eur Respir J 2000; 16:677–83.

16. Greenberg SB, Allen M, Wilson J, Atmar RL. Respiratory viral infections in adults with and without chronic obstructive pulmonary disease. Am J Respir Crit Care Med 2000; 162:167–73.

17. McManus TE, Coyle PV, Kidney JC. Childhood respiratory infections and hospital admissions for COPD. Respir Med 2006;100:512–8.

18. Papi A, Bellettato CM, Braccioni F, et al. Infections and airway inflammation in chronic obstructive pulmonary disease severe exacerbations. Am J Respir Crit Care Med 2006; 173:1114–21.

19. Tan WC, Xiang X, Qiu D, et al. Epidemiology of respiratory viruses in patients hospitalized with near-fatal asthma, acute exacerbations of asthma, or chronic obstructive pulmonary disease. Am J Med 2003;115:272–7.

20. Qiu Y, Zhu J, Bandi V, et al. Biopsy neutrophilia, neutrophil chemokine and receptor gene expression in severe exacerbations of chronic obstructive pulmonary disease. Am J Respir Crit Care Med 2003;168:968–75.

21. Cameron RJ, de Wit D, Welsh TN, et al. Virus infection in exacerbations of chronic obstructive pulmonary disease requiring ventilation. Intensive Care Med 2006;32:1022–9.

22. van den Hoogen BG, de Jong JC, Groen J, et al. A newly discovered human pneumovirus isolated from young children with respiratory tract disease. Nat Med 2001;7:719–24.

23. Falsey AR, Erdman D, Anderson LJ, Walsh EE. Human metapneumovirus infections in young and elderly adults. J Infect Dis 2003;187:785–90.

24. Williams JV, Harris PA, Tollefson SJ, et al. Human metapneumovirus and lower respiratory tract disease in otherwise healthy infants and children. N Engl J Med 2004; 350:443–50.

25. Martinello RA, Esper F, Weibel C, et al. Human metapneumovirus and exacerbations of chronic obstructive pulmonary disease. J Infect 2006;53:248–54.

26. Rohde G, Borg I, Arinir U, et al. Relevance of human metapneumovirus in exacerbations of COPD. Respir Res 2005;6:150.

27. Hamelin ME, Cote S, Laforge J, et al. Human metapneumovirus infection in adults with community-acquired pneumonia and exacerbation of chronic obstructive pulmonary disease. Clin Infect Dis 2005;41:498–502.

28. Allander T, Tammi MT, Eriksson M, et al. Cloning of a human parvovirus by molecular screening of respiratory tract samples. Proc Natl Acad Sci U S A 2005;102:12891–6.

29. Jones MS, Kapoor A, Lukashov VV, et al. New DNA viruses identified in patients with acute viral infection syndrome. J Virol 2005;79:8230–6.

30. Manning A, Russell V, Eastick K, et al. Epidemiological profile and clinical associations of human bocavirus and other human parvoviruses. J Infect Dis 2006;194:1283–90.

31. Kesebir D, Vazquez M, Weibel C, et al. Human bocavirus infection in young children in the United States: molecular epidemiological profile and clinical characteristics of a newly emerging respiratory virus. J Infect Dis 2006; 194:1276–82.

32. Cohen S, Tyrrell DA, Russell MA, et al. Smoking, alcohol consumption, and susceptibility to the common cold. Am J Public Health 1993;83:1277–83.

33. Cate TR, Couch RB, Fleet WF, et al. Production of tracheobronchitis in volunteers with rhinovirus in a small-particle aerosol. Am J Epidemiol 1965;81:95–105.

34. Couch RB, Cate TR, Douglas RG Jr, et al. Effect of route of inoculation on experimental respiratory viral disease in volunteers and evidence for airborne transmission. Bacteriol Rev 1966;30:517–31.

35. Anderson MJ, Higgins PG, Davis LR, et al. Experimental parvoviral infection in humans. J Infect Dis 1985;152:257–65.

36. Lee FE, Walsh EE, Falsey AR, et al. Experimental infection of humans with A2 respiratory syncytial virus. Antiviral Res 2004;63:191–6.

37. Baccam P, Beauchemin C, Macken CA, et al. Kinetics of influenza A virus infection in humans. J Virol 2006; 80:7590–9.

38. Bardin PG, Fraenkel DJ, Sanderson G, et al. Peak expiratory flow changes during experimental rhinovirus infection. Eur Respir J 2000;16:980–5.

39. Bardin PG, Sanderson G, Robinson BS, et al. Experimental rhinovirus infection in volunteers. Eur Respir J 1996;9:2250–5.

40. Gern JE, Vrtis R, Grindle KA, et al. Relationship of upper and lower airway cytokines to outcome of experimental rhinovirus infection. Am J Respir Crit Care Med 2000;162:2226–31.

41. Mallia P, Message SD, Kebadze T, et al. An experimental model of rhinovirus induced chronic obstructive pulmonary disease exacerbations: a pilot study. Respir Res 2006;7:116.

42. Hament JM, Kimpen JL, Fleer A, Wolfs TF. Respiratory viral infection predisposing for bacterial disease: a concise review. FEMS Immunol Med Microbiol 1999;26:189–95.

43. McCullers JA. Insights into the interaction between influenza virus and pneumococcus. Clin Microbiol Rev 2006; 19:571–82.

44. Lehtinen P, Jartti T, Virkki R, et al. Bacterial coinfections in children with viral wheezing. Eur J Clin Microbiol Infect Dis 2006;25:463–9.

45. Korppi M, Launiala K, Leinonen M, Hakela PH. Bacterial involvement in laryngeal infections in children. Acta Paediatr Scand 1990;79:564–5.

46. Kleemola M, Nokso-Koivisto J, Herva E, et al. Is there any specific association between respiratory viruses and bacteria in acute otitis media of young children? J Infect 2006;52:181–7.

47. Makela MJ, Puhakka T, Ruuskanen O, et al. Viruses and bacteria in the etiology of the common cold. J Clin Microbiol 1998;36:539–42.

48. Pitkaranta A, Roivainen M, Blomgren K, et al. Presence of viral and bacterial pathogens in the nasopharynx of otitis-prone children. A prospective study. Int J Pediatr Otorhinolaryngol 2006;70:647–54.

49. Ishizuka S, Yamaya M, Suzuki T, et al. Effects of rhinovirus infection on the adherence of *Streptococcus pneumoniae* to cultured human airway epithelial cells. J Infect Dis 2003;188:1928–39.

50. Passariello C, Schippa S, Conti C, et al. Rhinoviruses promote internalisation of *Staphylococcus aureus* into non-fully permissive cultured pneumocytes. Microbes Infect 2006; 8:758–66.

51. Sajjan US, Jia Y, Newcomb DC, et al. H. influenzae potentiates airway epithelial cell responses to rhinovirus by increasing ICAM-1 and TLR3 expression. FASEB J 2006;20:2121–3.

52. Monso E, Ruiz J, Rosell A, et al. Bacterial infection in chronic obstructive pulmonary disease. A study of stable and exacerbated outpatients using the protected specimen brush. Am J Respir Crit Care Med 1995;152(4 Pt 1):1316–20.

53. Smith CB, Golden C, Klauber MR, et al. Interactions between viruses and bacteria in patients with chronic bronchitis. J Infect Dis 1976;134:552–61.

54. Wilkinson TM, Hurst JR, Perera WR, et al. Effect of interactions between lower airway bacterial and rhinoviral infection in exacerbations of COPD. Chest 2006;129:317–24.

55. Hurst JR, Perera WR, Wilkinson TM, et al. Systemic and upper and lower airway inflammation at exacerbation of chronic obstructive pulmonary disease. Am J Respir Crit Care Med 2006;173:71–8.

56. Bandi V, Jakubowycz M, Kinyon C, et al. Infectious exacerbations of chronic obstructive pulmonary disease associated with respiratory viruses and non-typeable *Haemophilus influenzae*. FEMS Immunol Med Microbiol 2003;37:69–75.

57. Monto AS, Bryan ER. Susceptibility to rhinovirus infection in chronic bronchitis. Am Rev Respir Dis 1978;118:1101–3.

58. Ireland DC, Kent J, Nicholson KG. Improved detection of rhinoviruses in nasal and throat swabs by seminested RT-PCR. J Med Virol 1993;40:96–101.

59. Nicholson KG, Kent J, Hammersley V, Cancio E. Risk factors for lower respiratory complications of rhinovirus infections in elderly people living in the community: prospective cohort study. BMJ 1996;313:1119–23.

60. Hurst JR, Donaldson GC, Wilkinson TM, et al. Epidemiological relationships between the common cold and exacerbation frequency in COPD. Eur Respir J 2005; 26:846–52.

61. Fujimoto K, Yasuo M, Urushibata K, et al. Airway inflammation during stable and acutely exacerbated chronic obstructive pulmonary disease. Eur Respir J 2005;25:640–6.

62. Roland M, Bhowmik A, Sapsford RJ, et al. Sputum and plasma endothelin-1 levels in exacerbations of chronic obstructive pulmonary disease. Thorax 2001;56:30–5.

63. Bhowmik A, Seemungal TA, Sapsford RJ, Wedzicha JA. Relation of sputum inflammatory markers to symptoms and lung function changes in COPD exacerbations. Thorax 2000;55:114–20.

64. Sethi S, Muscarella K, Evans N, et al. Airway inflammation and etiology of acute exacerbations of chronic bronchitis. Chest 2000;118:1557–65.

65. Gompertz S, O'Brien C, Bayley DL, et al. Changes in bronchial inflammation during acute exacerbations of chronic bronchitis. Eur Respir J 2001;17:1112–9.

66. Aaron SD, Angel JB, Lunau M, et al. Granulocyte inflammatory markers and airway infection during acute exacerbation of chronic obstructive pulmonary disease. Am J Respir Crit Care Med 2001;163:349–55.

67. Stockley RA, O'Brien C, Pye A, Hill SL. Relationship of sputum color to nature and outpatient management of acute exacerbations of COPD. Chest 2000;117:1638–45.

68. Rosell A, Monso E, Soler N, et al. Microbiologic determinants of exacerbation in chronic obstructive pulmonary disease. Arch Intern Med 2005;165:891–7.

69. van der Valk P, Monninkhof E, van der Palen J, et al. Clinical predictors of bacterial involvement in exacerbations of chronic obstructive pulmonary disease. Clin Infect Dis 2004;39:980–6.

70. Stolz D, Christ-Crain M, Bingisser R, et al. Antibiotic treatment of exacerbations of COPD: a randomized, controlled trial comparing procalcitonin-guidance with standard therapy. Chest 2007;131:9–19.

71. Christ-Crain M, Jaccard-Stolz D, Bingisser R, et al. Effect of procalcitonin-guided treatment on antibiotic use and outcome in lower respiratory tract infections: cluster-randomised, single-blinded intervention trial. Lancet 2004;363(9409):600–7.

72. Bardin PG, Johnston SL, Sanderson G, et al. Detection of rhinovirus infection of the nasal mucosa by oligonucleotide in situ hybridization. Am J Respir Cell Mol Biol 1994; 10:207–13.

73. Mosser AG, Brockman-Schneider R, Amineva S, et al. Similar frequency of rhinovirus-infectible cells in upper and lower airway epithelium. J Infect Dis 2002;185:734–43.

74. Kim J, Sanders SP, Siekierski ES, et al. Role of NF-kappa B in cytokine production induced from human airway epithelial cells by rhinovirus infection. J Immunol 2000;165:3384–92.

75. Papadopoulos NG, Papi A, Meyer J, et al. Rhinovirus infection up-regulates eotaxin and eotaxin-2 expression in bronchial epithelial cells. Clin Exp Allergy 2001;31:1060–6.

76. Zalman LS, Brothers MA, Dragovich PS, et al. Inhibition of human rhinovirus-induced cytokine production by AG7088, a human rhinovirus 3C protease inhibitor. Antimicrob Agents Chemother 2000;44:1236–41.

77. Sanders SP, Siekierski ES, Porter JD, et al. Nitric oxide inhibits rhinovirus-induced cytokine production and viral replication in a human respiratory epithelial cell line. J Virol 1998;72:934–42.

78. Subauste MC, Jacoby DB, Richards SM, Proud D. Infection of a human respiratory epithelial cell line with rhinovirus. Induction of cytokine release and modulation of susceptibility to infection by cytokine exposure. J Clin Invest 1995;96:549–57.

79. Griego SD, Weston CB, Adams JL, et al. Role of p38 mitogen-activated protein kinase in rhinovirus-induced cytokine production by bronchial epithelial cells. J Immunol 2000;165:5211–20.

80. Edwards MR, Johnson MW, Johnston SL. Combination therapy: synergistic suppression of virus-induced chemokines in airway epithelial cells. Am J Respir Cell Mol Biol 2006; 34:616–24.

81. Johnston SL, Papi A, Bates PJ, et al. Low grade rhinovirus infection induces a prolonged release of IL-8 in pulmonary epithelium. J Immunol 1998;160:6172–81.

82. Schroth MK, Grimm E, Frindt P, et al. Rhinovirus replication causes RANTES production in primary bronchial epithelial cells. Am J Respir Cell Mol Biol 1999;20:1220–8.

83. Zhu Z, Tang W, Gwaltney JM Jr, et al. Rhinovirus stimulation of interleukin-8 in vivo and in vitro: role of NF-kappaB. Am J Physiol 1997;273(4 Pt 1):L814–24.

84. Suzuki T, Yamaya M, Sekizawa K, et al. Effects of dexamethasone on rhinovirus infection in cultured human tracheal epithelial cells. Am J Physiol Lung Cell Mol Physiol 2000;278:L560–71.

85. Terajima M, Yamaya M, Sekizawa K, et al. Rhinovirus infection of primary cultures of human tracheal epithelium: role of ICAM-1 and IL-1beta. Am J Physiol 1997;273(4 Pt 1):L749–59.

86. Fleming HE, Little FF, Schnurr D, et al. Rhinovirus-16 colds in healthy and in asthmatic subjects: similar changes in upper and lower airways. Am J Respir Crit Care Med 1999; 160:100–8.

87. Turner RB, Weingand KW, Yeh CH, Leedy DW. Association between interleukin-8 concentration in nasal secretions and severity of symptoms of experimental rhinovirus colds. Clin Infect Dis 1998;26:840–6.

88. de Kluijver J, Grunberg K, Pons D, et al. Interleukin-1beta and interleukin-1ra levels in nasal lavages during experimental rhinovirus infection in asthmatic and non-asthmatic subjects. Clin Exp Allergy 2003;33:1415–8.

89. Jarjour NN, Gern JE, Kelly EA, et al. The effect of an experimental rhinovirus 16 infection on bronchial lavage neutrophils. J Allergy Clin Immunol 2000;105(6 Pt 1):1169–77.

90. Teran LM, Johnston SL, Schroder JM, et al. Role of nasal interleukin-8 in neutrophil recruitment and activation in children with virus-induced asthma. Am J Respir Crit Care Med 1997;155:1362–6.

91. Grunberg K, Smits HH, Timmers MC, et al. Experimental rhinovirus 16 infection. Effects on cell differentials and soluble markers in sputum in asthmatic subjects. Am J Respir Crit Care Med 1997;156(2 Pt 1):609–16.

92. Pizzichini MM, Pizzichini E, Efthimiadis A, et al. Asthma and natural colds. Inflammatory indices in induced sputum: a feasibility study. Am J Respir Crit Care Med 1998;158:1178–84.

93. Konno S, Grindle KA, Lee WM, et al. Interferon-gamma enhances rhinovirus-induced RANTES secretion by airway epithelial cells. Am J Respir Cell Mol Biol 2002;26:594–601.

94. Papi A, Stanciu LA, Papadopoulos NG, et al. Rhinovirus infection induces major histocompatibility complex class I and costimulatory molecule upregulation on respiratory epithelial cells. J Infect Dis 2000;181:1780–4.

95. Teran LM, Seminario MC, Shute JK, et al. RANTES, macrophage-inhibitory protein 1alpha, and the eosinophil product major basic protein are released into upper respiratory secretions during virus-induced asthma exacerbations in children. J Infect Dis 1999;179:677–81.

96. Pacifico L, Iacobini M, Viola F, et al. Chemokine concentrations in nasal washings of infants with rhinovirus illnesses. Clin Infect Dis 2000;31:834–8.

97. Grissell TV, Powell H, Shafren DR, et al. Interleukin-10 gene expression in acute virus-induced asthma. Am J Respir Crit Care Med 2005;172:433–9.

98. Zhu Z, Tang W, Ray A, et al. Rhinovirus stimulation of interleukin-6 in vivo and in vitro. Evidence for nuclear factor kappa B-dependent transcriptional activation. J Clin Invest 1996;97:421–30.

99. Gentile DA, Villalobos E, Angelini B, Skoner D. Cytokine levels during symptomatic viral upper respiratory tract infection. Ann Allergy Asthma Immunol 2003;91:362–7.

100. Calhoun WJ, Dick EC, Schwartz LB, Busse WW. A common cold virus, rhinovirus 16, potentiates airway inflammation after segmental antigen bronchoprovocation in allergic subjects. J Clin Invest 1994;94:2200–8.

101. Spurrell JC, Wiehler S, Zaheer RS, et al. Human airway epithelial cells produce IP-10 (CXCL10) in vitro and in vivo upon rhinovirus infection. Am J Physiol Lung Cell Mol Physiol 2005;289:L85–95.

102. Greiff L, Andersson M, Andersson E, et al. Experimental common cold increases mucosal output of eotaxin in atopic individuals. Allergy 1999;54:1204–8.

103. Donninger H, Glashoff R, Haitchi HM, et al. Rhinovirus induction of the CXC chemokine epithelial-neutrophil activating peptide-78 in bronchial epithelium. J Infect Dis 2003;187:1809–17.

104. Sanders SP, Kim J, Connolly KR, et al. Nitric oxide inhibits rhinovirus-induced granulocyte macrophage colony-stimulating factor production in bronchial epithelial cells. Am J Respir Cell Mol Biol 2001;24:317–25.

105. Einarsson O, Geba GP, Zhu Z, et al. Interleukin-11: stimulation in vivo and in vitro by respiratory viruses and induction of airways hyperresponsiveness. J Clin Invest 1996;97:915–24.

106. Barrett B, Brown R, Voland R, et al. Relations among questionnaire and laboratory measures of rhinovirus infection. Eur Respir J 2006;28:358–63.

107. Grunberg K, Kuijpers EA, de Klerk EP, et al. Effects of experimental rhinovirus 16 infection on airway hyperresponsiveness to bradykinin in asthmatic subjects in vivo. Am J Respir Crit Care Med 1997;155:833–8.

108. Grunberg K, Timmers MC, Smits HH, et al. Effect of experimental rhinovirus 16 colds on airway hyperresponsiveness to histamine and interleukin-8 in nasal lavage in asthmatic subjects in vivo. Clin Exp Allergy 1997;27:36–45.

109. Laza-Stanca V, Stanciu LA, Message SD, et al. Rhinovirus replication in human macrophages induces NF-kappaB-dependent tumor necrosis factor alpha production. J Virol 2006;80:8248–58.

110. He SH, Zheng J, Duan MK. Induction of mucin secretion from human bronchial tissue and epithelial cells by rhinovirus and lipopolysaccharide. Acta Pharmacol Sin 2004;25:1176–81.

111. Inoue D, Yamaya M, Kubo H, et al. Mechanisms of mucin production by rhinovirus infection in cultured human airway epithelial cells. Respir Physiol Neurobiol 2006;154:484–99.

112. Yuta A, Doyle WJ, Gaumond E, et al. Rhinovirus infection induces mucus hypersecretion. Am J Physiol 1998;274 (6 Pt 1):L1017–23.

113. Corne JM, Marshall C, Smith S, et al. Frequency, severity, and duration of rhinovirus infections in asthmatic and non-asthmatic individuals: a longitudinal cohort study. Lancet 2002;359(9309):831–4.

114. Takaoka A, Hayakawa S, Yanai H, et al. Integration of interferon-alpha/beta signalling to p53 responses in tumour suppression and antiviral defence. Nature 2003;424:516–23.

115. Wark PA, Johnston SL, Bucchieri F, et al. Asthmatic bronchial epithelial cells have a deficient innate immune response to infection with rhinovirus. J Exp Med 2005;201:937–47.

116. Contoli M, Message SD, Laza-Stanca V, et al. Role of deficient type III interferon-lambda production in asthma exacerbations. Nat Med 2006;12:1023–6.

117. Sonnenfeld G, Hudgens RW. Effect of sidestream and mainstream smoke exposure on in vitro interferon-alpha/beta production by L-929 cells. Cancer Res 1986;46:2779–83.

118. Sanders SP, Siekierski ES, Richards SM, et al. Rhinovirus infection induces expression of type 2 nitric oxide synthase in human respiratory epithelial cells in vitro and in vivo. J Allergy Clin Immunol 2001;107:235–43.

119. Sanders SP, Proud D, Permutt S, et al. Role of nasal nitric oxide in the resolution of experimental rhinovirus infection. J Allergy Clin Immunol 2004;113:697–702.

120. de Gouw HW, Grunberg K, Schot R, et al. Relationship between exhaled nitric oxide and airway hyperresponsiveness following experimental rhinovirus infection in asthmatic subjects. Eur Respir J 1998;11:126–32.

121. Rytila P, Rehn T, Ilumets H, et al. Increased oxidative stress in asymptomatic current chronic smokers and GOLD stage 0 COPD. Respir Res 2006;7:69.

122. Kanner RE, Anthonisen NR, Connett JE, The Lung Health Study Research Group. Lower respiratory illnesses promote FEV(1) decline in current smokers but not ex-smokers with mild chronic obstructive pulmonary disease: results from the Lung Health Study. Am J Respir Crit Care Med 2001;164:358–64.

123. Donaldson GC, Seemungal TA, Bhowmik A, Wedzicha JA. Relationship between exacerbation frequency and lung function decline in chronic obstructive pulmonary disease. Thorax 2002;57:847–52.

124. Keicho N, Elliott WM, Hogg JC, Hayashi S. Adenovirus E1A upregulates interleukin-8 expression induced by endotoxin in pulmonary epithelial cells. Am J Physiol 1997;272 (6 Pt 1):L1046–52.

125. Keicho N, Elliott WM, Hogg JC, Hayashi S. Adenovirus E1A gene dysregulates ICAM-1 expression in transformed pulmonary epithelial cells. Am J Respir Cell Mol Biol 1997;16:23–30.

126. Fujii T, Hogg JC, Keicho N, et al. Adenoviral E1A modulates inflammatory mediator expression by lung epithelial cells exposed to PM10. Am J Physiol Lung Cell Mol Physiol 2003;284:L290–7.

127. Higashimoto Y, Elliott WM, Behzad AR, et al. Inflammatory mediator mRNA expression by adenovirus E1A-transfected bronchial epithelial cells. Am J Respir Crit Care Med 2002;166:200–7.

128. Ogawa E, Elliott WM, Hughes F, et al. Latent adenoviral infection induces production of growth factors relevant to airway remodeling in COPD. Am J Physiol Lung Cell Mol Physiol 2004;286:L189–97.

129. Higashimoto Y, Yamagata Y, Iwata T, et al. Adenoviral E1A suppresses secretory leukoprotease inhibitor and elafin secretion in human alveolar epithelial cells and bronchial epithelial cells. Respiration 2005;72:629–35.

130. Vitalis TZ, Kern I, Croome A, et al. The effect of latent adenovirus 5 infection on cigarette smoke-induced lung inflammation. Eur Respir J 1998;11:664–9.

131. Meshi B, Vitalis TZ, Ionescu D, et al. Emphysematous lung destruction by cigarette smoke. The effects of latent adenoviral infection on the lung inflammatory response. Am J Respir Cell Mol Biol 2002;26:52–7.

132. Matsuse T, Hayashi S, Kuwano K, et al. Latent adenoviral infection in the pathogenesis of chronic airways obstruction. Am Rev Respir Dis 1992;146:177–84.

133. Retamales I, Elliott WM, Meshi B, et al. Amplification of inflammation in emphysema and its association with latent adenoviral infection. Am J Respir Crit Care Med 2001; 164:469–73.

134. Falsey AR, Walsh EE. Respiratory syncytial virus infection in adults. Clin Microbiol Rev 2000;13:371–84.

135. Wilkinson TM, Donaldson GC, Johnston SL, et al. Respiratory syncytial virus, airway inflammation, and FEV1 decline in patients with chronic obstructive pulmonary disease. Am J Respir Crit Care Med 2006;173:871–6.

136. Borg I, Rohde G, Loseke S, et al. Evaluation of a quantitative real-time PCR for the detection of respiratory syncytial virus in pulmonary diseases. Eur Respir J Suppl 2003;21:944–51.

137. Falsey AR, Formica MA, Hennessey PA, et al. Detection of respiratory syncytial virus in adults with chronic obstructive pulmonary disease. Am J Respir Crit Care Med 2006;173:639–43.

138. Diaz PT, Clanton TL, Pacht ER. Emphysema-like pulmonary disease associated with human immunodeficiency virus infection. Ann Intern Med 1992;116:124–8.

139. Diaz PT, King MA, Pacht ER, et al. Increased susceptibility to pulmonary emphysema among HIV-seropositive smokers. Ann Intern Med 2000;132:369–72.

140. Crothers K, Butt AA, Gibert CL, et al. Increased COPD among HIV-positive compared to HIV-negative veterans. Chest 2006;130:1326–33.

141. Kanazawa H, Hirata K, Yoshikawa J. Accelerated decline of lung function in COPD patients with chronic hepatitis C virus infection: a preliminary study based on small numbers of patients. Chest 2003;123:596–9.

142. Kubo K, Yamaguchi S, Fujimoto K, et al. Bronchoalveolar lavage fluid findings in patients with chronic hepatitis C virus infection. Thorax 1996;51:312–4.

143. Guillon JM, Autran B, Denis M, et al. Human immunodeficiency virus-related lymphocytic alveolitis. Chest 1988;94:1264–70.

144. Saetta M, Di Stefano A, Turato G, et al. CD8+ T-lymphocytes in peripheral airways of smokers with chronic obstructive pulmonary disease. Am J Respir Crit Care Med 1998;157(3 Pt 1):822–6.

145. Twigg HL, Soliman DM, Day RB, et al. Lymphocytic alveolitis, bronchoalveolar lavage viral load, and outcome in human immunodeficiency virus infection. Am J Respir Crit Care Med 1999;159(5 Pt 1):1439–44.

146. Wang Z, Zheng T, Zhu Z, et al. Interferon gamma induction of pulmonary emphysema in the adult murine lung. J Exp Med 2000;192:1587–600.

147. Morris AM, Huang L, Bacchetti P, et al. Permanent declines in pulmonary function following pneumonia in human immunodeficiency virus-infected persons. The Pulmonary Complications of HIV Infection Study Group. Am J Respir Crit Care Med 2000;162(2 Pt 1):612–6.

148. Morris A, Sciurba FC, Lebedeva IP, et al. Association of chronic obstructive pulmonary disease severity and *Pneumocystis* colonization. Am J Respir Crit Care Med 2004;170:408–13.

CHAPTER 16

SMALL ANIMAL MODELS OF EMPHYSEMA

PIERO A. MARTORANA, DVM, ELEONORA CAVARRA, PHD, STEVEN D. SHAPIRO, MD, AND GIUSEPPE LUNGARELLA, MD

IN THE FIRST EDITION of this book, two of the present authors (P.A.M. and G.L.), together with Gordon Snider and Edgar Lucey of the Boston University School of Medicine, wrote a comprehensive review of all animal models of emphysema relating to the pathogenesis of this disease.[1] At that time, the review was guided by the great experience and knowledge of Gordon Snider, who had written his first review on animal models of emphysema in 1978,[2] and by Edgar Lucey, who collaborated with Snider in his second review in 1986.[3] In the first edition, the reader can find information on practically all of the models of experimental emphysema published to that date in the English literature.

Since the appearance of the first edition, a number of more selective reviews on this theme have been published.[4–9]

The present chapter takes a different approach in an attempt to selectively and critically review small animal models of chronic obstructive pulmonary disease (COPD) induced by cigarette smoke exposure. Because cigarette smoke has been identified as the most important risk factor for the development of COPD,[10] these models may provide the basis for the understanding of the complex pathogenetic cellular and molecular mechanisms involved in the development of the disease. In addition, pharmacologic studies of cigarette smoke–induced models of COPD are also considered here since the results could be of interest for future potential therapeutical approaches in humans.

Animal Species: Susceptibility to Emphysema

Relatively few animal species have been used in studies of cigarette smoke exposure. The species most commonly used are the mouse, the rat, and the guinea pig. It is interesting to note that the hamster, which has very often been used as a model of elastase-induced emphysema, probably because of its relatively low level of serum α_1-antitrypsin (A1AT),[11] is not commonly used in models of COPD involving cigarette smoke.

In recent years, studies of cigarette smoke–induced COPD have mainly focused on the mouse as the animal of choice. The advantage of this species is the relatively low cost, their rapid reproductive cycle and large litter sizes, the availability of antibodies and probes for the mouse, and the fact that mouse genes can be manipulated and that the mouse genome

has been sequenced and shows a large degree of homology with the human genome.

However, the mouse has some limitations as an animal model of COPD in that it does not fully model the human condition. This limitation should be kept in mind when interpreting studies of cigarette smoke exposure carried out in this species. The major limitations are listed in Table 1.

Additionally, not all inbred strains of mice develop emphysema following cigarette smoke exposure, and, in the susceptible strains, the severity of this lesion is limited and never reaches the extent seen in human smokers or in other models of emphysema in mice (Figure 1).

The susceptibility of various inbred strains of mice for the development of emphysema following cigarette smoke exposure is shown in Table 2.

As shown in Table 2, three strains were found to be resistant to the effect of cigarette smoke: the ICR, NZWLac/J, and 129J. ICR mice have been reported to increase lung antioxidant defenses when acutely exposed to cigarette smoke and failed to develop emphysema when exposed to cigarette smoke for 7 months.[12] The reason for this may be an upregulation of the enzyme peroxyredoxin 6,[13] possibly owing to upregulation of the nuclear factor erythroid-derived 2, like 2 (Nrf2) pathway.[14] In fact, disruption of the Nrf2 gene in the ICR mice leads to extensive emphysema following chronic cigarette smoke exposure.[15]

NZWLac/J mice did not develop emphysema following 6 months' exposure to cigarette smoke. The reason for this is thought to result from downregulation of proinflammatory cytokines and chemokines after cigarette smoke exposure.[16]

The 129J mouse strain is also resistant to the effects of chronic cigarette smoke exposure (GL, unpublished results, 2004). In addition, these mice did not show an inflammatory response to smoke in an acute model of cigarette smoke exposure,[17] presumably because they produce only low levels of tumor necrosis factor α (TNF-α).[18]

Additionally, four other strains of mice were reported to be susceptible to the development of emphysema. Among these, the strain C57Bl/6J is the most commonly studied. The C57Bl/6J mice have moderately low levels of serum A1AT and of serum elastase inhibitory capacity (EIC) (−24% and −25%, respectively)[19] and are sensitive to oxidants.[12] This sensitivity to oxidants may be the result of a reduced expression level of Nrf2-mediated antioxidant genes.[14] Nrf2 is a redox-sensitive

Table 1 Anatomic and Physiologic Characteristics of the Mouse and their Consequences as a Model of Cigarette Smoke–Induced Chronic Obstructive Pulmonary Disease	
Characteristics	*Consequence as a Model of Cigarette Smoke–Induced COPD*
Mice are obligate nose breathers	This results in a different pattern of particle filtration than in humans (mouth breathers) Thus, it does not make much difference the way (by nose only or by whole body) the animals are exposed to cigarette smoke
Mice have fewer branching airways (6 airway generations) than humans (23 airway generations)	This may result in a different handling of cigarette smoke. Specific information is still lacking
Mice do not have respiratory bronchioles	Thus, they lack the anatomic basis for the development of centrilobular emphysema
Mouse submucosal glands are restricted to the trachea	Thus, mice lack the anatomic basis for the development of bronchial submucosal glands hyperplasia
Mice practically do not have goblet cells in their bronchi and bronchioles	Thus, the appearance of clusters of goblet cells in their bronchi/bronchioles should be considered metaplasia
Mice do not develop mucus hypersecretion following cigarette smoke exposure	Thus, a major component of COPD is missing in the murine model
Mice have a different profile of proteinase expression than humans (ie, mice do not express MMP-1, but they express MMP-12 more prominantly than humans)	Thus, results obtained in mice should be extrapolated with caution to the human condition

COPD = chronic obstructive pulmonary disease; MMP = matrix metalloproteinase.

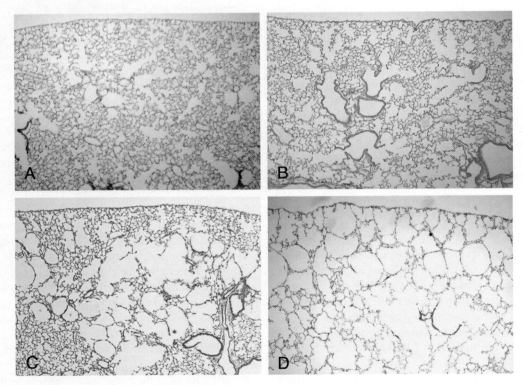

FIGURE 1. *A*, Lung of a mouse of the strain ICR (a strain not susceptible to cigarette smoke–induced emphysema) 6 months after cigarette smoke exposure showing a normal parenchyma. *B*, Lung of a mouse of the strain C57Bl/6J (a strain susceptible to cigarette smoke–induced emphysema) 6 months after cigarette smoke exposure showing disseminated foci of a moderate panlobular emphysema. *C*, Lung of a mouse of the strain C57Bl/6J 21 days after intratracheal administration of porcine pancreatic elastase at the dose of 100 µg, showing large areas of severe panlobular emphysema. *D*, Lung of a tight-skin mouse with spontaneous genetic emphysema (a mutation on a C57Bl/6J background) showing massive diffuse panlobular emphysema at 4 months of age (hematoxylin-eosin stain; ×40 original magnification).

Strain	Susceptibility to Emphysema	Potential Mechanism of Action	Reference
ICR	Not susceptible	Resistant to oxidants High Nrf2 activity	12 14
NZWLac/J	Not susceptible	Downregulation of inflammatory mediators	16
129J	Not susceptible	Low levels of TNF-α	Unpublished results
C57BL/6J	Susceptible	Serum A1AT deficiency (−24%) Sensitivity to oxidants Low Nrf2 activity	12, 19 12 14
DBA/2	Susceptible	Sensitive to oxidants Apoptosis	12 20
A/J	Susceptible	Loss cell survival genes	16, 23, 24
SJ/L	Susceptible	Unknown	16
Pallid (C57Bl/6J pa/pa)	Very susceptible	Serum A1AT deficiency (−55%)	12, 25
AKR/J	Very susceptible	Upregulation of inflammatory mediators	16
AKR/J (SAM 1 and 8)	Very susceptible	Premature senescence	26, 27

Table 2 Susceptibility to Cigarette Smoke–Induced Emphysema of Various Strains of Mice

A1AT = α$_1$-antitrypsin; Nrf2 = nuclear factor erythroid-derived 2, like 2; SAM = senescence-accelerated mouse; TNF-α = tumor necrosis factor α.

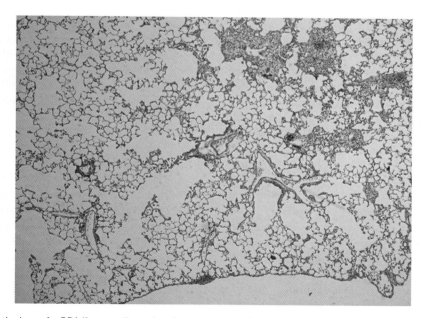

FIGURE 2. Micrograph of the lung of a DBA/2 mouse 7 months after exposure to cigarette smoke. Foci of emphysema and fibrosis are seen either in different areas or in the same area of the lung parenchyma (hematoxylin-eosin stain; ×40 original magnification).

basic leucine zipper protein transcription factor that is involved in the regulation of many detoxification and antioxidant genes.

DBA/2 is also a susceptible strain. DBA/2 mice are sensitive to oxidants,[12] and their alveoli develop uniform dilation that is preceded by the appearance of apoptotic cells in areas with a low expression of vascular endothelial growth factor (VEGF) receptor 2.[20] They also develop some fibrotic areas scattered throughout the parenchyma.[20] Emphysema and fibrosis may coexist either in different areas or in the same area of the lung (Figure 2).[21] The reason for the latter changes could depend on the activation of transforming growth factor (TGF)-α and TGF-β by neutrophil elastase.[21] However, a downregulation of the receptor for advanced glycation end products (RAGE) cannot be excluded as a mechanism.[13] Thus, this strain may be considered the mouse counterpart of a recently described syndrome in humans, combined pulmonary fibrosis and emphysema.[22]

A/J mice were also found to be susceptible to cigarette smoke,[16] and female mice of this strain were reported to be more susceptible than the males.[23] A recent study revealed that emphysema in A/J mice chronically exposed to cigarette smoke was associated with increased inflammation, oxidative stress, apoptosis, and global loss of various cell survival and cytoprotective genes.[24]

Mice of the strain SJ/L were also reported susceptible to cigarette smoke; however, an investigation into the reason for this susceptibility was not carried out.[16]

Three strains were found to be very susceptible: *pallid* (C57Bl/6J *pa/pa*), AKR/J, and the senescence-accelerated mouse (SAM). The cause of the high sensitivity of the *pallid* mouse may be the low levels of serum A1AT (approximately −55% when compared with other strains with "normal" levels) and of serum EIC (−67%).[19,25]

In AKR/J mice, the great sensitivity to cigarette smoke has been attributed to a broad upregulation of inflammatory mediators indicating a T-helper 1 (Th1)-adaptive inflammatory response.[16] Exposure of the AKR/J mice to cigarette smoke by "whole body" technique (ie, in groups) may be a problem because of their aggressive behavior, defined as high intrastrain aggression (<http://jaxmice.jax.org/index.html>).

The SAM group of mice consists of 14 senescence-prone (SAM-P) inbred strains with features of accelerated aging and 4 senescence-resistant (SAM-R) inbred strains with features of normal aging. The SAM has been under development since 1970 through selective inbreeding of the AKR/J strain. One reason for the high susceptibility to the effects of cigarette smoke may be the premature senescence in these mice.[26,27]

Susceptibility of the various strains to the development of bronchial changes such as goblet cell metaplasia (GCM) following cigarette smoke exposure has not been systematically investigated. Two strains of mice have been reported to develop GCM, A/J[23] and C57Bl/6J,[20] whereas mice of the strain DBA/2 strain have been found to develop only very few, if any, clusters of GCM.[20] It is of interest that the mean tracheal mucociliary transport rate is almost six times greater in the C57Bl/6J mice than in the DBA/2 mice. This difference was shown to be heritable, resulting from genetic polymorphism, which affects the mucociliary epithelium.[28] In addition, slow-transporting DBA/2 mice are highly susceptible to the airway pathogen Senday virus, whereas fast-transporting C57Bl/6J mice are highly resistant.[29] It is thus possible that the degree of mucociliary clearance and of cell adaptation in the bronchial tree is also strain dependent.

Since it is likely that genetic factors play an important role in the susceptibility to cigarette smoke in humans, these and future studies carried out in inbred strains of mice with different susceptibility to cigarette smoke may be of value for the investigation of susceptibility and resistance to cigarette smoke–induced COPD in humans.

Inflammatory Response

Recently, COPD was defined by the Global Initiative for Chronic Obstructive Lung Disease (GOLD) as a disease characterized by progressive, not fully reversible, flow limitation and "associated with an abnormal inflammatory response of the lungs to noxious particles and gases."[30] Thus, a central role has been attributed to the chronic inflammatory response that in humans is present throughout the airways and parenchyma and that is thought to participate in the progression and exacerbation of this disease.[31]

Lung Infiltration: Inflammatory Cells

It is of interest that early studies in which mice, rats, and hamsters were exposed to cigarette smoke resulted in the recruitment of inflammatory cells, mainly macrophages and lymphocytes, into the lungs of the exposed animals but not overt bronchial or parenchymal changes.[32–34] The first report of an unequivocal animal model of smoking-related emphysema appeared in 1990,[35] and since then, a large number of studies have investigated in animal models of cigarette smoke–induced COPD/emphysema the role and the kinetics of the inflammatory cells in the development of smoke–induced lesions. This is of particular interest since in COPD patients, the relationship between the inflammatory cell types, the sequence of their appearance, and their persistence remain unknown.

Table 3 summarizes studies characterizing the cell types infiltrating the lung in COPD patients and in animal models of smoke exposure.

In COPD patients, an increased number of neutrophils is recovered from sputum and bronchoalveolar lavage fluids (BALFs) compared with smokers without COPD. However, only a relatively small increase in these cells is present in the airways or parenchyma.[36,37] The lack of significantly increased numbers of neutrophils in the lung parenchyma may be due to the fact that these cells rapidly transit through the airways and the lung parenchyma.[38]

In mice, neutrophil recruitment in BALF occurs following the first cigarette. In an acute study, C57Bl/6J mice were exposed to the smoke from one to three cigarettes. Six hours after the exposure, the BALF neutrophil count was already increased, although the difference when compared with controls was not statistically significant. At 24 hours, the number of neutrophils significantly increased with the number of cigarettes smoked, but with a plateau after two cigarettes. By 48 hours, the neutrophil count started to decrease.[39] Neutrophils have the potential to secrete proteases, including

Table 3   Cell Type Infiltrating the Lung in Chronic Obstructive Pulmonary Disease Patients and Mouse Models of Smoke Exposure

Immune System	Cell Type	COPD Patients	Reference	Mouse Model	Results in Model	Reference
Innate	Neutrophils	Increase in BALF No or small increase in lung	34, 35, 36	Acute Chronic	Increase in BALF Increase in BALF; no increase in lung	17, 39–41 42, 43
	Alveolar macrophages	Increase in BALF and lung	44	Acute Chronic	No or small increase in BALF Increase in BALF and/or lung	17, 39–41 41, 42
Adaptive	CD8+	Increase	48, 49	Chronic	No change Increase	57, 58 16, 23, 42, 65
	CD4+	Increase	50, 64	Chronic	No change Increase	57, 58 16, 23, 42, 65
	B cells	Increase	48, 52, 64	Chronic	Increase	23, 65
	Dendritic cells	Increase	55	Chronic	Reduction Increase	58 42, 62

BALF = bronchoalveolar fluid lavage; COPD = chronic obstructive pulmonary disease.

neutrophil elastase, cathepsin G, and proteinase 3, as well as matrix metalloproteinases (MMPs). These proteinases may contribute to extracellular matrix destruction. Indeed, in the above-mentioned studies, BALF serine and metalloelastase-like activity was increased 24 hours after smoke exposure. Additionally, desmosine (a marker of elastin degradation) and hydroxyproline (a marker of collagen degradation) increased at 6 and 24 hours, with a decrease at 48 hours.[39] Subsequent studies in C57Bl/6J mice confirmed the early increase in BALF neutrophils following acute exposure to cigarette smoke.[17,40,41]

A recent study investigated the dynamics of neutrophil influx in BALF in C57Bl/6J mice during a 6-month cigarette smoke exposure. Smoke–exposed animals developed progressive neutrophilia; the number of neutrophils was significantly increased after 3 days and increased further up to 6 months. However, it is of interest that neutrophil numbers were not increased in the lung tissue.[42] These results were subsequently confirmed in a more recent study.[43] Significant emphysema was always present at 6 months and in the latter study was already evident at 3 months.[43] In this context, the smoking mouse is a good model of the human diseases.

Alveolar macrophages play a pivotal role in the pathophysiology of COPD as they are activated by cigarette smoke and secrete inflammatory proteins that may orchestrate the inflammatory processes associated with COPD.[44] In patients with COPD, there is a marked increase in the number of macrophages in BALF and in the lung parenchyma.[45]

In mice, acute exposure to cigarette smoke induces only modest increases in BALF macrophages.[17,40,41] The numbers of BALF macrophages depend largely on the number of cigarettes smoked; however, it has been suggested that the activation of macrophages rather than the increase in the macrophage number is crucial to initiating the acute inflammatory response.[40,46] In an elegant acute study in mice, it was shown that cigarette smoke activates macrophages to release MMP-12 (macrophage metalloelastase). This protease then mediates cigarette smoke–induced inflammation by releasing TNF-α from macrophages, with subsequent endothelial activation, neutrophil influx, and proteolytic matrix breakdown caused by neutrophil-derived proteases.[47]

Chronic exposure (6 months) of C57Bl/6J mice to cigarette smoke resulted in a progressive biphasic increase in BALF macrophages. There was a slight but significant increase after 7 days and a marked increase after 6 months. In the lungs, the number of macrophages increased significantly after 12 weeks and remained elevated for up to 6 months.[42] A morphometric study of the lung volume density of macrophages also showed a significant increase in these cells after 6 months of smoke exposure.[41]

In COPD patients, chronic inflammation is characterized not only by an increased number of inflammatory cells of the innate immune system (neutrophils and macrophages) but also by an increase in the number of cells of the adaptive immune system (B lymphocytes, T lymphocytes, dendritic cells), suggesting the involvement of antigen-presenting cells in the development of COPD.[44,48,49] CD8[+] lymphocyte numbers have been related to the progressive reduction of pulmonary function in both COPD and asthma.[49,50] CD4[+] lymphocytes have also been found to be increased in severe COPD.[51] These T cells, which may accumulate in the lung following antigen stimulation, could be involved in the pulmonary inflammation even after cessation of cigarette smoking.[52]

Little is known about the role of B cells in COPD. B cells organize in lymphoid follicles in the airways of smokers,[53] and there is a marked increase in lymphoid follicles in patients with severe COPD.[49] The role and importance of these follicles remain unclear. Dendritic cells are not only antigen-presenting cells but also play a role in linking the innate and adaptive immune response.[54,55] There is an increase in the number of dendritic cells in the airways and alveolar walls of smokers.[56]

A number of studies have investigated the presence and/or the role of cells of the adaptive immune system in models of cigarette smoke exposure. Some studies did not find an association between an increase in the number of cells of the adaptive immune system and the development of lung lesions following cigarette smoke exposure. For instance, in a subchronic exposure study, lungs from Balb/c mice exposed to smoke generated from 3, 6, and 9 cigarettes/day for 4 days showed macrophage- and neutrophil-rich inflammation in lung tissue and BALF but only a very small number of CD4[+] and CD8[+] lymphocytes. Quantitative real-time polymerase chain reaction showed upregulation of genes encoding chemokines, inflammatory mediators, and growth factors.[57] Thus, in this subchronic study, the cells of the adaptive immune system did not appear to play a major role in the induction of the inflammatory response.

The impact of cigarette smoke exposure on respiratory immune defense mechanisms was investigated in C57Bl/6 mice. Mice were exposed to two cigarettes daily, 5 days/week, for 2 to 4 months. Cigarette smoke exposure dramatically reduced the number of dendritic cells in the lung. These changes were observed following 2 months of tobacco smoke exposure and preceded the formation of emphysematous lesions. Furthermore, cigarette smoke exposure resulted in fewer dendritic cells expressing the costimulatory molecule B7.1. No differences were observed in the percentage of CD4[+] and CD8[+] T cells in the lungs of smoke–exposed mice compared with naive animals. Furthermore, the activation status of T cells was unchanged by tobacco smoke exposure, as assessed by expression of the early activation marker CD69. In addition, smoke exposure prevented the specific expansion and maximal activation of CD4[+] T cells and reduced the number of both activated CD4[+] and CD8[+] T cells in response to experimental adenovirus infection. Finally, marked reductions were observed in serum levels of adenovirus-specific immunoglobulins that were associated with diminished viral neutralizing capacity. Because both cellular and humoral immunity provide protection against viral and bacterial

pathogens, these findings may, at least in part, explain the increased prevalence of infections in COPD.[58]

Additionally, the role of the adaptive immune system in the development of cigarette smoke–induced emphysema was investigated in a chronic study in scid mice. These mice lack functional B and T cells and peribronchial lymphoid follicles. In these mice, cigarette smoke induced a progressive increase in the cells of the innate immune system in BALF (neutrophils and macrophages), augmented several epithelium-derived chemokines, and induced significant emphysema. Thus, this study suggests that the adaptive immune system does not play a major role in the development of cigarette smoke–induced emphysema.[59]

On the other hand, other experimental studies suggest an association between an increase in the number of the cells of the adaptive immune system and the development of lung lesions following cigarette smoke exposure. It is likely that the lung dendritic cell network is acutely sensitive to smoke inhalation. Dendritic cells would then take up, process, and present cigarette component antigens to CD8[+] cytotoxic T cells.[60] The finding of T cells in the lung would confirm that these cells are responding to an antigen challenge originating in the lung since naive, nonstimulated T cells do not enter the lung because their homing receptors make them relocate to the lymphatic tissue.[61]

Already in 1995, a study reported a 20-fold increase in dendritic cells in the lungs in mice after exposure to tobacco smoke. GCM also developed. After cessation of the exposure to tobacco smoke, the density of the dendritic cells returned to that of the control level, but the bronchial metaplasia did not reverse.[62] Recently, in C57Bl/6J mice, a clear infiltration of dendritic cells was observed in airways (10-fold increase) and lung parenchyma (1.5-fold increase) after 6 months of cigarette smoke exposure. In addition, smoke–exposed animals developed a progressive increase in T lymphocytes in the airways. The total number of CD4[+] T lymphocytes in the lungs at 6 months increased twofold, whereas CD8[+] T lymphocytes increased by 43%. Activation of CD4[+] and CD8[+] T cells was also assessed. After 14 days of smoke exposure, an increased number of activated CD4[+] and CD8[+] T cells was present in lung digests, and at 6 months, the number of activated CD4[+] and CD8[+] T cells was further increased.[42]

A recent study suggested a potentially new role for the dendritic cells in the development of cigarette smoke–induced emphysema in mice. After 1, 3, and 6 months' smoke exposure, there was a significant increase in MMP-12 and cathepsin D messenger ribonucleic acid (mRNA) in the lungs of mice exposed to cigarette smoke compared with air-exposed mice. To determine the cellular origin of MMP-12 and cathepsin D, dendritic cells and macrophages were isolated from the lungs of mice that showed an increase in MMP-12 mRNA after smoke exposure in both macrophage and dendritic cell populations, whereas cathepsin D was predominantly expressed in macrophages. These results indicate that cigarette smoke increases the expression of MMP-12 and cathepsin D in the lungs of mice and that not only macrophages but also dendritic cells produce MMP-12.[63]

In another study in mice of different strains, T cell inflammation and Th1 cytokine profile were present only in the lungs of the susceptible animals that developed emphysema. The authors suggested that an adaptive immune inflammatory reaction with CD4+ and CD8+ T cells and a Th1 chemokine-cytokine profile may be an important contribution to the development of emphysema in the susceptible strains of mice.[16] A recent article reported that the development of emphysema after chronic smoke exposure in female A/J mice was associated with an increase in the number of cells of the innate immune system (neutrophils, macrophages) and of the adaptive immune system (B cells and activated CD4+- and CD8+ T cells).[23]

Another recent work compared B-cell lung infiltration in patients with emphysema and in C57Bl/6J mice exposed to cigarette smoke.[64] Lymphoid follicles were detected in both the airway walls and the parenchyma in lung sections of the patients, where the majority (>80%) of these follicles were seen in the parenchyma of the lung rather than in the airway walls. The majority of cells in the follicles were B cells. The B-cell follicle core was surrounded by T cells, the majority being CD4+. The B cells were interspaced by follicular dendritic cells. The predominant immunoglobulin expressed on the surface of the B cells was immunoglobulin M (IgM). In mice, smoke exposure produced progressive emphysema over time. Starting at 4 months of exposure, a progressive increase in both the size and the number of similar lymphoid follicles was found. As in humans, the follicles contained B cells surrounded by CD4+ and CD8+ T cells and centrally located dendritic cells. IgM was present on the B cells. The authors suggested that a putative role for these B cells could include a reaction to either cigarette smoke components or extracellular matrix degradation products.[64] These findings are of interest, particularly when assessed in the light of a recent report on transgenic mice. Mice were generated that express TNF-α in the lungs under the control of a doxycycline-inducible promoter. The results obtained indicated that TNF-α gene expression was induced and was associated with focal lymphoid tissue formation in the lungs. In addition, mice administered doxycycline for 1 to 9 months developed significant increases in airspace size indicative of emphysema.[65]

All of these results underline the important role played by the animal models in the investigation of the lung cellular inflammatory responses to cigarette smoke.

Oxidative Stress

Oxidative stress occurs when the balance between oxidants and antioxidants shifts in favor of the oxidants, either from an excess of oxidants or from a depletion of antioxidants. Cigarette smoke is the main factor in the development of COPD. Cigarette smoke contains 10^{17} oxidant molecules per puff; this, together with the evidence of an increased

oxidative stress in smokers and in patients with COPD, strongly suggests that an oxidant/antioxidant imbalance plays a major role in the pathogenesis of COPD.[66] Oxidative stress may amplify the lung inflammatory response through the upregulation of redox-sensitive transcription factors, such as nuclear factor κB (NF-κB) and activator protein 1 (AP-1), and other signal transduction pathways, such as mitogen-activated protein (MAP) kinase and phosphoinositide-3-kinase (PI-3K), leading to enhanced gene expression of proinflammatory mediators. It was recently shown that oxidative stress and the redox status of the cells can regulate nuclear histone modifications (acetylation, methylation, and phosphorylation), leading to chromatin remodeling, the induction of proinflammatory mediators, and corticosteroid resistance.[67]

The oxidant burden in the lung is enhanced in smokers by the release of reactive oxygen species (ROS) from macrophages and neutrophils. Oxidants present in cigarette smoke can stimulate alveolar macrophages to produce ROS and to release mediators that attract neutrophils and other inflammatory cells into the lungs. Both neutrophils and macrophages can generate ROS via the nicotinamide adenine dinucleotide phosphate oxidase system. Additionally, cigarette smoking is associated with increased content of myeloperoxidase in neutrophils (H_2O_2 generated from O_2^- is metabolized by myeloperoxidase in the presence of chloride ions to hypochlorous acid, a strong oxidant), and this correlates with the degree of pulmonary dysfunction.[67]

Oxidative stress may also induce apoptosis in endothelial and epithelial cells, and this could contribute to the development of emphysema.[68] Several markers of oxidative stress can be detected in the breath of COPD patients, and several studies have demonstrated increased production of oxidants in exhaled air or breath condensate.[44]

In comparison with the large number of studies carried out in humans on cigarette smoke–induced oxidative stress, relatively few articles deal with this subject in animal models.

An immunohistochemical study was carried out to evaluate oxidative stress in the lung after acute cigarette smoke exposure in mice. The results showed that acute cigarette smoke exposure imposes oxidative stress predominantly on bronchiolar epithelial and alveolar type II cells, and markers of deoxyribonucleic acid (DNA) oxidation and lipid peroxidation were shown to be elevated in BALF.[69]

In another acute study in C57Bl/6J mice, cigarette smoke caused a significant and reversible decrease in total antioxidant capacity measured as Trolox equivalent antioxidant capacity (TEAC) and significant changes in oxidized glutathione, ascorbic acid, protein thiols, and 8-epi-prostaglandin F2 alpha (8-epi-PGF$_2\alpha$) in BALF. When the human recombinant secretory leukoprotease inhibitor (hrSLPI), which is sensitive to oxidative inactivation, was given intratracheally to the mice, cigarette smoke induced a 50% drop in the inhibitory activity of this agent. Pretreatment with N-acetylcysteine prevented the loss of hrSLPI activity. Thus, cigarette smoke may cause transient but repeated oxidative stress, resulting in oxidative inactivation of antiproteases. This can render smokers particularly susceptible to a proteolytic attack, with subsequent development of emphysema.[70]

The effect of oxidative stress on chromatin modifications and the consequent resistance to corticosteroids were investigated in the rat. Rats were exposed to cigarette smoke for either 3 days or 8 weeks. Cigarette smoke exposure resulted in an influx of neutrophils in BALF at both 3 days and 8 weeks. Neutrophils were also increased in the lung at 3 days, and macrophages were augmented at 8 weeks. Histone modification was seen at 8 weeks. This was associated with increased NF-κB, AP-1, and p38 MAP kinase activation and was accompanied by increased histone 3 phosphoacetylation and histone 4 acetylation. Decreased histone deacetylase 2 activity, related to protein modification by aldehydes and nitric oxide products, was also observed and correlated with a lack of corticosteroid suppression of smoke–induced proinflammatory mediator release.[71]

A recent study investigated cigarette smoke–induced apoptosis in the rat. It was suggested that cigarette smoke–induced apoptosis may result from two main mechanisms: one is the activation of p38/JNK-Jun-FasL signaling, and the other is stimulated by the stabilization of p53, an increase in the ratio of Bax to Bcl-2, release of cytochrome-c, and activation of the caspase cascade.[72]

There are strains of mice such as the ICR that are genetically resistant to oxidative stress (induced by cigarette smoke) and when chronically exposed to cigarette smoke do not develop emphysema and other lung changes. Other strains of inbred mice, such as the C57Bl/6J and DBA/2, are sensitive to oxidative stress and develop extensive emphysema and other lung changes when chronically exposed to cigarette smoke. These genetic differences have been presented and are discussed above under "Animal Species." The resistance to oxidative stress of the ICR mice had been attributed to an upregulated Nrf2 pathway since the disruption of the Nrf2 gene in the ICR mice leads to extensive emphysema following chronic cigarette smoke exposure.[13,15] Nrf2 belongs to the cap'n'collar/basic region leucine zipper transcription factor family and is activated by diverse oxidants, pro-oxidants, and antioxidant agents. After phosphorylation and dissociation from the cytoplasmic inhibitor, Nrf2 translocates to the nucleus and binds to an antioxidant response element (ARE). Through transcriptional induction of ARE-bearing genes that encode antioxidant-detoxifying proteins, Nrf2 activates cellular rescue pathways against oxidative injury, inflammation/immunity, apoptosis, and carcinogenesis.[73]

Recently, the importance of the Nrf2 gene in the protection against cigarette smoke–induced emphysema has been confirmed and extended in a new study. In this investigation, the mice in which the Nrf2 gene was deleted were of an ICR/129sv mixed genetic background backcrossed with Balb/c mice for nine generations, and wild-type mice were of the Balb/c strain. In Nrf2 knockout mice, emphysema was first observed at 8 weeks and was more extensive by 16 weeks following cigarette smoke exposure, whereas no pathologic abnormalities were observed in wild-type mice. In Nrf2-knockout mice, neutrophilic lung inflammation, permeability, lung damage, and elastase activity in BALF were significantly greater than in wild-type mice 8 weeks after smoke exposure. The expression of secretory leukoprotease inhibitor was inducible in wild-type but not in Nrf2 knockout mice. The authors concluded that Nrf2 protects against the development of emphysema not only by regulating the oxidant/antioxidant balance but also by affecting inflammation and the protease/antiprotease balance.[74]

Senescence marker protein 30 (SMP30) is a novel protein that decreases with age, suggesting a possible role in age-related physiologic and pathologic conditions.[75] In mice, SMP30 transcripts are detected in various organs, including the lung. SMP30 knockout (SMP30Y/–) mice have a shorter life span than wild-type mice. Additionally, they develop peripheral airspace enlargement without alveolar destruction and may thus be a novel model for senile lung.[76] SMP30Y/– and wild type mice were exposed to cigarette smoke for 8 weeks. Cigarette smoke exposure induced marked airspace enlargement with significant parenchymal destruction in the SMP30Y/– but not in the wild-type mice. Protein carbonyls, malondialdehyde, total glutathione, and apoptosis of lung cells were significantly increased only in the SMP30Y/– mice after 8 weeks' exposure to cigarette smoke. These results suggest that SMP30 protects mice lungs from oxidative stress associated with aging and smoking.[77]

The lung, given its direct exposure to oxygen, experiences enhanced oxidative stress compared with other organs. Also, cigarette smoke contributes additional oxidants, further augmenting free radical production. The first ROS produced in the reduction pathway of oxygen to water is superoxide anion. This free radical participates in the generation of other potent oxidants, such as hydrogen peroxide, hydroxyl radical, and peroxynitrite. Thus, it plays a critical role in oxidative metabolism in the lung. Superoxide dismutases (SODs) are a primary class of enzymes ($N = 3$) that initiate the process of detoxifying superoxide anion by converting it into hydrogen peroxide. Copper-zinc SOD (CuZnSOD) is mainly located in cytosol of bronchial epithelium, alveolar epithelium, mesenchymal cells, and endothelial cells of lung arterioles. Transgenic mice were generated with the human CuZnSOD gene in the genetic background C57Bl/6xCBA/J and exposed to cigarette smoke for 1 year. Wild-type littermates served as controls. In the wild-type mice, smoke exposure caused a marked increase in neutrophil count in BALF and doubled lung myeloperoxidase activity. This inflammatory response did not occur in the smoke–exposed CuZnSOD mice. Similarly, CuZnSOD expression prevented a 58% increase in lung lipid peroxidation products that occurred after smoke exposure. Finally, wild-type mice developed emphysema after smoke exposure, whereas CuZnSOD prevented the onset of emphysema in the smoke–exposed animals. These results show that an antioxidant manipulation can prevent smoke–induced inflammation and thus the development of emphysema.[78]

All of these experimental studies taken together strongly support a major role for oxidative stress in the development of cigarette smoke–induced lung changes.

Protease Burden

The protease-antiprotease hypothesis for the development of emphysema originated in the early 1960s. At that time, an experimental study reported that intratracheal administration of the protease papain to rats resulted in emphysema.[79] Almost at the same time, a clinical investigation indicated that patients with a deficiency of serum antiprotease A1AT developed severe, early-onset emphysema.[80]

The protease-antiprotease hypothesis suggested that emphysema may result from an imbalance, either inborn (A1AT deficiency) or acquired (cigarette smoke–induced oxidative inactivation of A1AT), of the elastase-antielastase homeostasis in the lung. Since human neutrophil elastase was also found to induce emphysema when instilled in the lung of laboratory animals,[81] this protease has been considered to be the main culprit (even though not the only one) in the pathogenesis of emphysema for more than 30 years.

In the late 1990s, experimental evidence was presented that an MMP, macrophage metalloelastase, was necessary for the development of emphysema in mice after chronic inhalation of cigarette smoke.[82]

Thus, the idea that neutrophil elastase was the major culprit had been challenged. Also, evidence was put forward that a variety of macrophage-derived MMPs, including gelatinases A and B, matrilysin, and macrophage metalloelastase, could all degrade elastin and thus may play a major role in the development of emphysema.

A recent study examined the relationship between neutrophils and macrophages and their proteases in an acute model of cigarette smoke–induced tissue breakdown. Mice with knockout genes for macrophage metalloelastase (MME$^{-/-}$ mice) and MME$^{+/+}$ mice were exposed to the smoke of four cigarettes. Twenty-four hours later, MME$^{+/+}$ mice showed elevation in BALF neutrophils, desmosine, and hydroxyproline. These changes were not observed in MME$^{-/-}$ mice. Both neutrophil influx and increased levels of desmosine and hydroxyproline could be restored by the administering alveolar macrophages from MME$^{+/+}$ mice to MME$^{-/-}$ mice and then exposing them to cigarette smoke. RS113456, a metalloproteinase inhibitor, also prevented neutrophil influx and connective tissue breakdown. Western blots against mouse A1AT showed that this antiprotease was not protected in MME$^{-/-}$ mice or by the administration of RS113456. It was thus concluded that, in mice, acute smoke–induced connective tissue breakdown, the precursor to emphysema, requires both neutrophils and MME. Neutrophil influx appears to be secondary to macrophage activation in this model. This process initially does not involve protection of A1AT from metalloproteinase attack.[40]

The link between MME (MMP-12) and neutrophil elastase has been the subject of a subsequent study again in an acute model of smoke exposure. Both mice lacking MMP-12 (MMP-12$^{-/-}$) and wild-type mice (MMP-12$^{+/+}$) demonstrated rapid increases in whole-lung NF-κB activation and gene expression of proinflammatory cytokines after acute cigarette smoke exposure. This indicated that the lack of MMP-12 did not produce a global failure to upregulate inflammatory mediators. However, only MMP-12$^{+/+}$ mice demonstrated an increase in TNF-α protein. Similarly, levels of whole-lung E-selectin, a marker of endothelial activation, were increased only in MMP-12$^{+/+}$ mice. These findings suggested that MMP-12 mediates cigarette smoke–induced inflammation acutely by releasing TNF-α from macrophages, with subsequent endothelial activation, neutrophil influx, and proteolytic matrix breakdown by neutrophil-derived proteases. TNF-α release may be a general mechanism whereby metalloproteinases drive cigarette smoke–induced inflammation.[47]

In a subsequent study in a chronic model of cigarette smoke exposure, it was postulated that in C57Bl/6J mice, TNF-α-driven proteolytic processes may account for approximately 70% of emphysema, whereas the remaining 30% of matrix breakdown and emphysema may be related to a second TNF-α-independent process, possibly related to a direct MMP attack on the extracellular matrix.[83] With regard to these figures, it is of interest that in another study, approximately 60% of neutrophil elastase–deficient mice when exposed to long-term cigarette smoke were protected from the development of emphysema.[84]

Thus, it appears that the final lesion of the matrix that results in emphysema is the end result of a crosstalk between MMPs and neutrophil elastase.

Pharmacologic Interventions

There is a pressing need for the development of new therapies for COPD, particularly as no existing treatment has been shown to reduce disease progression. Presently, two main approaches are being considered and investigated in experimental studies.[85–88]

The first approach consists of pharmacologic interventions designed to slow down the rate at which alveolar wall is lost in emphysema. This approach has used anti-inflammatory agents, protease inhibitors, and antioxidants. The second approach is an attempt to reverse the process of alveolar loss by inducing alveolar growth. To our knowledge, here only the effects of retinoids and/or retinoid receptor agonists have been investigated in rodents.

Table 4 summarizes some of the studies carried out with these agents in animal models of cigarette smoke exposure with regard to their effect on emphysema.

Strategies to reduce lung inflammatory cell infiltration are most appealing since such an effect would also reduce the lung burden of both proteases and oxidants.

The phosphodiesterases are a large family of intracellular enzymes that degrade cyclic nucleotides. The phosphodiesterase 4 (PDE$_4$) subtype specifically targets cyclic 3′,5′-adenosine monophosphate, a second messenger that exerts inhibitory effects on many inflammatory effects. Thus, substances that prevent the degradation of cyclic 3′,5′-adenosine monophosphate by inhibiting the activity of PDE$_4$ will potentiate the anti-inflammatory action of this second messenger. In a recent study, groups of C57Bl/6J mice were dosed daily with the PDE$_4$ inhibitor roflumilast at two dose levels (1 and 5 mg/kg orally) and were exposed to cigarette smoke for 7 months. In control animals, chronic smoke exposure caused a 1.8-fold increase in lung macrophage volume density. Emphysema was produced, as shown by an increase in the mean linear intercept (+21%), a decrease in the internal surface area (−13%), and a drop (−13%) in lung desmosine content, the latter indicating elastin degradation. The low dose of roflumilast did not have any effect, whereas the high dose prevented the increase in lung macrophage density by 70% and completely abrogated the other changes.[41]

In another study, A/J mice were treated with the selective PDE$_4$ inhibitor CI-1044 (10 or 30 mg/kg orally daily) and were exposed to cigarette smoke for 6 months. Chronic smoke exposure resulted in an increase in the mean linear intercept (+16%) and in the number of macrophages in lung tissue (+55%). CI-1044 reduced macrophage accumulation by 79% and 95% at doses of 10 and 30 mg/kg, respectively.

Furthermore, CI-1044 significantly inhibited airspace enlargement by 59% and 89% at 10 and 30 mg/kg doses, respectively.[89]

Thus, both of these studies support the role of inflammation in the development of cigarette smoke–induced matrix destruction and emphysema and suggest the potential use of PDE$_4$ inhibitors as new potential therapies.

Statins are 3-hydroxy-3-methyl-glutaryl-coenzyme-A reductase inhibitors that are used clinically as lipid-lowering agents. Statins, however, have other additional pharmacologic properties, including anti-inflammatory, antioxidant actions and effects on vascular function. All of these additional activities could potentially counteract the harmful effects of cigarette smoking. The activity of the statin simvastatin was investigated in a rat model of smoke exposure. Simvastatin was given daily at the dose of 5 mg/kg orally to Sprague-Dawley rats, and the animals were exposed to cigarette smoke for 4 months. Simvastatin almost completely inhibited lung parenchymal destruction and development of pulmonary hypertension and also inhibited peribronchial and perivascular infiltration of inflammatory cells and the induction of MMP-9 activity in lung tissue. The amelioration by simvastatin of the structural derangements caused by cigarette smoking may be attributed to the anti-inflammatory activity of this compound.[90]

As a consequence of the protease-antiprotease hypothesis for the development of emphysema, interest was expressed in the development of an antiprotease therapy as a way of either retarding, or stopping, the progression of emphysema. A1AT is used in humans with A1AT deficiency; however, little is known of the effects of this antiprotease in cigarette smoke–induced emphysema. In a recent study, CD-1 mice, transgenic for human A1AT, were used. These mice expressed extremely low levels of human A1AT; however, they were

Table 4	Synopsis of Pharmacologic Studies in Animal Models of Cigarette Smoke Exposure				
Approach	*Pharmacologic Class*	*Agent*	*Model*	*Effect on Emphysema*	*Reference*
Prevention of alveolar loss	Anti-inflammatory agents: PDE4 inhibitors	Roflumilast CI-1044	Mouse Mouse	100% prevention 89% prevention	41 89
	Statins	Simvastatin	Rat	100% prevention	90
	Serine elastase inhibitors	ZD0892 A1AT	Guinea pig Mouse	45% prevention 63% prevention	92 91
	MMP inhibitors	CP-471,474 Ilomastat	Guinea pig Mouse	100% prevention 96% prevention	93 94
	Antioxidants ECM components	Lycopene Hyluronan	SAM mouse Mouse	100% prevention 100% prevention	27 96
Formation of new alveoli	Retinoids	ATRA and RAR agonist	Rat	Partially reversed	94
		ATRA	Guinea pig	Failed to reverse	95

A1AT = human α$_1$-antitrypsin; ATRA= all-*trans* retinoic acid; ECM = extracellular matrix; MMP = matrix metalloproteinase; PDE$_4$ = phosphodiesterase 4; RAR = retinoic acid receptor γ-agonist; SAM = senescence-accelerated mouse.

made tolerant of exogenous human A1AT. Mice received 20 mg of human A1AT intraperitoneally every 48 hours and were exposed to cigarette smoke for 6 months. Treatment with A1AT produced an approximate twofold increase in serum A1AT levels and abolished cigarette smoke–induced neutrophilia and matrix product increase in BALF measured at 30 days. It is of interest that A1AT, which was oxidized to remove its antiproteolytic activity, also prevented BALF neutrophil influx. Additionally, A1AT provided 63% protection against emphysema and abolished a smoke–mediated increase in plasma TNF-α, which suggests that the protective effect of A1AT included an anti-inflammatory effect related to TNF-α suppression.[91]

In another study, a synthetic, orally active inhibitor of serine elastases (ZD0892) was tested in guinea pigs exposed to cigarette smoke for 6 months. Smoke exposure in the control animals produced emphysema and an increase in neutrophils, desmosine, and hydroxyproline in BALF and in plasma TNF-α. ZD0892 treatment prevented BALF increases in neutrophils, desmosine, and hydroxyproline and decreased TNF-α by 30% and emphysema by 45%. Thus, a synthetic serine elastase inhibitor was found to ameliorate both the inflammatory and the destructive effects of cigarette smoke.[92]

The potential protective effect of MMP inhibitors has been investigated in the guinea pig and in the mouse. In the first study, guinea pigs were treated subcutaneously with CP-471,474, a broad-spectrum MMP inhibitor, and exposed to cigarette smoke for 1, 2, and 4 months. In control animals, a moderate peribronchial, alveolar, and interstitial lung inflammation was present at 1 month. Interstitial inflammation consisted mainly of lymphocytes and macrophages, although polymorphonuclear cells were also observed. Macrophages were the primary intra-alveolar cells and often contained pigmented cytoplasm with finely granular iron-stained particles. These changes progressed and peaked at 2 months but regressed at 4 months. Significant emphysema was present at 2 and 4 months. At 2 months, the inhibitor significantly reduced both the extent and the severity of lung inflammation and completely prevented the development of emphysema. However, emphysema was reduced only by 30% at 4 months. This study supports a role for MMPs in the early inflammatory response and emphysematous lesions provoked by cigarette smoking and justifies the use of MMP inhibitors in pharmacologic studies. However, these studies suggest that other proteolytic enzymes were responsible for the late emphysematous changes.[93]

In a mouse study, ilomastat, a broad-spectrum MMP inhibitor, was given by inhalation to mice and the animals were exposed to daily cigarette smoke for 6 months. In control animals, cigarette smoke significantly increased the recruitment of macrophages into the lungs and resulted in alveolar airspace enlargement and emphysema. In animals treated daily with nebulized ilomastat for 6 months, lung macrophage levels were greatly reduced, and neutrophil accumulation was also inhibited. Corresponding reductions in airspace enlargement of up to 96% were observed. These observations suggest that delivery of ilomastat directly into the lungs of smoke–treated mice not only can inhibit lung tissue damage mediated by metalloproteases but may also reduce that component of tissue degeneration mediated by excess neutrophil-derived product.[94]

To our knowledge, there have been no recent reports on synthetic agents with antioxidant activity in models of cigarette smoke exposure. Recently, a Japanese group investigated the effect of lycopene, a natural compound given as tomato juice, on cigarette smoke–induced emphysema. They used SAM-prone 1 mice, a naturally occurring animal model of accelerated aging. At age 12 weeks, SAM-prone 1 mice inhaled either air or tobacco smoke for 8 weeks. After smoke exposure, the mean linear intercept and destructive index of the lungs were significantly increased. However, cigarette smoke induced no significant changes in SAM-resistant 1 mice (control mice that show normal aging). Smoke–induced emphysema was completely prevented by concomitant ingestion of lycopene. Also, in SAM-prone 1 mice, smoke exposure increased apoptosis and active caspase-3 of airway and alveolar septal cells and reduced VEGF in lung tissues, and lycopene ingestion significantly reduced apoptosis and increased the tissue VEGF level. Thus, ingestion of the antioxidant lycopene, given as tomato juice, was effective in preventing cigarette smoke–induced lung changes.[27]

A few years ago, it was reported that intratracheally administered hyaluronic acid was capable of ameliorating elastase-induced emphysema and that its mechanism of action may depend on an interaction with elastic fibers.[95] More recently, studies were undertaken to determine if aerosolized hyaluronic acid could prevent airspace enlargement and elastic fiber injury in a mouse model of cigarette smoke–induced pulmonary emphysema. Compared with untreated/smoked controls, hyaluronic acid–treated animals showed statistically significant reductions in mean linear intercept and elastic fiber breakdown products (desmosine and isodesmosine) in BALF. As in previous studies, aerosolized hyaluronic acid showed preferential binding to elastic fibers, suggesting that it may protect them from injury. Thus, these findings support further investigation of the potential use of hyaluronic acid as a treatment for pulmonary emphysema.[96]

The second therapeutic approach, new alveolar formation, is based on the knowledge that in COPD small conductive airways, alveoli and alveolar surface area are lost, with the consequence that the patients have too few alveoli and too little alveolar surface area for adequate gas exchange. This situation, combined with novel information on retinoids indicating an association of these agents with the process of alveologenesis, led to the hypothesis that retinoids could be importantly involved in the regulation and formation of new alveoli and thus be of therapeutic value in COPD patients.[97] A series of experiments in rodents had shown that exogenous all-*trans* retinoic acid (ATRA) induced the formation of extra alveoli in newborn rats and partially rescued pharmacologically and genetically impaired alveoli formation.[98–100]

The effects of ATRA and of a retinoic acid receptor γ-agonist (RO44753) were investigated in a rat model of cigarette smoke exposure. Rats were exposed daily to 10 cigarettes a day for 6 months. This resulted in biochemical and morphometric changes consistent with emphysema. Thereafter, smoke exposure was stopped and either ATRA (at one dose level) or RO44753 (at three dose levels) was given orally for 1 month. In ATRA-treated cigarette-exposed rats, a decrease in tissue desmosine, an increase in BALF elastin peptides, and increases in destructive index and mean linear intercept were reduced by 125%, 51%, 68%, and 74%, respectively. Similarly, in RO44753-treated rats, the cigarette smoke–induced changes were reduced dose-dependently, with the highest dose inducing a reduction in the same parameters as above of 145%, 72%, 80%, and 75%, respectively. It was concluded that ATRA and a specific retinoic acid receptor γ-agonist, given after cigarette smoke exposure, can reverse cigarette smoke–induced matrix breakdown and emphysematous lung damage.[101]

Another study was carried out in guinea pigs also to determine whether cigarette smoke–induced emphysema could be reversed by ATRA treatment. The animals were exposed either to air or cigarette smoke for 13 weeks. Either ATRA or the diluent was given daily intraperitoneally to a certain number of animals in both treatment groups. Smoking increased lung volume and airspace volume and reduced tissue volume and lung surface area to volume ratio. Histologically, smoke–exposed guinea pigs showed enlargement of the airspaces and destruction of the centrilobular regions of alveolar tissue. ATRA treatment did not affect the histologic picture of emphysema and did not reverse the cigarette smoke–induced changes in lung volume, airspace volume, tissue volume, or lung surface area to volume ratio. Thus, in this study, ATRA treatment failed to either prevent or reverse the smoke–induced changes.[102]

It is difficult to interpret the difference between these two studies. The difference in animal species is obvious and may indeed be important. As pointed out in a recent commentary on these findings, cigarette smoke per se depletes retinol in rat lungs while markedly increasing it in the guinea pig lungs.[97] Thus, these basal changes in the opposite direction may have influenced the effects of exogenously administered retinoids.

Further studies are thus necessary to investigate the hypothesis of new alveolar formation for the therapy of emphysema.

Conclusions

This selective review of the literature of recent years clearly shows a real explosion of studies involving small animal models of cigarette smoke exposure. These models have been used to evaluate hypotheses relating to the human disease and to assess potential therapeutic interventions. All of these are model studies; thus, only studies in humans will provide the definitive answer to any of these pathophysiologic hypotheses and/or therapeutic issues. However, awareness of the limitations of the animal models should be taken into account. These are all imperfect models in an imperfect world, and as long as the limits of the models are known, accepted, and openly discussed, the results obtained in any model can be translated in part or in toto to the human condition.

References

1. Snider GL, Martorana PA, Lucey EC, Lungarella G. Animal models of emphysema. In: Voelkel NF, MacNee W, editors. Chronic obstructive lung disease. Hamilton (ON): BC Decker;2002. p. 237–56.
2. Karlinsky JB, Snider GL. Animal models of emphysema. Am Rev Respir Dis 1978;117:1109–13.
3. Snider GL, Lucey EC, Stone PJ. Animal models of emphysema. Am Rev Respir Dis 1986;133:149–69.
4. Mahadeva R, Shapiro SD. Chronic obstructive pulmonary disease 3: experimental animal models of pulmonary emphysema. Thorax 2002;57:908–14.
5. Tuder RM, McGrath S, Neptune E. The pathobiological mechanisms of emphysema models: what do they have in common? Pulm Pharmacol Ther 2003;16:67–78.
6. Brusselle GG, Brake KR, Maes T, et al. Murine models of COPD. Pulm Pharmacol Ther 2006;19:155–65.
7. van der Vaart H, Postma DS, Timens W, ten Hacken NH. Acute effects of cigarette smoke on inflammation and oxidative stress: a review. Thorax 2004;59:713–21.
8. Martorana PA, Cavarra E, Lucattelli M, Lungarella G. Models for COPD involving cigarette smoke. Drug Discov Today 2006;3:225–30.
9. Martorana PA, Lucattelli M, Bartalesi B, Lungarella G. Animal models. In: Stockley RA, Rennard S, Rabe K, Celli B, editors. Chronic obstructive pulmonary disease. London: Blackwell; 2007. p. 341–8.
10. American Thoracic Society. Cigarette smoking and health. Am J Respir Crit Care Med 1996;153:861–5.
11. Ihrig J, Kleinerman J, Rynbrandt DJ. Serum antitrypsins in animals. Study of species variations, components, and the influence of certain irritants. Am Rev Respir Dis 1971; 103:377–89.
12. Cavarra E, Bartalesi B, Lucattelli M, et al. Effects of cigarette smoke in mice with different levels of proteinase inhibitor and sensitivity to oxidants. Am J Respir Crit Care Med 2001; 164:886–90.
13. Fineschi S, Cianti R, Bini L, et al. Differential protein expression in lungs of mouse strains with different sensitivity to cigarette smoke. Proc Am Thorac Soc 2006;3:A627.
14. Rangasamy T, Misra V, Lee H, et al. Differences in Nrf2 activity between emphysema resistant (ICR) and susceptible (C57Bl/6J) mice strains in response to acute cigarette smoke exposure. Proc Am Thorac Soc 2006;3:A129.
15. Rangasamy T, Cho CY, Thimmulappa RK, et al. Genetic ablation of Nrf2 enhances susceptibility to cigarette smoke–induced emphysema in mice. J Clin Invest 2004; 114:1248–59.

16. Guerassimov A, Hoshino Y, Takubo Y, et al. The development of emphysema in cigarette smoke–exposed mice is strain dependent. Am J Respir Crit Care Med 2004;170:974–80.

17. Churg A, Dai J, Tai H, et al. Tumor necrosis factor-α is central to acute cigarette smoke–induced inflammation and connective tissue breakdown. Am J Respir Crit Care Med 2002; 166:849–54.

18. Brass DM, Hoyle GW, Poovey HG, et al. Reduced tumor necrosis factor-α and transforming growth factor-β₁ expression in the lungs of inbred mice that fail to develop fibroproliferative lesions consequent to asbestos exposure. Am J Pathol 1999;154:853–62.

19. Gardi C, Cavarra E, Calzoni P, et al. Neutrophil lysosomal dysfunctions in mutant C57Bl/6J mice: interstrain variations in content of lysosomal elastase, cathepsin G and their inhibitors. Biochem J 1994;299:237–45.

20. Bartalesi B, Cavarra E, Fineschi S, et al. Different lung responses to cigarette smoke in two strains of mice sensitive to oxidants. Eur Respir J 2005;25:15–22.

21. Lucattelli M, Bartalesi B, Cavarra E, et al. Is neutrophil elastase the missing link between emphysema and fibrosis? Evidence from two mouse models. Respir Res 2005;6:83–97.

22. Cottin V, Nunes H, Brillet PY, et al. Combined pulmonary fibrosis and emphysema: a distinct underrecognized entity. Eur Respir J 2005;26:586–93.

23. March TH, Wilder JA, Esparza DC, et al. Modulators of cigarette smoke–induced emphysema in A/J mice. Toxicol Sci 2006;92:545–59.

24. Rangasamy T, Misra V, Lee H, et al. Oligonucleotide microarray analysis reveals global loss of expression of genes in emphysematous lung tissues of A/J mice. Proc Am Thorac Soc 2006;3:A627.

25. Martorana PA, Brand T, Gardi C, et al. The pallid mouse. A model of genetic α₁-antitrypsin deficiency. Lab Invest 1993;68:233–41.

26. Uejima Y, Fukuchi Y, Nagase T, et al. Influences of inhaled tobacco smoke on the senescence accelerated mouse (SAM). Eur Respir J 1990;3:1029–36.

27. Kasagi S, Seyama K, Mori H, et al. Tomato juice prevents senescence-accelerated mouse P1 strain from developing emphysema induced by chronic exposure to tobacco smoke. Am J Physiol Lung Cell Mol Physiol 2006;290:L396–404.

28. Brownstein DG. Tracheal mucociliary transport in laboratory mice: evidence for genetic polymorphism. Exp Lung Res 1987;13:185–91.

29. Brownstein DG. Genetics of natural resistance to Sendai virus in mice. Infect Immun 1983;41:308–12.

30. Fabbri L, Pauwels RA, Hurd SS. Global strategy for the diagnosis, management and prevention of chronic obstructive pulmonary disease: GOLD executive summary updated 2003. J COPD 2004;1:105–41.

31. Saetta M, Turato G, Lupi F, Fabbri LM. Inflammation in the pathogenesis of chronic obstructive pulmonary disease. In: Voelkel NF, MacNee W, editors. Chronic obstructive lung disease. Hamilton (ON): BC Decker;2002. p. 114–26.

32. Matulionis DH. Chronic cigarette smoke inhalation and aging in mice: 1. Morphologic and functional lung abnormalities. Exp Lung Res 1984;7:237–56.

33. Dalbey WE, Nettesheim P, Griesemer R, et al. Chronic inhalation of cigarette smoke by F-344 rats. J Natl Cancer Inst 1980;64:383–8.

34. Bernfield P, Homburger F, Soto E, Pai KJ. Cigarette smoke inhalation studies in inbred Syrian golden hamsters. J Natl Cancer Inst 1980;63:675–89.

35. Wright JL, Churg A. Cigarette smoke causes physiologic and morphologic changes of emphysema in the guinea pig. Am Rev Respir Dis 1990;142:1422–8.

36. Finkelstein R, Fraser RS, Ghezzo H, Cosio MG. Alveolar inflammation and its relation to emphysema in smokers. Am J Respir Crit Care Med 1995;152:1666–72.

37. Keating VM, Collins PD, Scott DM, Barnes PJ. Differences in interleukin-8 and tumor necrosis factor-α in induced sputum from patients with chronic obstructive pulmonary disease or asthma. Am J Respir Crit Care Med 1996; 153:530–4.

38. Selby C, MacNee W. Factors affecting neutrophil transit during acute pulmonary inflammation: minireview. Exp Lung Res 1993;19:407–28.

39. Dhami R, Gilks B, Xie C, et al. Acute smoke–induced connective tissue breakdown is mediated by neutrophils and prevented by α-1 antitrypsin. Am J Respir Cell Mol Biol 2000; 22:244–52.

40. Churg A, Zay K, Shay S, et al. Acute cigarette smoke–induced connective tissue breakdown requires both neutrophils and macrophage metalloelastase in mice. Am J Respir Cell Mol Biol 2002;27:368–74.

41. Martorana PA, Beume R, Lucattelli M, et al. Roflumilast fully prevents emphysema in mice chronically exposed to cigarette smoke. Am J Respir Crit Care Med 2005;172:848–53.

42. D'hulst AI, Vermaelen KY, Brusselle GG, et al. Time course of cigarette smoke–induced pulmonary inflammation in mice. Eur Respir J 2005;26:204–13.

43. D'hulst AI, Bracke KR, Maes T, et al. Role of tumor necrosis factor-α receptor p75 in cigarette smoke–induced pulmonary inflammation and emphysema. Eur Respir J 2006;28:102–12.

44. Barnes PJ, Shapiro SD, Pauwels RA. Chronic obstructive pulmonary disease : molecular and cellular mechanisms. Eur Respir J 2003;22:672–88.

45. MacNee W. Pathogenesis of chronic obstructive pulmonary disease. Proc Am Thorac Soc 2005;2:258–66.

46. Leclerc O, Lagente V, Planquois J-M, et al. Involvement of MMP-12 and phosphodiesterase type 4 in cigarette smoke–induced inflammation in mice. Eur Respir J 2006;27:1102–9.

47. Churg A, Wang RD, Tai H, et al. Macrophage metalloelastase mediates acute cigarette smoke–induced inflammation via tumor necrosis factor-α release. Am J Respir Crit Care Med 2003;167:1083–9.

48. Di Stefano A, Caramori G, Ricciardolo FL, et al. Cellular and molecular mechanisms in chronic obstructive pulmonary disease: an overview. Clin Exp Allergy 2004;34:1156–67.

49. Hogg JC, Chu F, Utokaparch S, et al. The nature of small airway obstruction in chronic obstructive pulmonary disease. N Engl J Med 2004;350:2645–53.

50. van Rensen EL, Sont JK, Evertse CE, et al. Bronchial CD8+ infiltrate and lung function decline in asthma. Am J Respir Crit Care Med 2005;172:837–41.

51. Hogg JC. Pathophysiology of airflow limitation in chronic obstructive pulmonary disease. Lancet 2004;364:709–21.

52. Willemse BW, ten Hacken NH, Rutgers B, et al. Effect of 1-year smoking cessation on airway inflammation in COPD and asymptomatic smokers. Eur Respir J 2005; 26:835–45.

53. Bosken CH, Hards J, Gatter K, Hogg JC. Characterization of the inflammatory reaction in the peripheral airways of cigarette smokers using immunocytochemistry. Am Rev Respir Dis 1992;145:911–7.

54. Bancherau J, Steinman RM. Dendritic cells and the control of immunity. Nature 1998;392:245–52.

55. Lipscomb MF, Masten BJ. Dendritic cells: immune regulators in health and disease. Physiol Rev 2002;82:97–130.

56. Soler P, Moreau A, Basset F, Hance AJ. Cigarette smoking induced changes in the number and differentiated state of pulmonary dendritic cells/Langerhans cells. Am Rev Respir Dis 1989;139:1112–7

57. Thatcher TH, McHug NA, Egan RW, et al. Role of CXCR2 in cigarette smoke–induced lung inflammation. Am J Physiol Lung Cell Mol Physiol 2005;289:L322–8.

58. Robbins CS, Dawe DE, Goncharova ST, et al. Cigarette smoke decreases pulmonary dendritic cells and impacts antiviral immune responsiveness. Am J Respir Cell Mol Biol 2004; 30:202–11.

59. D'hulst AI, Maes T, Bracke KR, et al. Cigarette smoke–induced pulmonary emphysema in scid-mice. Is the acquired immune system required? Respir Res 2005;6:147.

60. Vermaelen K, Pauwels R. Pulmonary dendritic cells. Am J Respir Crit Care Med 2005;172:530–51.

61. Cosio MG. Autoimmunity, T-cells and STAT-4 in the pathogenesis of chronic obstructive pulmonary disease. Eur Respir J 2004;24:3–5.

62. Zeid NA, Muller HK. Tobacco smoke induced lung granulomas and tumors: association with pulmonary Langerhans cells. Pathology 1995;27:247–54.

63. Brake K, Cataldo D, Maes T, et al. Matrix metalloproteinase-12 and cathepsin D expression in pulmonary macrophages and dendritic cells of cigarette smoke–exposed mice. Int Arch Allergy Immunol 2005;138:169–79.

64. van der Strate BWA, Postma DS, Brandsma C-A, et al. Cigarette smoke–induced emphysema. A role for the B cell? Am J Respir Crit Care Med 2006;173:751–8.

65. Vuillemenot BR, Rodriguez JF, Hoyle GW. Lymphoid tissue and emphysema in the lungs of transgenic mice inducibly expressing tumor necrosis factor-α. Am J Respir Cell Mol Biol 2004;30:438–48.

66. MacNee W. Treatment of stable COPD: antioxidants. Eur Respir Rev 2005;14:12–22.

67. Rahman I, Adcock IM. Oxidative stress and redox regulation of lung inflammation in COPD. Eur Respir J 2006; 28:219–42.

68. Shapiro SD, Ingenito EP. The pathogenesis of chronic obstructive pulmonary disease. Advances in the past 100 years. Am J Respir Cell Mol Biol 2005;32:367–72.

69. Aoshiba K, Koinuma M, Yokohori N, Nagai A. Immunohistochemical evaluation of oxidative stress in murine lungs after cigarette smoke exposure. Inhal Toxicol 2003;15:1029–38.

70. Cavarra E, Lucattelli M, Gambelli F, et al. Human SLPI inactivation after cigarette smoke exposure in a new in vivo model of pulmonary oxidative stress. Am J Physiol Lung Cell Mol Physiol 2001;281:L412–7.

71. Marwick JA, Kirkham PA, Stevenson CS, et al. Cigarette smoke alters chromatin remodeling and induces proinflammatory genes in rat lungs. Am J Respir Cell Mol Biol 2004; 31:633–42.

72. Kuo WH, Chen JH, Lin HH, et al. Induction of apoptosis in the lung tissue from rats exposed to cigarette smoke involves p38/JNK MAPK pathway. Chem Biol Interact 2005; 155:31–42.

73. Cho Y, Reddy SP, Kleeberger SR. Nrf2 defends the lung from oxidative stress. Antioxid Redox Signal 2006;8:76–87.

74. Iizuka T, Ishii Y, Itoh K, et al. Nrf2 deficient mice are highly susceptible to cigarette smoke–induced emphysema. Genes Cells 2005;10:1113–25.

75. Fujita T, Shirasawa T, Uchida K, Maruyama N. Gene regulation of senescence marker protein-30 (SMP30): coordinated upregulation with tissue maturation and gradual down-regulation with ageing. Mech Ageing Dev 1996;87:219–29.

76. Mori T, Ishigami A, Seyama K, et al. Senescence marker protein-30 knockout mouse as a novel murine model of senile lung. Pathol Int 2004;54:167–73.

77. Sato T, Seyama K, Sato Y, et al. Senescence marker protein-30 protects mice lungs from oxidative stress, aging, and smoking. Am J Respir Crit Care Med 2006;174:530–7.

78. Foronjy RF, Mirochnitchenko O, Prpokenko O, et al. Superoxide dismutase expression attenuates cigarette smoke– or elastase-generated emphysema in mice. Am J Respir Crit Care Med 2006;173:623–31.

79. Gross P, Pfitzer EA, Toker A, et al. Experimental emphysema: its production with papain in normal and silicotic rats. Arch Environ Health 1965;11:50–8.

80. Laurell CB, Eriksson S. The electrophoretic alpha-1-globulin pattern of serum alpha-1-antitrypsin deficiency. Scand J Clin Invest 1963;15:132–40.

81. Senior RM, Tegner H, Kuhn C, et al. The induction of pulmonary emphysema with human leukocyte elastase. Am Rev Respir Dis 1977;116:469–75.

82. Hautamaki RD, Kobayashi DK, Senior RM, Shapiro SD. Requirement for macrophage elastase for cigarette smoke–induced emphysema in mice. Science 1997; 277:2002–4.

83. Churg A, Wang R, Thai H, et al. Tumor necrosis factor-alpha drives 70% of cigarette smoke-induced emphysema in the mouse. Am J Respir Crit Care Med 2004;170:492–8.

84. Shapiro SD, Goldstein NM, McGarry Houghton A, et al. Neutrophil elastase contributes to cigarette smoke-induced emphysema in mice. Am J Pathol 2003;163:2329–35.

85. Barnes PJ, Stockley RA. COPD: current therapeutic interventions and future approaches. Eur Respir J 2005; 25:1084–106.

86. Barnes PJ. New approaches to COPD. Eur Respir Rev 2005; 14:2–11.

87. Owen C. Proteinases and oxidants as targets in the treatment of chronic obstructive pulmonary disease. Proc Am Thorac Soc 2005;2:373–85.

88. Rennard SI. Chronic obstructive pulmonary disease. Linking outcomes and pathobiology of disease modification. Proc Am Thorac Soc 2006;3:276–80.

89. Pruniaux M-P, Xu J, Bertrand CP, Shapiro SD. Efficacy of a selective phosphodiesterase 4 inhibitor, CI-1044, on cigarette smoke-induced emphysema development in mice. Am J Respir Crit Care Med 2003;167:A874.

90. Lee J-H, Lee D-S, Kim E-K, et al. Simvastatin inhibits cigarette smoking-induced emphysema and pulmonary hypertension in rat lungs. Am J Respir Crit Care Med 2005; 172:987–91.

91. Churg A, Wang RD, Xie C, Wright JL. α-1-Antitrypsin ameliorates cigarette smoke–induced emphysema in the mouse. Am J Respir Crit Care Med 2003;168:199–207.

92. Wright JL, Farmer S, Churg A. Synthetic serine elastase inhibitor reduces cigarette smoke–induced emphysema in guinea pigs. Am J Respir Crit Care Med 2002;166:954–60.

93. Selman M, Cisneros-Lira J, Gaxiola M, et al. Matrix metalloproteinases attenuates tobacco smoke–induced emphysema in guinea pigs. Chest 2003;123:1633–41.

94. Pemberton PA, Cantwell JS, Kim KM, et al. An inhaled matrix protease inhibitor prevents cigarette smoke–induced emphysema in the mouse. COPD 2005;2:303–10.

95. Cantor JO, Cerreta JM, Armand G, Turino GM. Further investigation of the use of intratracheally administered hyaluronic acid to ameliorate elastase-induced emphysema. Exp Lung Res 1997;23:229–44.

96. Cantor JO, Cerreta JM, Ochoa M, et al. Aerosolized hyaluronan limits airspace enlargement in a mouse model of cigarette smoke–induced pulmonary emphysema. Exp Lung Res 2005;31:417–30.

97. Massaro D, De Carlo Massaro G. Retinoids, alveolus formation, and alveolar deficiency. Clinical implications. Am J Respir Cell Mol Biol 2003;28:271–4.

98. Massaro G, Massaro D. Postnatal treatment with retinoic acid increases the number of pulmonary alveoli in rats. Am J Physiol 1996;270:L305–10.

99. Massaro G, Massaro D. Retinoic acid treatment partially rescues failed septation in rats and mice. Am J Physiol Lung Cell Mol Physiol 2000;278:L955–60.

100. Hind A, Maden M. A mouse model of alveolar regeneration. Am J Respir Crit Care Med 2002;165:A223.

101. Ofulue AF, Xiang AF, Yang Y, Belloni P. Retinoids reverse cigarette smoke–induced emphysema in the rat. Am J Respir Crit Care Med 2002;165:A137.

102. Meshi M, Vitalis TZ, Ionescu D, et al. Emphysematous lung destruction by cigarette smoke. The effects of latent adenoviral infection on the lung inflammatory response. Am J Respir Cell Mol Biol 2002;26:52–7.

CHAPTER 17

CHRONIC AIRWAY DISEASE IN NONHUMAN PRIMATES

DALLAS M. HYDE, PhD, LISA A. MILLER, PhD, EDWARD S. SCHELEGLE, PhD, MICHELLE V. FANUCCHI, PhD, LAURA S. VAN WINKLE, PhD, NANCY K. TYLER, PhD, MARK V. AVDALOVIC, MD, MICHAEL J. EVANS, PhD, RADHIKA KAJEKAR, PhD, ALAN R. BUCKPITT, PhD, KENT E. PINKERTON, PhD, JESSE P. JOAD, MD, LAUREL J. GERSHWIN, DVM, PhD, REEN WU, PhD, AND CHARLES G. PLOPPER, PhD

OUR GOAL IN THIS CHAPTER is to assess the utility of nonhuman primates as a model for chronic airways disease in humans. We address the current status of our understanding of a series of critical issues regarding the utility of the nonhuman primate model and its appropriateness for defining mechanisms as they relate to disease processes in human airways. Two diseases we focus on are asthma and chronic obstructive pulmonary disease (COPD). We address the biology of the airway within the conceptual framework of the epithelial mesenchymal trophic unit (EMTU). The basis of this concept is that all of the cellular and acellular compartments within the airway wall have a close interaction through a series of extracellular signaling cascades, which establish a dynamic homeostatic state. The homeostatic state of the EMTU responds to injury of one component by altering the signaling patterns and basic functions of the remaining components. We provide an evaluation of the differences between species in the organization of the airway wall in adults, compare differences in postnatal development of the airways by species, and compare airway specific remodeling and airway specific inflammation associated with asthma and COPD. Finally, we address the current status of our understanding of a series of critical issues regarding the utility of these animal models and their appropriateness for defining mechanisms as they relate to allergic airways disease in humans.

Asthma is the most common chronic disease of childhood.[1] Asthma is a worldwide health problem affecting both developed and developing countries that affects 300 million people, as estimated by the World Health Organization (WHO).[2] Specific age ranges and ethnicities are disproportionately affected. Asthma hospitalization rates have been highest among African Americans and children, whereas death rates for asthma have been consistently highest among African Americans aged 15 to 24 years (Centers for Disease Control and Prevention, 2007).[3] The WHO predicts that asthma deaths will increase by almost 20% in the next 10 years if urgent action is not taken.[2] Asthma is characterized by chronic inflammation, obstruction, and remodeling of the airways coupled with breathlessness and wheezing. Episodes

of recurrent wheezing, breathlessness, chest tightness, and cough are usually associated with airflow obstruction that is often reversible either spontaneously or with treatment. There is also increased bronchial hyperresponsiveness to a variety of stimuli.

COPD is the most common respiratory disease of adults and is characterized by the progressive development of airflow limitation that is not fully reversible.[4] COPD is a major cause of death and illness and is the fourth leading cause of death in the United States and throughout the world.[4] Chronic bronchitis, with obstruction of small airways, and emphysema, with enlargement of airspaces and destruction of lung parenchyma, loss of lung elasticity, and closure of small airways, are the diseases most commonly associated with the term *COPD*. There has been a worldwide increase in the prevalence of and mortality from COPD.[4] A marked increase in cigarette smoking and environmental pollution in industrialized countries are in large part responsible for the dramatic increase in COPD counterbalancing the reduced mortality from other causes, such as cardiovascular diseases in industrialized countries and infectious diseases in developing countries. The signs and symptoms of COPD include cough, excess sputum or mucus production, shortness of breath, especially with exercise, wheezing, and chest tightness.

Architecture of the Tracheobronchial Airways

As illustrated in Figure 1, the tracheobronchial conducting airways form a complex series of branching tubes from the trachea that extends to the gas exchange area of the parenchyma. The more proximal and larger branches, the bronchi, are usually characterized by the presence of mucous and basal cells in the epithelium, some mucosal glands in the interstitium, and abundant cartilage in the interstitial space. Distally, the smaller bronchioles have thinner walls with little to no cartilage, a less complex airway epithelial population, and a greater percentage of smooth muscle compared with the bronchi. In humans and nonhuman primates, cartilage is found in the walls of the

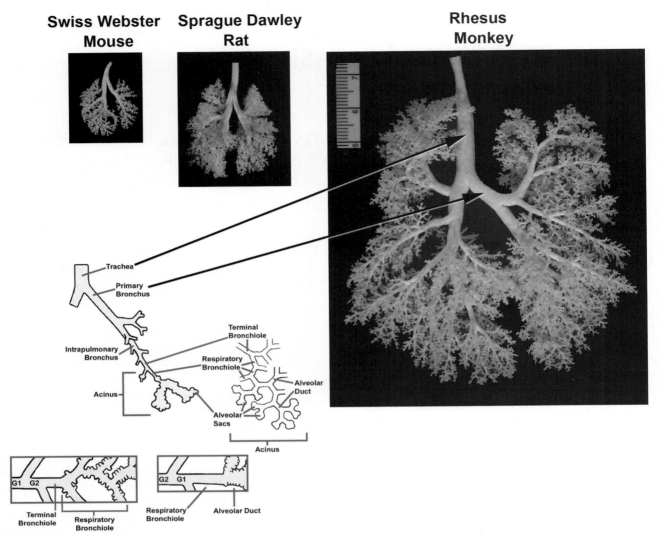

FIGURE 1. Silicone casts of representative mouse, rat, and rhesus monkey tracheobronchial airways are shown along with diagrammatic representations of the organization of airspaces in the mammalian respiratory system, including the trachea, primary bronchi, intrapulmonary bronchi, and acinus. Primates, including rhesus monkeys and humans, have an extensive area of transition between alveolar ducts and the most distal conduction airway, the terminal bronchiole, in the central portions of the acinus. This zone of transition is termed "respiratory bronchiole" because the majority of the wall is structured like a bronchiole, and bronchiolar epithelium is interrupted by alveolar outpockets organized for gas exchange with epithelial and endothelial cell composition of interalveolar septa in the alveolar ducts (*bottom left*). Note that the distal airway in mice and rats lacks the extensive respiratory bronchioles in the transition zone and is usually characterized with a terminal bronchiole branching directly into alveolar ducts (*bottom right*). The mouse, rat, and rhesus monkey were at approximately weaning age when the lungs were fixed and the casting material introduced by negative pressure to fill down to the respiratory bronchioles. Reproduced with permission from Hyde DM et al, © European Respiratory Society Journals Ltd.[170]

tracheobronchial airways, from the trachea distally to the smallest bronchioles (Table 1) In contrast, cartilage is only found predominantly in the trachea of mice and rats.

The average number of airway generations from the trachea to an alveolarized bronchiole is approximately the same for most mammalian species (see Table 1). Branching, in contrast, is relatively unique in primates, with branches separating from the parent airway at approximately 45° and being almost uniformly equal in size and in diameter (ie, dichotomous branching). Branching is monopodial in mice and rats.

The organization of the transition zone, the area where the conducting airways end and the gas exchange area begins, also differs between species (see Figure 1). Primates and carnivores have many respiratory bronchioles, which have a mixture of bronchiolar and alveolar epithelium, compared with other species, such as mice (see Table 1). As such, the size of the acinus, defined as the terminal (last conducting) bronchiole and all of its distal respiratory airways, is much larger in primates than mice and rats because of the numerous generations of respiratory bronchioles. In fact, there is an approximate 50-fold increase in acinar number

Parameter	Human	Monkey	Mouse
Cartilage in wall	Trachea to distal bronchiole	Trachea to distal bronchiole	Trachea
Nonrespiratory bronchioles	Several generations	Several generations	Several generations
Respiratory bronchioles	Several generations	Several generations	None or one
Generations to alveolarized bronchiole (axial path)	17–21	13–17	13–17
Branching pattern	Dichotomous	Dichotomous/tricotomous	Monopodial

Table 1 Comparison of Species Differences in Tracheobronchial Airway Organization

Adapted from McBride JT,[41] Tyler WS and Julian MD,[42] Plopper CG and Hyde DM,[44] and Mariassy AT.[171]

and a 170-fold increase in acinar volume over the range from the mouse to human lung.[5]

Within the gas exchange area of the lung, the ventilatory unit, alveoli and alveolar ducts distal to a single bronchiole-alveolar duct junction, changes with species. The diameter of the ventilatory unit is threefold greater in humans than in mice.[5] The ventilatory unit is the smallest common denominator in determining the distribution of inspired gas to the gas exchange surfaces of the lung. Weibel and colleagues suggested that the mean capillary oxygen partial pressure (PO_2) is lower in small species because of their relatively large cardiac output.[6] Hence, the mean transit time for blood in alveolar capillaries of a mouse would be shorter than for a human, in whom the path length is longer. Conversely, oxygen partial pressure in arterial blood (PaO_2) is probably higher in a mouse than in a human because of better alveolar ventilation through a higher breathing rate. Another reason would be that the distance for O_2 diffusion through the airways is shorter in mice because their ventilatory units are about threefold smaller than those of humans. Figure 2 is a model that shows how different acinar pathway lengths could result in differences in mean alveolar PO_2 in a size-dependent manner.[6] This concept becomes important when distal airway obstruction or destruction limits O_2 diffusion in a species such as humans or nonhuman primates, in which there is not as much reserve as exists in a mouse.

EMTU Concept

The concept of the EMTU was developed as a framework for defining the cellular and metabolic mechanisms regulating the response to injury in a complex biologic structure such as the tracheobronchial airway tree.[6,7] Each segment, or airway generation, within the branching tracheobronchial airway tree is addressed as a unique biologic entity whose properties may differ from those of neighboring branches and the intervening branch points. The portions of the airways between branch points are treated as separate biologic entities from each other. All of the components of the airway wall, both cellular and acellular, are assumed to play a role in both injury and repair responses and are thought of as compartments (Figure 3). The epithelial compartment of the airway wall is composed of surface epithelium and submucosal glands. The interstitial compartment includes the basement membrane zone (BMZ), fibroblasts, smooth muscle, cartilage, and vasculature. The nervous compartment includes the nerve processes that interdigitate between the vasculature, smooth muscle, subepithelial matrix, and epithelium and includes both the afferent and efferent limbs of the nervous system and the central regulating neurons in the brainstem. The vascular compartment includes capillaries, arterioles, and venules, primarily from the bronchial circulation, and lymphatic vessels. The immunologic compartment includes both migratory and resident inflammatory and immune cells.

The basic assumption of the EMTU is that all of the compartments interact with each other; that is, the biologic function of cells in one compartment is regulated by the functions of the cell populations in the other compartments. In the homeostatic state, these compartments establish a baseline trophic interaction that is disrupted during acute injury and repair and is reset by successive cycles of injury, inflammation, and repair characteristic of chronic airway diseases.

Perturbation of one compartment creates an imbalance in all compartments.[7,8] Baseline trophic interactions can be disrupted during acute injury and repair and can be altered by successive cycles of injury, inflammation, and repair typical of chronic airway diseases. Asthma and COPD manifest themselves by altering not only the epithelial compartment or the airway smooth muscle but also other compartments (eg, interstitial, vascular, immunologic, and nervous).[9,10]

The concept that cellular populations that comprise the conducting airway are a biologic entity unique to a particular branch of the airway tree emphasizes the number of factors by which they differ in their pathobiologic responses. Within the airway tree, the cellular response to toxic injury, including susceptibility to acute injury, the pattern of repair, and the development of tolerance vary markedly by airway level. Issues to be considered include airway microenvironment, the status of differentiation based on animal age, the history of previous exposure to injurants and inflammatory agents, the influence of anatomy on local dose of injurant delivered, and differences in airway wall organization between species and strains.

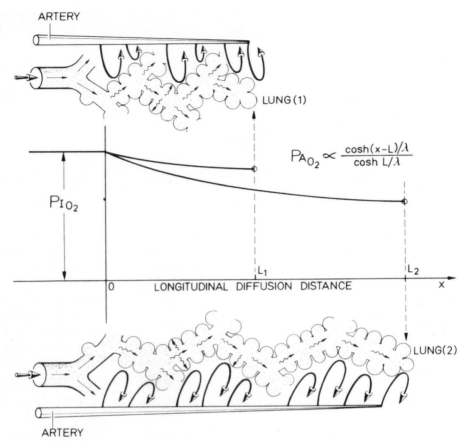

FIGURE 2. A model that shows how different acinar pathway lengths could result in differences in mean alveolar PO_2 in a size-dependent manner. Reproduced with permission from Weibel ER, Taylor CR, Gehr P, et al. Respir Physiol 1981;44:151–64.[6]

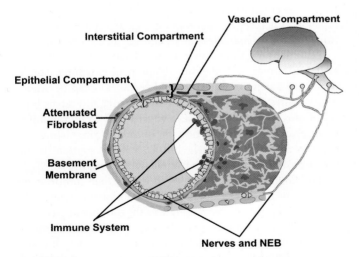

FIGURE 3. Diagrammatic representation of the wall of a tracheo-bronchial airway with the compartments that vary by species: epithelium, interstitium, nerves (including connections to the central nervous system and neuroepithelial cell bodies [NEB]), and immune or inflammatory cells. The interstitial compartment includes smooth muscle, fibroblasts, blood vessels, cartilage, and an extensive basement membrane zone, as found in primates. Reproduced with permission from Hyde DM et al, © European Respiratory Journals Ltd.[170]

Cellular Composition of the Tracheobronchial Airways

Tracheobronchial airway walls are highly complex cellular structures consisting of many different cell types that vary in their organization and cellular composition depending on species (Figure 4). The interstitium of the tracheal wall of all species contains C-shaped cartilage, and a band of smooth muscle joins the open end of the cartilages. However, the trachea and proximal airways of rhesus monkeys and humans have extensive submucosal glands beneath the epithelium, although these glands are present to a variable extent in smaller laboratory species (Table 2), usually confined to the most proximal portions of the trachea. There is also a substantial difference in the amount of epithelium that lines the luminal surface in the trachea between species (see Figure 3 and Table 2). The thickness of the epithelium in the trachea of rhesus monkeys is approximately twice that of mice and one-third to half that in humans (see Table 2).

The trachea demonstrates other major differences between species: the composition of the epithelium (see Table 2). Mucous cells are a substantial percentage of the airway in primates but are generally not present in the trachea of healthy, pathogen-free mice and rats. The proportion of ciliated cells

Rhesus Monkey

Swiss-Webster Mouse

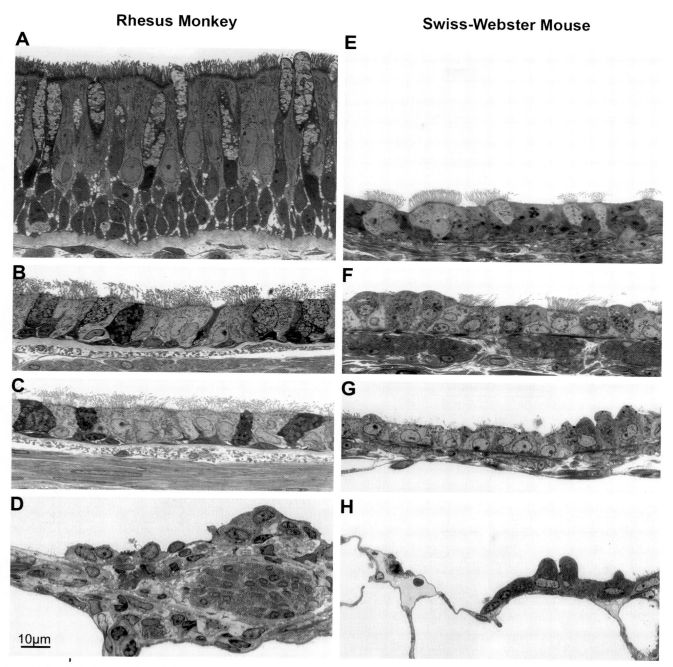

FIGURE 4. Histologic comparison of the airspace walls in the same airway generations of an adult male rhesus monkey (A–D) and an adult male Swiss Webster mouse (E–H). The luminal airspace (*at the top*) and the epithelium are set so that the basal lamina matches for both species. The epithelium is more complex and taller in the proximal airways of monkeys than at the same site in mice. Smooth muscle occupies a larger portion of the interstitium in monkeys than mice at all airway levels. All micrographs are at the same magnification with the magnification bar = μm. Toluidine blue staining. Reproduced with permission from Hyde DM et al, © European Respiratory Society Journals Ltd.[170]

in the epithelium is relatively similar in all species, yet the proportion of basal cells found in the epithelial surface differs. In general, the taller the epithelial surface, the more basal cells are present. As would be expected with the differences in secretory cell populations that line the trachea of different species, there is considerable variation in the carbohydrate content of the secretory product (Table 3). Alcian blue

(pH 2.5)—periodic acid—Schiff sequence staining was used to demonstrate acid (blue) and neutral (red) mucosubstances. The acidic mucins were characterized as being sulfated using high-iron diamine on an adjacent section.[11] Primates, in general, have a more heavily sulfated secretory product that is not usually found in laboratory mammals (see Table 3). The difference in secretory product composition is

Table 2	Comparison of Species Differences in Cells of the Trachea		
Parameter	*Human*	*Monkey*	*Mouse*
Wall			
Smooth muscle	Present	Present	Present
Cartilage	Present	Present	Present
Submucosal glands	Present	Present	Present (proximal third)
Epithelium			
Thickness (µm)	50–100	20–30	11–14
Cells/mm basement membrane	303 ± 20	181 ± 51	215
Mucous goblet cells (%)	9	17	< 1
Serous cells (%)		<1	< 1
Clara cells (%)		<1	49
Ciliated cells (%)	49	33	39
Basal cells (%)	33	42	10
Other cells (%)		8	1

Adapted from Van Winkle LS et al,[27] Harkema JR et al,[77] Hyde DM et al,[80] Plopper CG et al,[81] Mariassy AT,[171] Mercer RR et al,[172] and St George JA et al.[173]

also reflected, to some degree, in the composition of the carbohydrates in trachea (Figure 5)[12] and other conducting airway submucosal glands (Figure 6).[13]

Besides the trachea, other airways of the lung demonstrate species differences in their cellular composition. Although smooth muscle is present in the proximal intrapulmonary bronchi of all mammalian species, there is a substantial variation in the extent of cartilage and submucosal glands found in the lobar bronchus of primates and laboratory mammals (Table 4). In the most distal conducting airways, the bronchioles, the major differences between species are related primarily to the epithelial surface lining (Table 5). Throughout the tracheobronchial airways, mucous cells and basal cells predominate in primates, whereas Clara cells predominate in rodents (see Tables 2, 4, and 5).

In the most distal conducting airways, the bronchioles, the major differences between species are related primarily to the epithelial surface lining (see Table 4). In laboratory mammals, the Clara cell is the primary secretory cell phenotype, and there are no mucous cells. The extent of basal cells in the epithelium varies by the extent of alveolarization but is rare in the distal airways of laboratory rodents compared with primates. The bronchioles of rhesus monkeys have an extensive smooth muscle portion that is arranged in large bundles and is interspersed with extensive connective tissue not generally observed in other laboratory mammals (see Figure 4).

Mucociliary Epithelium in Rhesus Monkeys

The tracheobronchial airways of rhesus monkeys have been used extensively to define the biology of mucociliary epithelium. The capability of the airways to metabolically activate xenobiotics has been evaluated for both the cytochrome P-450 monooxygenases[14,15] and flavin-containing monooxygenases.[16,17] The composition of secretory products has been defined for complex carbohydrates in surface epithelium and glands throughout the airway tree in adults for

complex carbohydrates (see Figures 5 and 6)[12,13,18–21] and mucin antigens.[19] The expression and distribution of the cystic fibrosis transmembrane receptor[22] and keratins[23] have been characterized in airway epithelium. The pattern for differentiation of tracheobronchial epithelium[24–27] and submucosal glands has been defined.[28] Although regulatory control of epithelial differentiation has been studied *in vivo*,[29] the majority of the work has been done using biphasic epithelial cultures. The role of vitamin A in regulation of epithelial differentiation has been established for mucin genes,[30] cytokeratins,[31] markers of squamous cell differentiation,[31] small proline-rich protein,[32–34] an antioxidant, thioredoxin,[35] the cytokine interleukin (IL)-8,[36] epithelial growth factor,[37] and heterogeneous nuclear protein AI.[38] Extracellular calcium also plays a role in epithelial differentiation *in vitro*.[39]

Postnatal Development

During the first year of postnatal development in the rhesus monkey, the airways themselves are in active phases of growth; the epithelium, basement membrane, and smooth muscle of the airways are differentiating; the mucosal immune system of the airways is being established; the nerve networks within the airway are being established; the capillary beds in the airway and the parenchyma are forming; and alveolarization of the parenchyma is active.

Airway Growth

The number of conducting airways is completely developed by birth in humans, but airway size increases with lung growth.[40,41] Comparison of lung morphology in macaques and humans shows that there are similarities in segmental arrangement, structure and branching pattern of airways, arterial structure, and arterial changes after birth.[41,42] Although there are differences in the number of lobes, the number of generations of different types of airways and the overall structure in the monkey are more similar to those in humans than is the structure of the

Table 3 Comparison of Species Differences in Carbohydrate Content of Clara and Mucous Cells in Tracheal Epithelium

Parameter	Human	Monkey	Mouse
Abundance	+ + +	+ +	+/_
Periodic acid—Schiff	+(M)	+(M)	+(M) ±/−(C)
Alcian blue	+	+(M)	+(M) − (C)
High-iron diamine	+ and −(M)	+ and − (M) and − (M)	(M) −(C)

Adapted from St George JA and Wang S,[29] Harkema JR et al,[77] and St George JA et al.[173] C = Clara cells; M = mucous cells.

lung of other laboratory animals.[42] In the transition zone, the area where the conducting airways end and the gas exchange area begins, humans and rhesus monkeys have numerous generations of respiratory bronchioles. In humans, since terminal bronchioles are formed prenatally and only increase in size postnatally, we would expect that the number of respiratory bronchioles would also be formed by birth.[40] Terminal bronchioles in rhesus monkeys increase by a third in diameter and twice in length between 1 and 6 months of age (Figure 7).[43]

Epithelial Differentiation

In adult mammals, at least eight cell phenotypes line the tracheobronchial conducting airways, including ciliated cells, basal cells, mucous goblet cells, serous cells, Clara cells, small

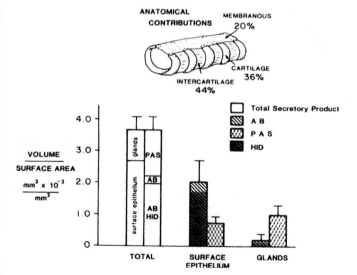

FIGURE 5. The percentage of total surface area contributed by each anatomic region was used to sum the results into volume per surface of total stainable mucosubstance for the entire trachea. Each bar represents group mean ± 1 SD of eight animals. Reproduced with permission, from Heidsiek JG, Hyde DM, Plopper CG, St George JA. J Histochem Cytochem 35:435–42;1987.[12] AB = Alcian blue positive; HID = high-iron diamine positive; PAS = periodic acid—Schiff positive/Alcian blue negative.

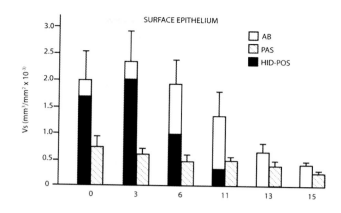

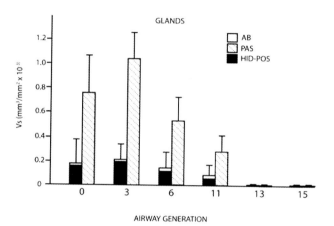

FIGURE 6. Graphs of the amount of secretory product (as mm³ × 10⁻³) stored per unit surface area (mm²) of basal lamina in tracheobronchial airways. The material for the surface epithelium (A) and submucosal glands (B) is summarized for the trachea (airway generation 0), the lobar bronchus of the right middle lobe (airway generation 3), and four generations of intrapulmonary airways (6, 11, 13, and 15). The largest amount of material stored per unit of surface is found in the lobar bronchus and the least amount on the pulmonary artery side of the respiratory bronchiole (generation 15). Reproduced with permission from Plopper CG, Heidsiek JG, Weir AJ, et al. Am J Anat 1989;184:31–40.[13]

mucous granule cells, brush cells, neuroendocrine cells, and a number of undifferentiated or partially differentiated phenotypes that have not been well characterized. Humans and other primates share a mixture of cell phenotypes not found in nonprimate species, primarily of the secretory cell types (Figure 8).[44] Epithelial differentiation (especially the secretory cell types and glandular elements) occurs postnatally for both rhesus monkeys[24,27,28] and humans.[45,46] The secretory cell population differentiates in a proximal to distal pattern, with nearly mature cells lining proximal airways and immature cells in more distal portions. This pattern is also found in the secretory cells of rodents, where it is quite extensive. Glandular mucous cells and serous cells differentiate at different times during pre- and postnatal development and through a different sequence of events (Figure 9).[27,28] This may occur on a different timetable in animals housed in ultraclean environments.[7]

Table 4	Comparison of Species Differences in Proximal Intrapulmonary Airways		
Parameter	*Human*	*Monkey*	*Mouse*
Wall			
Smooth muscle	Present	Present	Present
Cartilage	Present	Present	Absent
Submucosal glands	Present	Present	Absent
Epithelium			
Thickness (μm)	40–50	27	8–16
Cells/mm basement membrane	NA	175	109
Mucous goblet cells (%)	10	15	< 1
Serous cells (%)	3	5	< 1
Clara cells (%)	3	5	61
Ciliated cells (%)	37	47	36
Basal cells (%)	32	32	< 1
Other (%)	18	2	2

Adapted from Van Winkle LS et al,[27] Harkema JR et al,[77] Hyde DM et al,[80] Plopper CG et al,[81] and Mariassy AT,[171] and St George JA et al.[173]

Basement Membrane Zone

The BMZ develops postnatally in the airways of nonhuman primates (see Figures 9 and 10).[27,47] Changes include reorganization of collagen types I, III, and V (Figure 11); a three- to fourfold increase in thickness; and shifts in the deposition of perlecan (see Figure 11) and its storage of fibroblast growth factor 2 (FGF-2) (Figure 12).[47]

Smooth Muscle Development

Smooth muscle develops from myoblasts present in the mesenchyme of the developing lung.[48,49] The bulk of smooth muscle growth and differentiation in large bronchi occurs after birth, where it increases fourfold.[43,50] The process observed in the rhesus monkey as the airways grow postnatally involves changes in orientation of smooth muscle bundles and increases in total bundle number within an airway branch (Figure 13)[43]: this maintains the relative density of bundle content. Bundle size is also constant and therefore decreases in relation to airway size as each airway grows. Preterm infants with chronic lung disease have significantly increased amounts of smooth muscle in the larger airways.[49]

Mucosal Immune System

Newborn infant airways without pulmonary lesions contain few leukocytes. It has been suggested that in healthy infants, leukocyte "seeding" within the airways must be initiated following birth and exposure to environmental stimuli; this process likely continues during the first 2 years of life.[51] There are no significant changes in lavage cell profile from children between 3 to 8 and 8 to 14 years, suggesting that accumulation of resident immune or inflammatory cells within airways is essentially complete after the age of 3 years.[52] In a small study of 18 healthy children (3 months to 10 years), age significantly correlated with the frequency of lymphocytes within lavage; however, there was no correlation with other lavage cell phenotypes.[53] Several groups have reported striking differences in the CD4 to CD8 ratio of lavage lymphocytes from children

Table 5	Comparison of Species Differences in Terminal Bronchioles		
Parameter	*Human*	*Monkey*	*Mouse*
Wall			
Cartilage	Absent (bifurcation)	Absent (bifurcation)	Absent
Smooth muscle	Present	Present	Present
Submucosal glands	Absent	Absent	Absent
Epithelium			
Thickness (μm)	?	?	7–8
Cells/mm	?	?	?
Mucous goblet (%)			0
Serous cells (%)	35	≈20	0
Clara cells (%)			60–80
Ciliated cells (%)	52	≈50	40–20
Basal cells (%)	< 1	≈10	< 1
Other(%)	13	≈5	0

Adapted from Tyler WS and Julian MD,[42] Plopper CG and Hyde DM,[44] Harkema JR et al,[77] Mercer RR et al,[172] and Plopper CG et al.[174]

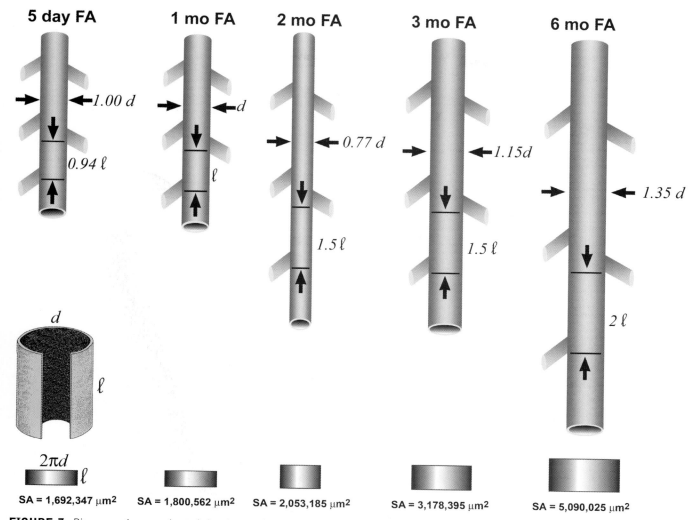

5 day FA   **1 mo FA**   **2 mo FA**   **3 mo FA**   **6 mo FA**

1.00 d

d

0.77 d

1.15d

1.35 d

0.94 ℓ

ℓ

1.5 ℓ

1.5 ℓ

2 ℓ

d

ℓ

2πd

ℓ

SA = 1,692,347 μm2   SA = 1,800,562 μm2   SA = 2,053,185 μm2   SA = 3,178,395 μm2   SA = 5,090,025 μm2

FIGURE 7. Diagrammatic comparison of size changes in the bronchiole 1 generation proximal to the terminal bronchiole of rhesus monkeys starting at 5 days of age and ending at 6 months. Scaling for length (*l*) and diameter (*d*) is based on setting the value for 30-day-old animals equal to 1. Luminal surface area (SA) was calculated from the values. Used with permission from Tran MU et al.[43] FA = filtered air.

(3 months to 16 years of age) compared with adults; CD4 to CD8 ratios ranged from 0.6 to 0.8 for children, in contrast with 1.8 to 2.7 for adults.[54-57] The lower CD4 to CD8 values for bronchoalveolar lavage in children appear to be owing to a higher number of CD8 cells.[57]

Bronchial Vasculature

Although the postnatal development of the bronchial system has not been described in primates, we do know that in adult rhesus monkeys, the subgross anatomic distribution is similar to that of humans, but there are differences in the supply to the pleura similar to other laboratory animals that have a thin pleura.[58,59]

Nerves

Along with anatomic development processes of the lung, the respiratory nervous system proliferates and innervates the developing respiratory tract. We believe that normal sensory innervation of the airway appears first in the large conducting airway and then progresses down the airway tree to more

distal airways. Based on our observation of midlevel airway epithelial innervation, we believe that this process is incomplete at 30 days of age but is complete at 180 days of age in infant rhesus monkeys.[60]

Neural regulation of airway smooth muscle lower airways (trachea and bronchi), and consequently airway caliber, is primarily parasympathetic in nature. Preganglionic axons are carried to the airways by the vagus nerves, where these axons form the preganglionic component of synapses on principal neurons within ganglia located within or near the airway wall.[61,62] The parasympathetic ganglia are located mainly in the trachea and larger bronchi, but postganglionic fibers innervate cells all the way to the bronchioles.[62,63] In the airways, the parasympathetic nervous system mediates both cholinergic contractions and nonadrenergic, noncholinergic (NANC) relaxations of the airway smooth muscle. In human airways, excitatory cholinergic nerves are the predominant bronchoconstrictor pathway. Although several putative neurotransmitters have been proposed for the inhibitory NANC system, vasoactive intestinal peptide (VIP) and nitric oxide (NO) have been suggested as the only neural bronchodilator

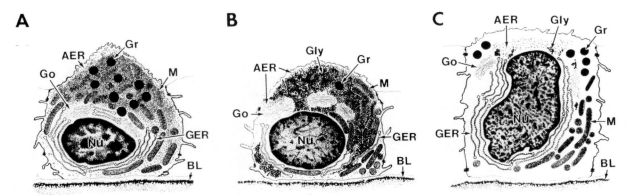

FIGURE 8. Comparison of the ultrastructural appearance of Clara cells in species with abundant agranular endoplasmic reticulum (AER) (A) such as most laboratory mammals; with species (B) in which cytoplasmic glycogen (GLY) predominates, such as carnivores; and with primates (C) in which neither component is abundant. From Plopper CG and Hyde DM.[44] BL = basal lamina; GER = granular endoplasmic reticulum; Go = Golgi apparatus; Gr = secretory granules; M = mitochondria; Nu = nucleus.

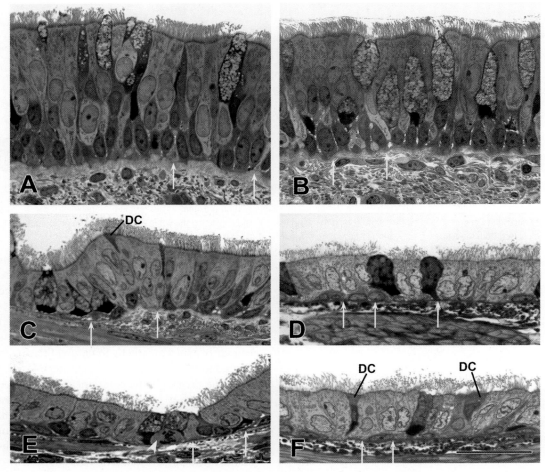

FIGURE 9. High-resolution light micrograph of representative airway epithelium from a 5-day-old monkey (A, C, E) and a 6-month-old monkey (B, D, F). Three airway generations are illustrated: trachea (A and B), proximal bronchus (C and D), and distal bronchus (E and F). The airway epithelium contained ciliated, mucous goblet, and basal cells in abundance, but total epithelial thickness decreases as the airways decrease in size. Dark ciliated cells (DC) were infrequent. Cells with mitotic figures (*arrowhead*) were more common in younger animals. The basement membrane became more distinct with age (*arrows*). Bar in *F* is 30 μ. Toluidine blue staining. Used with permission from Van Winkle LS et al.[27]

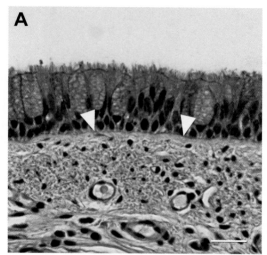

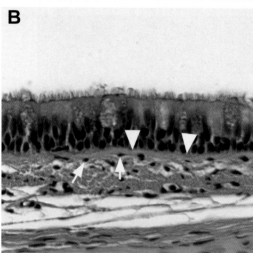

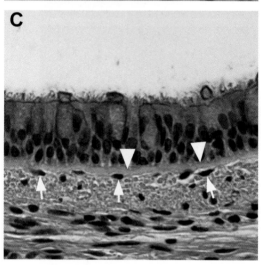

FIGURE 10. Hematoxylin and eosin—stained sections of tracheal rings from 1- to 6-month-old monkeys. Bar = 20 μm. *A*, At 1 month, the basement membrane zone (BMZ) is not apparent (*arrowheads*), and the layer of attenuated fibroblasts beneath the epithelium is not present. *B*, At 2 months, the BMZ is present (*arrowheads*), and the attenuated fibroblast sheath beneath the epithelium is organized (*arrows*). *C*, At 6 months, the tissue has the characteristics of the adult. Used with permission from Evans MJ et al.[47]

pathway in human airways.[64–66] It is now believed that the contractile and relaxant parasympathetic nerves are derived from distinct autonomic pathways.[67–69] Findings in normal ferret trachea suggest reciprocal innervation between ganglia that synthesize cholinergic neurotransmitters and those that synthesize NANC neurotransmitters, VIP, and NO.[70]

Alveolar Development

Stages of human lung development show alveolarization by formation of secondary interalveolar septa from about 36 weeks of gestation to about 1 to 2 years of age and microvascular maturation by remodeling of interalveolar septa and restructuring of the capillary bed from birth to 2 to 3 years of age.[71,72] The majority of alveoli are produced postnatally in humans to reach the adult number of about 450 million alveoli.[73] Using design-based stereologic methods in rhesus monkey lungs, it was recently shown that alveoli increase in number (Figure 14) but not volume (Figure 15) throughout all of the postnatal developmental or growth stages (infant, 1–12 months; juvenile, 12–24 months; adolescent, 2–4 years; and young adult, 4–8 years).[74]

Cellular Microenvironment Response to Injury

Two aspects of the microenvironment are critical when defining the pathobiology of the response to injury. The first is that all of the cellular populations in the airway wall are vital for maintaining differentiated function of the epithelium.[75] The three-dimensional configuration of the airway (an intact tubular structure including all components of the wall) is necessary, and absence of airway wall integrity results in a transformation of the epithelial populations.[75] In addition, the entire repair process after acute injury, including proliferation and migration to reestablish cell density and differentiation of epithelial phenotypes, occurs *in vitro* in intact airways under normal growth conditions independent of other extraneous factors in the animal.[76] The second feature is that the injury and the accompanying inflammatory response vary markedly by the position of the target cells within the tracheobronchial airway tree.[10,44,77–79] This is true for a wide variety of stressors, including oxidant gases[10,80,81] bioactivated hydrocarbons,[82–84] and allergens.[85] Regardless of the agent or the phenotype of the target cell population, the sensitivity varies widely between proximal and distal airways.

Airway-Specific Responses to Inhaled Allergens

Over the past 10 years, experimental induction of airway remodeling using immune-based models of allergic asthma has increased, especially in mice.[86] However, caution has been raised concerning the extrapolation of findings from experimentally induced mouse models to naturally occurring human asthma.[87,88] The immunologic basis of both human allergic and mouse models of asthma is an exuberant T-helper 2 (Th2) response to one or more allergens. However, there are notable differences between the two species, including airway development and structure, cellular composition, techniques for measuring pulmonary function, the chronic nature of the disease process, and expression of key cytokines

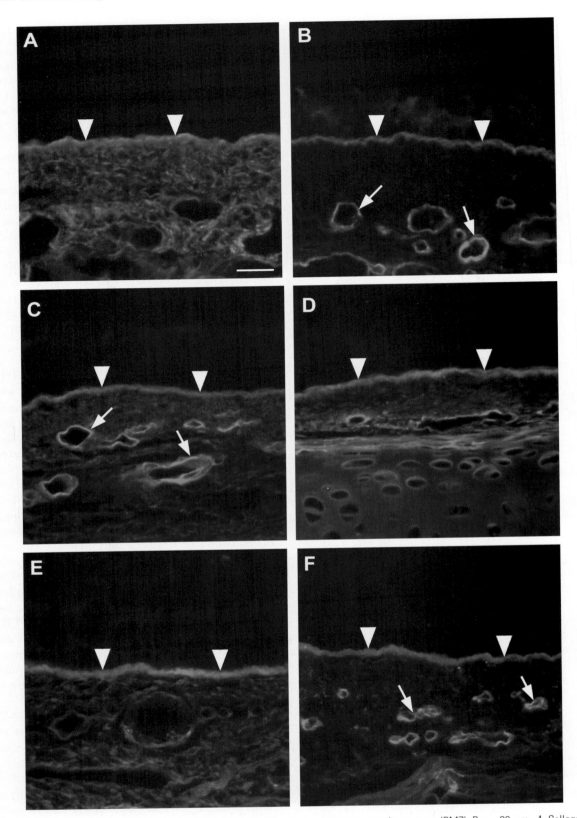

FIGURE 11. Immunohistochemistry of collagen and perlecan in the developing basement membrane zone (BMZ). Bar = 20 μm. *A*, Collagen III BMZ at 1 month (*arrowheads*). *B*, Perlecan BMZ is present at 1 month (*arrowheads*). There is also strong perlecan immunoreactivity in the walls of blood vessels (*arrows*). *C*, Collagen V BMZ at 2 and 3 months is similar (*arrowheads*). There is also strong immunoreactivity in the walls of blood vessels (*arrows*). *D*, Perlecan BMZ is similar at 2 and 3 months (*arrowheads*). *E*, Collagen I BMZ at 6 months is similar to that at 2 and 3 months (*arrowheads*). *F*, Perlecan BMZ at 6 months is similar to that at 2 and 3 months (*arrowheads*); however, the immunoreactivity is less intense compared with the walls of blood vessels (*arrows*). Primary antibodies to Collagen I, III, V, or Perlecan followed by a secondary antibody (Alexa Fluor 568). Used with permission from Evans MJ et al.[47]

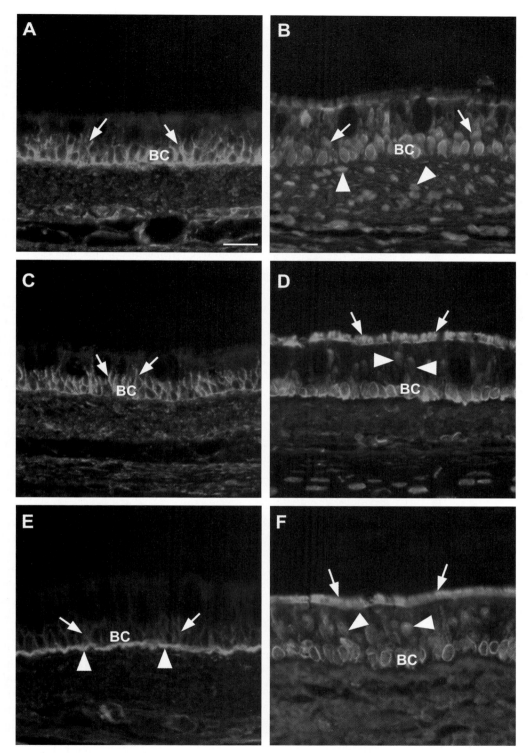

FIGURE 12. Immunohistochemisry of fibroblast growth factor (FGF)-2 and FGF receptor 1 in the developing epithelial mesenchymal trophic unit. Bar = 20 µm. *A*, FGF-2 immunoreactivity at 1 month is associated mainly with basal cells (BC) and the lateral intercellular space (*arrows*). It is not apparent in the basement membrane zone (BMZ) or extracellular matrix. *B*, FGF receptor 1 immunoreactivity at 1 month is associated mainly with basal cells and their nuclei and columnar cell nuclei (*arrows*). Immunoreactivity was also present in the nuclei of mesenchymal cells (*arrowheads*). *C*, FGF-2 immunoreactivity at 2 and 3 months is associated with BC and the lateral intercellular space (*arrows*). *D*, FGF receptor 1 immunoreactivity at 2 and 3 months is associated mainly with BC and cilia (*arrows*). Weak immunoreactivity is associated with the nuclei of columnar cells (*arrowheads*). Only a few mesenchymal cells expressed FGF receptor 1 at this time. *E*, FGF-2 immunoreactivity at 6 months is now present mainly in the BMZ (*arrowheads*). Weak immunoreactivity is associated with BC and the lateral intercellular space (*arrows*). *F*, FGF receptor 1 immunoreactivity at 6 months is associated mainly with BC and cilia (*arrows*). Weak immunoreactivity is associated with the nuclei of columnar cells (*arrowheads*). There was very little immunoreactivity in mesenchymal cells. Primary antibodies to FGF-2 or FGF receptor 1 followed by a secondary antibody (Alexa Fluor 568). Used with permission from Evans MJ et al.[47]

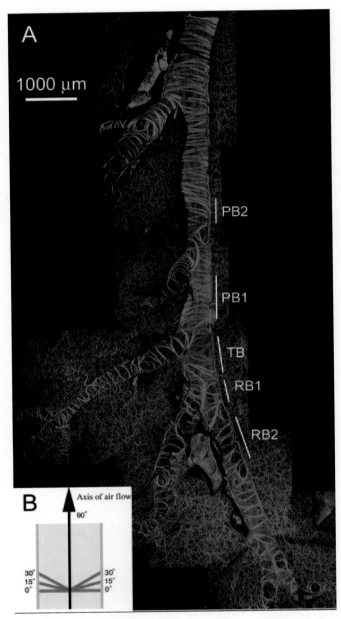

FIGURE 13. *A,* Composite map of laser scanning confocal images of smooth muscle in distal bronchioles of the rhesus monkey. Smooth muscle is identified with Alexa Fluor 568 phalloidin, a probe for filamentous actin. The following distal airways were evaluated in this study: bronchiole one generation proximal to the terminal bronchiole (PB1); bronchiole two generations proximal to the terminal bronchiole (PB2); first generation of respiratory bronchiole distal to the terminal bronchiole (RB1); second generation of respiratory bronchiole distal to the terminal bronchiole (RB2); and terminal bronchiole (TB). Twenty-five images were used to make this map. *B,* Diagram illustrating the basis of measurement of smooth muscle bundle orientation in an airway. The *arrow* depicts the axis of airflow. Bundle angles (θ) were measured from a line perpendicular to the axis of the airway, at which $\theta = 0$. Used with permission from Tran MU et al.[43]

and mediators.[89] Further, most mice lack intrinsic airway hyperresponsiveness (AHR). In humans, increases in airway smooth muscle are likely the primary mechanism causing AHR, and changes in the extracellular matrix may stimulate smooth muscle growth and contribute to the mechanics of airway obstruction. The classic chicken egg ovalbumin (OVA) intraperitoneal immunization with alum, followed by repetitive challenge with OVA intranasally, produces a robust eosinophilic inflammatory response around bronchi and allergen-dependent AHR, dependent on CD4[+] T lymphocytes via IL-4, but independent of IL-5, immunoglobulin E (IgE), or both.[90,91] However, other unique features of allergic airways disease are found in humans but not mice: lack of intrinsic AHR (except A/J mouse strain), smooth muscle hypertrophy in the more distal bronchi and respiratory bronchioles, exfoliation of epithelial sheets, and mast cell infiltration of airway smooth muscle.[89]

Uniqueness of the Rhesus Monkey Model of Asthma

Large animal models of asthma have been developed in sheep,[92] dogs,[93] and nonhuman primates (macaques).[94-98] The rhesus monkey model of asthma is used because of the genetic and physiologic similarity to humans that allows pulmonary function measurements commonly used in humans.[95] The airway anatomy and especially the similarities during postnatal development of the lung are another major advantage in using rhesus monkeys.[99] The rhesus monkey also has more specific reagents available for use compared with other nonhuman primates (NIH Nonhuman Primate Reagent Resource; <http://NHPreagents.bidmc.harvard.eud>). The model involves injection of a common human allergen, followed by intranasal instillation and repeated aerosol challenges of the allergen. The rhesus monkey model shares many of the key features of human allergic asthma, including: allergen-specific IgE and skin test positivity, eosinophils and IgE[+] cells in airways, a Th2 cytokine profile in airways, mucous cell hyperplasia, subepithelial fibrosis, basement membrane thickening, and persistent baseline hyperreactivity to histamine or methacholine.[95,96,100]

The house dust mite (HDM) allergen-rhesus monkey model shows the following: Th2-associated cytokine and chemokine induction; migration of eosinophils, lymphocytes, and dendritic cells into airways; early and late bronchoconstriction responses; and enhanced reactivity to histamine challenge in response to HDM challenge.[95,100]

The HDM—rhesus monkey model was developed by a multidisciplinary group of investigators at the California National Primate Research Center to address the problem of environmental enhancement of the induction of asthma, particularly in children. A number of discoveries about asthma using the rhesus monkey model have been made.

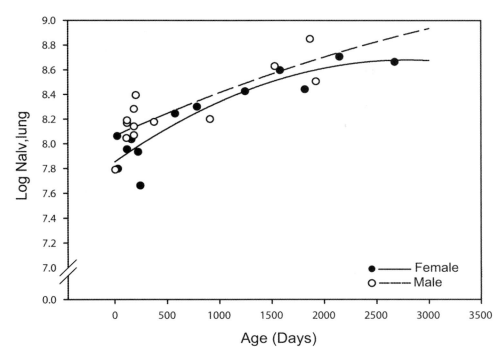

FIGURE 14. The log of the number of alveoli in the lung versus age (days) for females (*solid line* and *filled circles*) and males (*dashed line* and *open circles*) is plotted according to a quadratic function. Used with permission from Hyde DM et al.[74]

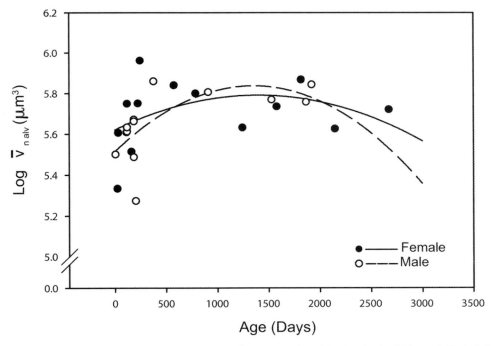

FIGURE 15. The log of the mean alveolar number-weighted volume (μm^3) versus age (days) for females (*solid line* and *filled circles*) and males (*dashed line* and *open circles*) is plotted according to a quadratic function. Used with permission from Hyde DM et al.[74]

A

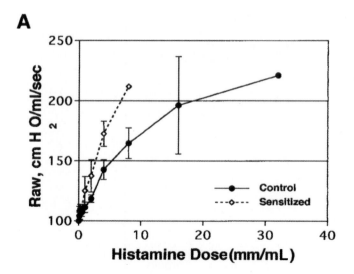

B

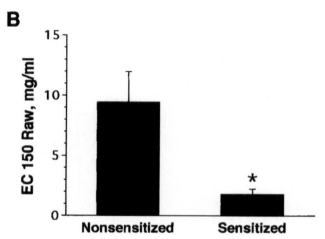

FIGURE 16. *A,* Comparison of percentage change in Raw as a function of increasing inhaled histamine concentrations (mg/mL) in sensitized and non-sensitized (control) rhesus monkeys. *B,* Comparison of effective concentration of histamine to produce a 150% (EC150) increase in Raw in sensitized and nonsensitized (control) rhesus monkeys. Reprinted from Am J Pathol 2001;158:333-41, with permission from the American Society for Investigative Pathology.[95] Raw = airway resistance.

Airway Physiology

Following aerosol challenge with HDM, sensitized rhesus monkeys show cough, rapid shallow breathing, and increased airway resistance, which can be reversed by albuterol aerosol treatment. Compared with nonsensitized monkeys, there is a fourfold reduction in the dose of histamine aerosol necessary to produce a 150% increase in airway resistance in sensitized monkeys (Figure 16).[95]

Airway Generation—Specific Immune and Inflammatory Cells and Cytokines

After aerosol challenge, serum levels of histamine are elevated in sensitized monkeys. Sensitized monkeys also exhibit increased levels of HDM-specific IgE in serum, numbers of eosinophils and exfoliated cells within lavage, and elevated

CD25 expression on circulating CD4+ lymphocytes.[95] In HDM-challenged monkeys, the volume of CD1a+ dendritic cells (Figure 17), CD4+ T helper lymphocytes and CD25+ cells (Figure 18), IgE+ cells (Figure 19), eosinophils (Figure 20), and proliferating cells (Figure 21) is significantly increased in the airways. All of these cell types accumulate within airways in unique patterns of distribution, suggesting compartmentalized responses with regard to trafficking. Although cytokine messenger ribonucleic acid levels are elevated throughout the conducting airway tree of HDM-challenged animals, the distal airways (terminal and respiratory bronchioles) exhibit the most pronounced upregulation.[85]

Airway Generation—Specific Remodeling

Intrapulmonary proximal and distal bronchi of sensitized and challenged monkeys have focal mucous goblet cell hyperplasia, thickening of the BMZ, hypercellularity in the epithelium and subepithelial connective tissue, and increases in smooth muscle and bronchial microvessels.[9,95] These changes are site specific and vary greatly within various portions of the airway wall in the same airway generation, between airway generations in an individual sensitized and challenged animal, and from animal to animal in the sensitized and challenged group. A mouse model of allergic airways did not show airway generation-specific remodeling using airway microdissection-based sampling but did show changes in the proximal airways that were significantly different from control mice.[101]

Epithelial Changes in Asthma

A characteristic of asthma is the sloughing of sheets of columnar epithelium from the airways leaving basal cells attached to the basal lamina.[102–104] The desmosomal attachments between sloughed epithelial cells are intact, suggesting that failure of the desmosomal attachment between basal and columnar cells is responsible for sloughing of airway epithelium in asthmatic subjects.[105-108] There is a reduction in the anchoring mechanisms between columnar cells and basal cells in the airways of asthmatic humans.[109,110] Whether this change, combined with the inflammatory and immune cell trafficking, is responsible for cell sloughing is not known. To study this response, one must use an animal model that includes a multilayered epithelium, resembling the human epithelium, with abundant basal cells throughout the majority of the airway tree. Basal cells are more sparsely distributed in mice than in the rhesus monkey.

Goblet cell hyperplasia is also a characteristic of asthmatic airways (Figure 22).[95,111] Goblet cells are generally not sloughed from the airways as are the ciliated cells, suggesting that they are more firmly attached to the basal cells. In asthma and other chronic airway diseases, the number of goblet cells increases and ciliated cells decreases, suggesting that the process of differentiation following repair of cell loss has been compromised. A mouse model of allergic airways showed

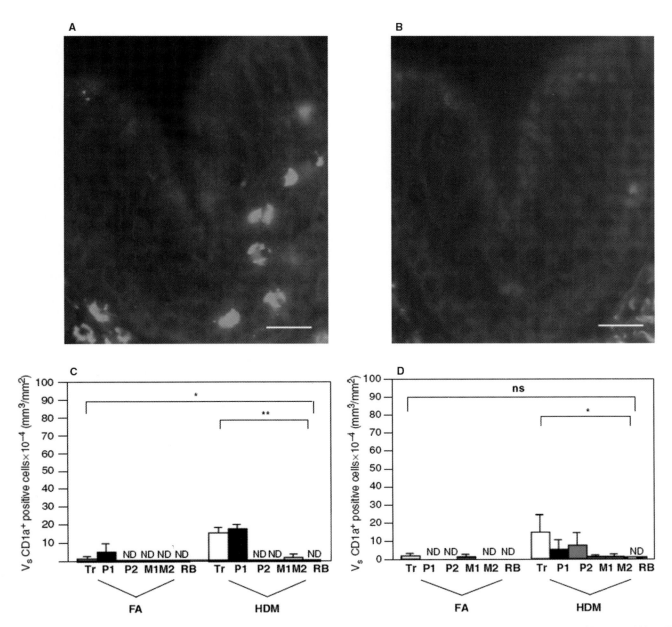

FIGURE 17. Distribution of CD1a+ dendritic cells within airway mucosa of house dust mite (HDM)-challenged rhesus monkeys. CD1a+ dendritic cells were identified by immunofluorescence staining of trachea and left caudal lobe sections obtained from HDM-challenged monkeys. Tr, P1, P2, M1, M2, and RB represent cryosections obtained from tissue blocks of trachea and regions progressively representing the most proximal (P1) to distal (RB) intrapulmonary airways of the lobe. Columns represent the average volume ± standard error of CD1a+ staining cells (mm^3) with respect to the surface area of basal lamina (mm^2). FA = filtered air control; HDM = house dust mite challenged; RB = respiratory bronchiole. *A*, CD1a+ immunofluorescence staining of trachea from a representative HDM monkey. Bar = 20 μm. *B*, Control staining of an adjacent section using a fluorescein isothiocyanate-conjugated mouse immunoglobulin G1 isotype control. Bar = 20 μm. *C*, Abundance of CD1a+ cells within the epithelial compartment of conducting airways. ND = none detected. *$p <$. 0001 by analysis of variance (block effect); **p = .0005 by analysis of variance (treatment effect). *D*, Abundance of CD1a+ cells within the interstitial compartment of conducting airways. *p = .0284 by analysis of variance (treatment effect). Reproduced with permission from Miller LA, Hurst SD, Coffman RL, et al. Airway generation-specific differences in the spatial distribution of immune cells and cytokines in allergen-challenged rhesus monkeys. Clin Exp Allergy 2005;35:894-906; Wiley-Blackwell, publishers.[85] ns = not significant.

that a 75% decrease in Clara cells and a 25% decrease in ciliated cells were completely compensated for by an increase in mucous cells.[101] Consequently, by day 22, 70% of the total epithelial cell population in the proximal airways was mucous cells (Figure 23). Electron microscopy illustrated that Clara cells were undergoing metaplasia to mucous cells and 1:5 to

1:10 of the mucous cells were proliferating. Epithelial cell death (necrosis or apoptosis) did not appear to be the stimulus driving epithelial proliferation, and the increase in mucous cell numbers was primarily a result of Clara cell metaplasia. These epithelial changes were not significant in the distal midlevel airway and bronchiole. In contrast, chronic

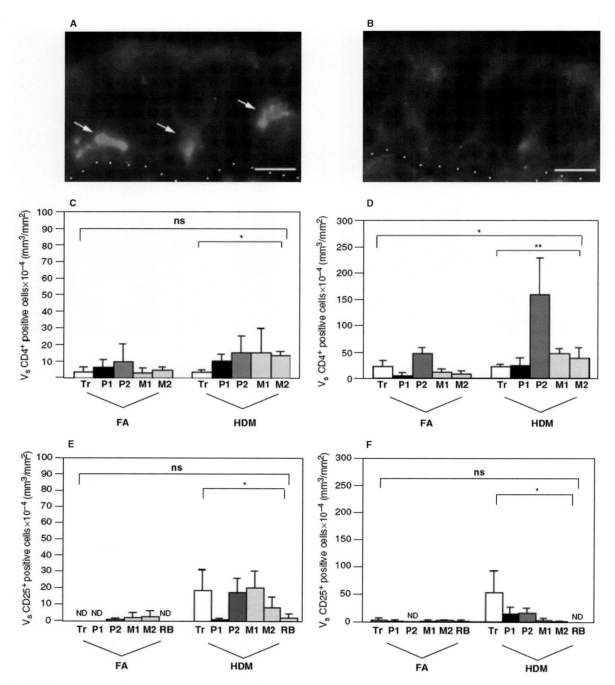

FIGURE 18. Distribution of CD4+ lymphocytes and CD25+ cells within airway mucosa of house dust mite (HDM)-challenged rhesus monkeys. CD3+/CD4+ lymphocytes and CD25+ cells were quantitated by immunofluorescence staining of trachea and left caudal lobe sections obtained from HDM-challenged monkeys. Tr, P1, P2, M1, M2, and RB represent cryosections obtained from tissue blocks of trachea and regions progressively representing the most proximal (P1) to distal (RB) intrapulmonary airways of the lobe. Columns represent the average volume ± standard error of CD3+/CD4+ or CD25+ staining cells (mm³) with respect to the surface area of basal lamina (mm²). FA = filtered air control; HDM = house dust mite challenged; RB = respiratory bronchiole. *A*, CD25+ immunofluorescence staining of a midlevel intrapulmonary airway (M1) from a representative HDM monkey. The *dotted line* defines the basement membrane of the region; the epithelium is above the line, and the interstitium is below the line. The *arrows* point to three CD25+ cells within the epithelium. Bar = 10 μm (B) Control staining of an adjacent section using a fluorescein isothiocyanate-conjugated mouse immunoglobulin G1 isotype control. Bar = 10 μm (C) Abundance of CD3+/CD4+ fluorescence double-positive lymphocytes within the epithelial compartment of conducting airways. *p = .07 by analysis of variance (treatment effect). *D*, Abundance of CD3+/CD4+ fluorescence double-positive lymphocytes within the interstitial compartment of conducting airways. *p = .0007 by analysis of variance (block effect); **p = .0037 by analysis of variance (treatment effect). *E*, Abundance of CD25+ cells within the epithelial compartment of conducting airways. *p = .0044 by analysis of variance (treatment effect). *F*, Abundance of CD25+ cells within the interstitial compartment of conducting airways. *p = .0818 by analysis of variance (treatment effect). Reproduced with permission from Miller LA, Hurst SD, Coffman RL, et al. Airway generation-specific differences in the spatial distribution of immune cells and cytokines in allergen-challenged rhesus monkeys. Clin Exp Allergy 2005;35:894–906; Wiley-Blackwell, publishers.[85] ns = not significant.

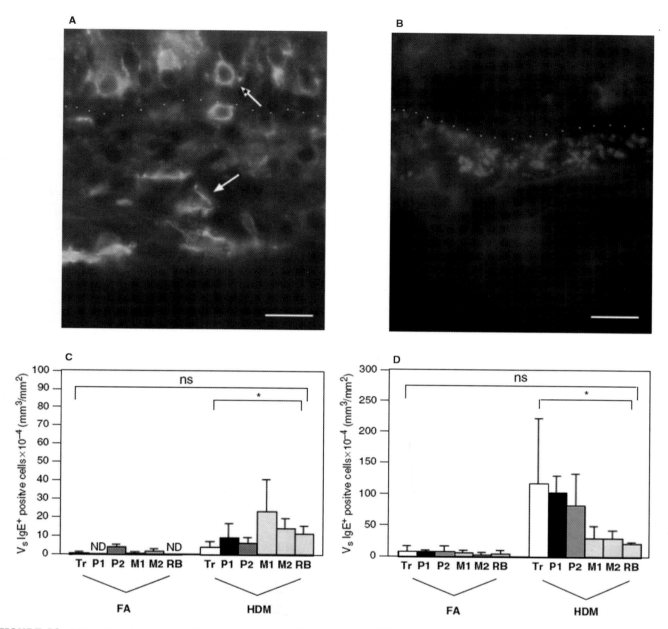

FIGURE 19. Distribution of IgE+ cells within airway mucosa of house dust mite (HDM)-challenged rhesus monkeys. IgE+ cells were quantitated by immunofluorescence staining of trachea and left caudal lobe sections obtained from HDM-challenged monkeys. Tr, P1, P2, M1, M2, and RB represent cryosections obtained from tissue blocks of trachea and regions progressively representing the most proximal (P1) to distal (RB) intrapulmonary airways of the lobe. Columns represent the average volume ± standard error of IgE+ staining cells (mm³) within the specified compartment with respect to the surface area of basal lamina (mm²). FA = filtered air control; HDM = house dust mite challenged; RB = respiratory bronchiole. *A*, IgE+ immunofluorescence staining of an intrapulmonary airway (block P2) from a representative HDM-challenged monkey. The *dotted line* defines the basement membrane; the epithelium is above the line, and the interstitium is below the line. The *normal arrow* points to an interstitial IgE+ cell; the **arrow* points to an epithelial IgE+ cell. Bar = 20 μm (B) Control staining of an adjacent section using nonspecific goat IgG and Alexa Fluor 488 secondary antibody. Bar = 20 μm. *C*, Abundance of IgE+ cells within the epithelial compartment of conducting airways. *p = .0088 by analysis of variance (treatment effect). *D*, Abundance of IgE+ cells within the interstitial compartment of conducting airways. *p = .0125 by analysis of variance (treatment effect). Reproduced with permission from Miller LA, Hurst SD, Coffman RL, et al. Airway generation-specific differences in the spatial distribution of immune cells and cytokines in allergen-challenged rhesus monkeys. Clin Exp Allergy 2005;35:894–906; Wiley-Blackwell, publishers.[85] ns = not significant.

exposure to OVA (2 consecutive days per week for 12 weeks) results in goblet cell hyperplasia into the distal airways of mice.[91] It does appear, however, that the epithelial changes in the airways of allergic mice are unique to the high number of Clara cells in their epithelium.

Airway Wall Matrix/Basement Membrane

A characteristic of asthma is a massive increase in BMZ thickness (Figures 24 and 25).[112] The BMZ is the central structure of the EMTU.[7,113] Exchange of information between the epithelium and fibroblasts occurs via the basal lamina: the

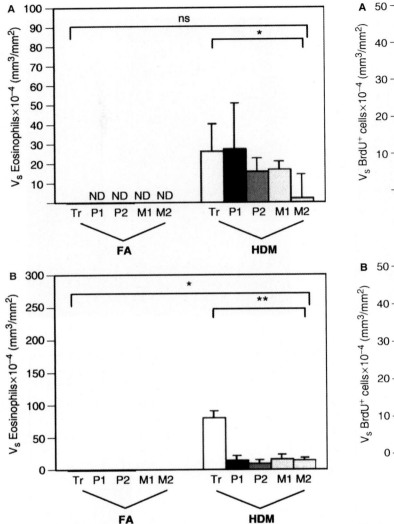

FIGURE 20. Distribution of eosinophils within airway mucosa of house dust mite (HDM)-challenged rhesus monkeys. Eosinophils were quantitated from hematoxylin-eosin staining of trachea and right middle lobe sections obtained from HDM-challenged monkeys. Tr, P1, P2, M1, and M2 represent cryosections obtained from tissue blocks of trachea and regions progressively representing the most proximal (P1) to midlevel intrapulmonary airways of the lobe. Columns represent the average volume ± standard error of eosinophils (mm^3) within the specified compartment with respect to the surface area of basal lamina (mm^2). FA = filtered air control; HDM = house dust mite challenged. *A*, Abundance of eosinophils within the epithelial compartment of conducting airways. $*p = .0046$ by analysis of variance (treatment effect). *B*, Abundance of eosinophils within the interstitial compartment of conducting airways. $*p < .0001$ by analysis of variance (block effect); $**p < .0001$ by analysis of variance (treatment effect). Reproduced with permission from Miller LA, Hurst SD, Coffman RL, et al. Airway generation-specific differences in the spatial distribution of immune cells and cytokines in allergen-challenged rhesus monkeys. Clin Exp Allergy 2005;35:894–906; Wiley-Blackwell, publishers.[85] ns = not significant.

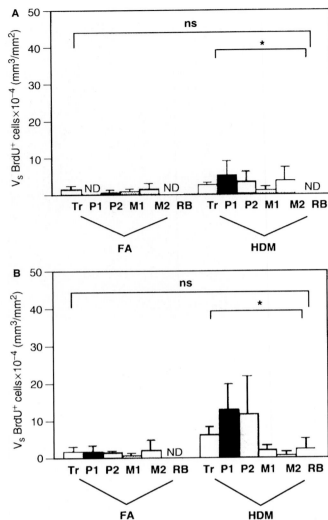

FIGURE 21. Distribution of proliferating cells within airway mucosa of house dust mite (HDM)-challenged rhesus monkeys. Proliferating cells were quantitated by immunostaining for 5-bromo-20-deoxyuridine (BrdU) incorporation in the trachea and left caudal lobe sections obtained from HDM-challenged monkeys. Tr, P1, P2, M1, M2, and RB represent cryosections obtained from tissue blocks of the trachea and regions progressively representing the most proximal (P1) to distal (RB) intrapulmonary airways of the lobe. Columns represent the average volume ± standard error of BrdU+ cells (mm^3) within the specified compartment with respect to the surface area of basal lamina (mm^2). FA = filtered air control; HDM = house dust mite challenged; RB = respiratory bronchiole. *A*, Abundance of BrdU1 cells within the epithelial compartment of conducting airways. $*p = .0708$ by analysis of variance (treatment effect). *B*, Abundance of BrdU+ cells within the interstitial compartment of conducting airways. $*p = .0410$ by analysis of variance (treatment effect). Reproduced with permission from Miller LA, Hurst SD, Coffman RL, et al. Airway generation-specific differences in the spatial distribution of immune cells and cytokines in allergen-challenged rhesus monkeys. Clin Exp Allergy 2005;35:894–906; Wiley-Blackwell, publishers.[85] ns = not significant.

lamina lucida, the lamina densa, and the lamina reticularis. The BMZ is a region specialized for the attachment of the epithelium with the matrix.[114,115] Epithelial cells are attached

to the lamina densa, which, in turn, is attached to the underlying collagen of the lamina reticularis. The lamina reticularis is especially pronounced under the respiratory epithelium of

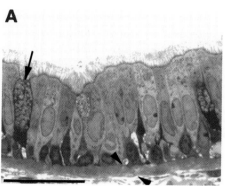 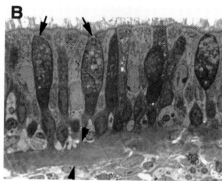

FIGURE 22. Histopathologic comparison of the epithelial composition in the intrapulmonary bronchi of a nonsensitized (A) and sensitized (B) rhesus monkey. High-resolution histopathologic comparison of a control monkey (A) and an area of heavy inflammatory cell infiltration with epithelial hypertrophy and mucous goblet cell (*arrows*) hyperplasia of sensitized monkey (B) (scale bar = 20 μm). Toluidine blue staining. The basement membrane (arrowheads) is thickened in the sensitized monkey. Reprinted from Am J Pathol 2001;158:333–41, with permission from the American Society for Investigative Pathology.[95]

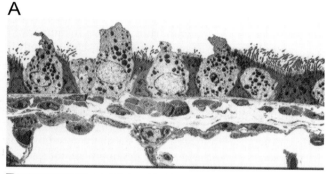 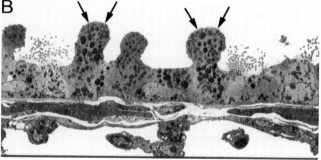 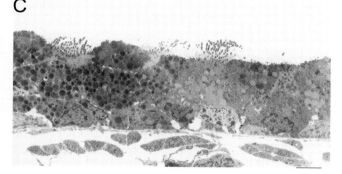

FIGURE 23. Electron micrographs from nonsensitized (A) and sensitized (B) mice 12 hours after the first ovalbumin (OVA) challenge and sensitized mice on protocol day 22 (C) (after the third OVA challenge). Mucus droplets can be seen within the apical projections of Clara cells at 12 hours (*arrows*), and by day 22, the epithelium was packed with mucus droplets. Scale bar = 5 μm. Reprinted from Am J Pathol 2003;162:2069–78, with permission from the American Society for Investigative Pathology.[101]

large conducting airways, where it may be several microns thick and composed of heterogeneous fibers (collagens type I, III, and V). Attenuated fibroblasts beneath the BMZ are thought to synthesize the collagen components of the BMZ.[7,8,113]

Remodeling of the epithelial BMZ, such as occurs in asthma, involves increased deposition of collagen in the BMZ.[116–118] Thickening of the BMZ is thought to protect against airway narrowing and air trapping.[119]

The BMZ has a number of functions in the EMTU. Besides being specialized for attachment of epithelium with the extracellular matrix, it also (a) serves as a barrier; (b) binds specific growth factors, hormones, and ions; (c) is involved with electrical charge; and (d) plays a critical role in cell-cell communication.[120,121] Heparan sulfate proteoglycans (perlecan) and chondroitin sulfate proteglycans (bamacan) are an intrinsic part of the BMZ that are involved with most of its functions.[122] Binding and storage of growth factors by perlecan (mainly FGF-2) are also important functions of the BMZ. FGF-2 is the main growth factor stored in the BMZ through binding with perlecan, an intrinsic constituent of the BMZ. FGF-2 is a ubiquitous multifunctional growth factor that has a variety of functions as a regulator of growth and differentiation. It is thought to be stored in the BMZ for rapid cellular responses to changes in local environmental conditions. FGF-2 forms a ternary signaling complex with the cell surface receptors FGFR-1 and syndecan-4. In the airway, these receptors are found only on basal cells.[123]

In the rhesus monkey, (1) FGF-2 is associated with synthesis of the BMZ in development and injury; (2) perlecan regulates FGF-2 and is necessary for normal development of the BMZ; and (3) the molecular signal associated with a thick BMZ persists during recovery[124]; however, the role of FGF-2 released from the BMZ and its interactions with basal cells of the airway epithelium has not been determined.

Fibroblasts

Attenuated fibroblasts are a distinct morphologic category of cells lying directly under the epithelium of the conducting airways of humans and rhesus monkeys.[113,116] They exist as a layer of large flat cells covering about 70% of the BMZ

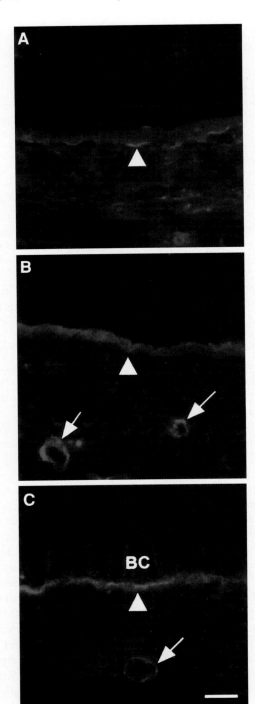

FIGURE 24. *A to C*, From a filtered-air control group. The magnification is the same in (A) to (C). Bar = 10 μ (B) Collagen I immunoreactivity in the basement membrane zone (BMZ) (*arrowhead*). Both the epithelial and mesenchymal surfaces are irregular. The mean width of the BMZ was 4.4 ± 0.5 μm (B) Perlecan immunoreactivity in the BMZ (*arrowhead*) and walls of blood vessels (*arrows*). The intensity was greater in the walls of blood vessels compared with the BMZ. The mean width of the BMZ was 4.3 ± 0.4 μm. *C*, Fibroblast growth factor 2 immunoreactivity was present in the BMZ (*arrowhead*), within and on the surface of basal cells (BC), and around the walls of blood vessels (*arrow*). The mean width of the BMZ was 4.6 ± 0.6 μm. Reprinted by permission from Macmillan Publishers Ltd: Lab Invest 82:1747–54; © 2002.[117]

(Figure 26).[113] In the bronchi of normal humans, these cells also exist as a discontinuous layer composed of attenuated fibroblasts and myofibroblasts. In asthmatics, the number of myofibroblasts in this fibroblast layer is more than double that of normal individuals and the cell layer is more than twice as far from the epithelial basal lamina owing to subepithelial fibrosis.[116] The functional role of this layer of cells is not known. Attenuated fibroblasts play a pivotal role in the pathogenesis of asthma based on morphologic evidence of subepithelial fibrosis in asthmatic human airways and the well-known role of collagen produced by these cells in tissue compliance and mechanics. The same appears to be the case for the rhesus monkey.

Smooth Muscle

The mechanism of increased smooth muscle associated with asthma in humans is unknown. Smooth muscle hypertrophy and hyperplasia are characteristics of the distribution of airway smooth muscle in remodeling airways in humans.[125] Type 1 asthmatics have increased smooth muscle mass only in large bronchi, largely owing to hyperplasia. Type II asthmatics have smooth muscle thickening from large bronchi to small bronchioles owing to both hypertrophy and hyperplasia. It is not known whether these differences are due to coexposure to air pollution, a phenotypic difference in myocytes by airway level, or differences in the impact of the allergen response on different stages of postnatal airway development. Increases in airway smooth muscle may increase airway contractility, as is found in AHR[126,127] and in airways taken from asthmatic patients.[128] The same is true for infant rhesus monkeys with allergic airways disease that also exhibit altered orientation and increases in muscle bundle mass (Figure 27).[129] Increased airway smooth muscle is a hallmark of asthma, but whether environmental factors such as HDM allergen or O_3 exposure can cause this increase, by altering development in neonates or repair in adults, can best be defined in a species with an extensive period of postnatal airway development such as the rhesus monkey.

Bronchial Vasculature

Bronchial and pulmonary vasculatures are important pathways through which growth factors and nutrients that are needed for lung growth and maturation and inflammatory cells are delivered to the lung. The bronchial vasculature of the EMTU contributes to the development of the human asthma phenotype via microvascular leakage and delivery of inflammatory mediators and leukocytes in the airways, and is a prerequisite for airway remodeling in bronchial asthma. Studies in patients with asthma have described an increase in bronchovascular density; in conjunction with this finding, patients with asthma have been shown to have elevated vascular endothelial growth factor (VEGF) in their sputum and VEGF-producing cells in the mucosa assessed by endobronchial biopsy.[130] Transgenic mice that overproduce VEGF have a twofold increase in tracheal vascular density and an enhanced Th2 immune response to allergen.[131] Although

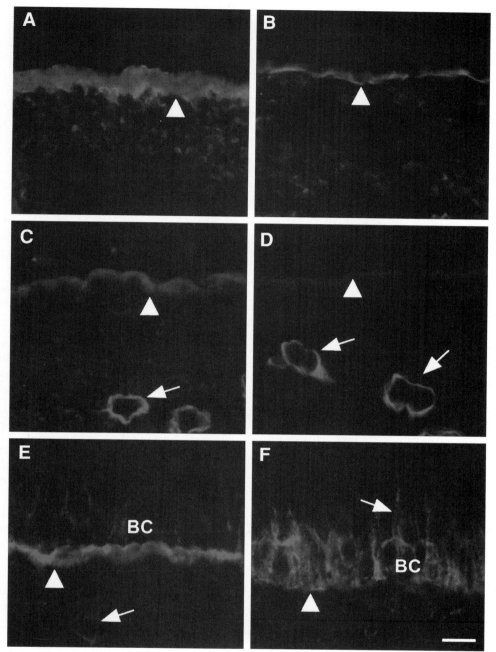

FIGURE 25. *A* to *F*, From tracheal rings of a house dust mite allergen (HDMA)-treated monkey. *B, D,* and *F,* From focal thin areas of the basement membrane zone (BMZ) associated with leukocyte trafficking. *A, C,* and *E,* From areas without leukocytes. Bar = 10 μm. *A,* Collagen I immunoreactivity in the BMZ (*arrowhead*). Both the epithelial and mesenchymal surfaces are irregular. The mean width of the BMZ, 6.3 ± 0.8 μm, was significantly greater ($p < .05$) than that of the filtered-air group. *B,* Collagen I immunoreactivity was much less in the thin regions of the BMZ associated with leukocyte trafficking (*arrowhead*). *C,* Perlecan immunoreactivity in the BMZ (*arrowhead*) and walls of blood vessels (*arrow*). The intensity was greater in the walls of blood vessels compared with the BMZ. The mean width of the BMZ, 5.5 ± 1.0 μm, was significantly greater ($p < .05$) than that of the filtered-air control group. *D,* Perlecan immunoreactivity was much less in the BMZ associated with leukocyte trafficking (*arrowhead*); however, the intensity was normal in the walls of blood vessels (*arrows*). *E,* From the same region of the tracheal ring as *B*. There was more fibroblast growth factor 2 (FGF-2) immunoreactivity in the BMZ from the HDMA group than the filtered-air group owing to its greater width (*arrowhead*). The immunoreactivity associated with basal cells (*BC*) was also greater in the HDMA group. The intensity was less in the walls of blood vessels compared with the BMZ (*arrow*). The width of the HDMA group, 6.2 ± 0.8 μm, was significantly greater ($p < .05$) than that of the filtered-air group. *F,* From the same region as Figure (C) illustrating the focal nature of the changes we observed in FGF-2 distribution around the tracheal ring. FGF-2 immunoreactivity is weak or absent in regions of the BMZ associated with leukocyte trafficking (*arrowhead*). However, strong FGF-2 immunoreactivity was associated with basal cells (*BC*) and the lateral intercellular space between columnar cells (*arrow*). Reprinted by permission from Macmillan Publishers Ltd: Lab Invest 82:1747–54; © 2002.[117]

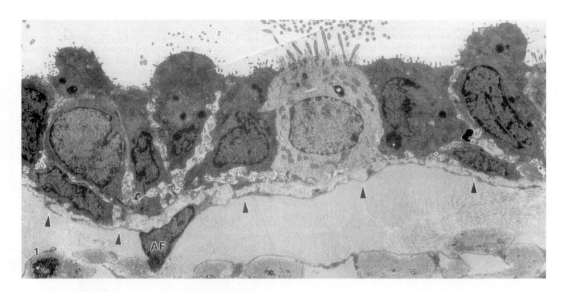

FIGURE 26. Transverse section of rat trachea. The surface epithelium is composed of ciliated, secretory, and basal cells. Beneath the basal lamina are the nucleus of an attenuated fibroblast (AF) and a portion of the attenuated cell (*arrowheads*). The area between the AF and the basal lamina represents the basement membrane zone (× 5,600 original magnification). Reproduced with permission from Evans MJ et al.[113]

the role of VEGF as an important mediator for the angiogenic events in allergic asthma is established, the cellular and molecular mechanisms that regulate VEGF and its receptors' expression are not well defined. Airway physiology and vascular density have been linked in multiple different studies. It is thought that increased vascularity leads to bronchial constriction and airway narrowing.[132,133] Even patients with impaired left ventricular function have been shown to have increased AHR[134] Rhesus monkeys with HDM-induced allergic airways also show an increase in bronchovascular density that was airway generation specific (Figure 28).[9]

Airway Nerves

Substantial reductions in sensory nerve innervation of midlevel intrapulmonary airways of infant rhesus monkeys episodically exposed for 6 months to HDM allergen and/or ozone were observed,[60] followed by a compensatory hyperinnervation after a 6-month recovery period. One explanation is that the initial reduction and consequent hyperinnervation are the result of the disruption of normal growth factors and cues during the postnatal development of airway epithelial innervation and the consequent overexpression of growth factors within the airway EMTU. Paralleling these observations of altered midlevel airway epithelial nerve density and distribution are the observations of Evans and colleagues of disruption of the conducting airway basement membrane and the associated grow factor FGF-2 after exposure for 6 months to HDM allergen and/or O_3.[117] Also paralleling changes in mid-level airway epithelial innervation are the observations of Evans and colleagues that the disruption of basement membrane and FGF-2 continue to be overexpressed during a 6-month recovery period.[124] Given that FGF-2 has been shown to be a potent nerve growth factor in the lung[135] and other organ systems,[136,137] we propose that FGF-2 released from the basement membrane directly affects nerve density and morphology within the airways.

These studies demonstrate that allergic asthma can be produced experimentally in a nonhuman primate, the rhesus macaque monkey, using a recognized human allergen, HDM, and provide a valuable model for human asthma.

Chronic Obstructive Pulmonary Disease

COPD is characterized by airflow limitation that is usually progressive and is associated with an abnormal inflammatory response of the lungs to noxious particles or gases, primarily caused by cigarette smoking. The site of airflow obstruction in COPD is predominantly the membranous bronchiole, devoid of cartilage and submucosal glands. Chronic respiratory bronchiolitis in young human smokers,[138] diesel-exposed cats[139] and ozone-exposed monkeys (Figure 29)[140,141] has similar increases in alveolar macrophages, interstitial inflammatory cells, and fibrosis. The respiratory bronchiolitis seen in lungs exposed to ozone is similar but less severe than that reported in lungs of smokers. The relative length of the smoking history compared with the exposure periods and the concentrations of pollutants may be factors in the relative severity. It is noteworthy that extended recovery periods in filtered air up to a year showed substantial resolution of cellular inflammation but a persistence of the respiratory bronchiole narrowing, epithelial metaplasia, and a progression of peribronchiolar fibrosis. These observations imply a common response of the proximal acinar region to inhaled irritants that results in chronic inflammation in species with extensive respiratory bronchioles, such as humans and rhesus monkeys.

Response to Oxidant Stress

The rhesus monkey via exposure to the air pollutant ozone has been used as a model of short-term oxidant-induced inflammation and lung injury.[81,142] The role that neutrophils

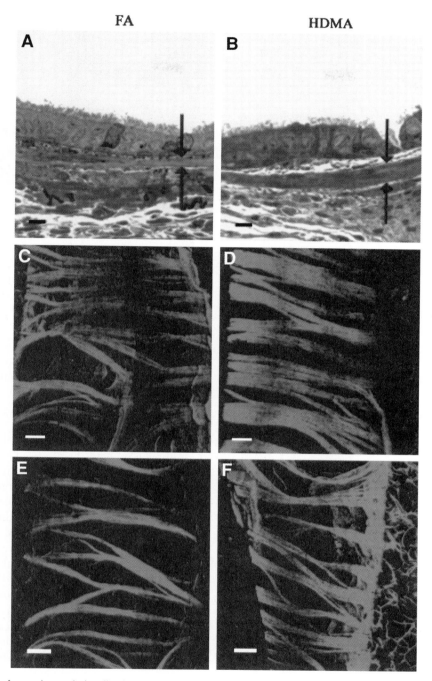

FIGURE 27. Comparison of smooth muscle bundles in 6-month-old rhesus monkeys exposed to filtered air (FA) (A, C, E) or house dust mite allergen (HDMA) (B, D, F). Smooth muscle bundle width (*between arrows*) was greater in midlevel cartilaginous airway generation in seven or eight of HDMA animals (B) compared with FA (A) animals. Bar = 10 mm. Smooth muscle bundles stained with Alexa Fluor 568 phalloidin in laser confocal images in PG1 (a nonalveolarized bronchiole) (C, D) and RB1 (a alveolarized bronchiole) (E, F). Bar = 100 μm. Reproduced with permission from Tran MU, Weir AJ, Fanucchi MV, et al. Smooth muscle hypertrophy in distal airways of sensitized infant rhesus monkeys exposed to house dust mite allergen. Clin Exp Allergy 2004;34:1627–33; Wiley-Blackwell, publishers.[129]

play in the acute ozone-induced injury,[80] repair of epithelial injury,[143] and the mechanism by which neutrophils migrate[144-146] and adhere to injured areas[147] have been defined. The induction of protective mechanisms by ozone exposure has been defined for heat shock proteins[148] and glutathione pools.[81,149]

In long-term ozone inhalation in rats and monkeys, the central acinus shows a dose-dependent response of increased numbers of cuboidal ozone-resistant epithelial cells, accumulation of alveolar macrophages, and interstitial thickening characterized by accumulation of smooth muscle cells, fibroblasts, interstitial macrophages, and mast cells (Figure

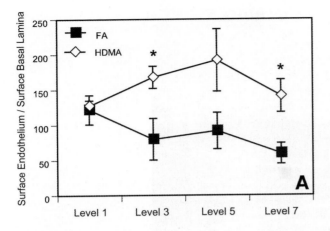

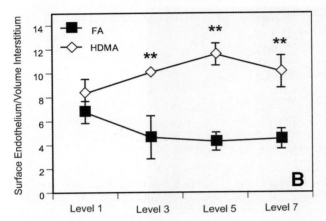

FIGURE 28. Morphometry. *A,* Surface of endothelium to surface of the epithelial basement membrane. Random intersections of bronchial vessel as a ratio to intersections of epithelial basement membrane at each airway generation. *Error bars* designate variability within each group at that airway generation. Significant values represented by *single asterisks* and include $p = .039$ (airway generation 3) and $p = .025$ (airway generation 7). *B,* Surface of endothelium to the volume of interstitium determined by quantitating intersection of endothelium expressed in a ratio with random point density of interstitium at each airway generation. Values are means ± standard error and represent variation of the group at each airway generation. Significant values are represented by *double asterisks* and include surface of endothelium to volume of interstitium, $p = .024$ (airway generation 3), $p = .009$ (airway generation 5), and $p = .012$ (airway generation 7). Reproduced with permission from Avdalovic MV et al.[9]

30).[140,150,151] Exposures of rhesus monkeys (8 hours/day) for 6 or 90 days to 0.15 or 0.30 ppm ozone resulted in ciliated cell necrosis, shortened cilia, and secretory cell hyperplasia with less stored glycoconjugates in the nasal region. Respiratory bronchiolitis was also observed in these monkeys at 6 days that persisted to 90 days of exposure.[152] Even at the lower concentration of 0.15 ppm ozone, nonciliated bronchiolar cells appeared hypertrophied and increased in abundance in respiratory bronchioles.[152] The principal lesion in monkeys in response to 0.25 ppm ozone (8 hours/day) daily or episodes (nine cycles of 1 month of ozone followed by 1 month of filtered air) for 18 months was respiratory bron-

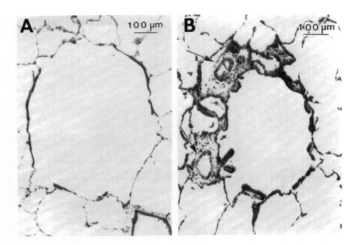

FIGURE 29. Light micrographs of respiratory bronchiole cross sections from control (A) and ozone-exposed monkeys at the same magnification. Note the thickened arteriole walls, enlarged connective tissue space surrounding vessels (*arrows*), and narrowed lumen in exposed respiratory bronchioles. Hematoxylin and eosin staining. From Fujinaka LE et al.[140]

chiolitis.[141] Our conclusions from these long-term monkey studies are as follows: (1) there is persistent epithelial injury in the anterior nasal cavity and respiratory bronchiole produced by exposure levels as low as 0.15 ppm ozone, (2) there is a worsening of the respiratory bronchiole lesion in monkeys during the postexposure period, and (3) episodic exposures cause more severe injury than daily exposures.

Although we have characterized the inflammatory process in the nonhuman primate lung with short-term exposure,[80] we cannot provide a simplistic outline of an inflammatory process in the lung with long-term daily exposure because of the lack of experimental data. Further, it is perplexing that when the epithelium of the central acinus is adaptive and resistant to long-term ozone exposure, the interstitium is reactive and marked by progressive inflammation and fibrosis. There is a need to gain an understanding of the inflammatory basis of the resolution process on lung injury after multiple episodes of ozone exposure before we can begin to understand what makes the long-term lesion not resolve.

In a comparative study of (1) long-term daily exposures (rats exposed to 0.95 ppm ozone, 8 hours daily for a total of 90 days) and (2) long-term episodic exposures (rats exposed to 0.95 ppm ozone, 8 hours daily in seven successive 5-day episodes separated by 9-day postexposure periods in filtered air), we observed a cumulative effect of repeated exposures on the interstitium while respiratory bronchiolar and alveolar duct epithelium was in a more dynamic state of injury and repair.[153,154] We selected the 9-day postexposure interval because the inflammatory process resolves by 6 to 9 days after the end of a 7-day ozone exposure in the rat.[155] We also noted that the injury in the central acinus shifted to more distal locations as evidenced by an increase in the volume of damaged centriacinar alveoli and in the volume of the alveolar duct/sac compartment in the lung in episodically compared

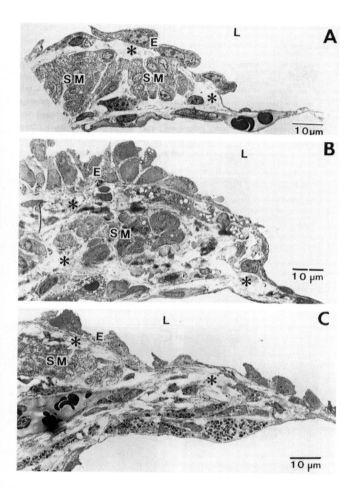

FIGURE 30. Montages of transmission electron micrographs of respiratory bronchioles from monkeys exposed for 1 year to filtered air (A) to 0.64 ppm ozone (B) or to 0.64 ppm ozone plus 3 months in filtered air (C). E = epithelium; L = respiratory bronchiole lumen; SM = smooth muscle. *Extracellular fibers. Bar = 10 μm. From Hyde DM et al.[151], with permission. This article was published in the chapter: Ozone-induced structural changes in monkey respiratory system. In: Schneider T, Lee SD, Wolters PJ, Grant MB, editors. Atmospheric ozone research and its policy implications. New York: Elsevier; 1989. p. 523–32. © Elsevier 1989.

with daily exposed rats. We also observed a significant decrease in the final body weight of the episodic group of rats compared with that of controls, implying depressed growth and appetite. This difference was not observed in the daily exposed rats. It seems likely that repeated episodes of ozone exposure produce repeated episodes of airway necrosis and inflammation. The injury induced by each episode following acclimation in air may exceed that produced by continuous exposure. There was increased interstitial collagen formation, suggesting fibrosis and smooth muscle hypertrophy in the central acinus following episodic exposure, which has not been observed following acute ozone exposure.

To understand how episodic ozone exposure can be a bridge between the acute and chronic ozone-induced lesion, we exposed rats to four 2-week cycles of 5 days of ozone (8 hours/day) followed by 9 days in filtered air, evaluating

epithelial injury and repair at numerous times during the experiment.[156] After four episodes, we observed a depressed epithelial cell proliferative response to ozone-induced injury that may in part be the result of a decreased neutrophil inflammation and/or release of mitogenic neuropeptides in response to ozone-induced injury (Figure 31).[156]

These findings are in good agreement with a study that compared monthly or seasonal exposure regimens to daily exposures in monkeys.[141] It is noteworthy that the seasonal or episodic ozone exposure caused significant lesions at 0.25 ppm ozone, a dose that causes little injury in rats. A comparative review of the greater sensitivity of the primate (macaque monkey) lung than the rodent (Sprague-Dawley rat) lung to ozone exposure showed that collagen metabolism following identical high levels of ozone exposure (1.5 ppm, 23 hours/day, 7 days) was increased an average of 200% above control rats, but in monkeys, there was an 800% increase.[157] Exposure of rats to 0.25 ppm ozone (8 hours/day, 42 days) produced less than a 10% increase in epithelial thickness or number of cells/mm² of epithelial basal lamina. By comparison, exposure of monkeys to 0.15 ppm ozone (8 hours/day for 6 or 90 days) produced a 150% increase in thickness and a 700% increase in the number of cells of the epithelium.[152] These data suggest that at environmentally relevant concentrations, ozone is much more toxic to the primate lung than to the rodent lung.

Since environmental pollution is in part responsible for the dramatic increase in COPD, what are the potential mechanisms of the oxidant contribution? Emphysema, one of the major causes of COPD, is defined as "a condition of the lung characterized by abnormal, permanent enlargement of airspaces distal to the terminal bronchiole, accompanied by destruction of their walls with or without obvious fibrosis."[158] Inflammation and excessive proteolysis via an elastase/antielastase imbalance has been proposed for over 35 years to be the downstream consequence of chronic cigarette smoking resulting in interalveolar septal destruction, but animal models have yielded variable results.[159] The downstream consequences of direct injury to interalveolar septal cells by cigarette smoke have not been fully explained by elastase/antielastase imbalance (inflammatory cell hypothesis).[160] The presence of apoptosis and decreased VEGF protein levels in human emphysematous lungs[161,162] and the induction of emphysema in rats by blocking VEGF receptors that is associated with increased apoptosis have provided additional data for a more attractive hypothesis.[163] Direct induction of interalveolar septal cell apoptosis in mice by instillation of active caspase-3 also resulted in emphysema.[164]

Together the studies of Kasahara and colleagues and Aoshiba and colleagues support the interdependence of interalveolar septal structure on both epithelial and endothelial integrity and that disruption of either leads to the same result of an imbalance in homeostasis with the consequence of emphysema.[163,164] There is also considerable evidence of markers of oxidative stress in smokers' lungs, presumably a direct effect of cigarette smoke or by

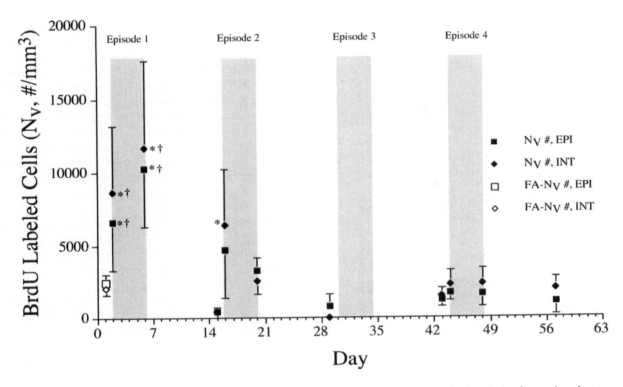

FIGURE 31. Number per volume of cell (N_V #/mm³) labeled with 5-bromo-20-deoxyuridine at selected points during four cycles of ozone exposure consisting of 5 days (8 h/d) of ozone (1 ppm) inhalation followed by 9 days of filtered air. EPI = epithelium; INT = interstitium. *Significant difference from filtered air (FA) control ($p \leq .05$). †Significant difference from day 14 of the same cycle ($p \leq .05$). Reprinted from Toxicol Appl Pharmacol: Schelegle ES, Walby WF, Alfaro MF et al. Repeated episodes of ozone inhalation attenuates airway injury/repair and release of substance P, but not adaptation. pp. 127–42, © 2003, with permission from Elsevier.[156]

chronic inflammation.[165,166] Since oxidative stress alters cellular signaling, particularly those involved in apoptosis and elastase/antielastase imbalance, it is also an important component of the pathogenesis of COPD.

Oxidative stress and apoptosis, which cause lung cellular destruction in emphysema, were induced by VEGF receptor blockade with destructive emphysema in focal areas of rat lungs.[167] In this model of emphysema, both a caspase inhibitor and a superoxide dismutase mimetic blocked the development of emphysema and reduced markers of oxidative stress and apoptosis, thereby implying an additive effect between apoptosis and oxidative stress.[167] In support of this concept, administration of the antioxidant N-acetyl-L-cysteine in rats protects interalveolar septal cells against apoptosis and against emphysema.[168] Overexpression of the human serine protease inhibitor α_1-antitrypsin in lung cells suppressed caspase-3 activation and oxidative stress in mouse lungs treated with a VEGF receptor blocker (SU5416) or with VEGF receptor 1 and 2 antibodies.[169] Similar results were obtained in SU5416-treated rats given human α_1-antitrypsin intravenously, and the development of emphysema was prevented.[169] The relationships among interalveolar septal cell destruction and apoptosis, oxidant injury, elastase/antielastase imbalance, and inflammation are emerging as important and unifying processes in COPD. In this context, the chronic ozone-induce injury model of the rhe-

sus monkey may serve as an important animal model in future investigations on the pathogenic mechanisms of COPD.

We have identified some critical issues regarding the utility of the nonhuman primate model and its appropriateness for defining mechanisms as they relate to disease processes in human airways. Using examples of nonhuman primate models of human asthma and COPD, we addressed the biology of the airway within the conceptual framework of the EMTU. This concept is that all of the cellular and acellular compartments within the airway wall have a close interaction through a series of extracellular signaling cascades that establish a dynamic homeostatic state. The homeostatic state of the EMTU responds to injury of one component by altering the signaling patterns and basic functions of the remaining components. We have highlighted differences between species in the organization of the airway wall in adults, compared differences in postnatal development of the airways by species, and compared airway-specific remodeling and airway-specific inflammation associated with asthma and COPD. Our current understanding of the utility of these animal models and their appropriateness for defining mechanisms as they relate to allergic airways disease and COPD in humans and compared with other laboratory animals has been highlighted in this chapter. We conclude that nonhuman primates remain one of the most appropriate models for chronic airway disease in humans.

References

1. American Thoracic Society. Adult asthma and asthma and children fact sheet. American Thoracic Society; 2005. <_http://www.lungusa.org/site/pp.asp?c=dvLUK9O0E&b=44352>_. Accessed October 24, 2005.

2. World Health Organization. Bronchial asthma. Fact sheet number 307. <http://www.who.int /mediacentre/ factsheets/ fs307/ en/index.html>. Accessed 2/1/08.

3. Centers for Disease Control and Prevention, National Center for Health Statistics. Asthma Prevalence, Health Care Use and Mortality, 2002. <www.cdc.gov/nchs/ products/pubs/ pubd/hestats/asthma/asthma.htm>. Date last updated: January 11, 2007. Accessed: February 2, 2008.

4. National Heart, Lung, and Blood Institute. Diseases and conditions index; COPD. <http:// www.nhlbi.nih.gov/health/ dci/Diseases/Copd/Copd_WhatIs.html>., Accessed 2/1/08.

5. Mercer RR, Crapo JD. Architecture of the acinus. In: Parent RP, editor. Comparative biology of the normal lung. Boca Raton (FL): CRC Press; 1991. p. 109–19.

6. Weibel ER, Taylor CR, Gehr P, et al. Design of the mammalian respiratory system. IX. Functional and structural limits for oxygen flow. Respir Physiol 1981;44:151–64.

7. Evans MJ, Van Winkle LS, Fanucchi MV, Plopper CG. The attenuated fibroblast sheath of the respiratory tract epithelial-mesenchymal trophic unit. Am J Respir Cell Mol Biol 1999;21:655–7.

8. Holgate ST, Davies DE, Lackie PM, et al. Epithelial-mesenchymal interactions in the pathogenesis of asthma. J Allergy Clin.Immunol 2000;105:193–204.

9. Avdalovic MV, Putney LF, Schelegle ES, et al. Vascular remodeling is airway generation-specific in a primate model of chronic asthma. Am J Respir Crit Care Med 2006;174:1069-76.

10. Paige R, Plopper C. Acute and chronic effects of ozone in animal models. In: Holgate ST, editor. Air pollution and health. New York: Academic Press; 1999. p. 531–57.

11. Spicer SS. Diamine methods for differentialing mucosubstances histochemically. J Histochem Cytochem 1965;13:211–34.

12. Heidsiek JG, Hyde DM, Plopper CG, St George JA. Quantitative histochemistry of mucosubstance in tracheal epithelium of the macaque monkey. J Histochem Cytochem 1987;35:435–42.

13. Plopper CG, Heidsiek JG, Weir AJ, et al. Tracheobronchial epithelium in the adult rhesus monkey: a quantitative histochemical and ultrastructural study. Am J Anat 1989;184:31–40.

14. Daniel FB, Schut HAJ, Sandwisch DW, et al. Interspecies comparisons of benzo(a)pyrene metabolism and DNA-adduct formation in cultured human and animal bladder and tracheobronchial tissues. Cancer Res 1983;43:4723–9.

15. Lee C, Watt KC, Chang AM, et al. Site-selective differences in cytochrome P450 isoform activities. Comparison of expression in rat and rhesus monkey lung and induction in rats. Drug Metab Dispos 1998;26:396–400.

16. Yueh MF, Krueger SK, Williams DE. Pulmonary flavin-containing monooxygenase (FMO) in rhesus macaque: expression of FMO2 protein, mRNA and analysis of the cDNA. Biochim Biophys Acta 1997;1350:267–71.

17. Krueger SK, Martin SR, Yueh MF, et al. Identification of active flavin-containing monooxygenase isoform 2 in human lung and characterization of expressed protein. Drug Metab Dispos 2002;30:34–41.

18. Choi HK, Finkbeiner WE, Widdicombe JH. A comparative study of mammalian tracheal mucous glands. J Anat 2000;197(Pt 3):361–72.

19. St George JA, Cranz DL, Zicker S, et al. An immunohistochemical characterization of rhesus monkey respiratory secretions using monoclonal antibodies. Am Rev Respir Dis 1985;132:556–63.

20. St George JA, Nishio SJ, Plopper CG. Carbohydrate cytochemistry of the rhesus monkey tracheal epithelium. Anat Rec 1984;210:293–302.

21. St George JA, Nishio SJ, Cranz DL, Plopper CG. Carbohydrate cytochemistry of rhesus monkey submucosal glands. Anat Rec 1986;216:60–7.

22. Dupuit F, Bout A, Hinnrasky J, et al. Expression and localization of CFTR in the rhesus monkey surface airway epithelium. Gene Ther 1995;2:156–63.

23. Huang TH, St George JA, Plopper CG, Wu R. Keratin protein expression during the development of conducting airway epithelium in nonhuman primates. Differentiation 1989;41:78–86.

24. Plopper CG, Alley JL, Weir AJ. Differentiation of tracheal epithelium during fetal lung maturation in the rhesus monkey *Macaca mulatta*. Am J Anat 1986;175:59–71.

25. Tyler NK, Hyde DM, Hendrickx AG, Plopper CG. Morphogenesis of the respiratory bronchiole in rhesus monkey lungs. Am J Anat 1988;182:215–23.

26. Tyler NK, Hyde DM, Hendrickx AG, Plopper CG. Cytodifferentiation of two epithelial populations of the respiratory bronchiole during fetal lung development in the rhesus monkey. Anat Rec 1989;225:297–309.

27. Van Winkle LS, Fanucchi MV, Miller LA, et al. Epithelial cell distribution and abundance in rhesus monkey airways during postnatal lung growth and development. J Appl Physiol 2004;97:2355–63.

28. Plopper CG, Weir AJ, Nishio SJ, et al. Tracheal submucosal gland development in the rhesus monkey, *Macaca mulatta*: ultrastructure and histochemistry. Anat Embryol 1986;174:167–78.

29. St George JA, Wang S. Secretory glycoconjugates of trachea and bronchi. In: Parent RA, editor. Treatise on pumonary toxicology. Comparative biology of the normal lung. Boca Raton (FL): CRC Press; 1991. p. 77–83.

30. An G, Luo G, Wu R. Expression of MUC2 gene is down-regulated by vitamin A at the transcriptional level in vitro in tracheobronchial epithelial cells. Am J Respir Cell Mol Biol 1994;10:546–51.

31. Huang TH, Ann DK, Zhang YJ, et al. Control of keratin gene expression by vitamin A in tracheobronchial epithelial cells. Am J Respir Cell Mol Biol 1994;10:192–201.

32. An G, Huang TH, Tesfaigzi J, et al. An unusual expression of a squamous cell marker, small proline-rich protein gene, in tracheobronchial epithelium: differential regulation and gene mapping. Am J Respir Cell Mol Biol 1992;7:104–11.

33. An G, Tesfaigzi J, Carlson DM, Wu R. Expression of a squamous cell marker, the spr1 gene, is posttranscriptionally down-regulated by retinol in airway epithelium. J Cell Physiol 1993;157:562–8.

34. An G, Tesfaigzi J, Chuu YJ, Wu R. Isolation and characterization of the human spr1 gene and its regulation of expression by phorbol ester and cyclic AMP. J Biol Chem 1993;268:10977–82.

35. An G, Wu R. Thioredoxin gene expression is transcriptionally up-regulated by retinol in monkey conducting airway epithelial cells. Biochem Biophys Res Commun 1992;183:170–5.

36. Chang MM, Harper R, Hyde DM, Wu R. A novel mechanism of retinoic acid-enhanced interleukin-8 gene expression in airway epithelium. Am J Respir Cell Mol Biol 2000;22:502–10.

37. Miller LA, Cheng LZ, Wu R. Inhibition of epidermal growth factor-like growth factor secretion in tracheobronchial epithelial cells by vitamin A. Cancer Res 1993;53:2527–33.

38. An G, Wu R. cDNA cloning of a hnRNP A1 isoform and its regulation by retinol in monkey tracheobronchial epithelial cells. Biochim Biophys Acta 1993;1172:292–300.

39. Martin WR, Brown C, Zhang YJ, Wu R. Growth and differentiation of primary tracheal epithelial cells in culture: regulation by extracellular calcium. J Cell Physiol 1991;147:138–48.

40. Beech DJ, Sibbons PD, Howard CV, van Velzen D. Terminal bronchiolar duct ending number does not increase postnatally in normal infants. Early Hum Dev 2000;59:193–200.

41. McBride JT. Architecture of the tracheobronchial tree. In: Parent RA, editor. Treatise on pulmonary toxicology: comparative biology of the normal lung. Boca Raton (FL): CRC Press; 1991. p. 49–61.

42. Tyler WS, Julian MD. Gross and subgross anatomy of lungs, pleura, connective tissue septa, distal airways, and structural units. In: Parent RA, editor. Treatise on pulmonary toxicology: comparative biology of the normal lung. Boca Raton (FL): CRC Press; 1991. p. 37–48.

43. Tran MU, Weir AJ, Fanucchi MV, et al. Smooth muscle development during postnatal growth of distal bronchioles in infant rhesus monkeys. J Appl Physiol 2004;97:2364–71.

44. Plopper CG, Hyde DM. Epithelial cells of bronchioles. In: Parent RA, editor. Treatise on pulmonary toxicology: comparative biology of the normal lung. Boca Raton (FL): CRC Press; 1991. p. 85–92.

45. Bucher U, Reid L. Development of the mucus-secreting elements in human lung. Thorax 1961;16:219–25.

46. Thurlbeck WM, Benjamin B, Reid L. Development and distribution of mucous glands in the foetal human trachea. Br J Dis Chest 1961;55:54–64.

47. Evans MJ, Fanucchi MV, Van Winkle LS, et al. Fibroblast growth factor-2 during postnatal development of the tracheal basement membrane zone. Am J Physiol Lung Cell Mol Physiol 2002;283:L1263–70.

48. Gaultier C, Girard F. [Normal and pathological lung growth: structure-function relationships]. Bull Eur Physiopathol Respir 1980;16:791–842.

49. Sward-Comunelli SL, Mabry SM, Truog WE, Thibeault DW. Airway muscle in preterm infants: changes during development. J Pediatr 1997;130:570–6.

50. Hislop AA, Haworth SG. Airway size and structure in the normal fetal and infant lung and the effect of premature delivery and artificial ventilation. Am Rev Respir Dis 1989;140:1717–26.

51. Grigg J, Riedler J. Developmental airway cell biology. The "normal" young child. Am J Respir Crit Care Med 2000;162:S52-5.

52. Heaney LG, Stevenson EC, Turner G, et al. Investigating paediatric airways by non-bronchoscopic lavage: normal cellular data. Clin Exp Allergy 1996;26:799–806.

53. Riedler J, Grigg J, Stone C, et al. Bronchoalveolar lavage cellularity in healthy children. Am J Respir Crit Care Med 1995;152:163–8.

54. Clement A, Chadelat K, Masliah J, et al. A controlled study of oxygen metabolite release by alveolar macrophages from children with interstitial lung disease. Am Rev Respir Dis 1987;136:1424–8.

55. Costabel U, Bross KJ, Ruhle KH, et al. Ia like antigens on T-cells and their subpopulations in pulmonary sarcoidosis and in hypersensitivity pneumonitis. Am Rev Respir Dis 1985;131:337–42.

56. Hunninghake GW, Crystal RG. Pulmonary sarcoidosis: a disorder mediated by excess helper T-lymphocyte activity at sites of disease activity. N Engl J Med 1981;305:429–34.

57. Ratjen F, Bredendiek M, Zheng L, et al. Lymphocyte subsets in bronchoalveolar lavage fluid of children without bronchopulmonary disease. Am J Respir Crit Care Med 1995;152:174–8.

58. McLaughlin RF, Tyler WS, Canada RO. A study of the subgross pulmonary anatomy in various mammals. Am J Anat 1961;108:149–65.

59. McLaughlin RF, Tyler WS, Canada RO. Subgross pulmonary anatomy of the rabbit, rat, and guinea pig, with additional notes on the human lung. Am Rev Respir Dis 1966; 94:380–7.

60. Larson SD, Schelegle ES, Walby WF, et al. Postnatal remodeling of the neural components of the epithelial-mesenchymal trophic unit in the proximal airways of infant rhesus monkeys exposed to ozone and allergen. Toxicol Appl Pharmacol 2004;194:211–20.

61. Honjin R. On the ganglia and nerves of the lower respiratory tract of the mouse. J Comp Neurol 1954;95:263–88.

62. Myers AC. Transmission in autonomic ganglia. Respir Physiol 2001;125:99–111.

63. Richardson JB. Nerve supply to the lungs. Am Rev Respir Dis 1979;119:785–802.

64. Barnes PJ, Belvisi MG. Nitric oxide and lung disease. Thorax 1993;48:1034–43.

65. Ward JK, Barnes PJ, Springall DR, et al. Distribution of human i-NANC bronchodilator and nitric oxide-immunoreactive nerves. Am J Respir Cell Mol Biol 1995;13:175–84.

66. van der Velden V, Hulsmann AR. Autonomic innervation of human airways: structure, function, and pathophysiology in asthma. Neuroimmunomodulation 1999;6:145–59.

67. Canning BJ, Undem BJ. Evidence that distinct neural pathways mediate parasympathetic contractions and relaxations of guinea-pig trachealis. J Physiol 1993;471:25–40.

68. Canning BJ, Fischer A. Localization of cholinergic nerves in lower airways of guinea pigs using antisera to choline acetyltransferase. Am J Physiol 1997;272:L731–8.

69. Dey RD, Altemus JB, Rodd A, et al. Neurochemical characterization of intrinsic neurons in ferret tracheal plexus. Am J Respir Cell Mol Biol 1996;14:207–16.

70. Zhu W, Dey RD. Projections and pathways of VIP- and nNOS-containing airway neurons in ferret trachea. Am J Respir Cell Mol Biol 2001;24:38–43.

71. Burri PH. Postnatal development and growth. In: Crystal RG, West JB, Barnes PJ, et al, editors. The lung scientific foundations. New York: Raven; 1991. p. 677–87.

72. Thurlbeck WM. Postnatal human lung growth. Thorax 1982;37:564–71.

73. Ochs M, Nyengaard JR, Jung A, et al. The number of alveoli in the human lung. Am J Respir Crit Care Med 2004;169:120–4.

74. Hyde DM, Blozis SA, Avdalovic MV, et al. Alveoli increase in number but not size from birth to adulthood in rhesus monkeys. Am J Physiol Lung Cell Mol Physiol 2007; 293:L570–79.

75. Van Winkle LS, Buckpitt AR, Plopper CG. Maintenance of differentiated murine Clara cells in microdissected airway cultures. Am J Respir Cell Mol Biol 1996;14:586–98.

76. Van Winkle LS, Isaac JM, Plopper CG. Repair of naphthalene-injured microdissected airways in vitro. Am J Respir Cell Mol Biol 1996;15:1–8.

77. Harkema JR, Mariassy AT, St George JA, et al. Epithelial cells of the conducting airways: a species comparison. In: Farmer SG, Hay DW, editors. The airway epithelium: physiology, pathophysiology and pharmacology. New York: Marcel Dekker; 1991. p. 3–39.

78. Plopper CG. Pulmonary bronchiolar epithelial cytotoxicity: microanatomical considerations. In: Gram TE, editor. Metabolic activation and toxicity of chemical agents to lung tissue and cells. Oxford (UK): Pergamon Press; 1993. p. 1–24.

79. Pinkerton KE, Avadhanam KP, Peake JL, Plopper CG. Tracheobronchial airways. In: Roth RA, editor. Toxicology of the respiratory system. New York: Pergamon Press; 1997. p. 23–44.

80. Hyde DM, Hubbard WC, Wong V, et al. Ozone-induced acute tracheobronchial epithelial injury: relationship to granulocyte emigration in the lung. Am J Respir Cell Mol Biol 1992;6:481–97.

81. Plopper CG, Hatch GE, Wong V, et al. Relationship of inhaled ozone concentration to acute tracheobronchial epithelial injury, site-specific ozone dose, and glutathione depletion in rhesus monkeys. Am J Respir Cell Mol Biol 1998;19:387–99.

82. Plopper CG, Macklin J, Nishio SJ, et al. Relationship of cytochrome P-450 activity to Clara cell cytotoxicity: III. Morphometric comparison of changes in the epithelial populations of terminal bronchioles and lobar bronchi in mice, hamsters, and rats after parenteral administration of naphthalene. Lab Invest 1992;67:553–65.

83. Plopper CG, Suverkropp C, Morin D, et al. Relationship of cytochrome P-450 activity to Clara cell cytotoxicity. I. Histopathologic comparison of the respiratory tract of mice, rats and hamsters after parenteral administration of naphthalene. J Pharmacol Exp Ther 1992;261:353–63.

84. Paige R, Wong V, Plopper C. Dose-related airway-selective epithelial toxicity of 1-nitronaphthalene in rats. Toxicol Appl Pharmacol 1997;147:224–33.

85. Miller LA, Hurst SD, Coffman RL, et al. Airway generation-specific differences in the spatial distribution of immune cells and cytokines in allergen-challenged rhesus monkeys. Clin Exp Allergy 2005;35:894–906.

86. Lloyd CM, Gonzalo JA, Coyle AJ, Gutierrez-Ramos JC. Mouse models of allergic airway disease. Adv Immunol 2001;77:263–95.

87. Bates J, Irvin C, Brusasco V, et al. The use and misuse of Penh in animal models of lung disease. Am J Respir Cell Mol Biol 2004;31:373–4.

88. Wagers S, Lundblad LK, Ekman M, et al. The allergic mouse model of asthma: normal smooth muscle in an abnormal lung? J Appl Physiol 2004;96:2019–27.

89. Boyce JA, Austen KF. No audible wheezing: nuggets and conundrums from mouse asthma models. J Exp Med 2005;201:1869–73.

90. Corry DB, Grunig G, Hadeiba H, et al. Requirements for allergen-induced airway hyperreactivity in T and B cell-deficient mice. Mol Med 1998;4:344–55.

91. Wegmann M, Fehrenbach H, Fehrenbach A, et al. Involvement of distal airways in a chronic model of experimental asthma. Clin Exp Allergy 2005;35:1263–71.

92. Snibson KJ, Bischof RJ, Slocombe RF, Meeusen EN. Airway remodelling and inflammation in sheep lungs after chronic airway challenge with house dust mite. Clin Exp Allergy 2005;35:146–52.

93. Out TA, Wang SZ, Rudolph K, Bice DE. Local T-cell activation after segmental allergen challenge in the lungs of allergic dogs. Immunology 2002;105:499–508.

94. Gundel RH, Wegner CD, Letts LG. Antigen-induced acute and late-phase responses in primates. Am Rev Respir Dis 1992;146:369–73.

95. Schelegle ES, Gershwin LJ, Miller LA, et al. Allergic asthma induced in rhesus monkeys by house dust mite (Dermatophagoides farinae). Am J Pathol 2001;158:333–41.

96. van Scott MR, Hooker JL, Ehrmann D, et al. Dust mite-induced asthma in cynomolgus monkeys. J Appl Physiol 2004;96:1433–44.

97. Weiszer I, Patterson R, Pruzansky JJ. Ascaris hypersensitivity in the rhesus monkey. I. A model for the study of immediate type hypersensivity in the primate. J Allergy 1968;41:14–22.

98. Yasue M, Nakamura S, Yokota T, et al. Experimental monkey model sensitized with mite antigen. Int Arch Allergy Immunol 1998;115:303–11.

99. Fanucchi MV, Plopper CG, Evans MJ, et al. Cyclic exposure to ozone alters distal airway development in infant rhesus monkeys. Am J Physiol Lung Cell Mol Physiol 2006;291:L644–50.

100. Coffman RL, Hessel EM. Nonhuman primate models of asthma. J Exp Med 2005;201:1875–9.

101. Reader JR, Tepper JS, Schelegle ES, et al. Pathogenesis of mucous cell metaplasia in a murine asthma model. Am J Pathol 2003;162:2069–78.

102. Cutz E, Levinson H, Cooper DM. Ultrastructure of airways in children with asthma. Histopathology 1978;2:407–21.

103. Laitinen LA, Heino M, Laitinen A, et al. Damage of the airway epithelium and bronchial reactivity in patients with asthma. Am Rev Respir Dis 1985;131:599–606.

104. Hogg JC. The pathology of asthma. Clin Chest Med 1984;5:567–71.

105. Evans MJ, Van Winkle LS, Fanucchi MV, Plopper CG. Cellular and molecular characteristics of basal cells in airway epithelium. Exp Lung Res 2001;27:401–15.

106. Evans MJ, Moller PC. Biology of airway basal cells. Exp Lung Res 1991;17:513–31.

107. Montefort S, Herbert CA, Robinson C, Holgate ST. The bronchial epithelium as a target for inflammatory attack in asthma. Clin Exp Allergy 1992;22:511–20.

108. Erjefalt JS, Persson CG. Airway epithelial repair: breathtakingly quick and multipotentially pathogenic. Thorax 1997;52:1010–2.

109. Shebani E, Shahana S, Janson C, Roomans GM. Attachment of columnar airway epithelial cells in asthma. Tissue Cell 2005;37:145–52.

110. Shahana S, Bjornsson E, Ludviksdottir D, et al. Ultrastructure of bronchial biopsies from patients with allergic and non-allergic asthma. Respir Med 2005;99:429–43.

111. Ordonez CL, Khashayar R, Wong HH, et al. Mild and moderate asthma is associated with airway goblet cell hyperplasia and abnormalities in mucin gene expression. Am J Respir Crit Care Med 2001;163:517–23.

112. Evans MJ, Fanucchi MV, Plopper CG. The basement membrane zone in asthma. Curr Respir Med Rev 2006;2:331–7.

113. Evans MJ, Guha SC, Cox RA, Moller PC. Attenuated fibroblast sheath around the basement membrane zone in the trachea. Am J Respir Cell Mol Biol 1993;8:188–92.

114. Fine JD. Structure and antigenicity of the skin basement membrane zone. J Cutan Pathol 1991;18:401–9.

115. Uitto J, Pulkkinen L. Molecular complexity of the cutaneous basement membrane zone. Mol Biol Rep 1996;23:35–46.

116. Brewster CE, Howarth PH, Djukanovic R, et al. Myofibroblasts and subepithelial fibrosis in bronchial asthma. Am J Respir Cell Mol Biol 1990;3:507–11.

117. Evans MJ, Van Winkle LS, Fanucchi MV, et al. Fibroblast growth factor-2 in remodeling of the developing basement membrane zone in the trachea of infant rhesus monkeys sensitized and challenged with allergen. Lab Invest 2002;82:1747–54.

118. Bousquet J, Jeffery PK, Busse WW, et al. Asthma. From bronchoconstriction to airways inflammation and remodeling. Am J Respir Crit Care Med 2000;161:1720–45.

119. Milanese M, Crimi E, Scordamaglia A, et al. On the functional consequences of bronchial basement membrane thickening. J Appl Physiol 2001;91:1035–40.

120. Adachi E, Hopkinson I, Hayashi T. Basement-membrane stromal relationships: interactions between collagen fibrils and the lamina densa. Int Rev Cytol 1997;173:73–156.

121. Sannes PL, Wang J. Basement membranes and pulmonary development. Exp Lung Res 1997;23:101–8.

122. Sannes PL, Burch KK, Khosla J, et al. Immunohistochemical localization of chondroitin sulfate, chondroitin sulfate proteoglycan, heparan sulfate proteoglycan, entactin, and laminin in basement membranes of postnatal developing and adult rat lungs. Am J Respir Cell Mol Biol 1993;8:245–51.

123. Evans MJ, Fanucchi MV, Baker GL, et al. Atypical development of the tracheal basement membrane zone of infant rhesus monkeys exposed to ozone and allergen. Am J Physiol Lung Cell Mol Physiol 2003;285:L931–9.

124. Evans MJ, Fanucchi MV, Baker GL, et al. The remodelled tracheal basement membrane zone of infant rhesus monkeys after 6 months of recovery. Clin Exp Allergy 2004;34:1131–6.

125. Ebina M, Takahashi T, Chiba T, Motomiya M. Cellular hypertrophy and hyperplasia of airway smooth muscles underlying bronchial asthma. A 3–D morphometric study. Am Rev Respir Dis 1993;148:720–6.

126. Stephens NL, Jiang H, Xu J, Kepron W. Airway smooth muscle mechanics and biochemistry in experimental asthma. Am Rev Respir Dis 1991;143:1182–8.

127. Stephens NL, Jiang H, Halayko A. Role of airway smooth muscle in asthma: possible relation to the neuroendocrine system. Anat Rec 1993;236:152–63.

128. Bramley AM, Thomson RJ, Roberts CR, Schellenberg RR. Hypothesis: excessive bronchoconstriction in asthma is due to decreased airway elastance. Eur Respir J 1994;7:337–41.

129. Tran MU, Weir AJ, Fanucchi MV, et al. Smooth muscle hypertrophy in distal airways of sensitized infant rhesus monkeys exposed to house dust mite allergen. Clin Exp Allergy 2004;34:1627–33.

130. Hoshino M, Nakamura Y, Hamid QA. Gene expression of vascular endothelial growth factor and its receptors and angiogenesis in bronchial asthma. J Allergy Clin Immunol 2001;107:1034–8.

131. Lee CG, Link H, Baluk P, et al. Vascular endothelial growth factor (VEGF) induces remodeling and enhances T(H)2-mediated sensitization and inflammation in the lung. Nat Med 2004;10:1095–103.

132. Hogg JC, Pare PD, Moreno R. The effect of submucosal edema on airways resistance. Am Rev Respir Dis 1987;135:S54–6.

133. McFadden ER Jr. Hypothesis: exercise-induced asthma as a vascular phenomenon. Lancet 1990;335:880–3.

134. Cabanes LR, Weber SN, Matran R, et al. Bronchial hyperresponsiveness to methacholine in patients with impaired left ventricular function. N Engl J Med 1989;320:1317–22.

135. Shimada J, Fushiki S, Tsujimura A, Oka T. Fibroblast growth factor-2 expression is up-regulated after denervation in rat lung tissue. Brain Res Mol Brain Res 1997;49:295–8.

136. Jungnickel J, Claus P, Gransalke K, et al. Targeted disruption of the FGF-2 gene affects the response to peripheral nerve injury. Mol Cell Neurosci 2004;25:444–52.

137. Sapieha PS, Peltier M, Rendahl KG, et al. Fibroblast growth factor-2 gene delivery stimulates axon growth by adult retinal ganglion cells after acute optic nerve injury. Mol Cell Neurosci 2003;24:656–72.

138. Cosio MG, Guerassimov A. Chronic obstructive pulmonary disease. Inflammation of small airways and lung parenchyma. Am J Respir Crit Care Med 1999;160:S21–5.

139. Hyde DM, Plopper CG, Weir AJ, et al. Peribronchiolar fibrosis in lungs of cats chronically exposed diesel exhaust. Lab Invest 1985;52:195–206.

140. Fujinaka LE, Hyde DM, Plopper CG, et al. Respiratory bronchiolitis following long-term ozone exposure in bonnet monkeys: a morphometric study. Exp Lung Res 1985;8:167–90.

141. Tyler WS, Tyler NK, Last JA, et al. Comparison of daily and seasonal exposures of young monkeys to ozone. Toxicology 1988;50:131–44.

142. Sterner-Kock A, Kock M, Braun R, Hyde DM. Ozone-induced epithelial injury in the ferret is similar to nonhuman primates. Am J Respir Crit Care Med 2000;162:1152–6.

143. Hyde DM, Miller LA, McDonald RJ, et al. Neutrophils enhance clearance of necrotic epithelial cells in ozone- induced lung injury in rhesus monkeys. Am J Physiol 1999;277:L1190–8.

144. Miller LA, Usachenko J, McDonald RJ, Hyde DM. Trafficking of neutrophils across airway epithelium is dependent upon both thioredoxin- and pertussis toxin-sensitive signaling mechanisms. J Leukoc Biol 2000;68:201–8.

145. Miller LA, Barnett NL, Sheppard D, Hyde DM. Expression of the beta6 integrin subunit is associated with sites of neutrophil influx in lung epithelium. J Histochem Cytochem 2001;49:41–8.

146. Oslund KL, Miller LA, Usachenko JL, et al. Oxidant-injured airway epithelial cells upregulate thioredoxin but do not produce interleukin-8. Am J Respir Cell Mol Biol 2004;30:597–604.

147. McDonald RJ, St. George JA, Pan LC, Hyde DM. Neutrophil adherence to airway epithelium is reduced by antibodies to the leukocyte CD11/CD18 complex. Inflammation 1993;17:145–51.

148. Wu R, Zhao YH, Plopper CG, et al. Differential expression of stress proteins in nonhuman primate lung and conducting airway after ozone exposure. Am J Physiol 1999; 277:L511–22.

149. Duan X, Buckpitt AR, Pinkerton KE, et al. Ozone-induced alterations in glutathione in lung subcompartments of rats and monkeys. Am J Respir Cell Mol Biol 1996;14:70–5.

150. Moffatt RK, Hyde DM, Plopper CG, et al. Ozone-induced adaptive and reactive cellular changes in respiratory bronchioles of Bonnet monkeys. Exp Lung Res 1987;12:57–74.

151. Hyde DM, Plopper CG, Harkema JR, et al. Ozone-induced structural changes in monkey respiratory system. In: Schneider T, Lee SD, Wolters PJ, Grant MB, editors. Atmospheric ozone research and its policy implications. New York: Elsevier; 1989. p. 523–32.

152. Harkema JR, Plopper CG, Hyde DM, et al. Response of macaque bronchiolar epithelium to ambient concentrations of ozone. Am J Pathol 1993;143:857–66.

153. Barr BC, Hyde DM, Plopper CG, Dungworth DL. Distal airway remodeling in rats chronically exposed to ozone. Am Rev Respir Dis 1988;137:924–38.

154. Barr BC, Hyde DM, Plopper CG, Dungworth DL. A comparison of terminal airway remodeling in chronic daily versus episodic ozone exposure. Toxicol Appl Pharmacol 1990;106:384–407.

155. Plopper CG, Chow CK, Dungworth DL, et al. Effect of low level of ozone on rat lungs. II. Morphological responses during recovery and re-exposure. Exp Mol Pathol 1978;29:400–11.

156. Schelegle ES, Walby WF, Alfaro MF, et al. Repeated episodes of ozone inhalation attenuates airway injury/repair and release of substance P, but not adaptation. Toxicol Appl Pharmacol 2003;186:127–42.

157. Plopper CG, Harkema JR, Last JA, et al. The respiratory system of non-human primates responds more to ambient concentrations of ozone than does that of rats. In: Bergland R, Lawson DR, McKee DJ, editors. Tropospheric ozone and the environment. Pittsburgh (PA): Air and Waste Management Association; 1991. p. 137–50.

158. Snider GL, Kleinerman J, Thurlbeck WM. The definition of emphysema. Report of a National Heart, Lung, and Blood Institute Division of Lung Diseases workshop. Am Rev Respir Dis1985;132:182–5.

159. Snider GL, Martorana PA, Lucey EC, Lungarella G. Animal models of emphysema. In: Voelkel NF, MacNee W, editors. Chronic obstructive lung diseases. Hamilton (ON): BC Decker; 2002. p. 237–56.

160. Shapiro SD. Vascular atrophy and VEGFR-2 signaling: old theories of pulmonary emphysema meet new data. J Clin Invest 2000;106:1309–10.

161. Kasahara Y, Tuder RM, Cool CD, et al. Endothelial cell death and decreased expression of vascular endothelial growth factor and vascular endothelial growth factor receptor 2 in emphysema. Am J Respir Crit Care Med 2001;163:737–44.

162. Majo J, Ghezzo H, Cosio MG. Lymphocyte population and apoptosis in the lungs of smokers and their relation to emphysema. Eur Respir J 2001;17:946–53.

163. Kasahara Y, Tuder RM, Taraseviciene-Stewart L, et al. Inhibition of VEGF receptors causes lung cell apoptosis and emphysema. J Clin Invest 2000;106:1311–9.

164. Aoshiba K, Yokohori N, Nagai A. Alveolar wall apoptosis causes lung destruction and emphysematous changes. Am J Respir Cell Mol Biol 2003;28:555–62.

165. MacNee W, Rahman I. Is oxidative stress central to the pathogenesis of chronic obstructive pulmonary disease? Trends Mol Med 2001;7:55–62.

166. MacNee W. Oxidants and COPD. Curr Drug Targets Inflamm Allergy 2005;4:627–41.

167. Tuder RM, Zhen L, Cho CY, et al. Oxidative stress and apoptosis interact and cause emphysema due to vascular endothelial growth factor receptor blockade. Am J Respir Cell Mol Biol 2003;29:88–97.

168. Demura Y, Taraseviciene-Stewart L, Scerbavicius R, et al. N-Acetylcysteine treatment protects against VEGF-receptor blockade-related emphysema. COPD 2004;1:25–32.

169. Petrache I, Fijalkowska I, Zhen L, et al. A novel antiapoptotic role for alpha1-antitrypsin in the prevention of pulmonary emphysema. Am J Respir Crit Care Med 2006;173:1222–8.

170. Hyde DM, Miller LA, Schelegle ES, et al. Asthma: a comparison of animal models using stereologic methods. Eur Respir Rev 2006;15:122–135.

171. Mariassy AT. Epithelial cells of trachea and bronchi. In: Parent RA, editor. Treatise on pulmonary toxicology: comparative biology of the normal lung. Boca Raton (FL): CRC Press; 1991. p. 63–76.

172. Mercer RR, Russell ML, Roggli VL, Crapo JD. Cell number and distribution in human and rat airways. Am J Respir Cell Mol Biol 1994;10:613–24.

173. St George JA, Harkema JR, Hyde DM, Plopper CG. Cell populations and structure/function relationships of cells in the airways. In: Gardner DE, Crapo JD, Massaro EJ, editors. Toxicology of the lung. New York: Raven Press; 1988. p. 71–102.

174. Plopper CG, Weir A, St George JA, et al. Cell populations and the respiratory system: interspecies diversity in composition, distribution, and morphology. In: Dungworth D, Kimmerle G, Lewkowski R, et al, editors. Inhalation toxicology. New York: Springer; 1988. p. 25–40.

CHAPTER 18

IMAGING OF CHRONIC OBSTRUCTIVE PULMONARY DISEASE

DAVID A. LYNCH, MD, AND HARVEY O. COXSON, PHD

THE TERM *CHRONIC OBSTRUCTIVE PULMONARY DISEASE* (COPD) encompasses asthmatic bronchitis, chronic bronchitis, chronic obstructive bronchitis, and emphysema.[1] Imaging provides important clues to the presence and extent of each of these entities. Some patients with COPD may have extensive emphysema, whereas others with equal functional impairment have little or no emphysema. To provide a comprehensive evaluation of the patient with COPD, the imager must document the presence and severity of emphysema, bronchial wall thickening, and air trapping.

In addition to identifying emphysema, high-resolution chest computed tomography (CT) can identify other smoking-related lung diseases, such as respiratory bronchiolitis, desquamative interstitial pneumonitis, and Langerhans histiocytosis. Imaging may also be used to identify complications of COPD, including lobar atelectasis, pulmonary hypertension, and lung cancer, and to evaluate patients before and after lung volume reduction surgery (LVRS).

In this chapter, we review the current and evolving imaging modalities available for assessment of COPD, describe the imaging features of emphysema and other smoking-related lung diseases, and discuss the role of imaging in identifying complications of COPD and of LVRS.

Imaging Modalities
Chest Radiography

Conventional chest radiography is usually the first imaging procedure performed in the patient with known or suspected COPD. Variation in the quality of analog (hard copy) chest images obtained in outpatient offices may lead to misdiagnoses. Overexposure of the radiograph may simulate emphysema, whereas underexposure may lead to a false diagnosis of interstitial lung disease. Digital imaging of the thorax, using either a photostimulable phosphor plate, selenium drum, or selenium plate, in combination with a picture archiving and communication system (PACS), allows immediate dissemination of the patient's images to radiology reading areas and clinics. Two recent innovations in digital imaging may be important for detection of nodules in patients with COPD. Dual-energy imaging allows "subtraction" of overlying bones to create an image composed almost entirely of soft tissues. The technique of temporal subtraction electronically subtracts a previous radiograph from the current image to enhance detection of changes. These techniques require further evaluation but may ultimately rival CT as cost-effective modalities for screening for lung cancer.

Computed Tomography

CT is increasingly used to provide phenotypic characterization of COPD. Typically, the entire lung is imaged in a single breath-hold (5–20 seconds), using spiral CT, producing a three-dimensional volumetric data set. This type of acquisition allows construction of overlapping images, multiplanar images (Figure 1), and three-dimensional models. It also facilitates quantitative evaluation of lung volumes, extent of emphysema, and airway abnormalities. Thin-section (high resolution computed tomography [HRCT]) images may be reconstructed from the same data set to allow precise characterization of emphysema and small airways abnormality.

CT imaging during expiration is useful for identification of air trapping (Figure 2) and may accentuate subtle areas of centrilobular emphysema. Expiratory images are typically obtained at end-expiration. Some institutions obtain only a few expiratory images at selected levels, whereas others acquire a full volumetric expiratory scan to evaluate the entire lung. More recently, the technique of dynamic expiration (imaging during a forced expiration) has been introduced as a complementary technique to evaluate for tracheomalacia. Dynamic imaging during coughing may also be used for the same purpose.

Inspiratory and expiratory spiral CT can be used to calculate total lung capacity (TLC) and residual volume (RV). In a study by Kauczor and colleagues, the volume of the lungs measured on inspiratory helical CT, performed without spirometric control, was approximately 12% less than TLC but was highly correlated with TLC.[2] The volume of the lungs on deep expiration was highly correlated with thoracic gas volume but correlated less well with RV. These findings suggest that the level of inspiration for inspiratory helical CT is approximately 12% lower than TLC, whereas on expiratory CT, the level of expiration is closer to functional residual capacity than to RV. Similarly, in a study of patients before and after LVRS, the TLC calculated by CT correlated very well with plethysmographic TLC, but calculated RV tended to overestimate the plethysmographic RV.[3]

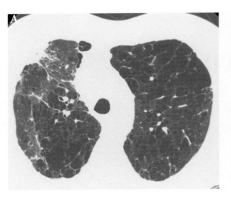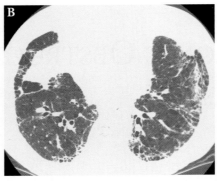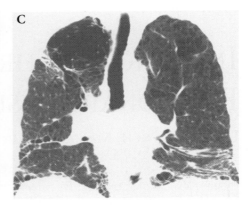

FIGURE 1. Axial and coronal computed tomography (CT) in a patient with emphysema and lung fibrosis. *A*, CT through the upper lobes shows moderate centrilobular emphysema. Subpleural scarring is present in the right upper lobe. *B*, Axial CT through the lower lobes shows subpleural reticular abnormality and honeycombing, typical for usual interstitial pneumonia. *C*, Coronal CT provides an excellent depiction of the relative extent of emphysema and lung fibrosis.

ACQUISITION TECHNIQUES FOR QUANTITATIVE CT

New fast spiral CT scanners allow imaging of the entire lung volume within a 10- to 20-second inspiratory breath-hold. From this volumetric data set, contiguous thick-section images and noncontiguous thin-section images may be reconstructed. The thick sections (3–5 mm) allow visualization of the entire lung, detecting nodules and other significant pathology, whereas the thinner sections allow better evaluation of emphysema and airways disease. Images can also be reconstructed in multiple planes, and three-dimensional models can be created. The large airways can be segmented from the lungs, using a region-growing technique.[4]

Standardization of the inspired volume of air can be important in ensuring reproducibility of quantitative CT measurements on lung CT. Several authors have used spirometric triggering devices, but these are not widely available. If spiral CT is used to acquire volumetric information in a single breath-hold, the achieved lung volumes can be measured directly,[2] obviating the need for spirometric gating.

LIMITATIONS

On occasion, even with modern scanners, respiratory or cardiac motion can result in low-attenuation areas adjacent to pulmonary vessels that may simulate emphysema. Inappropriate photography may cause emphysema to be invisible.

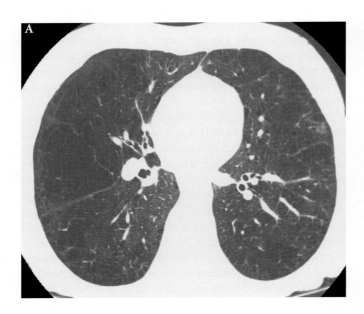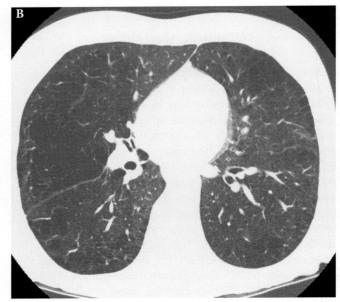

FIGURE 2. Inspiratory and expiratory computed tomography (CT) in emphysema. *A*, Inspiratory axial CT through the midlungs shows confluent emphysema in the right lung and centrilobular emphysema elsewhere. *B*, End-expiratory CT shows marked air trapping in the areas of emphysema. The more normal lung has increased in attenuation.

Limitations of measuring lung density with CT include variability owing to patient size, patient positioning within the scanner, location and environment of the lung area being assessed, type of CT scanner, kilovoltage, and reconstruction algorithm.

Lung attenuation measurements also remain critically dependent on imaging in full inspiration. Because lung density can change by 200 HU between full inspiration and full expiration,[5] some authors have advocated routine spirometric gating to verify the depth of inspiration.[6]

Mean lung density is decreased with hyperinflation in the absence of emphysema,[7] so the observation of decreased mean lung density is not specific for emphysema. Localized areas of emphysema less than 0.4 cm in diameter often cannot be seen on CT; mild centrilobular emphysema (CLE) and mild panlobular emphysema (PLE) may both be missed using 1.0 and 10 mm CT techniques.[8–10]

Lung Magnetic Resonance Imaging

Magnetic resonance imaging (MRI) of the lung is a very attractive technique, particularly because of the lack of ionizing radiation that is associated with most other imaging modalities and because it moves beyond simple anatomic imaging and provides functional information as well. However, factors such as the small nuclear spin polarization at thermal equilibrium and the field inhomogeneity problems associated with the lung have greatly limited the application of this technique.[11] Conventional proton MRI of the lungs is difficult because of the low concentration of hydrogen in the lung parenchyma, airspaces, and airways and the multiple fine air—soft tissue interfaces within the lung causing susceptibility artifacts. Respiratory and cardiac motion artifacts are a common problem and are accentuated by higher field strengths.

Fast gradient echo breath-hold MRI has been used at full inspiration and expiration to evaluate changes in lung volumes and thoracic dimensions following LVRS.[12] Lung volumes derived from the magnetic resonance data using a semiautomated computerized method of delineating the lungs and cross-sectional areas were compared with volumes measured on plethysmography and CT at 8 to 10 mm collimation. The authors found that magnetic resonance measurements of lung volumes were comparable to those derived from CT data but different from volumes derived from plethysmography, which remains the gold standard.[12] Gradient echo MRI can also be used to evaluate the abnormalities of diaphragmatic movement in patients with emphysema. Dynamic contrast-enhanced MRI using gadolinium has been used to quantify the extent of emphysema in an animal model.[13]

Investigators have pursued differing paths in the quest to image the airspaces by MRI. Misselwitz and colleagues obtained relatively homogeneous enhancement of the lungs in a rat model using an aerosolized formulation of gadolinium—diethylenetriamine pentaacetic acid (DTPA)

and T_1-weighted spin echo images at a field strength of 2 T.[14] Other researchers have performed limited flip angle gradient echo three-dimensional volume acquisition imaging using perfluorocarbon (PFC) aerosols for simultaneous analysis of lung structure and mapping of the partial pressure of oxygen (pO_2) within the lungs.[15,16] The pO_2 measurement method is based on the paramagnetic effect of dissolved molecular oxygen, which reduces the T_1 properties of PFC 19-F. This may lead, at some future stage, to clinical human in vivo oxygen-sensitive imaging in the pulmonary system.

Regional ventilation has also been assessed using oxygen-enhanced MRI. Although molecular oxygen is only weakly paramagnetic, it produces substantial signal changes in the lungs because of their large surface areas. Edelman and colleagues used inhaled molecular oxygen as a contrast agent, directly depicting transfer of oxygen across the alveolus into the pulmonary vasculature.[17] The degree of enhancement using dynamic oxygen-enhanced MRI in patients with COPD provided excellent correlation with lung diffusion capacity.[18] A limitation of this technique is the requirement for patients to inhale 100% oxygen, which may be dangerous for patients with blunted respiratory drives.

NOBLE GAS MRI OF THE LUNGS

The advent of hyperpolarized gas MRI techniques has opened up whole new avenues of research into ventilation of the lung[19,20] and the measurement of airspace[21] and airway dimensions.[22,23] One of the most important advances came with the development of a measurement of alveolar size known as the apparent diffusion coefficient (ADC). The ADC is a measurement of movement of a molecule of helium within an enclosed space, like the alveolus of the lung. In the normal lung, the movement of helium is restricted, but in emphysema, where the airspaces become much larger, the ADC is increased. Several studies have correlated the ADC with spirometry measurements in normal volunteers and in subjects with airflow limitation, emphysema, and animal models.[20–22,24–29] These studies show that the ADC measurement is a very valuable tool in assessing emphysema, and, in fact, Woods and colleagues recently showed that there was a very good correlation between the ADC and alveolar size measured using either the surface area to volume ratio of the lung parenchyma or the mean linear intercept and that the ADC was able to separate emphysematous lung from normal lung with greater sensitivity than histology.[21]

Other investigators have shown that it is possible to use hyperpolarized helium to create three-dimensional reconstruction of the airway lumen to the seventh generation of airways.[22,23] Although this is an interesting technique, it does not provide measurements of airway wall thickness, so the applicability is still uncertain.

In conclusion, there is substantial evidence that hyperpolarized gas MRI has some very powerful applications in the study of COPD. However, the limited availability of sources for hyperpolarized helium or xenon 129 makes the widespread use of this method problematic, and it is likely that this will remain a research tool for the immediate future.

Emphysema
Classification

Emphysema is classified radiologically as centrilobular, panlobular, distal acinar, and paracicatricial.[30] Each of these entities has a distinct appearance on HRCT of the chest.

DISTAL ACINAR EMPHYSEMA

Distal acinar emphysema, also called paraseptal emphysema, is focal enlargement of distal airspaces in an otherwise normal lung; this is almost always peripheral and usually most prominent at the lung apices (Figure 3). The areas of emphysema may range in size from 5 mm to 15 cm. Areas of distal acinar emphysema can involve the lung circumferentially or may be clustered along the fissures. Larger areas of distal acinar emphysema are usually termed bullae. Massive bullae can result in the entity called "vanishing lung," discussed below.[31–33]

CENTRILOBULAR EMPHYSEMA

CLE is the most common form of emphysema and is usually related to cigarette smoking. Because destruction of lung parenchyma in CLE is concentrated around proximal respiratory bronchioles, located near the center of the acinus, the characteristic findings are well-defined or poorly defined low-attenuation areas with invisible or very thin (< 1 mm) walls surrounded by apparently normal lung parenchyma, close to the centers of secondary lobules (Figure 4).[34,35] The areas of emphysema range in size from 1 to 10 mm. The centrilobular location of the emphysema may sometimes be confirmed by the fact that a centrilobular pulmonary arteriole courses

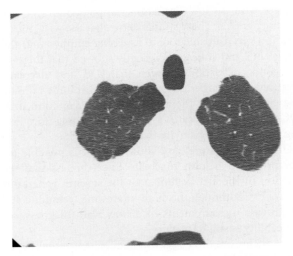

FIGURE 3. Distal acinar emphysema in a young male. Axial computed tomography through the upper lungs shows predominantly subpleural emphysema.

through the emphysematous area. CLE is distinguished from lung cysts by the absence of a defined wall.

PANLOBULAR EMPHYSEMA

In panlobular emphysema, the entire secondary pulmonary lobule is involved uniformly by emphysema. It may occur in patients with smoking-related emphysema who have complete destruction of the secondary lobule (Figure 5) and more typically in patients with α_1-antitrypsin deficiency (Figure 6). The process usually involves many adjoining lobules, resulting in large confluent areas of decreased lung attenuation on HRCT.[30] Residual interlobular septa are variably seen.

CICATRICIAL EMPHYSEMA

Cicatricial emphysema is the least common form of emphysema. It differs from other forms of emphysema because the overdistention of airspaces is due to adjacent lung fibrosis exerting a traction effect.[30] The associated fibrosis makes this an easy diagnosis on chest radiography or chest CT (Figure 7). Patients with progressive massive fibrosis owing to silicosis often have extensive cicatricial emphysema peripheral to the perihilar masslike fibrosis.

Imaging Diagnosis

Accurate diagnosis and quantification of emphysema in vivo are important because many patients with emphysema are asymptomatic and have normal spirometry.

CHEST RADIOGRAPHIC DIAGNOSIS

On the chest radiograph, emphysema may be identified either directly as irregular, asymmetric areas of decreased lung density associated with an abnormal vascular pattern or indirectly by identifying signs of hyperinflation (see Figure 5). In mild emphysema, both chest radiographs and pulmonary function tests correlate poorly with pathologic grading, but with more advanced disease, there is closer correlation and improved accuracy of diagnosis.[36] The overall accuracy of a chest radiograph in the diagnosis of severe emphysema is estimated at 60 to 75%, with a significant false-negative rate but a very low false-positive rate. Some authors reported better results,[37] but these do not seem to be widely reproducible.[38]

HYPERINFLATION

The term *overinflation* or *hyperinflation*, as used by radiologists, does not specifically imply air trapping, which is defined physiologically as an increase in RV. In emphysema, the radiographic observation of hyperinflation reflects increased lung compliance and air trapping. Patients with emphysema may not appear to be hyperinflated if they are markedly obese or scoliotic or if there is coexisting restrictive lung disease, particularly pulmonary fibrosis. Conversely, in elderly individuals, kyphosis may cause substantial diaphragmatic

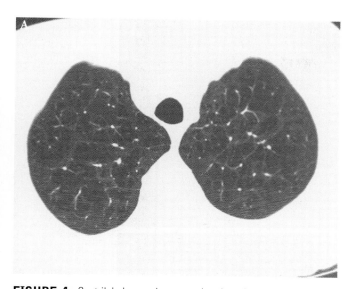
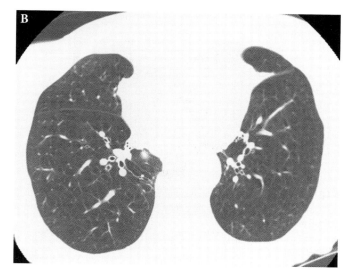

FIGURE 4. Centrilobular emphysema related to cigarette smoking. (*A*), Axial computed tomography (CT) through the upper lungs shows poorly defined "holes" of varying sizes, typical for centrilobular emphysema. (*B*), Axial CT through the lower lungs shows less profuse emphysema.

flattening, simulating hyperinflation on the lateral view. Hyperinflation is not specific for emphysema as it may be seen as obstructive airway disease, such as asthma and bronchiolitis.

Flattening of the diaphragmatic contour is the single most accurate sign of hyperinflation and has been shown to correlate well with clinically significant degrees of airflow obstruction.[36,39,40] With progressive hyperinflation, the diaphragmatic silhouette on the lateral projection becomes increasingly flattened and then inverted, with pseudoblunting of the costophrenic angles when it is displaced below the costal attachments. In extreme hyperinflation, the costal attachments of the diaphragm may be visible on the frontal chest radiograph.

Other signs of hyperinflation, such as increased anteroposterior (AP) diameter of the chest, increased retrosternal space, decreased heart size, and increased intercostal distance, are much less specific. For instance, osteopenic kyphosis is a common cause of increased AP diameter of the chest and increased retrosternal space.

Direct Radiographic Signs

The direct signs of emphysema on the chest radiograph are vascular deficiency and bullae. Vascular deficiency is a pattern of rapidly attenuating peripheral pulmonary arteries, which branch abnormally, are of irregular and smaller than expected caliber, and may be absent peripherally.[41] The pattern is due to stretching of vessels around an area of emphysema. This

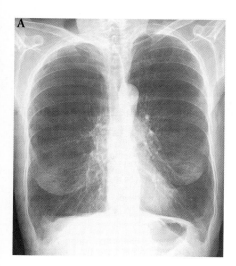
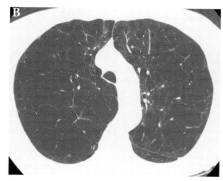
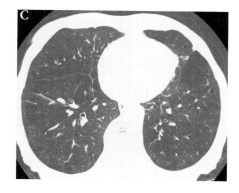

FIGURE 5. Panlobular emphysema in a cigarette smoker. (*A*), Posteroanterior chest radiograph shows marked hyperinflation. The pulmonary vasculature is decreased, particularly in the right upper lobe, and the vessels are straightened and thinned. (*B*), Axial computed tomography (CT) through the upper lungs shows large areas of confluent emphysema. (*C*), Axial CT through the lower lungs shows moderate centrilobular emphysema.

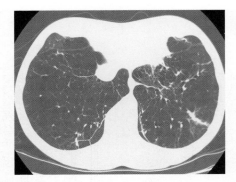

FIGURE 6. Panlobular emphysema in a patient with α₁-antitrypsin deficiency. Axial computed tomography through the lung bases shows a homogeneous decrease in lung attenuation. Multiple linear abnormalities are present; these may represent distorted interlobular septa related to hyperinflated pulmonary lobules.

radiographic pattern is more subjective than signs of hyperinflation and is also subject to greater intraobserver variation. The pattern is best appreciated in the upper lobes in CLE and in the lower lobes in PLE. It is a relatively specific sign, but it lacks sensitivity as it is a manifestation of more advanced confluent disease.

Direct signs of parenchymal destruction include local or diffuse areas of decreased lung density. Bullae are well-circumscribed avascular hyperlucent areas greater than 1 cm diameter with a scarcely visible pencil-thin wall (Figure 8). Bullae are often located in the upper lobes in both CLE and in paraseptal emphysema but are more evenly distributed in the lungs of patients with PLE.[42] Small or large bullae may be found as a manifestation of paraseptal emphysema in individuals with no other CT or physiologic evidence of emphysema, particularly in an apical location where they predispose patients to spontaneous pneumothorax.[43] Other common sites for subpleural bullae are the azygoesophageal recess behind the right main bronchus, adjacent to the left ventricle, and adjacent to the anterior junction line.

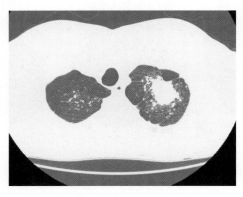

FIGURE 7. Cicatricial emphysema in a patient with silicosis and progressive massive fibrosis. Axial computed tomography through the upper lungs shows a left upper lobe mass with peripheral cicatricial emphysema.

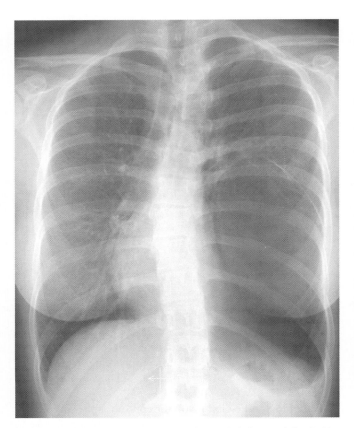

FIGURE 8. Young woman with large left lower lobe bulla. Posteroanterior chest radiograph shows a hyperlucent left lower lung with a thin well-defined wall. The bulla occupies more than half of the left hemithorax and causes substantial rightward mediastinal shift. The patient subsequently underwent bullectomy.

The natural history of bullae is variable, but they usually enlarge slowly and progressively over a period of years. Rapid symptomatic enlargement is recognized but uncommon and is an indication for bullectomy.[44] Bullae may resolve spontaneously[45] or may decompress by causing a pneumothorax. They may also disappear following an episode of hemorrhage or infection, so-called "autobullectomy."[45–47] Infection and, less commonly, hemorrhage may result in an air-fluid level within the bulla.[46–48]

VANISHING LUNG (GIANT IDIOPATHIC BULLOUS EMPHYSEMA)

The term *vanishing lung* was first used by Burke in 1937 to describe progressive enlargement of an area of localized emphysema with symptomatic compression of surrounding lung, typically seen in young males who are dyspneic (Figure 9).[31] The specific pathogenesis is unknown, but bullae are typically large (5-10 cm in diameter), with an asymmetric upper lobe distribution.[34–36]

CT DIAGNOSIS

CT is ideally suited for the diagnosis of emphysema because emphysema results in a decrease in lung attenuation. Both CT and HRCT techniques have an advantage over pathology

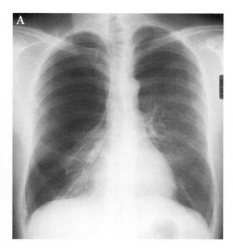
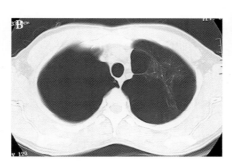
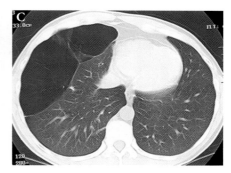

FIGURE 9. Young man with "vanishing lung." (*A*), Posteroanterior chest radiograph shows large lucency in the right hemithorax, with compression of the right lower lung. (*B*), Axial computed tomographic (CT) image through the upper lung shows multiple subpleural bullae at both apices. (*C*), Axial CT image through the lower lungs shows that the bullae extend down almost to the level of the diaphragm. The underlying right lung appears compressed but otherwise normal, indicating that the patient may be a suitable candidate for bullectomy. The patient underwent bullectomy, with a good postoperative response.

grading of emphysema as they are less prone to sampling errors intrinsic within pathology techniques. CT can also provide unilateral, regional, and lobar/segmental anatomic information compared with pulmonary function tests, which provide global assessments of function only. CT findings of emphysema are often disproportionate to spirometry, and, indeed, emphysema may be present with normal spirometry. Patients with similar forced expiratory volume in 1 second (FEV$_1$) values and Global Initiative for Chronic Obstructive Lung Disease (GOLD) stage may have very different extents of emphysema on CT, probably because of a different degree of small airways disease (Figure 10).

Multiple independent studies have shown good correlation between the grading of emphysema on CT and the pathology gold standard.[8,30,34,35,49] HRCT demonstrates improved sensitivity when compared with conventional (10 mm) CT in the diagnosis of mild emphysema.[49,50]

Several authors have demonstrated that CT and HRCT images obtained in full expiration may show areas of emphysema and air trapping with increased clarity.[37,51–53] Furthermore, Zwirewich and colleagues showed that low-dose (20 mA) HRCT provides information similar to that of high-dose (200 mA) HRCT with respect to diagnosis of emphysema, although low-dose HRCT is rarely used in clinical practice.[54]

α$_1$-ANTITRYPSIN DEFICIENCY

Most patients with α$_1$-antitrypsin deficiency have basal-predominant PLE, often associated with significant bullae and multiple linear opacities at the bases (see Figure 6). Thirty to 40% of patients with α$_1$-antitrypsin deficiency have bronchiectasis evident on CT (Figure 11).[9,42,55] In α$_1$-antitrypsin deficiency, the secondary pulmonary lobules

show homogeneously decreased attenuation on HRCT, with little remaining normal parenchyma in affected lobules. There is an associated decrease in the size, number, and side branches of pulmonary vessels in more advanced disease. The CT findings are maximal in the lower lobes. PLE related to α$_1$-antitrypsin deficiency is quite often associated with long linear densities in the lower lungs (see Figure 6).[56] These may represent thickened interlobular septa surrounding hyperinflated pulmonary lobules and may be a useful clue to the diagnosis in patients with moderate or advanced disease. Early emphysema owing to α$_1$-antitrypsin deficiency may be remarkably difficult to detect and may be hard to distinguish from obliterative bronchiolitis.

The presence of bronchiectasis and associated air trapping in α$_1$-antitrypsin deficiency may confound quantitative CT evaluation of emphysema. Therefore, any quantitative protocol should be accompanied by careful visual inspection of chest CT scans to detect bronchiectasis and other parenchymal abnormalities, which may influence lung density. Bronchiectasis is usually either cylindrical or varicose in type, evident in areas of maximal lung destruction, and occasionally severe but often not appreciated on routine radiographs.

Although most CT/HRCT study populations have been composed of patients with smoking-related emphysema, Spouge and colleagues studied the ability of CT and HRCT to diagnose pathologically proven panacinar emphysema in patients with α$_1$-antitrypsin deficiency.[9] They found that visual assessment of disease severity on CT correlated closely with the pathologic extent of panacinar emphysema ($r = .90$ for 10 mm CT and $r = .96$ for 1 mm HRCT). The authors also noted less interobserver variation in grading emphysema with HRCT when compared with conventional 10 mm CT.

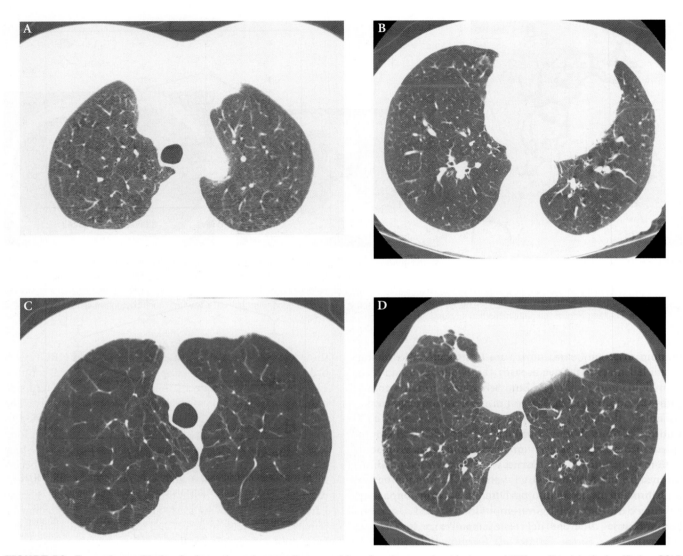

FIGURE 10. Two patients with chronic obstructive pulmonary disease and forced expiratory volume in 1 second 60% predicted, both classified as GOLD stage II. (*A*) and (*B*), This patient has minimal emphysema in the upper lungs (*C*) and (*D*), This patient has marked upper lobe predominant emphysema.

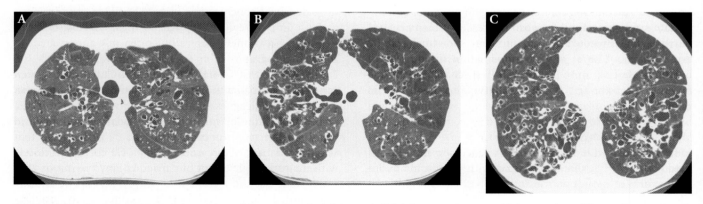

FIGURE 11. Severe bronchiectasis in a patient with α_1-antitrypsin deficiency. *A–C*, Axial computed tomographic images show diffuse varicose and cystic bronchiectasis. Decreased attenuation in the anterior lungs is probably due to panlobular emphysema.

Other Forms of Emphysema

EMPHYSEMA AND INTRAVENOUS DRUG ABUSE

Bullous changes have been noted in the lungs of users of illicit intravenous drugs, predominantly drugs intended for oral use, which often contain talc as a binding agent. Goldstein and colleagues found the overall incidence of bullous disease in intravenous drug abusers to be 2% (6 of 387).[57] When compared with a control group of patients with bullous disease, they noted that the drug users were significantly younger than the nonusers and that their bullae were larger and confined to the upper lobes. None of the drug abusers had α1-antitrypsin deficiency.

Weisbrod and colleagues documented four patients with a history of intravenous drug abuse who had combined obstructive airway disease and early emphysema on clinical, physiologic, and radiologic examinations.[58] Three of the four had bullae, and all had radiologic changes of intravenous talc granulomatosis (mainline granulomatosis). The authors concluded that although the pathogenesis of the disease is uncertain, it may involve synergism between cigarette smoke, direct toxic effects of the abused drugs, or induced intravascular leukocyte sequestration, causing local proteolytic injury.

Stern and colleagues retrospectively evaluated chest radiographs and CT findings in 21 patients with PLE caused by intravenous methylphenidate (Ritalin) abuse.[59] On chest radiographs, all patients had demonstrable emphysema, predominantly basal and symmetric in distribution. In 11 patients who had serial chest radiographs, basal emphysema progressed over a 2- to 7-year period. These authors concluded that the chest radiographic and CT findings in patients who inject methylphenidate are similar to those in patients with α1-antitrypsin deficiency and different from those seen in other forms of intravenous drug abuse. Sherman and colleagues also identified six patients with severe obstructive lung disease with a history of intravenous methylphenidate use for at least 4 years.[60] The finding of basal emphysema with normal α1-antitrypsin levels should alert the radiologist to the possibility of intravenous methylphenidate abuse.

Gurney and Bates compared 10 intravenous drug abusers with bullous disease and 8 nonabusers with pneumatoceles secondary to *Pneumocystis carinii* pneumonia (PCP).[61] The authors noted that in the small subset of eight patients who had CT scans, patients with bullous disease had peripheral abnormalities with sparing of the central portions of the lungs, and, in contrast, PCP pneumatoceles were located relatively uniformly throughout the lungs. These patterns of disease may help differentiate between the two etiologies.

PREMATURE EMPHYSEMA IN AIDS

Tasaka and colleagues noted marked progression of low-attenuation areas consistent with severe centrilobular emphysema in a human immunodeficiency virus (HIV)-positive patient treated for PCP with pulmonary function tests consistent with emphysema.[62] They postulated that emphysema-like lesions associated with PCP might be due to lung parenchyma destruction induced by HIV itself or increased elastase release from HIV-infected macrophages. Kuhlman and colleagues found that 42% of 55 patients with acquired immune deficiency syndrome (AIDS), who had a mean age of 37 years, had CT evidence of bullous changes, whereas the frequency of bullous changes in a comparable number of immunocompromised patients with acute leukemia was substantially lower.[63] Premature emphysema in patients with AIDS must be distinguished from the cystic lung lesions that result from PCP.

OTHER SYNDROMES ASSOCIATED WITH EMPHYSEMA

Santamaria and colleagues described subpleural cysts on the chest radiographs and HRCT scans of five of nine patients (56%) with lysinuric protein intolerance, an autosomal recessive disorder caused by defective transport of cationic amino acids.[64] Other conditions rarely reported to be associated with CT evidence of emphysema in the lungs include phakomatoses[65] and angiomatoses.[66]

Other Smoking-Related Lung Diseases

Saber-Sheath Trachea

Patients with COPD and emphysema may have a "saber-sheath" trachea evident on both AP and lateral radiographs and CT. In this condition, the trachea is normal down to the level of the thoracic inlet, but below this point, the coronal diameter is narrowed with a fixed deformity, often associated with dense ossification within the intrathoracic tracheal rings. The tracheal index is the ratio of the coronal to sagittal tracheal diameters, measured 1 cm above the aortic arch. When this ratio is less than 0.67, saber-sheath trachea is diagnosed.[67,68]

Chronic Bronchitis

Thickening of airway walls is the most common imaging finding in chronic bronchitis. On the chest radiograph, thickening of airway walls is common. Saber-sheath trachea may be seen. On chest CT, thickening of airway walls is seen in 26% of patients who are chronic cigarette smokers.[69]

Respiratory Bronchiolitis

Respiratory bronchiolitis related to cigarette smoking is probably the most common form of smoking-related lung disease. Abnormalities are seen on HRCT in at least 50% of cigarette smokers.[69] The typical smoking-related abnormalities are prominence of the centrilobular structures (Figure 12) owing to inflammatory thickening of airway walls and patchy ground-glass opacity owing to accumulation of pigmented macrophages in the alveoli. Airway wall thickening from chronic bronchitis may also be seen. The extent and severity of respiratory bronchiolitis range from asymptomatic minor abnormalities discovered in chronic smokers to the

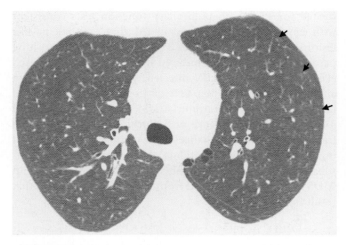

FIGURE 12. Respiratory bronchiolitis. Axial chest computed tomography through the upper lungs shows widespread poorly defined centrilobular nodules of ground-glass attenuation (*arrows*).

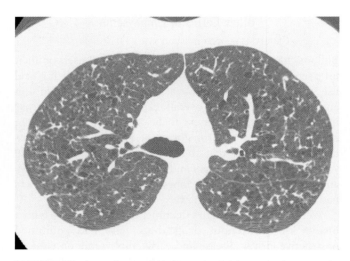

FIGURE 13. Langerhans cell histiocytosis. Axial computed tomography through the upper lungs shows widespread thin-walled cysts and irregular centrilobular nodules.

symptomatic diffuse abnormality found in patients with respiratory bronchiolitis—interstitial lung disease (RB-ILD).[70] In patients with RB-ILD, the salient features are ground-glass abnormality, centrilobular nodules, and areas of hypoattenuation, presumably representing air trapping.[71–73] The CT features of asymptomatic smokers' lung, symptomatic RB-ILD, and desquamative interstitial pneumonitis overlap significantly.[70]

The imaging features of respiratory bronchiolitis may be difficult to differentiate from hypersensitivity pneumonitis, but most patients with hypersensitivity pneumonitis are nonsmokers.[74]

Langerhans Cell Histiocytosis

Langerhans cell histiocytosis of the lung is an uncommon lung disease occurring almost exclusively in cigarette smokers. The chest radiographic appearance is often strongly suggestive of this diagnosis.[75] The chest radiograph usually shows a combination of cysts and nodules (the nodules are usually easier to see than the cysts), with mid- and upper zone predominance, sparing of the costophrenic sulci, and preservation of lung volumes.

HRCT contributes greatly to the accuracy of diagnosis of Langerhans cell histiocytosis. Grenier and colleagues showed that a first-choice diagnosis of Langerhans cell histiocytosis had a 60% likelihood of being correct when made from the chest radiograph but had a 90% likelihood of correctness on CT scanning.[76] The combination of pulmonary nodules and cysts is virtually diagnostic of Langerhans cell histiocytosis (Figure 13).[77,78] The nodules of Langerhans histiocytosis are usually poorly defined or irregular and may appear cavitary, whereas the cysts are commonly irregular or tubular in outline. A study by Bonelli and colleagues showed that Langerhans histiocytosis can be confidently diagnosed in 84% of cases: confident diagnoses were correct in 100% of cases.[79]

Imaging of Complications of COPD

Clinical deterioration in patients with emphysema usually manifests as worsening dyspnea and may be caused by benign or malignant collapse, pneumonia, pulmonary edema, bronchitis and bronchospasm, pneumothorax (Figure 14), pneumomediastinum, pulmonary thromboembolic disease, or a combination of these entities. Many of these conditions can be identified radiographically, particularly with use of comparison radiographs. Because up to 95% of patients will show no radiographic change, some question the cost-effectiveness of routine radiographs of patients with exacerbations of COPD. Others have proposed, based on their clinical experience, that radiographs should be obtained only in those patients with leukocytosis, chest pain, peripheral edema, or known cardiovascular disease, criteria that identified that subset of patients in whom the radiograph altered clinical management.[80]

Lobar/Segmental Atelectasis

Although new lung collapse in a smoker always raises concern for an endobronchial neoplasm, nonobstructive lobar collapse is quite common in patients with advanced COPD, particularly in the right middle lobe. The lobar collapse in these patients may simulate a mass (Figure 15).[81] In some patients, this is a recurrent, symptomatic event, not limited to a given segment or lobe. Potential causes of lobar collapse in COPD include compression by an adjacent overdistended emphysematous lung and acquired bronchomalacia.

Pneumothorax

Although pneumothorax is relatively uncommon in emphysema, it accounts for almost half of all cases of secondary pneumothorax.[82] The incidence of spontaneous pneumothorax is also increased in smokers, the majority

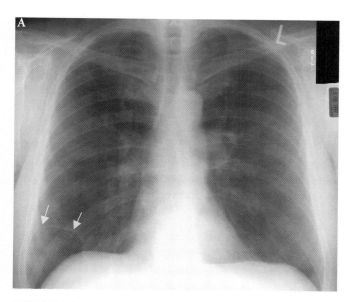
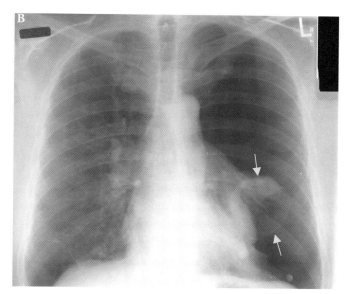

FIGURE 14. Spontaneous pneumothorax in a 58-year-old male with smoking-related emphysema. (*A*), Posteroanterior chest radiograph shows a right lower lobe bulla (*arrows*). (*B*), Subsequent chest radiograph shows a large left pneumothorax, with near-complete collapse of the left lung and pleural air outlining a noncollapsed bulla (*arrows*).

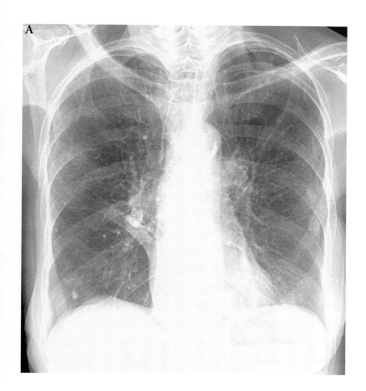
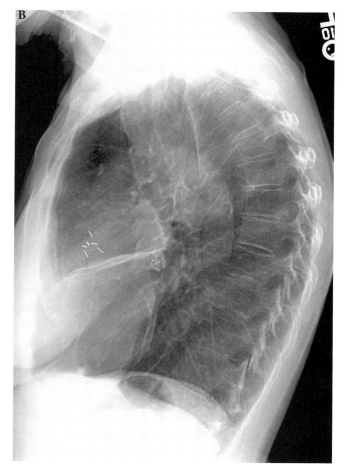

FIGURE 15. Nonobstructive lobar collapse in a patient with emphysema. (*A*), (*B*), Posteroanterior and lateral chest radiographs show hyperinflation with complete right middle lobe collapse.

of whom have emphysema.[82] The recurrence rate of pneumothorax in COPD patients is approximately 40.5% in the subsequent 3 to 5 years.[83,84] Subtle emphysema-like changes also may be found on CT in nonsmoking patients with verified spontaneous pneumothorax.[85]

It is critical to differentiate between a pneumothorax and a large bulla as management of these two conditions is distinct and placement of a thoracostomy tube into a large bulla will inevitably result in a chronic bronchopleural fistula. Comparison with old radiographs, decubitus views, and CT scanning may all be required to differentiate between a loculated pneumothorax and a large bulla.[86] The primary differentiating factor is that the white line of a pneumothorax will usually conform to the shape of the lung, whereas the edge of a bulla will commonly form an acute angle with the lung.

Pulmonary Hypertension

Patients with emphysema commonly develop pulmonary arterial hypertension with associated right ventricular hypertrophy. When the transverse diameter of the right interlobar pulmonary artery exceeds 17[87–89] or 18 mm,[90] pulmonary hypertension is likely. Pulmonary artery cross-sectional diameter on CT is predictive of mean pulmonary arterial pressure.[91]

Marked pulmonary arterial enlargement is unusual until CLE is advanced and involves the lower lobes (Figure 16). It is more commonly seen in patients with PLE, usually secondary to α_1-antitrypsin deficiency, in part related to the pattern of lung destruction and also to the greater physiologic importance of the lower lobes. Marked pulmonary arterial enlargement in CLE is a very late finding and in the absence of severe parenchymal disease should raise the possibility of coexisting pulmonary thromboembolic disease or sleep apnea.

Imaging and LVRS

LVRS has stimulated interest in imaging uncomplicated emphysema to identify those patients who will obtain maximal benefit from the procedure and to exclude those who are unsuitable for the procedure. Chest radiographs and CT scans are both useful in identifying relative or absolute contraindications to LVRS. These include previous thoracic surgery; pleural disease or other chest wall deformities, such as scoliosis and kyphosis, that might limit chest wall reconfiguration; bronchiectasis; active inflammatory lung disease or severe bronchitis; coronary artery disease manifest as cardiomegaly or coronary artery calcification; and malignancy. Chest radiographs and CT will also identify patients with inadequate hyperinflation, preserved respiratory mechanics (diaphragm excursion greater than 3 cm), or an insufficient residual normal lung.

Predicting Satisfactory Outcome/Patient Benefit

Maki and colleagues suggested that the chest radiograph may be a useful predictor of outcome following LVRS.[92] They found that the presence of markedly heterogeneous disease and of lung compression was the strongest predictor of an improvement in FEV_1 at 3 to 6 months after LVRS. Lando and colleagues found that LVRS resulted in a significant decrease in the AP diameter of the lower thorax, which correlated with a decrease in lung volumes.[93]

Certain CT criteria have been used and evaluated both prospectively and retrospectively in patients with severe emphysema considered for LVRS. Slone and colleagues at

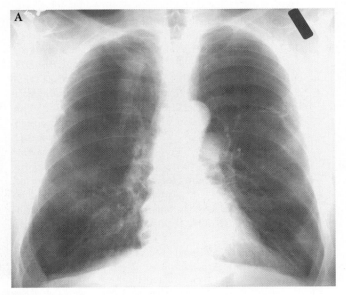
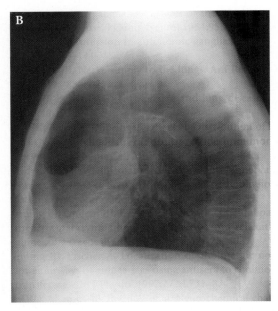

FIGURE 16. Masslike partial right upper lobe atelectasis in a 49-year-old man with steroid-dependent chronic obstructive pulmonary disease. Posteroanterior and lateral chest radiographs (*A, B*) show a bandlike mass in the right upper lobe, along with marked pulmonary arterial enlargement.

Washington University used 5-point grading scales for lung heterogeneity, used to define target areas of locally severe emphysema, and for lung atelectasis/compression, predominantly manifest as crowding of vascular markings in nonemphysematous regions of the lungs.[94] In the first 50 patients who underwent LVRS at Washington University, multivariate regression analysis identified regional heterogeneity, predominance of upper lobe disease, and compression of remaining lung areas as the most important predictors of good outcome. Postoperative performance indices, including 6-minute walking distance and partial pressure of oxygen in arterial blood, were statistically significantly better in those patients with grade 4 lung heterogeneity on CT images compared with those patients graded 1 and 2 for heterogeneity on CT scans.[95] Gierada and colleagues found that patients selected for surgery had higher quantitative emphysema severity (using the density mask technique) and a higher ratio of upper lobe to lower lobe disease than those who were not selected for surgery, suggesting that quantitative CT might be useful to increase consistency of surgical decisions.[95] Several independent studies have now confirmed the ability of CT to predict positive outcome from LVRS,[96–98] although Szekely and colleagues found that preoperative chest radiography and CT were not good predictors for length of hospital stay, hospital course, and mortality in LVRS patients.[99] Other quantitative indices that may predict outcome include the core to rind ratio of emphysema[100] and power law analysis of the relationship between the number and size of emphysematous areas.[101] In the National Emphysema Treatment Trial (NETT), the presence of non-upper lobe emphysema on visual evaluation was the only independent predictor of operative mortality.[102] In the medical arm of this randomized study, the ratio of emphysema in the lower lung zone compared with the upper lung zone was a predictor of mortality on multivariate analysis.[103]

Quantitative Measurements of the Lung in COPD

As investigators look for new ways to study the potential different COPD phenotypes, pathogenesis of COPD, and response to new interventions, there has been increasing interest in using radiologic imaging to quantify the lung structure. This research has followed two different tracks, focused on the extent of emphysema in the lung parenchyma or the airway wall structure.

Emphysema Analysis

CT is currently the most widely used technique to measure the structure of the lung. This is because once CT technology became accessible, investigators quickly realized that CT scans provided noninvasive images that were not only superior to chest radiographs but also provided densitometry data about the underlying lung structure. Today, most institutions have multidetector row CT scanners that produce exquisite images of the lung with submillimeter isotropic voxels, often in less than 10 seconds, well within the time that most subjects can hold their breath.

Quantitative CT analysis completely relies on the fact that the lung absorbs x-rays in direct correlation to the density of the lung tissue present.[104] Therefore, although the normal human lung has a distribution of x-ray attenuation values around a mean of approximately −800 HU, changes in the quantity of tissue and gas in the lung will cause a change in both the shape of this distribution and the percentage of lung voxels with a given x-ray attenuation value. The most common method to quantify emphysema applies a threshold, or density mask, to the x-ray attenuation curve and states that any voxels beyond this cutoff are "emphysematous" (Figure 17).[105–109] The initial studies correlated the extent of emphysema measured using pathology with different threshold cutoffs and found that for conventional thick-slice

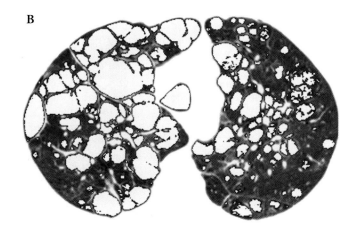

FIGURE 17. Density mask technique for evaluation of emphysema. (*A*), This figure shows the frequency distribution of x-ray attenuation values from a computed tomographic (CT) scan. Cutoff values of −910 and −950 HU are shown by the *dotted line.* The intersection of these lines on the y-axis indicates the percentage of emphysema in the CT scan using this technique, and this percentage of emphysema is used to compare between or within subjects. (*B*), The voxels with attenuation values less than −950 HU are highlighted on the CT scan.

CT images, a value of −910 HU compared the best with pathology.[110] As CT scanners and protocols have changed, this cutoff has been redefined first to −950 HU using HRCT[107] and, more recently, to −960 HU using multislice CT.[108] The second important technique to quantify emphysema is the percentile technique, whereby a percentile point on the x-ray distribution curve is predefined and the x-ray attenuation value at this point is compared between subjects.[111–116] Once again, the first investigators compared percentile values to gross pathology and showed that the lowest 5th percentile correlated well with pathology.[111,112] Lately, investigators have proposed that the lowest 15th percentile point is a robust threshold and allows subjects to be compared over time and is less susceptible to minor changes that may be induced by the CT scanner or the size of the breath the subject takes during the scan.[113–115] Recently, a careful correlation of pathology and multislice CT scanners showed that all percentile points below the lowest 18th percentile correlated with macroscopic and microscopic measures of emphysema, although the strongest correlation was with the lowest first percentile.[108]

Although the threshold cutoff and percentile techniques are the most common techniques used to quantify the extent of emphysema, they do not provide any information on the size or location of the emphysematous hole (Figure 18) or the effect the destruction has on the gas exchange surface of the lung. The most simple method to assess emphysematous hole size is a "fractal" or "cluster" analysis.[101,116] This technique correlates the size of low-attenuation areas, as defined by the number of connected voxels below a given threshold, to the number of these areas. Although limited studies have been published using this technique, studies have shown that as emphysematous holes grow in size they decrease in number[116] and that subjects with large upper lung region

lesions have the best outcome following LVRS.[101] In fact, this finding was one of the few positive correlations with outcome in the NETT and compared favorably with the qualitative assessment of emphysema distribution as assessed by a trained reader.[103] More complex techniques that quantify multiple features within the CT scan, such as the adaptive multiple feature method, have reported decent results in disease stratification, including the ability to separate smokers from nonsmokers in the absence of other disease.[117] The disadvantage of these new "texture" analysis techniques is that they often use complex mathematical terminology to describe the lung rather than the anatomic or physiologic terminology more commonly used in medicine and have not been validated using pathologic assessment of the underlying lung structure.

The early applications of quantitative CT techniques to clinical studies were restricted to small cross-sectional studies and outcome studies of LVRS. For example, Rogers and colleagues showed that the preoperative volume of severe emphysema predicts improved exercise capacity following surgery,[118] and Flaherty and colleagues showed that emphysema distributed in the upper regions of the lung compared with the lower regions was the best predictor of an increase in FEV_1 as measured by spirometry following surgery.[119] The first large-scale application of quantitative CT was in the NETT conducted in the United States.[103,120] This study confirmed the early findings that outcome following surgery is best for patients with both predominantly upper lobe emphysema and low baseline exercise capacity.[120]

Recently, attention has shifted to pharmaceutical studies of disease treatment and longitudinal disease progression. Dirksen and colleagues studied α_1-antitrypsin-deficient individuals but could not show a significant change in lung structure or function with treatment.[121] Similarly, Mao and

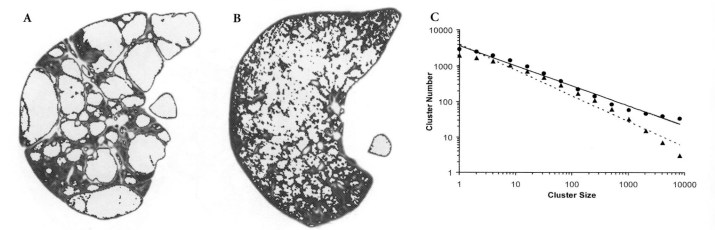

FIGURE 18. Density mask in two different subjects. This figure shows the voxels identified as below −950 HU in two different subjects, one with predominantly large holes (*A*) and one with more diffuse low-attenuation areas (*B*). Both of these subjects have approximately the same percentage of the lung occupied by these low-attenuation areas (≈65%), but the size of the holes differs substantially between the two subjects. A cluster analysis can separate these two subjects by comparing the slope of the regression line comparing low-attenuation area size to the number of connected low-attenuation areas (*C*). The regression line for subject A is shown as the *solid line*, and the regression line for subject B is shown as the *dotted line*.

colleagues, in a pilot study of all-*trans* retinoic acid treatment of human emphysema, could not measure a difference in emphysema defined by a density mask using a small group of subjects and a short study design.[122] However, in Dirksen and colleagues study, the author conducted a power analysis of the results and concluded that only 130 patients would have to be assessed using CT compared with the 550 patients needed to measure a functional change.[113]

As the use of quantitative CT in longitudinal and multicenter studies has become more popular, it has become obvious that changes in the CT image acquisition protocol can produce very different values. For example, Parr and colleagues noticed a drift in density mask measurements that was directly related to a difference in the air calibration of the CT scanners.[123] They found that although the water calibration of the scanner was performed routinely, there was no attempt to calibrate the scanner to air. Because of this drift in the x-ray attenuation values, the investigators developed a correction factor to correct the CT densitometry measurements.[123] Furthermore, Boedeker and colleagues found that even when all other aspects, such as scanner type and size of breath, were carefully controlled, the reconstruction algorithm could make up to a 15% (average 9.4%) difference in the extent of emphysema measured using a density mask technique.[124] Their data showed that some reconstruction algorithms, described as "overenhancing," improve spatial resolution by overenhancing the difference between lung voxels, thereby changing the frequency distribution of the apparent x-ray attenuation values within the CT image and, ultimately, the number of voxels below a certain cutoff value.[124]

The conclusion from these studies is that the lung densitometry values obtained using properly calibrated multislice CT scanners are within the variation observed for measurement of FEV$_1$ and can be used for longitudinal analysis of emphysema progression.[113,123,125] However, although the density mask and histogram techniques are well-validated hallmarks of disease activity, careful attention to detail is necessary to ensure that CT values can be compared between institutions and studies.

Airway Analysis

Since the major site of airflow obstruction in COPD is the small airway, no anatomic study of the lung would be complete without an assessment of the airway wall structure. Investigators first attempted to manually trace the airways seen using CT images; however; this technique was quickly abandoned because, in addition to being tedious and time consuming, numerous studies showed that the airway dimensions were very dependent on the display parameters of the printed image.[126–128]

Therefore, numerous computer algorithms have been developed to measure the airway lumen and wall area either automatically or semiautomatically. One of the more common techniques is the full-width-at-half-maximum ("half-max") method (Figure 19), whereby the distribution of apparent x-ray attenuation values along a ray projected from a central point of the lumen to the parenchyma is measured. The distance between the point at which the attenuation is halfway between the local minimum in the lumen or parenchyma and the maximum within the wall is considered to be wall thickness.[129,130] Unfortunately, the shape of this curve is dependent on various parameters, including the reconstruction algorithm used to create the image, partial volume averaging owing to field of view and orientation of the airway within the CT image, and the inevitable blurring of edges that occurs owing to the point spread function of the CT scanner, and validation studies show that the CT scans overestimate airway wall area and underestimate lumen area and that these

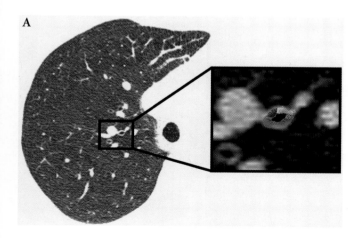
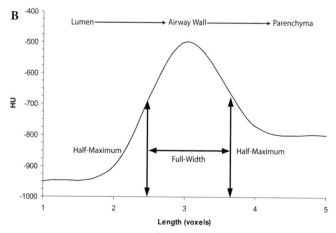

FIGURE 19. Measurement of airway wall thickness. This figure shows a magnified view of an airway from a computed tomographic scan (*A*) and the measurement of the airway wall dimensions using the full-width-at-half-maximum method (*B*). The length of the rays is determined by choosing the halfway point between the minimum x-ray attenuation value in the lumen or lung parenchyma and the maximum value within the airway wall. The lumen area and the internal perimeter of the airway wall are measured using the internal boundary of the rays and the wall area and the outer perimeter are measured by the external boundary of the rays.

errors become very large in small airways.[129,131] For these reasons, investigators have developed numerous other algorithms to measure these airways, such as the maximum-likelihood method, whereby the attenuation threshold along each ray is matched to an ideal calculated ray;[131] the score-guided erosion algorithm, where airway wall edges are found using an edge-finding algorithm that assumes that airways are circular and have a relatively high density compared with the surrounding parenchyma;[132] and an algorithm where ellipses are fit to the airway lumen and wall.[133]

The above techniques were all developed and validated using single-slice CT scanners, and although these techniques are important, they are difficult to apply across multiple centers and subjects because they can be applied only to airways that are perpendicular to the scan plane and therefore can be used to measure only a sample of the airways within the lung.

As with the lung parenchyma measurements, multislice row CT scanners that acquire (volumetric) thin-slice images of the whole chest with 0.5 to 1 mm slice thickness have changed the way that people analyze airways. Because the CT images now contain true isotropic voxels in which the z resolution (slice thickness) is the same dimension as the x and y (in plane), investigators can now use sophisticated airway segmentation and multiplanar reformat techniques to reconstruct and measure the airway in three dimensions (Figure 20).[134–136] This is an important advance because it

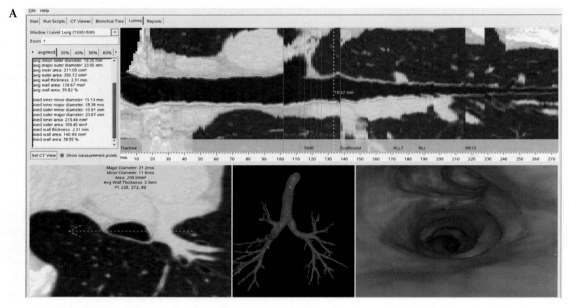

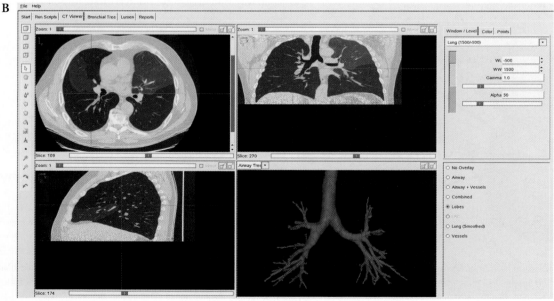

FIGURE 20. This figure shows multiplanar reformatted reconstructions of the lung and the airway tree. Using these new tools, it is now possible to segment the airway tree from the lung parenchyma and, using a predefined pathway, reconstruct it as a long straight tube and obtain measurements at a cross section to the center line of the airway at any point along the pathway (*A*). It is also possible not only to accurately segment the lung from the thoracic cavity but also to divide the lung into the five main lobes (*B*). Images courtesy of VIDA Diagnostics Inc.

now allows researchers to identify and track an individual airway at a specific location within the bronchial tree over time to study the natural history of a disease and possibly the effect of an intervention.[137]

Even though there is great interest in airways within the pulmonary community, the applications of airway measurement to COPD have been very limited. Nakano and colleagues evaluated the right apical segmental bronchus of 114 smokers using the "half-max" method.[130] The data from this study showed that the thickening in this large airway correlated with FEV_1 percent predicted, forced vital capacity percent predicted, and the ratio of RV to TLC. Furthermore, a multiple regression analysis suggested that, for a given FEV_1, subjects with more extensive emphysema had less airway wall thickening than those with less extensive emphysema. However, all symptomatic smokers had thicker walls than asymptomatic smokers.[130] A criticism of this article is that the important site of airflow obstruction in COPD is the small airways,[138,139] so to answer this question, Nakano and colleagues recently compared airway measurements from CT scans and histologic examination of excised lungs of smokers who had various degrees of airway obstruction.[140] They compared the wall area percentage of small airways (mean diameter 1.27 mm), measured histologically, with CT measurements of the wall area percentage of larger airways with a mean internal diameter of approximately 3.2 mm. These data show a significant association ($R^2 = .57$, $p = .001$) between the dimensions of the small and larger airways. The authors concluded that, at least for COPD, measuring airway dimensions in the larger bronchi, which are more accurately assessed by CT, can provide an estimate of small airway remodeling. It is likely that the same pathophysiologic process, which causes small airway obstruction, also takes place in larger airways, where it has less functional effect. Recently, Hasegawa and colleagues used multislice CT scans to measure the right apical and basal segmental bronchus at different branch points along its pathway.[141] Although the authors found a correlation with FEV_1 similar to the findings of Nakano and colleagues, they showed that if they moved more distally to the sixth generation of the airway, the correlation with FEV_1 improved. These data confirm that the airflow limitations are more strongly associated with the dimensions of the distal airways than the proximal ones and demonstrate that these new three-dimensional techniques can be used to obtain measurements from a specific location within a specific airway.

Summary

Imaging remains central to the diagnosis of emphysema and investigation of acute exacerbations in emphysema-COPD. Radiographs and pulmonary function tests remain relatively insensitive in detecting early stages of emphysema. However, CT has proven accuracy for in vivo detection and characterization of all types of emphysema. CT has a central role in evaluation and quantification of emphysema prior to surgical treatment. Newer magnetic resonance techniques, particularly noble gas imaging, are now providing both anatomic and functional imaging of the lungs in research and clinical settings and may well have a place in future imaging algorithms. Quantitative CT is emerging as a powerful tool in evaluation of the extent of emphysema and, more recently, of airways disease.

References

1. Petty TL, Weinmann GG. Building a national strategy for the prevention and management of and research in chronic obstructive pulmonary disease. National Heart, Lung, and Blood Institute workshop summary, Bethesda, Maryland, August 29–31, 1995. JAMA 1997;277:246–53.
2. Kauczor HU, Heussel CP, Fischer B, et al. Assessment of lung volumes using helical CT at inspiration and expiration: comparison with pulmonary function tests. AJR Am J Roentgenol 1998;171:1091–5.
3. Becker MD, Berkmen YM, Austin JH, et al. Lung volumes before and after lung volume reduction surgery: quantitative CT analysis. Am J Respir Crit Care Med 1998;157:1593–9.
4. Wood SA, Zerhouni EA, Hoford JD, et al. Measurement of three–dimensional lung tree structures by using computed tomography. J Appl Physiol 1995;79:1687–97.
5. Stern EJ, Webb WR. Dynamic imaging of lung morphology with ultrafast high-resolution computed tomography. J Thorac Imaging 1993;8:273–82.
6. Lamers RJ, Kemerink GJ, Drent M, van Engelshoven JM. Reproducibility of spirometrically controlled CT lung densitometry in a clinical setting. Eur Respir J 1998; 11:942–5.
7. Newman KB, Lynch DA, Newman LS, et al. Quantitative computed tomography detects air trapping due to asthma. Chest 1994;106:105–9.
8. Bergin C, Muller N, Nichols DM, et al. The diagnosis of emphysema. A computed tomographic-pathologic correlation. Am Rev Respir Dis 1986;133:541–6.
9. Spouge D, Mayo JR, Cardoso W, Muller NL. Panacinar emphysema: CT and pathologic findings. J Comput Assist Tomogr 1993;17:710–3.
10. Miller RR, Muller NL, Vedal S, et al. Limitations of computed tomography in the assessment of emphysema. Am Rev Respir Dis 1989;139:980–3.
11. Mayo JR. Magnetic resonance imaging of the chest. Where we stand. Radiol Clin North Am 1994;32:795–809.
12. Gierada DS, Hakimian S, Slone RM, Yusen RD. MR analysis of lung volume and thoracic dimensions in patients with emphysema before and after lung volume reduction surgery. AJR Am J Roentgenol 1998;170:707–14.
13. Morino S, Toba T, Araki M, et al. Noninvasive assessment of pulmonary emphysema using dynamic contrast-enhanced magnetic resonance imaging. Exp Lung Res 2006;32:55–67.
14. Misselwitz B, Muhler A, Heinzelmann I, et al. Magnetic resonance imaging of pulmonary ventilation. Initial experiences with a gadolinium-DTPA-based aerosol. Invest Radiol 1997;32:797–801.

15. Thomas SR, Gradon L, Pratsinis SE, et al. Perfluorocarbon compound aerosols for delivery to the lung as potential 19F magnetic resonance reporters of regional pulmonary pO₂. Invest Radiol 1997;32:29–38.

16. Pratt RG, Zheng J, Stewart BK, et al. Application of a 3D volume 19F MR imaging protocol for mapping oxygen tension (pO₂) in perfluorocarbons at low field. Magn Reson Med 1997;37:307–13.

17. Edelman RR, Hatabu H, Tadamura E, et al. Noninvasive assessment of regional ventilation in the human lung using oxygen-enhanced magnetic resonance imaging. Nat Med 1996;2:1236–9.

18. Ohno Y, Hatabu H, Takenaka D, et al. Dynamic oxygen-enhanced MRI reflects diffusing capacity of the lung. Magn Reson Med 2002;47:1139–44.

19. Salerno M, Altes TA, Brookeman JR, et al. Dynamic spiral MRI of pulmonary gas flow using hyperpolarized (3)He: preliminary studies in healthy and diseased lungs. Magn Reson Med 2001;46:667–77.

20. Swift AJ, Woodhouse N, Fichele S, et al. Rapid lung volumetry using ultrafast dynamic magnetic resonance imaging during forced vital capacity maneuver: correlation with spirometry. Invest Radiol 2007;42:37–41.

21. Woods JC, Choong CK, Yablonskiy DA, et al. Hyperpolarized 3He diffusion MRI and histology in pulmonary emphysema. Magn Reson Med 2006;56:1293–300.

22. Tooker AC, Hong KS, McKinstry EL, et al. Distal airways in humans: dynamic hyperpolarized 3He MR imaging—feasibility. Radiology 2003;227:575–9.

23. Lewis TA, Tzeng YS, McKinstry EL, et al. Quantification of airway diameters and 3D airway tree rendering from dynamic hyperpolarized 3He magnetic resonance imaging. Magn Reson Med 2005;53:474–8.

24. Fain SB, Panth SR, Evans MD, et al. Early emphysematous changes in asymptomatic smokers: detection with 3He MR imaging. Radiology 2006;239:875–83.

25. Fichele S, Woodhouse N, Swift AJ, et al. MRI of helium-3 gas in healthy lungs: posture related variations of alveolar size. J Magn Reson Imaging 2004;20:331–5.

26. Ley S, Zaporozhan J, Morbach A, et al. Functional evaluation of emphysema using diffusion-weighted ³helium-magnetic resonance imaging, high-resolution computed tomography, and lung function tests. Invest Radiol 2004;39:427–34.

27. Salerno M, de Lange EE, Altes TA, et al. Emphysema: hyperpolarized helium 3 diffusion MR imaging of the lungs compared with spirometric indexes—initial experience. Radiology 2002;222:252–60.

28. Swift AJ, Wild JM, Fichele S, et al. Emphysematous changes and normal variation in smokers and COPD patients using diffusion 3He MRI. Eur J Radiol 2005;54:352–8.

29. Mata JF, Altes TA, Cai J, et al. Evaluation of emphysema severity and progression in a rabbit model: comparison of hyperpolarized 3He and 129Xe diffusion MRI with lung morphometry. J Appl Physiol 2007;102:1273–80.

30. Foster WL Jr, Gimenez EI, Roubidoux MA, et al. The emphysemas: radiologic-pathologic correlations. Radiographics 1993;13:311–28.

31. Burke RM. Vanishing lungs: a case report of bullous emphysema. Radiology 1937;28:367–71.

32. Roberts L, Putman CE, Chen JTT, et al. Vanishing lung syndrome; upper lung bullous pneumonopathy. Rev Int Am Radiol 1987;2:249–55.

33. Stern EJ, Webb WR, Weinacker A, Muller NL. Idiopathic giant bullous emphysema (vanishing lung syndrome): imaging findings in nine patients. AJR Am J Roentgenol 1994;162:279–82.

34. Foster WL Jr, Pratt PC, Roggli VL, et al. Centrilobular emphysema: CT-pathologic correlation. Radiology 1986;159:27–32.

35. Hruban RH, Meziane MA, Zerhouni EA, et al. High resolution computed tomography of inflation-fixed lungs. Pathologic-radiologic correlation of centrilobular emphysema. Am Rev Respir Dis 1987;136:935–40.

36. Reich SB, Weinshelbaum A, Yee J. Correlation of radiographic measurements and pulmonary function tests in chronic obstructive pulmonary disease. AJR Am J Roentgenol 1985;144:695–9.

37. Miniati M, Filippi E, Falaschi F, et al. Radiologic evaluation of emphysema in patients with chronic obstructive pulmonary disease. Chest radiography versus high resolution computed tomography. Am J Respir Crit Care Med 1995;151:1359–67.

38. Takasugi JE, Godwin JD. Radiology of chronic obstructive pulmonary disease. Radiol Clin North Am 1998;36:29–55.

39. Nicklaus TM, Stowell DW, Christiansen WR, Renzetti AD Jr. The accuracy of the roentgenologic diagnosis of chronic pulmonary emphysema. Am Rev Respir Dis 1966;93:889–99.

40. Reid L, Millard FJC. Correlation between radiological diagnosis in structural lung changes in emphysema. Clin Radiol 1964;15:307.

41. Simon G. Radiology and emphysema. Clin Radiol 1964;15:293.

42. Guest PJ, Hansell DM. High resolution computed tomography (HRCT) in emphysema associated with alpha-1-antitrypsin deficiency. Clin Radiol 1992;45:260–6.

43. Putman CE, Godwin JD, Silverman PM, Foster WL. CT of localized lucent lung lesions. Semin Roentgenol 1984;19:173–88.

44. Boushy SF, Kohen R, Billig DM, Heiman MJ. Bullous emphysema: clinical, roentgenologic and physiologic study of 49 patients. Dis Chest 1968;54:327–34.

45. Douglas AC, Grant IWB. Spontaneous closure of large pulmonary bullae: a report on 3 cases. Br J Tuberc 1957;51:335–8.

46. McCluskie RA. Unusual fate of emphysematous bullae. Thorax 1981;36:77.

47. Stone DJ, Schwartz A, Feltman JA. Bullous emphysema: a long-term study of the natural history and the effects of therapy. Am Rev Respir Dis 1960;82.

48. Jay SJ, Johanson WG. Massive intrapulmonary hemorrhge: an uncommon complication of bullous emphysema. Am Rev Respir Dis 1974;110:497–501.

49. Kuwano K, Matsuba K, Ikeda T, et al. The diagnosis of mild emphysema. Correlation of computed tomography and pathology scores. Am Rev Respir Dis 1990;141:169–78.

50. Sanders C, Nath PH, Bailey WC. Detection of emphysema with computed tomography. Correlation with pulmonary function tests and chest radiography. Invest Radiol 1988;23:262–6.

51. Knudson RJ, Standen JR, Kaltenborn WT, et al. Expiratory computed tomography for assessment of suspected pulmonary emphysema. Chest 1991;99:1357–66.

52. Heremans A, Verschakelen JA, Van fraeyenhoven L, Demedts M. Measurement of lung density by means of quantitative CT scanning. A study of correlations with pulmonary function tests. Chest 1992;102:805–11.

53. Lamers RJ, Thelissen GR, Kessels AG, et al. Chronic obstructive pulmonary disease: evaluation with spirometrically controlled CT lung densitometry. Radiology 1994; 193:109–13.

54. Zwirewich CV, May JR, Muller NL. Low-dose high-resolution CT of lung parenchyma. Radiology 1991;180:413–7.

55. King MA, Stone JA, Diaz PT, et al. Alpha 1-antitrypsin deficiency: evaluation of bronchiectasis with CT. Radiology 1996;199:137–41.

56. Copley SJ, Wells AU, Muller NL, et al. Thin-section CT in obstructive pulmonary disease: discriminatory value. Radiology 2002;223:812–9.

57. Goldstein DS, Karpel JP, Appel D, Williams MH Jr. Bullous pulmonary damage in users of intravenous drugs. Chest 1986;89:266–9.

58. Weisbrod GL, Rahman M, Chamberlain D, Herman SJ. Precocious emphysema in intravenous drug abusers. J Thorac Imaging 1993;8:233–40.

59. Stern EJ, Frank MS, Schmutz JF, et al. Panlobular pulmonary emphysema caused by i.v. injection of methylphenidate (Ritalin): findings on chest radiographs and CT scans. AJR Am J Roentgenol 1994;162:555–60.

60. Sherman CB, Hudson LD, Pierson DJ. Severe precocious emphysema in intravenous methylphenidate (Ritalin) abusers. Chest 1987;92:1085–7.

61. Gurney JW, Bates FT. Pulmonary cystic disease: comparison of *Pneumocystis carinii* pneumatoceles and bullous emphysema due to intravenous drug abuse. Radiology 1989;173:27–31.

62. Tasaka S, Takagi H, Oguma T, Aoki T, Soejima K, Kanazawa M, et al. [Pulmonary emphysematous changes associated with Pneumocystis carinii pneumonia in an AIDS patient]. Nihon Kokyuki Gakkai Zasshi 1998;36:283–7.

63. Kuhlman JE, Knowles MC, Fishman EK, Siegelman SS. Premature bullous pulmonary damage in AIDS: CT diagnosis. Radiology 1989;173:23–6.

64. Santamaria F, Parenti G, Guidi G, et al. Early detection of lung involvement in lysinuric protein intolerance: role of high-resolution computed tomography and radioisotopic methods. Am J Respir Crit Care Med 1996;153:731–5.

65. Volpini E, Convertino G, Fulgoni P, et al. Pulmonary changes in a man affected by von Recklinghausen's disease. Monaldi Arch Chest Dis 1996;51:123–4.

66. Jafri SZ, Bree RL, Glazer GM, et al. Computed tomography and ultrasound findings in Klippel-Trenaunay syndrome. J Comput Assist Tomogr 1983;7:457–60.

67. Greene R, Lechner GL. "Saber-sheath" trachea: a clinical and functional study of marked coronal narrowing of the intrathoracic trachea. Radiology 1975;115:265–8.

69. Remy-Jardin M, Remy J, Boulenguez C, et al. Morphologic effects of cigarette smoking on airways and pulmonary parenchyma in healthy adult volunteers: CT evaluation and correlation with pulmonary function tests. Radiology 1993;186:107–15.

70. Heyneman LE, Ward S, Lynch DA, et al. Respiratory bronchiolitis, respiratory bronchiolitis-associated interstitial lung disease, and desquamative interstitial pneumonia: different entities or part of the spectrum of the same disease process? AJR Am J Roentgenol 1999;173:1617–22.

71. Park JS, Brown KK, Tuder RM, et al. Respiratory bronchiolitis-associated interstitial lung disease: radiologic features with clinical and pathologic correlation. J Comput Assist Tomogr 2002;26:13–20.

72. Gruden J, Webb WR. CT findings in a proved case of respiratory bronchiolitis. Am J Roentgenol 1993;161:44–46.

73. Holt R, Schmidt R, Godwin J, Raghu G. High resolution CT in respiratory bronchiolitis-associated interstitial lung disease. J Comput Assist Tomogr 1993;1993:46–50.

74. Warren C. Extrinsic allergic alveolitis: a disease commoner in nonsmokers. Thorax 1977;32:567–73.

75. Kulwiec E, Lynch D, Aguayo S, et al. Imaging of pulmonary histiocytosis X. Radiographics 1992;12:515–26.

76. Grenier P, Chevret S, Beigelman C, et al. Chronic diffuse infiltrative lung disease: determination of the diagnostic value of clinical data, chest radiography, and CT and Bayesian analysis. Radiology 1994;191:383–90.

77. Moore A, Godwin J, Muller N, al e. Pulmonary histiocytosis X: comparison of radiographic and CT findings. Radiology 1989;172:249–54.

78. Brauner MW, Grenier P, Mouelhi MM, et al. Pulmonary histiocytosis X: evaluation with high-resolution CT. Radiology 1989;172:255–8.

79. Bonelli FS, Hartman TE, Swensen SJ, Sherrick A. Accuracy of high-resolution CT in diagnosing lung diseases. AJR Am J Roentgenol 1998;170:1507–12.

80. Sherman S, Skoney JA, Ravikrishnan KP. Routine chest radiographs in exacerbations of chronic obstructive pulmonary disease. Diagnostic value. Arch Intern Med 1989;149:2493–6.

81. Gierada DS, Glazer HS, Slone RM. Pseudomass due to atelectasis in patients with severe bullous emphysema. AJR Am J Roentgenol 1997;168:85–92.

82. O'Rourke JP, Yee ES. Civilian spontaneous pneumothorax. Treatment options and long-term results. Chest 1989;96:1302–6.

83. Videm V, Pillgram-Larsen J, Ellingsen O, et al. Spontaneous pneumothorax in chronic obstructive pulmonary disease: complications, treatment and recurrences. Eur J Respir Dis 1987;71:365–71.

84. Light RW, O'Hara VS, Moritz TE, et al. Intrapleural tetracycline for the prevention of recurrent spontaneous pneumothorax. Results of a Department of Veterans Affairs cooperative study. JAMA 1990;264:2224–30.

85. Bense L, Lewander R, Eklund G, et al. Nonsmoking, non-alpha 1-antitrypsin deficiency-induced emphysema in nonsmokers with healed spontaneous pneumothorax, identified by computed tomography of the lungs. Chest 1993;103:433–8.

86. Phillips GD, Trotman-Dickenson B, Hodson ME, Geddes DM. Role of CT in the management of pneumothorax in patients with complex cystic lung disease. Chest 1997;112:275–8.

87. Chang CH. The normal roentgenographic measurement of the right descending pulmonary artery in 1,085 cases. Am J Roentgenol Radium Ther Nucl Med 1962;87:929–35.

88. Chang CH. The normal roentgenographic measurement of the right descending pulmonary artery in 1,085 cases and its clinical application. II. Clinical application of the measurement of the right descending pulmonary artery in the radiological diagnosis of pulmonary hypertensions from various causes. Nagoya J Med Sci 1965;28:67–80.

89. Matthay RA, Schwarz MI, Ellis JH Jr, et al. Pulmonary artery hypertension in chronic obstructive pulmonary disease: determination by chest radiography. Invest Radiol 1981;16:95–100.

90. Teichmann V, Jezek V, Herles F. Relevance of width of right descending branch of pulmonary artery as a radiological sign of pulmonary hypertension. Thorax 1970;25:91–6.

91. Kuriyama K, Gamsu G, Stern RG, et al. CT-determined pulmonary artery diameters in predicting pulmonary hypertension. Invest Radiol 1984;19:16–22.

92. Maki DD, Miller WT Jr, Aronchick JM, et al. Advanced emphysema: preoperative chest radiographic findings as predictors of outcome following lung volume reduction surgery. Radiology 1999;212:49–55.

93. Lando Y, Boiselle P, Shade D, et al. Effect of lung volume reduction surgery on bony thorax configuration in severe COPD. Chest 1999;116:30–9.

94. Slone RM, Gierada DS. Radiology of pulmonary emphysema and lung volume reduction surgery. Semin Thorac Cardiovasc Surg 1996;8:61–82.

95. Gierada DS, Yusen RD, Villanueva I, et al. Patient selection for lung volume reduction surgery: an objective model based on prior clinical decisions and quantitative CT analysis. Chest 2000;117:991–8.

96. Holbert JM, Brown ML, Sciurba FC, et al. Changes in lung volume and volume of emphysema after unilateral lung reduction surgery: analysis with CT lung densitometry. Radiology 1996;201:793–7.

97. Bae KT, Slone RM, Gierada DS, et al. Patients with emphysema: quantitative CT analysis before and after lung volume reduction surgery. Work in progress. Radiology 1997;203:705–14.

98. Weder W, Thurnheer R, Stammberger U, Burge M, Russi EW, Bloch KE. Radiologic emphysema morphology is associated with outcome after surgical lung volume reduction. Ann Thorac Surg 1997;64:313–9; discussion 319–20.

99. Szekely LA, Oelberg DA, Wright C, Johnson DC, Wain J, Trotman-Dickenson B, et al. Preoperative predictors of operative morbidity and mortality in COPD patients undergoing bilateral lung volume reduction surgery. Chest 1997;111:550–8.

100. Nakano Y, Coxson HO, Bosan S, Rogers RM, Sciurba FC, Keenan RJ, et al. Core to rind distribution of severe emphysema predicts outcome of lung volume reduction surgery. Am J Respir Crit Care Med 2001;164:2195–9.

101. Coxson HO, Whittall KP, Nakano Y, Rogers RM, Sciurba FC, Keenan RJ, et al. Selection of patients for lung volume reduction surgery using a power law analysis of the computed tomographic scan. Thorax 2003;58:510–4.

102. Naunheim KS, Wood DE, Krasna MJ, DeCamp MM, Jr., Ginsburg ME, McKenna RJ, Jr., et al. Predictors of operative mortality and cardiopulmonary morbidity in the National Emphysema Treatment Trial. J Thorac Cardiovasc Surg 2006;131:43–53.

103. Martinez FJ, Foster G, Curtis JL, et al. Predictors of mortality in patients with emphysema and severe airflow obstruction. Am J Respir Crit Care Med 2006;173:1326–34.

104. Hedlund LW, Vock P, Effmann EL. Evaluating lung density by computed tomography. Semin Respir Med 1983;5:76–87.

105. Müller NL, Staples CA, Miller RR, Abboud RT. "Density mask." An objective method to quantitate emphysema using computed tomography. Chest 1988;94:782–7.

106. Gevenois PA, de Maertelaer V, De Vuyst P, et al. Comparison of computed density and macroscopic morphometry in pulmonary emphysema. Am J Respir Crit Care Med 1995;152:653–7.

107. Gevenois PA, De Vuyst P, de Maertelaer V, et al. Comparison of computed density and microscopic morphometry in pulmonary emphysema. Am J Respir Crit Care Med 1996;154:187–92.

108. Madani A, Zanen J, de Maertelaer V, Gevenois PA. Pulmonary emphysema: objective quantification at multi-detector row CT—comparison with macroscopic and microscopic morphometry. Radiology 2006;238:1036–43.

109. Coxson HO, Rogers RM, Whittall KP, et al. A quantification of the lung surface area in emphysema using computed tomography. Am J Respir Crit Care Med 1999;159:851–6.

110. Hayhurst MD, Flenley DC, McLean A, et al. Diagnosis of pulmonary emphysema by computerized tomography. Lancet 1984;2:320–2.

111. Gould GA, MacNee W, McLean A, et al. CT measurements of lung density in life can quantitate distal airspace enlargement—an essential defining feature of human emphysema. Am Rev Respir Dis 1988;137:380–92.

112. Dirksen A. A randomized clinical trial of a-1 antitrypsin augmentation therapy. Am J Respir Crit Care Med 1999;160:1468–72.

113. Dirksen A, Friis M, Olesen KP, et al. Progress of emphysema in severe a1-antitrypsin deficiency as assessed by annual CT. Acta Radiol 1997;38:826–32.

114. Stolk J, Dirksen A, van der Lugt AA, et al. Repeatability of lung density measurements with low-dose computed tomography in subjects with alpha-1-antitrypsin deficiency-associated emphysema. Invest Radiol 2001;36:648–51.

115. Newell JD Jr, Hogg JC, Snider GL. Report of a workshop: quantitative computed tomography scanning in longitudinal studies of emphysema. Eur Respir J 2004;23:769–75.

116. Mishima M, Hirai T, Itoh H, et al. Complexity of terminal airspace geometry assessed by lung computed tomography in normal subjects and patients with chronic obstructive pulmonary disease. Proc Natl Acad Sci U S A 1999; 96: 8829–34.

117. Uppaluri R, Mitsa T, Sonka M, et al. Quantification of pulmonary emphysema from lung computed tomography images. Am J Respir Crit Care Med 1997;156:248–54.

118. Rogers RM, Coxson HO, Sciurba FC, et al. Preoperative severity of emphysema predictive of improvement after lung volume reduction surgery: use of CT morphometry. Chest 2000;118:1240–7.

119. Flaherty KR, Kazerooni EA, Curtis JL, et al. Short–term and long-term outcomes after bilateral lung volume reduction

surgery: prediction by quantitative CT. Chest 2001;119:1337–46.

120. Fishman A, Martinez F, Naunheim K, et al. A randomized trial comparing lung-volume-reduction surgery with medical therapy for severe emphysema. N Engl J Med 2003; 348:2059–73.

121. Dirksen A, Dijkman JH, Madsen F, Stoel B, Hutchison DC, Ulrik CS, et al. A randomized clinical trial of alpha(1)-antitrypsin augmentation therapy. Am J Respir Crit Care Med 1999;160:1468–72.

122. Mao JT, Goldin JG, Dermand J, et al. A pilot study of all-trans-retinoic acid for the treatment of human emphysema. Am J Respir Crit Care Med 2002;165:718–23.

123. Parr DG, Stoel BC, Stolk J, et al. Influence of calibration on densitometric studies of emphysema progression using computed tomography. Am J Respir Crit Care Med 2004;170:883–90.

124. Boedeker KL, McNitt-Gray MF, Rogers SR, et al. Emphysema: effect of reconstruction algorithm on CT imaging measures. Radiology 2004;232:295–301.

125. Stoel BC, Bakker ME, Stolk J, et al. Comparison of the sensitivities of 5 different computed tomography scanners for the assessment of the progression of pulmonary emphysema: a phantom study. Invest Radiol 2004;39:1–7.

126. Webb WR, Gamsu G, Wall SD, et al. CT of a bronchial phantom: factors affecting appearance and size measurements. Invest Radiol 1984;19:394–8.

127. McNamara AE, Muller NL, Okazawa M, et al. Airway narrowing in excised canine lung measured by high-resolution computed tomography. J Appl Physiol 1992;73:307–16.

128. Okazawa M, Muller NL, McNamara AE, et al. Human airway narrowing measured using high resolution computed tomography. Am J Respir Crit Care Med 1996;154:1557–62.

129. Nakano Y, Whittall KP, Kalloger SE, et al. Development and validation of human airway analysis algorithm using multi-detector row CT. Proc SPIE 2002;4683:460–9.

130. Nakano Y, Muro S, Sakai H, et al. Computed tomographic measurements of airway dimensions and emphysema in smokers. Correlation with lung function. Am J Respir Crit Care Med 2000;162:1102–8.

131. Reinhardt JM, D'Souza ND, Hoffman EA. Accurate measurement of intrathoracic airways. IEEE Trans Med Imaging 1997;16:820–7.

132. King GG, Muller NL, Whittall KP, et al. An analysis algorithm for measuring airway lumen and wall areas from high-resolution computed tomographic data. Am J Respir Crit Care Med 2000;161:574–80.

133. Saba OI, Hoffman EA, Reinhardt JM. Maximizing quantitative accuracy of lung airway lumen and wall measures obtained from x-ray CT imaging. J Appl Physiol 2003;95:1063–75.

134. Ferretti GR, Bricault I, Coulomb M. Virtual tools for imaging of the thorax. Eur Respir J 2001;18:381–92.

135. Ferretti GR, Vining DJ, Knoplioch J, Coulomb M. Tracheobronchial tree: three-dimensional spiral CT with bronchoscopic perspective. J Comput Assist Tomogr 1996; 20:777–81.

136. Aykac D, Hoffman EA, McLennan G, Reinhardt JM. Segmentation and analysis of the human airway tree from three-dimensional x-ray CT images. IEEE Trans Med Imaging 2003;22:940–50.

137. Niimi A, Matsumoto H, Amitani R, et al. Effect of short-term treatment with inhaled corticosteroid on airway wall thickening in asthma. Am J Med 2004;116:725–31.

138. Hogg JC, Macklem PT, Thurlbeck WM. Site and nature of airway obstruction in chronic obstructive lung disease. N Engl J Med 1968;278:1355–60.

139. Hogg JC, Chu F, Utokaparch S, et al. The nature of small-airway obstruction in chronic obstructive pulmonary disease. N Engl J Med 2004;350:2645–53.

140. Nakano Y, Wong JC, de Jong PA, et al. The prediction of small airway dimensions using computed tomography. Am J Respir Crit Care Med 2005;171:142–6.

141. Hasegawa M, Nasuhara Y, Onodera Y, et al. Airflow limitation and airway dimensions in chronic obstructive pulmonary disease. Am J Respir Crit Care Med 2006;173:1309–15.

Airway Circulation in Chronic Obstructive Pulmonary Disease

Adam Wanner, MD

Chronic obstructive pulmonary disease (COPD) is characterized by structural and functional changes in the conducting airways and the alveolar region of the lung. The two parts of the respiratory system are not supplied by the same circulation: the airways receive their blood supply primarily from bronchial branches of the bronchial arteries, whereas the alveolar structures are invested by the pulmonary vasculature. There are anatomic and hemodynamic differences between the two circulations, and their respective contributions to the physiopathology of COPD differ.

Although the role of the pulmonary circulation in COPD has been extensively studied and well characterized, the same cannot be said for the airway circulation. It is technically difficult to assess the function of the airway circulation in intact humans, and this has limited the amount of information on the airway vasculature in airway disease, including COPD. In particular, specific data on transudative and exudative processes and inflammatory cell diapedesis in the airway microvasculature are scarce. However, with the recent advent of noninvasive methods to measure airway blood flow, a better understanding of the local regulation of the airway circulation in COPD is slowly emerging. Such information has clinical relevance, considering that in the context of COPD, the airway circulation is the conduit for inflammatory cell recruitment and the source of airway edema, is involved in the vascular clearance of locally released inflammatory mediators and inhaled drugs that are deposited in the airway, and regulates the distribution of systemically administered drugs to the airway tissue.

The purpose of this chapter is to review (1) the structure of the airway vasculature and the alterations in airway blood flow in COPD; (2) the airway vascular effects of cigarette smoke, a major cause of COPD; and (3) the actions of pharmacologic agents on airway blood flow. For comparison, data on the normal structure and function of the airway circulation are also provided.

Normal Airway Circulation

The bronchial circulation is a high-pressure, small-volume system that derives arterial blood from the systemic circulation. Its main function is to provide nutrition to the walls of the airway (airway circulation), to the large pulmonary blood vessels, to hilar structures such as lymph nodes, and to the visceral pleura.[1] Moreover, most of the blood supply to the intraparenchymal airways down to 1 mm in diameter is derived from the airway circulation.[2] In the intraparenchymal airways, the airway circulation anastomoses with the pulmonary circulation and is also known as "pulmonary collateral circulation" or "systemic blood supply to the lungs."[3,4]

Structure

In humans, bronchial arteries usually arise from the aorta.[5] Other sources include the intercostal arteries, the internal mammary artery, and the coronary arteries.[5] On reaching the main bronchus on each side, the vessels surround the airway wall as an annulus forming the peribronchial plexus, which supplies branches to the bronchi and vasa vasorum. Smaller branches of the bronchial artery penetrate the bronchial muscular layer and form an extensive subepithelial vascular plexus.[6–9] This design permits individual blood flow control through parallel resistors with the possibility of shunting flow from one airway vascular bed to the other.[6,10]

The two interconnected plexuses follow the airways as far as the terminal bronchioles, where the bronchial capillaries anastomose freely with the pulmonary circulation at precapillary, capillary, and postcapillary levels.[11,12] Within the airway wall, the majority of blood flow is distributed to the subepithelial tissue, where the microvasculature occupies 10 to 30% of tissue volume[13,14]; subepithelial blood flow has been shown to comprise up to 80% of total airway blood flow (Figure 1).[6,15–20]

From the dense subepithelial capillary network in the airway,[11,17,21,22] blood drains through a complicated system. Venous blood from the proximal (extrapulmonary) airways drains successively through bronchial veins, azygos, and hemiazygos veins to the superior vena cava and the right heart; therefore, this drainage is subject to right atrial pressure. In contrast, the remaining intrapulmonary bronchial venous blood drains through postcapillary pulmonary vessels into the left atrium.[6,23–27]

Function

A major function of the subepithelial vascular network presumably is to meet the high metabolic rate of the epithelium and submucosal glands.[28] The epithelium is active in both ciliary beating and active transport of ions

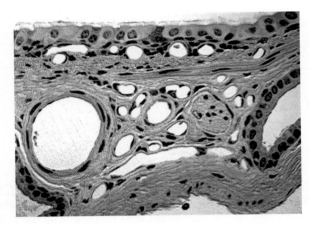

FIGURE 1. Subepithelial microvasculature in a large airway (sheep). Intravascular fixation at physiologic systemic and pulmonary arterial pressures. Note the microvascular volume, including arterioles, capillaries, and venule (H and E, 400x). Courtesy of Dr. Andrew Mariassy.

and macromolecules. The metabolic rate of cultured sheets of tracheal epithelia is high, corresponding to an oxygen consumption of 5.13 μmol.min^{-1}.g^{-1}. This value may be compared with 1.0 μmol.min^{-1}.g^{-1} for liver and 4.5 μmol.min^{-1}.g^{-1} for the beating heart.[11]

Under physiologic conditions, total bronchial blood flow comprises 0.5 to 1% of cardiac output.[4,6,9,28–33] Using various techniques, absolute values of airway mucosal blood flow, usually normalized for wet tissue weight, have been reported in different species, including humans.[34–39] Tracheal blood flow has been reported to range from 30 to 95 mL/min per 100 g of wet tissue in different animal models, with most values ranging between 30 and 50 mL/min per 100 g.[2,4,16,20,40] In healthy human adults, subepithelial blood flow in the tracheobronchial tree to a 200 μm depth from the epithelial surface ($\dot{Q}_{aw}$) amounts to between 25 and 40 μL.min^{-1}.mL^{-1}, where mL reflects the anatomic deadspace lined by the epithelium.[35,36,39]

Since the upstream and downstream pressures of the airway circulation are the aortic and left/right atrial pressures, respectively, those pressures are likely to have an effect on total airway blood flow.[41] Consequently, systemic arterial and left and right atrial hypertension, conditions that can exist in COPD patients who have pulmonary hypertension or cardiovascular comorbidity, could affect airway blood flow; thus far, this has not been investigated.

Although both adrenergic and cholinergic nerves have been demonstrated in the airway wall,[11] physiologic and pharmacologic studies suggest that the main nervous control of the airway circulation is by the sympathetic (adrenergic) nervous system.[6,10,11,19,27,42] α-Adrenergic agonists have been shown to induce vasoconstriction, whereas β_2-adrenergic agonists increase bronchial blood flow (Figure 2).[4,12,16,43–4] The site where the control occurs must be taken into account because large and small arteries show different levels of

responsiveness to the autonomic agonist. Subepithelial blood flow appears to lack local cholinergic control, whereas total airway blood flow is increased by vagal nerve stimulation and by intra-arterial or intravenous infusion of exogenous cholinergic agonists.[19,43,47,48] This suggests that subepithelial blood flow is regulated independently of total airway blood flow, as previously evidenced by Elsasser and colleagues, who demonstrated the presence of a local α-adrenergic control of $\dot{Q}_{aw}$.[49]

Autonomic nonadrenergic and noncholinergic mechanisms have also been described. Vasoactive intestinal peptide, histidine isoleucine, and histidine methionine released by parasympathetic nerves are vasodilators.[42,50] In contrast, neuropeptide Y released by sympathetic nerves is a vasoconstrictor in the bronchial circulation.[42,50] Sensory neuropeptides, such as substance P, neurokinin A and B, and calcitonin gene-related peptide released by unmyelinated sensory afferents, induce vasodilatation.[50,51] To what extent these and other inflammatory mediators have a role in the regulation of airway blood flow in COPD presently remains speculative.

Airway Circulation in COPD

Although the principal site of lung remodeling in COPD is at the alveolar level and therefore involves the pulmonary circulation, the conducting airways also participate in the physiopathology of the disease. The airway circulation relates to this component of COPD.

Structure

Early reports on the structure of the airway vasculature in COPD suggested that intrapulmonary bronchial artery branches are obliterated or narrowed in emphysematous regions of the lungs and that the bronchial venous system is greatly expanded.[52,53] These findings have not been supported by recent studies that showed some increase in airway wall vascularity in stable COPD with a slight increase in the number of vessels in small airways, but to a much lesser degree than in asthma, where there is an increased vascularity throughout the bronchial tree.[54,55] Thus, in contrast to asthma, angiogenesis in the airway wall does not appear to be a typical feature of COPD.

However, in patients with COPD accompanied by bronchiectasis, there is an extensive remodeling of the airway circulation with a marked proliferation and enlargement of the bronchial arteries and numerous precapillary anastomoses between the pulmonary and bronchial circulation.[4,45,56] This vascular remodeling is a likely cause of hemoptysis encountered by patients with bronchiectasis. It is also likely that the primary stimuli for the development of bronchiectasis and airway vascular hypertrophy are suppurative airway infections that typically are seen in these patients. In support of this assumption, chronic lung abscesses also have been shown to lead to a localized hypertrophy and hyperplasia of the airway circulation.[45]

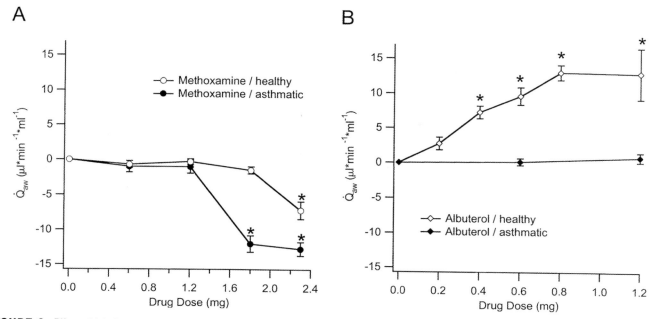

FIGURE 2. Effect of inhaled methoxamine (A) and albuterol (B) on subepithelial airway blood flow ($\dot{Q}_{aw}$) in asthmatic and healthy subjects. Mean ± standard error ($n = 11$ in each group). Data shown as change from respective baseline. *$p < .05$ versus baseline.

Baseline Airway Blood Flow

Using a soluble inert gas uptake technique, we found no significant difference in $\dot{Q}_{aw}$ among ex-smokers with COPD (51 ± 3 μL.min⁻¹.mL⁻¹), healthy ex-smokers (41 ± 3 μL.min⁻¹.mL⁻¹), healthy current smokers (46 ± 2 μL.min⁻¹.mL⁻¹), and healthy lifetime nonsmokers (41 ± 4 μL.min⁻¹.mL⁻¹), although the values tended to be higher in COPD patients.[57] In contrast, Paredi and colleagues reported a slower rise in exhaled breath temperature in COPD patients than in healthy subjects; they interpreted this as reflecting a decrease in airway blood flow.[58] The difference between the studies could be explained by differences in methodology or in patient populations with varying degrees of chronic bronchitis. Nonetheless, these findings are consistent with the morphologic observations that do not support the presence of significant new vessel formation in stable COPD in contrast to asthma. On the other hand, airway blood flow is likely increased in patients with COPD accompanied by bronchiectasis, reflecting the above-described hyperplasia of the airway circulation.[45]

Airway Blood Flow Reactivity

We have found that albuterol-induced vasodilation is blunted in ex-smokers with COPD (Figure 3),[58] similarly to patients with asthma.[35] Albuterol-induced vasodilation has been used as an index of endothelium-dependent vasodilation and endothelial function, especially in current smokers.[58] Since the COPD patients were ex-smokers and the asthmatics lifetime nonsmokers, it cannot be assumed that the abnormal albuterol responsiveness was due to endothelial dysfunction.

However, inasmuch as oxidative stress has been closely associated with endothelial dysfunction[59,60] and endogenously generated oxidants have been implicated in the pathogenesis of both COPD and asthma, it is conceivable that the blunted albuterol responsiveness of $\dot{Q}_{aw}$ reflects an abnormality in endothelium-dependent relaxation. To what extent the

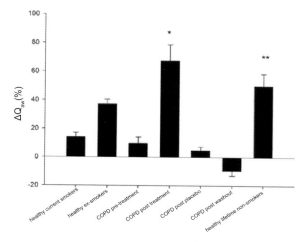

FIGURE 3. Subepithelial airway blood flow ($\dot{Q}_{aw}$) response to albuterol in healthy current smokers ($n = 10$), healthy ex-smokers ($n = 10$), ex-smokers with chronic obstructive pulmonary disease (COPD) treated with fluticasone-salmeterol combination (ie, pretreatment, posttreatment, postplacebo, and postwashout period) ($n = 10$), and healthy lifetime nonsmokers ($n = 10$). Data are expressed as the mean (± standard error) percent change from pre-albuterol value. The respective baseline values for ($\dot{Q}_{aw}$) were comparable among the groups.

defective vascular reactivity contributes to the development of COPD is unknown. It could be speculated that the blunted vasodilator response in the airways reflects systemic vascular disease such as systemic atherosclerosis that coexists with COPD.

Acute Respiratory Failure

Acute respiratory failure in COPD may be associated with increased pressure swings in the airway, dynamic hyperinflation, hypoxia and hypercarbia, and pulmonary hypertension. Measurements of the airway circulation during acute respiratory failure in patients with COPD have not been reported. However, the individual effects on the airway circulation of the mechanical and chemical stresses associated with acute respiratory failure have been investigated in animals, with human data confirming the findings in some instances.

The bronchial circulation is subject to the mechanical effects of airway pressure and lung inflation. Bruner and Schmidt were the first to investigate the effects of airway pressure on the bronchial circulation in dogs.[61] They found that an intratracheal pressure between 4 and 8 cm H_2O lowers bronchial blood flow independently of systemic blood pressure. Breitenbücher and colleagues found an inverse relationship between $\dot{Q}_{aw}$ and lung volume at zero airway pressure and between $\dot{Q}_{aw}$ and intrathoracic pressure.[62] Thus, acute respiratory failure-associated increases in both expiratory airway pressure and lung volume seem to decrease airway blood flow.

Increases in airway luminal pressures exceeding those encountered during quiet tidal breathing may also occur with coughing and with the use of cuffed tracheal tubes; increased coughing and the occasional need for tracheal intubation and mechanical ventilation are features of acute respiratory failure. This has been investigated with the application of positive end-expiratory pressure in dogs and sheep.[23,31,41,63–66] In those studies, an inverse relationship was found between tracheobronchial blow flow and airway luminal pressure, confirming the findings of Bruner and colleagues.[61] An interesting effect was seen at higher end-expiratory pressures when blood flow was diverted from the pulmonary vascular anastomotic route to the bronchial venous return via the systemic venous system.[66] These effects do not involve vascular smooth muscle contraction.[67] They probably are purely mechanical and due to stretching and compression of the bronchopulmonary anastomotic vessels.[60]

In the mucosa, under steady-state conditions, airway blood flow and blood volume are governed by arterial and venous pressure and interstitial pressure, which, in turn, is influenced by the pressure inside the airway lumen. Using a micropipette technique, microvascular pressure in the mucosa of the exposed rabbit trachea has been measured.[68] Values of 28, 17, and 14 mm Hg in the beginning, middle, and end of the capillaries, respectively, were reported. During tidal breathing, that is, normal spontaneous respiration, airway pressure is unlikely to influence vascular pressures[6] and hence blood flow in the mucosa of large airways. However, in the most peripheral bronchioles, where bronchial and pulmonary capillaries anastomose, microvascular pressure is probably lower than in large bronchi and airway blood flow may be subject to respiratory swings.[10]

Systemic arterial pressure, pulmonary capillary and venous vascular pressure, and bronchial venous pressure also determine bronchial blood flow. Several studies in dogs and sheep have demonstrated that bronchial blood flow is directly related to mean systemic blood pressure[32,61,69] and inversely related to mean pulmonary vascular pressures (pulmonary artery and pulmonary vein pressure).[14,69–71] A drop in mean systemic arterial pressure below 40 to 60 mm Hg[30,72,73] and an increase in pulmonary vascular pressure to above ≈ 44 cmH_2O[71] both decrease bronchial blow flow. Furthermore, Agostoni and colleagues demonstrated that when the pulmonary arterial pressure is increased over ≈ 46 cmH_2O and the pulmonary venous pressure is increased over ≈ 44 cmH_2O, the normal systemic to pulmonary blood flow is reversed.[71]

In most systemic regional vascular beds, hypoxia and hypercarbia increase blood flow. In contrast, these stimuli cause vasoconstriction in the pulmonary circulation, thereby reducing the perfusion of regions of alveolar hypoxia and hypercarbia.[29] The responses of the bronchial circulation to hypoxia and hypercarbia are still being debated.[23] Although there is little argument about the reported increase in total bronchial blood flow during systemic arterial hypercarbia and acidosis,[1,9,74] conflicting observations have appeared in the literature on the effect of hypoxia. Moderate to severe systemic hypoxemia has been reported to either increase[75] or decrease[74] bronchial perfusion in dogs. Sahin and colleagues studied tracheal vascular resistance in a dog preparation; they found that local arterial hypoxemia and hypercarbia increased tracheal vascular resistance, whereas systemic arterial hypoxemia and hypercarbia decreased it, an effect mediated by the central nervous system.[76]

Hypoxemia seems to have different effects on bronchial (total) blood flow and subepithelial blood flow ($\dot{Q}_{aw}$), as demonstrated in sheep by Elsasser and colleagues.[49] They found that hypoxemia caused by ventilation with a low-oxygen gas mixture increased bronchial blood flow by 41% while decreasing $\dot{Q}_{aw}$ by 27%. This could be interpreted as an appropriate physiologic response to hypoxemia whereby blood is diverted from the airway mucosa to the lung parenchyma via bronchopulmonary anastomoses, thereby promoting gas exchange.

Cigarette Smoking
Acute Effects

In several extrapulmonary vascular beds, smoking a cigarette has been shown to decrease blood flow transiently.[77–80] The airway circulation is one of the first systemic vascular beds to come in contact with cigarette smoke directly and is exposed to the highest concentration of cigarette smoke constituents. Their effects on airway blood flow therefore may be different from their systemic vascular effects. In anesthetized pigs, cigarette smoke increases airway blood flow transiently during the duration of inhalation, an effect that resembles inhalation challenge with nitric oxide.[81,82] This could be interpreted as indicating a vasodilator effect of nitric oxide contained in cigarette smoke. Inasmuch as cigarette smoke is an irritant, more prolonged vascular effects could be expected in conscious humans. Furthermore, cigarette smoke contains nicotine, a sympathomimetic that has variable hemodynamic actions in different vascular beds.[83,84]

We found that $\dot{Q}_{aw}$ increased by a mean of 81% at 5 minutes after healthy smokers smoked a cigarette[85]; the values were no longer different from baseline after 30 and 180 minutes. Cigarette smoke had no effect on forced expiratory volume in 1 second (FEV_1). Nicotine administered by nasal spray (systemic action) or oral inhalation (local and systemic action) had no effect on $\dot{Q}_{aw}$ or FEV_1, suggesting a pharmacologic or irritant effect of other cigarette smoke constituents. Thus, smoking a cigarette seems to cause transient vasodilation in the airway and vasoconstriction in extrapulmonary systemic vascular beds. Whether repetitive vasodilator responses to cigarette smoking have a role in the pathogenesis of COPD is not known.

Long-Term Effects

Although healthy current and ex-smokers have a near-normal baseline $\dot{Q}_{aw}$, as mentioned above, they have an abnormal vasodilator response to albuterol, presumably as a manifestation of endothelial dysfunction, as shown by Mendes and colleagues.[57] In that study, inhaled albuterol increased mean $\dot{Q}_{aw}$ by 50% in healthy lifetime nonsmokers and by 37% in healthy ex-smokers. In contrast, albuterol failed to increase mean $\dot{Q}_{aw}$ significantly in healthy current smokers (+14%) (see Figure 3). There was no correlation between the magnitude of albuterol responsiveness on the one hand and the amount of smoking in current and ex-smokers or the elapsed time after smoking cessation in ex-smokers on the other. The mean smoking-free time was the same in the healthy nonsmokers as in ex-smokers with COPD who were also studied and had a blunted response to albuterol. Yet, there was a partial recovery of albuterol responsiveness in healthy ex-smokers, whereas albuterol responsiveness remained blunted in the ex-smokers with COPD. The partial reversibility of albuterol responsiveness after smoking cessation in healthy ex-smokers but not in ex-smokers with COPD suggests that the abnormal vascular reactivity is sustained by the ongoing airway inflammation in COPD.

It may well be that the abnormal albuterol responsiveness in smokers reflects systemic endothelial dysfunction and that there is a correlation between systemic endothelial dysfunction and albuterol-induced vascular relaxation in the airway among healthy smokers. This remains to be investigated.

Pharmacologic Modification of Airway Blood Flow
Basic Considerations

As the principal source of blood supply to the conducting airways, the airway circulation can influence the metabolism and clearance of biologically active, locally released molecules, the distribution of systemically administered drugs to the airways, and the absorption of inhaled pharmacologic agents from the airway.[6,12,17,86,87] Therefore, alteration of airway perfusion may have important consequences in terms of the therapeutic effect of aerosol medications in the airway.[86] Pharmacologic agents that enhance airway blood flow, that is, vasodilators, may be rapidly cleared from the airway, thereby producing local effects of short duration compared with similar agents that lack a vascular effect. Conversely, augmenting airway blood flow may improve the distribution of systemically administered pharmacologic agents to the airway. Theoretically, an inhaled vasodilator may enhance the effect of a systemically administered drug by increasing its effective delivery to its final target, that is, the airway.[6] In contrast, combining an inhaled airway drug with a vasoconstrictor could enhance and prolong the local action of the airway drug.[38] Csete and colleagues showed that the magnitude and duration of the airway smooth muscle response to an aerosol antigen challenge in sheep could be increased or decreased with pharmacologic agents that decrease or increase airway blood flow, respectively.[88] Similarly, Wagner and Mitzner reported that the bronchoconstrictor response to inhaled methacholine can be enhanced by reducing blood flow to the bronchi.[89]

The mucosal barrier consist of at least five components: (1) the airway surface liquid; (2) the epithelium, which is the major component of the mucosal barrier for diffusion; (3) the basement membrane under the epithelium; (4) the interstitium of the airway mucosa; and (5) the subepithelial vascular network. Only after most of these components have been traversed will an active inhaled agent reach smooth muscle or glands and modify their function. For hydrophilic agents, but not for lipophilic ones, the epithelium is the major barrier for diffusion.[87,90] This means that among the commonly used inhaled airway medications, the lipophilic glucocorticoids and salmeterol can reach their deeper targets by diffusion, whereas the hydrophilic positively charged albuterol, formoterol, ipratropium, and tiotropium require epithelial organic cation transporters to be absorbed.[91] These transporters are pH sensitive, meaning that they transport less effectively at low pH. This may become a factor when treating COPD patients experiencing respiratory acidosis with these drugs administered by inhalation.

It has been suggested that an inflammatory increase in airway blood flow could favor the recruitment of inflammatory cells to the airway wall while increasing the clearance of locally released inflammatory substances (eg, spasmogens) and decreasing the magnitude and duration of the effect of inhaled bronchoactive drugs.[42] One might speculate that these opposing effects may be operative during acute exacerbations of COPD.

The bronchial circulation has an influence on airway mucociliary transport, as demonstrated by Wagner and Foster.[92] They found that by an unknown mechanism, the clearance of small insoluble radiolabeled aerosol particles from the airway was impaired when bronchial blood flow was stopped in sheep. Inasmuch as airway mucociliary transport is impaired in COPD, inhaled vasoconstrictors may further compromise this airway defense function.

Taken together, these observations do not provide a therapeutic rationale for selecting drugs based on their action on vasomotion because of the complex effects of airway blood flow on the physiopathology of stable and acutely exacerbated COPD. An exception may be the pharmacologic interaction between glucocorticoids and β2-adrenergic agonists.

Glucocorticoid-Adrenergic Interaction in the Regulation of Airway Blood Flow

Glucocorticoids and adrenergic agonists are stress hormones whose derivatives continue to form the basis of airway therapy not only in asthma but in COPD as well. These hormones have been shown to potentiate each other's effect in target tissues, including the airway. It has been known for some time that through a genomic action, glucocorticoids can upregulate the synthesis and G protein coupling of β2-adrenergic receptors, thereby enhancing the tissue responsiveness to β2-adrenergic agonists.[93] Indeed, we have shown that in patients with COPD, a 4-week treatment with an inhaled glucocorticoid-long-acting β2-adrenergic agonist combination restored β2-adrenergic responsiveness of airway blood flow (see Figure 3).[57] It is likely that the effect was driven by the glucocorticoid component of the treatment.

In addition, glucocorticoids have been shown to have acute, nongenomic actions in the airway that can potentiate the effects of β2-adrenergic agonists. Inhaled β2-adrenergic agonists are cleared from the airway tissue by local metabolism and vascular clearance. Glucocorticoids inhibit, within minutes, the uptake of organic cations including adrenergic agonists into non-neuronal cells containing the agonists' metabolizing enzymes.[94–96] This could increase the concentration of adrenergic agonists at adrenergic receptor sites in airway tissue, thereby potentiating the agonists' effects on airway and airway vascular smooth muscle. Presumably by acting through this mechanism on locally released norephinephrine, inhaled glucocorticoids also have been shown to cause an acute, dose-dependent decrease in $\dot{Q}_{aw}$ that can be blocked with an α2-adrenergic receptor antagonist.[97] The observation was made in healthy subjects and patients with asthma. It can be assumed that the acute vasoconstrictor response to an inhaled glucocorticoid would also be seen in patients with COPD. Thus far, this has not been tested. However, the glucocorticoid-induced vasoconstriction could further potentiate the pharmacologic effect of β2-adrenergic agonists by diminishing their vascular clearance.

The genomic and nongenomic interaction between glucocorticoids and β2-adrenergic agonists could become a relevant consideration in the treatment of obstructive lung diseases, including COPD. For example, the glucocorticoid-dependent potentiation of β2-adrenergic effects in the airway could have implications in terms of the timing of concomitantly administered glucocorticoids and β2-adrenergic agonists.

Conclusions

Patients with stable COPD and lung-healthy current smokers have baseline airway blood flow in the normal range but blunted endothelium-dependent airway vascular relaxation, possibly as an expression of endothelial dysfunction. Endothelium-dependent airway vascular relaxation can be restored with an inhaled glucocorticoid-long-acting β2-adrenergic agonist combination in COPD. It is likely that the glucocorticoid is the active ingredient. These findings suggest that inhaled glucocorticoids have beneficial systemic vascular effects in COPD and possibly in lung-healthy smokers as well. This remains to be shown.

Theoretically, restoring β2-adrenergic vasodilation and increasing the vascular clearance of the β2-adrenergic agonist with long-term inhaled glucocorticoid treatment could adversely influence the β2-adrenergic agonist's effect on other airway targets, such as airway smooth muscle. However, the clinical significance of this drug interaction is unproven and possibly mitigated by glucocorticoid's acute, transient vasoconstrictor effect.

References

1. Deffebach ME, Charan NB, Lakshminarayan S, et al. The bronchial circulation. Small, but a vital attribute of the lung. Am Rev Respir Dis 1987;135:463–81.
2. Ashley KD, Herndon DN, Traber LD, et al. Systemic blood flow to sheep lung: comparison of flow probes and microspheres. J Appl Physiol 1992;73:1996–2003.
3. Fishman AP, Turino GM, Brandfonbrener M, et al. The "effective" pulmonary collateral blood flow in man. J Clin Invest 1958;37:1071–86.
4. Fishman AP. The clinical significance of the pulmonary collateral circulation. Circulation 1961;24:677–90.
5. Liebow AA. Patterns of origin and distribution of the major bronchial arteries in man. Am J Anat 1965;117:19–32
6. Chediak AD, Wanner A. The circulation of the airways: anatomy, physiology and potential role in drug delivery to the respiratory tract. Adv Drug Deliv Rev 1990;5:11–8.
7. Charan NB, Carvalho PG. Anatomy of the normal bronchial circulatory system in humans and animals. In: Butler J, editor. The bronchial circulation. New York: Marcel Dekker; 1992. p. 45–77.
8. Bernard SL, Glenny RW, Polissar NL, et al. Distribution of pulmonary and bronchial blood supply to airways measured by fluorescent microspheres. J Appl Physiol 1996;80:430–6.
9. Laitinen LA, Laitinen A. The bronchial circulation. Histology and electron microscopy. In: Butler J, editor. The bronchial circulation. New York: Marcel Dekker; 1992. p. 79–98.
10. Wanner A. Circulation of the airway mucosa. J Appl Physiol 1989;67:917–25.
11. Widdicombe J. The airway vasculature. Exp Physiol 1993;78:433–52.
12. Lockhart A, Marthan R, Charan N, et al. Airway circulation in health and disease. Eur Respir J 1996;9:1105–10.
13. Baile EM, Sotres-Vega A, Parè PD. Airway blood flow and bronchovascular congestion in sheep. Eur Respir J 1994;7:1300–7.

14. Mariassy AT, Gazeroglu H, Wanner A. Morphometry of the subepithelial circulation in sheep airways. Am Rev Respir Dis 1991;143:162–6.

15. Wagner EM, Brown RH. Blood flow distribution within the airway wall. J Appl Physiol 2002;92:1964–9.

16. Parsons GH, Kramer GC, Link DP, et al. Studies of reactivity and distribution of bronchial blood flow in sheep. Chest 1985;87:180S–2S.

17. Wanner A. Clinical perspectives: role of the airway circulation in drug therapy. J Aerosol Med 1996;9:19–23.

18. Baile EM, Minshall D, Dodek PM, et al. Blood flow to the trachea and bronchi: the pulmonary contribution. J Appl Physiol 1994;76:2063–9.

19. Scuri M, McCaskill V, Chediak AD, et al. Effect of inhaled and intravenous acetylcholine on bronchial blood flow in anesthetized sheep. J Appl Physiol 1996;80:341–4.

20. Scuri M, McCaskill V, Chediak AD, et al. Measurement of airway mucosal blood flow with dimethylether: validation with microspheres. J Appl Physiol 1995;79:1386–90.

21. Laitinen A, Laitinen L, Moss R, et al. Organization and structure of the tracheal and bronchial blood vessels in the dog. J Anat 1989;166:133–40.

22. Beasley R, Roche WR, Roberts JA, et al. Cellular events in the bronchi in mild asthma and after bronchial provocation. Am Rev Respir Dis 1989;139:806–17.

23. Charan NB, Turk GM, Dhand R. Gross and subgross anatomy of bronchial circulation in sheep. J Appl Physiol 1984;57:658–64.

24. Charan NB, Turk GM, Czartolomny J, et al. Systemic arterial blood supply to the trachea and lung in sheep. J Appl Physiol 1987;62:2283–7.

25. Lumb A. The pulmonary circulation. In: Nunn's applied respiratory physiology. AB Lumb, ed. 5th ed. Oxford: Butterworth–Heinemann; 2000. p. 138–55.

26. Martinez L, de Letona J, Castro De la Mata R, Aviado DM. Local and reflex effects of bronchial arterial injection of drugs. J Pharmacol Exp Ther 1961;133:295–303.

27. Widdicombe JG. Tracheobronchial vasculature. Br Med Bull 1992;48:108–19.

28. Butler J. The bronchial circulation. NIPS 1991;6:21–5.

29. Link DP, Parsons GH, Lantz BMT. Measurement of bronchial blood flow in the sheep by videodilution technique. Thorax 195;40:143–9.

30. Baier H, Long WM, Wanner A. Bronchial circulation in asthma. Respiration 1985;48:199–205.

31. Salisbury PF, Weil P, State D. Factors influencing collateral blood flow to the dog's lung. Circ Res 1957;5:303–9.

32. Berne RM, Levy MN. Structure and function of the respiratory system In: Physiology. 4th ed. Berne RM, Levy MN, Koeppen BM, Tanton BA, eds. St. Louis: Mosby, 1998. p. 517–33.

33. Berry JL, Daly IB. The relation between the pulmonary and bronchial vascular systems. Proc R Soc Lond Ser B 1931;109:319–36.

34. Onorato DJ, Demirozu MC, Breitenbucher A, et al. Airway mucosal blood flow in humans. Response to adrenergic agonists. Am J Respir Crit Care Med 1994;149:1132–7.

35. Brieva J, Wanner A. Adrenergic airway vascular smooth muscle responsiveness in healthy and asthmatic subjects. J Appl Physiol 2001;90:665–9.

36. Kumar SD, Emery MJ, Atkins ND, et al. Airway mucosal blood flow in bronchial asthma. Am J Respir Crit Care Med 1998;158:153–6.

37. Brieva JL, Danta I, Wanner A. Effect of an inhaled glucocorticosteroid on airway mucosal blood flow in mild asthma. Am J Respir Crit Care Med 2000;161:293–6.

38. Kumar SD, Brieva JL, Danta I, et al. Transient effect of inhaled fluticasone on airway mucosal blood flow in subjects with and without asthma. Am J Respir Crit Care Med 2000;161:918–21.

39. Mendes ES, Pereira A, Danta I, et al. Comparative bronchial vasoconstrictive efficacy of inhaled glucocorticosteroids. Eur Respir J 2003;21:989–93.

40. Wanner A, Barker JA, Long WM, et al. Measurement of airway mucosal perfusion and water volume with an inert soluble gas. J Appl Physiol 1988;65:264–71.

41. Baier H, Yerger L, Moas R, Wanner A. Vascular and airway effects of endogenous cyclooxigenase products during lung inflation. J Appl Physiol 1985;59:884–9.

42. Horvath G, Wanner A. Tracheobronchial circulation. In: Barnes P, Drazen J, et al, editors. Asthma and COPD. Basic mechanisms and clinical management. San Diego: Academic Press, 2002. p. 1–6.

43. Wanner A, Chediak AD, Csete ME. Airway mucosal blood flow: response to autonomic and inflammatory stimuli. Eur Respir J 1990;3 Suppl 12:618s–23s.

44. Grollman A. The determination of the cardiac output of man by the use of acetylene. J Biol Chem 1929;88:432–45.

45. Charan NB, Turk GM, Dhand R. The role of bronchial circulation in lung abscess. Am Rev Respir Dis 1985;131:121–4.

46. Wetzel RC, Herold CJ, Zerhouni EA, et al. Intravascular volume loading reversibly decreases airway cross sectional area. Chest 1993;103:865–70.

47. Laitinen LA, Laitinen A, Widdicombe JG. Parasympathetic nervous control of tracheal vascular resistance in the dog. J Physiol (Lond) 1987;385:135–46.

48. Baile EM, Osborne S, Paré PD. Effect of autonomic blockade on tracheobronchial blood flow. J Appl Physiol 1986;62:520–5.

49. Elsasser S, Long WM, Baier HJ, et al. Independent control of mucosal and total airway blood flow during hypoxemia. J Appl Physiol 1991;71:223–8.

50. Laitinen LA, Laitinen A, Salonen RO, et al. Vascular actions of airway neuropeptides. Am Rev Respir Dis 1987;136:S59–64.

51. Widdicombe JG, Webber SE. Neuroregulation and pharmacology of the tracheobronchial circulation. In: Butler J, editor. The bronchial circulation. New York: Marcel Dekker; 1992. p. 249–89.

52. Cudkowicz L, Armstrong JB. The bronchial arteries in pulmonary emphysema. Thorax 1953;8:46–58.

53. Liebow AA. The bronchopulmonary venous collateral circulation with special reference to emphysema. Am J Pathol 1953;29:251–63.

54. Hashimoto M, Tanaka H, Shoshaku A. Quantitative analysis of bronchial wall vascularity in the medium and small airways of patients with asthma and COPD. Chest 2005;127:965–72.

55. Jeffrey P. Remodeling and inflammation of bronchi in asthma and chronic obstructive pulmonary disease. Proc Am Thorac Soc 2004;1:176–83.

56. Liebow AA, Hales MR, Lindskog GE. Enlargement of the bronchial arteries, and their anastomoses with the pulmonary arteries in bronchiectasis. Am J Pathol 1949;25:211–31.

57. Mendes ES, Campos M, Wanner A. Airway blood flow reactivity in healthy smokers and in ex-smokers with or without COPD. Chest 2006;129:893–8.

58. Paredi P, Caramori G, Cramer D, et al. Slower rise of exhaled breath temperature in chronic obstructive pulmonary disease. Eur Respir J 2003;21:439–43.

59. Schindler C, Dobrev D, Grossmann M, et al. Mechanisms of beta-adrenergic receptor-mediated vasodilation. Clin Pharmacol Ther 2004;75:49–59.

60. Zeiher AM, Schächinger V, Minners J.. Long-term cigarette smoking impairs endothelium-dependent coronary arterial vasodilator function. Circulation 1995;92:1094–100.

61. Bruner HD, Schmidt CF. Blood flow in the bronchial artery of the anesthetized dog. Am J Physiol 1947;148:648–66.

62. Breitenb‚cher A, Chediak AD, Wanner A. Effect of lung volume and intrathoracic pressure on airway mucosal blood flow in man. Respir Physiol 1994;10:316–21.

63. Modell HI, Beck K, Butler J. Functional aspects of canine bronchial-pulmonary vascular communications. J Appl Physiol Respir Environ Exerc Physiol 1981;50:1045–50.

64. Wagner EM, Mitzner WA, Bleecker ER. Effects of airway pressure on bronchial blood flow. J Appl Physiol 1987;62:561–6.

65. Cassidy SS, Haynes MS. The effects of ventilation with positive end-expiratory pressure on the bronchial circulation. Respir Physiol 1986;66:269–78.

66. Baile EM, Albert RK, Kirk W, et al. Positive end-expiratory pressure decreases bronchial blood flow in the dog. J Appl Physiol 1984;56:1289–93.

67. Wanner A. The airway circulation in bronchial asthma. Med Thorac 1989;42:189–94.

68. Nordin U, Kallskog O, Lindholm CE, et al. Transvascular fluid exchange in the tracheal mucosa. Acta Otolaryngol Suppl (Stockh) 1977;345:19–22.

69. Aramendia P, Martinez L, de Letona J, Aviado DM. Responses of the bronchial veins in a heart-lung-bronchial preparation. With special reference to a pulmonary to bronchial shunt. Circ Res 1962;10:3–10.

70. Charan NB, Turk GM, Ripley R. Measurement of bronchial arterial blood flow and bronchovascular resistance in sheep. J Appl Physiol 1985;59:305–8.

71. Agostoni PG, Deffebach ME, Kirk W, et al. Upstream pressure for systemic to pulmonary flow from bronchial circulation in dogs. J Appl Physiol 1987;63:485–91.

72. Auld PAM, Rudolph AM, Golinko RJ. Factors affecting bronchial collateral flow in the dog. Am J Physiol 1960;198:1166–70.

73. Magno MG, Fishman AP. Origin, distribution, and blood flow of bronchial circulation in anesthetized sheep. J Appl Physiol 1982;53:272–9.

74. Baile EM, Paré PD. Response of the bronchial circulation to acute hypoxemia and hypercarbia in the dog. J Appl Physiol 1983;55:1474–9.

75. Lilker ES, Nagy EJ. Gas exchange in the pulmonary collateral circulation of dogs. Am Rev Respir Dis 1975;112:615–20.

76. Sahin G, Webber SE, Widdicombe JG. Chemical control of tracheal vascular resistance in dogs. J. Appl Physiol 1987;63:988–95.

77. Czernin J, Waldherr C. Cigarette smoking and coronary blood flow. Prog Cardiovasc Dis 2003;45:395–404

78. Yamamoto Y, Nishiyama Y, Monden T, et al. A study of the acute effect of smoking on cerebral blood flow using 99mTc-ECD SPECT. Eur J Nucl Med Mol Imaging 2003;30:612–4.

79. Morgado PB, Chen HC, Patel V, et al. The acute effect of smoking on rertinal blood flow in subjects with and without diabetes. Ophthalmology 1994;101:1220–6.

80. Monfrecola G, Riccio G, Savarese C, et al. The acute effect of smoking on cutaneous microcirculation blood flow in habitual smokers and and nonsmokers. Dermatology 1998;197:115–8.

81. Alving K, Fornhem C, Weitzberg E, Lundberg JM. Nitric oxide mediates cigarette smoke-induced vasodilatory responses in the lung. Acta Physiol Scand 1992;146:407–8.

82. Alving K, Fornhem C, Lundberg JM. Pulmonary effects of endogenous and exogenous nitric oxide in the pig: relation to cigarette smoke inhalation. Br J Pharmacol 1993;110:739–46.

83. Benowitz NL. Cigarette smoking and cardiovascular disease: pathophysiology and implications for treatment. Prog Cardiovasc Dis 2003;46:91–111.

84. Vleeming W, Rambali B, Opperhuizen A. The role of nitric oxide in cigarette smoking and nicotine addiction. Nicotine Tob Res 2002;4:341–8.

85. Randhawa K, Mendes E, Wanner A. Acute effect of cigarette smoke and nicotine on airway blood flow and airflow in healthy smokers. Lung 2006;184:363–8.

86. Wagner EM. The role of the tracheobronchial circulation in aerosol clearance. J Aerosol Med 1995;8:1–5.

87. Widdicombe J. Drug uptake in the trachea. J Aerosol Med 1996;9:11–7.

88. Csete ME, Chediak AD, Abraham WM, et al. Airway blood flow modifies allergic airway smooth muscle contraction. Am Rev Respir Dis 1991;144:59–63.

89. Wagner EM, Mitzner WA. Bronchial circulatory reversal of methacholine-induced bronchoconstriction. J Appl Physiol 1990;64:1220–4.

90. Hanafi Z, Corfield DR, Webber SE, et al. Tracheal blood flow and luminal clearance of 99mTc-DTPA in sheep. J Appl Physiol 1992;73:1273–81.

91. Horvath G, Schmid N, Fragoso M, et al. Epithelial OCTN1/2 organic cation/carnitin transporters ensure pH dependent drug absorption in the airway. Am J Respir Cell Mol Biol 2007;36:53–60.

92. Wagner EM, Foster WM. Importance of airway blood flow on particle clearance from the lung. J Appl Physiol 1996;81:1878–83.

93. Mak JC, Nishikawa M, Barnes PJ. Glucocorticosteroids increase beta-2 adrenergic receptor transcription in human lung. Am J Physiol 1995;268:L41–6.

94. Celermajer DS, Sorensen KE, Georgakopoulos D, et al. Cigarette smoking is associated with dose-dependent and potentially reversible impairment of endothelium-dependent dilatation in healthy young adults. Circulation 1993;88:2146–55.

95. Butler R, Morris AD, Struthers AD. Cigarette smoking in men and vascular responsiveness. Br J Clin Pharmacol 2001;52:145–9.

96. Wiesmann F, Petersen SE, Leeson PM, et al. Global impairment of brachial, carotid, and aortic vascular function in young smokers. J Am Coll Cardiol 2004;44:2056–64.

97. Dawes M, Sienawska C, Delves T, et al. Quantitative aspects of the inhibition of (N)G-monomethyl-L-arginine responses to endothelium-dependent vasodilators in human forearm vasculature. Br J Pharmacol 2001;134:939–44.

CHAPTER 20

Pulmonary Hypertension in Chronic Obstructive Pulmonary Disease

Emmanuel Weitzenblum, MD, Ari Chaouat, MD, and
Matthieu Canuet, MD

The term *cor pulmonale* is still very popular in the medical literature, but its definition varies, and there is presently no consensual definition. Pathologic and clinical definitions have been successively proposed,[1,2] but it seems more appropriate to define *cor pulmonale* by the presence of pulmonary hypertension (PH),[3] which can be measured by right heart catheterization and noninvasively estimated, by Doppler echocardiography, and it seems justified to substitute for the concept of cor pulmonale that of PH.

Owing to its frequency, chronic obstructive pulmonary disease (COPD) is by far the most common cause of PH, far more common than restrictive lung disease, obesity-hypoventilation syndrome, pulmonary thromboembolic disease, and "idiopathic" pulmonary arterial hypertension. With time, PH may lead to the development of right ventricular enlargement, which may result in right ventricular failure, but it should be emphasized that PH is only one among other complications of advanced COPD and that the prognosis of COPD is linked to the severity of respiratory insufficiency rather than to the occurrence of PH, which is essentially a "marker" of long-standing hypoxemia. Indeed, this does not apply to "disproportionate" PH, but few COPD patients exhibit this severe degree of PH.[4]

Here we provide an overview of PH resulting from hypoxic COPD and try to cover all aspects of PH in COPD, from epidemiology to therapy.

Definitions

Forty years ago, an expert committee of the World Health Organization (WHO) defined cor pulmonale as "hypertrophy of the right ventricle resulting from diseases affecting the function and/or structure of the lungs, except when these pulmonary alterations are the result of diseases that primarily affect the left side of the heart or of congenital heart disease."[1] This pathologic definition is, in fact, of limited value in clinical practice since the diagnosis of right ventricular hypertrophy (RVH) is difficult to make during the patients' lifetime. It has been proposed to define cor pulmonale clinically by the presence of edema in patients with respiratory failure, but, again, this definition is far from satisfactory.[2] Finally, as PH is the sine qua non of cor pulmonale,[5] the best definition of cor pulmonale is the following: PH resulting from diseases affecting the structure and/or the function of the lungs; PH results in right ventricular enlargement (hypertrophy

and/or dilatation) and may lead with time to right heart failure (RHF).[3]

PH complicating chronic respiratory disease, particularly COPD, is generally defined by the presence of a pulmonary artery mean pressure (PAP) >20 mm Hg.[6] This is slightly different from the definition of idiopathic PH (PAP >25 mm Hg).[7] In young (<50 years) healthy subjects, PAP is most often between 10 and 15 mm Hg.[8,9] With aging, there is a slight increase in PAP but not exceeding 1 mm Hg/10 years as a mean.[8] A resting PAP >20 mm Hg is always abnormal, even in elderly subjects. In the "natural history" of COPD, PH is often preceded by an abnormally large increase in PAP during exercise,[10] defined by a pressure >30 mm Hg for a mild level of steady-state exercise. The term *exercising pulmonary hypertension* has been used, but the term *pulmonary hypertension* should be reserved for resting PH.

In the recent classification of PH, which was adopted following the WHO meeting held in Evian, France, in September 1998[7] and recently updated,[11] Chapter 3 deals with pulmonary hypertension associated with disorders of the respiratory system and/or hypoxemia. The etiologies are COPD, interstitial lung disease, sleep-disordered breathing, and alveolar hypoventilation disorders, but, again, owing to its frequency, COPD is the most common cause of PH, far more common than interstitial lung disease, sleep-disordered breathing (obstructive sleep apnea syndrome [OSAS]), and alveolar hypoventilation disorders (which include kyphoscoliosis, neuromuscular diseases, and the obesity-hypoventilation syndrome).

Epidemiology: Magnitude of the Problem

There are, in fact, few data on the incidence and prevalence of PH resulting from COPD. The main reason is that right heart catheterization cannot be performed on a large scale in patients at risk. An alternative is the use of noninvasive methods,[12] particularly Doppler echocardiography, which is presently the best method.

Another way of facing the problem is to determine the prevalence of patients at risk of developing PH, that is, patients with hypoxemic COPD. This was done in the United Kingdom by Williams and Nicholl, who observed that in the Sheffield population aged ≥45 years, an estimated 0.3% had both a partial pressure of arterial oxygen (PaO_2) <55 mm Hg and a forced expiratory volume in 1 second (FEV_1) <50% of the predicted value.[13] For England and Wales, this would represent 60,000 subjects at risk of PH and eligible for long-term oxygen therapy (LTOT). Extrapolating these results to the population of the United States, one arrives at a figure of approximately 300,000 COPD patients at risk of PH. Most patients with PH secondary to COPD are over 50 years of age, and about two-thirds are male.

The mortality related to PH complicating COPD is also difficult to assess. We do have data about the mortality resulting from COPD (100,000/yr in the United States, 20,000/yr in France), but we do not know the impact of PH on mortality. PH is a complication among others of advanced COPD, and it is not possible to separate it accurately from respiratory failure.

Pathology

The structural basis of PH in COPD includes three potential mechanisms: pulmonary vascular remodeling, reduction in the total number of pulmonary vessels, and thrombosis. Thrombosis was observed only in one study[14] and is probably negligible in most patients. Rarefaction of the pulmonary vessels could be expected in severe emphysema but has been documented only in idiopathic pulmonary arterial hypertension[15] and in animal models of chronic hypoxic PH.[16] Accordingly, the only demonstrated morphologic basis of PH in COPD is the remodeling of pulmonary arteries and arterioles.

Few studies using necropsy material have investigated the pulmonary vasculature in advanced COPD patients.[17–19] These studies have shown a muscularization of pulmonary arterioles (<80 μm in diameter). Pulmonary arterioles exhibit a distinct media of circularly oriented smooth muscle, whereas in normal subjects, there is no muscular layer. This muscularization of pulmonary arterioles can extend to the periphery in precapillary vessels as little as 20 μm in diameter. The muscularization of nonmuscular pulmonary arteries is due to hypertrophy, proliferation, and phenotypic transformation of contractile cells.

Changes in the intima are an important part of the remodeling of pulmonary arteries in COPD patients. Intimal thickening is observed in muscular pulmonary arteries and in pulmonary arterioles.[17,20] These intimal lesions are characterized by the development of longitudinal muscle, fibrosis, and elastosis. The other component of intimal thickness is the occurrence of inner muscular tubes, which correspond to a new layer of circular smooth muscle sandwiched between distinct internal and external lamina in pulmonary arterioles.[17]

It has been known for many years that pulmonary vascular remodeling is present not only in end-stage COPD patients but also in patients with mild COPD and even in smokers with normal lung function.[20–22] More recently, the Barcelona group showed that smokers with normal lung function may also develop intimal thickening in pulmonary muscular arteries associated with an increased proportion of muscularized small pulmonary arteries.[23] This observation suggests that pulmonary vascular lesions appear very early in the natural history of COPD even if PH is a late complication

and that hypoxia is an unlikely cause of these alterations. These structural abnormalities could be the consequences of an endothelial dysfunction of pulmonary arteries probably induced by cigarette smoke.[23,24] However, it must be underlined that the smokers and COPD patients included in these studies had no PH and that the clinical relevance of these early abnormalities is presently unknown.

Pathophysiology: Mechanisms of PH in COPD

PAP represents the sum of the pulmonary artery "capillary" (or wedge) pressure (PCWP) and of the driving pressure across the pulmonary circulation.[25] The latter is the product of cardiac output ($\dot{Q}$) and pulmonary vascular resistance (PVR). Accordingly, PAP = PCWP + ($\dot{Q} \times$ PVR) (Table 1).

Thus, three variables can contribute to an elevation of PAP: PCWP, cardiac output, and PVR (see Table 1). In chronic respiratory disease, particularly COPD, the role of an elevated cardiac output and of an increase of the wedge pressure is almost negligible. An increased cardiac output has been observed during episodes of acute respiratory failure in some but not all studies.[26–28] An abnormally high wedge pressure has been observed during severe acute exacerbations of COPD[26] and during a steady state of the disease.[29,30] However, cardiac output and wedge pressure are generally at normal levels in COPD patients, and PH is precapillary (Figure 1),[30] almost exclusively accounted for by the increased PVR.

Predominant Role of Alveolar Hypoxia

The factors leading to an increased PVR in COPD are listed in Table 2. These factors are numerous, but alveolar hypoxia is by far the predominant factor.[5,31] Anatomic factors (pruning of the pulmonary vascular bed) are classically distinguished from functional factors. In fact, alveolar hypoxia, the most potent functional factor, may have long-term morphologic consequences.

Two distinct mechanisms of action of alveolar hypoxia must be considered: acute hypoxia causes pulmonary vasoconstriction, and chronic long-standing hypoxia induces

Table 1	Possible Causes of Pulmonary Hypertension		
PAP	=	PCWP	+	driving pressure
PAP	=	PCWP	+	$\dot{Q} \times$ PVR

An increased PAP may result from
- an increased PCWP (postcapillary pulmonary hypertension: left heart diseases)
- an increased $\dot{Q}$ (shunts, hyperkinetic states)
- an increased PVR (precapillary pulmonary hypertension: respiratory diseases)

PAP = pulmonary artery mean pressure; PCWP = pulmonary "capillary" wedge pressure; PVR = pulmonary vascular resistance; $\dot{Q}$ = cardiac output.

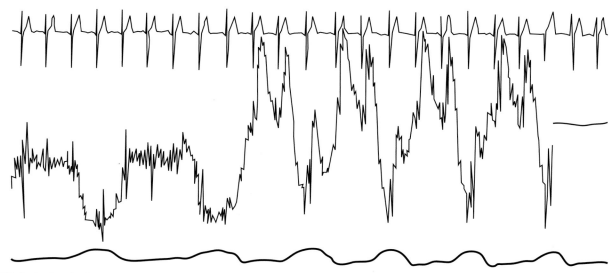

FIGURE 1. In chronic obstructive pulmonary disease (COPD), pulmonary hypertension is "precapillary": the pulmonary "capillary" wedge pressure (*left part of the trace*) is normal (9 mm Hg), whereas pulmonary artery pressure (*right part of the trace*) is elevated (25 mm Hg) owing to the elevation of pulmonary vascular resistance. In COPD patients, important swings of systolic and diastolic pulmonary artery pressure from inspiration to expiration are observed, which simply reproduce the elevated intrathoracic pressure changes.

(with time) structural changes in the pulmonary vascular bed, the so-called "remodeling" of the pulmonary vasculature.[32]

EFFECTS OF ACUTE ALVEOLAR HYPOXIA

Since the historic studies in 1946 by Von Euler and Liljestrand,[33] it has been known that acute hypoxia induces a rise of PVR and PAP in humans, as well as in almost all species of mammals, that is accounted for by hypoxic pulmonary vasoconstriction.[34,35]

Table 2   Factors Leading to Increased Pulmonary Vascular Resistance in Chronic Respiratory Diseases
Anatomic factors:
Reduction (destruction, obstruction) of the pulmonary vascular bed
Thromboembolic lesions
Fibrosis
Emphysema
Functional factors
Alveolar hypoxia*
Acute hypoxia (pulmonary vasoconstriction)
Chronic hypoxia ("remodeling" of the pulmonary vascular bed)
Acidosis, hypercapnia
Hyperviscosity (polycythemia)
Hypervolemia (polycythemia)
Mechanical factors (compression of alveolar vessels)

*The most important factor

This vasoconstriction is localized to the small pulmonary arteries. Its precise mechanism is now better understood. There has been, in particular, a marked increase in knowledge of the factors involved in the regulation of the vasomotor tone: smooth muscle cell potassium channels,[36] endothelium-derived mediators, principally nitric oxide (NO),[37] and endothelin.[38]

In normal humans, the reactivity of the pulmonary circulation to acute hypoxia varies from one individual to another,[39] and this interindividual variability is also found in COPD patients.[40,41] This means that some patients are "responders" to acute hypoxia, exhibiting a marked increase in PVR and PAP during the hypoxic challenge, whereas others are "poor responders" or even "nonresponders,"[41] as illustrated in Figure 2. The clinical situation that bears the closest analogy with acute hypoxic challenges is probably an exacerbation of COPD leading to acute respiratory failure and the sleep-related episodes of worsening hypoxemia (see below).

EFFECTS OF CHRONIC ALVEOLAR HYPOXIA

PH is generally observed in COPD patients exhibiting chronic hypoxemia (PaO_2 <55–60 mm Hg). On the other hand, a natural experiment of the effects of chronic hypoxia does exist: the PH that develops in healthy people living at altitudes >3,500 m who have a PaO_2 in the range of 45 to 60 mm Hg. These individuals have a mild to moderate degree of precapillary PH,[42,43] very similar to that observed in COPD. Morphologic studies performed in these highlanders have shown remodeling of the pulmonary vascular bed, with hypertrophy of the muscular media of the small pulmonary arteries, muscularization of pulmonary arterioles, and intimal fibrosis.[32,43] Importantly, this remodeling is potentially reversible since PH disappears when native highlanders spend a sufficient time at sea level.[43]

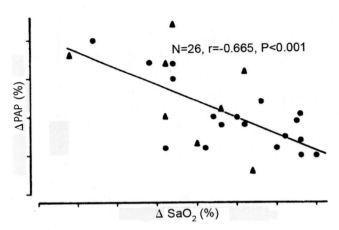

FIGURE 2. Variability of the pulmonary vascular response to a hypoxic challenge (fraction of inspired oxygen [FiO_2] = 0.13) in 26 chronic obstructive pulmonary disease patients. X axis: Δ SaO_2 = changes in arterial oxygen saturation; y axis: Δ PAP = changes in pulmonary arterial pressure during the challenge.

There is some degree of similarity between the structural changes in the pulmonary circulation in highlanders and those observed in COPD patients with PH,[18,43] and it has been deduced by analogy that the latter changes were a result of chronic hypoxia. However, the concept that the pulmonary vascular remodeling in healthy native highlanders and in hypoxemic COPD patients is similar has been challenged by Wilkinson and colleagues, who observed that the vascular remodeling in advanced COPD is not fully reversible with LTOT.[17] However, another morphologic study led to different conclusions.[19]

It should be emphasized that in COPD patients, chronic alveolar hypoxia is not the only factor producing an elevated PVR. These patients have marked morphologic changes of the lung parenchyma, particularly when emphysema is severe, and these changes could partly account for the increased PVR.[17] This probably explains why the remodeling of the pulmonary vasculature in COPD is not reversible with LTOT, which is different from high-altitude PH.

OTHER FUNCTIONAL FACTORS

The role of other anatomic and functional factors listed in Table 2, namely, the destruction of the pulmonary capillary bed by emphysema, hypercapnic acidosis,[44,45] hyperviscosity owing to polycythemia,[46] and mechanical factors (effects of marked respiratory pressure swings (see Figure 1) on the pulmonary circulation,[47] appears small when compared with the effects of alveolar hypoxia.[48]

Daily Duration of Alveolar Hypoxia Required to Induce PH

In COPD, hypoxemia is frequently permanent and is observed during both daytime and nighttime. Hypoxemia is subject to fluctuations and may worsen during exercise and sleep.

Sleep-related hypoxemia may be present in the early stages of COPD when daytime hypoxemia is not yet observed.[49,50] This has raised the question: can isolated nocturnal hypoxemia induce PH in humans? In other words, what is the minimum daily duration of hypoxemia that is required to generate permanent (nighttime and daytime) PH?

Studies performed in rats have shown that intermittent hypoxia (2–8 h/d) induces RVH.[51–56] In humans, we have two "models" of intermittent hypoxemia: sleep-related hypoxemia in COPD patients not exhibiting significant daytime hypoxemia and OSAS. It has been hypothesized that in COPD patients, sleep-related hypoxemia could lead to permanent PH.[57] Initial studies have shown that nocturnal desaturators had a higher PAP than nondesaturators, the daytime PaO_2 being > 60 mm Hg in all patients.[50,58] However, more recent studies included a larger number of patients and showed no difference in PAP between desaturators and nondesaturators[59,60]; PAP also did not correlate with the degree and duration of nocturnal hypoxemia.[59] Similarly, the great majority of OSAS patients do not exhibit permanent (diurnal) PH.[61,62] However, there is still controversy, and Sajkov and colleagues noted the presence of PH in some OSAS patients without associated pulmonary or heart disease.[63,64]

It thus appears that there is some discrepancy between the experimental data and the results of clinical studies and that observations made in animals cannot be transposed to the human condition. In most COPD (and OSAS) patients, isolated nocturnal hypoxemia does not appear to be sufficient to induce permanent PH. On the other hand, marked interindividual differences in the response of the pulmonary circulation to hypoxia have been observed in healthy individuals,[65,66] as well as in COPD[40,41] and OSAS patients.[66] In patients who are marked "responders" to alveolar hypoxia, repetitive elevations of PAP during sleep may lead, with time, to pulmonary vascular remodeling, even in the absence of daytime hypoxemia.[64]

Hemodynamic Features: Characteristics of PH in COPD
At Rest during the Stable State of COPD

PH in COPD is precapillary, with an increased pressure difference between PAP and the PCWP (see Figure 1) reflecting the increased PVR. In almost all COPD patients, marked oscillations of systolic and diastolic pulmonary pressures are observed with respiration (see Figure 1); these oscillations reflect the elevated intrathoracic pressure changes owing to increased airway resistance.

The main characteristic of PH in COPD is probably its mild to moderate degree, resting PAP in the stable state of the disease usually ranging between 20 and 35 mm Hg.[4,67,68] This modest degree of PH, also observed in OSAS patients,[62] is very different from other causes of PH, such as left heart disease, congenital heart disease, pulmonary thromboembolic disease, and, particularly, idiopathic PH, in which mean PAP

Table 3 Comparison of Pulmonary Hypertension Observed in Chronic Hypoxic Lung Diseases (Chronic Obstructive Pulmonary Disease, Obstructive Sleep Apnea Syndrome), and Idiopathic Pulmonary Arterial Hypertension

Variables	Idiopathic Pulmonary Arterial Hypertension[69]	COPD[67]	OSAS[62]
Number of patients	187	62	37
Number of women	110	2	2
Age (yr)	36 ± 15	55 ± 8	52 ± 11
FEV_1 (mL)	—	1,170 ± 390	1,830 ± 790
TLC (% of the predicted)	—	110 ± 15	80 ± 12
PaO_2 (mm Hg)	—	60 ± 9	64 ± 9
$PaCO_2$ (mm Hg)	—	45 ± 6	44 ± 5
PAP (mm Hg)	60 ± 15	26 ± 6	26 ± 6
PCWP (mm Hg)	8 ± 4	8 ± 2	8 ± 3
$\dot{Q}$(L/min/m²)	2.27 ± 0.90	3.8 ± 1.1	2.8 ± 0.6
PVR (mm Hg/L/min/m²)	26 ± 14	4.8 ± 1.4	3 ± 2.0

COPD = chronic obstructive pulmonary disease; FEV_1 = forced expiratory volume in 1 second; OSAS = obstructive sleep apnea syndrome; $PACO_2$ = partial pressure of arterial carbon dioxide; PAO_2 = partial pressure of arterial oxygen; PAP = pulmonary artery mean pressure; PCWP = pulmonary capillary wedge pressure; PVR = pulmonary vascular resistance; $\dot{Q}$ = cardiac output; TLC = total lung capacity.
Mean values ± standard deviation.

is usually >40 mm Hg and may exceed 80 mm Hg in some patients. Table 3 compares the pulmonary hemodynamic data of COPD[67] and OSAS[62] patients exhibiting PH with a large series of "primary" PH.[69] It can be seen that PAP is markedly elevated in primary PH (60 ± 15 mm Hg) but is modestly increased in COPD (26 ± 6 mm Hg) and in OSAS (26 ± 6 mm Hg) patients.

A PAP of ≥40 mm Hg is unusual in COPD patients,[4,70–72] except when measurements are made during an acute exacerbation[27,73] or when there is an associated cardiopulmonary disease, such as left heart disease, collagen vascular disease, or obesity-hypoventilation syndrome.[4] Special attention will be paid to severe or "disproportionate" PH in COPD, which has been investigated in recent studies (see below).[4,71,72]

The consequences of the (generally) modest level of PH in COPD include the absence or the late occurrence of RHF and the frequent inability of noninvasive methods to make a diagnosis of PH. Even Doppler echocardiography, which is by far the best method,[12] is not reliable in COPD[74] when compared with left heart disease or idiopathic pulmonary arterial hypertension.

Again, even if baseline PH is generally mild in COPD, it may worsen, sometimes markedly and abruptly, during exercise and sleep and during acute exacerbations of the disease.

Acute Exacerbations of the Disease

In patients with advanced COPD, acute exacerbations can lead to acute respiratory failure, which is characterized by a worsening of hypoxemia and hypercapnia. There is, simultaneously, at least in patients with PH, an increase in PAP from its baseline value during a steady state of the disease.[27,28] PAP may increase by as much as 20 mm Hg but usually returns to its baseline on recovery.[75]

Figure 3 shows the results observed by our group in 24 COPD patients investigated during an acute exacerbation with severe respiratory failure (mean $PaO_2 \approx 38$ mm Hg) and 3 weeks following recovery (mean $PaO_2 \approx 53$ mm Hg). The mean baseline PAP was 27 mm Hg, which increased to a mean of 44 mm Hg during acute respiratory failure. There was a striking parallel between changes in PaO_2 and PAP.

During Exercise

In advanced COPD patients with resting PH, PAP increases markedly during steady-state exercise. As illustrated in Figure 4, a COPD patient whose baseline mean PAP is modestly elevated (25–30 mm Hg) may exhibit severe PH (50–60 mm Hg) during moderate (30–40 watt) exercise.

Of interest, the behavior of pulmonary hemodynamics is identical in the two other groups (groups 1 and 2) shown in Figure 4, who are less severely disabled since they do not exhibit resting PH: in the three groups, PAP rises to about twice the level of its resting value. This is explained by the fact that PVR does not decrease during exercise in these advanced COPD patients,[29,76,77,79] whereas it does in healthy subjects. As the cardiac output is doubled for this level of exercise, PAP increases by about 100% (see Figure 4). From a practical

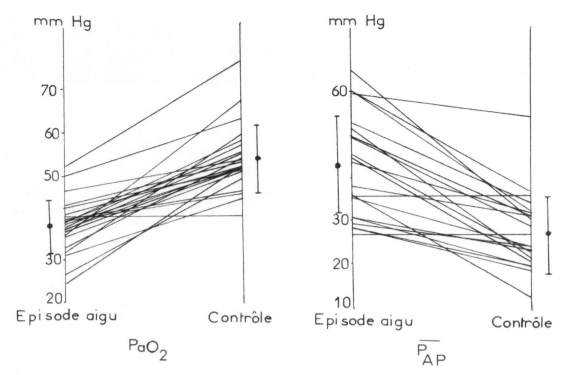

FIGURE 3. Changes in arterial partial pressure of oxygen (PaO2) and pulmonary artery pressure (PAP) in 24 chronic obstructive pulmonary disease patients investigated during an episode of acute respiratory failure ("episode aigu") and after recovery ("contrôle"). With recovery, PaO2 rose and PAP fell: the parallelism of these changes suggests the intervention of hypoxic vasoconstriction during acute exacerbations of chronic obstructive pulmonary disease (personal data, 1974).

viewpoint, this means that daily activities, such as climbing stairs or even walking, can induce marked PH. Raeside and colleagues showed that patients with severe COPD treated with oxygen could tolerate invasive hemodynamic assessment, including 24-hour ambulatory monitoring of PAP.[80] The highest levels of PAP were observed during exercise (and sleep), but performing normal daily activities also led to a significant increase in PAP.

During Sleep

COPD patients who are hypoxemic resting and awake become more hypoxemic during sleep.[81–83] The most severe episodes of nocturnal desaturation generally occur during rapid eye movement (REM) sleep.[83–85] The fall of saturation of oxygen (SaO2) during sleep from its baseline value during wakefulness may be as high as 20 to 30%.[83] These episodes of sleep-related desaturation are not due to apneas, except if COPD is associated with an OSAS, but to alveolar hypoventilation and/or ventilation-perfusion mismatching.[84,85] These episodes are often accompanied by peaks of PH.[86–89] The more profound the dips of hypoxemia, the more severe the peaks of PH.[88] PAP can increase by as much as 15 to 20 mm Hg from its baseline value.[80,86,88] There is generally a close relationship between changes in SaO2 and PAP during

sleep,[87,88] likely reflecting hypoxic pulmonary vasoconstriction. Sleep-related episodes of PH are of short duration,[89] and PAP returns to its baseline level with morning awakening.[88]

Thus, even though PH is usually mild (20–35 mm Hg) in COPD patients, it may increase markedly during exercise, sleep, and exacerbations of the disease. These acute increases of afterload can favor the development of right ventricular failure, especially during exacerbations of the disease.[73]

Diagnosis of PH in COPD
Clinical Diagnosis

Symptoms and physical signs are of little help in the diagnosis of PH in COPD. Symptoms such as dyspnea and fatigue are generally present in advanced COPD patients with or without PH; they are probably the consequence of airflow limitation and pulmonary hyperinflation rather than PH.

Physical signs that are observed in severe PH and particularly in idiopathic PH (a loud pulmonary component of the second heart sound, best audible at the pulmonary area; pansystolic murmur owing to tricuspid regurgitation) are rarely present in COPD patients with PH. This can be explained by the presence of mild to moderate PH in most patients, by the late occurrence (or no occurrence at all) of RHF, and hyperinflation.

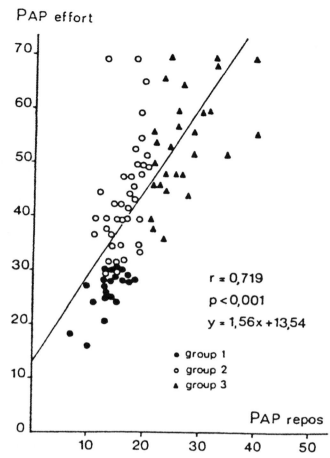

FIGURE 4. Resting pulmonary arterial pressure (PAP) and exercising (30–40 watts, steady state) PAP in a large series of chronic obstructive pulmonary disease patients ($n = 92$) (personal data, 1972). For comments, see the text. PAP effort = exercising PAP; PAP repos = resting PAP. Group 1: no resting pulmonary hypertension and exercising PAP < 30 mm Hg; group 2: no resting pulmonary hypertension, but exercising PAP >30 mm Hg; group 3: resting pulmonary hypertension.

Finally, peripheral edema occurs rather late in the course of COPD, and it is not synonymous with RHF in these patients: peripheral edema may simply indicate the presence of secondary hyperaldosteronism induced by renal insufficiency.[90]

Noninvasive Diagnostic Methods

The sensitivity of the electrocardiogram (ECG) for the diagnosis of PH is poor,[91,92] whereas the specificity of signs of RVH is high. Electrical signs of RVH occur late in the evolution of COPD patients and are absent in many patients. It is accepted that in COPD, the sensitivity of ECG for the diagnosis of PH does not exceed 20 to 40%.

The radiologic prediction of PH is even more problematic: the radiologic signs lack both sensitivity and specificity.[91] The diameter of the right descending branch of the pulmonary artery is often increased in cases of PH, but the specificity of an enlarged right descending branch is good only if the cutoff value is high and the sensitivity is generally low.

Magnetic resonance imaging (MRI) allows measurements of the right ventricular wall and chamber volume and of the diameter of the pulmonary artery and may prove useful for the diagnostis of PH and altered right ventricular structure and function.[93–95] The problem is that MRI is not routinely used in COPD patients suspected of exhibiting PH.

Doppler echocardiography is by far the best method for the noninvasive diagnosis of PH.[12,96,97] A technique that allows estimation of PAP from the measurement of the maximum velocity of the regurgitant jet in patients with tricuspid regurgitation (TR), using continuous wave Doppler echocardiography, was described in 1984.[98] The maximum velocity of the TR jet allows the calculation of the right ventricle to right atrial gradient from the Bernouilli equation: the gradient is equal to $4 \times V^2$ (V = maximum velocity of TR). The calculated gradient is then added to the right atrial pressure (5 or 10 mm Hg according to the clinical status) to give an estimated value of right ventricular systolic pressure that is equal to the pulmonary artery systolic pressure. With the same technique, in case of pulmonary regurgitation, it is possible to estimate the pulmonary artery diastolic pressure.

In cardiac patients, the values obtained are closely correlated with those found at right heart catheterization.[99] Although a TR signal can be recorded in 90 to 100% of patients with clinical signs of RHF,[98] the rate of success decreases in the absence of these signs.[100] In COPD patients, the chance of obtaining TR signals of sufficient quality is generally low.[74,101,102] Arcasoy and colleagues investigated a large series ($n = 374$) of candidates for lung transplantation (patients), most of them exhibiting COPD.[103] The estimation of systolic PAP by echocardiography was possible in only 44% of the patients (hyperinflation precluded optimal visualization of the heart), and 52% of pressure estimations were found to be inaccurate (more than 10 mm Hg difference compared with measured pressure obtained during right heart catherization).

Plasma brain natriuretic peptide (BNP) may be a biomarker of PH. BNP is a cardiac hormone that is synthesized by the ventricles and secreted into the circulation in response to increased wall stretch and tension as occurs during elevations in end-diastolic pressure. BNP appears to be a good marker for PH in chronic lung disease patients,[104] but further studies are needed to determine whether BNP is a useful diagnostic tool in COPD patients.

Is There Still a Place for Right Heart Catheterization?

Right heart catheterization continues to be the gold standard for the diagnosis of PH.[2,105,106] It allows the direct measurement of PAP, PCWP, right heart filling pressures, and cardiac output (by thermodilution or according to the Fick principle). Pressures and the cardiac output are measured at rest, in the supine position, during steady-state exercise, and, in some cases, after therapeutic interventions (oxygen, NO, and other vasodilators). From PAP, PCWP, and cardiac output, it is possible to calculate PVR (PVR = PAP – PCWP/Q). Right heart catheterization is generally performed with Swan-Ganz catheters,[107] but small-diameter floated catheters can also be used in COPD patients[75]; they are easily introduced percutaneously and are well tolerated.

Right heart catheterization has two main drawbacks: first, it is an invasive procedure, has some risks, and cannot be routinely performed in COPD patients. The second drawback is the inherent methodologic limitation of this technique: the fluid-filled catheter is incapable of measuring instantaneous pressures and does not give information about the natural pulsatility of the pulmonary circulation.[12,96] Micromanometer-tipped, high-fidelity catheters have been developed to overcome this problem.[96] However, these catheters are expensive and less flexible than the usual fluid-filled catheters.[96]

In most COPD patients, Doppler echocardiography should be attempted when PH is suspected. The indications for right heart catheterization should be limited when there is a suspicion of severe PH (systolic pressure estimated from Doppler echocardiography >50 to 60 mm Hg), in particular when COPD is associated with other respiratory diseases (eg, sleep apnea syndrome, interstitial disease, severe obesity); when there is a marked discordance between the results of Doppler echocardiography and the clinical and pulmonary function data; when an associated left heart failure is suspected in patients with severe dyspnea; and when preoperative evaluation of patients who are candidates for lung transplantation or lung volume reduction surgery is required.

Severe or "Disproportionate" PH in COPD

We have seen that in most COPD patients, PH, when present, is mild to moderate, with a resting PAP in a stable state of the disease ranging between 20 and 35 mm Hg. A minority of COPD patients exhibit severe PH, which can be defined by a resting PAP >35 to 40 mm Hg. This level of PH is considered "disproportionate" or severe PH in COPD and has promoted recent studies that aimed to evaluate its frequency, understand its mechanisms, and consider possible therapies.[4,70,72]

In 120 COPD patients who were evaluated for participation in the National Emphysema Treatment Trial, Scharf and colleagues observed that only 6 patients (5%) had a PAP >35 mm Hg.[71] Thabut and colleagues investigated 215 COPD patients who had undergone right heart catheterization as candidates for lung volume reduction surgery or lung transplantation and observed that the occurrence of moderately severe (35–45 mm Hg) and severe (>45 mm Hg) PH was rather infrequent, being 9.8 and 3.7%, respectively.[72]

Our group observed that of 998 COPD patients who underwent right heart catheterization between 1990 and 2002, during a period of disease stability, only 27 had a resting PAP ≥40 mm Hg.[4] Of the 27 patients, 16 had another disease possibly causing PH (eg, sleep apnea syndrome). The remaining 11 patients (11 of 998; 1.1%) had COPD as the only cause of PH. It is clear that severe PH is very uncommon in COPD.

Of interest, Thabut and colleagues identified by statistical analysis ("cluster" analysis) a particular subgroup of 16 "atypical" patients (7.4%) who were characterized by moderately severe bronchial obstruction (mean FEV_1 = 48.5 ± 11.8%) contrasting with severe PH (PAP = 39.8 ± 10.2 mm Hg) and profound hypoxemia (PaO_2 = 46.2 ± 15.7 mm Hg) but without hypercapnia ($PaCO_2$ = 39.7 ± 10.9 mm Hg).[72] In many regards, these 16 "atypical" patients are similar to our small subgroup of 11 patients with COPD as the unique cause of severe PH. Table 4 indicates that these patients had less severe bronchial obstruction than the remainder (COPD patients with severe PH and an associated disease; COPD patients with "usual" PH, and COPD patients without PH), and their mean FEV_1 was 50%. They had profound hypoxemia (mean PaO_2 = 46 mm Hg), hypocapnia (mean $PaCO_2$ = 32 mm Hg), and, by definition, a markedly elevated PAP (mean = 48 mm Hg). Thabut and colleagues' "atypical" patients and our own subgroup represent a subset of COPD patients in whom pulmonary vascular disease is predominant, and, interestingly, these patients present with hypocapnia.

How can the presence of severe PH in COPD patients with moderate airflow obstruction (but with pronounced hypoxemia) be explained? Two hypotheses can be proposed.[108] Some COPD patients could have an increased reactivity of pulmonary arteries and arterioles to stimuli such as hypoxia. We have seen that the response of the pulmonary circulation to acute hypoxia in COPD patients is characterized by a marked interindividual variability (see Figure 2).[40,41] The "high responders" to hypoxia could be expected to develop a marked pulmonary vascular remodeling when exposed to persistent alveolar hypoxia.[108]

The pulmonary vascular response to hypoxia may be inherited, and the study by Eddahibi and colleagues suggested a role for a genetic predisposition to PH in COPD patients since the 5HTT gene polymorphism appears to determine the severity of PH.[109] In 67 hypoxemic COPD patients who had undergone right heart catheterization, those (n = 21) who carried the LL genotype, which is associated with higher levels of 5HTT expression in pulmonary artery smooth muscle cells, had a significantly higher PAP than the 34 LS patients (p < .002) and the 12 SS patients (p < .005), whereas bronchial obstruction and hypoxemia were similar in the three groups (Table 5). Thus, the severity of PH could be determined by genetic factors.

The second hypothesis is the fortuitous coexistence of COPD and a pulmonary vascular disease somewhat similar to idiopathic pulmonary arterial hypertension. Some characteristics of the COPD subgroup with severe PH, such as hypocapnia and a low cardiac output, are similar to those observed in idiopathic pulmonary arterial hypertension. This hypothesis of an associated pulmonary vascular disease needs to be better documented, particularly by adequate morphologic studies.

It seems necessary to detect these COPD patients with severe PH because they have a poor prognosis when compared with COPD patients with "usual" PH (20–40 mm Hg) or without PH (< 20 mm Hg), as demonstrated in the study by Chaouat and colleagues.[4] Furthermore, they need an adequate

Table 4 Comparison of Four Subgroups of Chronic Obstructive Pulmonary Disease Patients Classified According to the Presence and Severity of Pulmonary Hypertension

Variables	Severe PH without Associated Disease (n = 11)	Severe PH with Associated Disease (n = 16)	Control Subgroup (PAP ≥ 20 mm Hg) (n = 16)	Control Subgroup (PAP < 20 mm Hg) (n = 16)
Age (yr)	67 (62–68)	61 (56–68)	66 (63–73)	62 (53–75)
FEV₁ (% predicted)	50 (44–56)	41 (35–63)	27 (23–34)	35 (29–50)
FEV₁/VC (%)	49 (39–53)	49 (43–55)	34 (26–38)	39 (31–52)
DLCO (mL/min/mm Hg)	4.6 (4.2–6.7)	10.4 (8.2–16.6)	10.3 (8.9–12.8)	13 (11.0–17.0)
PaO₂ (mm Hg)	46 (41–53)	54 (42–67)	56 (54–64)	72 (68–76)
PaCO₂ (mm Hg)	32 (28–37)	47 (34–51)	47 (44–49)	40 (37–42)
A-aO₂ (mm Hg)	56 (50–68)	37 (20–49)	30 (27–37)	28 (25–34)
PAP (mm Hg)	48 (46–50)	43 (42–49)	25 (22–37)	16 (13–18)
PCWP (mm Hg)	6 (4–7)	9 (4–18)	7 (6.5–7.5)	7.5 (7–7.5)
Q̇ (L/min/m²)	2.3 (1.8–2.5)	2.8 (1.9–3.8)	2.8 (2.4–3.1)	3.3 (2.9–4.0)
TPR (IU/m²)	21.3 (17.6–36.6)	14.9 (11.0–28.4)	9.0 (7.4–9.9)	4.0 (3.7–5.5)

Adapted from Chaouat A et al.[4]

A-aO₂ = alveolar-arterial PO₂ difference; DLCO = diffusion capacity for carbon monoxide; FEV₁ = forced expiratory volume in 1 second; PACO₂ = partial pressure of arterial carbon dioxide; PAO₂ = partial pressure of arterial oxygen; PAP = pulmonary artery mean pressure; PCWP = pulmonary capillary wedge pressure; PH = pulmonary hypertension; TPR = total pulmonary resistance; VC = vital capacity.
Values are median (interquartile range).
Severe PH (groups 1 and 2) is defined by PAP ≥40 mm Hg. In group 3, PAP ranges between 20 and 40 mm Hg ("usual" PH). In group 4, PAP is < 20 mm Hg (no PH). Group 1 is characterized by less severe bronchial obstruction, a marked decrease in DLCO, profound hypoxemia, and marked hypocapnia; the differences are statistically significant when compared with the three other subgroups.

Table 5 Characteristics of Chronic Obstructive Pulmonary Disease Patients Classified According to their *5HTT* Expression Genotype (LL, LS, SS)

Variables	All	LL	LS	SS	LL vs LS	LL vs SS
Patients (n)	67	21	34	12	—	
Age (yr)	62 ± 9	64 ± 8	62 ± 9	60 ± 8	NS	NS
Sex (F/M)	9/58	5/16	2/32	2/10	NS	NS
Tobacco (pack-years)	48 ± 18	42 ± 20	52 ± 15	46 ± 22	NS	NS
FEV₁ (L)	1.04 ± 0.40	1.21 ± 0.46	0.98 ± 0.37	0.89 ± 0.26	NS	NS
FEV₁ (% predicted)	37 ± 15	45 ± 16	34 ± 15	31 ± 9	< .01	< .01
FEV₁/VC (%)	47 ± 14	52 ± 15	46 ± 14	42 ± 9	NS	NS
PaO₂ (mm Hg)	60 ± 8	58 ± 7	60 ± 8	63 ± 8	NS	NS
PaCO₂ (mm Hg)	45 ± 7	42 ± 7	46 ± 7	46 ± 7	NS	NS
PAP (mm Hg)	27 ± 9	34 ± 13	23 ± 5	22 ± 4	< .002	< .005
Q̇ (L/min/m²)	2.94 ± 0.60	2.86 ± 0.67	3.00 ± 0.50	3.06 ± 0.58	NS	NS
PVR (IU)	5.9 ± 4.2	10.2 ± 6.2	4.6 ± 1.7	4.2 ± 2.3	< .01	< .05

Adapted from Eddahabi S et al.[109]

FEV₁ = forced expiratory volume in 1 second; NS = not significant; PACO₂ = partial pressure of arterial carbon dioxide; PAO₂ = partial pressure of arterial oxygen; PAP = pulmonary artery mean pressure; PVR = pulmonary vascular resistance; Q̇ = cardiac output; VC = vital capacity.
Values are mean ± SD.
LL genotype is associated with higher levels of *5HTT* expression.
For the interpretation of these results, see the text.

treatement: LTOT in those patients who are markedly hypoxemic (PaO$_2$ ≤55–60 mm Hg). Oxygen therapy may prove to be insufficient to stabilize PH or to reduce its progression, and other therapies must be proposed. Lung transplantation could be a choice in some patients. Pulmonary vasodilators and antiproliferative drugs, including prostanoids, endothelin receptor antagonists, and phosphodiesterase inhibitors, could be tested in COPD patients with severe PH, particularly in those who share some characteristics with idiopathic pulmonary arterial hypertension.

Evolution and Prognosis of PH in COPD

"Natural History" of PH in COPD

The progression of PH is slow in COPD patients, and several studies have shown that PAP may remain stable over periods of 2 to 5 years.[75,110,111] In all of these studies devoted to the "natural history" of PH, investigations were performed during a stable clinical state. A further study in which 93 COPD patients were followed for 5 to 12 years, with a mean of 90 months, confirmed that the changes in PAP were rather small: + 0.5 mm Hg/yr for the group as a whole.[112] Of interest, the evolution of PAP was identical in the patients with and without initial PH. This means that in the majority of COPD patients whose PAP was initially normal, it will not exceed 20 mm Hg after 3 to 5 years. A more recent article on the "natural history" of pulmonary hemodynamics in COPD patients with an initial PAP <20 mm Hg showed that only 33 of 121 developed PH after a mean interval of 6.8 ± 2.9 years.[10] This study also showed that patients with PAP >30 mm Hg on exercise at the onset (so-called "exercising PH") have a significantly increased risk of developing PH with the passage of time.

Nevertheless, a minority (about 30%) of advanced COPD patients exhibit a marked worsening of PAP during follow-up.[112] These patients do not differ from the others at the onset, but they are characterized by a progressive deterioration of PaO$_2$ and PaCO$_2$ during the evolution.[75,112] A significant correlation between changes in PaO$_2$ and PAP during the follow-up has been observed.[112] Thus, regular measurements of arterial blood gases are recommended for advanced COPD patients, particularly those with PH.[10,75] The longitudinal evolution of PH is favorably influenced by LTOT (see the Treatment section).

From PH to RHF

RIGHT VENTRICULAR FUNCTION IN COPD PATIENTS WITH PH

The classic view of the development of RHF in COPD patients is the following[2]: PH increases the work of the right ventricle, which leads more or less rapidly to right ventricular enlargement (associating hypertrophy and dilatation), which can result in right ventricular dysfunction (systolic, diastolic). Later, RHF, characterized by the presence of peripheral edema, can be observed in some COPD patients. The interval between the onset of PH and the appearance of RHF is not known and

may vary from patient to patient. Even if there is a relationship between the severity of PH and the development of RHF, marked differences can be observed in individual patients. Some patients with well-documented PH never develop clinical signs of RHF, whereas other patients with a similar degree of PH soon exhibit peripheral edema. The classic notion that peripheral edema reflects RHF has, in fact, been questioned,[2,113,114] and it has even been suggested that the occurrence of true RHF in COPD is unlikely, taking into account the modest level of PH.[114]

RVH, which is present in most patients with prolonged PH, is, in fact, a beneficial adaptation that enables the ventricle to face an increased workload (increased afterload) while maintaining adequate function. Similarly, right ventricular dilatation allows an increase in preload, which contributes to maintaining the cardiac output within physiologic limits according to the Frank-Starling mechanism.

Systolic ventricular dysfunction is generally defined by a decreased (< 40–45%) right ventricular ejection fraction (RVEF). RVEF is measured by isotopic methods and cannot be (presently) assessed by echocardiography. A decreased RVEF is most often the consequence of an increased afterload (increased PAP or PVR or both). However, variable correlations between RVEF and PAP have been observed in COPD patients.[68,115–117] RVEF also depends on preload. Accordingly, RVEF is not a good measurement of intrinsic right ventricular contractility,[2] and the presence of a decreased RVEF does not mean that there is a true right ventricular dysfunction.[118,119] The investigation of the diastolic right ventricular function is very difficult to perform and cannot be proposed as a routine procedure.

One way of assessing right ventricular performance is to measure right ventricular contractility. Indices of contractility were initially developed to assess left ventricular function; they are based on the relationship between the pressure and the volume of the ventricle at end-systole. The slope of this relationship has been called ventricular elastance, and it reflects ventricular contractility.[120] The end-systolic pressure-volume relationship of the right ventricle has rarely been investigated in COPD patients.[68,116,118,121] Burghuber and Bergmann observed that right ventricular contractility was identical and within normal limits in COPD patients both with and without PH, whereas patients with PH exhibited, as expected, a lower RVEF.[116,118] These results are in good agreement with those of the Edinburgh group.[68]

It thus appears that myocardial contractility is generally well preserved in COPD patients with PH, even though their RVEF is found to be low. The only circumstances in which a diminished right ventricular contractility could be documented in COPD were acute exacerbations with the presence of marked peripheral edema.[121] MacNee and colleagues showed that the right ventricular end-systolic pressure to volume ratio was decreased in six edematous COPD patients but not in eight COPD patients with similar levels of PVR but who did not exhibit peripheral edema.[121]

RIGHT VENTRICULAR FAILURE: CAN IT OCCUR IN COPD PATIENTS?

Peripheral edema is frequently observed in patients with advanced COPD and is considered to reflect RHF, but it may simply indicate the presence of secondary hyperaldosteronism[90] induced by functional renal insufficiency, which is, in turn, a consequence of hypercapnic acidosis and/or hypoxemia.[90,122] In COPD patients, the presence of edema is not synonymous with heart failure.[2,113,114]

The usual definition of cardiac failure (insufficient cardiac output) does not apply to COPD patients in whom cardiac output is preserved or even increased during acute exacerbations associated with clinical signs of RHF (peripheral edema).[26] It is practical to document RHF by the presence of elevated right ventricular filling pressures (right atrial pressure, right ventricular end-diastolic pressure).[26,73]

The role of pressure overload in the development of RHF in these patients has been debated. MacNee and colleagues found no difference in PAP between six COPD patients with marked peripheral edema and hemodynamic signs of RHF (PAP = 33 ± 6 mm Hg) and eight other similar patients without edema and hemodynamic signs of RHF (PAP = 30 ± 8 mm Hg), and they concluded that RHF in these patients was probably due to causes other than PH.[121] On the other hand, some COPD patients with peripheral edema do have RHF, which is best explained by a worsening of pressure overload during acute exacerbations of the disease.[73] This is illustrated in Table 6, which shows data in 16 COPD patients investigated before and during an episode of marked peripheral edema.[73] In 9 of 16 patients, hemodynamic signs of RHF (elevated [≥ 12 mm Hg] right ventricular end-diastolic pressure) were present during the episode of edema and were probably accounted for by a significant worsening of PH (from 27 ± 5 to 40 ± 6 mm Hg; $p < .001$), which, in turn, was explained by a worsening of hypoxemia (from 63 ± 4 to 49 ± 7 mm Hg; $p < .001$). Seven of 16 patients with edema had no hemodynamic signs of RHF and no significant changes in PAP from baseline (see Table 6); the origin of edema in these patients is unclear.

The occurrence of RHF was previously considered an indicator of poor prognosis in COPD,[123] but further studies have clearly shown that a prolonged survival of 10 years and more can be observed after the first episode of peripheral edema.[75] The prevalence of clinical RHF has markedly decreased with the implementation of long-term oxygen therapy for the most hypoxemic COPD patients.

Prognosis of PH in COPD

The level of PAP is a good indicator of prognosis in COPD patients with PH[67,110,124]: the prognosis is worse in patients with PH when compared with patients without PH. The prognosis is particularly poor for patients with a severe degree of PH,[110,124] but, as mentioned above, PAP measured in a stable state of the disease is most often < 35 to 40 mm Hg in COPD.[4]

The 5-year survival rate is about 50%.[67,110,124] LTOT significantly improves the survival of hypoxemic (PaO2 < 55–60 mm Hg) COPD patients, as demonstrated by the Nocturnal Oxygen Therapy Trial (NOTT) and the Medical Research Council (MRC) trial, which included a majority of patients with PH.[125,126] Consequently, it can be expected that the prognosis of PH will improve with LTOT, as suggested by Cooper and colleagues.[127] PAP is still an excellent prognostic indicator in COPD patients treated with LTOT.[128–130] Our group observed that in COPD patients given LTOT, the 5-year survival rate was 66% in those whose initial PAP was < 25 mm Hg but only 36% when the initial PAP was > 25 mm Hg ($p < .001$).[130] The prognostic value of PAP may be explained by the fact that it is perhaps a marker of both the duration and the severity of alveolar hypoxia.[130]

Treatment

The treatment of RHF in COPD relies on diuretics and oxygen therapy. The treatment of PH includes oxygen therapy and vasodilators, both of which are considered below. An important question is: is it necessary to treat PH in COPD? As we know, PH is mild to moderate in COPD, and the necessity for treatment can be questioned.[131] The main argument in

Table 6 Evolution of Arterial Blood Gases and Hemodynamic Variables in 16 COPD Patients Investigated Before and During an Episode of Peripheral Edema

Group	RVEDP (mm Hg)		PAP (mm Hg)		Q̇ (L/min/m²)		PaO2 (mm Hg)		PaCO2 (mm Hg)	
	T1	T2	T1	T2	T1	T2	T1	T2	T1	T2
1 (n = 9)	7.5 ± 3.9	13.4 ± 1.2*	27 ± 5	40 ± 6*	3.23 ± 0.82	3.19 ± 1.07	63 ± 4	49 ± 7*	46 ± 7	59 ± 14*
2 (n = 7)	5.5 ± 2.4	5.1 ± 1.5	20 ± 6	21 ± 5	3.63 ± 0.36	3.29 ± 1.32	66 ± 7	59 ± 7	42 ± 6	45 ± 6

Adapted from Weitzenblum E et al.[73]

PAP = pulmonary artery mean pressure; Q̇ = cardiac output; RVEDP = right ventricular end-diastolic pressure; T1 = stable state of the disease; T2 = episode of edema.
*Difference between T1 and T2 statistically significant, $p < .001$.
Group 1 = patients with hemodynamic signs of right heart failure (elevated RVDEP); group 2 = patients without hemodynamic signs of right heart failure.

favor of treatment is that PH, even when modest, may worsen, particularly during acute exacerbations, and these acute increases in PAP can contribute to the development of RHF.[73]

Long-Term Oxygen Therapy

Alveolar hypoxia is considered the major determinant of the elevation of PVR and PAP in COPD patients. One of the aims of LTOT is the improvement in PH induced by chronic alveolar hypoxia, but can this be achieved? Experimental data in animals, quoted above,[51,52] have raised the hope that pulmonary vascular changes can be reversed in COPD patients on LTOT. In fact, whether the structural changes of the small pulmonary vessels, which are observed in patients with advanced COPD, are potentially reversible on LTOT and whether these structural changes are fully accounted for by chronic alveolar hypoxia is at present unknown.[17,19] The well-known NOTT and MRC LTOT studies were not principally devoted to pulmonary hemodynamics; however, pulmonary hemodynamic data were available at the onset in all patients, and follow-up right heart catheterization was performed in a relatively high number of patients.[125,126] In the MRC study, 42 patients who survived >500 days from the onset of the study were catheterized again after at least 1 year of follow-up.[126] PAP was stable in the subgroup of 21 patients given LTOT, whereas it increased significantly (+ 2.8 mm Hg/yr) in the control group of 21 patients. In the NOTT study, hemodynamic data at the onset and after 6 months of LTOT were available in 117 patients.[125,132] Continuous ($\geq$18 h/d) LTOT decreased slightly but significantly resting (– 3 mm Hg as a mean) and exercising PAP (– 6 mm Hg as a mean) and PVR, whereas nocturnal oxygen therapy (10–12 h/d) did not.

We have compared pulmonary hemodynamics before and after the onset of O_2 therapy in patients ($n = 16$) as their own controls.[133] A reversal in the progression of PH was observed on LTOT; PAP was not normalized but returned to its baseline level 6 years (as a mean) earlier. When changes in PAP were expressed as changes/year, the difference was also statistically significant, with an increase of 1.5 mm Hg/yr before the onset of LTOT versus a decrease of 2.1 mm Hg/yr after the initiation of LTOT ($p <.01$).

More recently, Zielinski and colleagues investigated COPD patients given LTOT (15 h/d).[134] In 12 patients who completed 6 years of LTOT, PAP fell from 25 ± 7 to 21 ± 4 mm Hg after 2 years but increased slightly to 26 ± 6 mm Hg after 6 years. On average, there was long-term stabilization of PH with LTOT.

The best hemodynamic results have been obtained in the continuous oxygen group of the NOTT[125,132] and in our own study (17–18 h O_2/d),[133] that is, in the studies in which the daily duration of oxygen therapy was the longest. Accordingly, one should recommend continuous oxygen therapy.

In summary, LTOT stabilizes or at least attenuates and sometimes reverses the progression of PH, but PAP seldom returns to normal. The longer the daily duration of LTOT, the better are the pulmonary hemodynamic results.

Nocturnal Oxygen Therapy in Patients with Isolated Sleep-Related Hypoxemia: Is It Recommended?

COPD patients who are hypoxemic while awake will also be hypoxemic during sleep. In most COPD patients, hypoxemia does, in fact, worsen during sleep, especially during REM sleep, as already mentioned. It follows that it is particularly important to reverse hypoxia in these patients during sleep, and it is sometimes recommended to add 1 L/min of oxygen flow to the daytime resting prescription.[135]

Some COPD patients do not have significant hypoxemia when awake ($PaO_2 > 60$ mm Hg) but are hypoxemic during sleep, with a mean nocturnal transcutaneous $SaO_2 < 88$ to 90%.[49,50] It has been hypothesized that sleep-related hypoxemia, occurring in COPD patients without significant daytime hypoxemia, could lead to permanent (daytime) PH.[57,136] If this was the case, it would be justified to prescribe nocturnal oxygen therapy to these patients. In fact, this hypothesis has not been proven,[50,58,59] and a multicenter study, which included 105 COPD patients, showed that daytime PAP was identical in nocturnal desaturators and nondesaturators (Figure 5).[59] These data do not support the hypothesis that isolated sleep-related hypoxemia induces the development of (permanent) PH.

Two controlled studies investigated the effects of nocturnal oxygen therapy given to COPD patients exhibiting sleep-related hypoxemia but without significant daytime hypoxemia. Fletcher and colleagues compared 19 desaturators receiving nocturnal oxygen with 19 comparable desaturators treated with room air.[137] In fact, only 16 patients could complete the study (3 years):

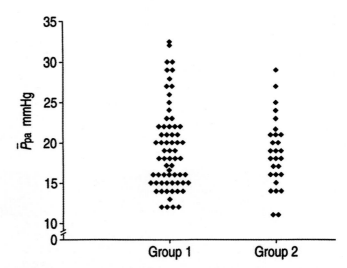

FIGURE 5. Comparison of pulmonary artery mean pressure (PAP) in two groups of chronic obstructive pulmonary disease patients whose daytime arterial partial pressure of oxygen (PaO_2) is >60 mm Hg. Group 1 patients ($n = 29$) have no significant nocturnal desaturation; group 2 patients ($n = 76$) have significant nocturnal desaturation. It can be seen that PAP is almost identical in the two groups. Nocturnal hypoxemia does not favor the development of pulmonary hypertension. Adapted from Chaouat A et al.[59]

PAP increased by 3.9 mm Hg as a mean in the control group ($n = 9$) and decreased by 3.7 mm Hg in patients ($n = 7$) treated with nocturnal oxygen ($p < .02$). The authors concluded that nocturnal oxygen therapy had favorable effects on pulmonary hemodynamics. A more recent European multicenter study compared the evolution of PAP in 41 nocturnal desaturators randomly allocated to nocturnal oxygen and 35 similar patients receiving no nocturnal oxygen.[60] The duration of the study was 2 years. Twenty-four patients in the nocturnal oxygen group and 22 in the control group completed the study. Nocturnal oxygen therapy did not modify the evolution of pulmonary hemodynamics, which was the same in the two groups.

Thus, studies at present, particularly those related to the evolution of pulmonary hemodynamics, do not justify the use of nocturnal oxygen in COPD patients who do not qualify for conventional oxygen therapy according to current criteria.[137]

Vasodilator Drugs

Experience with vasodilators has come from the treatment of idiopathic and severe pulmonary arterial hypertension. It is based on the belief that pulmonary vasoconstriction is an important component of PH. In fact, vasodilators have rarely been prescribed in COPD patients. The acute effects of some drugs, such as calcium channel blockers and urapidil, have been somewhat favorable,[138,139] but there have been few long-term studies, and the results of these studies were disapointing.[140] What is needed is a selective pulmonary vasodilator that lowers PAP and PVR without decreasing cardiac output and that does not worsen ventilation-perfusion mismatch, as do many vasodilators and particularly calcium channel blockers.

NO is a selective and potent pulmonary vasodilator. It improves pulmonary hemodynamics and hypoxemia acutely in some studies in COPD,[141] but other studies have shown that it worsens ventilation-perfusion mismatch and hypoxemia.[142,143] There has been one long-term study of NO in 40 COPD patients already on LTOT.[144] Patients were randomly assigned to receive either oxygen alone or "pulsed" inhalation of NO with oxygen over a period of 3 months. The addition of NO produced a significant improvement in PAP, PVR, and cardiac output (Table 7). These results are promising, but the technological and toxicologic problems related to the prolonged use of inhaled NO are far from being solved, and, clearly, we need further studies in this field.

Prostanoids (epoprostenol and other derivatives of prostacyclin), endothelin receptor antagonists (bosentan, sitaxsentan, ambrisentan), and phosphodiesterase inhibitors (sildenafil) are presently used for the treatment of idiopathic pulmonary arterial hypertension and other forms of severe pulmonary arterial hypertension. They have vasodilator and may have antiproliferative properties. They have been shown to improve survival, symptoms (dyspnea), quality of life, and pulmonary hemodynamics. Such agents could be tested in COPD patients with severe PH, particularly in those who share some characteristics with idiopathic pulmonary arterial hypertension patients. To our knowledge, there has been no controlled study with any of these drugs in COPD. Since COPD patients with severe or "disproportionate" PH are few, the possibility of a multicentric controlled study should be considered.[108]

Other Therapies in Advanced COPD: Lung Volume Reduction Surgery and Lung Transplantation

LUNG VOLUME REDUCTION SURGERY

Patients with advanced emphysema may benefit from lung volume reduction surgery (LVRS).[145] Generally, COPD patients with moderate to severe PH (PAP $\geq$ 35 mm Hg) are not candidates for LVRS and should rather be considered for lung transplantation. LVRS may have favorable pulmonary hemodynamic effects since it improves pulmonary function and arterial blood gases. On the other hand, it could have deleterious effects since it may cause a reduction in the pulmonary vascular tree.

Table 7 Comparison of the Long-Term (3 months) Pulmonary Hemodynamic Effects of Inhalation of Oxygen Alone versus Oxygen + Nitric Oxide

Variables	Oxygen Alone (n = 17)		Oxygen + NO (n = 15)		p Value
	Baseline	3 mo	Baseline	3 mo	
PAP (mm Hg)	24.6 ± 5.7	25.2 ± 6.5	27.6 ± 4.4	20.6 ± 4.9	< .001
PVR (dynes/s/cm-5)	259.5 ± 101.7	264.0 ± 109.2	276.9 ± 96.6	173.1 ± 87.9	.001
Q(L/min/m^2)	2.7 ± 0.5	2.7 ± 0.6	2.7 ± 0.6	3.0 ± 0.4	.138
PCWP (mm Hg)	9.6 ± 2.9	9.4 ± 2.6	10.4 ± 3.3	8.4 ± 2.8	.168
SAP (mm Hg)	92.1 ± 16.2	90.6 ± 14.2	94.3 ± 13.2	94.9 ± 9.2	.308

Adapted from Vonbank K et al.[144]

NO = nitric oxide; PAP = pulmonary artery mean pressure; PCWP = pulmonary capillary wedge pressure; PVR = pulmonary vascular resistance; $\dot{Q}$ = cardiac output; SAP = systemic arterial mean pressure.
Values are mean ± SD.

There have been few studies on pulmonary hemodynamics before and after LVRS.[146–148] These studies have included small series of patients and have shown conflicting results with increases in PAP after LVRS in one study[148] but not in others.[146,147] Thus, it has not been established whether LVRS has adverse effects on pulmonary hemodynamics or whether the reduction in the vascular bed owing to the resection of lung tissue can be offset by the better mechanical properties of the respiratory system (see Chapter 27).

Lung Transplantation

Lung transplantation is performed in selected COPD patients with end-stage disease. Bjortuft and colleagues investigated a group of 24 patients, including 19 COPD patients, who underwent single-lung transplantation.[149] The majority of patients (15 of 24) had mild to moderate PH at the onset (there was only one case of severe PH [45 mm Hg] in COPD patients), and in these patients, PAP significantly decreased from 28 ± [SEM] 1 to 18 ± 1 mm Hg after transplantation; there was a similar decrease in PVR. These results were maintained after 2 years of follow-up. Thus, COPD patients with PH normalize pulmonary hemodynamics after single-lung transplantation.

Conclusions

PH is frequently observed in patients with advanced COPD, but the actual prevalence of PH in COPD is still unknown. PH is probably more a marker of both the duration and the severity of chronic alveolar hypoxia than a true "complication" of COPD. Alveolar hypoxia plays a central role in the pathogenesis of PH even though the precise mechanisms of (acute) hypoxic vasoconstriction and of (chronic) pulmonary vascular remodeling are not fully understood. In humans, there is a marked interindividual variability in the pulmonary vascular response to hypoxia, which may be inherited, and recent studies suggest that a *5HTT* gene polymorphism appears to determine the severity of PH in hypoxemic COPD patients.

The main characteristic of PH in COPD is probably its mild to moderate degree, resting PAP in a stable state of the disease usually ranging between 20 and 35 mm Hg. However, PH may worsen during exercise, sleep, and exacerbations of the disease. This acute increase in the afterload can favor the development of right ventricular failure, which is observed in some COPD patients, most often during acute exacerbations.

At present, LTOT is the logical treatment of PH since alveolar hypoxia is considered to be the major determinant of the elevation of PVR and PAP in COPD patients. LTOT stabilizes or at least attenuates and sometimes reverses the progression of PH, but PAP seldom returns to normal. The longer the daily duration of LTOT, the better are the pulmonary hemodynamic results. Vasodilators (prostacyclin, endothelin receptor antagonists, sildenafil, NO) may be considered in patients with severe PH (PAP >40 mm Hg), but such a level of PH is unusual (< 5% of patients with advanced COPD), and the indications of vasodilators have not been precisely defined. In the future, the treatment might combine LTOT and specific vasodilators.

References

1. Chronic cor pulmonale. Report of an expert committee. Circulation 1963;27:594–615.
2. MacNee W. Pathophysiology of cor pulmonale in chronic obstructive pulmonary disease. Am J Respir Crit Care Med 1994;150:833–52; 1158–68.
3. Weitzenblum E. Chronic cor pulmonale. Heart 2003; 89:225–30.
4. Chaouat A, Bugnet AS, Kadaoui N, et al. Severe pulmonary hypertension and chronic obstructive pulmonary disease. Am J Respir Crit Care Med 2005;172:189–94.
5. Fishman AP. Chronic cor pulmonale. Am Rev Respir Dis 1976;114:775–94.
6. Bishop JM. Cardiovascular complications of chronic bronchitis and emphysema. Med Clin North Am 1973;57:771–80.
7. Fishman AP. Clinical classification of pulmonary hypertension. Clin Chest Med 2001;22:385–91.
8. Tartulier M, Bourret M, Deyrieux F. Les pressions artérielles pulmonaires chez l'homme normal. Effets de l'âge et de l'exercice musculaire. Bull Physiopathol Respir 1972;8:1295–321.
9. Naeije R. Pulmonary vascular function. In: Peacock AJ, Rubin LJ, editors. Pulmonary circulation. Diseases and their treatment. London: Arnold; 2004. p. 3–13.
10. Kessler R, Faller M, Weitzenblum E, et al. "Natural history" of pulmonary hypertension in a series of 131 patients with chronic obstructive lung disease. Am J Respir Crit Care Med 2001;164:219–24.
11. Simonneau G, Galie N, Rubin LJ, Langleben D. Clinical classification of pulmonary hypertension. J Am Coll Cardio 2004;43:5S–12S
12. Naeije R, Torbicki A. More on the noninvasive diagnosis of pulmonary hypertension: Doppler echocardiography revisited. Eur Respir J 1995;8:1445–9.
13. Williams BT, Nicholl JP. Prevalence of hypoxaemic chronic obstructive lung disease with reference to long-term oxygen therapy. Lancet 1985;1:369–72.
14. Bignon J, Khoury F, Even P, et al. Morphometric study in chronic obstructive bronchopulmonary disease. Pathologic, clinical, and physiologic correlations. Am Rev Respir Dis 1969;99:669–95.
15. Rabinovitch M, Keane JF, Fellows KE, et al. Quantitative analysis of the pulmonary wedge angiogram in congenital heart defects. Correlation with hemodynamic data and morphometric findings in lung biopsy tissue. Circulation 1981;63:152–64.
16. Meyrick B, Reid L. The effect of continued hypoxia on rat pulmonary arterial circulation. An ultrastructural study. Lab Invest 1978;38:188–200.
17. Wilkinson M, Langhome CA, Heath D, et al. A pathophysiological study of 10 cases of hypoxic cor pulmonale. Q J Med 1988;66:65–85.
18. Wright JL, Petty T, Thurlbeck WM. Analysis of the structure of the muscular pulmonary arteries in patients with pulmonary hypertension and COPD: National Institutes of Health Nocturnal Oxygen Therapy Trial. Lung 1992; 170:109–24.

19. Calverley PM, Howatson R, Flenley DC, Lamb D. Clinicopathological correlations in cor pulmonale. Thorax 1992;47:494–8.
20. Magee F, Wright JL, Wiggs BR, et al. Pulmonary vascular structure and function in chronic obstructive pulmonary disease. Thorax 1988;43:183–9.
21. Hale KA, Niewoehner DE, Cosio MG. Morphologic changes in the muscular pulmonary arteries: relationship to cigarette smoking, airway disease, and emphysema. Am Rev Respir Dis 1980;122:273–8.
22. Wright JL, Lawson L, Pare PD, et al. The structure and function of the pulmonary vasculature in mild chronic obstructive pulmonary disease. The effect of oxygen and exercise. Am Rev Respir Dis 1983;128:702–7.
23. Santos S, Peinado VI, Ramirez J, et al. Characterization of pulmonary vascular remodelling in smokers and patients with mild COPD. Eur Respir J 2002;19:632–8.
24. Peinado VI, Barbera JA, Abate P, et al. Inflammatory reaction in pulmonary muscular arteries of patients with mild chronic obstructive pulmonary disease. Am J Respir Crit Care Med 1999;159:1605–11.
25. Fishman AP. Pulmonary circulation. In: Fishman AP, editor. Handbook of physiology. The respiratory system. Circulation and nonrespiratory functions. Vol 1, sect 3. Bethesda (MD): American Physiological Society; 1985. p. 93–166.
26. Lockhart A, Tzareva M, Schrijen F, Sadoul P. Etudes hémodynamiques des décompensations respiratoires aiguës des bronchopneumopathies chroniques. Bull Eur Physiopathol Respir 1967;3:645–67.
27. Abraham AS, Cole RB, Green ID, et al. Factors contributing to the reversible pulmonary hypertension of patients with acute respiratory failure studied by serial observations during recovery. Circ Res 1969;24:51–60.
28. Weitzenblum E, Hirth C, Roeslin N, et al. Les modifications hémodynamiques pulmonaires au cours de l'insuffisance respiratoire aiguë des bronchopneumopathies chroniques. Respiration 1971;28:539–54.
29. Lockhart A, Tzareva M, Nader F, et al. Elevated pulmonary artery wedge pressure at rest and during exercise in chronic bronchitis: fact or fancy. Clin Sci 1969;37:503–17.
30. Lockhart A. Hémodynamique pulmonaire dans la bronchite chronique. Bull Physiopathol Respir 1973;9:1069–99.
31. Fishman AP. Hypoxia on the pulmonary circulation. How and where it acts. Circ Res 1976;38:221–31.
32. Heath D. Remodeling of the pulmonary vasculature in hypoxic lung disease. In: Peacock AJ, editor. Pulmonary circulation. London: Chapman & Hall; 1996. p. 71–9.
33. Von Euler US, Liljestrand G. Observation of the pulmonary arterial blood pressure in the cat. Acta Physiol Scand 1946;12:301–20.
34. Motley HL, Cournand A, Werko L, et al. The influence of short periods of induced acute hypoxia upon pulmonary artery pressure in man. Am J Physiol 1947;150:315–20.
35. Fishman AP, McClement J, Himmelstein A, Cournand A. Effects of acute anoxia on the circulation and respiration in patients with chronic pulmonary disease studied during the steady state. J Clin Invest 1952;31:770–81.
36. Archer S, Michelakis E. The mechanism(s) of hypoxic pulmonary vasoconstriction: potassium channels, redox O_2 sensors, and controversies. News Physiol Sci 2002;17:131–7.
37. Dinh-Xuan AT, Higenbottam TW, Clelland CA, et al. Impairment of endothelium-dependent pulmonary-artery relaxation in chronic obstructive lung disease. N Engl J Med 1991;324:1539–47.
38. Giaid A, Yanagisawa M, Langleben D, et al. Expression of endothelin-1 in the lungs of patients with pulmonary hypertension. N Engl J Med 1993;328:1732–9.
39. Grover RF. Chronic hypoxic pulmonary hypertension. In: Fishman A, editor. The pulmonary circulation: normal and abnormal. Philadelphia: University of Pennsylvania Press; 1990. p. 283–99.
40. Ashutosh K, Mead G, Dunsky M. Early effects of oxygen administration and prognosis in chronic obstructive pulmonary disease and cor pulmonale. Am Rev Respir Dis 1983;127:399–404.
41. Weitzenblum E, Schrijen F, Mohan-Kumar T, et al. Variability of the pulmonary vascular response to acute hypoxia in chronic bronchitis. Chest 1988;94:772–8.
42. Penaloza D, Sime F, Banchero N, Gamboa R. Pulmonary hypertension in healthy men born and living at high altitude. Med Thorac 1962;19:449–60.
43. Harris P, Heath D. The pulmonary circulation at high altitude. In: Harris P, Heath D, editors. The human pulmonary circulation. Edinburgh: Churchill Livingstone; 1986. p. 493–506.
44. Bergofsky EH, Lehr DE, Fishman AP. The effect of changes in hydrogen ion concentration on the pulmonary circulation. J Clin Invest 1962;41:1492–502.
45. Enson Y, Giuntini C, Lewis ML, et al. The influence of hydrogen ion concentration and hypoxia on the pulmonary circulation. J Clin Invest 1964;43:1146–62.
46. Segel N, Bishop JM. The circulation in patients with chronic bronchitis and emphysema at rest and during exercise, with special reference to the influence of changes in blood viscosity and blood volume on the pulmonary circulation. J Clin Invest 1966;45:1555–68.
47. Harris P, Segel N, Green I, Housley E. The influence of the airways resistance and alveolar pressure on the pulmonary vascular resistance in chronic bronchitis. Cardiovasc Res 1968;2:84–92.
48. Lockhart A, Nader F, Tzareva M, Schrijen F. Comparative effects of exercise and isocapnic voluntary hyperventilation on pulmonary haemodynamics in chronic bronchitis and emphysema. Eur J Clin Invest 1970;1:69–76.
49. Fletcher EC, Miller J, Divine GW. Nocturnal oxyhemoglobin desaturation in COPD patients with arterial oxygen tensions above 60 torr. Chest 1987;92:604–8.
50. Levi-Valensi P, Weitzenblum E, Rida Z, et al. Sleep-related oxygen desaturation and daytime pulmonary haemodynamics in COPD patients. Eur Respir J 1992;5:301–7.
51. Kay JM. Effect of intermittent normoxia on chronic hypoxic pulmonary hypertension, right ventricular hypertrophy and polycythemia in rats. Am Rev Respir Dis 1980;121:993–1001.
52. Kay JM, Suyma KL, Keane PM. Effect of intermittent normoxia on muscularisation of pulmonary arterioles induced by chronic hypoxia in rats. Am Rev Respir Dis 1981;123:454–8.
53. Widimsky J, Ostadal B, Urbanova D, et al. Intermittent high altitude hypoxia. Chest 1980;77:383–9.
54. Nattie EE, Doble EA. Threshold of intermittent hypoxia-induced right ventricular hypertrophy in the rat. Respir Physiol 1984;56:253–9.

55. Moore-Gillon JC, Cameron JR. Right ventricular hypertrophy and polycythaemia in rats after intermittent exposure to hypoxia. Clin Sci 1985;6:595–9.

56. McGuire M, Bradford A. Chronic intermittent hypercapnic hypoxia increases pulmonary arterial pressure and haematocrit in rats. Eur Respir J 2001;18:279–85.

57. Block AJ, Boysen PG, Wynne JW. The origins of cor pulmonale: a hypothesis. Chest 1979;75:109–10.

58. Fletcher EC, Luckett RA, Miller T, et al. Pulmonary vascular hemodynamics in chronic lung disease patients with and without oxyhemoglobin desaturation during sleep. Chest 1989;95:757–64.

59. Chaouat A, Weitzenblum E, Kessler R, et al. Sleep-related O_2 desaturation and daytime pulmonary haemodynamics in COPD patients with mild hypoxaemia. Eur Respir J 1997;10:1730–5.

60. Chaouat A, Weitzenblum E, Kessler R, et al. A randomized trial of nocturnal oxygen therapy in chronic obstructive pulmonary disease patients. Eur Respir J 1999;14:1002–8.

61. Bradley TD, Rutherford R, Grossmann RF, et al. Role of daytime hypoxemia in the pathogenesis of right heart failure in the obstructive sleep apnea syndrome. Am Rev Respir Dis 1985;131:835–9.

62. Chaouat A, Weitzenblum E, Krieger J, et al. Pulmonary hemodynamics in the obstructive sleep apnea syndrome. Results in 220 consecutive patients. Chest 1996;109:380–6.

63. Sajkov D, Cowie RJ, Thornton AT, et al. Pulmonary hypertension and hypoxemia in obstructive sleep apnea syndrome. Am J Respir Crit Care Med 1994;149:416–22.

64. Sajkov D, Wang T, Saunders NA, et al. Daytime pulmonary hemodynamics in patients with obstructive sleep apnea without lung disease. Am J Respir Crit Care Med 1999;159:1518–26.

65. Grover RF, Voelkel JHK, Voigt GC, Blount SG. Reversal of high altitude pulmonary hypertension. Am J Cardiol 1966;18:928–32.

66. Laks L, Lehrhaft B, Grunstein RR, Sullivan CE. Pulmonary artery pressure responses to hypoxia in sleep apnea. Am J Respir Crit Care Med 1997;155:193–8.

67. Weitzenblum E, Hirth C, Ducolone A, et al. Prognostic value of pulmonary artery pressure in chronic obstructive pulmonary disease. Thorax 1981;36:752–8.

68. Biernacki W, Flenley DC, Muir AL, MacNee W. Pulmonary hypertension and right ventricular function in patients with COPD. Chest 1988;94:1169–75.

69. Rich S, Dantzker DR, Ayres SM, et al. Primary pulmonary hypertension: a national prospective study. Ann Intern Med 1987;107:216–23.

70. Stevens D, Sharma K, Szidon P, et al. Severe pulmonary hypertension associated with COPD. Ann Transplant 2000;5:8–12.

71. Scharf S, Igbal M, Keller C, et al. Hemodynamic characterization of patients with severe emphysema. Am J Respir Crit Care Med 2002;166:314–22.

72. Thabut G, Dauriat G, Stern JB, et al. Pulmonary hemodynamics in advanced COPD candidates for lung volume reduction surgery or lung transplantation. Chest 2005;127:1531–6.

73. Weitzenblum E, Apprill A, Oswald M, et al. Pulmonary hemodynamics in patients with chronic obstructive pulmonary disease before and during an episode of peripheral edema. Chest 1994;105:1377–82.

74. Tramarin R, Torbicki A, Marchandise B, et al. Doppler echocardiographic evaluation of pulmonary artery pressure in chronic obstructive pulmonary disease. A European multicentre study. Eur Heart J 1991;12:103–11.

75. Weitzenblum E, Loiseau A, Hirth C, et al. Course of pulmonary hemodynamics in patients with chronic obstructive pulmonary disease. Chest 1979;75:656–62.

76. Horsfield K, Segel N, Bishop JM. The pulmonary circulation in chronic bronchitis at rest and during exercise breathing air and 80% oxygen. Clin Sci 1968;43:473–83.

77. Burrows B, Kettel LJ, Niden AH, et al. Patterns of cardiovascular dysfunction in chronic obstructive lung disease. N Engl J Med 1972;286:912–8.

78. Weitzenblum E, El Gharbi T, Vandevenne A, et al. L'hémodynamique pulmonaire au cours de l'exercice musculaire dans la bronchite chronique non «décompensée». Bull Physiopathol Respir 1972;8:49–71.

79. Jezek V, Schrijen F, Sadoul P. Right ventricular function and pulmonary hemodynamics during exercise in patients with chronic obstructive bronchopulmonary disease. Cardiology 1973;58:20–31.

80. Raeside AD, Brown A, Patel KR, et al. Ambulatory pulmonary artery pressure monitoring during sleep and exercise in normal individuals and patients with COPD. Thorax 2002;57:1050–9.

81. Wynne JW, Block AJ, Hemenway J, et al. Disordered breathing and oxygen desaturation during sleep in patients with chronic obstructive lung disease. Am J Med 1979;66:573–9.

82. Douglas NJ, Calverley PMA, Leggett RJE, et al. Transient hypoxaemia during sleep in chronic bronchitis and emphysema. Lancet 1979;1:1–4.

83. Catterall JR, Douglas NJ, Calverley PMA, et al. Transient hypoxemia during sleep in chronic obstructive pulmonary disease is not a sleep apnea syndrome. Am Rev Respir Dis 1983;128:24–9.

84. Hudgel DW, Martin RJ, Capheart M, et al. Contribution of hypoventilation to sleep oxygen desaturation in chronic obstructive pulmonary disease. J Appl Physiol 1983;55:669–77.

85. Fletcher EC, Gray BA, Levin DC. Non-apneic mechanism of arterial oxygen desaturation during rapid-eye-movement sleep. J Appl Physiol 1983;54:632–9.

86. Coccagna G, Lugaresi E. Arterial blood gases and pulmonary and systemic arterial pressure during sleep in chronic obstructive pulmonary disease. Sleep 1978;1:117–24.

87. Boysen PG, Block AJ, Wynne JW, et al. Nocturnal pulmonary hypertension in patients with chronic obstructive pulmonary disease. Chest 1979;76:538–42.

88. Weitzenblum E, Muzet A, Ehrhart M, et al. Variations nocturnes des gaz du sang et de la pression artérielle pulmonaire chez les bronchitiques chroniques insuffisants respiratoires. Nouv Presse Méd 1982;11:1119–22.

89. Fletcher EC, Levin DC. Cardiopulmonary hemodynamics during sleep in subjects with chronic obstructive pulmonary disease: the effect of short and long-term oxygen. Chest 1984;85:6–14.

90. Farber MO, Weinberger MH, Robertson GL, et al. Hormonal abnormalities affecting sodium and water balance in acute respiratory failure due to chronic obstructive lung disease. Chest 1984;85:49–54.

91. Oswald-Mammosser M, Oswald T, Nyankiye E, et al. Non-invasive diagnosis of pulmonary hypertension in chronic obstructive pulmonary disease. Comparison of ECG, radiological measurements, echocardiography and myocardial scintigraphy. Eur J Respir Dis 1987;71:419–29.

92. Bernard R, Smets P, Nicaise J, et al. Corrélation entre l'électrocardiogramme et la pression artérielle pulmonaire dans les pneumopathies chronique (étude de 274 observations). Bull World Health Organ 1973;49:155–65.

93. Turnbull LW, Ridgway JP, Biernacki W, et al. Assessment of the right ventricle by magnetic resonance imaging in chronic obstructive lung disease. Thorax 1990;45:597–601.

94. Hiroyuki S, Takashi D, Miyoji A, et al. Evaluation of cor pulmonale on a modified short-axis section of the heart by magnetic resonance imaging. Am Rev Respir Dis 1992;146:1576–81.

95. Kruger S, Haage P, Hoffmann R, et al. Diagnosis of pulmonary arterial hypertension and pulmonary embolism with magnetic resonance angiography. Chest 2001;120:1556–61.

96. Raeside D, Peacock A. Making measurements in the pulmonary circulation: when and how? Thorax 1997;52:9–11.

97. Burghuber OC. Doppler assessment of pulmonary haemodynamics in chronic hypoxic lung disease. Thorax 1996;51:9–12.

98. Yock P, Popp R. Non-invasive estimation of right ventricular systolic pressure by Doppler ultrasound in patients with tricuspid regurgitation. Circulation 1984;70:657–62.

99. Berger M, Haimowitz A, Van Tosh, et al. Quantitative assessment of pulmonary hypertension in patients with tricuspid regurgitation using continuous wave Doppler ultrasound. J Am Coll Cardiol 1985;6:359–65.

100. Chan KL, Currie PJ, Seward JB, et al. Comparison of three ultrasound methods in the prediction of pulmonary artery pressure. J Am Coll Cardiol 1987;9:549–54.

101. Torbicki A, Skwarski K, Hawrylkiewicz I, et al. Attempts at measuring pulmonary arterial pressure by means of Doppler echocardiography in patients with chronic lung disease. Eur Respir J 1989;2:856–60.

102. Laaban JP, Diebold B, Zelinski R, et al. Noninvasive estimation of systolic pulmonary artery pressure using Doppler echocardiography in patients with chronic obstructive pulmonary disease. Chest 1989;96:1258–62.

103. Arcasoy SM, Christie JD, Ferrari VA, et al. Echocardiographic assessment of pulmonary hypertension in patients with advanced lung disease. Am J Respir Crit Care Med 2003;167:735–40.

104. Leuchte HH, Baumgartner RA, Nounou ME, et al. Brain natriuretic peptide is a prognostic parameter in chronic lung disease. Am J Respir Crit Care Med 2006;173:744–50.

105. Naeije R. Should pulmonary hypertension be treated in chronic obstructive pulmonary disease? In: Weir EK, Archer SL, Reeves JT, editors. The diagnosis and treatment of pulmonary hypertension. Mount Kisco (NY): Futura Publishing; 1992. p. 209–39.

106. Barbera JA, Peinado VI, Santos S. Pulmonary hypertension in chronic obstructive pulmonary disease. Eur Respir J 2003;21:892–905.

107. Swan HJC, Ganz W, Forrester JS, et al. Catheterization of the heart in man with the use of a flow directed catheter. N Engl J Med 1970,283:447–51.

108. Weitzenblum E, Chaouat A. Severe pulmonary hypertension in COPD. Is it a distinct disease? Chest 2005;127:1480–2.

109. Eddahibi S, Chaouat A, Morrell N, et al. Polymorphism of the serotonin transporter gene and pulmonary hypertension in chronic obstructive pulmonary disease. Circulation 2003;108:1839–44.

110. Ourednik A, Susa Z. How long does the pulmonary hypertension last in chronic obstructive bronchopulmonary disease? In: Widimsky J, editor. Progress in respiration research. Pulmonary hypertension. Basel: Karger; 1975. p. 24–8.

111. Schrijen F, Uffholtz H, Polu JM, et al. Pulmonary and systemic hemodynamic evolution in chronic bronchitis. Am Rev Respir Dis 1978;117:25–31.

112. Weitzenblum E, Sautegeau A, Ehrhart M, et al. Long-term course of pulmonary arterial pressure in chronic obstructive pulmonary disease. Am Rev Respir Dis 1984;130:993–8.

113. Edema in cor pulmonale [editorial]. Lancet 1975;ii:1289–90.

114. Richens JM, Howard P. Oedema in cor pulmonale. Clin Sci 1982;62:255–9.

115. Brent BN, Berger HJ, Matthay RA, et al. Physiologic correlates of right ventricular ejection fraction in chronic obstructive pulmonary disease: a combined radionuclide and hemodynamic study. Am J Cardiol 1982;50:255–62.

116. Burghuber OC, Bergmann H. Right ventricular contractility in chronic obstructive pulmonary disease. A combined radionuclide and haemodynamic study. Respiration 1988;53:1–12.

117. Mols P, Huynh CH, Dechamps P, et al. Prediction of pulmonary pressure in chronic obstructive pulmonary disease by radionuclide ventriculography. Chest 1989;96:1280–4.

118. Burghuber OC. Right ventricular contractility is preserved and preload increased in patients with chronic obstructive pulmonary disease and pulmonary artery hypertension. In: Jezek V, Morpurgo M, Tramarin R, editors. Current topics in rehabilitation. Right ventricular hypertrophy and function in chronic lung disease. Berlin: Springer-Verlag; 1992. p. 135–41.

119. Weitzenblum E, Chaouat A. Right ventricular function in COPD. Can it be assessed reliably by the measurement of right ventricular ejection fraction? Chest 1998;113:567–9.

120. Crottogini AJ, Willshaw P. Calculating the end-systolic pressure/volume relation. Circulation 1991;83:1121–2.

121. MacNee W, Wathen C, Flenley DC, et al. The effects of controlled oxygen therapy on ventricular function in patients with stable and decompensated cor pulmonale. Am Rev Respir Dis 1988;137:1289–95.

122. Aber GM, Bishop JM. Serial changes in renal function, arterial gas tension and the acid-base state in patients with chronic bronchitis and oedema. Clin Sci 1965;28:511–25.

123. Vandenbergh E, Clement J, Van De Woestijne KP. Course and prognosis of patients with advanced chronic obstructive pulmonary disease. Am J Med 1973;55:736–46.

124. Bishop JM, Cross KW. Physiological variables and mortality in patients with various categories of chronic respiratory disease. Bull Eur Physiopathol Respir 1984;20:495–500.

125. Nocturnal Oxygen Therapy Trial Group. Continuous or nocturnal oxygen therapy in hypoxemic chronic obstructive lung disease. Ann Intern Med 1980;93:391–8.

126. Report of the Medical Research Council Working Party. Long-term domiciliary oxygen therapy in chronic hypoxic

cor pulmonale complicating chronic bronchitis and emphysema. Lancet 1981;1:681–6.

127. Cooper CB, Waterhouse J, Howard P. Twelve year clinical study of patients with hypoxic cor pulmonale given long term domiciliary oxygen therapy. Thorax 1987;42:105–10.

128. Keller A, Ragaz A, Borer P. Predictors for early mortality in patients with long-term oxygen home therapy. Respiration 1985;48:216–21.

129. Skwarsky K, MacNee W, Wraith PK, et al. Predictors of survival in patients with chronic obstructive pulmonary disease treated with long-term oxygen therapy. Chest 1991; 100:1522–7.

130. Oswald-Mammosser M, Weitzenblum E, Quoix E, et al. Prognostic factors in COPD patients receiving long-term oxygen therapy. Chest 1995;107:1193–8.

131. Weitzenblum E, Kessler R, Oswald M, et al. Medical treatment of pulmonary hypertension in chronic lung disease. Eur Respir J 1994;7:148–52.

132. Timms RM, Khaja FU, Williams GW, and the Nocturnal Oxygen Therapy Trial Group. Hemodynamic response to oxygen therapy in chronic obstructive pulmonary disease. Ann Intern Med 1985;102:29–36.

133. Weitzenblum E, Sautegeau A, Ehrhart M, et al. Long term oxygen therapy can reverse the progression of pulmonary hypertension in patients with chronic obstructive pulmonary disease. Am Rev Respir Dis 1985;131:493–8.

134. Zielinski J, Tobiasz M, Hawrylkiewicz I, et al. Effects of long-term oxygen therapy on pulmonary hemodynamics in COPD patients. A 6-year prospective study. Chest 1998;113:65–70.

135. American Thoracic Society. Standards for the diagnosis and care of patients with chronic obstructive pulmonary disease. Am J Respir Crit Care Med 1995;152:S77–120.

136. Flenley DC. Clinical hypoxia: causes, consequences and correction. Lancet 1978;1:542–6.

137. Fletcher EC, Luckett RA, Goodnight-White S, et al. A double-blind trial of nocturnal supplemental oxygen for sleep desaturation in patients with chronic obstructive pulmonary disease and a daytime PaO_2 above 60mmHg. Am Rev Respir Dis 1992;145:1070–6.

138. Adnot S, Defouilloy C, Brun-Buisson C, et al. Hemodynamic effects of urapidil in patients with pulmonary hypertension. Am Rev Respir Dis 1987;135:288–93.

139. Saadjian A, Philip-Joet F, Bun H, et al. Effects of nicardipine on pulmonary and systemic vascular reactivity to oxygen in patients with pulmonary hypertension secondary to chronic obstructive lung disease. J Cardiovasc Pharmacol 1991;17:731–7.

140. Saadjian A, Philip-Joet F, Vestri R, et al. Long term treatment of chronic obstructive lung disease by nifedipine: an 18 month hemodynamic study. Eur Respir J 1988;1:716–20.

141. Adnot S, Kouyoumdjan C, Defouilloy C, et al. Hemodynamic and gas exhange responses to infusion of acetylcholine and inhalation of nitric oxide in patients with chronic obstructive lung disease and pulmonary hypertension. Am Rev Respir Dis 1993;148:310–6.

142. Katayama Y, Higenbottam TW, Diaz De Atauri MJ, et al. Inhaled nitric oxide and arterial oxygen tension in patients with chronic obstructive pulmonary disease and severe pulmonary hypertension. Thorax 1997;52:120–4.

143. Roger N, Barbera JA, Roca J, et al. Nitric oxide inhalation during exercise in chronic obstructive pulmonary disease. Am J Respir Crit Care Med 1997;156:800–6.

144. Vonbank K, Ziesche R, Higenbottam TW, et al. Controlled prospective randomised trial on the effects on pulmonary haemodynamics of the ambulatory long-term use of nitric oxide and oxygen in patients with severe COPD. Thorax 2003;58:289–93.

145. National Emphysema Treatment Trial Research Group. A randomized trial comparing lung-volume-reduction surgery with medical therapy for severe emphysema. N Engl J Med 2003;348:2059–73.

146. Oswald-Mammosser M, Kessler R, Massard G, et al. Effects of lung volume reduction surgery on gas exchange and pulmonary hemodynamics at rest and during exercise. Am J Respir Crit Care Med 1998;158:1020–5.

147. Kubo K, Koizumi T, Fujimoto K, et al. Effects of lung volume reduction surgery on exercise pulmonary hemodynamics in severe emphysema. Chest 1998;114:1575–82.

148. Weg IL, Rossoff L, McKeon K, et al. Development of pulmonary hypertension after lung volume reduction surgery. Am J Respir Crit Care Med 1999;159:552–6.

149. Bjortuft O, Simonsen S, Geiran OR, et al. Pulmonary haemodynamics after single-lung transplantation for end-stage pulmonary parenchymal disease. Eur Respir J 1996; 10:2007–11.

CHAPTER 21

Muscle Involvement in Chronic Obstructive Pulmonary Disease

Xavier Busquets, PhD, Montse Morlá, PhD, Amanda Iglesias, PhD, and Alvar G. N. Agustí, MD, FRCP

In the past several years, a number of studies have provided evidence that chronic obstructive pulmonary disease (COPD) is often associated with extrapulmonary abnormalities, the so-called "systemic effects" of the disease.[1–7] One of the best-characterized systemic effects of COPD involves abnormalities of skeletal muscle structure and function that cause both skeletal muscle dysfunction[8–20] and muscle wasting.[21–30] These muscle effects contribute to limit exercise capacity in these patients and to influence their prognosis negatively.[9] These observations have boosted the interest in skeletal muscle pathobiology in COPD, and, as a consequence, a number of molecular mechanisms involved in injury and repair processes in muscles have been identified. In addition, this research has contributed to a better definition of rehabilitation strategies in the clinical management of these patients.[9,31] This chapter reviews the normal skeletal muscle structure and function, the cellular mechanisms involved in normal muscle repair, the potential mechanisms underlying skeletal muscle injury in patients with COPD, and the resulting muscle abnormalities observed in these patients.

Overview of Skeletal Muscle Structure and Function

Skeletal Muscle Contraction

The fibers forming skeletal muscle are huge cells formed by the fusion of many separate smaller cells. The individual nuclei of the contributing cells lie just beneath the plasma membrane. The bulk of the cytoplasm is made up of myofibrils, the contractile elements of the muscle cells.[32,33] These cylindrical structures are 1 to 2 µm in diameter and may be as long as the muscle cell itself. A myofibril consists of a chain of identical contractile units, or sarcomeres. Each sarcomere is about 2.5 µm long. Sarcomeres are highly organized assemblies of a variety of proteins. Among them, three types of filaments (actin, myosin II, and titin filaments) are the key components. Myosin filaments are centrally positioned in each sarcomere, whereas the actin filaments extend inward from each end of the sarcomere (where they are anchored to an structure known as the Z disk). The titin filaments (also known as connectins) are giant filamentous polypeptide-containing tandem immunoglobulin-like domains that span half of the striated muscle sarcomere. Titin extends as the sarcomere is stretched, developing what is known as passive force, which prevents overextension of muscular fibers.[32,33]

The contraction of a muscle cell is caused by simultaneous shortening of all sarcomeres, which, in turn, is caused by the actin filaments sliding past the myosin filaments. The sliding motion is generated by myosin heads that project from the sides of the myosin filament and interact with adjacent actin filament. During each cycle of contraction, a single myosin head hydrolyzes one molecule of adenosine triphosphate. After a contraction is completed, the myosin heads lose contact with the actin filament and the muscle relaxes (Figure 1).[32,33]

The force-generating molecular interaction between myosin and actin takes place only when the skeletal muscle receives a signal from the nervous system. The total force generated by a muscle depends on the number of motor units activated and the amount of force contributed by each motor unit. The central nervous system has two levels of control of the force generated by the muscle: (1) the number of activated motor units (ie, recruitment) and (2) the action potential discharge frequency of motoneurons (frequency modulation). This simple model assumes that all muscle fibers within a motor unit are activated by the motoneuron in an all-or-none fashion and that each muscle fiber belongs to only one motor unit.[32,33]

The electrical signal triggered by the motoneuron is relayed to the sarcoplasmic reticulum. The latter contains a very high concentration of Ca^{2+}, and in response to the electrical excitation, this Ca^{2+} is released into the cytosol through ion channels that open in the sarcoplasmic reticulum. Muscle contraction is triggered by the rise of cytoplasmic Ca^{2+} concentration. When the level of Ca^{2+} rises, Ca^{2+} binds to troponin, inducing a change in its shape. This, in turn, causes the tropomyosin molecules to shift their position, allowing myosin heads to bind the actin filament and initiating contraction.[32,33]

The increase in Ca^{2+} in the cytosol ceases as soon as the nerve signal stops because the Ca^{2+} is rapidly pumped back into the sarcoplasmic reticulum by the sarcoendoplasmic calcium pump adenosine triphosphatase (ATPase) (SERCA).[32,33]

Fiber Types

The skeletal muscle cells (fibers) can vary considerably in their mechanical, histochemical, and biochemical properties, providing the basis for its classification in a number of subtypes. The most common classification is according to the histochemical staining of myofibrillar ATPase as type I, IIa, IIb, and IIx.[34]

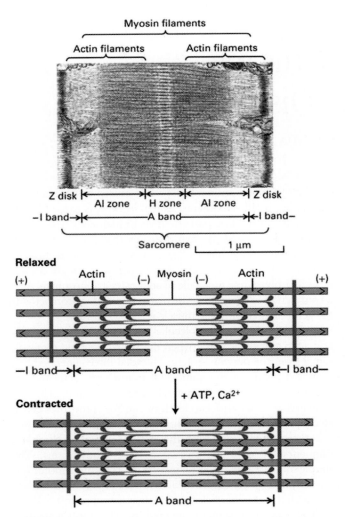

FIGURE 1. Electron microscopic image of a sarcomere (*top*). The sliding motion within the sarcomere (*bottom*) is generated by myosin heads, which interact with adjacent actin filaments. Adapted from Lodish H, Berk A, Matsudaira P, et al. Molecular cell biology, 5e. New York: W.H. Freeman and Co., 2005. ATP = adenosine triphosphate.

Skeletal muscle fibers have also been classified based on differences in myosin heavy-chain (MHC) isoforms.[35,36] Several studies have confirmed a general correspondence between the histochemical classification of fibers as type I, IIa, IIb, and IIx with MHC_{slow}, MHC_{2A}, MHC_{2X}, and MHC_{2B}, respectively.[35–39]

Regulation of Muscle Mass

Skeletal muscle tissue mass (as all other tissues) represents a balance between protein synthesis and protein degradation (protein turnover). Turnover rates for specific proteins in the skeletal muscle depend on their function.[40,41] The regulation of protein turnover in skeletal muscle is, in fact, of great importance since muscle mass accounts for about 40 to 45% of total body mass. About 40% of skeletal muscle amino acids originate from endogenous protein breakdown, whereas the rest is derived from food intake.[40] Therefore, positive regulators of muscle mass (protein synthesis) and negative regulators of muscle mass (protein breakdown) should be distinghished.

POSITIVE REGULATORS

Somatomedins, a family of polypeptide growth factors produced in the skeletal muscle and in other tissues that mediate the action of anabolic hormones, such as growth hormone (GH) or testosterone, are generally considered positive regulators of muscle mass.[42,43]

The main somatomedin is insulin-like growth factor I (IGF-I), which stimulates both proliferation and differentiation of myoblasts throughout a number of signal transduction pathways. Studies carried out with L6A1 myoblasts demonstrate that the mitogenic response of IGF-I is mediated by the mitogen-activated protein kinase (MAPK) pathway, whereas IGF-stimulated differentiation is mediated by the phosphatidylinositol 3 (PI3)-kinase/p70(S6k) pathway.[44]

In humans, IGF-I enhances muscle protein synthesis[45] and suppresses protein breakdown via ubiquitin-dependent pathways.[45] In fact, IGF-I inversely regulates a number of proteins termed atrogins,[46] which include members of the ubiquitin ligases (as atrogin-1/MAFbx).[47] These atrogin-dependent protein changes induced by IGF-I occur via the Akt/FOXO and the Akt/mTOR signal transduction pathways.[47–49]

Studies in mouse myoblast C2C12 cells demonstrate that IGF-I can mobilize intracellular calcium, activates the Ca^{2+}/calmodulin-dependent phosphatase calcineurin, and induces the nuclear translocation of the transcription factor NF-ATc1, which, in turn, regulates the expression of muscle-specific genes.[50]

In skeletal muscles, the hypertrophic effects of IGF-I can also be mediated by satellite cell proliferation.[51,52]

NEGATIVE REGULATORS

Proinflammatory cytokines are considered important negative regulators of skeletal muscle mass because they can induce under some circumstances protein degradation and apoptosis. Among them, tumor necrosis factor (TNF-α cachectin) plays a central role.[53]

TNF-α signals through two distinct receptors, TNF-R1 (also known as p55TNFR) and TNF-R2 (also known as p75TNFR).[54–56] The cytoplasmic tail of TNF-R1 contains a death domain, which is essential for induction of apoptosis.[57] TNF-R1 occupancy triggers a signaling pathway, resulting in the activation of the transcription factor nuclear factor κB (NF-κB).[58] Direct administration of TNF-α in rats is effective in accelerating muscle protein breakdown.[59,60] Below we review the molecular mechanism by which TNF-α causes protein loss.

TNF-α exerts its effect in muscle cells in a number of ways. *In-vitro* studies carried out in C2C12-differentiated myotubes demonstrated that the loss of total protein content (some of these proteins are muscle specific, such as fast-type

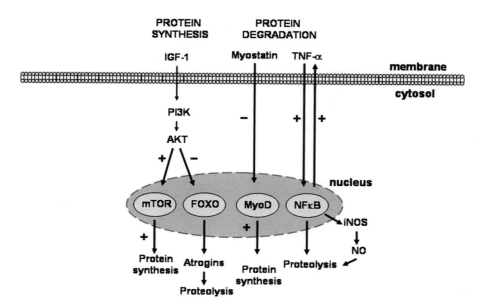

FIGURE 2. Overview of the main signal transduction pathways controlling protein synthesis and protein degradation in skeletal muscle. Growth factors (such as insulinlike growth factor I [IGF-1]) enhance protein synthesis by activation of mammalian target of rapamycin (mTOR) transcription factor and inhibiting Forkhead box O (FOXO) transcription factor via the PI3K/Akt signal transduction pathway. Cytokines such as tumor necrosis factor α (TNF-α) or myostatin inhibit protein synthesis by inhibiting MyoD transcription factor activity (myostatin) or activating the proinflammatory nuclear factor κB (NF-κB) transcription factor. iNOS = inducible nitric oxide synthase; NO = nitric oxide.

myosin heavy chain) is mediated by a rapid activation of NF-κB.[61] These effects appear to be related to the activation of (1) the ubiquitin-proteasome system since TNF-α stimulates UbcH2 (ubiquitin carrier protein) expression in mouse limb muscles both in vivo and in cultured myotubes[62] and (2) the general activation of the MAPKs p38, extracellular signal related kinase (ERK) 1/2, and Jun-N terminal kinase (JNK), leading to an upregulation of atrogin1/muscle atrophy F-box (MAFbx) gene expression.[63]

TNF-α-induced apoptotic cell death also represents a potential mechanism by which muscle wasting can occur. Exposure of C2C12-derived myotubes to TNF-α induced apoptosis characterized by enhanced caspase-3 activity, which resulted in poly(adenosine diphosphate–ribose) polymerase (PARP) cleavage and increased histone-associated deoxyribonucleic acid (DNA) fragmentation.[64] In line with the above in-vitro results, intraperitoneal administration of TNF-α to rats showed enhanced DNA laddering in the skeletal muscle, which indicate DNA damage consistent with apoptosis.[65]

TNF-α can exert its catabolic effects to skeletal muscle throughout a variety of other cellular mechanisms. Studies in C2C12-derived myotubes demonstrate that TNF-α inhibits insulin-induced stimulation of protein synthesis through a decrease in the ribosomal initiation factor eIF4F in a MEK1-sensitive signaling pathway.[66] Additional studies in the same experimental model suggest that TNF-α can cause insulin resistance in skeletal muscle by inhibiting insulin receptor substrate-1 (IRS-1) and IRS-2-mediated PI3-kinase activation, as well as p42(MAPK) and p44(MAPK) tyrosine phosphorylation.[67] In this regard, insulin resistance in

skeletal muscle associated with impaired phosphorylation of Akt substrate 160 has been demonstrated after TNF-α infusion in healthy humans.[68]

Finally, downregulation of the IGF-I receptor by TNF-α has also been proposed as a mechanism influencing protein degradation.[69]

An overview of the main signal transduction pathways controlling protein synthesis and protein degradation in skeletal muscle is shown in Figure 2.

Cellular Mechanisms of Muscle Repair

Muscle injury is mediated by increased intracellular Ca²⁺ levels inhibiting mitochondrial respiration and activating Ca²⁺-dependent proteases. In addition, skeletal muscle cell membrane lysis activates macrophages, which, in turn, secrete a number of mitotic factors for muscle satellite cells.[70] The activation and proliferation of the satellite cells are key events for muscle repair after injury (see below).

Satellite Cells

Satellite cells are muscle precursor cells placed between the cell membrane of myofibers and the basal lamina of skeletal muscle fibers. In young muscle, satellite cells have many ribosomes, extended rough endoplasmic reticulum, and Golgi complexes, indicative of metabolically active cells. In normal adult muscle, satellite cells are mitotically and metabolically quiescent, with a reduced concentration of the above organelles.[71]

Activated satellite cells can be identified by immunostaining and immunoblotting for various gene transcripts and proteins. These include members of the family of nuclear proteins

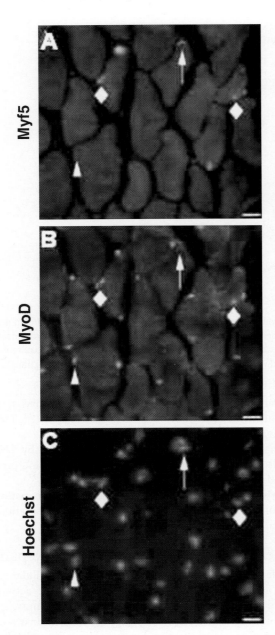

FIGURE 3. Triple immunofluorescence staining visualizing A, β-galactosidase (Myf5) (Texas Red), B, MyoD (fluorescein isothiocyanate), and C, the nuclei, Hoechst). The *arrow* points to a β-galactosidase (Myf5)-positive satellite cell that is negative for MyoD. The *arrowhead* marks an example of a MyoD-positive nucleus that is negative for β-galactosidase (Myf5). The *diamonds* mark two nuclei as examples, which are positive for both MyoD and β-galactosidase (Myf5). Bars = 5 μm. Adapted from Cooper RN et al.[72]

expressed by the muscle regulatory factor (MRF) as myf5, MyoD, myogenin, and MRF4 (Figure 3).[72–74] Extracellular matrix proteins secreted by satellite cells as syndecan-3 and syndecan-4 are also markers of satellite cells.[75,76]

Activation of Satellite Cells

During muscle regeneration, satellite cells exit their normal quiescent state and proliferate, as observed by changes in their morphology and contents. As indicated above, a quiescent satellite cell presents little cytoplasm and few organelles, whereas an activated satellite cell has hypertrophied organelles and an expanded cytoplasm.[77] Satellite cell proliferation is not restricted to a damage site. Damage of a muscle fiber will activate satellite cells all along the fiber, leading to the proliferation and migration of satellite cells to the damaged area.[78] In some conditions, recruitment of satellite cells also requires damage to the connective tissue that separates muscles.[78,79]

On exposure to signals from the damaged environment, quiescent satellite cells are activated and start proliferating; those cells are referred to as myogenic precursor cells (MPCs) or adult myoblasts. At the molecular level, activation of MPC is characterized by the rapid upregulation of two MRFs: Myf5 and MyoD. MyoD upregulation appears within 12 hours of activation and is detectable prior to any sign of cellular division.[80,81] Accordingly, MyoD$^{-/-}$ mice have a reduced regenerative capacity characterized by an increase in MPC population and a decrease in regenerated myotubes.[82]

After the MPC proliferation phase, expression of myogenin and MRF4 (MRF members) is upregulated concomitant with the onset of a terminal differentiation program. The differentiation program is completed with the activation of muscle-specific proteins, such as MHC, and the fusion of MPC.[83]

At the end of regeneration, MPCs fuse to each other to form syncytial muscle fibers. Intercellular junction structures that mediate cell-cell adhesion play an important role in this process. In this regard, classic cadherins such as M-cadherin are essential molecules for the specific fusion of myoblasts with each other during muscle regeneration.[84] Other molecules, such as m-calpain, and intermediary filament members, such as vimentin, desmin, and nestin, have also been implicated in myoblast fusion during muscle regeneration.[85]

Satellite Cell Activators

Growth factors play an important role in a number of muscle regeneration mechanisms. These include satellite cell activation, migration to the injury site, proliferation of satellite cell–derived MPCs, and differentiation to myotubes and myofibers. Hepatocyte growth factor (HGF) is considered to be one of the most important growth factors involved in organ regeneration because of its mitogenic properties.[86] The released HGF binds to the c-met receptor, which initiates signals that lead to DNA synthesis.[80]

HGF isolated from extracts of injured muscles can induce quiescent satellite cell activation.[87] In-vitro, HGF can stimulate quiescent satellite cells to enter the cell cycle and increase MPC proliferation and inhibit MPC differentiation.[87,88] In addition, HGF plays a role in promoting satellite cell migration to the site of injury via activation of the Ras/Ral pathway.[89]

Fibroblast growth factors (FGFs) are potent activators of MPC proliferation and inhibitors of MPC differentiation.[90,91] FGF-6 is expressed in muscle and is upregulated during muscle regeneration.[91] FGF-2 is a potent myoblast activator *in vitro*.[92]

As discussed previously, different IGFs play a role in the maintenance of muscle mass. In the context of muscle repair, *in-vitro* studies show that both IGF-I and IGF-II are able to alter MRF expression and induce proliferation, differentiation, and fusion of myoblasts.[92] IGFs may, in particular, be implicated in promoting reinnervation during muscle repair since motoneurons also respond to IGFs.[93]

Transforming growth factor β (TGF-β) family members have been recognized as modulators of myoblast activity by inhibiting proliferation and differentiation.[90] The roles of TGF-β$_1$, -β$_2$, and -β$_3$ during muscle regeneration are still not well understood and involve several mechanisms, such as myoblast fusion, regulation of immune responses, and motoneuron survival.[94]

Self-Renewal of Muscle Satellite Cells

Several models have been proposed to explain the maintenance of the quiescent satellite cell population in adult skeletal muscle. In one of them, satellite cells divide to produce two daughter cells, one activated and the other quiescent.[95] This asymmetric cell division may be explained by the observation that the plasma membrane–associated protein Numb is segregated asymmetrically in activated MPCs. Cells expressing high levels of Numb were found to undergo differentiation, whereas low or absent expression of Numb resulted in continued proliferation and inhibition of differentiation.[96]

Differential expression of the myogenic regulatory factors following activation supports a model in which activated satellite cells can return to a quiescent state and repopulate the satellite cell compartment. Activation of satellite cells results in upregulation of Myf-5 or MyoD (Figure 4). In the absence of MyoD, activated MPCs show enhanced proliferation and fail to differentiate, and these cells represent an intermediate stage between activated MPCs and quiescent satellite cells.[97,98] When Pax7 is overexpressed, MyoD is downregulated; therefore, inhibition of differentiation and cell-cycle withdrawal in myogenic cells occur.[99] Moreover, Pax7 is never detected in cells expressing myogenin (a marker of terminal differentiation).[100]

Activated satellite cells are able to return to a quiescent state and repopulate the satellite cell compartment. In this model, activated satellite cells enter a proliferative stage by expressing Myf-5 and/or MyoD. Symmetric division gives rise to a population of daughter cells, some of which downregulate MyoD and repopulate the quiescent satellite cell compartment, whereas other cells maintain MyoD expression, finish the differentiation, and contribute to muscle repair.[100]

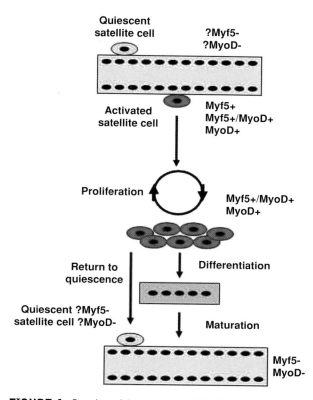

FIGURE 4. Overview of the expression of MyoD and Myf5 during skeletal muscle regeneration processes in a mouse model. Adapted from Cooper RN et al.[72]

Mechanisms of Muscle Injury in COPD
Sedentarism

Owing to shortness of breath during exercise, patients with COPD often adopt a sedentary lifestyle. Physical inactivity causes net loss of muscle mass, reduces the force-generating capacity of muscle, and decreases its resistance to fatigue.[101] In this context, exercise training is known to improve muscle function in COPD patients.[101–106] However, some of the biochemical abnormalities found in the muscles of COPD patients are unlikely to be explained just by sedentarism. For instance, sedentarism is characterized by low cytochrome oxidase activity,[107] whereas an increased activity of cytochrome oxidase has been observed in the skeletal muscle of patients with COPD.[108] Furthermore, this same abnormality occurs in circulating lymphocytes in COPD patients,[109] and, given that these cells are not influenced by muscle inactivity, other explanations need to be entertained. Finally, at variance with the normal training response, exercise in patients with COPD enhances the release of amino acids from skeletal muscle, particularly alanine and glutamine.[110–113] All of the above suggest the presence of intrinsic amino acid metabolic abnormalities in COPD skeletal muscles, which are discussed below.

Metabolic Abnormalities

Skeletal muscle of COPD patients is characterized by an altered amino acid metabolism, as shown by a loss of the aminoacid alanine[114] and a reduction in transaminase activities[115] during exercise.

The skeletal muscle oxidative capacity measured by the activity of oxidative enzymes as citrate synthase (CS) and 3-hydroxyacyl CoA dehydrogenase (HADH) seems to be significantly reduced in COPD patients.[116–118] These results are in concordance with the early onset of lactic acidosis in COPD.[118,119] In contrast with this reduced oxidative capacity observed in the skeletal muscles of COPD patients, increased activity of mitochondrial cytochrome oxidase has been reported in COPD patients.[108]

On the other hand, creatine kinase (CK) activity was significantly greater in the muscles of patients with COPD.[120] Mechanistically, this upregulation of CK activity has been identified as oxidative protein modification involving carbonylation.[120]

Skeletal muscular uncoupling protein 3 (UCP3) has been implicated in the regulation of energy metabolism. UCP3 content is decreased in the peripheral skeletal muscle of patients with COPD, and this is related to disease severity.[121]

Catabolic/anabolic disturbances were found in COPD patients, leading to a shift toward catabolism.[122] Phosphofructokinase activity was higher in COPD patients, whereas succinic acid dehydrogenase and HADH activities were decreased.[117]

Tissue Hypoxia

Several observations support the role for tissue hypoxia in COPD. It has been reported that hypoxia affects the contractile properties of respiratory and hind limb muscles[123,124]; induces hypoxia-inducible transcription factor 1 expression[125] and angiogenesis,[126,127]; suppresses protein synthesis; causes net loss of amino acids; and reduces expression of MHC isoforms[128,129] and loss of muscle mass.[130,131]

Systemic Inflammation

Systemic inflammation is likely an important pathogenic mechanism affecting skeletal muscles in COPD. COPD patients show increased plasma levels of a variety of proinflammatory cytokines, particularly TNF-α.[132–136] Circulating monocytes and bronchoalveolar lavage T lymphocytes harvested from COPD patients produce more TNF-α and other cytokines than in healthy controls.[137–139] Accumulation of neutrophils in the skeletal muscle of patients with COPD has been also reported.[140]

Proinflammatory cytokines are also produced by human skeletal cells and can exert autocrine effects.[141] As indicated above, the most important effect of TNF-α is proteolysis in skeletal muscle throughout a number of mechanisms, which include the upregulation of atrogins,[62,63] apoptosis,[65] and inhibition of ribosomal initiation of protein synthesis.[67,142]

In addition, TNF-α can induce the expression of a variety of genes, such as those encoding the inducible form of nitric oxide synthase (iNOS) (see next section), creating a closed loop and contributing to the persistence and amplification of the inflammatory cascade.[143]

Oxidative and Nitrosative Stress

Over the past decade, reactive oxygen species (ROS) and nitric oxide (NO) derivatives have been established as physiologic modulators of skeletal muscle function.[144,145] Total antioxidant capacity is enhanced in the peripheral muscles of COPD patients, suggesting that the antioxidant system may be exposed to and subsequently triggered by elevated levels of ROS.[144] This might be particularly relevant since regulation of glutathione, the most important intracellular antioxidant,[18] is abnormal in the skeletal muscle of patients with COPD.[110,111,146] Oxidative stress affects muscles, causing enhanced fatigue[147–149] and proteolysis.[150]

NO is a free radical synthesized from the amino acid L-arginine by the action of three nitric oxide synthases (NOSs),[151,152] all of which are expressed in human skeletal muscle.[153] Two NOS isoforms, the so-called type I neuronal or brain NOS and type III or endothelial NOS, are expressed constitutively in skeletal muscle, whereas the third isoform, type II NOS or iNOS, is expressed in response to a variety of stimuli, including cytokines, oxidants, and/or hypoxia. Among the three isoforms, type I seems to play a central role in the regulation of contractile properties of skeletal muscles in mammals.[148]

In this regard, the type I NOS isoform is upregulated in the quadriceps femoris of COPD patients (Figure 5), and this correlates with elevated 3-nitrotyrosine levels in the same muscles. These results indicate the development of nitrosative stress in the quadriceps of patients with COPD, suggesting its involvement in muscle dysfunction.[154]

Systemic inflammation can upregulate the expression of iNOS in myotubes,[155] and iNOS overexpression has been reported in COPD patients who lose weight.[156,157] In turn, the increased NO production resulting from NOS upregulation can cause protein nitrotyrosination,[154,157,158] which, in turn, can alter the function of key proteins in the regulation of skeletal muscle performance, such as SERCA2, and facilitate protein degradation through the U/P system[150] and/or enhance skeletal muscle apoptosis. Finally, NOS induction can also impair skeletal muscle contractility.[159,160]

In addition, ROS and NO activities impact on the aging of skeletal muscle,[161] characterized, among other things, by loss of muscle mass.[162] In this context, a premature and/or accelerated aging process seems to occur in smokers.[163]

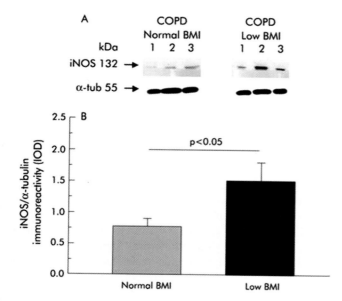

FIGURE 5. *A,* Representative Western blot of inducible nitric oxide synthase (iNOS) in the quadriceps femoris muscle of three patients with chronic obstructive pulmonary disease (COPD) with a normal body mass index (BMI) and three patients with low BMI. *B,* Mean (standard error) iNOS expression (normalized by α-tubulin content) in each group. Adapted from Agusti A et al.[156]

Tobacco Smoke

Although it is accepted that tobacco smoke is the main risk factor for COPD,[3] much less attention has been paid to the direct potential effects of tobacco smoke on skeletal muscle structure and function. Components of tobacco smoke clearly reach the systemic circulation, as shown by the increased prevalence of coronary artery disease and endothelial dysfunction in smokers,[164,165] and contain many substances that are potentially harmful to skeletal muscle. For instance, nicotine alters the expression of important growth factors, such as TGF-β_1, which, together with myostatin signal transduction pathways, potently repress skeletal muscle cell differentiation.[166] On the other hand, nicotine competes with acetylcholine for its receptor at the neuromuscular junction, thus having the potential to affect muscle contraction directly. Furthermore, nicotine also interferes with postsynaptic receptor scaffold formation by preventing the tyrosine phosphorylation of acetylcholine receptors (AChRs), which precedes AChR clustering.[167]

Skeletal Muscle Abnormalities in COPD
Fiber Type Changes

Patients with COPD and chronic respiratory failure exhibit skeletal muscle structural alterations, characterized by a decrease in type I fibers[168–172] and an increase in the proportion and cross-sectional area of type IIb fibers.[170] These

findings suggest an adaptation of the muscle fibers to a low partial pressure of oxygen in arterial blood.[170] Loss of muscle mass in COPD patients is associated specifically with fiber types IIA and IIX and IIX atrophy.[173]

Effects on Respiratory Muscles

Proteolysis/apoptosis-related mechanisms also occur in respiratory muscles. 20S (Svelberg) proteasome activity was increased approximately threefold in the diaphragm of patients with COPD, together with increased messenger ribonucleic acid (mRNA) levels of the muscle-specific ubiquitin-ligase MAFbx and caspase-3.[174]

Metabolic changes have been also described in respiratory muscles. Biopsies of the diaphragm from COPD demonstrated increased activities of L(+)HADH (a marker of the β-oxidation capacity). These results suggest that in COPD, the diaphragm adapts to a higher workload by increasing the oxidative capacity and mitochondrial function.[175,176] In COPD patients, the metabolic activities of hexokinase, CS, and HADH were higher in intercostal muscles when compared with latissimus dorsi.[177] These data support the hypothesis that the internal and external intercostal muscles play a more important role in COPD patients than in normal subjects and are consistent with the hypothesis that COPD has an endurance training effect on both intercostal muscles.[177] In this context, biopsies of diaphragm and intercostal muscles placed in an oxygraphic chamber to measure maximal oxygen uptake show that the maximal oxidative capacity of the diaphragm and external intercostal muscles was increased significantly in emphysematous COPD patients.[178] This is consistent with an increased mitochondrial capacity and efficiency in the inspiratory muscles, supporting an endurance training-like effect.[178]

Accordingly, oxidative stress may also occur in respiratory muscles. In fact, the diaphragms of patients with severe COPD showed both higher protein carbonyl groups and hydroxynonenal-protein adducts than control subjects.[179] NOS induction was found in COPD limb muscles in which nitrossative stress occurs.[156,157] However changes in neuronal NOS and iNOS were not found in the diaphragm of COPD patients,[179] indicating that oxidative stress, rather than NO, occurs in the diaphragm of COPD patients. In this context, the reduced levels of glutamate and glutathione reported in the quadriceps femoris of patients with COPD[110,111,146] do not affect the diaphragm.[180] Other alterations have been reported in the diaphragms of COPD patients. Interestingly, COPD patients show an upregulation of mRNA levels of vascular endothelial growth factor in the diaphragm, suggesting an enhancement of angiogenesis.[181] Finally, a number of structural changes have also been observed in respiratory muscles. The previously described changes in fiber composition in limb muscles (a decrease in type I and an increase in type II proportion) have also been described in the

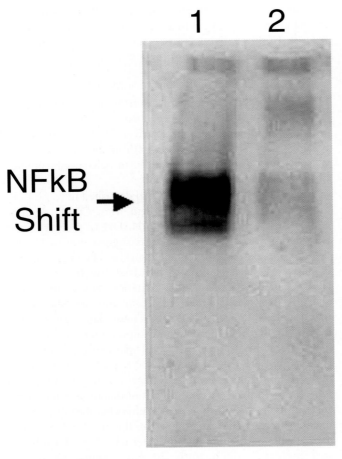

FIGURE 6. A representative electrophoretic mobility shift assay showing nuclear factor κB (NF-κB) binding to nuclear extracts from biopsy specimens of the quadriceps femoris muscle obtained from patients with chronic obstructive pulmonary disease with a normal body mass index (BMI) (*lane 1*) or a low BMI (*lane 2*). For details, see Agusti A et al.[157]

diaphragm, together with changes in the titin protein in COPD costal diaphragm biopsies.[77,175,182,183] Other structural changes reveal extensive collagen accumulation in the COPD diaphragm, as shown by postmortem diaphragm studies.[184]

Muscle Wasting

One of the most important systemic effects occurring in patients with COPD is muscle wasting.[21–30] Muscle wasting is particularly prevalent in patients with advanced disease.[185] Muscle mass, not body weight, predicts the outcome in patients with COPD[186] and has important clinical implications because it not only worsens their prognosis[187] but also affects their exercise capacity and health status.[188] It is therefore important to develop rational and effective new treatments to palliate weight loss in COPD.[29] To this end, a better understanding of the underlying cellular mechanism is essential.[29]

In broad terms, cachexia is characterized by increased myofibrillar protein breakdown.[189] Muscle protein breakdown in COPD is associated with a number of other tissue alterations that have been discussed above, in particular a shift in muscle fiber type,[168–172] a reduction in oxidative enzymes and oxidative capacity,[116–118] and alterations in the amino acid profile.[114,115] It is difficult to establish which abnormalities are, in fact, causes or effects of the cachectic condition. However, it is well established that systemic inflammation is an important pathogenic mechanism in COPD muscle waste. COPD patients show elevated plasma levels of TNF-α.[132–136] As indicated above, TNF-α can cause muscle wasting through a number of mechanisms. One of these mechanisms, an activation of the transcription factor NF-κB identified in C2C12 cells,[61] readily occurs in cachectic COPD patients (Figure 6).[157] NF-κB regulates the transcription of a number of genes, including iNOS. Elevated levels of iNOS protein[156,157] and nitrosination of key proteins such as SERCA2 have also been observed in cachectic COPD patients.

TNF-α-induced skeletal muscle DNA damage and apoptotic features have been identified in myotube cultures and in animal models.[64,65] In this regard, apoptotic features, such as DNA damage and PARP proteolysis, have also been observed in COPD patients who lose weight (Figure 7).[190]

Other causative factors of cachexia identified in COPD patients include protein degradation enhanced by increased ubiquination and neurohormonal effects, such as leptin production.[191] In this regard, it is worth mentioning that novel neurohormonal mechanisms were identified recently.

Ghrelin is a novel GH-releasing peptide that is an endogenous ligand for the GH secretagogue receptor. It is possible that release of GH from the pituitary gland might be regulated not only by hypothalamic GH-releasing hormone but also by ghrelin. Ghrelin stimulates food intake, induces adiposity, and acts directly on the central nervous system to decrease sympathetic nerve activity. Administration of ghrelin inhibits muscle wasting in cachectic patients with COPD.[192]

Other new factors include polyunsaturated fatty acids (PUFAs), which mediate several inflammatory pathways, including inhibition of iNOS and NO production.[193] Administration of PUFAs increased weight, fat-free mass, and muscle strength in patients with COPD.[194]

Conclusions

Skeletal muscle abnormalities are frequent and clinically relevant in patients with COPD, particularly in those with more severe disease. A better understanding of the cellular and molecular mechanisms underlying these alterations may facilitate the development of novel therapeutic strategies for this devastating disease. In this context, a number of these new therapeutic strategies are described in Chapter 29.

Healthy control   **COPD patient**

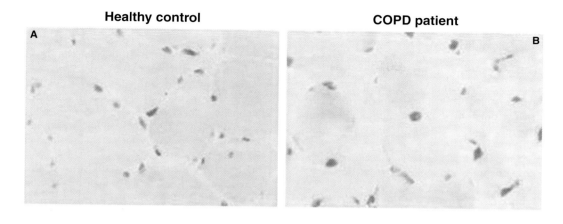

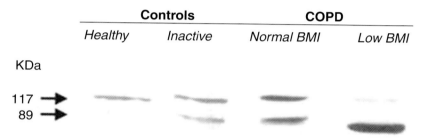

FIGURE 7. Deoxyribonucleic acid (DNA) damage in the skeletal muscle of low body weight patients with chronic obstructive pulmonary disease (COPD). *Top panel:* Representative example of a muscle biopsy (30x) obtained in a control subject (A) and in a patient with COPD and a low body mass index (BMI) (B). Apoptosis (TUNEL) assay: nuclei are small (blue in the original color picture) in the former (no DNA damage), whereas most of them are large (brown in the original color picture) (DNA damage) in the latter. *Bottom panel:* Western blot showing the relative intensities of the two poly(adenosine diphosphate–ribose) polymerase bands (89 and 117 kDa fragments) in a representative subject of each of the four groups studied. Adapted from Agusti A et al.[190]

References

1. Agusti AG. Systemic effects of chronic obstructive pulmonary disease. Novartis Found Symp 2001;234:242–9.
2. Andreassen H, Vestbo J. Chronic obstructive pulmonary disease as a systemic disease: an epidemiological perspective. Eur Respir J Suppl 2003;46:2s–4s.
3. Barnes PJ. Chronic obstructive pulmonary disease. N Engl J Med 2000;343:260–80.
4. Decramer M, De Benedetto F, Del Ponte A, Marinari S. Systemic effects of COPD. Respir Med 2005;99 Suppl B:S3–10.
5. Gross NJ. Extrapulmonary effects of chronic obstructive pulmonary disease. Curr Opin Pulm Med 2001;7:84–92.
6. Wouters EF. Chronic obstructive pulmonary disease 5: systemic effects of COPD. Thorax 2002;57:1067–70.
7. Wouters EF, Creutzberg EC, Schols AM. Systemic effects in COPD. Chest 2002;121:127S–30S.
8. Peripheral muscle function in COPD. Monaldi Arch Chest Dis 1997;52:303.
9. Skeletal muscle dysfunction in chronic obstructive pulmonary disease. A statement of the American Thoracic Society and European Respiratory Society. Am J Respir Crit Care Med 1999;159:S1–40.
10. Berton E, Antonucci R, Palange P. Skeletal muscle dysfunction in chronic obstructive pulmonary disease. Monaldi Arch Chest Dis 2001;56:418–22.
11. Casaburi R. Skeletal muscle function in COPD. Chest 2000;117:267S–71S.
12. Casaburi R. Skeletal muscle dysfunction in chronic obstructive pulmonary disease. Med Sci Sports Exerc 2001;33:S662–70.
13. Gosker HR, Wouters EF, van der Vusse GJ, Schols AM. Skeletal muscle dysfunction in chronic obstructive pulmonary disease and chronic heart failure: underlying mechanisms and therapy perspectives. Am J Clin Nutr 2000;71:1033–47.
14. Mador MJ, Bozkanat E. Skeletal muscle dysfunction in chronic obstructive pulmonary disease. Respir Res 2001;2:216–24.
15. Maltais F, LeBlanc P, Jobin J, Casaburi R. Peripheral muscle dysfunction in chronic obstructive pulmonary disease. Clin Chest Med 2000;21:665–77.
16. Maltais F, Debigare R. Biology of muscle impairment in COPD. Monaldi Arch Chest Dis 2003;59:338–41.
17. Polkey MI. Peripheral muscle weakness in COPD: where does it come from? Thorax 2003;58:741–2.
18. Reid MB. COPD as a muscle disease. Am J Respir Crit Care Med 2001;164:1101–2.

19. Troosters T, Gosselink R, Decramer M. Chronic obstructive pulmonary disease and chronic heart failure: two muscle diseases? J Cardiopulm Rehabil 2004;24:137–45.

20. Wagner PD. Is COPD also a disease of skeletal muscle? Am J Respir Crit Care Med 2002;165:1336–7.

21. Schols AM. Pulmonary cachexia. Int J Cardiol 2002;85:101–10.

22. Debigare R, Cote CH, Maltais F. Peripheral muscle wasting in chronic obstructive pulmonary disease. Clinical relevance and mechanisms. Am J Respir Crit Care Med 2001;164:1712–7.

23. Hasselgren PO, Fischer JE. Muscle cachexia: current concepts of intracellular mechanisms and molecular regulation. Ann Surg 2001;233:9–17.

24. Farber MO, Mannix ET. Tissue wasting in patients with chronic obstructive pulmonary disease. Neurol Clin 2000;18:245–62.

25. Morley JE, Thomas DR, Wilson MM. Cachexia: pathophysiology and clinical relevance. Am J Clin Nutr 2006;83:735–43.

26. Delano MJ, Moldawer LL. The origins of cachexia in acute and chronic inflammatory diseases. Nutr Clin Pract 2006;21:68–81.

27. Schols AM, Broekhuizen R, Weling-Scheepers CA, Wouters EF. Body composition and mortality in chronic obstructive pulmonary disease. Am J Clin Nutr 2005;82:53–9.

28. Schols AM. Pulmonary cachexia. Int J Cardiol 2002;85:101–10.

29. Debigare R, Cote CH, Maltais F. Peripheral muscle wasting in chronic obstructive pulmonary disease. Clinical relevance and mechanisms. Am J Respir Crit Care Med 2001;164:1712–7.

30. Farber MO, Mannix ET. Tissue wasting in patients with chronic obstructive pulmonary disease. Neurol Clin 2000;18:245–62.

31. Nici L, Donner C, Wouters E, et al. American Thoracic Society/European Respiratory Society statement on pulmonary rehabilitation. Am J Respir Crit Care Med 2006;173:1390–413.

32. Young B, Heath JW. Muscle. in: Young B, Heath JW, eds. Wheater's functional histology. New York: Harcourt; 2000. p. 97–115.

33. Alberts B, Bray D, Hopkins K, et al. Cytoskeleton. In: Alberts B, Bray D, Hopkins K. Essential cell biology. New York: Garland Science; 2000. p. 592–605.

34. Brooke MH, Kaiser KK. Three "myosin adenosine triphosphatase" systems: the nature of their pH lability and sulfhydryl dependence. J Histochem Cytochem 1970;18:670–2.

35. Ennion S, Sant'ana PJ, Sargeant AJ, et al. Characterization of human skeletal muscle fibres according to the myosin heavy chains they express. J Muscle Res Cell Motil 1995;16:35–43.

36. Schiaffino S, Gorza L, Sartore S, et al. Three myosin heavy chain isoforms in type 2 skeletal muscle fibres. J Muscle Res Cell Motil 1989;10:197–205.

37. Larsson L, Ansved T, Edstrom L, et al. Effects of age on physiological, immunohistochemical and biochemical properties of fast-twitch single motor units in the rat. J Physiol 1991;443:257–75.

38. Larsson L, Edstrom L, Lindegren B, et al. MHC composition and enzyme-histochemical and physiological properties of a novel fast-twitch motor unit type. Am J Physiol 1991;261:C93-101.

39. Sieck GC, Fournier M, Prakash YS, Blanco CE. Myosin phenotype and SDH enzyme variability among motor unit fibers. J Appl Physiol 1996;80:2179–89.

40. Stein TP, Buzby GP. Protein metabolism in surgical patients. Surg Clin North Am 1981;61:519–27.

41. Stein TP, Wade CE. Protein turnover in atrophying muscle: from nutritional intervention to microarray expression analysis. Curr Opin Clin Nutr Metab Care 2003;6:95–102.

42. Florini JR, Ewton DZ, Coolican SA. Growth hormone and the insulin-like growth factor system in myogenesis. Endocr Rev 1996;17:481–517.

43. Urban RJ, Bodenburg YH, Gilkison C, et al. Testosterone administration to elderly men increases skeletal muscle strength and protein synthesis. Am J Physiol 1995;269:E820–6.

44. Coolican SA, Samuel DS, Ewton DZ, et al. The mitogenic and myogenic actions of insulin-like growth factors utilize distinct signaling pathways. J Biol Chem 1997;272:6653–62.

45. Fryburg DA. Insulin-like growth factor I exerts growth hormone- and insulin-like actions on human muscle protein metabolism. Am J Physiol 1994;267:E331–6.

46. Lecker SH, Jagoe RT, Gilbert A, et al. Multiple types of skeletal muscle atrophy involve a common program of changes in gene expression. FASEB J 2004;18:39–51.

47. Sandri M, Sandri C, Gilbert A, et al. FOXO transcription factors induce the atrophy-related ubiquitin ligase atrogin-1 and cause skeletal muscle atrophy. Cell 2004;117:399–412.

48. Latres E, Amini AR, Amini AA, et al. Insulin-like growth factor-1 (IGF-1) inversely regulates atrophy-induced genes via the phosphatidylinositol 3-kinase/Akt/mammalian target of rapamycin (PI3K/Akt/mTOR) pathway. J Biol Chem 2005;280:2737–44.

49. Stitt TN, Drujan D, Clarke BA, et al. The IGF-1/PI3K/Akt pathway prevents expression of muscle atrophy-induced ubiquitin ligases by inhibiting FOXO transcription factors. Mol Cell 2004;14:395–403.

50. Semsarian C, Wu MJ, Ju YK, et al. Skeletal muscle hypertrophy is mediated by a Ca^{2+}-dependent calcineurin signalling pathway. Nature 1999;400:576–81.

51. Jacquemin V, Furling D, Bigot A, et al. IGF-1 induces human myotube hypertrophy by increasing cell recruitment. Exp Cell Res 2004;299:148–58.

52. Machida S, Booth FW. Insulin-like growth factor 1 and muscle growth: implication for satellite cell proliferation. Proc Nutr Soc 2004;63:337–40.

53. Agusti AG, Noguera A, Sauleda J, et al. Systemic effects of chronic obstructive pulmonary disease. Eur Respir J 2003;21:347–60.

54. Baud V, Karin M. Signal transduction by tumor necrosis factor and its relatives. Trends Cell Biol 2001;11:372–7.

55. Chen G, Goeddel DV. TNF-R1 signaling: a beautiful pathway. Science 2002;296:1634–5.

56. Wajant H, Pfizenmaier K, Scheurich P. Tumor necrosis factor signaling. Cell Death Differ 2003;10:45–65.

57. MacEwan DJ. TNF receptor subtype signalling: differences and cellular consequences. Cell Signal 2002;14:477–92.

58. Liu ZG, Hsu H, Goeddel DV, Karin M. Dissection of TNF receptor 1 effector functions: JNK activation is not linked to apoptosis while NF-kappaB activation prevents cell death. Cell 1996;87:565–76.

59. Llovera M, Garcia-Martinez C, Agell N, et al. TNF can directly induce the expression of ubiquitin-dependent proteolytic system in rat soleus muscles. Biochem Biophys Res Commun 1997;230:238–41.

60. Goodman MN. Tumor necrosis factor induces skeletal muscle protein breakdown in rats. Am J Physiol 1991;260:E727–30.

61. Li YP, Reid MB. NF-kappaB mediates the protein loss induced by TNF-alpha in differentiated skeletal muscle myotubes. Am J Physiol Regul Integr Comp Physiol 2000;279:R1165–70.

62. Li YP, Lecker SH, Chen Y, et al. TNF-alpha increases ubiquitin-conjugating activity in skeletal muscle by up-regulating UbcH2/E220k. FASEB J 2003;17:1048–57.

63. Li YP, Chen Y, John J, et al. TNF-alpha acts via p38 MAPK to stimulate expression of the ubiquitin ligase atrogin1/MAFbx in skeletal muscle. FASEB J 2005;19:362–70.

64. Tolosa L, Morla M, Iglesias A, et al. IFN-gamma prevents TNF-alpha-induced apoptosis in C2C12 myotubes through down-regulation of TNF-R2 and increased NF-kappaB activity. Cell Signal 2005;17:1333–42.

65. Carbo N, Busquets S, van Royen M, et al. TNF-alpha is involved in activating DNA fragmentation in skeletal muscle. Br J Cancer 2002;86:1012–6.

66. Williamson DL, Kimball SR, Jefferson LS. Acute treatment with TNF-alpha attenuates insulin-stimulated protein synthesis in cultures of C2C12 myotubes through a MEK1-sensitive mechanism. Am J Physiol Endocrinol Metab 2005;289:E95–104.

67. del Aguila LF, Claffey KP, Kirwan JP. TNF-alpha impairs insulin signaling and insulin stimulation of glucose uptake in C2C12 muscle cells. Am J Physiol 1999;276:E849–55.

68. Plomgaard P, Bouzakri K, Krogh-Madsen R, et al. Tumor necrosis factor-alpha induces skeletal muscle insulin resistance in healthy human subjects via inhibition of Akt substrate 160 phosphorylation. Diabetes 2005;54:2939–45.

69. Frost RA, Nystrom GJ, Lang CH. Tumor necrosis factor-alpha decreases insulin-like growth factor-I messenger ribonucleic acid expression in C2C12 myoblasts via a Jun N-terminal kinase pathway. Endocrinology 2003;144:1770–9.

70. Grounds MD. Towards understanding skeletal muscle regeneration. Pathol Res Pract 1991;187:1–22.

71. Schultz E, Gibson MC, Champion T. Satellite cells are mitotically quiescent in mature mouse muscle: an EM and radioautographic study. J Exp Zool 1978;206:451–6.

72. Cooper RN, Tajbakhsh S, Mouly V, et al. In vivo satellite cell activation via Myf5 and MyoD in regenerating mouse skeletal muscle. J Cell Sci 1999;112 (Pt 17):2895–901.

73. Grounds MD, Yablonka-Reuveni Z. Molecular and cell biology of skeletal muscle regeneration. Mol Cell Biol Hum Dis Ser 1993;3:210–56.

74. Sabourin LA, Rudnicki MA. The molecular regulation of myogenesis. Clin Genet 2000;57:16–25.

75. Brzoska E, Grabowska I, Wrobel E, Moraczewski J. Syndecan-4 distribution during the differentiation of satellite cells isolated from soleus muscle treated by phorbol ester and calphostin C. Cell Mol Biol Lett 2003;8:269–78.

76. Cornelison DD, Filla MS, Stanley HM, et al. Syndecan-3 and syndecan-4 specifically mark skeletal muscle satellite cells and are implicated in satellite cell maintenance and muscle regeneration. Dev Biol 2001;239:79–94.

77. Schultz E, McCormick KM. Skeletal muscle satellite cells. Rev Physiol Biochem Pharmacol 1994;123:213–57.

78. Schultz E, Jaryszak DL, Valliere CR. Response of satellite cells to focal skeletal muscle injury. Muscle Nerve 1985;8:217–22.

79. Schultz E, Jaryszak DL, Gibson MC, Albright DJ. Absence of exogenous satellite cell contribution to regeneration of frozen skeletal muscle. J Muscle Res Cell Motil 1986;7:361–7.

80. Cornelison DD, Wold BJ. Single-cell analysis of regulatory gene expression in quiescent and activated mouse skeletal muscle satellite cells. Dev Biol 1997;191:270–83.

81. Yablonka-Reuveni Z, Rivera AJ. Temporal expression of regulatory and structural muscle proteins during myogenesis of satellite cells on isolated adult rat fibers. Dev Biol 1994;164:588–603.

82. Cornelison DD, Olwin BB, Rudnicki MA, Wold BJ. MyoD(−/−) satellite cells in single-fiber culture are differentiation defective and MRF4 deficient. Dev Biol 2000;224:122–37.

83. Zhou Z, Bornemann A. MRF4 protein expression in regenerating rat muscle. J Muscle Res Cell Motil 2001;22:311–6.

84. Geiger B, Ayalon O. Cadherins. Annu Rev Cell Biol 1992;8:307–32.

85. Vaittinen S, Lukka R, Sahlgren C, et al. The expression of intermediate filament protein nestin as related to vimentin and desmin in regenerating skeletal muscle. J Neuropathol Exp Neurol 2001;60:588–97.

86. Zarnegar R, Michalopoulos GK. The many faces of hepatocyte growth factor: from hepatopoiesis to hematopoiesis. J Cell Biol 1995;129:1177–80.

87. Tatsumi R, Anderson JE, Nevoret CJ, et al. HGF/SF is present in normal adult skeletal muscle and is capable of activating satellite cells. Dev Biol 1998;194:114–28.

88. Miller KJ, Thaloor D, Matteson S, Pavlath GK. Hepatocyte growth factor affects satellite cell activation and differentiation in regenerating skeletal muscle. Am J Physiol Cell Physiol 2000;278:C174–81.

89. Suzuki J, Yamazaki Y, Li G, et al. Involvement of Ras and Ral in chemotactic migration of skeletal myoblasts. Mol Cell Biol 2000;20:4658–65.

90. Allen RE, Boxhorn LK. Regulation of skeletal muscle satellite cell proliferation and differentiation by transforming growth factor-beta, insulin-like growth factor I, and fibroblast growth factor. J Cell Physiol 1989;138:311–5.

91. Kastner S, Elias MC, Rivera AJ, Yablonka-Reuveni Z. Gene expression patterns of the fibroblast growth factors and their receptors during myogenesis of rat satellite cells. J Histochem Cytochem 2000;48:1079–96.

92. Lefaucheur JP, Sebille A. Muscle regeneration following injury can be modified in vivo by immune neutralization of basic fibroblast growth factor, transforming growth factor beta 1 or insulin-like growth factor I. J Neuroimmunol 1995;57:85–91.

93. Levinovitz A, Jennische E, Oldfors A, et al. Activation of insulin-like growth factor II expression during skeletal muscle regeneration in the rat: correlation with myotube formation. Mol Endocrinol 1992;6:1227–34.

94. McLennan IS, Koishi K. The transforming growth factor-betas: multifaceted regulators of the development and maintenance of skeletal muscles, motoneurons and Schwann cells. Int J Dev Biol 2002;46:559–67.

95. Charge SB, Rudnicki MA. Cellular and molecular regulation of muscle regeneration. Physiol Rev 2004;84:209–38.

96. Conboy IM, Rando TA. The regulation of Notch signaling controls satellite cell activation and cell fate determination in postnatal myogenesis. Dev Cell 2002;3:397–409.

97. Megeney LA, Kablar B, Garrett K, et al. MyoD is required for myogenic stem cell function in adult skeletal muscle. Genes Dev 1996;10:1173–83.

98. Sabourin LA, Girgis-Gabardo A, Seale P, et al. Reduced differentiation potential of primary MyoD$^{-/-}$ myogenic cells derived from adult skeletal muscle. J Cell Biol 1999;144:631–43.

99. Olguin HC, Olwin BB. Pax-7 up-regulation inhibits myogenesis and cell cycle progression in satellite cells: a potential mechanism for self-renewal. Dev Biol 2004;275:375–88.

100. Zammit PS, Golding JP, Nagata Y, et al. Muscle satellite cells adopt divergent fates: a mechanism for self-renewal? J Cell Biol 2004;166:347–57.

101. Maltais F, LeBlanc P, Simard C, et al. Skeletal muscle adaptation to endurance training in patients with chronic obstructive pulmonary disease. Am J Respir Crit Care Med 1996;154:442–7.

102. Casaburi R, Porszasz J, Burns MR, et al. Physiologic benefits of exercise training in rehabilitation of patients with severe chronic obstructive pulmonary disease. Am J Respir Crit Care Med 1997;155:1541–51.

103. Gosselin N, Lambert K, Poulain M, et al. Endurance training improves skeletal muscle electrical activity in active COPD patients. Muscle Nerve 2003;28:744–53.

104. Koppers RJ, Vos PJ, Boot CR, Folgering HT. Exercise performance improves in patients with COPD due to respiratory muscle endurance training. Chest 2006;129:886–92.

105. McKeough ZJ, Alison JA, Bye PT, et al. Exercise capacity and quadriceps muscle metabolism following training in subjects with COPD. Respir Med 2006;100:1817–25.

106. Sala E, Roca J, Marrades RM, et al. Effects of endurance training on skeletal muscle bioenergetics in chronic obstructive pulmonary disease. Am J Respir Crit Care Med 1999;159:1726–34.

107. Henriksson J, Reitman JS. Time course of changes in human skeletal muscle succinate dehydrogenase and cytochrome oxidase activities and maximal oxygen uptake with physical activity and inactivity. Acta Physiol Scand 1977;99:91–7.

108. Sauleda J, Garcia-Palmer F, Wiesner RJ, et al. Cytochrome oxidase activity and mitochondrial gene expression in skeletal muscle of patients with chronic obstructive pulmonary disease. Am J Respir Crit Care Med 1998;157:1413–7.

109. Sauleda J, Garcia-Palmer FJ, Gonzalez G, et al. The activity of cytochrome oxidase is increased in circulating lymphocytes of patients with chronic obstructive pulmonary disease, asthma, and chronic arthritis. Am J Respir Crit Care Med 2000;161:32–5.

110. Engelen MP, Schols AM, Does JD, et al. Altered glutamate metabolism is associated with reduced muscle glutathione levels in patients with emphysema. Am J Respir Crit Care Med 2000;161:98–103.

111. Engelen MP, Wouters EF, Deutz NE, et al. Effects of exercise on amino acid metabolism in patients with chronic obstructive pulmonary disease. Am J Respir Crit Care Med 2001;163:859–64.

112. Engelen MP, Schols AM. Altered amino acid metabolism in chronic obstructive pulmonary disease: new therapeutic perspective? Curr Opin Clin Nutr Metab Care 2003;6:73–8.

113. Engelen MP, Orozco-Levi M, Deutz NE, et al. Glutathione and glutamate levels in the diaphragm of patients with chronic obstructive pulmonary disease. Eur Respir J 2004;23:545–51.

114. Steiner MC, Evans R, Deacon SJ, et al. Adenine nucleotide loss in the skeletal muscles during exercise in chronic obstructive pulmonary disease. Thorax 2005;60:932–6.

115. Cepelak I, Dodig S, Romic D, et al. Enzyme catalytic activities in chronic obstructive pulmonary disease. Arch Med Res 2006;37:624–9.

116. Maltais F, LeBlanc P, Whittom F, et al. Oxidative enzyme activities of the vastus lateralis muscle and the functional status in patients with COPD. Thorax 2000;55:848–53.

117. Jakobsson P, Jorfeldt L, Henriksson J. Metabolic enzyme activity in the quadriceps femoris muscle in patients with severe chronic obstructive pulmonary disease. Am J Respir Crit Care Med 1995;151:374–7.

118. Maltais F, Simard AA, Simard C, et al. Oxidative capacity of the skeletal muscle and lactic acid kinetics during exercise in normal subjects and in patients with COPD. Am J Respir Crit Care Med 1996;153:288–93.

119. Maltais F, Jobin J, Sullivan MJ, et al. Metabolic and hemodynamic responses of lower limb during exercise in patients with COPD. J Appl Physiol 1998;84:1573–80.

120. Barreiro E, Gea J, Matar G, Hussain SN. Expression and carbonylation of creatine kinase in the quadriceps femoris muscles of patients with chronic obstructive pulmonary disease. Am J Respir Cell Mol Biol 2005;33:636–42.

121. Gosker HR, Schrauwen P, Hesselink MK, et al. Uncoupling protein-3 content is decreased in peripheral skeletal muscle of patients with COPD. Eur Respir J 2003;22:88–93.

122. Debigare R, Marquis K, Cote CH, et al. Catabolic/anabolic balance and muscle wasting in patients with COPD. Chest 2003;124:83–9.

123. Shiota S, Okada T, Naitoh H, et al. Hypoxia and hypercapnia affect contractile and histological properties of rat diaphragm and hind limb muscles. Pathophysiology 2004;11:23–30.

124. Ottenheijm CA, Heunks LM, Geraedts MC, Dekhuijzen PN. Hypoxia-induced skeletal muscle fiber dysfunction: role for reactive nitrogen species. Am J Physiol Lung Cell Mol Physiol 2006;290:L127–35.

125. Vogt M, Puntschart A, Geiser J, et al. Molecular adaptations in human skeletal muscle to endurance training under simulated hypoxic conditions. J Appl Physiol 2001;91:173–82.

126. Deveci D, Marshall JM, Egginton S. Chronic hypoxia induces prolonged angiogenesis in skeletal muscles of rat. Exp Physiol 2002;87:287–91.

127. Hoppeler H. Vascular growth in hypoxic skeletal muscle. Adv Exp Med Biol 1999;474:277–86.

128. Bigard AX, Sanchez H, Birot O, Serrurier B. Myosin heavy chain composition of skeletal muscles in young rats growing under hypobaric hypoxia conditions. J Appl Physiol 2000;88:479–86.

129. Rennie MJ, Edwards RH, Emery PW, et al. Depressed protein synthesis is the dominant characteristic of muscle wasting and cachexia. Clin Physiol 1983;3:387–98.

130. Green HJ, Sutton JR, Cymerman A, et al. Operation Everest II: adaptations in human skeletal muscle. J Appl Physiol 1989;66:2454–61.

131. Bigard AX, Brunet A, Guezennec CY, Monod H. Skeletal muscle changes after endurance training at high altitude. J Appl Physiol 1991;71:2114–21.

132. Rabinovich RA, Figueras M, Ardite E, et al. Increased tumour necrosis factor-alpha plasma levels during moderate-intensity exercise in COPD patients. Eur Respir J 2003;21:789–94.

133. Di Francia M, Barbier D, Mege JL, Orehek J. Tumor necrosis factor-alpha levels and weight loss in chronic obstructive pulmonary disease. Am J Respir Crit Care Med 1994;150:1453–5.

134. Schols AM, Buurman WA, Staal van den Brekel AJ, et al. Evidence for a relation between metabolic derangements and increased levels of inflammatory mediators in a subgroup of patients with chronic obstructive pulmonary disease. Thorax 1996;51:819–24.

135. Yasuda N, Gotoh K, Minatoguchi S, et al. An increase of soluble Fas, an inhibitor of apoptosis, associated with progression of COPD. Respir Med 1998;92:993–9.

136. Eid AA, Ionescu AA, Nixon LS, et al. Inflammatory response and body composition in chronic obstructive pulmonary disease. Am J Respir Crit Care Med 2001;164:1414–8.

137. de Godoy I, Donahoe M, Calhoun WJ, et al. Elevated TNF-α production by peripheral blood monocytes of weight-losing COPD patients. Am J Respir Crit Care Med 1996;153:633–7.

138. Barcelo B, Pons J, Fuster A, et al. Intracellular cytokine profile of T lymphocytes in patients with chronic obstructive pulmonary disease. Clin Exp Immunol 2006;145:474–9.

139. Barczyk A, Pierzchala W, Kon OM, et al. Cytokine production by bronchoalveolar lavage T lymphocytes in chronic obstructive pulmonary disease. J Allergy Clin Immunol 2006;117:1484–92.

140. Peterson JM, Feeback KD, Baas JH, Pizza FX. Tumor necrosis factor-alpha promotes the accumulation of neutrophils and macrophages in skeletal muscle. J Appl Physiol 2006;101:1394–9.

141. Plomgaard P, Penkowa M, Pedersen BK. Fiber type specific expression of TNF-alpha, IL-6 and IL-18 in human skeletal muscles. Exerc Immunol Rev 2005;11:53–63.

142. Williamson DL, Kimball SR, Jefferson LS. Acute treatment with TNF-α attenuates insulin-stimulated protein synthesis in cultures of C2C12 myotubes through a MEK1-sensitive mechanism. Am J Physiol Endocrinol Metab 2005;289:E95–104.

143. Rahman I, Morrison D, Donaldson K, Macnee W. Systemic oxidative stress in asthma, COPD, and smokers. Am J Respir Crit Care Med 1996;154:1055–60.

144. Gosker HR, Bast A, Haenen GR, et al. Altered antioxidant status in peripheral skeletal muscle of patients with COPD. Respir Med 2005;99:118–25.

145. Langen RC, Korn SH, Wouters EF. ROS in the local and systemic pathogenesis of COPD. Free Radic Biol Med 2003;35:226–35.

146. Rabinovich RA, Ardite E, Troosters T, et al. Reduced muscle redox capacity after endurance training in patients with chronic obstructive pulmonary disease. Am J Respir Crit Care Med 2001;164:1114–8.

147. Abraham RZ, Kobzik L, Moody MR, et al. Cyclic GMP is a second messenger by which nitric oxide inhibits diaphragm contraction. Comp Biochem Physiol A Mol Integr Physiol 1998;119:177–83.

148. Hirschfield W, Moody MR, O'Brien WE, et al. Nitric oxide release and contractile properties of skeletal muscles from mice deficient in type III NOS. Am J Physiol Regul Integr Comp Physiol 2000;278:R95–100.

149. Reid MB, Shoji T, Moody MR, Entman ML. Reactive oxygen in skeletal muscle. II. Extracellular release of free radicals. J Appl Physiol 1992;73:1805–9.

150. Mitch WE, Goldberg AL. Mechanisms of muscle wasting. The role of the ubiquitin-proteasome pathway. N Engl J Med 1996;335:1897–905.

151. Moncada S, Higgs A. The L-arginine-nitric oxide pathway. N Engl J Med 1993;329:2002–12.

152. Moncada S, Palmer RM, Higgs EA. Nitric oxide: physiology, pathophysiology, and pharmacology. Pharmacol Rev 1991;43:109–42.

153. Kobzik L, Reid MB, Bredt DS, Stamler JS. Nitric oxide in skeletal muscle. Nature 1994;372:546–8.

154. Barreiro E, Gea J, Corominas JM, Hussain SN. Nitric oxide synthases and protein oxidation in the quadriceps femoris of patients with chronic obstructive pulmonary disease. Am J Respir Cell Mol Biol 2003;29:771–8.

155. Williams G, Brown T, Becker L, et al. Cytokine-induced expression of nitric oxide synthase in C2C12 skeletal muscle myocytes. Am J Physiol 1994;267:R1020–5.

156. Agusti A, Morla M, Sauleda J, et al. NF-kappaB activation and iNOS upregulation in skeletal muscle of patients with COPD and low body weight. Thorax 2004;59:483–7.

157. Montes DO, Torres SH, De Sanctis J, et al. Skeletal muscle inflammation and nitric oxide in patients with COPD. Eur Respir J 2005;26:390–7.

158. Barreiro E, de la Puente B, Minguella J, et al. Oxidative stress and respiratory muscle dysfunction in severe chronic obstructive pulmonary disease. Am J Respir Crit Care Med 2005;171:1116–24.

159. Alloatti G, Penna C, Mariano F, Camussi G. Role of NO and PAF in the impairment of skeletal muscle contractility induced by TNF-alpha. Am J Physiol Regul Integr Comp Physiol 2000;279:R2156–63.

160. Lanone S, Mebazaa A, Heymes C, et al. Muscular contractile failure in septic patients: role of the inducible nitric oxide synthase pathway. Am J Respir Crit Care Med 2000;162:2308–15.

161. Reid MB, Durham WJ. Generation of reactive oxygen and nitrogen species in contracting skeletal muscle: potential impact on aging. Ann N Y Acad Sci 2002;959:108–16.

162. Woods K, Marrone A, Smith J. Programmed cell death and senescence in skeletal muscle stem cells. Ann N Y Acad Sci 2000;908:331–5.

163. Morla M, Busquets X, Pons J, et al. Telomere shortening in smokers with and without COPD. Eur Respir J 2006;27:525–8.

164. Celermajer DS, Adams MR, Clarkson P, et al. Passive smoking and impaired endothelium-dependent arterial dilatation in healthy young adults. N Engl J Med 1996;334:150–4.

165. Raitakari OT, Adams MR, McCredie RJ, et al. Arterial endothelial dysfunction related to passive smoking is potentially

reversible in healthy young adults. Ann Intern Med 1999;130:578–81.

166. Kollias HD, Perry RL, Miyake T, et al. Smad7 promotes and enhances skeletal muscle differentiation. Mol Cell Biol 2006;26:6248–60.

167. Ferayorni AJ, Gunville CF, Grow WA. Nicotine decreases agrin signaling and acetylcholine receptor clustering in C2C12 myotube culture. J Neurobiol 2004;60:51–60.

168. Hughes RL, Katz H, Sahgal V, et al. Fiber size and energy metabolites in five separate muscles from patients with chronic obstructive lung diseases. Respiration 1983;44:321–8.

169. Jakobsson P, Jorfeldt L, Brundin A. Skeletal muscle metabolites and fibre types in patients with advanced chronic obstructive pulmonary disease (COPD), with and without chronic respiratory failure. Eur Respir J 1990;3:192–6.

170. Pereira MC, Isayama RN, Seabra JC, et al. Distribution and morphometry of skeletal muscle fibers in patients with chronic obstructive pulmonary disease and chronic hypoxemia. Muscle Nerve 2004;30:796–8.

171. Jobin J, Maltais F, Doyon JF, et al. Chronic obstructive pulmonary disease: capillarity and fiber-type characteristics of skeletal muscle. J Cardiopulm Rehabil 1998;18:432–7.

172. Whittom F, Jobin J, Simard PM, et al. Histochemical and morphological characteristics of the vastus lateralis muscle in patients with chronic obstructive pulmonary disease. Med Sci Sports Exerc 1998;30:1467–74.

173. Gosker HR, Engelen MP, van Mameren H, et al. Muscle fiber type IIX atrophy is involved in the loss of fat-free mass in chronic obstructive pulmonary disease. Am J Clin Nutr 2002;76:113–9.

174. Ottenheijm CA, Heunks LM, Li YP, et al. Activation of ubiquitin-proteasome pathway in the diaphragm in chronic obstructive pulmonary disease. Am J Respir Crit Care Med 2006;174: 997–1002.

175. Wijnhoven JH, Janssen AJ, van Kuppevelt TH, et al. Metabolic capacity of the diaphragm in patients with COPD. Respir Med 2006;100:1064–71.

176. Doucet M, Debigare R, Joanisse DR, et al. Adaptation of the diaphragm and the vastus lateralis in mild-to-moderate COPD. Eur Respir J 2004;24:971–9.

177. Sanchez J, Brunet A, Medrano G, et al. Metabolic enzymatic activities in the intercostal and serratus muscles and in the latissimus dorsi of middle-aged normal men and patients with moderate obstructive pulmonary disease. Eur Respir J 1988;1:376–83.

178. Ribera F, N'Guessan B, Zoll J, et al. Mitochondrial electron transport chain function is enhanced in inspiratory muscles of patients with chronic obstructive pulmonary disease. Am J Respir Crit Care Med 2003;167:873-9.

179. Barreiro E, de la Puente B, Minguella J, et al. Oxidative stress and respiratory muscle dysfunction in severe chronic obstructive pulmonary disease. Am J Respir Crit Care Med 2005;171:1116–24.

180. Engelen MP, Orozco-Levi M, Deutz NE, et al. Glutathione and glutamate levels in the diaphragm of patients with chronic obstructive pulmonary disease. Eur Respir J 2004;23:545–51.

181. Alexopoulou C, Mitrouska I, Arvanitis D, et al. Vascular-specific growth factor mRNA levels in the human diaphragm. Respiration 2005;72:636–41.

182. Levine S, Nguyen T, Kaiser LR, et al. Human diaphragm remodeling associated with chronic obstructive pulmonary disease: clinical implications. Am J Respir Crit Care Med 2003;168:706–13.

183. Ottenheijm CA, Heunks LM, Hafmans T, et al. Titin and diaphragm dysfunction in chronic obstructive pulmonary disease. Am J Respir Crit Care Med 2006;173:527–34.

184. Scott A, Wang X, Road JD, Reid WD. Increased injury and intramuscular collagen of the diaphragm in COPD: autopsy observations. Eur Respir J 2006;27:51–9.

185. Schols AM, Broekhuizen R, Weling-Scheepers CA, Wouters EF. Body composition and mortality in chronic obstructive pulmonary disease. Am J Clin Nutr 2005;82:53–9.

186. Mador MJ. Muscle mass, not body weight, predicts outcome in patients with chronic obstructive pulmonary disease. Am J Respir Crit Care Med 2002;166:787–9.

187. Schols AM, Slangen J, Volovics L, Wouters EF. Weight loss is a reversible factor in the prognosis of chronic obstructive pulmonary disease. Am J Respir Crit Care Med 1998;157:1791–7.

188. Mostert R, Goris A, Weling-Scheepers C, et al. Tissue depletion and health related quality of life in patients with chronic obstructive pulmonary disease. Respir Med 2000;94:859–67.

189. Rutten EP, Franssen FM, Engelen MP, et al. Greater whole-body myofibrillar protein breakdown in cachectic patients with chronic obstructive pulmonary disease. Am J Clin Nutr 2006;83:829–34.

190. Agusti AG, Sauleda J, Miralles C, et al. Skeletal muscle apoptosis and weight loss in chronic obstructive pulmonary disease. Am J Respir Crit Care Med 2002;166:485–9.

191. Balasubramanian VP, Varkey B. Chronic obstructive pulmonary disease: effects beyond the lungs. Curr Opin Pulm Med 2006;12:106–12.

192. Nagaya N, Kojima M, Kangawa K. Ghrelin, a novel growth hormone-releasing peptide, in the treatment of cardiopulmonary-associated cachexia. Intern Med 2006;45:127–34.

193. Komatsu W, Ishihara K, Murata M, et al. Docosahexaenoic acid suppresses nitric oxide production and inducible nitric oxide synthase expression in interferon-gamma plus lipopolysaccharide-stimulated murine macrophages by inhibiting the oxidative stress. Free Radic Biol Med 2003;34:1006–16.

194. Broekhuizen R, Wouters EF, Creutzberg EC, et al. Polyunsaturated fatty acids improve exercise capacity in chronic obstructive pulmonary disease. Thorax 2005;60:376–82.

CHAPTER 22

OSTEOPOROSIS

SHERYL F. VONDRACEK, PHARMD, FCCP, BCPS, AND
MICHAEL T. MCDERMOTT, MD

OSTEOPOROSIS is "A SYSTEMIC skeletal disorder characterized by low bone mass and microarchitectural deterioration of bone tissue, with a consequent increase in bone fragility and susceptibility to fracture."[1] The gold standard method for diagnosing osteoporosis before a fragility fracture (low trauma fracture) occurs is measurement of bone mineral density (BMD) at the hip and/or lumbar spine using dual-energy x-ray absorptiometry (DXA). According to the World Health Organization (WHO), osteoporosis is defined as a T-score at or below −2.5, which equates to a BMD value that is 2.5 SD or more below the average value in a young healthy sex-matched reference population.[2] Osteopenia or low bone mass is defined as a T-score between −1.0 and −2.5. The WHO criteria for osteoporosis were developed based on data from cohorts of postmenopausal Caucasian women; however, they are often applied to other racial or ethnic groups and to men.[3] Based on these criteria, it is estimated that 44 million women and men aged 50 years or older have low bone mass or osteoporosis in the United States.[4] By 2010, these numbers are expected to increase to 52 million. Consequently, over 1.5 million osteoporotic or low trauma fractures occur annually in the United States. Osteoporosis-related fractures of the hip and spine have been shown to increase pain and disability, reduce quality of life and activities of daily living, and can increase the risk for death by two- to threefold.[5–9]

Patients with chronic obstructive pulmonary disease (COPD) are at high risk for developing osteoporosis, with a reported incidence ranging from 36 to 60%.[10–15] In a cross-sectional study, men with chronic lung disease receiving either oral, inhaled, or no glucocorticoids were compared with men without lung disease.[12] Overall, men with chronic lung disease had a fivefold higher prevalence of osteoporosis. This ranged from a ninefold higher prevalence in those subjects receiving chronic glucocorticoid therapies to fourfold in those not receiving steroids. The prevalence of osteoporosis was evaluated in another cross-sectional study of 44 elderly Japanese women (average age 72–77 years) with either COPD or asthma who had never received chronic systemic corticosteroids.[11] Of the women with COPD, 50% had osteoporosis compared with only 21% with asthma. In addition, the women with COPD had a higher prevalence of more than one vertebral fracture compared with patients with asthma (40% vs 15%, respectively). The prevalence of osteoporosis is especially high in patients with severe lung disease. In a cross-sectional study of 70 adult men and women with end-stage pulmonary disease awaiting lung transplantation, BMD in the osteoporosis range was present in 30% of patients when measured at the lumbar spine and 49% when measured at the femoral neck.[13] Twenty-eight patients had a diagnosis of COPD (average age 56 ± 1 years). The mean ± SD lumbar spine and femoral neck T-score was −2.0 ± 0.3 and −2.7 ± 0.3, respectively. Spinal radiographs obtained in 21 of the COPD patients revealed a 29% prevalence of vertebral fractures. Osteoporotic fractures are a serious problem for patients with COPD. These patients are uniquely sensitive to the negative outcomes related to fractures, especially vertebral fractures, as they have been shown to increase the risk for disease exacerbations and have been demonstrated to compromise lung function, specifically forced vital capacity (FVC), in this population.[16–18] For example, it has been estimated that each osteoporotic vertebral compression fracture can lead to a 9% loss in predicted FVC.

Multiple mechanisms may be involved in the underlying pathophysiology of osteoporosis in patients with COPD. It is important to understand the complex nature of osteoporosis in patients with COPD so that specific diagnostic and management strategies can be implemented in a timely fashion to reduce the risk for osteoporosis and subsequent fractures in this population.

Pathophysiology and Risk Factors

Patients with COPD are exposed to the same risk factors and secondary causes for osteoporosis as the general population (Table 1).[19–23] Several of these factors, such as cigarette smoking, exposure to glucocorticoids, impaired lung function, low body weight, and physical deconditioning, possibly contribute a greater degree to bone loss and fractures in patients with COPD and are worthy of a more in-depth discussion.

Glucocorticoid Use

Glucocorticoid use is the most common secondary cause of osteoporosis and the third most common cause of osteoporosis overall.[24] It is estimated that approximately 30 to 50% of patients taking chronic systemic glucocorticoids will experience a fracture.[24,25] Several studies have demonstrated a significant and rapid increase in bone loss and fracture risk in patients receiving chronic systemic glucocorticoid therapy.[26–28] Data have confirmed the negative effects of

Table 1 Risk Factors and Selected Secondary Causes for Osteoporosis in Patients with Chronic Obstructive Pulmonary Disease

Risk Factors	Secondary Causes
Current cigarette smoking*	Chronic systemic glucocorticoid use*
Low trauma fracture after age 45 yr*	Oversupplementation of thyroxine
Low body weight/body mass index*	Anticonvulsants (eg, phenytoin, carbamazepine or phenobarbital)
History of low trauma fracture in a first-degree relative*	Thyrotoxicosis
Inadequate calcium intake	Rheumatoid arthritis*
Impaired lung function	Chronic kidney or liver disease
Caucasian and Asian race	Malignancies
Physical inactivity	Hypogonadism
Advanced age*	Inflammatory bowel disease
	Transplantation
	Vitamin D deficiency

*Major risk factor for fracture (Independent of BMD).

chronic systemic glucocorticoid therapy in patients with COPD.[12,29–31]

The pathophysiology of glucocorticoid-induced osteoporosis is multifactorial. Glucocorticoids can negatively affect all aspects of bone remodeling. They directly decrease bone formation through inhibition of osteoblastic proliferation and differentiation and enhanced osteoblast apoptosis.[25,32–34] They interfere with the bone's natural repair mechanism through increased apoptosis of osteocytes, the bone's communication cells.[33] Glucocorticoids increase bone resorption by multiple mechanisms as well. They increase the expression of receptor activator of nuclear factor κB ligand (RANKL) and decrease the expression of osteoprotegerin, its soluble decoy receptor, both of which result in increased osteoclastogenesis.[32] They reduce estrogen and testosterone levels by decreasing the production of luteinizing hormone from the pituitary gland and through adrenal suppression, further enhancing osteoclastic bone resorption. Finally, they cause a negative calcium balance by decreasing intestinal calcium absorption and increasing urinary calcium excretion.[24,25,29,33–35]

Infrequently, patients with COPD may require chronic use of systemic glucocorticoids for the management of their disease. More commonly, patients with COPD are treated on a chronic basis with high-dose inhaled glucocorticoids and on an intermittent basis with high-dose systemic glucocorticoids for disease exacerbations. It is well documented that the chronic use of oral glucocorticoids can decrease BMD and increase fracture risk. Studies evaluating the effect of inhaled steroids on BMD and fracture risk have demonstrated conflicting results. Variations in study design, type and dose of inhaled steroid, duration of therapy, and, most importantly, the underlying respiratory disease process may account for the differences in results. A Cochrane Review of inhaled steroid use in patients with asthma or mild COPD

demonstrated no evidence that conventional doses of inhaled steroids given for 2 to 3 years decreased BMD or increased fracture risk.[36] In a separate meta-analysis of 14 studies, long-term inhaled steroid use was not associated with a decrease in BMD in patients with asthma or COPD.[37] In a retrospective cohort study of over 115,000 elderly women, inhaled glucocorticoids were not associated with an increased hip fracture risk (hazard ratio = 0.92; 95% confidence interval [CI] 0.75–1.12).[38] Data from a large retrospective cohort study using the United Kingdom General Practice Research Database demonstrated that the relative rates for nonvertebral, vertebral, and hip fractures were 15%, 51%, and 22% higher in inhaled steroids users ($n = 170,818$) compared with control patients ($n = 170,818$). These differences remained significant even after adjusting for potential confounding variables. However, when compared with a cohort of patients receiving only bronchodilators ($n = 108,786$), there was no statistically significant difference in the relative risk for fracture in the inhaled steroid group, possibly indicating that the increased risk was related to the severity of underlying pulmonary disease and not the inhaled steroids. One large nested case-control study in a cohort of Veterans Affairs patients with COPD did find an association between high-dose inhaled steroid use and nonvertebral fractures.[39,40] In this study, current high-dose inhaled steroid users had a 68% relative increased risk for nonvertebral fractures compared with nonusers of inhaled steroids.

Few prospective randomized trials have evaluated the effect of inhaled glucocorticoids on BMD and fractures. Osteoporosis risk was evaluated as a secondary end point in two large prospective randomized trials of inhaled steroids in patients with COPD. The Lung Health Study compared inhaled triamcinolone 600 μg twice daily with placebo in 1,116 patients with COPD. Bone density was evaluated in a subset of these patients. After 3 years, lumbar spine and femoral neck BMD was significantly lower in the inhaled triamcinolone group by 1.33% ($p = .007$) and 1.78% ($p < .001$), respectively, compared with the placebo group.[41] The European Respiratory Society Study on Chronic Obstructive Pulmonary Disease (EUROSCOP) compared inhaled budesonide 400 µg twice daily with placebo in 912 patients with mild COPD.[42] BMD and fracture risk were evaluated in 161 and 653 subjects, respectively. No significant differences in fracture or BMD were noted between the budesonide and placebo groups. At this time, evidence suggests that low to medium doses of inhaled glucocorticoids have no appreciable effect on bone density and fracture risk. The impact of long-term, high-dose inhaled glucocorticoid use on bone loss and fracture risk, specifically in patients with COPD, needs further evaluation.

Patients with COPD frequently receive short bursts (typically ≤ 2 weeks duration) of systemic glucocorticoids for the treatment of disease exacerbations. Multiple short courses of oral glucocorticoids may contribute to bone loss. A cross-sectional study of 86 white men with COPD compared BMD values in four groups of subjects (continuous oral glucocorticoids, multiple courses of systemic glucocorticoids totaling <1,000 mg of prednisolone, multiple courses of systemic glucocorticoids totaling ≥1,000 mg of prednisolone, and no systemic glucocorticoid exposure).[31] Subjects who had received short courses of prednisolone with a cumulative exposure of ≥1,000 mg prednisolone had significantly lower BMD values at all sites measured compared with the other groups. Patients with severe COPD can experience, on average, two to three exacerbations per year.[43,44] Over a several-year period, this can add up to significant glucocorticoid exposure. More information is needed on the potential negative bone effects of short courses of systemic corticosteroids in patients with COPD.

Although the harmful effects of glucocorticoids on bone health are well documented, the increased risk for osteoporosis in patients with COPD cannot be completely explained by glucocorticoid use as several cross-sectional studies have demonstrated low BMD and high fracture rates in patients with COPD not receiving systemic glucocorticoids.[11,12,30,31,42] Therefore, other factors must be taken into consideration when determining the risk for osteoporosis in a patient with COPD.

Cigarette Smoking

A past or current history of cigarette smoking accounts for a portion of the increased osteoporosis risk in patients with COPD. A long history of cigarette smoking is the primary cause for the development of COPD in up to 80 to 90% of patients, and smoking is considered an independent risk factor for the development of osteoporosis.[45] Several studies have demonstrated greater bone loss and higher fracture rates in smokers.[46–51] For example, a large meta-analysis estimated that smoking increases the lifetime risk for vertebral and hip fractures by 31% and 13% in women and 40% and 32% in men, respectively.[49] The effect of current and past smoking

on the risk of fracture was evaluated in another meta-analysis of 10 internationally representative prospective cohorts.[47] This study included 59,232 men and women. The results demonstrated that, after adjusting for BMD, current smoking was associated with a statistically significant increase in any osteoporotic fracture (relative risk [RR] = 1.29; 95% CI = 1.13–1.28). The increased relative risk for hip fracture, which was analyzed separately, was 60% (RR = 1.60; 95% CI = 1.27–2.02). A decrease in sex hormone concentrations, reduced intestinal calcium absorption, a direct toxic effect on osteoblasts, and detrimental effects of smoking on neurovascular function have all been implicated as possible mechanisms for bone loss and increased fracture risk.[46,48] Currently, cigarette smoking is considered a major risk factor for bone loss and fractures in patients with COPD. Smoking cessation may reduce the risk for fracture over time.[46–49] Therefore, reducing the risk for osteoporosis is one more reason to emphasize smoking cessation in patients with COPD.

Impaired Lung Function

Impaired lung function, as measured by forced expiratory volume in 1 second (FEV_1), has been shown to be an independent predictor of osteoporosis in several cross-sectional studies of patients with and without COPD.[52–56] The mechanism for this is unknown. A cohort study using the National Health and Nutrition Examination Survey (NHANES) III database evaluated the association between airflow obstruction and osteoporosis based on total hip BMD.[56] The study included 9,502 Caucasian subjects. The odds of having osteoporosis were twofold higher in those subjects with moderate or severe airflow obstruction compared with subjects with mild or no airflow obstruction independent of age, body mass index (BMI), smoking history, physical activity, and recent oral corticosteroid use. In another cross-sectional study of 4,830 women aged 45 to 76 years, there was a positive correlation between BMD and FEV_1, with the mean BMD decreasing with decreasing quartiles of FEV_1.[55] The prevalence of low BMD was about three times higher in the lowest FEV_1 quartile compared with the highest. This association remained significant after adjusting for age, weight, height, current smoking, past history of disease (COPD, asthma, coronary artery disease, or cancer), hormone replacement therapy, and steroid use. A similar study conducted in 947 men aged 65 to 76 years also demonstrated a positive and significant correlation between FEV_1 and hip BMD.[54] Patients in the highest FEV_1 quartile had the highest BMD values at all hip sites. Compared with the bottom quartile, the mean hip BMD in the top quartile was 2 to 3.5% higher. The association between respiratory function and BMD needs further evaluation.

Limited Physical Activity

As the severity of COPD worsens, dyspnea can limit a person's mobility and may lead to significant disability and deconditioning. Lack of physical activity has been associated with bone loss and increased fracture risk.[57] In addition, decreased activity can lead to muscle wasting and an increased risk for falls.[58] Data are lacking on the impact of deconditioning on osteoporosis risk in patients with COPD.

Low Body Weight and BMI

Low body weight and weight loss are strong predictors of bone loss in elderly men and women and independent predictors of increased fracture risk.[23,59–62] The link between body weight and osteoporosis is not completely understood. It is proposed that obesity protects against osteoporosis by several mechanisms, including an increased mechanical loading on the skeleton, increased aromatization of androgens to estrogens in the adipose tissue, lowered sex hormone–binding globulin levels, or an increase in circulating insulin caused by insulin resistance.[63,64]

Patients with advanced COPD frequently have a reduced BMI, and low BMI is one of the strongest predictors of osteoporosis in patients with COPD.[53,65–67] In several cross-sectional studies, a low BMI was the only factor independently correlated with osteoporosis risk in this population.[11,12,31,68] Weight loss in patients with COPD is also a common phenomenon, occurring in approximately 35 to 60% of patients with moderate to severe COPD.[69] Patients with severe pulmonary disease may lose weight because of an increased resting energy expenditure owing to an increased workload to breathe that is not balanced by an increase in caloric intake. It has also been suggested that weight loss may be due to systemic inflammation.[69] Cachexia and loss of BMD have been linked to an increase in cytokines in other disease states, such as cystic fibrosis and chronic heart failure.[70,71]

Possible Role of Systemic Inflammation

Clear evidence exists that patients with COPD have an increased risk for osteoporosis. Although many underlying factors contribute to this process, they do not completely explain the increased risk. One important factor that has not been fully evaluated is the role of inflammation in the development of osteoporosis in this population. Inflammation may start in the lungs owing to damage from smoking; however, evidence has shown that the localized inflammation can become systemic, leading to a generalized inflammatory reaction affecting multiple areas of the body. Several inflammatory mediators that are involved in lung tissue breakdown and repair also play a role in bone remodeling (Table 2). The evidence supporting their roles in the development of osteoporosis is briefly reviewed. For a more detailed discussion of the role of systemic inflammation in COPD, the reader is referred to Chapter 23.

Tumor Necrosis Factor α

Tumor necrosis factor α (TNF-α) is an important chemotactic protein for macrophages and neutrophils, the predominant inflammatory cells associated with COPD, and has been implicated in causing the ongoing parenchymal destruction seen in patients with COPD.[72–74] TNF-α also has a direct and indirect effect on epithelial barrier function via inducing cell death, as seen with emphysema, and replacing ciliated cells by goblet cells leading to mucus hypersecretion, as seen with chronic obstructive bronchitis.[72] Several studies have demonstrated that lung and serum levels of TNF-α are elevated in certain patients with COPD.[66,75–79]

Cachexia is characterized by anorexia and weight loss that involves the depletion of fat and fat-free mass (FFM).[80] Evidence suggests that weight loss in patients with COPD occurs largely because of a loss of FFM.[52,81] This loss of FFM may be due to increased protein breakdown caused by systemic inflammation. TNF-α can contribute to a reduction in FFM by decreasing muscle anabolism, increasing muscle catabolism, and causing direct structural damage.[81,82] TNF-α has been implicated as one of the cytokines contributing to cachexia in various other chronic disease populations, including those with congestive heart failure, cancer, and acquired immune deficiency syndrome (AIDS) and the frail elderly.[69,70,81–86] Elevated levels of TNF-α have been demonstrated in patients with COPD who have low body weight or reduced skeletal muscle.[66,67,78,87] In addition, a positive correlation between the loss of FFM and low BMD and an improvement in FFM and an increase in BMD has been demonstrated in patients with COPD.[14,52]

TNF-α acts as a potent stimulator of bone resorption by increasing the expression of RANKL, which is a key factor in the activation and differentiation of osteoclasts. Although no studies to date have directly correlated TNF-α levels with low BMD or bone loss in patients with COPD, elevated TNF-α levels have been implicated in contributing to bone loss in several other disease states, such as cystic fibrosis, rheumatoid arthritis, inflammatory bowel disease, and ankylosing spondylitis, in which systemic inflammation is central to the pathophysiology.[70,71,88–92] Studies are needed that evaluate the role of TNF-α in the development of osteoporosis in patients with COPD.

Leptin

Leptin, the peptide hormone encoded by the obese (*ob*) gene, is secreted by adipocytes and is involved in the regulation of growth and metabolism.[93] Leptin receptor can be found in peripheral tissues, such as the kidney, lung, and adrenal gland, and in various cells, including hematopoietic precursor cells and bone marrow, neutrophils, monocytes, and peripheral T cells.[93] It is involved in the regulation of hematopoiesis, angiogenesis, and the immune and inflammatory responses.[94,95]

It has been documented that damage to lung parenchyma in COPD is linked to inflammation and that the recruitment and survival of inflammatory cells within airways might be linked to leptin.[93,94] However, results from studies evaluating the relationship between leptin and other inflammatory markers have been conflicting.[75,94,96–98] In a small study of

Table 2 Inflammatory Mediators Possibly Involved in the Development of Osteoporosis

Inflammatory Mediator	Possible Mechanism for Bone Loss
Tumor necrosis factor α	Potent stimulator of osteoclastic bone resorption by increasing the expression of RANKL, which is a key factor in the activation and differentiation of osteoclasts
Leptin	Possibly stimulates bone formation by acting on human marrow stromal cells to enhance osteoblast differentiation and to inhibit adipocyte differentiation
Matrix metalloproteinase 9	Highly expressed in osteoclasts and are thought to be responsible for the degradation of the nonmineralized bone matrix. They may also be involved in the recruitment of osteoclasts to the resorptive site
Vascular endothelial growth factor	Stimulation of the production of osteotrophic growth factors from endothelial cells, in turn stimulating both the differentiation and activation of osteoblasts and osteoclasts
Adiponectin	Increase in RANKL and inhibition of the production of osteoprotegerin, which would enhance osteoclastogenesis and bone resorption

RANKL = receptor activator of nuclear factor-κB ligand

14 men with moderate to severe COPD, sputum leptin was significantly correlated with other inflammatory markers, such as TNF-α, in sputum.[94] Plasma leptin and sputum leptin were inversely correlated in these patients. In another study, serum leptin levels were significantly lower in 31 COPD patients compared with 15 age-matched controls but did not correlate with activation of the TNF-α system.[75]

More consistent has been the finding that leptin concentrations strongly correlate with BMI and body fat in patients with COPD.[75,96–98] In a small cross-sectional study, BMI (21.6 kg/m^2 vs 25.1 kg/m^2; $p = .001$), fat mass (15.7 kg vs 23.5 kg; $p = .001$), and plasma leptin concentrations (2.6 ng/mL vs 5.1 ng/mL; $p < .02$) were all significantly lower in men with emphysema, as determined by high-resolution computed tomography, compared with men with chronic bronchitis.[96] Leptin concentrations were significantly correlated with fat mass in both groups of patients. Similarly, leptin concentrations significantly correlated with BMI, body weight, and body fat percent in a cross-sectional study of 30 male patients with stable COPD and 20 healthy male controls.[99] A cross-sectional study conducted in China evaluated serum leptin and TNF-α levels in patients with an acute exacerbation of COPD or stable COPD, malnourished patients with stable COPD, and 34 control patients.[98] Serum leptin levels were significantly lower in the malnourished patients compared with the other groups.

The effect of leptin on bone turnover and osteoporosis is not clear. Both osteoblasts and adipocytes mature from bone marrow stromal cells.[100] In-vitro data suggest that leptin stimulates bone formation possibly by acting on human marrow stromal cells to enhance osteoblast differentiation and to inhibit adipocyte differentiation.[100,101] Data regarding the relationship between serum or plasma leptin concentrations and bone turnover markers or BMD in women are conflicting. In a cross-sectional evaluation of 139 postmenopausal Japanese women being evaluated for osteoporosis,

plasma concentrations of leptin were significantly positively correlated with total body ($p = .028$) and femoral neck BMD ($p = .027$) even after controlling for percent fat, age, years since menopause, and height.[101] In addition, plasma leptin levels were significantly lower in women with documented vertebral fractures ($n = 49$) than in those without ($n = 90$). In a study of 90 postmenopausal Egyptian women with osteoporosis, there was no significant correlation between serum leptin and lumbar spine BMD or markers of bone turnover.[102] Similarly, in an evaluation of 90 postmenopausal Turkish women with osteoporosis ($n = 36$), osteopenia ($n = 24$), or normal BMD ($n = 30$), there was no statistically significant difference in leptin levels between groups, nor did leptin concentrations correlate with lumbar spine or femoral neck BMD.[103] Interestingly, leptin did not correlate with BMI in this study.

No studies to date have demonstrated a statistically significant relationship between leptin and BMD in men after controlling for BMI.[102–106] Multiple regression analysis revealed a positive association between leptin and BMD only in women in a study of Caucasian men and postmenopausal women between 45 and 92 years of age.[105] In another study, serum leptin and fat mass were significantly correlated with BMD in premenopausal and postmenopausal women but not in men.[104] A population-based longitudinal study related baseline plasma leptin concentrations to bone mass over 4 years in a cohort of 302 men and women aged 60 to 75 years from the United Kingdom.[106] Baseline plasma leptin was strongly correlated with BMD at all sites in men and women ($p < .001$). However, this relationship did not remain significant after adjusting for baseline BMI. Lastly, in an evaluation of obese ($n = 285$) and nonobese ($n = 327$) healthy Danish men, linear regression analysis did not reveal a significant association between serum leptin and BMD.[63] It is unknown if there is a relationship between leptin and BMD in patients with COPD as no studies have been conducted in this population.

Others

Although less clear, there is some evidence linking changes in vascular endothelial growth factor (VEGF), matrix metallo-proteinase (MMP)-9, and adiponectin to the development of emphysema and possibly bone loss. VEGF plays a multifunctional role in both the development of vasculature and the maintenance of vascular function.[107] Decreases in VEGF or inhibition of the VEGF receptor can lead to endothelial cell apoptosis and have been shown to result in emphysematous changes in human and rat lung tissue.[107–110] VEGF may play an important role in bone remodeling through stimulation of the production of osteotrophic growth factors from endothelial cells, in turn stimulating both the differentiation and activation of osteoblasts and osteoclasts. Alterations in the balance of VEGF may lead to decreased bone formation or increased bone resorption.

MMPs are enzymes that play a critical role in the process of tissue remodeling, wound healing, and metastasis of tumors. MMP-9 and MMP-12 account for most of the macrophage-derived elastase activity in smokers, and the release of MMP-9 is under the influence of several inflammatory mediators and cytokines, in particular TNF-α.[111–113] Several researchers have shown increased concentrations of MMP-9 in brochoalveolar lavage fluid from patients with emphysema and an increased expression and activity of MMP-9 in lung parenchyma.[112,114] MMPs are also involved in the bone remodeling process.[115] They are highly expressed in osteoclasts and are thought to be responsible for the degradation of the nonmineralized bone matrix.[115] They may also be involved in the recruitment of osteoclasts to the resorptive site. More research is needed on the role of systemic inflammation in the development of osteoporosis.

Weight loss is a potent inducer of adiponectin synthesis.[116] In one study, elevated plasma adiponectin correlated with BMI, hyperinflation, and increased TNF-α levels in men with COPD.[117] Elevated levels of adiponectin may have a deleterious effect on bone through increasing the receptor activator of nuclear factor-κB ligand and inhibiting the production of osteoprotegerin, which would enhance bone resorption.[118] Several studies have demonstrated a significant negative relationship between adiponectin and BMD independent of body weight.[119–121]

Diagnosis and Management of Osteoporosis

All patients with a diagnosis of COPD should be evaluated for osteoporosis risk.[10,122] The diagnosis of osteoporosis can only be made based on the presence of a low trauma fracture or bone density results from the hip and/or spine using central DXA. Figure 1 summarizes the evaluation and management of osteoporosis in patients with COPD. All patients with COPD over the age of 65 years should have their BMD evaluated using central DXA. In addition, patients less than 65 years of age who are actively smoking or have a history of an osteoporotic fracture in a primary-degree family member, a low BMI (< 21 kg/m^2)/body weight (< 127 lb or 58 kg), a recent history of unintentional weight loss, severe disease (FEV$_1$ $< 50\%$ predicted), or multiple exposures to systemic corticosteroids should have central DXA testing. If low bone density is detected, it is important to rule out the more common potentially correctable secondary causes for osteoporosis. This can be accomplished by conducting selected routine laboratory tests.

The approach to the management of osteoporosis in patients with COPD is similar to that in other populations. Appropriate calcium and vitamin D intakes, modification of adverse lifestyle practices (such as excessive alcohol intake), and weight-bearing exercises should be recommended in all patients who have evidence of osteoporosis or are at risk for the disease. Since smoking is a significant contributor to bone loss in this population, educational efforts should be directed at smoking cessation in patients who continue to smoke. Multidisciplinary pulmonary rehabilitation programs are beneficial for patients with COPD and may have an added benefit in those with osteoporosis. Improvement in the level of physical activity and muscle strength can potentially increase bone strength and decrease the risk of falls. In addition, dietary counseling can improve caloric and nutritional intake, including appropriate consumption of calcium and vitamin D.

All patients should be educated to consume at least 1,200 mg of elemental calcium per day.[123] This can be accomplished through the consumption of foods naturally high in calcium, such as dairy products, or those fortified with calcium, such as orange juice or selected cereals. Calcium supplements should be recommended for patients who are unable to meet the recommended calcium intake from diet alone. Calcium supplements come in a variety of formulations to better meet the needs of patients. It is important to recommend that patients take calcium supplements in divided doses (no more than 500 mg at one time) for maximal absorption.

An adequate serum concentration of vitamin D is needed to reduce the risk for bone loss, falls, and fractures. Most experts agree that for optimal bone health, vitamin D concentrations should be kept at > 30 ng/mL.[124–127] Inadequate levels of vitamin D are common, especially in the elderly. The amount of vitamin D needed to maintain concentrations above 30 ng/mL is controversial and may differ among patient populations. Until more information is available, all patients with COPD should be recommended to consume at least 800 to 1,200 units per day of vitamin D$_3$ or cholecalciferol, which is well below the safe upper intake limit.[125,128] Unfortunately, this cannot be adequately achieved through dietary intake, so over-the-counter supplemental sources will need to be used. Most multivitamins contain 400 IU of vitamin D, and combination products with calcium are widely available.

Patients with COPD and no major risk factors for osteoporosis whose central bone density results indicate a T-score

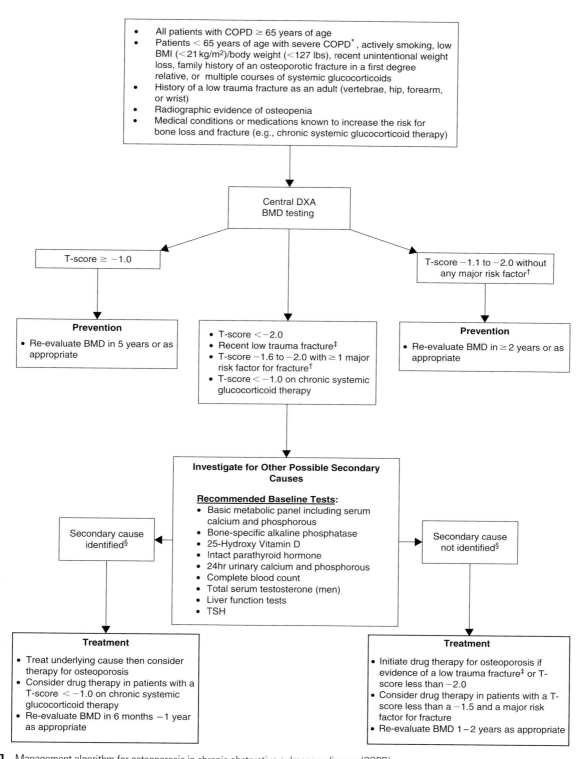

FIGURE 1. Management algorithm for osteoporosis in chronic obstructive pulmonary disease (COPD).
BMD = bone mineral density; BMI = body mass index; DXA = dual-energy x-ray absorptiometry; TSH = thyroid-stimulating hormone.
*Postbronchodilator forced expiratory volume in 1 second <50% predicted; †major risk factors (independent risk factors for fracture): current smoker, low body weight (<127 lb or 58 kg) or BMI (<21 kg/m²), history of osteoporotic fracture in a first-degree relative, and personal history of fracture as an adult after age 45 years, chronic systemic glucocorticoid therapy for ≥ 3 months; ‡hip, spine, wrist, or forearm; §examples of possible other secondary causes in patients with COPD: hypogonadism, vitamin D deficiency, malignancy, hyperthyroidism, inflammatory bowel disease, chronic kidney or liver disease, chronic systemic glucocorticoid therapy.

of −2.0 or better should be educated on appropriate calcium and vitamin intake and pertinent lifestyle modifications. Drug therapy for osteoporosis will not be necessary at this time. Repeat BMD testing should be recommended at 2 to 5 years depending on the T-score. Pharmacologic therapy should be considered in any patient with a T-score at the total hip or lumbar spine that is lower than −2.0 or lower than −1.5 if the patient has another major risk factor for osteoporosis.[23] Any patient with evidence of a low trauma fracture of the vertebrae, hip, wrist, or forearm should receive drug therapy for osteoporosis regardless of the T-score. Patients with COPD who are receiving chronic systemic glucocorticoid therapy should follow the guidelines for the management of glucocorticoid-induced osteoporosis.[35,129] In these patients, drug therapy may be considered at a T-score of −1.0 or lower.

There are several therapies currently indicated by the US Food and Drug Administration (FDA) for osteoporosis (Table 3). The bisphosphonates alendronate, risedronate, ibandronate, and zoledronic acid act as antiresorptive agents by reducing osteoclastic life span and function. The oral formulations are considered a first-line option for the treatment of osteoporosis because they have minimal side effects and have demonstrated efficacy in reducing fractures in a variety of patient populations, including glucocorticoid-induced osteoporosis.[130–137] Injectable ibandronate is FDA indicated only in postmenopausal women and may be best for patients who cannot take an oral formulation or have adherence problems.[138,139] A once-yearly infusion of zoledronic acid is approved for postmenopausal women with osteoporosis and has been shown to reduce fractures and all cause mortality in men and women post hip fracture.[140,141] Raloxifene, an estrogen agonist-antagonist, is also approved to reduce invasive breast cancer risk in postmenopausal women with osteoporosis.[142] Teriparatide is the only FDA-indicated therapy that acts as an anabolic agent, enhancing osteoblastic function and increasing new bone formation. It is considered a second-line option for men and women at high risk for fracture. It has demonstrated efficacy in a wide range of patients; however, it is very expensive, requires extensive patient education, and must be administered by subcutaneous injection once daily.[143,144] Although testosterone replacement therapy can be considered in men who are hypogonadal, its use is limited by potential side effects.[145] Alendronate, risedronate, and teriparatide have all been shown to improve BMD in men with hypogonadism and would be a better choice for the management of osteoporosis in this population.[143,146] Additionally, hormone replacement therapy should not be used for the treatment of osteoporosis in women with COPD as the risks outweigh the benefits.

Possible Future Therapies for Bone Loss in COPD

It is possible that in some patients with COPD, bone loss is enhanced by systemic inflammation. Therefore, therapies that target reducing the inflammatory mediators may be effective in reducing the bone loss seen in this patient population. There is evidence that therapies targeting TNF-α in patients with inflammatory diseases such as rheumatoid arthritis, Crohn's disease and ankylosing spondylitis can reduce bone loss in these patients.[147–153] In one study, 29 patients with ankylosing spondylitis were treated with infliximab, a monoclonal antibody to TNF-α.[151] Bone density was evaluated at baseline and after 6 months. Significant increases in BMD at the spine (3.6 ± 5.9%) and total hip (2.3 ± 3.4%) were demonstrated. Osteocalcin, a marker of bone formation, was also significantly increased at 6 weeks. In another study, 26 men and women with active rheumatoid arthritis received infliximab therapy for 12 months.[152] BMD significantly increased from baseline to 12 months at the lumbar spine (p < .001) and femoral neck (p < .001). Etanercept, a soluble, dimeric, recombinant human TNF receptor (p75 TNFR) developed for neutralization of TNF-α, has also been evaluated. A substudy of 40 patients from a larger double-blind, placebo-controlled phase 3 trial compared etanercept 25 mg subcutaneously twice daily and placebo for 24 weeks on hip and spine BMD in patients with ankylosing spondylitis. Etanercept treatment resulted in a significantly greater improvement in spinal BMD from baseline compared with placebo (3.19% vs 0.67%; p = .0267). There was no difference in hip BMD.[154] There are currently no studies that have evaluated the effects of anti-TNF therapy on bone density in patients with COPD. However, a study evaluating the impact of infliximab on lung function in patients with moderate to severe COPD demonstrated no benefit and more cases of cancer and pneumonia in the treatment group.[155]

Currently available therapies for osteoporosis, such as oral bisphosphonates and raloxifene, have been shown to alter cytokine production and reduce bone loss in patients with inflammatory diseases such as rheumatoid arthritis.[147,156–164] Alendronate 40 mg orally daily for 90 days was compared with placebo in 32 patients with mild rheumatoid arthritis. A significant decrease in interleukin-1, interleukin-6, and TNF-α was demonstrated in the alendronate-treated group.[163] A similar effect on cytokines was seen after 24 months of raloxifene therapy in 14 postmenopausal women with osteoporosis.[162] Interleukin-6 and TNF-α were decreased by 70% and 35%, respectively. Raloxifene is thought to suppress monocyte/macrophage production of cytokines, similar to estrogen. The mechanism by which bisphosphonates affect cytokines is unknown. However, one possible mechanism is the induction of the apoptosis of monocytes/macrophages, which stimulate the release of cytokines in the bone microenvironment.[157] Alendronate, risedronate, and pamidronate have all been shown to increase or preserve bone density in patients with rheumatoid arthritis.[156,159–161]

Other drugs that reduce circulating levels of TNF-α may prove to have a beneficial effect on bone density in patients with COPD and warrant investigation. Pentoxifylline limits TNF-α transcription through inhibition of phosphodiesterase IV,

Table 3 Pharmacologic Options for the Treatment of Osteoporosis in Chronic Obstructive Pulmonary Disease

Drug	Mechanism	Recommended Dosing	Role in Therapy	Comments
Bisphosphonates				
Alendronate (Fosamax)	Antiresorptive	70 mg orally once weekly	1st line option; FDA indicated for use in PMPW, men, and GIOP	Alendronate available in a combination product with 5600 units of vitamin D3; most common side effects are gastrointestinal (e.g., dyspepsia); not recommended in patients with a Clcr < 30–35 mL/min; special administration instruction*
Risedronate (Actonel)	Antiresorptive	35 mg orally once weekly	1st line option; FDA indicated for use in PMPW, men, and GIOP	
Ibandronate (Boniva)	Antiresorptive	150 mg orally once monthly	1st line option; FDA indicated for use in PMPW	
		3 mg IV every 3 mo	2nd line option; FDA indicated for use in PMPW; may be best for patients who cannot tolerate oral bisphosphonates or have adherence issues	Not recommended in patients with a Clcr < 30 mL/min; infusion-related, flu-like symptoms are most common; 15–30s IV injection administered by a health care provider
Zoledronic Acid (Reclast)	Antiresorptive	5 mg/100 mL IV infusion once yearly	1st line option; FDA indicated for use in PMPW; may be best for patients who cannot tolerate oral bisphosphonates or have adherence issues	Not recommended in patients with a Clcr < 35 mL/min; infusion-related, flu-like symptoms are most common; IV infusion administered over no less than 15 minutes
Parathyroid Hormone				
Teriparatide (Forteo)	Anabolic	20 μg SC daily	2nd line option; FDA indicated for use in PMPW and men at high risk for fracture	Expensive; extensive patient education; should not be prescribed for patients with hypercalcemia or a history of prior radiation therapy involving the skeleton
Estrogen Agonist-Antagonist				
Raloxifene (Evista)	Antiresorptive	60 mg orally once daily	2nd line option; FDA indicated for PMPW	Contraindicated in patients with a history of VTE; FDA-approved to reduce invasive breast cancer risk
Other				
Calcitonin (Miacalcin)	Antiresorptive	One spray (200 units) intranasally daily (alternate nostrils)	3rd line option; FDA indicated for PMPW	Minimal side effects; limited efficacy data

Clcr = creatinine clearance; FDA = US Food and Drug Administration; GIOP = glucocorticoid-induced osteoporosis; IV = intravenous; PMPW = postmenopausal women; SC = subcutaneously; VTE = venous thromboembolism.

*Must be taken on an empty stomach with 6 to 8 oz of plain water, first thing in the morning. Must remain upright for 30 minutes (60 minutes for ibandronate) and wait at least 30 minutes (60 minutes with ibandronate) before eating, drinking, or taking any other oral medication.

whereas thalidomide appears to enhance messenger ribonucleic acid destabilization of TNF-α.[165–166] Both have relatively modest effects on TNF concentrations.[165] Bupropion, an antidepressant used for smoking cessation, has been shown to lower TNF-α levels in patients with various inflammatory disease states such as Crohn's disease and hepatitis B.[167,168] This therapy could have a unique role in both preventing bone loss and assisting with smoking cessation in patients with COPD. If TNF-α proves to be an important

player in bone loss in patients with COPD, alternative therapies should be investigated to determine their effect on BMD in this population.

Conclusions

The reader is referred to Table 4 for a summary of key points. Osteoporosis occurs with significantly greater frequency in patients with COPD. The causes and mechanisms of bone loss in COPD are multifactorial and include cigarette smoking,

Table 4   Key Points
Patients with COPD are at high risk for osteoporosis
Systemic inflammation may contribute to the bone loss in this population
All patients with COPD should be evaluated for osteoporosis risk
All patients with COPD over the age of 65 yr and patients < 65 yr of age with severe disease or selected risk factors should undergo BMD testing using central DXA
To improve bone health, all patients with COPD should be educated on adequate intakes of calcium and vitamin D and smoking cessation and be enrolled in a pulmonary rehabilitation exercise program
Patients with COPD who have evidence of a low trauma fracture should receive pharmacologic therapy
Patients with COPD who have low bone density as evidenced by a T-score lower than −2.0 at the total hip or lumbar spine should be considered for pharmacologic therapy
Oral bisphosphonates are first-line options for the treatment of osteoporosis in patients with COPD

BMD = bone mineral density; COPD = chronic obstructive pulmonary disease; DXA = dual-energy x-ray absorptiometry.

glucocorticoid use, low body weight, physical deconditioning, and suboptimal calcium and vitamin D nutrition. The contribution of pulmonary inflammation, particularly the roles of altered circulating levels of inflammation-related cytokines, such as TNF-α, leptin, VEGF, MMP-9, and adiponectin is an intriguing and promising new area of investigation, although further work is clearly needed. Because of the significant deleterious effects osteoporotic fractures have on pulmonary function and overall prognosis, the diagnosis of osteoporosis should be considered and actively sought in most, if not all, patients with COPD. The diagnosis of osteoporosis is made when a patient has a typical low trauma fracture of the spine, hip, wrist, or forearm or has a BMD T-score of ≤ −2.5 (2.5 or more standard deviations below peak bone mass in young normals). Nonpharmacologic preventive measures, such as adequate intake of calcium (1,200 mg/d) and vitamin D (800–1,200 units/d), regular exercise, and smoking cessation, are appropriate for all COPD patients. Pharmacologic therapy with an antiresorptive or anabolic medication should be considered in any COPD patient who has sustained a low trauma fracture, has a T-score <−2.0, or has a T-score <−1.5 with another major risk factor.

References

1. Consensus development conference: diagnosis, prophylaxis, and treatment of osteoporosis. Am J Med 1993;94:646–50.
2. Kanis JA. Assessment of fracture risk and its application to screening for postmenopausal osteoporosis: synopsis of a WHO report. WHO Study Group. Osteoporos Int 1994;4:368–81.
3. Writing Group for ISCD Position Development Conference. Diagnosis of osteoporosis in men, premenopausal women, and children. J Clin Densitom 2004;7:17–26.
4. National Osteoporosis Foundation. America's bone health: the state of osteoporosis and low bone mass. 2004. Available at: <www.nof.org/advocacy/prevalence/index.htm> (accessed January 3, 2007).
5. Tosteson AN, Gabriel SE, Grove MR, et al. Impact of hip and vertebral fractures on quality-adjusted life years. Osteoporos Int 2001;12:1042–9.
6. Cooper C, Atkinson EJ, Jacobsen SJ, et al. Population-based study of survival after osteoporotic fractures. Am J Epidemiol 1993;137:1001–5.
7. Greendale GA, Barrett-Connor E, Ingles S, Haile R. Late physical and functional effects of osteoporotic fracture in women: the Rancho Bernardo Study. J Am Geriatr Soc 1995;43:955–61.
8. Trombetti A, Herrmann F, Hoffmeyer P, et al. Survival and potential years of life lost after hip fracture in men and age-matched women. Osteoporos Int 2002;13:731–7.
9. Center JR, Nguyen TV, Schneider D, et al. Mortality after all major types of osteoporotic fracture in men and women: an observational study. Lancet 1999;353:878–82.
10. Biskobing DM. COPD and osteoporosis. Chest 2002;121: 609–20.
11. Katsura H, Kida K. A comparison of bone mineral density in elderly female patients with COPD and bronchial asthma. Chest 2002;122:1949–55.
12. Iqbal F, Michaelson J, Thaler L, et al. Declining bone mass in men with chronic pulmonary disease: contribution of glucocorticoid treatment, body mass index, and gonadal function. Chest 1999;116:1616–24.
13. Shane E, Silverberg SJ, Donovan D, et al. Osteoporosis in lung transplantation candidates with end-stage pulmonary disease. Am J Med 1996;101:262–9.
14. Mineo TC, Ambrogi V, Mineo D, et al. Bone mineral density improvement after lung volume reduction surgery for severe emphysema. Chest 2005;127:1960–6.
15. Yeh SS, Phanumas D, Hafner A, Schuster MW. Risk factors for osteoporosis in a subgroup of elderly men in a Veterans Administration nursing home. J Investig Med 2002;50:452–7.
16. Schlaich C, Minne HW, Bruckner T, et al. Reduced pulmonary function in patients with spinal osteoporotic fractures. Osteoporos Int 1998;8:261–7.
17. Harrison RA, Siminoski K, Vethanayagam D, Majumdar SR. Osteoporosis-related kyphosis and impairments in pulmonary function: a systematic review. J Bone Miner Res 2006;22:447–57.
18. Leech JA, Dulberg C, Kellie S, et al. Relationship of lung function to severity of osteoporosis in women. Am Rev Respir Dis 1990;141:68–71.
19. Harper KD, Weber TJ. Secondary osteoporosis. Diagnostic considerations. Endocrinol Metab Clin North Am 1998;27:325–48.
20. Kanis JA, Oden A, Johnell O, et al. The use of clinical risk factors enhances the performance of BMD in the prediction of hip and osteoporotic fractures in men and women. Osteoporos Int 2007;18:1033–46.
21. Kanis JA, Johnell O, Oden A, et al. Ten year probabilities of osteoporotic fractures according to BMD and diagnostic thresholds. Osteoporos Int 2001;12:989–95.

22. Kanis JA, Borgstrom F, De Laet C, et al. Assessment of fracture risk. Osteoporos Int 2005;16:581–9.

23. National Osteoporosis Foundation. Physician's guide to prevention and treatment of osteoporosis. 2003. National Osteoporosis Foundation, Washington, D.C. Available at: http:// <www.nof.org/physguide/index.asp> (accessed January 3, 2007).

24. Rubin MR, Bilezikian JP. Clinical review 151: the role of parathyroid hormone in the pathogenesis of glucocorticoid-induced osteoporosis: a re-examination of the evidence. J Clin Endocrinol Metab 2002;87:4033–41.

25. Lane NE, Lukert B. The science and therapy of glucocorticoid-induced bone loss. Endocrinol Metab Clin North Am 1998;27:465–83.

26. Kanis JA, Johansson H, Oden A, et al. A meta-analysis of prior corticosteroid use and fracture risk. J Bone Miner Res 2004;19:893–9.

27. van Staa TP, Leufkens HG, Abenhaim L, et al. Use of oral corticosteroids and risk of fractures. J Bone Miner Res 2000;15:993–1000.

28. van Staa TP, Leufkens HG, Abenhaim L, et al. Oral corticosteroids and fracture risk: relationship to daily and cumulative doses. Rheumatology (Oxford) 2000;39:1383–9.

29. Goldstein MF, Fallon JJ Jr, Harning R. Chronic glucocorticoid therapy-induced osteoporosis in patients with obstructive lung disease. Chest 1999;116:1733–49.

30. McEvoy CE, Ensrud KE, Bender E, et al. Association between corticosteroid use and vertebral fractures in older men with chronic obstructive pulmonary disease. Am J Respir Crit Care Med 1998;157:704–9.

31. Dubois EF, Roder E, Dekhuijzen PN, et al. Dual energy x-ray absorptiometry outcomes in male COPD patients after treatment with different glucocorticoid regimens. Chest 2002;121:1456–63.

32. Canalis E, Bilezikian JP, Angeli A, Giustina A. Perspectives on glucocorticoid-induced osteoporosis. Bone 2004;34:593–8.

33. Mazziotti G, Angeli A, Bilezikian JP, et al. Glucocorticoid-induced osteoporosis: an update. Trends Endocrinol Metab 2006;17:144–9.

34. Delany AM, Pereira RM, Pereira RC, Canalis E. The cellular and molecular basis of glucocorticoid actions in bone. Front Horm Res 2002;30:2–12.

35. Recommendations for the prevention and treatment of glucocorticoid-induced osteoporosis. American College of Rheumatology Task Force on Osteoporosis Guidelines. Arthritis Rheum 1996;39:1791–801.

36. Jones A, Fay JK, Burr M, et al. Inhaled corticosteroid effects on bone metabolism in asthma and mild chronic obstructive pulmonary disease. Cochrane Database Syst Rev 2002;Issue 1:CD003537.

37. Halpern MT, Schmier JK, Van Kerkhove MD, et al. Impact of long-term inhaled corticosteroid therapy on bone mineral density: results of a meta-analysis. Ann Allergy Asthma Immunol 2004;92:201–7; quiz 7–8, 67.

38. Lau E, Mamdani M, Tu K. Inhaled or systemic corticosteroids and the risk of hospitalization for hip fracture among elderly women. Am J Med 2003;114:142–5.

39. Lee TA, Weiss KB. Fracture risk associated with inhaled corticosteroid use in chronic obstructive pulmonary disease. Am J Respir Crit Care Med 2004;169:855–9.

40. van Staa TP, Leufkens HG, Cooper C. Use of inhaled corticosteroids and risk of fractures. J Bone Miner Res 2001;16:581–8.

41. Scanlon PD, Connett JE, Wise RA, et al. Loss of bone density with inhaled triamcinolone in Lung Health Study II. Am J Respir Crit Care Med 2004;170:1302–9.

42. Johnell O, Pauwels R, Lofdahl CG, et al. Bone mineral density in patients with chronic obstructive pulmonary disease treated with budesonide Turbuhaler. Eur Respir J 2002;19:1058–63.

43. Seemungal TA, Donaldson GC, Paul EA, et al. Effect of exacerbation on quality of life in patients with chronic obstructive pulmonary disease. Am J Respir Crit Care Med 1998;157:1418–22.

44. Seemungal TA, Donaldson GC, Bhowmik A, et al. Time course and recovery of exacerbations in patients with chronic obstructive pulmonary disease. Am J Respir Crit Care Med 2000;161:1608–13.

45. Standards for the diagnosis and care of patients with chronic obstructive pulmonary disease. American Thoracic Society. Am J Respir Crit Care Med 1995;152(5 Pt 2): S77–121.

46. Hoidrup S, Prescott E, Sorensen TI, et al. Tobacco smoking and risk of hip fracture in men and women. Int J Epidemiol 2000;29:253–9.

47. Kanis JA, Johnell O, Oden A, et al. Smoking and fracture risk: a meta–analysis. Osteoporos Int 2005;16:155–62.

48. Cornuz J, Feskanich D, Willett WC, Colditz GA. Smoking, smoking cessation, and risk of hip fracture in women. Am J Med 1999;106:311–4.

49. Ward KD, Klesges RC. A meta-analysis of the effects of cigarette smoking on bone mineral density. Calcif Tissue Int 2001;68:259–70.

50. Kiel DP, Zhang Y, Hannan MT, et al. The effect of smoking at different life stages on bone mineral density in elderly men and women. Osteoporos Int 1996;6:240–8.

51. Burger H, de Laet CE, van Daele PL, et al. Risk factors for increased bone loss in an elderly population: the Rotterdam Study. Am J Epidemiol 1998;147:871–9.

52. Bolton CE, Ionescu AA, Shiels KM, et al. Associated loss of fat-free mass and bone mineral density in chronic obstructive pulmonary disease. Am J Respir Crit Care Med 2004;170:1286–93.

53. Vrieze A, de Greef MH, Wijkstra PJ, Wempe JB. Low bone mineral density in COPD patients related to worse lung function, low weight and decreased fat-free mass. Osteoporos Int 2007;18:1197–202.

54. Lekamwasam S, Trivedi DP, Khaw KT. An association between respiratory function and hip bone mineral density in older men: a cross-sectional study. Osteoporos Int 2005;16:204–7.

55. Lekamwasam S, Trivedi DP, Khaw KT. An association between respiratory function and bone mineral density in women from the general community: a cross sectional study. Osteoporos Int 2002;13:710–5.

56. Sin DD, Man JP, Man SF. The risk of osteoporosis in Caucasian men and women with obstructive airways disease. Am J Med 2003;114:10–4.

57. Henderson NK, White CP, Eisman JA. The roles of exercise and fall risk reduction in the prevention of osteoporosis. Endocrinol Metab Clin North Am 1998;27:369–87.

58. Wei TS, Hu CH, Wang SH, Hwang KL. Fall characteristics, functional mobility and bone mineral density as risk factors of hip fracture in the community-dwelling ambulatory elderly. Osteoporos Int 2001;12:1050–5.

59. Hannan MT, Felson DT, Dawson-Hughes B, et al. Risk factors for longitudinal bone loss in elderly men and women: the Framingham Osteoporosis Study. J Bone Miner Res 2000;15:710–20.

60. Espallargues M, Sampietro-Colom L, Estrada MD, et al. Identifying bone-mass-related risk factors for fracture to guide bone densitometry measurements: a systematic review of the literature. Osteoporos Int 2001;12:811–22.

61. Knoke JD, Barrett-Connor E. Weight loss: a determinant of hip bone loss in older men and women. The Rancho Bernardo Study. Am J Epidemiol 2003;158:1132–8.

62. Ensrud KE, Cauley J, Lipschutz R, Cummings SR. Weight change and fractures in older women. Study of Osteoporotic Fractures Research Group. Arch Intern Med 1997;157:857–63.

63. Morberg CM, Tetens I, Black E, et al. Leptin and bone mineral density: a cross–sectional study in obese and nonobese men. J Clin Endocrinol Metab 2003;88:5795–800.

64. Reid IR. Leptin deficiency–lessons in regional differences in the regulation of bone mass. Bone 2004;34:369–71.

65. Guerra S, Sherrill DL, Bobadilla A, et al. The relation of body mass index to asthma, chronic bronchitis, and emphysema. Chest 2002;122:1256–63.

66. Pitsiou G, Kyriazis G, Hatzizisi O, et al. Tumor necrosis factor-alpha serum levels, weight loss and tissue oxygenation in chronic obstructive pulmonary disease. Respir Med 2002;96:594–8.

67. Eid AA, Ionescu AA, Nixon LS, et al. Inflammatory response and body composition in chronic obstructive pulmonary disease. Am J Respir Crit Care Med 2001;164:1414–8.

68. Incalzi RA, Caradonna P, Ranieri P, et al. Correlates of osteoporosis in chronic obstructive pulmonary disease. Respir Med 2000;94:1079–84.

69. Berry JK, Baum C. Reversal of chronic obstructive pulmonary disease-associated weight loss: are there pharmacological treatment options? Drugs 2004;64:1041–52.

70. Anker SD, Clark AL, Teixeira MM, et al. Loss of bone mineral in patients with cachexia due to chronic heart failure. Am J Cardiol 1999;83:612–5, A10.

71. Ionescu AA, Nixon LS, Evans WD, et al. Bone density, body composition, and inflammatory status in cystic fibrosis. Am J Respir Crit Care Med 2000;162:789–94.

72. De Boer WI. Cytokines and therapy in COPD: a promising combination? Chest 2002;121:209S–18S.

73. Churg A, Dai J, Tai H, et al. Tumor necrosis factor-alpha is central to acute cigarette smoke–induced inflammation and connective tissue breakdown. Am J Respir Crit Care Med 2002;166:849–54.

74. Chung KF. Cytokines in chronic obstructive pulmonary disease. Eur Respir J Suppl 2001;34:50s–9s.

75. Takabatake N, Nakamura H, Abe S, et al. Circulating leptin in patients with chronic obstructive pulmonary disease. Am J Respir Crit Care Med 1999;159:1215–9.

76. Nguyen LT, Bedu M, Caillaud D, et al. Increased resting energy expenditure is related to plasma TNF-alpha concentration in stable COPD patients. Clin Nutr 1999;18:269–74.

77. Gan WQ, Man SF, Senthilselvan A, Sin DD. Association between chronic obstructive pulmonary disease and systemic inflammation: a systematic review and a meta-analysis. Thorax 2004;59:574–80.

78. Di Francia M, Barbier D, Mege JL, Orehek J. Tumor necrosis factor-alpha levels and weight loss in chronic obstructive pulmonary disease. Am J Respir Crit Care Med 1994;150:1453–5.

79. Takabatake N, Nakamura H, Abe S, et al. The relationship between chronic hypoxemia and activation of the tumor necrosis factor-alpha system in patients with chronic obstructive pulmonary disease. Am J Respir Crit Care Med 2000;161:1179–84.

80. Sharma R, Anker SD. Cytokines, apoptosis and cachexia: the potential for TNF antagonism. Int J Cardiol 2002;85:161–71.

81. Debigare R, Cote CH, Maltais F. Peripheral muscle wasting in chronic obstructive pulmonary disease. Clinical relevance and mechanisms. Am J Respir Crit Care Med 2001;164:1712–7.

82. Laghi F, Tobin MJ. Disorders of the respiratory muscles. Am J Respir Crit Care Med 2003;168:10–48.

83. Fearon KC, Moses AG. Cancer cachexia. Int J Cardiol 2002;85:73–81.

84. Argiles JM, Busquets S, Lopez-Soriano FJ. Cytokines in the pathogenesis of cancer cachexia. Curr Opin Clin Nutr Metab Care 2003;6:401–6.

85. Pfitzenmaier J, Vessella R, Higano CS, et al. Elevation of cytokine levels in cachectic patients with prostate carcinoma. Cancer 2003;97:1211–6.

86. Yeh SS, Schuster MW. Geriatric cachexia: the role of cytokines. Am J Clin Nutr 1999;70:183–97.

87. Wouters EF. Chronic obstructive pulmonary disease. 5: systemic effects of COPD. Thorax 2002;57:1067–70.

88. Rodan GA RL, Bilezikian JP. Pathophysiology of osteoporosis. In: Bilezikian JRL, Rodan GA, editors. Principles of bone biology. Vol 2. 2nd ed. San Diego (CA): Academic Press; 2002. p. 1275–89.

89. Lange U, Teichmann J, Stracke H. Correlation between plasma TNF-alpha, IGF-1, biochemical markers of bone metabolism, markers of inflammation/disease activity, and clinical manifestations in ankylosing spondylitis. Eur J Med Res 2000;5:507–11.

90. Chen G, Goeddel DV. TNF–R1 signaling: a beautiful pathway. Science 2002;296:1634–5.

91. Romas E, Gillespie MT, Martin TJ. Involvement of receptor activator of NFkappaB ligand and tumor necrosis factor-alpha in bone destruction in rheumatoid arthritis. Bone 2002;30:340–6.

92. Mundy GR, Chen D, Oyajobi BO. Bone remodeling. In: Flavus MJ, editor. Primer on the metabolic bone diseases and disorders of mineral metabolism. 5th ed. Washington (DC): American Society for Bone and Mineral Research; 2003. p. 46–57.

93. Bruno A, Chanez P, Chiappara G, et al. Does leptin play a cytokine-like role within the airways of COPD patients? Eur Respir J 2005;26:398–405.

94. Broekhuizen R, Vernooy JH, Schols AM, et al. Leptin as local inflammatory marker in COPD. Respir Med 2005;99:70–4.

95. Fantuzzi G, Faggioni R. Leptin in the regulation of immunity, inflammation, and hematopoiesis. J Leukoc Biol 2000;68:437–46.

96. Schols AM, Creutzberg EC, Buurman WA, et al. Plasma leptin is related to proinflammatory status and dietary intake in patients with chronic obstructive pulmonary disease. Am J Respir Crit Care Med 1999;160:1220–6.

97. Calikoglu M, Sahin G, Unlu A, et al. Leptin and TNF-alpha levels in patients with chronic obstructive pulmonary disease and their relationship to nutritional parameters. Respiration 2004;71:45–50.

98. Yang YM, Sun TY, Liu XM. The role of serum leptin and tumor necrosis factor-alpha in malnutrition of male chronic obstructive pulmonary disease patients. Chin Med J (Engl) 2006;119:628–33.

99. Karakas S, Karadag F, Karul AB, et al. Circulating leptin and body composition in chronic obstructive pulmonary disease. Int J Clin Pract 2005;59:1167–70.

100. Thomas T, Gori F, Khosla S, et al. Leptin acts on human marrow stromal cells to enhance differentiation to osteoblasts and to inhibit differentiation to adipocytes. Endocrinology 1999;140:1630–8.

101. Yamauchi M, Sugimoto T, Yamaguchi T, et al. Plasma leptin concentrations are associated with bone mineral density and the presence of vertebral fractures in postmenopausal women. Clin Endocrinol (Oxf) 2001;55:341–7.

102. Shaarawy M, Abassi AF, Hassan H, Salem ME. Relationship between serum leptin concentrations and bone mineral density as well as biochemical markers of bone turnover in women with postmenopausal osteoporosis. Fertil Steril 2003;79:919–24.

103. Yilmazi M, Keles I, Aydin G, et al. Plasma leptin concentrations in postmenopausal women with osteoporosis. Endocr Res 2005;31:133–8.

104. Thomas T, Burguera B, Melton LJ 3rd, et al. Role of serum leptin, insulin, and estrogen levels as potential mediators of the relationship between fat mass and bone mineral density in men versus women. Bone 2001;29:114–20.

105. Weiss NS, Liff JM, Ure CL, et al. Mortality in women following hip fracture. J Chronic Dis 1983;36:879–82.

106. Dennison EM, Syddall HE, Fall CH, et al. Plasma leptin concentration and change in bone density among elderly men and women: the Hertfordshire Cohort Study. Calcif Tissue Int 2004;74:401–6.

107. Koyama S, Sato E, Haniuda M, et al. Decreased level of vascular endothelial growth factor in bronchoalveolar lavage fluid of normal smokers and patients with pulmonary fibrosis. Am J Respir Crit Care Med 2002;166:382–5.

108. Kasahara Y, Tuder RM, Taraseviciene-Stewart L, et al. Inhibition of VEGF receptors causes lung cell apoptosis and emphysema. J Clin Invest 2000;106:1311–9.

109. Tuder RM, Petrache I, Elias JA, et al. Apoptosis and emphysema: the missing link. Am J Respir Cell Mol Biol 2003;28:551–4.

110. Kasahara Y, Tuder RM, Cool CD, et al. Endothelial cell death and decreased expression of vascular endothelial growth factor and vascular endothelial growth factor receptor 2 in emphysema. Am J Respir Crit Care Med 2001;163:737–44.

111. Lim S, Roche N, Oliver BG, et al. Balance of matrix metalloprotease-9 and tissue inhibitor of metalloprotease-1 from alveolar macrophages in cigarette smokers. Regulation by interleukin-10. Am J Respir Crit Care Med 2000;162:1355–60.

112. Daheshia M. Therapeutic inhibition of matrix metalloproteinases for the treatment of chronic obstructive pulmonary disease (COPD). Curr Med Res Opin 2005;21:587–94.

113. Russell RE, Culpitt SV, DeMatos C, et al. Release and activity of matrix metalloproteinase-9 and tissue inhibitor of metalloproteinase-1 by alveolar macrophages from patients with chronic obstructive pulmonary disease. Am J Respir Cell Mol Biol 2002;26:602–9.

114. Belvisi MG, Bottomley KM. The role of matrix metalloproteinases (MMPs) in the pathophysiology of chronic obstructive pulmonary disease (COPD): a therapeutic role for inhibitors of MMPs? Inflamm Res 2003;52:95–100.

115. Delaisse JM, Andersen TL, Engsig MT, et al. Matrix metalloproteinases (MMP) and cathepsin K contribute differently to osteoclastic activities. Microsc Res Tech 2003;61:504–13.

116. Tilg H, Moschen AR. Adipocytokines: mediators linking adipose tissue, inflammation and immunity. Nat Rev Immunol 2006;6:772–83.

117. Tomoda K, Yoshikawa M, Itoh T, et al. Elevated circulating plasma adiponectin in underweight patients with COPD. Chest 2007;132:135–40.

118. Luo XH, Guo LJ, Xie H, et al. Adiponectin stimulates RANKL and inhibits OPG expression in human osteoblasts through the MAPK signaling pathway. J Bone Miner Res 2006;21:1648–56.

119. Richards JB, Valdes AM, Burling K, et al. Serum adiponectin and bone mineral density in women. J Clin Endocrinol Metab 2007;92:1517–23.

120. Lenchik L, Register TC, Hsu FC, et al. Adiponectin as a novel determinant of bone mineral density and visceral fat. Bone 2003;33:646–51.

121. Jurimae J, Rembel K, Jurimae T, Rehand M. Adiponectin is associated with bone mineral density in perimenopausal women. Horm Metab Res 2005;37:297–302.

122. Pauwels RA, Buist AS, Calverley PM, et al. Global strategy for the diagnosis, management, and prevention of chronic obstructive pulmonary disease. NHLBI/WHO Global Initiative for Chronic Obstructive Lung Disease (GOLD) workshop summary. Am J Respir Crit Care Med 2001;163:1256–76.

123. NIH Consensus Development Panel on Optimal Calcium Intake. Optimal calcium intake. JAMA 1994;272:1942–8.

124. Heaney RP, Dowell MS, Hale CA, Bendich A. Calcium absorption varies within the reference range for serum 25-hydroxyvitamin D. J Am Coll Nutr 2003;22:142–6.

125. Bischoff-Ferrari HA. How to select the doses of vitamin D in the management of osteoporosis. Osteoporos Int 2007;18:401–7.

126. Bischoff-Ferrari HA, Willett WC, Wong JB, et al. Fracture prevention with vitamin D supplementation: a meta-analysis of randomized controlled trials. JAMA 2005;293:2257–64.

127. Dawson-Hughes B, Heaney RP, Holick MF, et al. Estimates of optimal vitamin D status. Osteoporos Int 2005;16:713–6.

128. Standing Committee on the Scientific Evaluation of Dietary Reference Intakes, Food and Nutrition Board, Institute of Medicine. Dietary reference intakes for calcium, phosphorus, magnesium, vitamin D, and fluoride. Washington (DC): National Academy Press; 1997.

129. Recommendations for the prevention and treatment of glucocorticoid-induced osteoporosis: 2001 update. American College of Rheumatology Ad Hoc Committee on Glucocorticoid-Induced Osteoporosis. Arthritis Rheum 2001;44:1496–503.

130. Black DM, Thompson DE, Bauer DC, et al. Fracture risk reduction with alendronate in women with osteoporosis: the Fracture Intervention Trial. FIT Research Group. J Clin Endocrinol Metab 2000;85:4118–24.

131. Chesnut IC, Skag A, Christiansen C, et al. Effects of oral ibandronate administered daily or intermittently on fracture risk in postmenopausal osteoporosis. J Bone Miner Res 2004;19:1241–9.

132. McClung MR, Geusens P, Miller PD, et al. Effect of risedronate on the risk of hip fracture in elderly women. Hip Intervention Program Study Group. N Engl J Med 2001;344:333–40.

133. Reginster J, Minne HW, Sorensen OH, et al. Randomized trial of the effects of risedronate on vertebral fractures in women with established postmenopausal osteoporosis. Vertebral Efficacy with Risedronate Therapy (VERT) Study Group. Osteoporos Int 2000;11:83–91.

134. Harris ST, Watts NB, Genant HK, et al. Effects of risedronate treatment on vertebral and nonvertebral fractures in women with postmenopausal osteoporosis: a randomized controlled trial. Vertebral Efficacy With Risedronate Therapy (VERT) Study Group. JAMA 1999;282:1344–52.

135. Reid DM, Hughes RA, Laan RF, et al. Efficacy and safety of daily risedronate in the treatment of corticosteroid-induced osteoporosis in men and women: a randomized trial. European Corticosteroid-Induced Osteoporosis Treatment Study. J Bone Miner Res 2000;15:1006–13.

136. Saag KG, Emkey R, Schnitzer TJ, et al. Alendronate for the prevention and treatment of glucocorticoid-induced osteoporosis. Glucocorticoid-Induced Osteoporosis Intervention Study Group. N Engl J Med 1998;339:292–9.

137. Orwoll ES, Klein R. Osteoporosis in men. Epidemiology, pathophysiology, and clinical characterization. In: Marcus R, Feldman D, Kelsey J, editors. Osteoporosis. Vol 1. 2nd ed. San Diego (CA): Academic Press;2001. p. 103–49.

138. Croom KF, Scott LJ. Intravenous ibandronate: in the treatment of osteoporosis. Drugs 2006;66:1593–601.

139. Delmas PD, Adami S, Strugala C, et al. Intravenous ibandronate injections in postmenopausal women with osteoporosis: one-year results from the Dosing Intravenous Administration Study. Arthritis Rheum 2006;54:1838–46.

140. Black DM, Delmas PD, Eastell R, et al. Once-yearly zoledronic acid for treatment of postmenopausal osteoporosis. N Engl J Med 2007;356:1809–22.

141. Lyles KW, Colon-Emeric CS, Magaziner JS, et al. Zoledronic acid and clinical fractures and mortality after hip fracture. N Engl J Med 2007;357:1799–809.

142. Barrett-Connor E, Mosca L, Collins P, et al. Effects of raloxifene on cardiovascular events and breast cancer in postmenopausal women. N Engl J Med 2006;355:125–37.

143. Orwoll ES, Scheele WH, Paul S, et al. The effect of teriparatide [human parathyroid hormone (1–34)] therapy on bone density in men with osteoporosis. J Bone Miner Res 2003;18:9–17.

144. Neer RM, Arnaud CD, Zanchetta JR, et al. Effect of parathyroid hormone (1–34) on fractures and bone mineral density in postmenopausal women with osteoporosis. N Engl J Med 2001;344:1434–41.

145. American Association of Clinical Endocrinologists Hypogonadism Task Force. American Association of Clinical Endocrinologists medical guidelines for clinical practice for the evaluation and treatment of hypogonadism in adult male patients - 2002 update. Endocr Pract 2002;8:439–56.

146. Orwoll E, Ettinger M, Weiss S, et al. Alendronate for the treatment of osteoporosis in men. N Engl J Med 2000;343:604–10.

147. Pazianas M, Rhim AD, Weinberg AM, et al. The effect of anti-TNF-alpha therapy on spinal bone mineral density in patients with Crohn's disease. Ann N Y Acad Sci 2006;1068:543–56.

148. Mauro M, Radovic V, Armstrong D. Improvement of lumbar bone mass after infliximab therapy in Crohn's disease patients. Can J Gastroenterol 2007;21:637–42.

149. Vis M, Havaardsholm EA, Haugeberg G, et al. Evaluation of bone mineral density, bone metabolism, osteoprotegerin and receptor activator of the NFkappaB ligand serum levels during treatment with infliximab in patients with rheumatoid arthritis. Ann Rheum Dis 2006;65:1495–9.

150. Seriolo B, Paolino S, Sulli A, et al. Bone metabolism changes during anti-TNF-alpha therapy in patients with active rheumatoid arthritis. Ann N Y Acad Sci 2006;1069:420–7.

151. Allali F, Breban M, Porcher R, et al. Increase in bone mineral density of patients with spondyloarthropathy treated with anti-tumour necrosis factor alpha. Ann Rheum Dis 2003;62:347–9.

152. Lange U, Teichmann J, Muller-Ladner U, Strunk J. Increase in bone mineral density of patients with rheumatoid arthritis treated with anti-TNF-alpha antibody: a prospective open-label pilot study. Rheumatology (Oxford) 2005;44:1546–8.

153. Briot K, Garnero P, Le Henanff A, et al. Body weight, body composition, and bone turnover changes in patients with spondyloarthropathy receiving anti-tumour necrosis factor α treatment. Ann Rheum Dis 2005;64:1137–40.

154. Davis JS, Fleischmann RM, Molitor J, et al. Effects of etanercept (ENBREL®) on spinal and hip bone mineral density in patients with ankylosing spondylitis: 24-week data. American College of Rheumatology Annual Meeting; October 2003: Orlando, FL. Abstract 365.

155. Rennard SI, Fogarty C, Kelsen S, et al. The safety and efficacy of infliximab in moderate to severe chronic obstructive pulmonary disease. Am J Respir Crit Care Med 2007;175:926–34

156. Eggelmeijer F, Papapoulos SE, van Paassen HC, et al. Increased bone mass with pamidronate treatment in rheumatoid arthritis. Results of a three-year randomized, double-blind trial. Arthritis Rheum 1996;39:396–402.

157. Van Offel JF, Schuerwegh AJ, Bridts CH, et al. Influence of cyclic intravenous pamidronate on proinflammatory monocytic cytokine profiles and bone density in rheumatoid arthritis treated with low dose prednisolone and methotrexate. Clin Exp Rheumatol 2001;19:13–20.

158. Gur A, Denli A, Cevik R, et al. The effects of alendronate and calcitonin on cytokines in postmenopausal osteoporosis: a 6-month randomized and controlled study. Yonsei Med J 2003;44:99–109.

159. Eastell R, Devogelaer JP, Peel NF, et al. Prevention of bone loss with risedronate in glucocorticoid-treated rheumatoid arthritis patients. Osteoporos Int 2000;11:331–7.

160. Yilmaz L, Ozoran K, Gunduz OH, et al. Alendronate in rheumatoid arthritis patients treated with methotrexate and glucocorticoids. Rheumatol Int 2001;20:65–9.

161. Tascioglu F, Colak O, Armagan O, et al. The treatment of osteoporosis in patients with rheumatoid arthritis receiving glucocorticoids: a comparison of alendronate and intranasal salmon calcitonin. Rheumatol Int 2005;26:21–9.

162. Gianni W, Ricci A, Gazzaniga P, et al. Raloxifene modulates interleukin-6 and tumor necrosis factor-alpha synthesis in vivo: results from a pilot clinical study. J Clin Endocrinol Metab 2004;89:6097–9.

163. Cantatore FP, Acquista CA, Pipitone V. Evaluation of bone turnover and osteoclastic cytokines in early rheumatoid arthritis treated with alendronate. J Rheumatol 1999;26:2318–23.

164. Redlich K, Gortz B, Hayer S, et al. Repair of local bone erosions and reversal of systemic bone loss upon therapy with anti-tumor necrosis factor in combination with osteoprotegerin or parathyroid hormone in tumor necrosis factor-mediated arthritis. Am J Pathol 2004;164:543–55.

165. Korzenik JR. Crohn's disease: future anti-tumor necrosis factor therapies beyond infliximab. Gastroenterol Clin North Am 2004;33:285–301.

166. von Haehling S, Genth-Zotz S, Anker SD, Volk HD. Cachexia: a therapeutic approach beyond cytokine antagonism. Int J Cardiol 2002;85:173–83.

167. Kast RE, Altschuler EL. Bone density loss in Crohn's disease: role of TNF and potential for prevention by bupropion. Gut 2004;53:1056.

168. Kast RE, Altschuler EL. Tumor necrosis factor-alpha in hepatitis B: potential role for bupropion. J Hepatol 2003;39:131–3.

CHAPTER 23

Systemic Manifestations of Chronic Obstructive Pulmonary Disease

Emile F.M. Wouters, PhD, MD

Chronic obstructive pulmonary disease (COPD) is largely caused by cigarette smoking and associated with airflow limitation and chronic inflammation in the lungs.[1] The burden of this progressive disease is evident from mortality figures and disability-adjusted life-years (DALYS). Reported as the sixth leading cause of death in 1990, it is currently ranked fourth cause and is projected to rank third by 2020.[2] Moreover, it is the only leading cause of death with increasing prevalence.[3] Similarly, from its ranking as the twelfth leading cause of DALYS in 1990, it is projected to become the fifth by 2020.[2]

Comorbid conditions are frequently observed in patients with COPD. There is no consensus definition for comorbidities that distinguish them from systemic consequences of COPD. Intuitively, an operational definition is that the systemic consequences are direct consequences of the disease with a cause-and-effect relationship, whereas comorbidities are diseases that occur associated with COPD, perhaps because of shared risk factors.

A limited number of studies have systematically reviewed comorbid conditions in COPD. A study conducted in UK General Practices reported that COPD is associated with many comorbidities, particularly those related to cardiovascular, bone, and other smoking-related conditions.[4] Another study revealed that patients with COPD had a higher prevalence of certain comorbid conditions, including coronary artery disease, congestive heart failure, other cardiovascular disease, local malignant neoplasm, neurologic disease other than stroke with hemiplegia, ulcers, and gastritis.[5] Other studies have evaluated comorbidity as part of the workup of patients hospitalized for acute exacerbations.[6,7] Comorbidity in these studies was checked by the Charlson index, an automated method to quantify comorbidity for analytic purposes.[8] These studies showed that the Charlson index is associated with reduced survival. A recent evaluation of the USA National Hospital discharge survey revealed that hospital diagnosis of COPD was associated with a higher rate of age-adjusted, in-hospital mortality for pneumonia, hypertension, heart failure, ventilatory failure, and thoracic malignancies and was not associated with a greater prevalence of hospitalization or in-hospital mortality for acute and chronic renal failure, human immunodeficiency virus (HIV), gastrointestinal hemorrhage, and cerebrovascular disease.[9]

COPD is increasingly recognized as an inflammatory disease not to be confined to chronic inflammation of the lungs but to be associated with systemic inflammation, potentially leading to these comorbidities or systemic consequences.[10,11] This systemic inflammation may be more pronounced in some stable COPD patients than in others.[12–15] Probably the main sources of systemic inflammation in COPD are exacerbations of the disease, which result in bursts of systemic inflammatory markers that are released into the systemic circulation.[16–19]

Patients with COPD have been observed, most notably during exacerbations, to have increases in systemic oxidative stress,[20,21] circulating levels of cytokines (tumor necrosis factor [TNF]-α,[12,13,15] interleukin [IL]-6,[18] IL-8,[16,17,19] C-reactive protein (CRP),[14] adhesion molecules,[17] fibrinogen,[14] and circulating activated inflammatory cells, particularly neutrophils.[22–24] Repetitive bursts of cytokines or cells released during exacerbations most probably play a major role in producing systemic consequences of COPD. The link between COPD and systemic consequences and comorbidities is poorly understood.

This chapter reviews current evidence with respect to muscle wasting, cardiovascular morbidity, and disturbances in bone metabolism.

Muscle Wasting

Typical symptoms of patients with COPD are shortness of breath, first only during exercise and in a later stage also at rest,[25,26] and exercise intolerance. The latter is related not only to the local impairment but also to systemic features such as weight loss and loss of fat-free mass (FFM). Because FFM gives a reflection of the metabolic active organs in which skeletal muscle is the largest, FFM depletion is associated with muscle weakness, reduced exercise tolerance,[27] and impaired health status.[28] Body mass index (BMI) and overall systemic inflammation appeared to be the major determinants for hospitalization and death risk in end-stage respiratory disease.[29] However, Schols and colleagues showed that the fat-free mass index (FFMI; FFM corrected for height squared) but not the fat mass index was an independent predictor for survival.[30] The authors concluded that FFMI provided information concerning disease prognosis that is beyond that provided by BMI. Confirming these data, measurement of the midthigh cross-sectional area with computed tomography gave a better prediction of survival than did the BMI.[31] Another study also reported that FFMI is a significant predictor of mortality, independent of covariates such as sex, smoking, lung function, and even BMI.[32] Since it is shown that the assessment of FFM and thus the prevalence of muscle wasting in COPD is an independent predictor of mortality, the systemic effects of the disease cannot be overlooked anymore. Therefore, the assessment of the body composition gains significance concerning both the quantity and the quality of patients with COPD. In addition, to develop effective therapies and rehabilitation programs to prevent or treat muscle wasting in COPD, it is of importance to learn about the factors and the mechanisms involved in the process of muscle wasting (see Chapter 21).

Prevalence

Weight loss commonly occurs in patients with COPD. A decreased body weight was reported in 49% of 253 patients with COPD referred to a center for pulmonary rehabilitation.[33] Besides the prevalence of weight loss, the actual prevalence of muscle wasting is probably underestimated when extrapolated from body weight measurements because FFM may be reduced despite preservation of body weight. In a study by Schols and colleagues, a group of 412 COPD patients was divided into four subgroups depending on their BMI and body composition: cachexia (low BMI, low FFMI), semistarvation (low BMI, normal FFMI), muscle atrophy (normal BMI, low FFMI), and patients with no impairment.[30] The results showed that the survival rate of patients suffering from cachexia or muscle atrophy did not differ significantly but was higher than that of those patients suffering from semistarvation. Thus, independent of the BMI and disease severity, FFMI can predict the mortality rate. From a recent study conducted in a large outpatient group, it was concluded that the prevalence of FFM depletion was about 30% in patients with a forced expiratory volume in 1 second (FEV_1) between 30 and 70% predicted[34] and was associated with impaired peripheral muscle strength.[35]

Pathogenesis

Whole body weight loss generally occurs when energy expenditure exceeds energy intake. Increased resting energy expenditure is indeed reported in patients with COPD,[36] which was independent of the severity of the COPD but influenced patients' physical performance.[37] However, in numerous patients, daily activity level decreases,[38] so their total energy expenditure is actually not different compared with that of healthy controls. Loss of body weight together with an excessive loss of skeletal muscle mass in chronic disease (cachexia) differs from loss of body weight alone by the presence of metabolic modifications related to the underlying disease. Inactivity per se contributes to a decrease in skeletal muscle mass via several adaptive changes, such as reduced proportion of type I fibers and oxidative enzyme

capacity, muscle fiber atrophy, and reduced muscle capillarization.[39] However, peripheral skeletal muscle wasting in COPD is due not only to muscle disuse but also to a form of myopathy that involves a whole cascade of factors contributing to the development of muscle wasting (Figure 1).

Wasting of skeletal muscle mass is always the result of an imbalance between muscle protein synthesis and breakdown. A higher myofibrillar protein breakdown is shown in cachectic COPD patients, despite no differences in whole body protein breakdown.[40] Various mechanisms are involved in the increased protein breakdown, but the ubiquitine-proteasome pathway is assumed to provide most of the proteolytic activity required for the degradation of myofibrillar protein.[41] The contribution of this pathway to the development of cachexia is very important, and a number of factors that play a crucial role in the activation of the ubiquitine-proteasome pathway have been detected. Animal studies have shown that the proinflammatory cytokines TNF-α and IL-6 stimulate the ubiquitine-proteasome pathway[42] via the activation of nuclear factor κB (NF-κB) that was increased in underweight COPD patients.[43] A direct effect of inflammation on muscle wasting has not been found so far in humans, but many data in the literature strongly support a causal relationship. Like other chronic diseases, COPD is characterized by low-grade systemic inflammation,[44,45] which was associated with an increased production of TNF-α[46] and IL-6.[47] In addition, it was recently shown that exercise induces more systemic inflammation in muscle-wasted patients with COPD than in non-muscle-wasted patients.[48]

Like inflammation, the presence of hypoxia is a common finding in COPD, and both factors contribute to the generation of reactive oxygen species (ROS).[49] Oxidative stress occurs during an imbalance between the ROS production and the antioxidant capacity to scavenge these ROS products. In COPD patients, both altered antioxidant

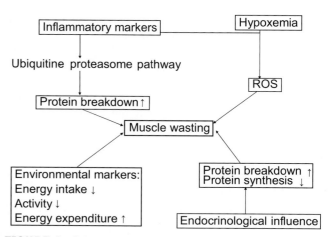

FIGURE 1. Schematic overview of various factors involved in the development of muscle wasting in patients with chronic obstructive pulmonary disease. ROS = reactive oxygen species.

status[50,51] and increased systemic oxidative stress[52] at rest and after low-intensity exercise[53] have been shown. Moreover, an impairment of the adaptive response to oxidative stress was also reported in COPD patients.[54,55] The exercise-induced oxidative stress was even more pronounced in muscle-wasted patients with COPD compared with non-muscle-wasted patients.[48] Although a relationship between systemic oxidative stress and muscle wasting was well described,[39] the mechanisms by which oxidative stress contributes to muscle wasting are not completely clear. ROS affect cellular metabolism by damaging deoxyribonucleic acid (DNA) and by affecting cellular oxidative capacity, resulting in apoptosis. On the other hand, ROS can induce the production of IL-6, assuming that oxidative stress can act as the cause rather than the effect of systemic inflammation.[48] More research has to clarify the exact mechanism of how a disturbed oxidant/antioxidant balance induces muscle wasting in COPD patients.

Muscle wasting is the result of an imbalance between protein breakdown and protein synthesis. Consequently, decreased muscle protein synthesis owing to disturbed cell regeneration capacity can also contribute to the muscle wasting syndrome. Satellite cells are myogenic precursor cells that play an essential role in the regeneration of injured muscle and maintenance of muscle mass. The myogenic regulatory factor MyoD appears to be important in satellite cell differentiation. A number of factors have been implicated in the activation and proliferation of satellite cells. On the other hand, inflammatory markers such as NF-κB and TNF-α have been shown to inhibit MyoD expression and can thus contribute to a disturbed regeneration capacity and thus to muscle wasting (see Chapter 21).

Amino acids are the building blocks of muscle proteins, and a disturbance in the amino acid metabolism can contribute to skeletal muscle wasting. In this view, plasma leucine concentration is often reduced in patients with COPD, and this was associated with decreased levels of FFM.[56] Moreover, skeletal muscle glutamate concentration is consistently decreased in patients with COPD.[44,57] Both amino acids are able to induce an insulin response, and leucine increases protein synthesis, whereas glutamate plays a central role in amino-transamination reactions. Therefore, disturbances in these amino acids can also contribute to muscle wasting.

Apart from the mechanical alterations in skeletal muscle of patients with COPD owing to inflammation or hypoxia, endocrinologic differences can also be a factor in the muscle wasting process in these patients. In this view, a reduced level of anabolic hormones in patients with COPD contributes to an impaired anabolic response needed for maintenance of skeletal muscle mass. In general, anabolic stimuli induce an increase in protein synthesis and a reduction in protein breakdown to stimulate muscle growth and development.

Bone Disturbances

In life, bone is a rigid yet dynamic organ that is continuously molded, shaped, and repaired. Bone microstructure is patterned to provide maximal strength with minimal mass, as determined by the physiologic needs of the organism. Once formed, bone undergoes a process termed remodeling that involves breakdown (resorption) and buildup (synthesis) of bone. Bone remodeling is the predominant metabolic process regulating bone structure and function during adult life, with the key participant being the osteoclast.[58,59]

Most adult skeletal diseases are due to excess osteoclastic activity, leading to an imbalance in bone remodeling that favors resorption.[60]

Osteoporosis has been recognized as one of the systemic effects of COPD (see Chapter 22). Osteoporosis is a systemic skeletal disease characterized by microarchitectural reduction of bone tissue leading to a low bone mass, increased bone fragility, and thereby increased fracture risk.[61] The preclinical state of osteoporosis is called osteopenia. Osteoporosis is commonly found in postmenopausal females and elderly subjects or as a consequence of chronic disease or medical treatment. Different methods of bone mineral density (BMD) measurements can be used. Dual-energy x-ray absorptiometry (DXA) is currently the most frequently used, is accurate and reproducible, and involves very low doses of radiation. BMD is expressed in standard deviation of means, the T- and Z-scores. The T-score is a standard deviation compared with a young adult sex-matched control population. The Z-score is a standard deviation compared with an age- and sex-matched control population.[62] One standard deviation reduction in the BMD increases the fracture risk by 1.5- to 3-fold.[63] Large epidemiologic studies aimed at assessing the incidence and prevalence of osteoporosis within populations of patients with COPD at various stages of disease severity are lacking. Depending on the study population, as many as 35 to 72% of patients with COPD have been reported to be osteopenic, and 36 to 60% of patients with COPD have osteoporosis.[64] In COPD patients admitted for pulmonary rehabilitation, in 56% there were indications of bone mineral loss, and osteoporosis was present in 36% of these patients.[65] Another study reported osteoporosis in 27.2% and osteopenia in 38.3% at the total lumbar site; at the total hip site, osteoporosis was present in 19.8% and osteopenia in 51.9% of the patients.[66] Frequency of bone loss at either the hip or lumbar spine was related to the severity of lung disease. Based on the data from participants in the Third National Health and Nutrition Examination Survey in the United States, Sin and colleagues reported that airflow limitation was associated with increased odds of osteoporosis compared with those without obstruction: airflow obstruction, independent of age, BMI, and medications, including recent use of corticosteroids, increased the risk of osteoporosis in a severity-dependent fashion.[67] These and other data suggest that osteoporosis is found in a proportion of patients with COPD and confirm the view that long-term epidemiologic studies are required to identify the patients who have a high risk of developing osteoporosis.

The etiology of osteoporosis in COPD is very complex, and various factors may contribute to its pathogenesis. Potential risk factors are extensively reviewed in recent papers.[62] In the context of the current review, BMI and body composition, hypogonadism, and endocrinologic abnormalities, as well as the potential role of chronic systemic inflammation, are important to discuss.

Studies have reported that in underweight elderly, the bone mineral content is reduced compared with age-matched subjects with normal BMI.[68,69] Others reported positive relationships between the BMI and bone mass in patients with COPD.[70,71] The possible relationship between weight loss and particularly loss of FFM and BMD in COPD is further explored in the study by Bolton and colleagues.[66] These authors reported that loss of FFM and loss of BMD were related, occurred commonly, and could be subclinical in patients with COPD. Furthermore, they demonstrated increased excretion of cellular and bone collagen protein breakdown products in those patients with low FFM and low BMD, indicating a protein catabolic state in these patients.

Hypogonadism and the reduced availability of sex hormones contribute to the development of osteoporosis. In addition to sex hormones, the insulinlike growth factors (IGFs) play a potential role in osteoporosis. IGF-I may influence bone mass directly or through its role in the preservation of skeletal muscle mass. Further studies are needed to analyze the potential link between IGF-I activity on the bone and skeletal muscles and the pathogenesis of osteoporosis.[62]

Systemic inflammation may have an association with loss of bone, with similar relationships reported in other chronic diseases.[62,72,73] In vitro, both IL-6 and TNF-α stimulate osteoclasts and increase bone resorption.[74–78]

Systemic inflammation is particularly linked to activation of the osteoclastogenesis by the OPG/RANK/RANKL system. Differentiation, activation, and survival of osteoclasts are regulated by the balance between RANKL (RANK ligand) and osteoprotegerin (OPG). OPG is also known as an osteoclast inhibitory factor and is a TNF receptor family member that functions as a decoy receptor. OPG regulates bone density and bone mass in animals[79,80] and on systemic administration can block pathologic bone resorption in various animal models.[79,81] OPG is also produced by osteoblasts in response to anabolic agents such as estrogens and transforming growth factor β-related bone morphogenetic proteins.[82,83]

RANKL is a TNF family member. RANKL exhibits its activity through RANK (receptor activator of NF-κB), another membrane-bound member of the TNF receptor family.[79,84,85] In bone marrow, RANKL is produced by osteoblasts and both osteoblastic and fibroblastic stromal cells. Known inducers of bone resorption and hypercalcemia, such as IL-1, TNF-α, parathyroid hormone (PTH), PTH-related peptide, vitamin D, and others act indirectly through production of RANKL, so OPG can be considered a natural RANKL antagonist of osteoclast activity independent of inducing cytokine (Figure 2).[86] Inhibition of RANKL signaling may be a viable therapeutic strategy for treatment of diseases in which excessive resorption or remodeling of bone prevails. Elucidation of the osteoclast biology may lead to the development of new therapeutics to preserve bone loss in a variety of clinical conditions.

Cardiovascular Morbidity and Mortality

Cardiovascular diseases form one of the most important comorbidities related to COPD.

In a cohort of mild COPD patients, the Lung Health Study showed that lung cancer and cardiovascular complications accounted for nearly two-thirds of all deaths during follow up. The main causes of death in mild or moderate COPD are lung cancer and cardiovascular diseases, whereas in more advanced COPD, respiratory failure becomes the most important cause of death.[87] Other studies confirmed these findings. A 3-year follow up study of 4,284 patients who received hospital treatment for coronary heart disease reported mortality rates of 21% for patients diagnosed with COPD versus 9% in those without COPD.[88] A cohort study including 11,943 COPD patients reported an approximately two- to fourfold increased risk of death at the 3-year follow up owing to cardiovascular diseases compared with an age- and sex-matched control group without COPD. Cardiovascular diseases accounted for 42% of first hospitalizations and 44% of second hospitalizations of patients with mild COPD followed up in the Lung Health Study.[87] The rate of hospitalizations for lower respiratory tract infection was only one-third of that for cardiovascular illnesses. For every 10% decrease in FEV_1, cardiovascular mortality increased by 28%, and nonfatal cardiovascular events increased by almost 20%, after adjustments for relevant confounders such as age, sex, smoking status, and treatment assignment.[89]

Strong epidemiologic evidence points to reduced FEV_1 as a marker of cardiovascular mortality. A longitudinal population-based study reported that patients with poor lung function had the highest risk of cardiovascular mortality. The risk of death from ischemic heart disease was more than fivefold higher for the lowest versus highest lung function quintiles.[90] An increased mortality with decreased lung function is confirmed by many other studies.[91–94] A systematic review and meta-analysis that included >80,000 patients identified an almost twofold risk of cardiovascular mortality in patients with the lowest versus highest lung function quintiles.[90] Another study assessed the role of lung function in cardiovascular mortality and reported that FEV_1 is a predictor of all-cause mortality after control for physical fitness and smoking status.[95] Others found that poor lung function accounted for approximately one-quarter of the attributable mortality risk related to ischemic heart disease.[96] Therefore, it can be concluded that COPD is an important risk factor for

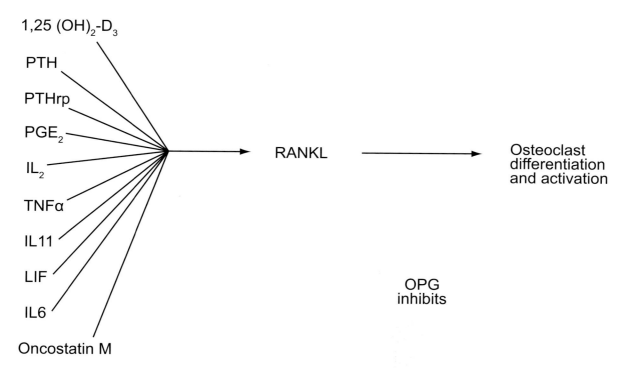

FIGURE 2. The balance of RANKL and osteoprotegerin (OPG) controls osteoclast activity. Most (all?) known inducers of bone resorption and hypercalcemia act indirectly through production of RANKL; hence, OPG can be used pharmacologically to control osteoclast activity independent of the inducing cytokine. IL = interleukin; LIF = leukemia inhibitory factor; PGE2 = prostaglandin E2; PTH = parathyroid hormone; PTHrp = parathyroid hormone–related peptide; TNFα = tumor necrosis factor α.

atherosclerosis, ischemic heart disease, stroke, and sudden cardiac death.

The underlying mechanisms contributing to this increased risk for atherosclerosis in COPD are poorly understood. The pathogenesis of atherosclerosis is complex and multifactorial. Persistent low-grade systemic inflammation is believed to be one of the centerpiece events leading to plaque formation, and there are compelling epidemiologic data linking systemic inflammation to atherosclerosis, ischemic heart disease, strokes, and coronary deaths.[97] COPD is characterized by systemic inflammation.[3] Interestingly, systemic inflammation is not solely associated with severe COPD but may also be present in those with mild and moderate COPD. In general, most of these data are obtained in cross-sectional study; the persistence of this systemic inflammation is poorly documented. Most studies in COPD have been conducted by evaluation of a limited number of molecules involved in the promotion or amplification of atherosclerosis. The most studied of these molecules in COPD is CRP.

Indeed, accumulating evidence suggests that circulating CRP represents one of the strongest independent predictors of vascular death. CRP influences vascular vulnerability directly by a variety of mechanisms.[98] In one study, an important interplay is suggested between systemic inflammation measured by CRP levels and airflow limitation in the development of cardiovascular morbidity by application of a cardiac infarction injury score based on an electrocardiographic scoring scheme.[99] Recently, increased arterial stiffness related to the severity of airflow limitation was reported in COPD patients.[100] This arterial stiffening was related to the level of systemic inflammation.

Fibrinogen was also evaluated in a limited number of studies demonstrating increased fibrinogen levels in COPD patients.

In addition to CRP and fibrinogen, many other factors can induce and promote inflammation or atherogenesis.[97] Low-density lipoprotein (LDL) is one of the principal risk factors for atherosclerosis. Indeed, LDL is a major cause of injury to the endothelium and underlying smooth muscle. When LDL particles become trapped in an artery, they can undergo progressive oxidation and be internalized by macrophages by means of the scavenger receptors on the surfaces of these cells. The internalization leads to the formation of lipid peroxides and facilitates the accumulation of cholesterol esters, resulting in the formation of foam cells. Homocysteine is another factor contributing to atherogenesis as it is toxic to the endothelium, is prothrombic, increases collagen production, and decreases the availability of nitric oxide. Limited data in COPD are available demonstrating elevated plasma homocysteine levels in COPD. An immunoregulatory molecule, CD40 ligand, can be expressed by macrophages, T cells, endothelium, and smooth muscle, and its receptor, CD40, is expressed on the same cells. Both are upregulated in lesions of atherosclerosis, providing evidence of the role of immune activation in the process of atherosclerosis. Ligation of CD40 mediates an array of proinflammatory effects, including the expression of cytokines, chemokines, adhesion molecules, matrix metalloproteinases, and growth factors. These activities are crucial to the process of atherogenesis and promote plaque instability. No data are yet available about upregulation of the CD40 system in COPD.[98]

At present, adipose tissue is no longer considered an inert tissue mainly devoted to energy storage but is emerging as an active participant in regulating physiologic and pathologic processes, including inflammation. Adipose tissue in the current view is that of an active secretory organ, sending out and responding to signals that modulate a variety of biologic processes. Adipokines are proteins produced by adipocytes: leptin and adiponectin are primarily produced by these cells and can therefore be properly classified as adipokines.[101,102]

Leptin, a 167–amino acid peptide hormone produced by white adipose tissue, is primarily involved in the regulation of food intake and energy expenditure. Leptin receptors are expressed in many tissues, including the cardiovascular system. Plasma leptin concentration is proportional to body adiposity and is markedly increased in obese individuals. Recent studies suggest that hyperleptinemia may play a role in cardiovascular diseases, including atherosclerosis.[103] Leptin exerts many potentially atherogenic effects, such as induction of endothelial dysfunction, stimulation of inflammatory reaction, oxidative stress, decrease in paraoxonase activity, platelet aggregation, migration, hypertrophy, and proliferation of vascular smooth muscle cells. Leptin-deficient and leptin receptor-deficient mice are protected from arterial thrombosis and neointimal hyperplasia in response to arterial wall injury. Several clinical studies have demonstrated that a high leptin level predicts acute cardiovascular events, restenosis after coronary angioplasty, and cerebral stroke independently of traditional risk factors. In addition, plasma leptin correlates with markers of subclinical atherosclerosis such as carotid artery intima thickness and coronary artery calcifications.

Adiponectin, the protein that is almost exclusively secreted from adipocytes, is a potent modulator of glucose and lipid metabolism and an indicator of metabolic disorders. Low plasma adiponectin levels are negatively associated with insulin resistance, are predictive of type 2 diabetes onset, and are related to increased risk for the development of cardiovascular disease. Underlying mechanisms include direct effects of adiponectin on fat oxidation and vasculature.[104] Fat tissue is also involved in the systemic inflammatory process by production of other cytokines and acute-phase response proteins such as IL-6 and plasminogen activator inhibitor 1 (PAI-1). PAI-1 is an important factor in the maintenance of vascular hemostasis, inhibiting the activation of plasminogen, the precursor of plasmin, which is involved in the breakdown of fibrin. To understand the underlying mechanisms of cardiovascular changes in COPD, it would be important to understand the interplay and relative contribution of the multifactorial factors involved.[101]

Conclusions

Nowadays, COPD is defined as a preventable and treatable disease with some significant extrapulmonary effects, which may contribute to the disease severity in individual patients. Some of these extrapulmonary effects are at present considered comorbid conditions. There is growing attention for causal relationships between one disorder and another or for an underlying vulnerability to different disorders. Better understanding of the role and consequences of systemic inflammation in certain phenotypes of COPD and understanding of the chronicity of underlying inflammatory processes will broaden our current approach to COPD as a single disease. A patient-oriented approach to COPD needs to take into account that several coexisting components of the chronic disease can contribute to the experienced symptomatology of the patient. Respiratory specialists need to extend their expertise to broader diagnostic and treatment approaches to optimally manage the patient suffering from COPD. This approach certainly will result in a better treatable disease condition and better health for the patient.

References

1. Pauwels RA, Buist AS, Calverley PM, et al. Global strategy for the diagnosis, management, and prevention of chronic obstructive pulmonary disease. NHLBI/WHO Global Initiative for Chronic Obstructive Lung Disease (GOLD) workshop summary. Am J Respir Crit Care Med 2001;163:1256–76.
2. Murray CJ, Lopez AD. Alternative projections of mortality and disability by cause 1990–2020: Global Burden of Disease study. Lancet 1997;349:1498–504.
3. Lopez AD, Shibuya K, Rao C, et al. Chronic obstructive pulmonary disease: current burden and future projections. Eur Respir J 2006;27:397–412.
4. Soriano JB, Visick GT, Muellerova H, et al. Patterns of comorbidities in newly diagnosed COPD and asthma in primary care. Chest 2005;128:2099–107.
5. Mapel DW, Hurley JS, Frost FJ, et al. Health care utilization in chronic obstructive pulmonary disease. A case-control study in a health maintenance organization. Arch Intern Med 2000;160:2653–8.
6. Groenewegen KH, Schols AM, Wouters EF. Mortality and mortality-related factors after hospitalization for acute exacerbation of COPD. Chest 2003;124:459–67.
7. Almagro P, Calbo E, Ochoa de Echaguen A, et al. Mortality after hospitalization for COPD. Chest 2002;121:1441–8.
8. Charlson ME, Pompei P, Ales KL, et al. A new method of classifying prognostic comorbidity in longitudinal studies: development and validation. J Chronic Dis 1987;40:373–83.
9. Holguin F, Folch E, Redd SC, et al. Comorbidity and mortality in COPD-related hospitalizations in the United States, 1979 to 2001. Chest 2005;128:2005–11.

10. Sin DD, Anthonisen NR, Soriano JB, et al. Mortality in COPD: role of comorbidities. Eur Respir J 2006;28:1245–57.

11. Sevenoaks MJ, Stockley RA. Chronic obstructive pulmonary disease, inflammation and co-morbidity—a common inflammatory phenotype? Respir Res 2006;7:70.

12. Di Francia M, Barbier D, Mege JL, et al. Tumor necrosis factor-alpha levels and weight loss in chronic obstructive pulmonary disease. Am J Respir Crit Care Med 1994;150:1453–5.

13. Schols AM, Buurman WA, Staal van den Brekel AJ, et al. Evidence for a relation between metabolic derangements and increased levels of inflammatory mediators in a subgroup of patients with chronic obstructive pulmonary disease. Thorax 1996;51:819–24.

14. Gan WQ, Man SF, Senthilselvan A, et al. Association between chronic obstructive pulmonary disease and systemic inflammation: a systematic review and a meta-analysis. Thorax 2004;59:574–80.

15. Broekhuizen R, Wouters EF, Creutzberg EC, et al. Raised CRP levels mark metabolic and functional impairment in advanced COPD. Thorax 2006;61:17–22.

16. Sauleda J. Systemic inflammation during exacerbations of chronic obstructive pulmonary disease. Lack of effect of steroid treatment [abstract]. Eur Respir J 1999;14:359s.

17. Asin J, Maesen B, van den Bosch, et al. Serum interleukin–8, circulating cell adhesion molecules and hydrogen peroxide in exhaled air in patients with unstable COPD during treatment with corticosteroids [abstract]. Eur Respir J 1998; 12:193S.

18. Wedzicha JA, Seemungal TA, MacCallum PK, et al. Acute exacerbations of chronic obstructive pulmonary disease are accompanied by elevations of plasma fibrinogen and serum IL-6 levels. Thromb Haemost 2000;84:210–5.

19. Spruit MA, Gosselink R, Troosters T, et al. Muscle force during an acute exacerbation in hospitalised patients with COPD and its relationship with CXCL8 and IGF-I. Thorax 2003; 58:752–6.

20. Rahman I, Morrison D, Donaldson K, et al. Systemic oxidative stress in asthma, COPD, and smokers. Am J Respir Crit Care Med 1996;154:1055–60.

21. Pratico D, Basili S, Vieri M, et al. Chronic obstructive pulmonary disease is associated with an increase in urinary levels of isoprostane F2alpha-III, an index of oxidant stress. Am J Respir Crit Care Med 1998;158:1709–14.

22. Burnett D, Chamba A, Hill SL, et al. Neutrophils from subjects with chronic obstructive lung disease show enhanced chemotaxis and extracellular proteolysis. Lancet 1987;2:1043–6.

23. Noguera A, Batle S, Miralles C, et al. Enhanced neutrophil response in chronic obstructive pulmonary disease. Thorax 2001;56:432–7.

24. Noguera A, Busquets X, Sauleda J, et al. Expression of adhesion molecules and G proteins in circulating neutrophils in chronic obstructive pulmonary disease. Am J Respir Crit Care Med 1998;158:1664–8.

25. Standards for the diagnosis and care of patients with chronic obstructive pulmonary disease. American Thoracic Society. Am J Respir Crit Care Med 1995;152:S77–121.

26. Feenstra TL, van Genugten ML, Hoogenveen RT, et al. The impact of aging and smoking on the future burden of chronic obstructive pulmonary disease: a model analysis in the Netherlands. Am J Respir Crit Care Med 2001;164:590–6.

27. Baarends EM, Schols AM, Mostert R, et al. Peak exercise response in relation to tissue depletion in patients with chronic obstructive pulmonary disease. Eur Respir J 1997;10:2807–13.

28. Mostert R, Goris A, Weling Scheepers C, et al. Tissue depletion and health related quality of life in patients with chronic obstructive pulmonary disease. Respir Med 2000;94:859–67.

29. Cano NJ, Pichard C, Roth H, et al. C-reactive protein and body mass index predict outcome in end-stage respiratory failure. Chest 2004;126:540–6.

30. Schols AM, Broekhuizen R, Weling-Scheepers CA, et al. Body composition and mortality in chronic obstructive pulmonary disease. Am J Clin Nutr 2005;82:53–9.

31. Marquis K, Debigare R, Lacasse Y, et al. Midthigh muscle cross-sectional area is a better predictor of mortality than body mass index in patients with chronic obstructive pulmonary disease. Am J Respir Crit Care Med 2002;166:809–13.

32. Vestbo J. Clinical assessment, staging, and epidemiology of chronic obstructive pulmonary disease exacerbations. Proc Am Thorac Soc 2006;3:252–6.

33. Schols AM, Slangen J, Volovics L, et al. Weight loss is a reversible factor in the prognosis of chronic obstructive pulmonary disease. Am J Respir Crit Care Med 1998;157:1791–7.

34. Vermeeren MA, Creutzberg EC, Schols AM, et al. Prevalence of nutritional depletion in a large out-patient population of patients with COPD. Respir Med 2006;100:1349–55.

35. Gosker HR, Lencer NH, Franssen FM, et al. Striking similarities in systemic factors contributing to decreased exercise capacity in patients with severe chronic heart failure or COPD. Chest 2003;123:1416–24.

36. Creutzberg EC, Schols AM, Bothmer-Quaedvlieg FC, et al. Prevalence of an elevated resting energy expenditure in patients with chronic obstructive pulmonary disease in relation to body composition and lung function. Eur J Clin Nutr 1998;52:396–401.

37. Sergi G, Coin A, Marin S, et al. Body composition and resting energy expenditure in elderly male patients with chronic obstructive pulmonary disease. Respir Med 2006;100:1918–24.

38. Baarends EM, Schols AM, Westerterp KR, et al. Total daily energy expenditure relative to resting energy expenditure in clinically stable patients with COPD. Thorax 1997;52:780–5.

39. Couillard A, Prefaut C. From muscle disuse to myopathy in COPD: potential contribution of oxidative stress. Eur Respir J 2005;26:703–19.

40. Rutten EP, Franssen FM, Engelen MP, et al. Greater whole-body myofibrillar protein breakdown in cachectic patients with chronic obstructive pulmonary disease. Am J Clin Nutr 2006;83:829–34.

41. Hasselgren PO, Fischer JE. Muscle cachexia: current concepts of intracellular mechanisms and molecular regulation. Ann Surg 2001;233:9–17.

42. Langen RC, Schols AM, Kelders MC, et al. Inflammatory cytokines inhibit myogenic differentiation through activation of nuclear factor-kappaB. FASEB J 2001;15:1169–80.

43. Agusti A, Morla M, Sauleda J, et al. NF-kappaB activation and iNOS upregulation in skeletal muscle of patients with COPD and low body weight. Thorax 2004;59:483–7.

44. Pouw EM, Schols AM, Deutz NE, et al. Plasma and muscle amino acid levels in relation to resting energy expenditure and inflammation in stable chronic obstructive pulmonary disease. Am J Respir Crit Care Med 1998;158:797–801.

45. Broekhuizen R, Wouters EF, Creutzberg EC, et al. Polyunsaturated fatty acids improve exercise capacity in chronic obstructive pulmonary disease. Thorax 2005; 60:376–82.

46. Takabatake N, Nakamura H, Abe S, et al. The relationship between chronic hypoxemia and activation of the tumor necrosis factor-alpha system in patients with chronic obstructive pulmonary disease. Am J Respir Crit Care Med 2000;161:1179–84.

47. Bolton CE, Broekhuizen R, Ionescu AA, et al. Cellular protein breakdown and systemic inflammation are unaffected by pulmonary rehabilitation in COPD. Thorax 2007;62:109–14.

48. van Helvoort HA, Heijdra YF, Heunks LM, et al. Supplemental oxygen prevents exercise-induced oxidative stress in muscle-wasted patients with chronic obstructive pulmonary disease. Am J Respir Crit Care Med 2006;173:1122–9.

49. Langen RC, Korn SH, Wouters EF. ROS in the local and systemic pathogenesis of COPD. Free Radic Biol Med 2003;35:226–35.

50. Engelen MP, Schols AM, Does JD, et al. Altered glutamate metabolism is associated with reduced muscle glutathione levels in patients with emphysema. Am J Respir Crit Care Med 2000;161:98–103.

51. Gosker HR, Bast A, Haenen GR, et al. Altered antioxidant status in peripheral skeletal muscle of patients with COPD. Respir Med 2005;99:118–25.

52. Mercken EM, Hageman GJ, Schols AM, et al. Rehabilitation decreases exercise-induced oxidative stress in chronic obstructive pulmonary disease. Am J Respir Crit Care Med 2005;172:994–1001.

53. Heunks LM, Dekhuijzen PN. Respiratory muscle function and free radicals: from cell to COPD. Thorax 2000;55:704–16.

54. Engelen MP, Wouters EF, Deutz NE, et al. Factors contributing to alterations in skeletal muscle and plasma amino acid profiles in patients with chronic obstructive pulmonary disease. Am J Clin Nutr 2000;72:1480–7.

55. Rabinovich RA, Ardite E, Troosters T, et al. Reduced muscle redox capacity after endurance training in patients with chronic obstructive pulmonary disease. Am J Respir Crit Care Med 2001;164:1114–8.

56. Engelen MP, Schols AM, Does JD, et al. Skeletal muscle weakness is associated with wasting of extremity fat-free mass but not with airflow obstruction in patients with chronic obstructive pulmonary disease. Am J Clin Nutr 2000; 71:733–8.

57. Porteu F, Hieblot C. Tumor necrosis factor induces a selective shedding of its p75 receptor from human neutrophils. J Biol Chem 1994;269:2834–40.

58. Chambers TJ. Regulation of the differentiation and function of osteoclasts. J Pathol 2000;192:4–13.

59. Teitelbaum SL. Bone resorption by osteoclasts. Science 2000;289:1504–8.

60. Rodan GA, Martin TJ. Therapeutic approaches to bone diseases. Science 2000;289:1508–14.

61. Johnston C, Slemenda C. Risk assessment: theoretical considerations. Am J Med 1993;95:2S–5S.

62. Ionescu AA, Schoon E. Osteoporosis in chronic obstructive pulmonary disease. Eur Respir J Suppl 2003;46:64s–75s

63. Marshall D, Johnell O, Wedel H. Meta-analysis of how well measures of bone mineral density predict occurrence of osteoporotic fractures. BMJ 1996;312:1254–9.

64. Biskobing DM. COPD and osteoporosis. Chest 2002;121:609–20.

65. Engelen MP, Schols AM, Heidendal GA, et al. Dual-energy x-ray absorptiometry in the clinical evaluation of body composition and bone mineral density in patients with chronic obstructive pulmonary disease. Am J Clin Nutr 1998;68:1298–303.

66. Bolton CE, Ionescu AA, Shiels KM, et al. Associated loss of fat-free mass and bone mineral density in chronic obstructive pulmonary disease. Am J Respir Crit Care Med 2004;170:1286–93.

67. Sin DD, Man JP, Man SF. The risk of osteoporosis in Caucasian men and women with obstructive airways disease. Am J Med 2003;114:10–4.

68. Aloia JF, Vaswani A, Ma R, et al. To what extent is bone mass determined by fat-free or fat mass? Am J Clin Nutr 1995;61:1110–4.

69. Coin A, Sergi G, Beninca P, et al. Bone mineral density and body composition in underweight and normal elderly subjects. Osteoporos Int 2000;11:1043–50.

70. Iqbal F, Michaelson J, Thaler L, et al. Declining bone mass in men with chronic pulmonary disease: contribution of glucocorticoid treatment, body mass index, and gonadal function. Chest 1999;116:1616–24.

71. Nishimura Y, Nakata H, Tsutsumi M, et al. Relationship between changes of bone mineral content and twelve-minute walking distance in men with chronic obstructive pulmonary disease: a longitudinal study. Intern Med 1997;36:450–3.

72. Anker SD, Coats AJ. Cardiac cachexia: a syndrome with impaired survival and immune and neuroendocrine activation. Chest 1999;115:836–47.

73. Espat NJ, Moldawer LL, Copeland EM 3rd. Cytokine-mediated alterations in host metabolism prevent nutritional repletion in cachectic cancer patients. J Surg Oncol 1995;58:77–82.

74. Bertolini DR, Nedwin GE, Bringman TS, et al. Stimulation of bone resorption and inhibition of bone formation in vitro by human tumour necrosis factors. Nature 1986;319:516–8.

75. Gowen M, Mundy GR. Actions of recombinant interleukin 1, interleukin 2, and interferon-gamma on bone resorption in vitro. J Immunol 1986;136:2478–82.

76. Raisz LG. Local and systemic factors in the pathogenesis of osteoporosis. N Engl J Med 1988;318:818–28.

77. Manolagas SC, Jilka RL. Bone marrow, cytokines, and bone remodeling. Emerging insights into the pathophysiology of osteoporosis. N Engl J Med 1995;332:305–11.

78. Neale SD, Schulze E, Smith R, et al. The influence of serum cytokines and growth factors on osteoclast formation in Paget's disease. QJM 2002;95:233–40.

79. Simonet WS, Lacey DL, Dunstan CR, et al. Osteoprotegerin: a novel secreted protein involved in the regulation of bone density. Cell 1997;89:309–19.

80. Yasuda H, Shima N, Nakagawa N, et al. Identity of osteoclastogenesis inhibitory factor (OCIF) and osteoprotegerin (OPG): a mechanism by which OPG/OCIF inhibits osteoclastogenesis in vitro. Endocrinology 1998;139:1329–37.

81. Morony S, Capparelli C, Lee R, et al. A chimeric form of osteoprotegerin inhibits hypercalcemia and bone resorption induced by IL-1beta, TNF-alpha, PTH, PTHrP, and 1, 25(OH)2D3. J Bone Miner Res 1999;14:1478–85.

82. Udagawa N, Takahashi N, Yasuda H, et al. Osteoprotegerin produced by osteoblasts is an important regulator in osteoclast development and function. Endocrinology 2000;141:3478–84.

83. Schoppet M, Preissner KT, Hofbauer LC. RANK ligand and osteoprotegerin: paracrine regulators of bone metabolism and vascular function. Arterioscler Thromb Vasc Biol 2002;22:549–53.

84. Morinaga T, Nakagawa N, Yasuda H, et al. Cloning and characterization of the gene encoding human osteoprotegerin/-osteoclastogenesis-inhibitory factor. Eur J Biochem 1998;254:685–91.

85. Anderson DM, Maraskovsky E, Billingsley WL, et al. A homologue of the TNF receptor and its ligand enhance T-cell growth and dendritic-cell function. Nature 1997;390:175–9.

86. Feige U. Osteoprotegerin. Ann Rheum Dis 2001;60 Suppl 3:iii81–4.

87. Anthonisen NR, Connett JE, Kiley JP, et al. Effects of smoking intervention and the use of an inhaled anticholinergic bronchodilator on the rate of decline of FEV1. The Lung Health Study. JAMA 1994;272:1497–505.

88. Berger JS, Sanborn TA, Sherman W, et al. Effect of chronic obstructive pulmonary disease on survival of patients with coronary heart disease having percutaneous coronary intervention. Am J Cardiol 2004;94:649–51.

89. Anthonisen NR, Connett JE, Murray RP. Smoking and lung function of Lung Health Study participants after 11 years. Am J Respir Crit Care Med 2002;166:675–9.

90. Sin DD, Wu L, Man SF. The relationship between reduced lung function and cardiovascular mortality: a population-based study and a systematic review of the literature. Chest 2005;127:1952–9.

91. Sorlie PD, Kannel WB, O'Connor G. Mortality associated with respiratory function and symptoms in advanced age. The Framingham Study. Am Rev Respir Dis 1989; 140:379–84.

92. Ebi-Kryston KL, Hawthorne VM, Rose G, et al. Breathlessness, chronic bronchitis and reduced pulmonary function as predictors of cardiovascular disease mortality among men in England, Scotland and the United States. Int J Epidemiol 1989;18:84–8.

93. Persson C, Bengtsson C, Lapidus L, et al. Peak expiratory flow and risk of cardiovascular disease and death. A 12–year follow up of participants in the population study of women in Gothenburg, Sweden. Am J Epidemiol 1986;124:942–8.

94. Truelsen T, Prescott E, Lange P, et al. Lung function and risk of fatal and non-fatal stroke. The Copenhagen City Heart Study. Int J Epidemiol 2001;30:145–51.

95. Stavem K, Aaser E, Sandvik L, et al. Lung function, smoking and mortality in a 26-year follow up of healthy middle-aged males. Eur Respir J 2005;25:618–25.

96. Hole DJ, Watt GC, Davey-Smith G, et al. Impaired lung function and mortality risk in men and women: findings from the Renfrew and Paisley prospective population study. BMJ 1996;313:711–5; discussion 715–6.

97. Epstein SE, Stabile E, Kinnaird T, et al. Janus phenomenon: the interrelated tradeoffs inherent in therapies designed to enhance collateral formation and those designed to inhibit atherogenesis. Circulation 2004;109:2826–31.

98. Szmitko PE, Wang CH, Weisel RD, et al. New markers of inflammation and endothelial cell activation: part I. Circulation 2003;108:1917–23.

99. Sin DD, Man SF. Why are patients with chronic obstructive pulmonary disease at increased risk of cardiovascular diseases? The potential role of systemic inflammation in chronic obstructive pulmonary disease. Circulation 2003;107:1514–9.

100. Sabit R, Bolton CE, Edwards PH, et al. Arterial stiffness and osteoporosis in chronic obstructive pulmonary disease. Am J Respir Crit Care Med 2007;175:1259–65.

101. Fantuzzi G. Adipose tissue, adipokines, and inflammation. J Allergy Clin Immunol 2005;115:911–9; quiz 920.

102. Trayhurn P, Wood IS. Adipokines: inflammation and the pleiotropic role of white adipose tissue. Br J Nutr 2004; 92:347–55.

103. Beltowski J. Leptin and atherosclerosis. Atherosclerosis 2006;189:47–60.

104. Kantartzis K, Rittig K, Balletshofer B, et al. The relationships of plasma adiponectin with a favorable lipid profile, decreased inflammation, and less ectopic fat accumulation depend on adiposity. Clin Chem 2006;52:1934–42

CHAPTER 24

Biomarkers in Chronic Obstructive Pulmonary Disease

Emile F.M. Wouters, PhD, MD, Scott Wagers, MD, and Jan Dallinga, PhD

Biomarkers of organ damage and dysfunction occupy a central position in the armamentarium of the clinician: biochemical and molecular markers have been used in medicine for disease characterization and diagnosis for centuries. Biomarkers are factors that are objectively measured and evaluated as indicators of normal biologic processes or pathogenic processes and/or as indicators of pharmacologic responses to therapeutic intervention. Clinical end points are variables that can be used to measure how patients feel, function, or survive. Surrogate end points are biomarkers that are intended to substitute for a clinical end point. Although several biomarkers may be needed to create an ideal surrogate end point cluster to truly characterize clinical end points, individual biochemical or molecular markers can be used as biomarkers to evaluate disease progression and to evaluate the effects of therapeutic intervention early in development.[1] Biomarkers need to represent mechanism-based processes and can provide exciting clues to the pathophysiology of diseases. Therefore, the ideal biomarker increases pathologically in the presence of the disease (high sensitivity), does not increase in the absence of disease (high specificity), offers information about the risk and prognosis, changes in accordance with the clinical evolution, creates opportunities to anticipate clinical changes, relates to disease burden and extent, needs to be reproducible, and optimally will be cheap and easy to measure.[2]

The need for biomarkers in chronic obstructive pulmonary disease (COPD) research to better diagnose and to assess phenotype, severity, and the effects of treatment is well recognized.[3,4] In this chapter, we discuss the more established and the more novel biomarkers that have been studied in COPD.

Pulmonary Biomarkers

Pulmonary biomarkers are perhaps the most studied biomarkers in COPD as a number of lung sampling techniques are in use: bronchoalveolar lavage, bronchial biopsy, induced sputum, and exhaled breath sampling. When considering a biomarker, thought has to be given to sampling techniques as they are not necessarily comparable.[5,6]

Bronchoalveolar lavage is thought to provide more of a distal airway sample, whereas induced sputum is considered a proximal airway sample.[7] Yet sputum induction can produce more of a distal sample if the time of induction is extended.[8] Exhaled breath condensate (EBC) has received much attention recently; however, the use of this technique is controversial as it produces samples with a substantial degree of dilution[9] compared with other techniques; it is thereby sensitive to collection technique errors and requires highly sensitive assays.

Distinguishing COPD

Numerous studies have compared biomarkers in COPD with biomarkers in other diseases, most commonly asthma. Cell differential would seem to be a likely candidate biomarker, particularly in regard to distinguishing COPD from asthma as COPD is thought to be characterized by neutrophilic inflammation and asthma by eosinophil inflammation. Indeed, studies that have compared these two diseases have found, in general, a higher percentage of neutrophils in the sputum and bronchoalveolar lavage fluid in patients with COPD and a higher percentage of eosinophils in patients with asthma.[10–13] However, this difference is not distinct as patients with asthma, in particular severe persistent asthma with fixed obstruction, can have substantial neutrophils in their sputum,[14] and some patients with COPD have been found to have elevated eosinophils in the sputum.[12,14,15] In studies that compared patients with COPD with controls, not directly comparing asthma and COPD, elevated numbers of eosinophils are also often found,[16–21] mostly during exacerbations but also in stable patients. There is limited evidence that some of the cell-specific markers may be distinguishing between asthma and COPD. Myeloperoxidase (MPO), a neutrophil marker, and eosinophilic cationic protein (ECP) have been shown to be both differentially elevated and equivalent in asthma and COPD.[22,23] Keatings and Barnes did find that another marker, human neutrophil lipocalin (HNL), was much higher in patients with COPD compared with those with asthma.[22] Better definition of the individual cell populations does hold promise as a useful biomarker, as evidenced by the study by Tsoumakidou and colleagues, in which significantly increased CD4/CD8 and CD4 interferon-γ to interleukin (IL)-4-positive cell ratios were found in patients with severe persistent asthma compared with those with COPD.[13] Cationic antimicrobial protein 18 (CAP18) has also been found in higher concentrations in the sputum of patients with COPD compared with asthma.[24] CAP18 is a member of the cathelicidin family of proteins; it functions as part of the innate immune system and is produced by many cell types, likely neutrophils in COPD. In the same study, however, CAP18 was found to be elevated also in patients with cystic fibrosis (CF), making it not unique to COPD.[24] Nonetheless, it seems less likely that one would face as much of a diagnostic quandary between CF and COPD as with asthma. Tumor necrosis factor α (TNF-α) and IL-8 have also been studied in terms of their ability to diagnose COPD. Although both are elevated in COPD,[11,23–27] TNF-α was found in a comparison study to be elevated also in the induced sputum of asthmatics.[11] A protease/antiprotease imbalance is central to the current thinking about the pathogenesis of COPD; accordingly, several studies have found that tissue inhibitors of metalloproteinase (TIMP) are elevated in patients with COPD but not in asthma.[28,29] This is contrary to what one would think of COPD as one would expect there to be more proteases, but it has been speculated that the elevation in TIMP is a consequence of elevated proteases in an attempt to compensate for the overall increased protease activity. Plymoth and colleagues were able to identify a subset of proteins in bronchoalveolar lavage samples that predicted in a longitudinal follow-up study which smokers went on to develop COPD.[30] Such an approach perhaps represents the state of the art and the future of biomarker research. Lastly, EBC samples have been compared between COPD, asthma, and bronchiectasis, and patients with COPD and bronchiectasis were found to have lower pH values than those with asthma.[31] However, it was also found in this study that EBC from patients with moderate asthma had a lower pH than those with mild asthma, suggesting that pH is a reflection of the degree of inflammation. In summary, although there are some intriguing possibilities, there is no obvious pulmonary biomarker that can distinguish COPD from other diseases. Whether there ever will be one is unclear because, to date, the studies that have been done have been relatively small, so even where there appears to be a distinguishing biomarker, it may simply be a type I error.

Characterizing COPD

The vast majority of the biomarker literature in COPD has focused more on comparison of patients with COPD with those without COPD, either healthy smokers or healthy controls. In effect, most studies have contributed to building up a biomarker profile of COPD, which is a necessary step but far from establishing a definitive biomarker. Cell counts from sputum, bronchoalveolar lavage, and biopsy studies are the most studied type of biomarker. Numerous studies have confirmed that neutrophils are elevated in the lungs of individuals with COPD,[6,10–13,15,16,18,19,22,27,32–39] and as mentioned above, there is ample evidence that eosinophils are also increased in COPD.[10–13,16,18–21] One study reported that as many as 38% of COPD patients have sputum eosinophilia.[17] Studies on macrophages focus mostly on the characteristics of sampled macrophages as sampled or evaluate macrophages in cell culture. Macrophage phenotype as determined by macrophage surface marker determination has been shown

to be different in COPD patients compared with smokers and nonsmokers[40,41]; however, the phenotypes identified are not the same in every study. This may reflect the sampling technique as Domagala-Kulawik and colleagues examined induced sputum and found elevated numbers of CD11b- and CD14-positive macrophages,[41] whereas Lofdahl and colleagues studied bronchoalveolar lavage and found higher expression of CD11c and lower expression of CD86 and CD11a.[40] Macrophages in bronchoalveolar lavage and bronchial biopsies express more MMP-12 than controls,[42,43] whereas macrophages removed from the lung, and then cultured, have been shown to produce more IL-6[44] and MMP-9[45] and less transforming growth factor β and TIMP-1[46] than controls. Macrophages from COPD patients have also been shown to have a greater ability to degrade elastin.[43] Lymphocyte populations sampled from the lungs of patients with COPD have higher CD8 expression in both bronchoalveolar lavage and sputum.[13,47–49] As for proteins, multiple studies have found elevations in TNF-α and IL-8 in sputum[11,16,27,50] and that these proteins are also released more by cells within the lung.[26,51] Whereas IL-8 has been studied in the bronchoalveolar lavage fluid and found to be elevated in patients with COPD,[6,25,52,53] there are no published reports of TNF-α levels in bronchoalveolar fluid, which is interesting in light of the published negative studies for anti-TNF-α therapy,[54,55] especially considering that the lung periphery, which is presumably assayed by bronchoalveolar lavage samples, is recognized as being an important site of pathophysiology in COPD.[56] TNF-α receptor expression, which is thought to be indicative of TNF-α activity, in sputum has been found to be inversely correlated to forced expiratory volume in 1 second (FEV_1) in a COPD population.[50] Monocyte chemotactic protein 1 was found to be elevated in bronchoalveolar lavage fluid from individuals with chronic bronchitis compared with nonsmoking controls but not with smoking controls.[57] In contrast, macrophage inflammatory protein 1β did show a significant differential rise in patients with chronic bronchitis compared with smokers, suggesting that it might be a smoke-induced inflammation-independent marker of COPD.[57] By-products of oxidative damage, nitrotyrosine, nitrogen oxides, aldehydes, nitrosothiols, and 8-isoprostane, have been found in elevated concentrations of sputum and EBC.[52,58–63] Of specific interest is that antioxidant levels have also been found to be reduced in patients with COPD[62] and that individual inflammatory cells in COPD patients had increased nitrotyrosine immunoreactivity,[64] indicating that individuals who develop COPD may be more prone to oxidative damage. Not surprisingly, proteases and the protease/antiprotease balance have been found to be deranged in patients with COPD compared with controls. Fujita and colleagues found in bronchoalveolar lavage fluid that the elastase/antielastase balance related directly to the presence of emphysema.[65] More recently, MMPs have been studied, and in sputum, MMP-1, -8, -9, and -12 have been reported to be elevated in patients with COPD compared with controls.[28,66–69] It is therefore not surprising that hyaluronan, an extracellular matrix breakdown product, has also been found in the sputum of patients with COPD and correlated with markers of inflammation.[70] Hyaluronan therefore reflects both the structural damage and ongoing inflammation in COPD, making it a potentially unique marker, but further studies are needed. Another potentially unique marker that could link the systemic consequences of COPD to the lung compartment is leptin. Leptin can be found in induced sputum and correlates with inflammatory markers in the sputum as well, but its relationship to systemic leptin is unclear as plasma and sputum leptin levels were inversely correlated.[71] An innovative method that may provide a biomarker is the measurement of exhaled breath temperature. Patients with COPD have a slower rise in exhaled breath temperature that correlates with exhaled nitric oxide (NO) but not sputum neutrophils.[72] This deficit in temperature change is thought to represent alterations in lung vascularity and thereby represents a unique biomarker that may allow us to assess an unmeasured aspect of COPD, pulmonary vascularity.

Disease Severity

Functioning as a marker of severity of disease is one of the potential uses of biomarkers in COPD.[3] A recent meta-analysis of 652 studies was conducted regarding clinical markers of COPD severity.[4] The pulmonary biomarkers that were examined included neutrophils, macrophages, eosinophils, CD8+ lymphocytes, IL-6, IL-8, TNF-α, C-reactive protein (CRP), fibrinogen, and exhaled NO and carbon monoxide (CO). Markers were related to disease stage as defined by the American Thoracic Society (ATS) guidelines.[73] Cell type analysis was possible only on sputum data as not enough studies included bronchoalveolar lavage or bronchial biopsies. Although both macrophages and neutrophils showed significant differences throughout all disease stages compared with healthy controls, only neutrophil numbers showed a trend toward an increase with successive stages. In terms of pulmonary biochemical markers, IL-8 in sputum showed a difference between mild and moderate stages and in lavage between healthy and mild stages. There were insufficient data to analyze samples for all other markers and exhaled breath data. This study highlights the lack of studies that establish any pulmonary biomarker as a marker of disease severity but perhaps suggests that sputum neutrophils and IL-8 are potential candidates of disease severity. However, the ATS disease classification is largely based on FEV_1, which itself is a marker and not an outcome measure, whereas symptom scales such as the St George Respiratory Questionaire (SGRQ) are outcome measures.[3] Snoeck-Stroband and colleagues were able to show in a group of 114 patients with COPD that the number of sputum macrophages relates to the SGRQ score and disease outcome.[74] In addition, a marker of oxidative stress, nitrogen oxide–peroxynitrite inhibitory capacity, relates to COPD severity, whereas vascular endothe-

lial growth factor (VEGF) levels decreased with increasing severity.[75] Another way to look at severity is the rate of disease progression, and Stanescu and colleagues, in a long-term longitudinal study, demonstrated that the percentage of neutrophils in the sputum was correlated with the rate of decline in FEV_1.[39]

Phenotype

Historically, two different phenotypes of COPD have been recognized: emphysema and chronic bronchitis.[76] Proteases, neutrophil elastase, and MMP-9 have been related to the degree of emphysema present on high-resolution computed tomographic (CT) images.[65,66,77,78] HNL and IL-8 are also elevated in the bronchoalveolar lavage fluid of smokers with emphysema compared with those without emphysema.[53,79] Kanazawa and colleagues found that VEGF levels in induced sputum increased with airflow limitation in patients with chronic bronchitis and decreased with airflow limitation in those with emphysema.[80] In addition, VEGF levels in induced sputum have also been reported to be related to the degree of pulmonary hypertension in patients with chronic bronchitis.[81] The number of neutrophils in bronchoalveolar lavage and bronchial biopsies, as shown by Lapperre and colleagues,[82] correlates with results from nitrogen washout testing, perhaps a test of small airway dysfunction, indicating that neutrophils may be useful for defining the extent of small airways involvement in COPD. Sputum eosinophils in COPD have been linked to airway hyperresponsiveness,[83] the degree of bronchodilator reversibility,[84] and the response to inhaled steroids.[17]

Exacerbations

Exacerbations provide an opportunity to demonstrate that a COPD biomarker is associated with at least a temporary worsening of the disease severity. However, concurrent infections complicate the interpretation of these associations. Saetta and colleagues found during exacerbation a marked increase in eosinophil counts in bronchial biopsies and in the sputum.[19] To a lesser extent, they found increases in neutrophils and CD3 lymphocytes but did not find an increase in macrophages or mast cells. This exacerbation-related increase of sputum neutrophils has been confirmed by other studies,[16,18,21,32] although the increase in eosinophils has not been found uniformly,[48] which indicates that sputum eosinophilia is the result of concomitant viral infections.[18] Soluble receptors for IL-5, a known eosinophil chemoattractant, have also been found to increase during exacerbations.[85] Increases in neutrophil counts, however, appear to be independent of whether or not the exacerbation is infectious, viral or bacterial.[18] Bhowmik and colleagues found that induced sputum cell counts did not predict the duration or degree of lung function derangements during an exacerbation,[86] yet a treatment strategy that aims to minimize eosinophils in the sputum resulted in a reduction of 62% of the incidence of severe exacerbations.[20] This is perhaps the best validation of the use of a biomarker as it demonstrates a change in an important outcome: exacerbation rate. Aaron and colleagues observed an increase in the levels of both TNF-α and IL-8 in the sputum of COPD patients during an exacerbation and observed a subsequent significant decline on follow-up 1 month later.[87] When bronchoalveolar lavage is examined, comparable increases in IL-8 levels are not observed.[25] Furthermore, a study in which treatment with tiotroprium reduced the exacerbation rate found no effect on sputum IL-6, CRP, or MPO and an increase in IL-8 in those treated with tiotroprium.[88] As for EBC, concentrations of IL-1β, IL-6, IL-8, IL-10p70, and TNF-α, as well as leukotriene B$_4$ (LTB$_4$) and 8-isoprostane, have been reported to increase during exacerbations in EBC.[52,89,90] Given the ease of use and portability of EBC, measuring biomarkers within EBC may be ideal for predicting exacerbations or guiding treatment.

Systemic Biomarkers

COPD is both a pulmonary and a systemic disease. The systemic complications of COPD include nutritional abnormal body composition (see Chapter 23), skeletal muscle wasting, and exercise limitation, as well as involvement of other organ systems (cardiovascular, neurologic, and skeletal).[91] Most of these complications are at least in part thought to be the consequence of systemic inflammation, and, accordingly, most of the systemic biomarkers are related to inflammatory processes. In contrast to the pulmonary biomarkers, the sampling technique is not as much of a concern; however, involving systemic inflammatory biomarkers can also be elevated by disease processes in other organ systems.

Characterizing COPD

A meta-analysis conducted in 2004 by Gan and colleagues selected 14 studies that evaluated systemic inflammatory markers in patients with COPD.[92] Levels of CRP, fibrinogen, TNF-α, and circulating leukocytes were higher in patients with COPD compared with controls. IL-8 and IL-6 did not show significant differences; however, at the time of analysis, there was only a limited number of studies on these cytokines. Since 2004, several studies have confirmed this COPD-related elevation in CRP,[93–97] and a relatively large study found that in a cohort of patients 70 to 79 years of age, IL-6 was higher in those with obstructive lung disease.[97] CRP levels have also been shown to relate to COPD severity both in terms of lung function and SGRQ score,[93] as well as mortality and disease progression.[95] Desmosine is a breakdown product of elastin, and Cardoso and colleagues found that in resected lung sections, desmosine levels were consistently expressed in areas of emphysema.[98] Desmosine can be measured in both blood and urine, and the concentration of desmosine in the urine[99–103] and plasma[101] of patients with COPD was higher than that in controls. Desmosine is also elevated in the urine of smokers,[102] but it is decreased in patients with severe emphysema,[99] presumably reflecting the lack of remaining elastin. There is some indication that desmosine levels are particularly elevated in patients

with α$_1$-antitrypsin deficiency,[103] and desmosine may thereby serve as a useful marker to follow treatment of these patients. Lastly, in what represents the state of the art in biomarker use in disease characterization, Pinto-Plata used a proteomics approach to identify a panel of 24 specific biomarkers in the blood of patients with COPD and demonstrated significant correlations of these biomarkers with FEV$_1$, diffusing capacity, 6-minute walking distance, and the Body-Mass Index, Airflow Obstruction, Dyspnea, Exercise Capacity (BODE) index.[104]

Phenotype

Patients with COPD who lose weight, particularly fat-free mass, represent a COPD phenotype that is in part the result of systemic inflammation. Pitsiou and colleagues divided COPD patients into a "pink puffer," low body weight, and a "blue bloater" category and found that TNF-α serum levels were increased in the pink puffers.[105] A similar result was obtained by Di Francia and colleagues when patients were divided into groups according to whether or not they had intentionally lost weight.[106] In addition, blood TNF receptor levels have been shown to be inversely correlated with the percentage of body fat.[107] In a similar manner, increased blood CRP levels have been shown to be related to resting energy expenditure and fat-free mass or body mass index.[93,108] Appetite-regulating biomolecules, leptin and ghrelin, have also been related to body composition in COPD. Broekhuizen and colleagues found that blood leptin levels were lower in cachectic patients with COPD compared with those who were not,[109] and plasma ghrelin was found to be significantly higher in underweight COPD patients.[110] What is not known is whether these markers predict who will become cachectic, which would make them very useful as a clinical biomarker. Pulmonary hypertension is also a phenotypic feature of COPD, more typically in the latter stages of disease. Joppa and colleagues found that patients with pulmonary hypertension had elevated blood levels of CRP and TNF-α and that CRP was an independent predictor of pulmonary systolic pressure.[111] Since the diagnosis of pulmonary hypertension requires at least an echocardiogram, CRP measurements may prove to be useful at least in determining who to screen for pulmonary hypertension.

Exacerbations

Increases in blood levels of CRP, IL-6, IL-8, LTB$_4$, procalcitonin, copeptin, leptin, ECP, MPO, and fibrinogen have all been reported during exacerbations.[111–121] CRP correlates with disease stage in patients experiencing an exacerbation[120] and improves with treatment of the exacerbation (see Chapter 25).[114] Perera and colleagues found that patients with elevated CRP levels did not recover as frequently as those with lower CRP levels and had a greater chance of recurrence within 50 days.[116] When coupled with clinical symptoms, CRP has also been shown to confirm the diagnosis of a COPD exacerbation with some degree of sufficient sensitivity and specificity.[115,116] Furthermore, the baseline level of CRP was found by Dahl and colleagues to be predictive of subsequent hospitalization and death.[112] Examination of the rate of rise of blood fibrinogen levels can also be helpful in predicting exacerbations.[116,121] During an exacerbation, blood procalcitonin levels may be useful for determining appropriate therapy. Procalcitonin release is stimulated by the presence of a bacterial infection, and, accordingly, three studies have now found that the measurement of procalcitonin can be used to safely determine which patients should be treated with antibiotics.[118,119,122]

Assessing Effectiveness: Biomarkers in Use

Ultimately, one would like to have biomarkers that have been validated as being accurate reflections of longer-term outcome measures in COPD. However, as is evident from the above review, no biomarker has been validated except for perhaps sputum eosinophilia as a marker of the risk of exacerbation.[20] Nonetheless, a number of pharmacologic intervention trials have reported on the effect of treatment on biomarkers in COPD.

Steroids

Inhaled steroids have been shown to reduce sputum neutrophils[123–125] and oral steroids have been shown to reduce concentrations of the neutrophil marker MPO.[126] Sputum eosinophils are also reduced by oral[127] and inhaled steroids,[128] as well as combination therapy with salmeterol and fluticasone.[128,129] Inhaled steroids can also reduce bronchoalveolar lavage fluid concentrations of IL-8.[123] Sin and colleagues demonstrated that withdrawal of inhaled steroids led to a rise in CRP and subsequent treatment led to a reduction.[130] Although steroids are clearly affecting CRP, what that means for outcomes is less clear. However, the TORCH study suggested that such changes may be highly significant for the most powerful of outcome measures, mortality.[131] This is particularly true in light of the results reported by Dahl and colleagues linking CRP levels to mortality.[112]

Bronchodilators

Bronchodilators are not typically thought of as anti-inflammatory agents. Yet Yildirim and colleagues demonstrated that different combinations of bronchodilators (theophylline, ipratropium, formoterol) all reduced sputum and blood levels of IL-8, TNF-α, and LTB$_4$ without affecting lung function tests or arterial blood gas measurements.[132] Theophylline alone has been shown to be anti-inflammatory in COPD patients by showing that it reduces sputum neutrophils, MPO, and IL-8.[67,88] Powrie and colleagues found that tiotropium significantly reduced exacerbations and, because of the lack of an effect on inflammatory biomarkers (serum CRP, sputum MPO, IL-6, and IL8), concluded that the reduction in exacerbations was not related to a reduction in inflammation.[88] In this way, biomarkers may help define the mechanism of pharmacotherapeutic agents, but we do not know that measuring a few inflammatory parameters is reflective of inflammation in a broader sense.

All-trans Retinoic Acid

Retinoids promote alveolar septal repair in animal models,[133] and, accordingly, there is interest in their use in patients with COPD.[134] In a patient study, measurement of MMP-9 and TIMP in the sputum at baseline and during all-trans retinoic acid (ATRA) treatment showed that ATRA favorably modifies the MMP-9 to TIMP ratio.[135] Most recently, a feasibility study of ATRA treatment in patients failed to show an overall improvement in the degree of CT scan–evaluated emphysema but did show some time-dependent improvements with the highest-dose regimen.[136] This is an example of how biomarkers can provide an intermediate evidentiary step in the process of proving efficacy for a therapeutic intervention and may even provide the impetus for further investigation when benefits in terms of outcomes are modest.

COPD and Volatile Compounds in Exhaled Breath

Gaseous and low-boiling compounds present in exhaled air prove to provide valuable information on the condition of the airway tract. In particular, NO has been the subject of many studies trying to relate NO levels in the exhaled air to inflammatory respiratory conditions. In addition, CO, ethane, and, more recently, various volatile organic compounds (VOCs) have been investigated and related to the health and conditions of people suffering from COPD.

Nitric Oxide

During the last decade, measurements of NO have become routine procedures for the diagnosis and monitoring of asthma. In addition, many articles have appeared dealing with the relationship between COPD and NO.

Olin and colleagues concluded that NO measurements can reflect inflammatory changes in the peripheral airways of nonsmokers, ex-smokers, and current smokers,[137] but whether these NO levels can predict early onset of COPD remains uncertain. This conclusion differs slightly from that of Tzortzaki and colleagues, who underlined the controversial results published with respect to the relationship between NO and COPD, NO and smoking, and NO and FEV$_1$.[138] These authors also stated that, formerly, smoking COPD patients showed elevated exhaled NO levels and that the NO levels were generally inversely correlated to FEV$_1$. Three of four cited articles indeed show the negative correlation between NO and FEV$_1$[139–141]; in one article, a positive correlation was presented.[142]

Bhowmik and colleagues reported increased NO levels in COPD patients during exacerbations compared with stable COPD, but they also reported increased NO levels when patients suffered from a cold or a sore throat.[143] The influence of inhaled corticosteroids was described by Zietkowski and colleagues.[144] They reported a decrease in NO when patients were stable in comparison with an exacerbation, albeit without a change in lung function (FEV$_1$). Recently, other researchers showed the usefulness of NO for the determination of disease severity by measuring the exhaled NO at different flows, thus distinguishing airway-derived NO, which is flow independent, from peripheral NO, derived from the alveoli.[145–147] The latter was related to disease severity and appears to be independent of smoking behavior.

Carbon Monoxide

CO can also be used as a biomarker in asthma and CF.[148–150] Its use has been demonstrated in pediatric asthma and CF, and this marker is even more increased during exacerbations. In formerly smoking COPD patients, higher levels of CO were found compared with nonsmoking controls.[139,151,152] CO was also elevated in smokers,[138,150] and environmental CO and CO from passive smoking complicate the use of CO as a reliable monitor for COPD.

Paredi and colleagues found that CO levels were higher in COPD patients compared with healthy controls; however, treatment of the patients with inhaled steroids appeared to have no effect on CO levels.[153]

Volatile Organic Compounds

An article by Paredi and colleagues describes the use of exhaled ethane as a marker of disease and as a marker of treatment effect.[153] When ethane levels in 22 ex-smoking COPD patients were compared with the levels in 14 non-smoking controls, the ethane levels in COPD patients were significantly higher. Treatment with steroids results in a significant lowering of the ethane levels compared with steroid-naive patients. An inverse correlation between ethane and FEV_1 was established in the nontreated patients.

Exhaled breath contains hundreds of VOCs per sample. Thousands of different compounds can be detected when breath samples are analyzed. This means that breath represents a high number of potential biomarkers, and a combination of several exhaled components may be used for high selectivity and specificity for various diseases.

From recent articles by Phillips and colleagues,[154,155] it is clear that measuring VOCs in exhaled breath followed by "fuzzy logic" data analysis can be used to classify patients and controls. Once a small number of components has been selected, a "leave one out" method can be applied to classify all subjects, based on the model built with all but that one subject's VOC profile. For tuberculosis, this leads to 96% sensitivity and 79% specificity[154]; for lung cancer, these figures are 80.5% and 81%, respectively.[155] Of course, these figures should be interpreted with great care. Similar studies on COPD and VOC have not yet been reported.

An interesting study involving the measurement of various VOC was published by Poli and colleagues.[156] In this study, a preselection of 13 biologically relevant VOCs is used to classify four different groups of subjects: healthy smokers, healthy nonsmokers, patients with non–small cell lung cancer, and COPD patients. Although the article is directed at distinguishing the cancer patients from the other three groups, data analysis (multinominal logistic regression analysis) reveals

that the COPD patients can be differentiated from the controls. However, the number of subjects in this study was rather small. In this study, 19 of 23 COPD patients were classified correctly (83%); 2 of 35 subjects from the group of smokers were classified as having COPD.

Conclusions

Although a multitude of studies have investigated various biomarkers in COPD, for the most part, these studies have been small and cross-sectional. Relatively little information has been published on the reproducibility, comparability, and reliability of biomarkers for COPD. Overall, specific biomarkers have been used to provide mechanistic insights. In this way, biomarkers have bolstered our understanding of the disease process. The transition from research to everyday clinical application requires replication in multiple settings, experimental evidence supporting a pathophysiologic role, and, ideally, intervention trials that demonstrate that alteration of the biomarker signal is associated with improved outcome.[2]

References

1. Colburn WA. Biomarkers in drug discovery and development: from target identification through drug marketing. J Clin Pharmacol 2003;43:329–41.
2. Manolio T. Novel risk markers and clinical practice. N Engl J Med 2003;349;17:1587–89.
3. Jones PW, Agusti AG. Outcomes and markers in the assessment of chronic obstructive pulmonary disease. Eur Respir J 2006;27:822–32.
4. Franciosi LG, Page CP, Celli BR, et al. Markers of disease severity in chronic obstructive pulmonary disease. Pulm Pharmacol Ther 2006;19:189–99.
5. Maestrelli P, Saetta M, Di Stefano A, et al. Comparison of leukocyte counts in sputum, bronchial biopsies, and bronchoalveolar lavage. Am J Respir Crit Care Med 1995;152(6 Pt 1):1926–31.
6. Rutgers SR, Timens W, Kaufmann HF, et al. Comparison of induced sputum with bronchial wash, bronchoalveolar lavage and bronchial biopsies in COPD. Eur Respir J 2000;15:109–15.
7. Kelly CA, Kotre CJ, Ward C, et al. Anatomical distribution of bronchoalveolar lavage fluid as assessed by digital subtraction radiography. Thorax 1987;42:624–8.
8. Belda J, Hussack P, Dolovich M, et al. Sputum induction: effect of nebulizer output and inhalation time on cell counts and fluid-phase measures. Clin Exp Allergy 2001;31:1740–4.
9. Effros RM, Peterson B, Casaburi R, et al. Epithelial lining fluid solute concentrations in chronic obstructive lung disease patients and normal subjects. J Appl Physiol 2005;99:1286–92.
10. Fabbri LM, Romagnoli M, Corbetta L, et al. Differences in airway inflammation in patients with fixed airflow obstruction due to asthma or chronic obstructive pulmonary disease. Am J Respir Crit Care Med 2003;167:418–24.
11. Keatings VM, Collins PD, Scott DM, Barnes PJ. Differences in interleukin-8 and tumor necrosis factor-alpha in induced sputum from patients with chronic obstructive pulmonary

disease or asthma. Am J Respir Crit Care Med 1996;153:530–4.

12. Louis RE, Cataldo D, Buckley MG, et al. Evidence of mast-cell activation in a subset of patients with eosinophilic chronic obstructive pulmonary disease. Eur Respir J 2002;20:325–31.

13. Tsoumakidou M, Tzanakis N, Kyriakou D, et al. Inflammatory cell profiles and T-lymphocyte subsets in chronic obstructive pulmonary disease and severe persistent asthma. Clin Exp Allergy 2004;34:234–40.

14. Tzanakis N, Chrysofakis G, Tsoumakidou M, et al. Induced sputum CD8+ T-lymphocyte subpopulations in chronic obstructive pulmonary disease. Respir Med 2004;98:57–65.

15. Balzano G, Stefanelli F, Iorio C, et al. Eosinophilic inflammation in stable chronic obstructive pulmonary disease. Relationship with neutrophils and airway function. Am J Respir Crit Care Med 1999;160(5 Pt 1):1486–92.

16. Fujimoto K, Yasuo M, Urushibata K, et al. Airway inflammation during stable and acutely exacerbated chronic obstructive pulmonary disease. Eur Respir J 2005;25:640–6.

17. Leigh R, Pizzichini MM, Morris MM, et al. Stable COPD: predicting benefit from high-dose inhaled corticosteroid treatment. Eur Respir J 2006;27:964–71.

18. Papi A, Bellettato CM, Braccioni F, et al. Infections and airway inflammation in chronic obstructive pulmonary disease severe exacerbations. Am J Respir Crit Care Med 2006;173:1114–21.

19. Saetta M, Di SA, Maestrelli P, et al. Airway eosinophilia in chronic bronchitis during exacerbations. Am J Respir Crit Care Med 1994;150(6 Pt 1):1646–52.

20. Siva R, Green RH, Brightling CE, et al. Eosinophilic airway inflammation and exacerbations of COPD: a randomised controlled trial. Eur Respir J 2007;29:906–13.

21. Zhu J, Qiu YS, Majumdar S, et al. Exacerbations of bronchitis: bronchial eosinophilia and gene expression for interleukin-4, interleukin-5, and eosinophil chemoattractants. Am J Respir Crit Care Med 2001;164:109–16.

22. Keatings VM, Barnes PJ. Granulocyte activation markers in induced sputum: comparison between chronic obstructive pulmonary disease, asthma, and normal subjects. Am J Respir Crit Care Med 1997;155:449–53.

23. Yamamoto C, Yoneda T, Yoshikawa M, et al. Airway inflammation in COPD assessed by sputum levels of interleukin-8. Chest 1997;112:505–10.

24. Xiao W, Hsu YP, Ishizaka A, et al. Sputum cathelicidin, urokinase plasminogen activation system components, and cytokines discriminate cystic fibrosis, COPD, and asthma inflammation. Chest 2005;128:2316–26.

25. Drost EM, Skwarski KM, Sauleda J, et al. Oxidative stress and airway inflammation in severe exacerbations of COPD. Thorax 2005;60:293–300.

26. Profita M, Chiappara G, Mirabella F, et al. Effect of cilomilast (Ariflo) on TNF-alpha, IL–8, and GM-CSF release by airway cells of patients with COPD. Thorax 2003;58:573–9.

27. Willemse BW, ten Hacken NH, Rutgers B, et al. Association of current smoking with airway inflammation in chronic obstructive pulmonary disease and asymptomatic smokers. Respir Res 2005;6:38.

28. Calikoglu M, Unlu A, Tamer L, Ozgur E. [MMP-9 and TIMP-1 levels in the sputum of patients with chronic obstructive pulmonary disease and asthma]. Tuberk Toraks 2006;54:114–21.

29. Culpitt SV, Rogers DF, Traves SL, et al. Sputum matrix metalloproteases: comparison between chronic obstructive pulmonary disease and asthma. Respir Med 2005;99:703–10.

30. Plymoth A, Lofdahl CG, Ekberg-Jansson A, et al. Protein expression patterns associated with progression of chronic obstructive pulmonary disease in bronchoalveolar lavage of smokers. Clin Chem 2007;53:636–44.

31. Kostikas K, Papatheodorou G, Ganas K, et al. pH in expired breath condensate of patients with inflammatory airway diseases. Am J Respir Crit Care Med 2002;165:1364–70.

32. Caramori G, Romagnoli M, Casolari P, et al. Nuclear localisation of p65 in sputum macrophages but not in sputum neutrophils during COPD exacerbations. Thorax 2003;58:348–51.

33. Hodge SJ, Hodge GL, Holmes M, Reynolds PN. Flow cytometric characterization of cell populations in bronchoalveolar lavage and bronchial brushings from patients with chronic obstructive pulmonary disease. Cytometry B Clin Cytom 2004;61:27–34.

34. Lusuardi M, Capelli A, Cerutti CG, et al. Airways inflammation in subjects with chronic bronchitis who have never smoked. Thorax 1994;49:1211–6.

35. Peleman RA, Rytila PH, Kips JC, et al. The cellular composition of induced sputum in chronic obstructive pulmonary disease. Eur Respir J 1999;13:839–43.

36. Pesci A, Balbi B, Majori M, et al. Inflammatory cells and mediators in bronchial lavage of patients with chronic obstructive pulmonary disease. Eur Respir J 1998;12:380–6.

37. Pesci A, Majori M, Cuomo A, et al. Neutrophils infiltrating bronchial epithelium in chronic obstructive pulmonary disease. Respir Med 1998;92:863–70.

38. Riise GC, Ahlstedt S, Larsson S, et al. Bronchial inflammation in chronic bronchitis assessed by measurement of cell products in bronchial lavage fluid. Thorax 1995;50:360–5.

39. Stanescu D, Sanna A, Veriter C, et al. Airways obstruction, chronic expectoration, and rapid decline of FEV1 in smokers are associated with increased levels of sputum neutrophils. Thorax 1996;51:267–71.

40. Lofdahl JM, Wahlstrom J, Skold CM. Different inflammatory cell pattern and macrophage phenotype in chronic obstructive pulmonary disease patients, smokers and non-smokers. Clin Exp Immunol 2006;145:428–37.

41. Domagala-Kulawik J, Maskey-Warzechowska M, Hermanowicz-Salamon J, Chazan R. Expression of macrophage surface markers in induced sputum of patients with chronic obstructive pulmonary disease. J Physiol Pharmacol 2006;57 Suppl 4:75–84.

42. Molet S, Belleguic C, Lena H, et al. Increase in macrophage elastase (MMP-12) in lungs from patients with chronic obstructive pulmonary disease. Inflamm Res 2005;54:31–6.

43. Russell RE, Thorley A, Culpitt SV, et al. Alveolar macrophage-mediated elastolysis: roles of matrix metalloproteinases, cysteine, and serine proteases. Am J Physiol Lung Cell Mol Physiol 2002;283:L867–73.

44. Song W, Zhao J, Li Z. Interleukin-6 in bronchoalveolar lavage fluid from patients with COPD. Chin Med J (Engl) 2001;114:1140–2.

45. Russell RE, Culpitt SV, DeMatos C, et al. Release and activity of matrix metalloproteinase-9 and tissue inhibitor of metallo-proteinase-1 by alveolar macrophages from patients with chronic obstructive pulmonary disease. Am J Respir Cell Mol Biol 2002;26:602–9.

46. Pons AR, Sauleda J, Noguera A, et al. Decreased macrophage release of TGF-beta and TIMP-1 in chronic obstructive pulmonary disease. Eur Respir J 2005;26:60–6.

47. Smyth LJ, Starkey C, Vestbo J, Singh D. CD4 regulatory cells in COPD patients. Chest 2007;132:156–63.

48. Tsoumakidou M, Tzanakis N, Chrysofakis G, et al. Changes in sputum T-lymphocyte subpopulations at the onset of severe exacerbations of chronic obstructive pulmonary disease. Respir Med 2005;99:572–9.

49. Costabel U, Maier K, Teschler H, Wang YM. Local immune components in chronic obstructive pulmonary disease. Respiration 1992;59 Suppl 1:17–9.

50. Vernooy JH, Kucukaycan M, Jacobs JA, et al. Local and systemic inflammation in patients with chronic obstructive pulmonary disease: soluble tumor necrosis factor receptors are increased in sputum. Am J Respir Crit Care Med 2002;166:1218–24.

51. Schulz C, Wolf K, Harth M, et al. Expression and release of interleukin-8 by human bronchial epithelial cells from patients with chronic obstructive pulmonary disease, smokers, and never-smokers. Respiration 2003;70:254–61.

52. Dekhuijzen PN, Aben KK, Dekker I, et al. Increased exhalation of hydrogen peroxide in patients with stable and unstable chronic obstructive pulmonary disease. Am J Respir Crit Care Med 1996;154(3 Pt 1):813–6.

53. Tanino M, Betsuyaku T, Takeyabu K, et al. Increased levels of interleukin-8 in BAL fluid from smokers susceptible to pulmonary emphysema. Thorax 2002;57:405–11.

54. Rennard SI, Fogarty C, Kelsen S, et al. The safety and efficacy of infliximab in moderate to severe chronic obstructive pulmonary disease. Am J Respir Crit Care Med 2007;175:926–34.

55. van der Vaart H, Koeter GH, Postma DS, et al. First study of infliximab treatment in patients with chronic obstructive pulmonary disease. Am J Respir Crit Care Med 2005;172:465–9.

56. Hogg JC. State of the art. Bronchiolitis in chronic obstructive pulmonary disease. Proc Am Thorac Soc 2006;3:489–93.

57. Capelli A, Di Stefano A, Gnemmi I, et al. Increased MCP-1 and MIP-1beta in bronchoalveolar lavage fluid of chronic bronchitics. Eur Respir J 1999;14:160–5.

58. Beeh KM, Beier J, Koppenhoefer N, Buhl R. Increased glutathione disulfide and nitrosothiols in sputum supernatant of patients with stable COPD. Chest 2004;126:1116–22.

59. Carpagnano GE, Kharitonov SA, Foschino-Barbaro MP, et al. Supplementary oxygen in healthy subjects and those with COPD increases oxidative stress and airway inflammation. Thorax 2004;59:1016–9.

60. Corradi M, Montuschi P, Donnelly LE, et al. Increased nitrosothiols in exhaled breath condensate in inflammatory airway diseases. Am J Respir Crit Care Med 2001;163:854–8.

61. Corradi M, Rubinstein I, Andreoli R, et al. Aldehydes in exhaled breath condensate of patients with chronic obstructive pulmonary disease. Am J Respir Crit Care Med 2003;167:1380–6.

62. Kanazawa H, Shiraishi S, Hirata K, Yoshikawa J. Imbalance between levels of nitrogen oxides and peroxynitrite inhibitory activity in chronic obstructive pulmonary disease. Thorax 2003;58:106–9.

63. Ko FW, Lau CY, Leung TF, et al. Exhaled breath condensate levels of 8-isoprostane, growth related oncogene alpha and monocyte chemoattractant protein-1 in patients with chronic obstructive pulmonary disease. Respir Med 2006;100:630–8.

64. Ichinose M, Sugiura H, Yamagata S, et al. Increase in reactive nitrogen species production in chronic obstructive pulmonary disease airways. Am J Respir Crit Care Med 2000;162(2 Pt 1):701–6.

65. Fujita J, Nelson NL, Daughton DM, et al. Evaluation of elastase and antielastase balance in patients with chronic bronchitis and pulmonary emphysema. Am Rev Respir Dis 1990;142:57–62.

66. Boschetto P, Quintavalle S, Zeni E, et al. Association between markers of emphysema and more severe chronic obstructive pulmonary disease. Thorax 2006;61:1037–42.

67. Culpitt SV, de Matos C, Russell RE, et al. Effect of theophylline on induced sputum inflammatory indices and neutrophil chemotaxis in chronic obstructive pulmonary disease. Am J Respir Crit Care Med 2002;165:1371–6.

68. Demedts IK, Morel-Montero A, Lebecque S, et al. Elevated MMP–12 protein levels in induced sputum from patients with COPD. Thorax 2006;61:196–201.

69. Vernooy JH, Lindeman JH, Jacobs JA, et al. Increased activity of matrix metalloproteinase-8 and matrix metalloproteinase-9 in induced sputum from patients with COPD. Chest 2004;126:1802–10.

70. Dentener MA, Vernooy JH, Hendriks S, Wouters EF. Enhanced levels of hyaluronan in lungs of patients with COPD: relationship with lung function and local inflammation. Thorax 2005;60:114–9.

71. Broekhuizen R, Vernooy JH, Schols AM, et al. Leptin as local inflammatory marker in COPD. Respir Med 2005;99:70–4.

72. Paredi P, Caramori G, Cramer D, et al. Slower rise of exhaled breath temperature in chronic obstructive pulmonary disease. Eur Respir J 2003;21:439–43.

73. Standards for the diagnosis and care of patients with chronic obstructive pulmonary disease. American Thoracic Society. Am J Respir Crit Care Med 1995;152(5 Pt 2):S77–121.

74. Snoeck-Stroband JB, Postma DS, Lapperre TS, et al. Airway inflammation contributes to health status in COPD: a cross-sectional study. Respir Res 2006;7:140.

75. Kanazawa H, Yoshikawa J. Elevated oxidative stress and reciprocal reduction of vascular endothelial growth factor levels with severity of COPD. Chest 2005;128:3191–7.

76. Filley GF, Beckwitt HJ, Reeves JT, Mitchell RS. Chronic obstructive bronchopulmonary disease. II. Oxygen transport in two clinical types. Am J Med 1968;44:26–38.

77. Vignola AM, Paganin F, Capieu L, et al. Airway remodelling assessed by sputum and high-resolution computed tomography in asthma and COPD. Eur Respir J 2004;24:910–7.

78. Yoshioka A, Betsuyaku T, Nishimura M, et al. Excessive neutrophil elastase in bronchoalveolar lavage fluid in subclinical emphysema. Am J Respir Crit Care Med 1995;152 (6 Pt 1):2127–32.

79. Ekberg-Jansson A, Andersson B, Bake B, et al. Neutrophil-associated activation markers in healthy smokers relates to a fall in DL(CO) and to emphysematous changes on high resolution CT. Respir Med 2001;95:363–73.

80. Kanazawa H, Asai K, Hirata K, Yoshikawa J. Possible effects of vascular endothelial growth factor in the pathogenesis of chronic obstructive pulmonary disease. Am J Med 2003;114:354–8.

81. Kanazawa H, Asai K, Nomura S. Vascular endothelial growth factor as a non-invasive marker of pulmonary vascular remodeling in patients with bronchitis-type of COPD. Respir Res 2007;8:22.

82. Lapperre TS, Willems LN, Timens W, et al. Small airways dysfunction and neutrophilic inflammation in bronchial biopsies and BAL in COPD. Chest 2007;131:53–9.

83. Rutgers SR, Timens W, Tzanakis N, et al. Airway inflammation and hyperresponsiveness to adenosine 5′-monophosphate in chronic obstructive pulmonary disease. Clin Exp Allergy 2000;30:657–62.

84. Papi A, Romagnoli M, Baraldo S, et al. Partial reversibility of airflow limitation and increased exhaled NO and sputum eosinophilia in chronic obstructive pulmonary disease. Am J Respir Crit Care Med 2000;162:1773–7.

85. Rohde G, Gevaert P, Holtappels G, et al. Soluble interleukin-5 receptor alpha is increased in acute exacerbation of chronic obstructive pulmonary disease. Int Arch Allergy Immunol 2004;135:54–61.

86. Bhowmik A, Seemungal TA, Sapsford RJ, Wedzicha JA. Relation of sputum inflammatory markers to symptoms and lung function changes in COPD exacerbations. Thorax 2000;55:114–20.

87. Aaron SD, Angel JB, Lunau M, et al. Granulocyte inflammatory markers and airway infection during acute exacerbation of chronic obstructive pulmonary disease. Am J Respir Crit Care Med 2001;163:349–55.

88. Powrie DJ, Wilkinson TM, Donaldson GC, et al. Effect of tiotropium on sputum and serum inflammatory markers and exacerbations in chronic obstructive pulmonary disease. Eur Respir J 2007;30:472–8.

89. Biernacki WA, Kharitonov SA, Barnes PJ. Increased leukotriene B4 and 8-isoprostane in exhaled breath condensate of patients with exacerbations of COPD. Thorax 2003;58:294–8.

90. Gessner C, Scheibe R, Wotzel M, et al. Exhaled breath condensate cytokine patterns in chronic obstructive pulmonary disease. Respir Med 2005;99:1229–40.

91. Agusti AG, Noguera A, Sauleda J, et al. Systemic effects of chronic obstructive pulmonary disease. Eur Respir J 2003;21:347–60.

92. Gan WQ, Man SF, Senthilselvan A, Sin DD. Association between chronic obstructive pulmonary disease and systemic inflammation: a systematic review and a meta-analysis. Thorax 2004;59:574–80.

93. Broekhuizen R, Wouters EF, Creutzberg EC, Schols AM. Raised CRP levels mark metabolic and functional impairment in advanced COPD. Thorax 2006;61:17–22.

94. de Torres JP, Cordoba-Lanus E, Lopez-Aguilar C, et al. C-reactive protein levels and clinically important predictive outcomes in stable COPD patients. Eur Respir J 2006;27:902–7.

95. Man SF, Connett JE, Anthonisen NR, et al. C-reactive protein and mortality in mild to moderate chronic obstructive pulmonary disease. Thorax 2006;61:849–53.

96. Pinto-Plata VM, Mullerova H, Toso JF, et al. C-reactive protein in patients with COPD, control smokers and non-smokers. Thorax 2006;61:23–8.

97. Yende S, Waterer GW, Tolley EA, et al. Inflammatory markers are associated with ventilatory limitation and muscle dysfunction in obstructive lung disease in well functioning elderly subjects. Thorax 2006;61:10–6.

98. Cardoso WV, Sekhon HS, Hyde DM, Thurlbeck WM. Collagen and elastin in human pulmonary emphysema. Am Rev Respir Dis 1993;147:975–81.

99. Cocci F, Miniati M, Monti S, et al. Urinary desmosine excretion is inversely correlated with the extent of emphysema in patients with chronic obstructive pulmonary disease. Int J Biochem Cell Biol 2002;34:594–604.

100. Ma S, Lin YY, Turino GM. Measurements of desmosine and isodesmosine by mass spectrometry in COPD. Chest 2007;131:1363–71.

101. Schriver EE, Davidson JM, Sutcliffe MC, et al. Comparison of elastin peptide concentrations in body fluids from healthy volunteers, smokers, and patients with chronic obstructive pulmonary disease. Am Rev Respir Dis 1992;145(4 Pt 1):762–6.

102. Stone PJ, Gottlieb DJ, O'Connor GT, et al. Elastin and collagen degradation products in urine of smokers with and without chronic obstructive pulmonary disease. Am J Respir Crit Care Med 1995;151:952–9.

103. Viglio S, Iadarola P, Lupi A, et al. MEKC of desmosine and isodesmosine in urine of chronic destructive lung disease patients. Eur Respir J 2000;15:1039–45.

104. Pinto-Plata V, Toso J, Lee K, et al. Profiling serum biomarkers in patients with COPD: associations with clinical parameters. Thorax 2007;62:595–601.

105. Pitsiou G, Kyriazis G, Hatzizisi O, et al. Tumor necrosis factor-alpha serum levels, weight loss and tissue oxygenation in chronic obstructive pulmonary disease. Respir Med 2002;96:594–8.

106. Di Francia M, Barbier D, Mege JL, Orehek J. Tumor necrosis factor-alpha levels and weight loss in chronic obstructive pulmonary disease. Am J Respir Crit Care Med 1994;150 (5 Pt 1):1453–5.

107. Takabatake N, Nakamura H, Abe S, et al. The relationship between chronic hypoxemia and activation of the tumor necrosis factor-alpha system in patients with chronic obstructive pulmonary disease. Am J Respir Crit Care Med 2000;161(4 Pt 1):1179–84.

108. Schols AM, Buurman WA, Staal van den Brekel AJ, et al. Evidence for a relation between metabolic derangements and increased levels of inflammatory mediators in a subgroup of patients with chronic obstructive pulmonary disease. Thorax 1996;51:819–24.

109. Broekhuizen R, Grimble RF, Howell WM, et al. Pulmonary cachexia, systemic inflammatory profile, and the interleukin 1beta -511 single nucleotide polymorphism. Am J Clin Nutr 2005;82:1059–64.

110. Itoh T, Nagaya N, Yoshikawa M, et al. Elevated plasma ghrelin level in underweight patients with chronic obstructive pulmonary disease. Am J Respir Crit Care Med 2004;170:879–82.

111. Joppa P, Petrasova D, Stancak B, Tkacova R. Systemic inflammation in patients with COPD and pulmonary hypertension. Chest 2006;130:326–33.

112. Dahl M, Vestbo J, Lange P, et al. C-reactive protein as a predictor of prognosis in chronic obstructive pulmonary disease. Am J Respir Crit Care Med 2007;175:250–5.

113. Dentener MA, Creutzberg EC, Schols AM, et al. Systemic anti-inflammatory mediators in COPD: increase in soluble interleukin 1 receptor II during treatment of exacerbations. Thorax 2001;56:721–6.

114. Donaldson GC, Seemungal TA, Patel IS, et al. Airway and systemic inflammation and decline in lung function in patients with COPD. Chest 2005;128:1995–2004.

115. Hurst JR, Donaldson GC, Perera WR, et al. Use of plasma biomarkers at exacerbation of chronic obstructive pulmonary disease. Am J Respir Crit Care Med 2006;174:867–74.

116. Perera WR, Hurst JR, Wilkinson TM, et al. Inflammatory changes, recovery and recurrence at COPD exacerbation. Eur Respir J 2007;29:527–34.

117. Pinto-Plata VM, Livnat G, Girish M, et al. Systemic cytokines, clinical and physiological changes in patients hospitalized for exacerbation of COPD. Chest 2007;131:37–43.

118. Stolz D, Christ-Crain M, Bingisser R, et al. Antibiotic treatment of exacerbations of COPD: a randomized, controlled trial comparing procalcitonin-guidance with standard therapy. Chest 2007;131:9–19.

119. Stolz D, Christ-Crain M, Morgenthaler NG, et al. Copeptin, C-reactive protein, and procalcitonin as prognostic biomarkers in acute exacerbation of COPD. Chest 2007;131:1058–67.

120. Tkacova R, Kluchova Z, Joppa P, et al. Systemic inflammation and systemic oxidative stress in patients with acute exacerbations of COPD. Respir Med 2007;101:1670–6.

121. Wedzicha JA, Seemungal TA, MacCallum PK, et al. Acute exacerbations of chronic obstructive pulmonary disease are accompanied by elevations of plasma fibrinogen and serum IL-6 levels. Thromb Haemost 2000;84:210–5.

122. Christ-Crain M, Jaccard-Stolz D, Bingisser R, et al. Effect of procalcitonin-guided treatment on antibiotic use and outcome in lower respiratory tract infections: cluster-randomised, single-blinded intervention trial. Lancet 2004;363:600–7.

123. Balbi B, Majori M, Bertacco S, et al. Inhaled corticosteroids in stable COPD patients: do they have effects on cells and molecular mediators of airway inflammation? Chest 2000;117:1633–7.

124. Confalonieri M, Mainardi E, Della PR, et al. Inhaled corticosteroids reduce neutrophilic bronchial inflammation in patients with chronic obstructive pulmonary disease. Thorax 1998;53:583–5.

125. Ozol D, Aysan T, Solak ZA, et al. The effect of inhaled corticosteroids on bronchoalveolar lavage cells and IL-8 levels in stable COPD patients. Respir Med 2005;99:1494–500.

126. Barczyk A, Sozanska E, Trzaska M, Pierzchala W. Decreased levels of myeloperoxidase in induced sputum of patients with COPD after treatment with oral glucocorticoids. Chest 2004;126:389–93.

127. Brightling CE, Monteiro W, Ward R, et al. Sputum eosinophilia and short-term response to prednisolone in chronic obstructive pulmonary disease: a randomised controlled trial. Lancet 2000;356:1480–5.

128. Brightling CE, McKenna S, Hargadon B, et al. Sputum eosinophilia and the short term response to inhaled mometasone in chronic obstructive pulmonary disease. Thorax 2005;60:193–8.

129. Barnes NC, Qiu YS, Pavord ID, et al. Antiinflammatory effects of salmeterol/fluticasone propionate in chronic obstructive lung disease. Am J Respir Crit Care Med 2006;173:736–43.

130. Sin DD, Lacy P, York E, Man SF. Effects of fluticasone on systemic markers of inflammation in chronic obstructive pulmonary disease. Am J Respir Crit Care Med 2004;170:760–5.

131. Calverley PM, Anderson JA, Celli B, et al. Salmeterol and fluticasone propionate and survival in chronic obstructive pulmonary disease. N Engl J Med 2007;356:775–9.

132. Yildirim E, Yildiz F, Kacar OS, et al. Effects of different combined bronchodilator therapies on airway inflammation in COPD. Clin Drug Investig 2005;25:453–61.

133. Massaro GD, Massaro D. Retinoic acid treatment abrogates elastase-induced pulmonary emphysema in rats. Nat Med 1997;3:675–7.

134. Mao JT, Goldin JG, Dermand J, et al. A pilot study of all-trans-retinoic acid for the treatment of human emphysema. Am J Respir Crit Care Med 2002;165:718–23.

135. Mao JT, Tashkin DP, Belloni PN, et al. All-trans retinoic acid modulates the balance of matrix metalloproteinase-9 and tissue inhibitor of metalloproteinase-1 in patients with emphysema. Chest 2003;124:1724–32.

136. Roth MD, Connett JE, D'Armiento JM, et al. Feasibility of retinoids for the treatment of emphysema study. Chest 2006;130:1334–45.

137. Olin AC, Andelid K, Vikgren J, et al. Single breath N2-test and exhaled nitric oxide in men. Respir Med 2006;100:1013–9.

138. Tzortzaki EG, Tsoumakidou M, Makris D, Siafakas NM. Laboratory markers for COPD in "susceptible" smokers. Clin Chim Acta 2006;364:124–38.

139. Montuschi P, Kharitonov SA, Barnes PJ. Exhaled carbon monoxide and nitric oxide in COPD. Chest 2001;120:496–501.

140. Ansarin K, Chatkin JM, Ferreira IM, et al. Exhaled nitric oxide in chronic obstructive pulmonary disease: relationship to pulmonary function. Eur Respir J 2001;17:934–8.

141. Maziak W, Loukides S, Culpitt S, et al. Exhaled nitric oxide in chronic obstructive pulmonary disease. Am J Respir Crit Care Med 1998;157(3 Pt 1):998–1002.

142. Corradi M, Majori M, Cacciani GC, et al. Increased exhaled nitric oxide in patients with stable chronic obstructive pulmonary disease. Thorax 1999;54:572–5.

143. Bhowmik A, Seemungal TA, Donaldson GC, Wedzicha JA. Effects of exacerbations and seasonality on exhaled nitric oxide in COPD. Eur Respir J 2005;26:1009–15.

144. Zietkowski Z, Kucharewicz I, Bodzenta-Lukaszyk A. The influence of inhaled corticosteroids on exhaled nitric oxide in stable chronic obstructive pulmonary disease. Respir Med 2005;99:816–24.

145. Barnes PJ, Chowdhury B, Kharitonov SA, et al. Pulmonary biomarkers in chronic obstructive pulmonary disease. Am J Respir Crit Care Med 2006;174:6–14.

146. Brindicci C, Ito K, Resta O, et al. Exhaled nitric oxide from lung periphery is increased in COPD. Eur Respir J 2005;26:52–9.

147. Kharitonov SA, Barnes PJ. Exhaled biomarkers. Chest 2006;130:1541–6.

148. Paredi P, Kharitonov SA, Barnes PJ. Analysis of expired air for oxidation products. Am J Respir Crit Care Med 2002;166 (12 Pt 2):S31–7.

149. Paredi P, Kharitonov SA, Barnes PJ. Exhaled carbon monoxide in lung disease. Eur Respir J 2003;21:197.

150. Kharitonov SA, Barnes PJ. Exhaled markers of inflammation. Curr Opin Allergy Clin Immunol 2001;1:217–24.

151. Yasuda H, Yamaya M, Nakayama K, et al. Increased arterial carboxyhemoglobin concentrations in chronic obstructive pulmonary disease. Am J Respir Crit Care Med 2005;171:1246–51.

152. Kharitonov SA, Barnes PJ. Biomarkers of some pulmonary diseases in exhaled breath. Biomarkers 2002;7:1–32.

153. Paredi P, Kharitonov SA, Leak D, et al. Exhaled ethane, a marker of lipid peroxidation, is elevated in chronic obstructive pulmonary disease. Am J Respir Crit Care Med 2000;162(2 Pt 1):369–73.

154. Phillips M, Cataneo RN, Condos R, et al. Volatile biomarkers of pulmonary tuberculosis in the breath. Tuberculosis (Edinb) 2007;87:44–52.

155. Phillips M, Altorki N, Austin JH, et al. Prediction of lung cancer using volatile biomarkers in breath. Cancer Biomark 2007;3:95–109.

156. Poli D, Carbognani P, Corradi M, et al. Exhaled volatile organic compounds in patients with non-small cell lung cancer: cross sectional and nested short-term follow-up study. Respir Res 2005;6:71.

Exacerbation of Chronic Obstructive Pulmonary Disease

Norbert F. Voelkel, MD

Context: To understand the scientific questions and—most importantly—acknowledge the prejudices of the time.

Just as COPD as an entity is heterogenous, so are exacerbations, and despite wide scientific interest in these episodes, there is still much debate regarding how exacerbations should be defined, their etiology and their prognostic significance.[1]

It appears that literally everything about chronic obstructive pulmonary disease (COPD) exacerbations—definition, pathogenesis, prevention and treatment—remains controversial and unclear. The executive summary provided by the Global Initiative for Chronic Obstructive Lung Disease (GOLD) Executive Committee in 2006 uses the following definition: "An exacerbation is defined as an event in the natural course of the disease characterized by a change in the patient's baseline dyspnea, cough, and/or sputum that is beyond the normal day-to-day variations, is acute in onset and may warrant a change in medication in a patient with underlying COPD."[2]

At the present time, there is no single definition—accepted by all stakeholders-of "the COPD exacerbation." Jørgen Vestbo recently collected and compared a number of definition statements and discussed the pros and cons of these attempts to define a COPD exacerbation.[1] Previously, when challenged with the task of defining a COPD exacerbation, young clinicians would resort to stating what it is not: a COPD exacerbation is not pneumonia, not an episode of heart failure, not pulmonary embolism, not a pneumothorax, etc. As we will see, this may not be entirely so.

Intuitively, it is central to all discussions regarding COPD exacerbations that we need to get the definition right; the analysis of outcomes and health care costs depends critically on this definition. If exacerbations are heterogeneous in nature, it follows that the working definitions are different, highlighting various facets of symptom presentation and manifestations of comorbidities.

During the last 5 years, a number of committees analyzed previously used definitions of COPD exacerbation or attempted to improve these definitions. Vestbo discussed the advantages and disadvantages of symptom- or action-driven definitions.[1] Very briefly, symptom-driven definitions can be problematic because patients perceive symptoms very differently, and we know that COPD exacerbations are underreported.[1] On the other hand, action-driven definitions also may be problematic because of regional differences in health care practice and changes in COPD management over time; for example, in some practice settings, patients are hospitalized, but not in others. Opinions on how to define COPD exacerbations still vary widely. For example, as Burge and Wedzicha stated, "there is no generally agreed upon definition for an exacerbation of COPD. It seems reasonable to use a definition that does not imply etiology or severity,"[3] whereas the group spearheaded by Romain Pauwels concluded, after examining 10 different definitions, that "despite efforts to describe COPD exacerbations and their associated symptoms, the continuing lack of a widely accepted and reproducible definition highlights the fact that *attempting to define and re-define exacerbations based on our current level of understanding may not be possible*"[4] (my italics). They further concluded that a "sign" or, better yet, several signs were needed that relate to a biologic mechanism. The reader will conclude for himself or herself the successfulness of striving for one uniformly accepted definition if there are several biologic mechanisms. Without any doubt, an exacerbation definition linked to a "sign" or supported by a biologic mechanism would be desirable.

Returning again to the symptom-driven definitions—as subjective as the perception of symptoms may be—worsening of the patient's condition is where it all starts.[5] But we recognize that exacerbation could be "more disease, a harsher COPD, or something entirely different"[6] and agree that a COPD exacerbation is also a diagnosis of exclusion. Excluded should be the worsening caused by pneumonia or heart failure but perhaps not the worsening caused by pulmonary embolism (see below).

Diagnosis

Despite uncertainties as to how to define COPD exacerbations, the diagnosis is arrived at by being practical. Andersson and colleagues studied the health care costs of COPD exacerbations in 202 patients after sending the patients a letter and asking them to answer the following questions[7]:

Did you:

- Take more medication for respiratory disease?
- Take time off work?
- Make an unplanned visit to a nurse or doctor?
- Visit an emergency care unit, or
- Stay overnight in a hospital?

Haughney and colleagues attempted to assess the attributes of exacerbations considered most important for patients.[8] They interviewed 125 patients using 12 question cards presenting paired scenarios of choices and preferences, for example, "Choose between the two alternatives the one that is the worse for you" and "Which of two descriptions of symptoms, treatment, and duration of illness would be the worst for you?" Using this instrument, the authors found that 20% of the patients considered the most important impact of an exacerbation the impact on everyday life and 16% the need for medical care, and for 11%, the impact was "breathlessness." An exacerbation was "diagnosed" based on "the worsening of respiratory symptoms so as to require medical intervention, that is, oral corticosteroids and/or antibodies and/or hospitalization."[5] Kessler and colleagues, again using trained interviewers, found in the same patient cohort that only 1.6% of the patients understood the term "exacerbation," preferring simpler terms such as "chest infection" (16%) or "crisis" (16%).[9] Approximately two-thirds of these patients recognized when an exacerbation was imminent, but the other third reported no warning signs. Spencer and colleagues examined the time course of recovery from an exacerbation based on a history of chronic bronchitis and presentation with purulent sputum, increased cough, and dyspnea.[10] In an attempt to assess the frequency and severity of exacerbations, Donaldson and colleagues used diary cards from 132 patients to report on the history of COPD exacerbations over 6 years.[11] The patients were asked to record postmedication peak expiratory flow and any increase over their normal, stable condition in dyspnea, sputum purulence or volume, wheezing, sore throat, and cough. In this group of patients, there were, over the 6-year period, 1,111 exacerbations, of which 81% were identified from the symptom data recorded on the diary cards. A symptom count index for these patients at their baseline was 0.36, which rose to 2.23 at the time of exacerbation onset, yet the peak expiratory flow did *not* decline at exacerbation onset.

Finally, Wouters, in his analysis of data from a large-scale international survey conducted in Canada, France, Italy, the Netherlands, Spain, the United Kingdom, and the United States, used treatment of patients with antibiotics as a possible indicator of an exacerbation in these COPD patients.[12] The use of antibiotics ranged from 38 to 57%, suggesting that exacerbations caused by respiratory infections were frequent events. However, the analysis of the causes of death, using data from the Copenhagen City Heart Study,[13] again illustrates the difficulties in making valid conclusions from death certificate studies because of misclassification. Jensen and colleagues concluded that COPD was both underreported and overreported on death certificates, making it difficult to decide how many patients died from COPD exacerbations.[13]

Mortality from COPD Exacerbations

It is apparent that understanding the pathogenesis of COPD exacerbations is central to the issues of the definition, diagnosis, and treatment of this condition. A greater investment in exacerbation research is still required. This investment is easily justified since exacerbations precede emergency department visits, hospitalizations, and death. A recent study from the Massachusetts General Hospital in Boston followed patients for 3 years after emergency department visits for COPD exacerbations.[14] At the end of the follow-up period, 46% of the patients had died, and the mortality was related to older age, comorbid conditions, and previous COPD exacerbations. A cross-sectional study of the 1996 Nationwide Inpatient Sample identified patients by *International Classification of Diseases* codes and excluded patients younger than 40 years of age.[15] Data from more than 70,000 patients were analyzed. The in-hospital mortality was 3%, but 30% of the intubated patients died. In contrast, a prospective Dutch study of 171 patients reported an in-hospital mortality of 8% after 1 year of follow-up, but 23% of these patients had died as outpatients.[16] Risk factors associated with higher mortality were oral use of corticosteroids, higher partial pressure of carbon dioxide in arterial blood, and older age. It has also been reported that the mortality increases with the frequency of severe exacerbations.[17,18]

Pathogenesis of COPD Exacerbations

A simple (but perhaps not too simple) way of categorizing exacerbations is depicted in Figure 1.

Infectious Exacerbations

Among the three components that can cause or contribute to exacerbations—infections, cardiovascular events, and systemic inflammation—the infectious etiology is supported by a large amount of data.[19–24] Both a flare-up of an existing chronic infection and a new acute infection need to be considered factors that can worsen lung inflammation. In COPD patients who are smokers and have chronic bronchitis, exacerbations occur more frequently than in patients without chronic bronchitis,[25] and uncleared mucus may provide a biofilm that provides the milieu for persistent bacterial growth.[26] The topic of airway bacterial colonization and antibiotic resistance of pathogens is discussed in Chapter 14. White and colleagues recently reviewed the pros and cons of

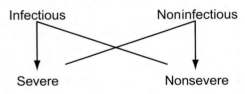

COPD Exacerbations

FIGURE 1. Exacerbations can be infectious or noninfectious. There is also the possibility that, in some patients, infectious and noninfectious causes are combined. COPD = chronic obstructive pulmonary disease.

bacteria playing an important role in COPD exacerbations of bronchitic patients.[27] Although the same bacteria are often found during the stable state and during exacerbations, the bacterial load increases in some patients during exacerbations.[21] The emergence of new bacterial strains during exacerbations has also been recently reported,[28,29] but whether "exacerbation strains" are indeed common is presently debated.[30,31] Certainly, the "worsening," whether or not caused by bacterial infections, is in daily medical practice treated with antibodies. The patient's improvement after a course of antibodies is then frequently used as evidence to argue that the worsening had indeed been caused by a bacterial infection. However, some controlled therapy trials show little or no benefit,[32] although antibiotic treatment of patients with purulent sputum showed a clinical improvement.[33] Lastly, Miravitlles proposed a "fall and rise" of bacterial load hypothesis of acute COPD exacerbations.[21]

Role of Viral Infections

Although viral infections can explain many of the worsening aspects of patients' conditions, such as mucus hypersecretion, increased bronchoconstriction, and eosinophilia, and can predispose individuals to bacterial infections, direct viral culture evidence is required for the diagnosis. Based on nasal, throat, and sputum culture results, on average, only a small number of COPD exacerbations are temporarily associated with positive viral culture results. Serologic studies have suggested that viral infections are the likely cause of 20% of COPD exacerbations.[23,24] Influenza, rhinovirus, and respiratory syncytial virus are being isolated at varying frequencies at the time of hospital admission (see Chapter 15).

Noninfectious Exacerbation

Two European studies reported pulmonary vascular thrombotic or embolic lesions in COPD patients. Russo and colleagues examined 25 COPD patients and 27 patients with left-sided heart disease with transesophageal echocardiography and found that 12 COPD patients, none of whom had the diagnosis of previous pulmonary embolism, showed central pulmonary arterial lesions, and many of these patients had evidence of pulmonary hypertension.[34] Only one of the heart failure patients had a pulmonary embolic event. The authors hypothesized that disordered coagulation and endothelial cell dysfunction might contribute to in situ thrombosis. Whereas this echocardiographic study was performed in clinically stable patients, a recent spiral chest computed tomographic study focused on COPD patients who had an exacerbation of "unknown origin."[35] Severe exacerbations in these patients were defined as "acute deterioration from a stable condition that required hospitalization."[5] Over 45 months at a single institution, 197 COPD patients were evaluated, and 25% of these patients had evidence of pulmonary embolism; of note, none of these patients had been treated with mechanical ventilation, and the exacerbations occurred without a history of a cold and without purulent sputum, yet the patients with

pulmonary embolism were more frequently hypoxemic.[35] This study is awaiting confirmation by a multicenter study and, if confirmed, would lend support to the concept depicted in Figure 1, that is, there are infectious and noninfectious exacerbations. Another facet of the noninfectious exacerbations was recently highlighted by Abroug and colleagues.[36] These authors measured troponin and amino-terminal pro—brain natriuretic peptide (NT-pro-BNP) in 148 consecutive patients admitted to the intensive care unit with the diagnosis of acute COPD exacerbation; patients with pneumonia, pneumothorax, or pulmonary embolism had been excluded from the study. The median age of these patients was 68 years, and 83% of the patients had a smoking history. In these patients admitted to the intensive care unit, 30% had previously not diagnosed echocardiographic evidence of left heart dysfunction. Troponin and NT-pro-BNP level were elevated in these patients who had been admitted with cough, dyspnea, and sputum production. Unfortunately, the authors did not attempt to correlate echocardiographic variables with the plasma biomarker levels.

Taken together, these very recent studies—why did it take so long?—send a clear message: COPD is not just an airway disease, and, most certainly, prevention and treatment of "cardiovascular COPD exacerbations" will differ from the prevention and treatment of infectious exacerbations.

Biomarkers

In very broad strokes, biomarkers are derived either from molecules or cells. There are three different kinds of biomarkers, and within the context of COPD exacerbations, we can posit that there are biomarkers that *identify* an exacerbation and distinguish between different kinds of exacerbations, for example, between infectious and noninfectious forms. A different set of biomarkers may *predict the development* of COPD exacerbations, and likely there are biomarkers that have *prognostic* value. They can predict whether a certain form of treatment will be effective (such markers can be based on pharmacogenomic information) or prolong survival.

In COPD, biomarkers have been searched for in plasma, urine, bronchoalveolar lavage, sputum, and bronchial samples.[37–39] A review of more than 600 publications indicates that few of the examined biomarkers of COPD activity or severity have been validated. Hurst and colleagues examined 36 potential biomarkers of acute COPD exacerbations in 90 patients with a mean age of 70 years and a baseline forced expiratory volume in 1 second of 44% predicted.[40] Plasma samples were examined at baseline and at some time during an exacerbation. The selected 36 plasma biomarkers were those that best discriminated patients with COPD from a matched cohort of subjects in a previously unpublished study. Presumably, 90 exacerbations occurred, and C-reactive protein (CRP) rose from a median baseline value of 4 to 15 mg/L and interleukin (IL)-6 from 1.5 to 3.25 pg/mL. Most of the other plasma markers either did not change or increased only by 3 to 20%. The increase in the levels of CRP was perhaps not unexpected given that this group of patients from East London typically develops infectious exacerbations, as reported previously. Most likely, this particular marker lacks specificity. Dev and colleagues measured CRP in 50 patients and found elevated plasma levels in 84% of them at the time of hospital admission for an exacerbation,[41] whereas Weis and Almdal showed that 30% of patients with a COPD exacerbation had normal CRP values.[42] Serum procalcitonin has been used by other groups as a marker of bacterial infections,[43] and Muller and Tamm, in an editorial, pointed out that highly sensitive CRP levels fluctuate wildly and are affected by steroid treatment.[44] Indeed, most of the patients in the study reported by Hurst and colleagues had been treated with inhaled corticosteroids.[40]

Aaron and colleagues examined sputum cytokine levels in 14 patients during a COPD exacerbation and found elevations of tumor necrosis factor α and IL-8.[45] However, regardless of the marker, the variability of the degree of change within a study cohort is large and apparently not connected with the severity of the exacerbation, but airway neutrophilia may be.[20] In conclusion, the ideal sensitive and specific COPD exacerbation biomarkers still remain to be described; this is perhaps not surprising as the presently considered biomarkers relate to infection and inflammation, whereas some exacerbations may not depend on an acute or chronic infection or on systemic inflammation (see above).

Risk Factors

The concept of an "exacerbation phenotype" led to the search for exacerbation risk factors. Again, relatively little information is available to predict which patient is prone to developing exacerbations. There appears to be some consensus that old age, previous exacerbations, severity of lung function impairment, and high levels of CRP may be predictors,[20,40,46,47] whereas the severity of exacerbations is associated with the presence of significant comorbidities. Current smoking and body mass index may not be exacerbation risk factors, but possibly chronic mucus hypersecretion is a risk factor.[47]

Comorbidities

Preliminary evidence suggests that anemia—perhaps anemia of chronic disease—is a frequent finding in elderly COPD patients. Similowski and colleagues searched a database of 2,524 patients on long-term oxygen therapy and found a prevalence of anemia in 12.6% of the men and 8.2% of the women.[48] Anemic patients required more hospitalizations when compared with nonanemic patients. We can perhaps assume that some of these hospitalizations were triggered by COPD exacerbations. Unrecognized heart failure also may be a risk factor for COPD exacerbations if the patient's worsening is contributed to by heart failure symptoms. Rutten and colleagues examined 1,186 patients who were older than 65 years and diagnosed with COPD but not heart failure by their general practitioners.[49] Of this group, 405

patients were investigated and 20% received a new diagnosis of heart failure.

Prevention and Treatment

As we are getting better at phenotyping patients with COPD (see Chapter 24) and expanding our knowledge of the etiologies of the exacerbations, it is hoped that we will arrive at treatment strategies that will prevent most of the exacerbations. Undoubtedly, many studies will be necessary to get to this point, but some of us think we can see light at the tunnel's end. A National Institutes of Health multicenter macrolide antibiotic exacerbations study is currently under way and enrolling patients.[50] The anti-inflammatory properties of the drug, rather than its antibiotic profile, were considered as this prevention trial was designed. Presumably, standard treatments of acute exacerbations do not prevent subsequent exacerbations; in fact, 1 in 27% of patients experienced a relapse after treatment and hospitalization.[51] However, several studies show a moderate reduction in the number of observed exacerbations. The long-acting anticholinergic tiotropium reduces exacerbations by 14% when compared with placebo,[52] and the inhaled corticosteroid fluticasone propionate reduces the exacerbation by 25% per year when compared with placebo. N-Acetylcysteine reduces the risk of rehospitalization for COPD by 80%.[53] A meta-analysis of data from eight randomized trials concluded that the use of N-acetylcysteine significantly reduced the odds of exacerbations in patients with COPD.[54] However, a critical analysis by Suissa cautioned that the statistical treatment of the data and their meta-analysis in recent inhaled corticosteroid trials assessing their effect on exacerbations may have been problematic.[55] Highly variable follow-up times and the lack of weighted analysis may account for the fact that the meta-analysis of some studies suggested a statistically significant treatment effect when the individual studies had reported nonsignificant effects.[55]

The Future

Kardos and colleagues reported a 35% reduction in COPD exacerbations with the addition of inhaled corticosteroids to long-acting bronchodilator therapy.[56] The idea that we will be able to understand COPD and the worsening of it can now be seriously entertained. Treatment targets are infection, inflammation, mucus secretion, immune responses, and endothelial cell dysfunction. Unfortunately, there are no animal models of COPD exacerbations to help with the evaluation of these treatment targets. A study by Wilkinson and colleagues collected daily symptoms and treatments of exacerbation data of 126 patients over a period of 6 years.[57] This interesting study showed that failure to report exacerbations was associated with an increased risk of hospitalizations and that prompt and early treatment improved the recovery after an exacerbation. More than 90% of all exacerbations were treated with antibiotics, and oral prednisolone therapy hastened the recovery by 2.6 days.[57] A different US study reported by

Adams and colleagues found that antibiotic treatment of exacerbations resulted in a reduced relapse rate; however, the choice of antibiotic was important.[58] Perhaps telemonitoring of COPD patients (see Chapter 31) combined with early treatment can be used in the future with the aim of reducing the severity and frequency of exacerbations. Finally, it is perhaps also possible to treat the systemic COPD manifestations and influence the cardiopulmonary comorbidities with agents such as statins and angiotensin-converting enzyme (ACE) inhibitors and reduce exacerbation rates. A retrospective cohort analysis by Mancini and colleagues suggested that statins, ACE inhibitors, and angiotensin receptor blockers reduced not only cardiac events in COPD patients but also COPD hospitalizations and mortality, irrespective of the patients' cardiovascular risk profile.[59] Indeed, a study from Norway supports this idea. Søyseth and colleagues analyzed— again retrospectively—a cohort of 854 patients with a diagnosis of COPD exacerbations and reported that the 118 "statin users," which included a higher number of patients with ischemic heart disease and arterial hypertension, had an improved survival after a COPD exacerbation, regardless of whether the patients had ischemic heart disease.[60]

References

1. Vestbo J. What is an exacerbation of COPD? Eur Respir Rev 2004;13:6–13.
2. Rabe KF, Hurd S, Anzueto A, et al. Global strategy for the diagnosis, management, and prevention of chronic obstructive pulmonary disease: GOLD executive summary. Am J Respir Crit Care Med 2007;176:532–55.
3. Burge S, Wedzicha JA. COPD exacerbations: definitions and classifications. Eur Respir J 2003;21 Suppl 41:46s–53s.
4. Pauwels R, Calverley P, Buist AS, et al. COPD exacerbations: the importance of a standard definition. Respir Med 2004;98:99–107.
5. Rodriguez-Rosin R. Toward a consensus definition for COPD exacerbations. Chest 2000;117:398–401S.
6. Voelkel NF, Tuder R. COPD exacerbation. Chest 2000;117(5 Suppl):376S–9S.
7. Andersson F, Borg S, Jansson SA, et al. The costs of exacerbations in chronic obstructive pulmonary disease (COPD). Respir Med 2002;96:700–8.
8. Haughney J, Partridge MR, Vogelmeier C, et al. Exacerbations of COPD: quantifying the patients perspective using discrete choice modeling. Eur Respir J 2005;26:623–9.
9. Kessler R, Stahl E, Vogelmeier C, et al. Patient understanding, detection and experience of COPD exacerbations: an observational, interview-based study. Chest 2006;130:133–42.
10. Spencer S, Jones PW, and the Globe Study Group. Time course of recovery of health status following an infective exacerbation of chronic bronchitis. Thorax 2003;58:589–93.
11. Donaldson GC, Seemungal TAR, Patel IS, et al. Longitudinal changes in the nature, severity and frequency of COPD exacerbations. Eur Respir J 2003;22:931–6.
12. Wouters EF. Economic analysis of the confronting COPD survey: an overview of results. Respir Med 2003;97 Suppl C:S3–14.
13. Jensen HH, Godtfredsen NS, Lange P, Vestbo J. Potential misclassification of causes of death from COPD. Eur Respir J 2006;28:781–5.
14. Kim S, Clark S, Camargo CA Jr. Mortality after an emergency department visit for exacerbation of chronic obstructive pulmonary disease. J COPD 2006;3:75–81.
15. Patil SP, Krishnan JA, Lechtzin N, et al. In-hospital mortality following acute exacerbations of chronic obstructive pulmonary disease. Arch Intern Med 2003;163:1180–6.
16. Groenewegen KH, Schols AM, Wouters EF. Mortality and mortality-related factors after hospitalization for acute exacerbation of COPD. Chest 2003;124:459–67.
17. Kim S, Emerman CL, Cydulka RK, et al. Prospective multicenter study of relapse following emergency department treatment of COPD exacerbation. Chest 2004;125:473–81.
18. Soler-Cataluna JJ, Martinez-Garcia MA, Roman Sanchez P, et al. Severe acute exacerbations and mortality in patients with chronic obstructive pulmonary disease. Thorax 2006;60:925–31.
19. Hurst JR, Perera WR, Wilkinson TMA, et al. Exacerbation of chronic obstructive pulmonary disease. Proc Am Thorac Soc 2006;3:481–2.
20. Papi A, Bellettato CM, Braccioni F, et al. Infections and airway inflammation in chronic obstructive pulmonary disease severe exacerbations. Eur J Respir Crit Care Med 2006;173:1114–21.
21. Miravitlles M. Exacerbations of chronic obstructive pulmonary disease: when are bacteria important? Eur Respir J 2002;20 Suppl 36:9s–19s.
22. Sapey E, Stockley RA. COPD exacerbations 2: aetiology. Thorax 2006;61:250–8.
23. Greenberg SB, Allen M, Wilson J, et al. Respiratory viral infections in adults with and without chronic obstructive pulmonary disease. Am J Respir Crit Care Med 2000;162:167–73.
24. Beckham JB, Cadena A, Lin J, et al. Respiratory viral infections in patients with chronic obstructive pulmonary disease. J Infect 2005;50:322–30.
25. Konner RE, Anthonisen NR, Connett JE. Lower respiratory illnesses promote FEV_1 decline in current smokers but not ex-smokers with mild chronic obstructive pulmonary disease. Results from the Lung Health Study. Am J Respir Crit Care Med 2001;164:358–64.
26. Gompertz S, O'Brien C, Bayley DL, et al. Changes in bronchial inflammation during acute exacerbations of chronic bronchitis. Eur Respir J 2001;17:1112–9.
27. White AJ, Gompertz S, Stockley RA. Chronic obstructive pulmonary disease 6: the aetiology of exacerbations of chronic obstructive pulmonary disease. Thorax 2005;58:73–80.
28. Murphy TF, Brauer AL, Schiffmacher AT, Sethy S. Persistent colonization by *Haemophilus influenzae* in chronic obstructive pulmonary disease. Am J Respir Crit Care Med 2004;170:266–72.
29. Chin CL, Manzel IJ, Lehman EE, et al. *Haemophilus influenzae* from COPD patients with exacerbation induce more inflammation than colonizers. Am J Respir Crit Care Med 2005;172:85–91.
30. Bresser P, Out TA, Van Alphen L, et al. Airway inflammation in nonobstructive and obstructive chronic bronchitis with chronic *Haemophilus influenzae* airway infection. Comparison

with noninfected patients with chronic obstructive pulmonary disease. Am J Respir Crit Care Med 2000;162:947–52.

31. Hirschmann JV. Do bacteria cause exacerbations of COPD? Chest 2000;118:193–203.

32. Ball P, Harris JM, Lowson D, et al. Acute infective exacerbations of chronic bronchitis. QJM 1995;88:61–8.

33. Stockley RA, O'Brien C, Pye A, et al. Relationship to sputum colour to nature and out-patient management of acute exacerbations of COPD. Chest 2000;117:1638–45.

34. Russo A, De Luca M, Vigna C, et al. Central pulmonary artery lesions in chronic obstructive pulmonary disease: a transesophogeal echocardiography study. Circulation 1999;100:1808–15.

35. Tillie-Leblond I, Marguette CH, Perez T, et al. Pulmonary embolism in patients with unexplained exacerbation of chronic obstructive pulmonary disease: prevalence and risk factors. Ann Intern Med 2006;144:390–6.

36. Abroug F, Ouanes-Besbes L, Nciri N, et al. Association of left-heart dysfunction with severe exacerbation of chronic obstructive pulmonary disease. Diagnostic performance of cardiac biomarkers. Am J Respir Crit Care Med 2006;174:990–6.

37. Pinto-Plata VM, Livnat G, Girish M, et al. Systemic cytokines, clinical and physiological changes in patients hospitalized for exacerbation of COPD. Chest 2006;131:37–43.

38. Boschetto P, Quintavalle S, Zeni E, et al. Association between markers of emphysema and more severe chronic obstructive pulmonary disease. Thorax 2006;61:1037–42.

39. Franciosi LG, Page CP, Celli BR, et al. Markers of exacerbation severity in chronic obstructive pulmonary disease. Respir Dis 2006;7:74.

40. Hurst JR, Donaldson GC, Perera WR, et al. Use of plasma biomarkers at exacerbation of chronic obstructive pulmonary disease. Am J Respir Crit Care Med 2006;174:867–74.

41. Dev D, Wallace E, Sankaran R, et al. Value of C-reactive protein measurements in exacerbations of chronic obstructive pulmonary disease. Respir Med 1998;92:664–7.

42. Weis N, Almdal T. C-reactive protein—can it be used as a marker of infection in patients with exacerbations of chronic obstructive pulmonary disease? Eur J Intern Med 2006;17:88–91.

43. Stolz D, Christ-Crain M, Morgenthaler NG, et al. Copeptin, C-reactive protein, and procalcitonin as prognostic biomarkers in acute exacerbation of COPD. Chest 2007;131:1058–67.

44. Muller B, Tamm M. Biomarkers in acute exacerbation of chronic obstructive pulmonary disease: among the blind, the one-eyed is king. Am J Respir Crit Care Med 2006;174:848–9.

45. Aaron SD, Angel JB, Lunau M, et al. Granulocyte inflammatory markers and airway infection during acute exacerbation of chronic obstructive pulmonary disease. Am J Respir Crit Care Med 2001;163:349–55.

46. Perera WR, Hurst JR, Wilkinson TM, et al. Inflammatory changes, recovery, and recurrence of COPD exacerbation. Eur Respir J 2007;29:527–34.

47. Miravitlles M, Guerrero T, Mayordomo C, et al. Factors associated with increased risk of exacerbation and hospital admission in a cohort of ambulatory COPD patients: a multiple logistic regression analysis. The EOLO Study Group. Respiration 2000;67:495–501.

48. Similowski T, Agusti A, MacNee W, Schonhofer B. The potential impact of anaemia of chronic disease in COPD. Eur Respir J 2006;27:390–6.

49. Rutten FH, Cramer MJ, Suithoff NP, et al. Comparison of B-type natriuretic peptide assays for identifying heart failure in stable elderly patients with a clinical diagnosis of chronic obstructive pulmonary disease. Eur J Heart Fail 2007 March 6 [Epub ahead of print].

50. Hodge S, Hodge G, Bronzyna S, et al. Azythromycin increases phagocytosis of apoptotic bronchial epithelial cells by alveolar macrophages. Eur Respir J 2006;28:486–95.

51. Vondracek SF, Hemstreet BA. Retrospective evaluation of systemic corticosteroids for the management of acute exacerbations of chronic obstructive pulmonary disease. Am J Health Syst Pharm 2006;63:645–52.

52. Dusser B, Bravo ML, Iacono P. The effect of tiotropium on exacerbations and airflow in patients with COPD. Eur Respir J 2006;27:547–55.

53. Dekhuijzen PN. Acetylcysteine in the treatment of severe COPD. Ned Tijdschr Geneeskd 2006;150:1222–6.

54. Sutherland ER, Crapo JD, Bowler RP. N-Acetylcysteine and exacerbations of chronic obstructive pulmonary disease. COPD 2006;3:195–202.

55. Suissa A. Effectiveness of inhaled corticosteroids in chronic obstructive pulmonary disease: immortal time bias in observational studies. Am J Respir Crit Care Med 2003;168:49–53.

56. Kardos P, Wencker M, Glaab T, Vogelmeier C. Impact of salmeterol/fluticasone propionate vs salmetrerol on exacerbations in severe chronic obstructive pulmonary disease. Am J Respir Crit Care Med 2007;175:144–9.

57. Wilkinson TMA, Donaldson GC, Hurst JA, et al. Early therapy improves outcomes of exacerbations of chronic obstructive pulmonary disease. Am J Respir Crit Care Med 2004;169:1298–303.

58. Adams SG, Melo J, Luther M, Anzueto A. Antiobiotics are associated with lower relapse rates in patients with acute exacerbations of COPD. Chest 2000;117:1345–42.

59. Mancini GB, Etminan M, Zhang B, et al. Reduction of morbidity and mortality by statins, angiotensin-converting enzyme inhibitors, and angiotensin receptor blockers in patients with chronic obstructive pulmonary disease. J Am Coll Cardiol 2006;47:2554–60.

60. Søyseth V, Brekke PH, Smith P, Omland T. Statin use is associated with reduced mortality in chronic obstructive pulmonary disease. ERJ 2007;29:279–83.

CHAPTER 26

Medical Therapy for Chronic Obstructive Pulmonary Disease

Bartolome R. Celli, MD

The airflow obstruction of chronic obstructive pulmonary disease (COPD), as defined by the forced expiratory volume in 1 second (FEV$_1$), is thought to be only partially irreversible.[1,2] This physiologic fact has generated an unjustified nihilistic therapeutic attitude in many health care providers. The evidence accumulated suggests otherwise, and an optimistic attitude toward these patients goes a long way in relieving patients' fears and misconceptions. In contrast to many other diseases, some forms of intervention, such as smoking cessation,[1,2] long-term oxygen therapy in hypoxemic patients,[3,4] lung volume reduction surgery in certain patients with inhomogeneous upper lobe emphysema,[5] and perhaps pharmacologic therapy,[6] improve survival, whereas others, such as pulmonary rehabilitation,[1–3,7] lung transplantation,[8] and bronchodilators,[1,2] improve symptoms and the quality of a patient's life once the diagnosis has been established. Table 1 summarizes the available therapeutic options for patients with COPD. This chapter reviews the medical management of COPD.

The overall goals of treatment are to prevent further deterioration in lung function, to alleviate symptoms, and to treat complications as they arise.[1,2] Once diagnosed, patients should be encouraged to participate actively in their management. This concept of collaborative management may improve self-reliance and esteem. Although not proven, it may also help improve compliance with treatment. All patients should be encouraged to lead a healthy life and exercise regularly. Preventive care is extremely important at this time, and all patients should receive immunizations, including pneumococcal vaccine every 5 years and yearly influenza vaccines.[1,2,9,10] An algorithm detailing this comprehensive approach is shown in Figure 1.

COPD: A Multicomponent Disease

There is increasing evidence that independent of the degree of airflow obstruction, lung volumes are important in the genesis of the symptoms and limitations of patients with more advanced disease. A series of elegant studies have demonstrated that dyspnea perceived during exercise, including walking, more closely relates to the development of dynamic hyperinflation than to changes in FEV$_1$.[11–16] Further, the improvement in exercise brought about by several therapies, including bronchodilators, oxygen, lung reduction surgery, and even rehabilitation, is more closely related to delaying dynamic hyperinflations than by changing the degree of airflow obstruction.[17,18] Casanova and colleagues showed that hyperinflation, expressed as the ratio of inspiratory capacity to total lung capacity, predicted survival better than the FEV$_1$.[19] This not only provides us with new insights into pathogenesis but also opens the door for new

Table 1 Therapy of Patients with Symptomatic Stable Chronic Obstructive Pulmonary Disease		
Improve Survival	*May Improve Survival*	*Improve Patient-Centered Outcomes*

Smoking cessation	Pharmacotherapy with salmeterol and fluticasone	Pharmacotherapy
		    Short-acting bronchodilators
		    Long-acting antimuscarinics
		    Long-acting β-agonists
		    Inhaled corticosteroids
		    Theophylline
		    α$_1$-Antitrypsin for selected patients
		    Antibiotics for selected patients

Lung volume reduction surgery for selected patients	Pulmonary rehabilitation	Oxygen therapy
Noninvasive ventilation for acute or chronic hypercapneic ventilatory failure		Surgery Lung volume reduction Lung transplantation
		Pulmonary rehabilitation

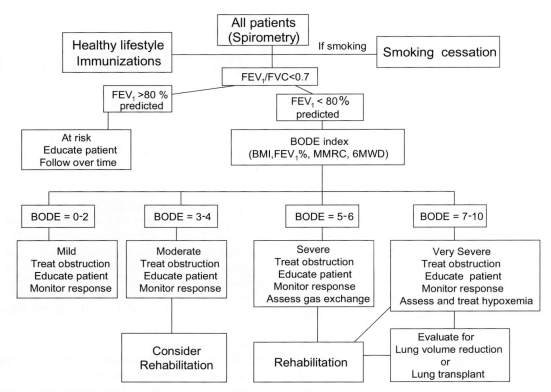

FIGURE 1. Algorithm describing the comprehensive management of patients with chronic obstructive pulmonary disease. BMI = body mass index; BODE = Body mass index, obstruction, dyspnea, and exercise capacity; FEV$_1$ = forced expiratory volume in 1 second; FVC = forced vital capacity; MMRC = Modified Medical Research Scale; 6MWD = six-minute walking distance.

imaginative ways to alter lung volumes and perhaps impact on disease progression.

That COPD may be associated with important systemic expressions in patients with more advanced disease is now accepted (see Chapter 23).[1,15,20] Perhaps as a consequence of a persistent systemic inflammatory state or due to other, yet unproven mechanisms, such as imbalanced oxidative stress or abnormal immunologic response, the fact is that many patients with COPD may have decreased free fat mass, impaired systemic muscle function, anemia, osteoporosis, depression, pulmonary hypertension, and cor pulmonale, all of which are important determinants of outcome. Indeed, dyspnea measured with a simple tool such as the Modified Medical Research Scale,[21] the body mass index obtained by dividing the weight in kilograms by the height in meters squared (kg/m^2),[22,23] and the timed walked distance in 6 minutes[24,25] are all better predictors of mortality than the FEV$_1$. The incorporation of these variables into the multi-dimensional body mass index, obstruction, dyspnea, and exercise capacity (BODE) index predicts survival even better.[26] The index is also responsive to exacerbations[27] and, more importantly, acts as a surrogate marker of future outcome after interventions,[28] thus providing clinicians with a useful tool to help determine the comprehensive severity of the disease. Several chapters in this book more amply detail each of these concepts.

Based on the multidimensional nature of the disease and the availability of multiple effective therapies, the approach shown in Figure 1 may more accurately help clinicians evaluate patients and choose therapies than the current approach using primarily the FEV$_1$ percentage from reference values.

COPD: A Treatable Disease

Current evidence suggests that besides smoking cessation,[29–32] long-term oxygen therapy in hypoxemic patients,[3,4] mechanical ventilation in acute respiratory failure, and lung volume reduction surgery for patients with upper lobe emphysema and poor exercise capacity[5] improve survival. The TORCH study (Towards a Revolution in COPD Health) in over 6,000 patients not only showed that the combination of salmeterol and fluticasone improved lung function and health status but also that the relative risk of dying over the 3 years of the study decreased by 17.5%.[6] Other therapies, such as pulmonary rehabilitation and lung transplantation, improve symptoms and the quality of a patient's life once the diagnosis has been established.[1,2,7,8] All of these modalities of therapies and their effects are summarized in Table 1.

Therapy is Effective for the Respiratory Manifestations of COPD

Once diagnosed, the patient should be encouraged to actively participate in disease management. This concept of collaborative management may improve self-reliance and esteem. All patients should be encouraged to lead a healthful lifestyle and exercise regularly. Preventive care is extremely important at this time, and all patients should receive immunizations, including pneumococcal vaccine and yearly influenza vaccines.[1,3]

Smoking Cessation and Decreased Exposure to Biomass Fuel

As smoking is the major cause of COPD, smoking cessation is the most important component of therapy for patients who still smoke[1,3] and should be provided to all patients who smoke. Because secondhand smoking is known to damage lung function, limitation of exposure to involuntary smoke, particularly in children, should be encouraged. The factors that cause patients to smoke include the addictive potential of nicotine, conditional responses to stimuli surrounding smoking, psychosocial problems such as depression, poor education and low income, and forceful advertising campaigns. As the causes that drive the patient to smoke are multifactorial, smoking cessation programs should also involve multiple interventions. The clinician should always participate in the treatment of smoking addiction because a physician's advice and intervention and use of the appropriate medications, including nicotine patch, gum, or inhalers, bupropion, and varencicline, help obtain successful results.[30–34] The significant burden of COPD in patients exposed to biomass fuel in certain areas of the world should improve by changing to more efficient and less polluting sources of energy.

Pharmacologic Therapy of Airflow Obstruction

Most patients with COPD require pharmacologic therapy. This should be organized according to the severity of symptoms, the degree of lung dysfunction, and the tolerance of the patient to specific drugs.[1,3] A stepwise approach similar in concept to that developed for systemic hypertension may be helpful since medications alleviate symptoms, improve exercise tolerance and quality of life, and may decrease mortality. Tables 2 and 3 provide a summary of the evidence supporting the effect of individual and combined therapies on outcomes of importance to patients with COPD. Because most patients with COPD are elderly, care must be taken when prescribing drugs for this population.[35]

Bronchodilators

Several important concepts guide the use of bronchodilators. In some patients, the changes in the FEV_1 may be small and the symptomatic benefit may be due to other mechanisms, such as a decrease in the hyperinflation of the lung.[11,13] Some older COPD patients cannot effectively activate metered-dose inhalers (MDIs), and we should work with the patient to achieve mastery of the MDI. If this is not possible, use of a spacer or nebulizers to facilitate inhalation of the medication will help achieve the desired results. Mucosal deposition in the mouth will result in local side effects (ie, thrush with inhaled steroids) or general absorption and its consequences (ie, tremor after β2-agonists). Finally, the inhaled route is preferred over the oral administration, and long-acting bronchodilators are more effective than short-acting ones.[1,2] The currently available bronchodilators are described below.

β2-Agonists

These drugs increase cyclic adenosine monophosphate (AMP) within many cells and promote airway smooth muscle relaxation. Other nonbronchodilator effects have been observed, but their significance is uncertain. In patients with mild intermittent symptoms, it is reasonable to initiate drug therapy with an MDI of a short-acting β2-agonist as needed for relief of symptoms.[1,2] In patients with persistent symptoms, it is indicated to use long-acting β2-agonists[1,2,11,13,36–39] twice daily. They prevent nocturnal bronchospasm, increase exercise endurance, and improve quality of life. The safety profile of salmeterol in the TORCH trial is reassuring to clinicians who frequently prescribe selective long-acting β2-agonists for their patients with COPD.

Anticholinergics

These drugs act by blocking muscarinic receptors that are known to be functional in COPD. The appropriate dosage of the short-acting ipratropium bromide is two to four puffs three or four times a day, but some patients require and tolerate larger dosages.[1,2] The therapeutic effect is a decrease in exercise-induced increased lung inflation or dynamic hyperinflation.[12] The long-acting tiotropium is very effective in inducing prolonged bronchodilation[14] and decreasing lung volume[15] in patients with COPD. In addition, it improves dyspnea, decreases exacerbations,[40] and improves health-related quality of life when compared with placebo and even ipratroprium bromide. The results of the large UPLIFT trial evaluating the potential role of tiotropium as a disease-modifying agent[41] will determine its place in the overall armamentarium of treatments for patients with COPD. Currently, tiotropium represents a first-line agent for patients with persistent symptoms.

Phosphodiesterase Inhibitors

Theophylline is a nonspecific phosphodiesterase inhibitor that increases intracellular cyclic AMP within airway smooth muscle. The bronchodilator effects of these drugs are best seen at high doses, where there is also a higher risk of toxicity. Its potential for toxicity has led to a decline in its popularity. Theophylline is of particular value for less compliant or less capable patients who cannot use aerosol therapy optimally. The previously recommended therapeutic serum levels of 15 to 20 mg/dL are too close to the toxic range and are frequently associated with side effects. Therefore, a lower target range of 8 to 13 mg/dL is safer and still therapeutic in nature.[1,3] The combination of two or more bronchodilators (theophylline, albuterol, and ipratropium) has some logical

Table 2 Effect of Individual Pharmacologic Agents on Important Outcomes of Patients with Chronic Obstructive Pulmonary Disease

	FEV_1	Lung Volume	Dyspnea	QoL	AE	Exercise Endurance	Disease Modifier by FEV_1	Mortality	Side Effects
Albuterol	Yes (A)	Yes (B)	Yes (B)	NA	NA	Yes (B)	NA	NA	Some
Ipratropium bromide	Yes (A)	Yes (B)	Yes (B)	No (B)	Yes (B)	Yes (B)	No	NA	Minimal
Long-acting beta-agonists	Yes (A)	Yes (A)	Yes (A)	Yes (A)	Yes (A)	Yes (B)	No	NA	Minimal
Tiotropium	Yes (A)	Yes (A)	Yes (A)	Yes (A)	Yes (A)	Yes (A)	NA	NA	Minimal
Inhaled corticosteroids	Yes (A)	NA	Yes (B)	Yes (A)	Yes (A)	NA	No	No	Some
Theophylline	Some (A)	Yes (B)	Yes (A)	Yes (B)	NA	Yes (B)	NA	NA	Important
PDE4 inhibitors	Some (B)	NA	NA	Yes (B)	NA	NA	NA	NA	Some

AE = ; FEV_1 = forced expiratory volume in 1 second; NA = not available; QoL = quality of life.
Level of evidence: A = more than one randomized trial; B = limited randomized trials.

Table 3 Effect of Some Combined Pharmacologic Agents on Important Outcomes of Patients with Chronic Obstructive Pulmonary Disease

	FEV_1	Lung Volume	Dyspnea	QoL	AE	Exercise Endurance	Disease Modifier by FEV_1	Mortality	Side Effects
Salmeterol + theophylline	Yes (B)	NA	Yes (B)	Yes (B)	NA	NA	NA	NA	Some
Formoterol + tiotropium	Yes (A)	NA	Yes (B)	Yes (B)	NA	NA	NA	NA	Minimal
Salmeterol + fluticasone	Yes (A)	Yes (B)	Yes (A)	Yes (A)	Yes (A)	Yes (B)	Yes	Some	Some
Formoterol + budesonide	Yes (A)	NA	Yes (A)	Yes (A)	Yes (A)	NA	NA	NA	Minimal
Tiotropium + salmeterol + fluticasone	Yes (A)	NA	Yes (B)	Yes (B)	Yes (A)	NA	NA	NA	Some

AE = ; FEV_1 = forced expiratory volume in 1 second; NA = not available; QoL = quality of life.
Level of evidence: A = more than one randomized trial; B = limited randomized trials.

rationale as they seem to have additive effects and can result in maximum benefit in stable COPD.[1,2,42] A possible action of theophylline on the expression of genes centrally controlling inflammation in COPD[43] deserves further investigation.

The specific phosphodiesterase E_4 inhibitors cilomilast and roflumilast may have an anti-inflammatory and bronchodilator effect but less gastrointestinal irritation and thus prove extremely useful if their theoretical advantages are clinically confirmed. The first 6-month studies show modest bronchodilation effects and some effect on quality of life.[44,45]

Anti-inflammatory Therapy

In contrast to their value in asthma management, anti-inflammatory drugs have not been documented to have a significant role in the routine treatment of patients with stable COPD.[1,2] Cromolyn and nedocromil have not been established as useful agents, although they could possibly be helpful if the patient has associated respiratory tract allergy. One study using monoclonal antibodies against interleukin-8[46] and another one against tumor necrosis factor α[47] failed to detect any response. However, patients were selected according to the degree of airflow obstruction and not based on the presence or level of the specific targeted molecule. The groups of leukotriene inhibitors that have proven useful in asthma have not been adequately tested in COPD, so a final conclusion about their potential use cannot be drawn.

Corticosteroids

Glucocorticoids act at multiple points within the inflammatory cascade, although their effects in COPD appear to be more modest compared with bronchial asthma. In outpatients, exacerbations necessitate a course of oral steroids, as we discuss later in this chapter, but it is important to wean patients quickly since the older COPD population is susceptible to complications such as skin damage, cataracts, diabetes, osteoporosis, and secondary infections. These risks do not accompany standard doses of inhaled corticosteroid aerosols, which may cause thrush but pose a negligible risk for other outcomes, such as cataract and osteoporosis. Several large multicenter trials evaluated the role of inhaled corticosteroids in preventing or slowing the progressive course of symptomatic COPD.[48–55] The results of these earlier studies showed minimal, if any, benefits in the rate of decline of lung function. On the other hand, in the one study in which it was evaluated, inhaled fluticasone decreased the rate of loss of health-related quality of life and the exacerbations.[6] Recent retrospective analysis of large databases suggesting a possible effect of inhaled corticosteroids on improving survival[51,52] was not confirmed in the TORCH trial, in which the inhaled corticosteroid–only arm did not show improved survival compared with placebo, whereas the combination arm was significantly more effective than inhaled corticosteroid alone.[6] In that trial, the combination was superior in terms of all outcomes evaluated. This, coupled with the more frequent development

of pneumonia in the patients receiving inhaled corticosteroid, suggests that inhaled corticosteroid should not be prescribed alone but rather associated with a long-acting β2-agonist.[6]

Combination Therapy

All of the studies that explored the value of a combination of different agents have shown significant improvements over single agents alone,[6,56] and it may be time to think of combination therapy as first-line therapy. Inititally, the combination of inhaled ipatroprium and albuterol proved effective in the management of COPD.[57] More recently, the combination of tiotropium and formoterol, even when administered once daily, was almost as effective as the administration of tiotropium once daily and the recommended twice-daily dose of formoterol.[58] Similarly, the combination of theophylline and salmeterol was significantly more effective than either agent alone. The TORCH study showed an effect of the salmeterol-fluticasone combination on survival, FEV_1, exacerbation rate, and quality of life compared with placebo and either of the individual components,[6] confirming earlier studies evaluating the combination of β-agonists and corticosteroids.[53,54] A recent trial compared tiotropium plus placebo with tiotropium plus salmeterol and with tiotropium plus the combination of salmeterol and fluticasone in over 400 patients.[56] Although the primary outcome, the exacerbation rate, was similar among the groups, the number of hospitalizations, health-related quality of life, and lung function were significantly better in the group receiving tiotropium plus salmeterol and fluticasone.

Depending on economic considerations, once symptoms become persistent, therapy should begin with a long-acting antimuscarinic agent such as tiotropium or long-acting β2-agonists twice daily. Once a patient reaches an FEV_1 lower than 60% of predicted and continues to be symptomatic, the evidence from the TORCH trial supports the addition of the combination of inhaled corticosteroid and long-acting β2-agonist. Continuation of tiotropium is reasonable, given its effectiveness and safety record. All of the trials support the concept that intense and aggressive therapy does modify the course of the disease, including the rate of decline of FEV_1, as was shown in the TORCH study.[6]

Mucokinetic Agents

These drugs aim to decrease sputum viscosity and adhesiveness to facilitate expectoration. The only controlled study in the United States suggesting a value for these drugs in the chronic management of bronchitis was a multicenter evaluation of organic iodide.[59] This study demonstrated symptomatic benefits. Oral acetylcysteine is favored in Europe for its antioxidant effects. A large trial recently reported failed to document any substantial benefit.[60] Genetically engineered ribonuclease seems to be useful in cystic fibrosis but is of no value in COPD.[1,2]

Antibiotics

In patients with evidence of respiratory tract infection, such as fever, leukocytosis, and a change in the chest radiograph, antibiotics have proven effective.[61–65] If recurrent infections occur, particularly in winter, continuous or intermittent prolonged courses of antibiotics may be useful.[1,2] The major bacterial strains to be considered are *Streptococcus pneumoniae*, *Haemophilus influenzae*, and *Moraxella catarrhalis* (see Chapter 14.). The antibiotic choice will depend on local experience, supported by sputum culture and sensitivities if the patient is moderately ill or needs to be admitted to hospital.[1,2]

α_1-Antitrypsin

Although supplemental weekly or monthly administration of this enzyme may be indicated in nonsmoking, younger patients with genetically determined emphysema, in practice, such therapy is difficult to initiate. There is evidence that the administration of α_1-antitrypsin is relatively safe.[1,3,66,67] Although not entirely clear, the most likely candidates for replacement therapy would be patients with mild to moderate COPD.

Vaccination

Ideally, infectious complications of the respiratory tract should be prevented in patients with COPD by using effective vaccines. Thus, routine prophylaxis with pneumococcal and influenza vaccines is recommended.[12,68,69]

Therapy is Effective for the Systemic Manifestations of COPD

The systemic manifestations of COPD are very important and include peripheral muscle dysfunction, malnutrition, cardiovascular compromise, osteoporosis, depression, anemia, and lung cancer. Some of them may be responsive to therapy. The rest of this chapter concentrates on those therapies that may beneficially influence the outcome in patients with COPD.

Pulmonary Rehabilitation

Pulmonary rehabilitation has gradually become the gold standard treatment for patients with severe lung disease, especially COPD.[1,2] This chapter reviews the basic definitions, objectives, components, and outcomes of pulmonary rehabilitation. By definition, rehabilitation services are provided to patients with symptoms, most of them with advanced lung disease. Although most of the data that have resulted in the acceptance of this therapeutic modality have been obtained from studies of patients with COPD, the basic principles and tools are applicable to patients with many other limiting chronic diseases of the respiratory system. As new therapeutic strategies such as surgical and nonsurgical lung volume reduction and lung transplantation require well-conditioned patients, pulmonary rehabilitation is becoming a crucial component of the overall treatment strategy of many patients who heretofore were deemed untreatable. The following discussion is both practical and inclusive and should provide the reader with a thorough overview of the topic.

Definition

The Council for Rehabilitation states that rehabilitation attempts to restore the individual to the fullest medical, mental, emotional, social, and vocational potential of which he or she is capable. The most important concept in the definition is that any program must attempt to treat each patient enrolled as an "individual." The variation that arises from the need to individualize therapy from one patient to another is one of the factors that makes the objective evaluation of each group of patients enrolled in a rehabilitation program difficult.

Pulmonary rehabilitation has been redefined by the American Thoracic Society and the European Respiratory Society as "an evidence-based, multidisciplinary, and comprehensive intervention for patients with chronic respiratory diseases who are symptomatic and often have decreased daily life activities. Integrated into the individualized treatment of the patient, pulmonary rehabilitation is designed to reduce symptoms, optimize functional status, increase participation, and reduce health care costs through stabilizing or reversing systemic manifestations of the disease."[7]

Because pulmonary rehabilitation is multidisciplinary and uses different therapeutic components, it is difficult to attribute improved global outcomes to the effect of individual elements of a program. Independent of the study design used, conventional pulmonary function tests do not usually change after pulmonary rehabilitation.[70,71] Nevertheless, well-controlled studies have shown significant improvement in different outcomes, including increased exercise capacity, improved health-related quality of life, decreased dyspnea, and hospital admissions.[70–80]

Objectives and Goals

It follows from the definition that pulmonary rehabilitation has three major objectives:

1. Control, alleviate, and, as much as possible, reverse the symptoms and pathophysiologic processes leading to respiratory impairment.
2. Improve the quality and attempt to prolong the patient's life.
3. Reduce health care use and costs.

In the broadest sense, pulmonary rehabilitation aims to provide good, comprehensive respiratory care for patients with pulmonary diseases.[1,2,7] In its practical sense, comprehensive care may be best provided by a multidisciplinary approach through a structured rehabilitation program.

Patient Selection

Any patient symptomatic from a respiratory disease with some functional limitation is a candidate for rehabilitation. It is preferable to choose patients with moderate to moderately severe disease in whom we hope to prevent the disabling effects of end-stage respiratory failure. This is an important issue because it seems intuitive that patients with minimal functional limitations may benefit little from programs designed to improve function. On the other hand, patients who are "too" far advanced along the course of their illness could be considered "unlikely to benefit" from rehabilitation. This is not true, as shown by the fact that patients with the most severe degree of lung disease, such as those awaiting lung transplantation and lung volume reduction surgery, have shown significant functional improvement and increased exercise endurance after pulmonary rehabilitation.[1,2,7]

Patients with mild disease may not justify the intense effort employed to rehabilitate disabled patients. Other factors that may hinder the ultimate success of rehabilitation for an individual are the presence of disabling diseases such as severe heart failure, arthritis, very low educational level, occupation, lack of support, and, above all, motivation.[7] Although it is customary to not consider patients with cancer candidates for rehabilitation, we have included selected patients with limited exercise performance who are otherwise candidates for surgery. This is particularly important as there are new reports of simultaneous resection of lung nodules in patients with severe COPD who were until now deemed inoperable because of very severe airflow obstruction. Likewise, the inclusion of pulmonary rehabilitation in the preoperative conditioning of patients undergoing lung transplantation or lung volume reduction surgery has expanded the list of indications for rehabilitation.[7]

The decision whether to have an inpatient or an outpatient program depends on the methods of reimbursement, patient population, available personnel, and hospital policy. The ideal system is one that provides an in-hospital treatment arm for patients who may benefit from the program while recovering from acute exacerbations and an outpatient arm (including home therapy) that could complete the program started in the hospital. This ensures good continuity of care.

Therapeutic Modalities that Improve Patients' Performance

EXERCISE CONDITIONING

Exercise conditioning is based on three physiologic principles[81]: specificity of training, which attributes improvement only for the type of exercise practiced; intensity of training, which establishes that only a load higher than baseline will induce a training effect; and reversal of the training effect, which states that once discontinued, the training effect will disappear. The first two have been extensively applied in the rehabilitation of patients with severe COPD. Extrapolation from the effects on normal volunteers and in populations such as patients selected from lung transplantation patients do give support to the inclusion of exercise in the rehabilitation of patients with diseases different from COPD.

Lower Extremity Exercise

Several controlled trials prove that pulmonary rehabilitation is better than regular treatment in symptomatic COPD patients. Goldstein and colleagues' study involved 89 patients randomized to either inpatient rehabilitation for 8 weeks, which was then followed by 16 weeks of outpatient treatment or to conventional care as provided by their physician.[71] At the end of the study, the patients in the rehabilitation group ($n = 45$) significantly improved their exercise endurance, that is, submaximal cycle time, compared with controls ($n = 44$). This was associated with a decrease in dyspnea, improvement in emotional function, and mastery. Wijkstra and colleagues reported the results of 12 weeks of rehabilitation in 28 COPD patients who were compared with 15 patients who received no treatment and served as controls.[72] This study is unique in that the rehabilitation was conducted at home, with the program supervised by nonspecialists. After rehabilitation, the treated patients showed a greater increase in walked distance, maximal work in watts, and oxygen uptake (VO_2) and a decrease in lactate production and perception of dyspnea when compared with controls. These two studies, one inpatient and one at home, as well as several others that have a similar design,[74–77] proved that rehabilitation is effective and that rehabilitation is better than other conventional treatments.

Exercise training is the most important component of a pulmonary rehabilitation program. Casaburi reviewed 36 uncontrolled studies that evaluated the effect of exercise training on exercise performance in over 900 patients with COPD. Exercise training improved exercise endurance in all of these patients.[82] This has been confirmed by controlled trials, which have shown that a rehabilitation program that includes lower extremity exercise is better than other forms of therapy, such as optimization of medication, education, breathing retraining, and group therapy.[79,80]

All of these studies hold in common an increase in exercise endurance, a modest but significant improvement in work rate or oxygen uptake, and a decrease in the perception of dyspnea. Perhaps the most complete of these reports is the one by Ries and colleagues.[79] They randomized 119 patients to education ($n = 62$) and education with exercise training ($n = 57$). After 6 months, the trained patients significantly increased their exercise endurance time and peak oxygen uptake and reported an improvement in the perception of dyspnea and self-assessed efficacy for walking when compared with controls. A subsequent followup of this cohort showed that the gains were lost after 1 year and that a once-a-month followup training visit was not sufficient to maintain the gained effects. In an unique report, O'Hara and colleagues enrolled 14 patients with COPD in a home program that included weight lifting.[83] After training, weight lifters had reduced their minute ventilation and increased by 16% their ergometry endurance when compared with controls. This study suggests that strength training may achieve results similar to those of specific endurance training and could be an alternative form of training. Indeed, more recent reports using strength training provide evidence that this form of training is effective in achieving and maintaining improvement.

It has been suggested that with exercise, patients with COPD become desensitized to the dyspnea induced by the ventilatory load. This was supported by studies such as the one by Belman and Kendregan, who randomized patients to upper or lower extremity exercise and obtained muscle biopsies of the trained limbs before and after training.[81] In spite of a significant increase in exercise endurance, there were no changes in the oxidative enzyme content of the trained muscle. In contrast, Maltais and colleagues documented evidence for a true training effect.[84] In this study, the muscle biopsies of trained patients, but not those of the controls, manifested significant increases in all enzymes responsible for oxidative muscle function. That these biochemical changes are associated with important physiologic outcomes is supported by a reduction in exercise lactic acidosis and minute ventilation after training.[85]

All symptomatic patients who are willing and capable of some exercise are candidates for rehabilitation. ZuWallack and colleagues evaluated 50 patients with severe COPD before and after exercise training.[84] They observed an inverse relationship between the baseline 12-minute walking distance, the oxygen uptake, and the improvement. The results in patients selected for lung transplantation show that rehabilitation improves performance to a degree not achieved with any other form of therapy. The data therefore support exercise as a crucial component in the rehabilitation of patients with very severe lung disease. There was a significant improvement in 6-minute walking distance in patients with severe COPD (mean FEV_1 of 0.78 L) who underwent preoperative pulmonary rehabilitation at our institution before lung volume reduction surgery.

Upper Extremity Exercise

Most of our knowledge about exercise conditioning is derived from programs emphasizing leg training. This is unfortunate because the performance of many everyday tasks requires not only the hands but also the concerted action of other muscle groups that are also used in upper torso and arm positioning. Some of these serve a dual function (respiratory and postural), and arm exercise will decrease their capacity to participate in ventilation.[87-89] These observations suggest that if the arms are trained to perform more work, or if the ventilatory requirement for the same work is decreased, as we have shown, this could improve the capacity to perform activities of daily living.[90]

Arm training results in improved performance, which is, for the most part, task specific. Ries and colleagues studied the effect of two forms of arm exercise, gravity resistance and modified proprioceptive neuromuscular facilitation, and compared them with no arm exercise in 45 patients with COPD.[90] The 20 patients who completed the program improved performance on the tests that were specific for the training. The patients also reported a decrease in fatigue for all tests performed.

Martinez and colleagues showed that unsupported arm training (against gravity) decreases oxygen uptake at the same workload when compared with arm cranking training.[91] They concluded that unsupported arm exercise may be more effective to train patients in activities that resemble those of daily living. A group of cystic fibrosis patients studied by Keens and colleagues underwent upper extremity training consisting of swimming and canoeing for 1.5 hours daily.[92] After 6 weeks, they exhibited increased upper extremity endurance; most importantly, their increase in maximal sustainable ventilatory capacity was similar to that obtained with ventilatory muscle training. This suggests that arm exercise training programs can train ventilatory muscles.

Because simple arm elevation results in significant increases in minute ventilation ($V_{[E]}$), oxygen uptake (VO_2), and carbon dioxide production (VCO_2), we studied 14 patients with COPD before and after 8 weeks of three-times-weekly 20-minute sessions of unsupported arm and leg exercise. Our study was part of a comprehensive rehabilitation program to test whether arm training decreases the ventilatory requirement for arm activity. There was a 35% decrease in the rise of VO_2 and VCO_2 brought about by arm elevation, associated with a significant decrease in VO_E.[93] Because the patients also trained their legs, we could not conclude that the improvement was due to the arm exercise. To answer this question, we had patients with COPD undergo either unsupported arm training ($n = 11$) or resistance breathing training ($n = 14$). After 24 sessions, arm endurance increased only for the unsupported arm training group. Interestingly, maximal inspiratory pressure increased significantly for both groups, indicating that by training the arms, we may induce ventilatory muscle training for those ribcage muscles that hinge on the shoulder girdle.[94]

PHYSICAL MODALITIES OF VENTILATORY THERAPY

These modalities include controlled breathing techniques (diaphragmatic breathing exercise, pursed-lip breathing, and bending forward), chest physical therapy (postural drainage, chest percussion, vibration position), and respiratory muscle endurance or strength training. The benefits of these modalities include less dyspnea, a decrement in anxiety and panic attacks, and improvement in sensation of well-being. Although strength and endurance training of the respiratory muscle is associated with an increase in exercise endurance, the clinical significance of these effects remains debatable. These modalities require careful instruction by specialists who are familiar with the techniques. They should be initiated under close supervision until the patient shows thorough understanding of the techniques. It is often necessary to involve relatives since more of these modalities require the help of another person (eg, chest percussion).

Breathing Training

Breathing training is aimed at controlling the respiratory rate and breathing pattern, thus decreasing air trapping. It also attempts to decrease the work of breathing and improve the position and function of the respiratory muscles. The easiest of these maneuvers is pursed-lip breathing. Patients inhale through the nose and exhale between 4 and 6 seconds through lips pursed in a whistling-kissing position. The exact mechanism by which this maneuver decreases dyspnea is unknown. It does not seem to change functional residual capacity or oxygen uptake, but it does decrease respiratory rate with an increase in tidal volume. Bending forward posture has been shown to result in a decrease in dyspnea in some patients with severe COPD, both at rest and during exercise. These changes can also be seen in the supine or Trendelenburg position. The best explanation for the improvement is that of improved diaphragmatic function as the increased gastric pressure in these positions places the diaphragm in a better contracting position.

Diaphragmatic breathing is a technique aimed at changing the breathing pattern from one in which the ribcage muscles are the predominant pressure generators to a more normal one, in which the pressures are generated with the diaphragm. It is usually practiced for at least 20 minutes two to three times daily. The patient should start the training in the supine position and, once familiar with it, perform it in the upright posture. The patient is instructed to breathe in while trying to outwardly displace his or her hand, which is placed on the abdomen. The patient then exhales with pursed lips while being encouraged to use the abdominal muscles in an attempt to return the diaphragm to a more lengthened resting position. Although most patients report improvement in dyspnea and perception of dyspnea, this technique results in minimal, if any, changes in oxygen uptake and resting lung volume.[95] Similar to pursed-lip breathing, there is usually a fall in respiratory rate, minute ventilation, and increased tidal volume.

Chest Physical Therapy

The goal of these techniques is that of removing airway secretions, thereby decreasing airflow resistance and bronchopulmonary infection. These techniques include postural drainage, chest percussion, vibration, and directed cough. Postural drainage uses gravity to help drain the individual lung segments. Chest percussion should be performed with care in patients with osteoporosis or bone problems.

Cough is also an effective technique for removing excess mucus from the larger airways. Unfortunately, patients with COPD have impaired cough mechanisms, maximum expiratory flow is reduced, ciliary beat is impaired, and the mucus itself has altered viscoelastic properties. Since cough spasms may lead to dyspnea, fatigue, and worsened obstruction, directed cough may be helpful by modulating the beneficial effects and preventing the untoward ones. With controlled coughs, patients are instructed to inhale deeply, hold their breath for a few seconds, and then cough two or three times with the mouth open. They are also instructed to compress their upper abdomen to assist in the cough. It seems clear that

pulmonary functions do not improve with any of these techniques. On the other hand, programs that include a combination of postural drainage, percussion, vibration, and cough do increase the clearance of inhaled radio tracers and increase sputum volume and weight. The single most important criterion for chest physical therapy is the presence of sputum production.

Ventilatory Muscle Strength and Endurance Training

Leith and Bradley first demonstrated that, like their skeletal counterparts, the respiratory muscles of normal individuals can be specifically trained to improve their strength or their endurance.[96] Subsequent to that observation, a number of studies have shown that a training response will occur if there is sufficient stimulus. An increase in inspiratory muscle strength (and perhaps endurance) should result in improved respiratory muscle function by decreasing the ratio of the pressure required to breathe (PI) and the maximal pressure that the respiratory system can generate (PImax). The PI to PImax ratio, which represents the effort required to complete each breath as a function of the force reserve, is the most important determinant of fatigue in loaded respiratory muscles.[97,98] Since patients with COPD have reduced inspiratory muscle strength, considerable efforts have been made to define the role of respiratory muscle training in these patients. In some cases, training ventilatory muscles is extremely effective. In others, it is of no use or even counterproductive. Every clinician should be well aware of situations when such training is or is not appropriate.

Strength Training

A high-intensity, low-frequency stimulus is needed to train respiratory muscles. Inspiratory muscles are trained by inspiratory maneuvers performed against a closed glottis or shutter.

Several studies have shown an increase in maximal inspiratory pressures when the respiratory muscles have been specifically trained for strength.[98-124] Decreasing PI/PImax through respiratory muscle strength training does not appear to be clinically important. Yet respiratory muscle strength often increases as a by-product of endurance training achieved with the use of resistive loads. It is possible that some of the benefits observed after endurance training may relate to the increased strength.

Endurance Training

Endurance is achieved through low-intensity, high-frequency training programs, of which there are three types: flow resistive loading, threshold loading, and voluntary isocapneic hyperpnea.

Flow Resistive Loading and Threshold Loading

In flow resistive training, the load is created primarily by decreasing the inspiratory breathing hole size, provided that frequency, tidal volume, and inspiratory time are held constant. Although most studies in patients with COPD have shown an improvement in the time that a given respiratory load can be maintained (ventilatory muscle endurance), the results must be interpreted with caution since it has been shown that endurance can be influenced and actually increased with changes in the pattern of breathing. Threshold loading can result in some muscle training by ensuring that at least the inspired pressure is high enough to ensure training, independent of the inspiratory flow rate. Although the breathing pattern is important (inspiratory time or T_I and respiratory rate), it is not as critically important as the inspired pressure.

Because many studies have not been controlled, it is difficult to attribute their results to the training. The many studies that have been published show an increase in the endurance time during which the ventilatory muscles could tolerate a known load; some show a significant increase in strength and a decrease in dyspnea during the performance of inspiratory load and exercise.[101–124] In the studies that evaluated systemic exercise performance, there was a minimal increase in walking distance or constant load exercise endurance.

It is clear that ventilatory muscle training with resistive breathing results in improved ventilatory muscle strength and endurance. In COPD, however, it is not clear whether this effort results in decreased morbidity or mortality or offers any clinical advantage that makes it worth the effort. In many studies, compliance has been low, with up to 50% of all pulmonary patients failing to complete the programs. Larger multicenter studies with clinical outcomes are needed to select the appropriate patients who may benefit from this labor-intensive form of therapy. Currently, ventilatory muscle training is recommended for patients with symptoms and evidence of ventilatory muscle weakness.

Ventilatory Isocapneic Hyperpnea

This is a training method by which patients maintain high levels of ventilation over time (15 minutes, two or three times daily). The oxygen and carbon dioxide are kept constant in the breathing circuit. In an uncontrolled study, patients with COPD not only increased their maximal sustained ventilatory capacity but also, after 6 weeks of training, increased arm and leg exercise performance after 6 weeks. Two controlled studies also reported an increase in maximal sustainable ventilatory capacity in COPD patients trained for 6 weeks, but their improvement in exercise endurance was no better than that of the control group.[113–124]

It seems that respiratory muscle training results in increased strength and capacity of the muscles to endure a respiratory load. There is debate as to whether it also results in improved exercise performance or improved performance in activities of daily living. Knowing the respiratory muscle factors that may contribute to ventilatory limitation in COPD, one might logically predict that increases in strength and endurance should help respiratory muscle function. But this is perhaps important only in the capacity of the patients to handle inspiratory loads, for example, during acute exacerbations of their disease. It is less likely that ventilatory muscle training will greatly affect systemic exercise performance.

Ventilatory Muscle Training for Intensive Care Patients

Few data exist to justify training the ventilatory muscles of patients in intensive care units. It is apparent that as soon as patients are left to breathe on their own (as during any form of weaning), their respiratory muscles are being retrained. We actually use this "training method" whenever we place patients on either a T-piece or low synchronized intermittent mandatory ventilation (SIMV), although we do not generally analyze the results as we would for a formal training method. More often we think of training in terms of additional, external loads in addition to spontaneous respiration. Few researchers have studied patients recovering from ventilatory failure. Belman reported improvement in two patients who had difficulty weaning from mechanical ventilation; after respiratory muscle threshold training, they were able to come off mechanical ventilation.[125] In a larger but still uncontrolled study, Aldrich and colleagues recruited 30 patients who had suffered from stable chronic respiratory failure for at least 3 weeks but who had failed repeated weaning attempts.[126] Patients with active infections or unstable cardiovascular, renal, or endocrine problems were excluded, as were those with gross malnutrition (albumin < 2.5 g/dL) or neuromuscular disease. Training consisted of intermittently breathing through an inspiratory resistor while either spontaneously breathing or being supported at two to eight breaths per minute with SIMV. The patients' PImax improved from 37 ± 15 to 46 ± 15 cm H_2O, whereas vital capacity increased from 561 ± 325 to 901 ± 480 mL. Of the 30 patients, 12 were weaned after 10 to 46 days of training (40% success). Because the study was uncontrolled and used a selected group of patients, its findings may not apply to all patients recovering from respiratory failure; furthermore, the success rate is little different from those reported in weaning facilities that have not used this training. Before ventilatory muscle training can be recommended as a form of treatment for patients with respiratory failure, more rigorous research is needed.

Caution is Necessary

It is important to understand that ventilatory muscle training, especially with resistive or threshold loading, may be deleterious. Breathing at a high tension time index with either a PI/PImax or prolonged inspiratory time over the total duration of a respiratory cycle (T_I/T_{TOT}) may induce muscle fatigue.[127] Because the respiratory muscles cannot be rested, as is customary in the training of peripheral muscles in athletes, fatigue may precipitate ventilatory failure in COPD patients. Increased PI is an intrinsic part of ventilatory muscle training; hence, it is possible that if an intense enough program is enforced, fatigue may actually be precipitated.

Respiratory Muscle Resting

When the respiratory muscles have to work against a large enough load, they may fatigue.[127] Experimentally, this has been shown to occur in both normal volunteers and patients with COPD. Clinically, it seems that respiratory muscle fatigue plays an important role in the acute respiratory failure of patients with COPD. It seems logical that noninvasive ventilation (NIV) may be helpful in cases of acute or chronic respiratory failure with impending respiratory muscle fatigue Several randomized trials have confirmed this assumption.[128–130] These trials evaluated different outcomes, including the rate of intubation, length of intensive care unit and hospital stay, dyspnea, and mortality. Although not all showed the same results in mortality, there was uniform agreement that positive pressure NIV was effective in reversing acute respiratory failure. The most successfully treated patients were those with elevated partial pressure of carbon dioxide in arterial blood ($PaCO_2$), who were able to cooperate with the caregivers and had no other important comorbid problems (sepsis, severe pneumonia). Because positive pressure NIV is potentially dangerous, patients considered for this therapy should be closely monitored and treated by individuals familiar with these ventilatory techniques.

The possibility that the respiratory muscles of patients with stable severe COPD were functioning close to the fatigue threshold led numerous investigators to explore the role of resting of the muscles with the use of negative and positive pressure NIV. All but one of the controlled trials using both forms of ventilation have shown no benefit in most of the outcomes studied.[131–138] Therefore, the routine use of NIV in stable COPD is not justified.

Nutritional Evaluation

Many patients with emphysema appear thin and emaciated and may have anemia, all of which confer a poor prognosis.[139,140] It was recently shown that, in fact, they may be protein-calorie malnourished. Although evidence is lacking as to the type of plan that would result in unequivocal benefits for the respiratory system, most authorities agree that an attempt should be made to correct deficiencies that may be present. Correction of factors such as anemia (to improve oxygen carrying capacity) and electrolyte imbalances (sodium, potassium, phosphorus, and magnesium) could result in improved cardiopulmonary performance. Similarly, simple measures such as encouraging the patient to take small amounts of food at more frequent intervals result in less abdominal distention and decrease dyspnea after meals. We also recommend evaluating oxygen saturation during meals. If present, this can be alleviated by supplementing O_2 at feeding time.

Psychological Support

Most patients with advanced lung disease have minor but frequently psychological problems, mainly reactive depression and anxiety. Fortunately, these problems are likely to improve as the patients become involved in a rehabilitation program that improves activity and performance. Simple measures, such as being able to exercise under the supervision of supportive specialists, frequently result in a desensitization to symptoms, including dyspnea and fear. It has been shown that 15 to 20 rehabilitation sessions that include education, exercise, modalities of physical therapy, breathing techniques, and relaxation are more effective in reducing anxiety than a similar number of psychotherapy sessions. Occasionally, patients will have major psychological problems that will receive primary psychiatric evaluation and treatment (see Chapter 30).

Home Oxygen Therapy

Therapeutic oxygen has been used systematically since Petty and Finigan recognized the association between hypoxemia and right heart failure and appreciated the benefit of continuous oxygen delivery to patients with severe COPD.[141] Since then, much has been learned about the effects of oxygen and hypoxemia, and progress has been made in the area of mechanical oxygen delivery devices.

The results of the Nocturnal Oxygen Therapy Trial and Medical Research Council studies established that continuous home oxygen improves survival in hypoxemic COPD and that survival is related to the number of hours of supplemental oxygen per day.[3,4] Other beneficial effects of long-term oxygen include reduction in polycythemia, perhaps related more to lowered carboxyhemoglobin levels than improved arterial saturation, reduction in pulmonary artery pressures, dyspnea, and rapid eye movement–related hypoxemia during sleep. Oxygen also improves sleep and may reduce nocturnal arrhythmias. Importantly, oxygen can also improve neuropsychiatric testing and exercise tolerance.[142–147] This has been attributed to central mechanisms causing reduced minute ventilation at the same workload, thereby delaying the time until ventilatory limitation is reached. The improved arterial oxygenation enables greater oxygen delivery, reversal of hypoxemia-induced bronchoconstriction and the effect of oxygen on respiratory muscle recruitment.[145]

Prescribing Home Oxygen

Patients are evaluated for long-term oxygen therapy by measuring the partial pressure of oxygen in arterial blood (PaO_2). It is therefore recommended that measurement of PaO_2, not pulse oximetry (oxygen saturation [SaO_2]), be the clinical standard for initiating long-term oxygen therapy, particularly during rest.[1,2] Oximetry SaO_2 may be used to adjust oxygen flow settings over time. If hypercapnia or acidosis is suspected, an arterial blood gas test must be performed. Some COPD patients who were not hypoxemic before the events leading to their exacerbation will eventually recover to the point that they will no longer need oxygen. It is therefore recommended that the need for long-term oxygen be reassessed in 30 to 90 days when the patient is clinically stable and receiving adequate medical management. Oxygen therapy can be discontinued if the patient does not meet blood gas criteria. To prescribe long-term oxygen therapy, a certificate of medical necessity must be completed. The Health Care Financing Administration (HCFA) form evolved in an attempt to insure that the physician, not the home medical equipment supplier, was in charge of decisions concerning therapy. HCFA requires the physician or an employee of the physician, rather than the home medical equipment supplier, to fill the form.

Like any drug, oxygen has potential deleterious effects that may be particularly relevant to older patients. The hazardous effects of oxygen therapy can be considered under three broad headings.[1,2,148–152] First, there are physical risks, such as fire hazard or tank explosion, trauma from catheters or masks, and drying of mucous membranes owing to high flow rates and inadequate humidification. Second, there are functional effects related to increased carbon dioxide retention and absorptive atelectasis. Elevated $PaCO_2$ in response to supplemental oxygen is a well-recognized complication in a minority of patients. The mechanism has traditionally been ascribed to reductions in the hypoxic ventilatory drive. However, in many patients, the decrease in minute ventilation is minimal. The most consistent finding is a worsening of the pulmonary ventilation to perfusion distribution with an increase in the dead space to tidal volume ratio. This presumably results from oxygen's blockage of local hypoxic vasoconstriction, thereby increasing perfusion of poorly ventilated areas. Third, although possible, cytotoxic effects and atelectasis have not clearly been demonstrated with the low flow rates (1–5 L/min, FiO_2 24–36%) typically used for chronic home oxygen therapy in COPD.

Oxygen Delivery Systems

Long-term home oxygen is available from three different delivery systems: oxygen concentrators, liquid systems, and compressed gas.[1] Each system has advantages and disadvantages, and the correct system for each patient depends on patient limitations and the clinical application. Oxygen systems were recently compared on the basis of weight, cost, portability, ease of refilling, and availability. The former three factors may be of particular importance in elderly, often debilitated patients. Compressed gas is stored in variably sized steel or aluminum cylinders that weigh 200, 16, 9, and 4 lb and last 2.4 days, 5.2 hours, 2 hours, and 1.2 hours at 2 L/min flow. The advantages of compressed gas oxygen are its low price, availability, and capacity to be stored for long periods. The disadvantages are its weight (with the large cylinders), short oxygen supply time (with the smaller cylinders), potential hazard of a torpedo-like effect if the valve becomes suddenly disconnected from the compressed gas cylinder, and inferior transfillability. Liquid oxygen is stored at very low temperatures that reduce the volume to less than 1% of the room temperature equivalent. Portable containers weigh up to 10 lb and last 4 to 8 hours at 2/min flow. A wheel-mounted, stationary unit is also available that can last up to 7 days at 1 L/min. The advantages of this system are its relative

portability and ease of transfillability. The disadvantages are its higher cost and requirements for intermittent pressure venting, resulting in oxygen "consumption" even when the system is not being used. Oxygen concentrators are electrical devices that extract oxygen by passing in air through a molecular sieve. The oxygen is delivered to the patient, and the nitrogen is returned to the atmosphere. They are typically used in a stationary capacity, such as in the car or a room, whereas liquid or gas is used to provide portability. The major advantage of the oxygen concentrator is its relative cost effectiveness; the disadvantages are its need for a power source, regular servicing, and relative lack of portability.

Administration Devices

Oxygen is typically administered with continuous flow by a nasal cannula; however, because alveolar delivery occurs during a small portion of a spontaneous respiratory cycle (approximately the first sixth), the rest of the cycle being used to fill dead space and for exhalation, the majority of continuously flowing oxygen is not used by the patient and is wasted into the atmosphere. To improve efficiency and increase patient mobility, several devices are available that focus on oxygen conservation and delivery during early inspiration. These devices include reservoir cannulas, demand-type systems, and transtracheal catheters.[152]

Reservoir nasal cannulas and pendants store oxygen during expiration and deliver a 20 mL bolus during early inspiration. Because more alveolar oxygen is delivered, flows may be reduced proportionally. This has been shown to result in a 2 to 4:1 oxygen savings at rest and with exercise. Cosmetic considerations have traditionally limited patient acceptance of these devices.

Demand valve systems have an electronic sensor that delivers oxygen only during early inspiration or provides an additional pulse early in inspiration as an adjuvant to the continuous flow. By restricting or accentuating oxygen during inspiration, wasted delivery into dead space or during exhalation is minimized. This results in a 2 to 7:1 oxygen savings. The effect of mouth breathing on efficacy is not yet clear. Transtracheal oxygen therapy employs a thin flexible catheter placed into the lower trachea for delivery of continuous (or pulsed) oxygen.[152–155] Because oxygen is delivered directly into the trachea, dead space is reduced and the upper trachea serves as a reservoir of undiluted oxygen. This provides a 2 to 3:1 oxygen savings over a nasal cannula.

Exacerbations, Hospitalization, and Discharge Criteria

Although acute exacerbations are difficult to define (see Chapter 25) and their pathogenesis is poorly understood, impaired lung function can lead to respiratory failure, requiring intubation and mechanical ventilation. In addition, repeated exacerbations are associated with poor outcome.[156–160] The purpose of acute treatment is to manage the patient's decompensation and comorbid conditions to prevent further deterioration and readmission. Table 4 lists the components of the history, physical examination, and laboratory evaluation that should be obtained during a moderate to severe acute exacerbation to assist the formulation of therapy and the decision for hospital admission.[1,2] Figure 2 describes an approach to patients with exacerbations.

The therapy of an exacerbation is based on the administration of the same medications that are given in the stable patient with preference for nebulized medications. In addition, the administration of systemic corticosteroids has resulted in improved outcomes.[162–165] If a bacterial infection is suspected, the administration of antibiotics based on the local prevalence of bacteria is indicated.[166–169]

Table 4	Emergency Room Evaluation of Exacerbations of Chronic Obstructive Pulmonary Disease
History	Baseline respiratory status, sputum volume and characteristics, duration and progression of symptoms
	Dyspnea severity, exercise limitations, sleeping and eating difficulty, home care resources, home therapeutic regimen
	Comorbid acute or chronic conditions
Physical	Evidence of cor pulmonale, tachypnea, bronchospasm, pneumonia
	Hemodynamic instability, altered mentation, respiratory muscle fatigue, excessive work of breathing.
Laboratory	ABG, chest radiograph (posteroanterior, lateral), ECG, theophylline level (if outpatient theophylline used)
	Pulse oximetry monitoring, ECG monitoring
	Additional studies including sputum or blood culture as clinically indicated

ABG = arterial blood gases; ECG = electrocardiogram.

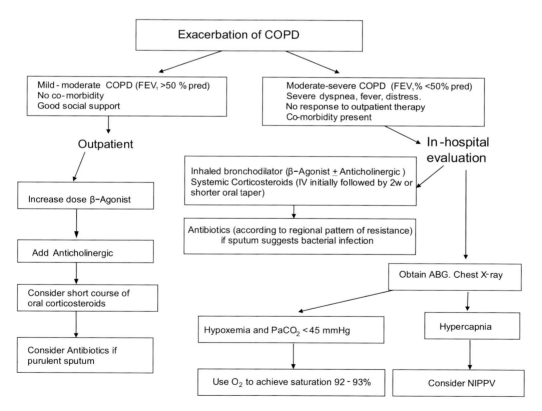

FIGURE 2. Algorithm to approach a patient with exacerbation of chronic obstructive pulmonary disease (COPD). ABG = arterial blood gases; FEV1 = forced expiratory volume in 1 second; IV = intravenous; NIPPV = noninvasive positive pressure ventilation; PaCO2 = partial pressure of carbon dioxide in arterial blood.

Table 5 Indications for Hospitalization of a Patient with Chronic Obstructive Pulmonary Disease

1. The patient has an acute exacerbation of COPD characterized by increase in dyspnea, cough, and sputum production with one or more of the following features:

   - Symptoms that do not adequately respond to outpatient management

   - Inability of a previously mobile patient to walk between rooms

   - Inability to eat or sleep owing to dyspnea

   - Family and/or physician assessment that the patient cannot manage at home and supplementary home care resources are not immediately available

   - Presence of high-risk comorbid pulmonary (eg, pneumonia) or nonpulmonary conditions

   - Prolonged, progressive symptoms before emergency room visit

   - Presence of worsening hypoxemia, new or worsening hypercarbia, or new or worsening cor pulmonale

2. Acute respiratory failure characterized by severe respiratory distress, uncompensated hypercarbia, or severe hypoxemia

3. The patient has new or worsening cor pulmonale unresponsive to outpatient management.

4. Invasive surgical or diagnostic procedures are planned requiring analgesics or sedatives that may worsen pulmonary function

5. Comorbid conditions, such as severe steroid myopathy or acute vertebral compression fractures with severe pain, have worsened pulmonary function

COPD=chronic obstructive pulmonary disease.

Traditionally, the decision to admit to a hospital derives from subjective interpretation of clinical features, such as the severity of dyspnea, determination of respiratory failure, short-term response to emergency room therapy, presence of

Table 6 Indications for Intensive Care Unit Admission of Patients with Acute Exacerbations of Chronic Obstructive Pulmonary Disease

1. Severe dyspnea; does not respond to initial emergency room therapy

2. Presence of confusion, lethargy, or respiratory muscle fatigue characterized by paradoxical diaphragmatic motion

3. Laboratory evidence demonstrates persistent/worsening hypoxemia despite supplemental oxygen or severe/worsening respiratory acidosis (eg, pH < 7.30)

4. Need for assisted mechanical ventilation by means of an endotracheal tube or noninvasive technique

right heart failure, and presence of complicating features, such as severe bronchitis, pneumonia, or other comorbid conditions.[1] This approach to decision making is less than ideal in that up to 28% of patients with an acute exacerbation of COPD discharged from an emergency room have recurrent symptoms within 14 days. Additionally, 17% of patients discharged after emergency room management of COPD will relapse and require hospitalization. Few clinical studies have investigated patient-specific objective clinical and laboratory features that identify patients with COPD who require hospitalization. A general consensus supports the need for hospitalization in patients with severe acute hypoxemia or acute hypercarbia; less extreme arterial blood gas abnormalities, however, do not assist with decision making. The posttreatment FEV_1 as a percentage of predicted, combined with the clinical assessment, identifies patients in need of admission. Asymptomatic patients with a posttreatment FEV_1 of less than 40% of predicted were successfully discharged from the emergency room; patients with a posttreatment FEV_1 of less than 40% of predicted accompanied by persistent respiratory symptoms require admission.

Other factors that identify high-risk patients include a previous emergency room visit within 7 days, the number of doses of nebulized bronchodilators, use of home oxygen, previous relapse rate, administration of aminophylline, and the use of corticosteroids and antibiotics at the time of emergency room discharge.

Once improved, clinical assessment plans for modifying drug regimens, use of home oxygen, or potential benefits from pulmonary rehabilitation programs should be prepared. The duration of hospitalization in COPD depends at least partially on the existence of a multidisciplinary team that directs respiratory management.

Because of the complex management issues in caring for COPD patients with impending or frank respiratory failure, physician specialists with extensive experience in and knowledge of COPD should participate in the care of hospitalized patients who present with underlying severe disease; those who require invasive or noninvasive modes of mechanical ventilation[129–131] develop hypoxemia unresponsive to fraction of inspired oxygen (FiO_2) 0.50 or new-onset hypercarbia, require steroids >48 hours to maintain adequate respiratory function, undergo thoracoabdominal surgery, or require specialized techniques to manage copious airway secretions.

The indications for hospital admission are summarized in Table 5. The experts' consensus considers the severity of the underlying respiratory dysfunction, progression of symptoms, response to outpatient therapy, existence of comorbid conditions, necessity of surgical interventions that may affect pulmonary function, and the availability of adequate home care. The severity of respiratory dysfunction dictates the need for admission to an intensive care unit (Table 6). Depending on the resources available within an institution, admission of patients with severe exacerbations of COPD to intermediate

Table 7 Discharge Criteria after Treatment for Acute Exacerbations of Chronic Obstructive Pulmonary Disease

1. Inhaled β-agonist therapy is required no more frequently than every 6 hours
2. Previously ambulatory patient is able to walk across the room
3. The patient is able to sleep without frequent awakening by dyspnea
4. Any component of reactive airway disease is under stable control
5. The patient is stable off parenteral therapy for 12 to 24 hours
6. The patient or home caregiver is educated as to correct use of medications
7. Arrangements for followup care and home care (eg, visiting nurse, home oxygen delivery, meal provisions) are completed

Patients who do not yet fulfill criteria for discharge to home may be successfully managed at non–acute care placement sites for observation during the final resolution of symptoms.

or special respiratory care units may be appropriate if personnel, skills, and equipment exist to identify and manage acute respiratory failure successfully. Limited data support the discharge criteria listed in Table 7.

Conclusion

Over the years, our knowledge of COPD has increased significantly. Smoking cessation campaigns have resulted in a significant decrease in smoking prevalence in the United States. Similar efforts in the rest of the world should have the same impact. The consequence should be a drop in the incidence of COPD in the years to come. The widespread application of long-term oxygen therapy for hypoxemic patients has resulted in increased survival. During this time, we have expanded our drug therapy armamentarium and have used it to effectively improve dyspnea and quality of life. Recent studies have documented the benefits of pulmonary rehabilitation. NIV has offered new alternatives for the patient with acute or chronic failure. Surgical and more innovative nonsurgical volume reduction may serve as an alternative to lung transplantation for those patients with severe COPD who are still symptomatic after maximal medical therapy. With all of these options, a nihilistic attitude toward the patient with COPD is not justified.[170]

References

1. Celli BR, MacNee W. Standards for the diagnosis and treatment of COPD. Eur Respir J 2004;23:932–46.
2. Global Initiative for Chronic Obstructive Lung Disease. Available at: http://www.GOLD.org (updated 2006). Accessed February 5, 2008.
3. Nocturnal Oxygen Therapy Trial Group. Continuous or nocturnal oxygen therapy in hypoxemic chronic obstructive lung disease. Ann Intern Med 1980;93:391–8.
4. Report of the Medical Research Council Working Party. Long-term domiciliary oxygen therapy in chronic hypoxic cor pulmonale complicating chronic bronchitis and emphysema. Lancet 1981;1:681–5.
5. National Emphysema Treatment Trial Research Group. A randomized trial comparing lung-volume-reduction surgery with medical therapy for severe emphysema. N Engl J Med 2003;348:2059–73.
6. Calverley PM, Anderson JA, Celli B, et al; TORCH Investigators. Salmeterol and fluticasone propionate and survival in chronic obstructive pulmonary disease. N Engl J Med 2007;356:775–89.
7. Nici L, Donner C, Wouters E, et al; ATS/ERS Pulmonary Rehabilitation Writing Committee. American Thoracic Society/European Respiratory Society statement on pulmonary rehabilitation. Am J Respir Crit Care Med 2006;173:1390–413.
8. Patterson G, Maurer J, Williams T, et al. Comparison of outcomes of double and single lung transplantation for obstructive lung disease. J Thorac Cardiovasc Surg 1999;110:623–32.
9. Nichol KL, Baken L, Nelson A. Relation between influenza vaccination and outpatient visits, hospitalization, and mortality in elderly persons with chronic lung disease. Ann Intern Med 1999;130:397–403.
10. Nichol KL, Mendelman PM, Mallon KP, et al. Effectiveness of live, attenuated intranasal influenza virus vaccine in healthy, working adults: a randomized controlled trial. JAMA 1999;282:137–44.
11. Belman MJ, Botnick WC, Shin JW. Inhaled bronchodilators reduce dynamic hyperinflation during exercise in patients with chronic obstructive pulmonary disease. Am J Respir Crit Care Med 1996;153:967–75.
12. O'Donnell D, Lam M, Webb K. Spirometric correlates of improvement in exercise performance after anticholinergic therapy in chronic obstructive pulmonary disease. Am J Respir Crit Care Med 1999;160:542–9.
13. O'Donnell D, Voduc N, Fitzpatrick M, Webb K. Effect of salmeterol on the ventilatory response to exercise in chronic obstructive pulmonary disease. Eur Respir J 2004;24:86–94
14. O'Donnell D, Flugre T, Gerken F, et al. Effects of tiotropium on lung hyperinflation, dyspnea and exercise tolerance in COPD. Eur Respir J 2004;23:832–40.
15. Celli B, ZuWallack R, Wang S, Kesten S. Improvement of inspiratory capacity and hyperinflation with tiotropium in COPD patients with severe hyperinflation. Chest 2003;124:1743–8.
16. O'Donnell DE, Sciurba F, Celli B, et al. Effect of fluticasone propionate/salmeterol on lung hyperinflation and exercise endurance in COPD. Chest 2006;130:647–56.
17. Marin J, Carrizo S, Gascon M, et al. Inspiratory capacity, dynamic hyperinflation, breathlessness and exercise performance during the 6 minute walk test in chronic obstructive pulmonary disease. Am J Respir Crit Care Med 2001;163:1395–400.
18. Martinez F, Montes de Oca M, Whyte R, et al. Lung-volume reduction surgery improves dyspnea, dynamic hyperinflation and respiratory muscle function. Am J Respir Crit Care Med 1997;155:2018–23.

19. Casanova C, Cote C, de Torres JP, et al. Inspiratory-to-total lung capacity ratio predicts mortality in patients with chronic obstructive pulmonary disease. Am J Respir Crit Care Med 2005;171:591–7.

20. Agustí AG, Noguera A, Sauleda J, et al. Systemic effects of chronic obstructive pulmonary disease. Eur Respir J 2003;21:347–60.

21. Nishimura K, Izumi T, Tsukino M, Oga T. Dyspnea is a better predictor of 5-year survival than airway obstruction in patients with COPD. Chest 2002;121:1434–40.

22. Schols AM, Slangen J, Volovics L, Wouters EF. Weight loss is a reversible factor in the prognosis of chronic obstructive pulmonary disease. Am J Respir Crit Care Med 1998;157:1791–7.

23. Landbo C, Prescott E, Lange P, et al. Prognostic value of nutritional status in chronic obstructive pulmonary disease. Am J Respir Crit Care Med 1999;160:1856–61.

24. Gerardi DA, Lovett L, Benoit-Connors ML, et al. Variables related to increased mortality following out-patient pulmonary rehabilitation. Eur Respir J 1996;9:431–5.

25. Pinto-Plata VM, Cote C, Cabral H, et al. The 6-minute walk distance: change over time and value as a predictor of survival in severe COPD. Eur Respir J 2004;23:28–33.

26. Celli BR, Cote CG, Marin JM, et al. The body mass index, airflow obstruction, dyspnea and exercise capacity index in chronic obstructive pulmonary disease. N Engl J Med 2004;350:1005–12.

27. Cote CG, Dordelly LJ, Celli BR. Impact of COPD exacerbations on patient centered outcomes. Chest 2007;131:696–704.

28. Imsfeld S, Bloch KE, Weder W, Russi EW. The BODE index after lung volume reduction surgery correlates with survival. Chest 2006;129:835–6.

29. Kottke TE, Battista RN, DeFriese GH. Attributes of successful smoking cessation interventions in medical practice: a meta-analysis of 39 controlled trials. JAMA 1988;259:2882–9.

30. Anthonisen NR, Connett JE, Kiley JP, et al, for the Lung Health Study Group. The effects of smoking intervention and the use of an inhaled anticholinergic bronchodilator on the rate of decline of FEV_1: the Lung Health Study. JAMA 1994;272:1497–505.

31. Anthonisen NR, Skeans MA, Wise RA, et al; Lung Health Study Research Group. The effects of a smoking cessation intervention on 14.5-year mortality: a randomized clinical trial. Ann Intern Med 2005;142:233–9.

32. Fiore M, Bailey W, Cohen S, et al. Treating tobacco use and dependence. Rockville (MD): US Department of Health and Human Services; June 2000.

33. Jorenby DE, Leischow SG, Nides MA, et al. A controlled trial of sustained release buproprion, a nicotine patch or both for smoking cessation. N Engl J Med 1999;340:685–91.

34. Keating GM, Siddiqui MA. Varenicline: a review of its use as an aid to smoking cessation therapy. CNS Drugs 2006;20:945–80.

35. Chalker R, Celli B. Special considerations in the elderly. Clin Chest Med 1993;14:437–52.

36. Dahl R, Greefhorst LA, Nowak D, et al. Inhaled formoterol dry powder versus ipratropium bromide in chronic obstructive pulmonary disease. Am J Respir Crit Care Med 2001;164:778–84.

37. Tantucci C, Duguet A, Similowski T, et al. Effect of salbutamol on dynamic hyperinflation in chronic obstructive pulmonary disease patients. Eur Respir J 1998;12:799–804.

38. Rennard SI, Anderson W, ZuWallack R, et al. Use of a long-acting inhaled beta2-adrenergic agonist, salmeterol xinafoate, in patients with chronic obstructive pulmonary disease. Am J Respir Crit Care Med 2001;163:1087–92.

39. Ramirez-Venegas A, Ward J, Lentine T, Mahler D. Salmeterol reduces dyspnea and improves lung function in patients with COPD. Chest 1997;112:336–40.

40. Niwehowener D, Rice K, Cote C, et al. Prevention of exacerbations of chronic obstructive pulmonary disease with tiotropium, a once daily anticholinergic: a randomized trial. Ann Intern Med 2005;143:317–26.

41. Decramer M, Celli B, Tashkin D, et al. Clinical trial design considerations in assessing long-term functional impacts of tiotropium. J COPD 2004;1:303–12.

42. Karpel JP, Kotch A, Zinny M, et al. A comparison of inhaled ipratropium, oral theophylline plus inhaled β-agonist, and the combination of all three in patients with COPD. Chest 1994;105:1089–94.

43. Barnes PJ, Ito K, Adcock IM. Corticosteroid resistance in chronic obstructive pulmonary disease: inactivation of histone deacetylase. Lancet 2004;363:731–3.

44. Rabe K, Bateman E, O'Donnell D, et al. Roflumilast-an oral anti-inflammatory treatment for chronic obstructive pulmonary disease: a randomized controlled trial. Lancet 2005;366:563–71.

45. Rennard S, Schachter N, Strek M, et al. Cilomilast for COPD: results of a 6-month, placebo controlled study of a potent, selective inhibitor of posphodiesterase 4. Chest 2006;129:56–66.

46. Mahler D, Huang S, Tabrizzi M, Bell G. Efficacy and safety of a monoclonal antibody recognizing interleukin-8 in COPD: a pilot study. Chest 2004;126:926–34.

47. Rennard S, Fogarty C, Kelsen S, et al. The safety and efficacy of infliximab in moderate to severe chronic obstructive pulmonary disease Am J Respir Crit Care Med 2007;175:926–34.

48. Vestbo J; TORCH Study Group. The TORCH (Towards a Revolution in COPD Health) survival study protocol. Eur Respir J 2004;24:206–10.

49. Pauwels R, Lofdahl C, Laitinen L, et al. Long-term treatment with inhaled budesonide in persons with mild chronic obstructive pulmonary disease who continue smoking. N Engl J Med 1999;340:1948–53.

50. Vestbo J, Sorensen T, Lange P, et al. Long-term effect of inhaled budesonide in mild and moderate chronic obstructive pulmonary disease: a randomised trial. Lancet 1999;353:1819–23.

51. Sin DD, Tu JV. Inhaled corticosteroids and the risk for mortality and readmission in elderly patients with chronic obstructive pulmonary disease. Am J Respir Crit Care Med 2001;164:580–4.

52. Soriano JB, Vestbo J, Pride N, et al. Survival in COPD patients after regular use of fluticasone propionate and salmeterol in general practice. Eur Respir J 2002;20:819–24.

53. Calverley PM, Boonsawat W, Cseke Z, et al. Maintenance therapy with budesonide and formoterol in chronic obstructive pulmonary disease. Eur Respir J 2003;22:912–9.

54. Szafranski W, Cukier A, Ramirez A, et al. Efficacy and safety of budesonide/formoterol in the management of COPD. Eur Respir J 2003;21:74–81.

55. Cazzola M, Dahl R. Inhaled combination therapy with inhaled long-acting beta-2-agonist and corticosteroids in stable COPD. Chest 2004;126:220–37.

56. Aaron S, Vandemheen KL, Fergusson D, et al. Tiotropium in combination with placebo, salmeterol or fluticasone-salmeterol for treatment of chronic obstructive pulmonary disease: a randomized trial. Ann Intern Med 2007;146:545–55.

57. COMBIVENT Inhalation Aerosol Study Group. In chronic obstructive pulmonary disease, a combination of ipratropium and albuterol is more effective than either agent alone. An 85-day multicenter trial. Chest 1994;105:1411–9.

58. Van Noord J, Aumann J, Jasnseens E, et al. Comparison of tiotropium q.d, formoterol bid and both combined qd in patients with COPD. Eur Respir J 2005;26:214–22.

59. Petty TL. The National Mucolytic Study: results of a randomized, double-blind, placebo-controlled study of iodinated glycerol in chronic obstructive bronchitis. Chest 1990;97:75–83.

60. Decramer M, Rutten-van Molken M, Dekhuijzen PN, et al. Effects of N-acetylcysteine on outcomes in chronic obstructive pulmonary disease (Bronchitis Randomized on NAC Cost-Utility Study, BRONCUS): a randomised placebo-controlled trial. Lancet 2005;365:1552–60.

61. Anthonisen NR, Manfreda J, Warren CPW, et al. Antibiotic therapy in exacerbations of chronic obstructive pulmonary disease. Ann Intern Med 1987;106:196–204.

62. Saint S, Bent S, Vittinghoff F, Grady D. Antibiotics in chronic obstructive pulmonary disease exacerbation. A metanalysis. JAMA 1995;273:957–60.

63. Stockley R, O'Bryan C, Pie A, Hill S. Relationship of sputum color to nature and outpatient management of acute exacerbation of COPD. Chest 2000;117:1638–45.

64. Miravitlles M. Epidemiology of chronic obstructive pulmonary disease exacerbations. Clin Pulm Med 2002;9:191–7.

65. Adams SG, Melo J, Luther M, Anzueto A. Antibiotics are associated with lower relapse rates in outpatients with acute exacerbations of COPD. Chest 2000;117:1345–52.

66. Dirksen A, Dijkman JH, Madsen F, et al. A randomized clinical trial of alpha(1)-antitrypsin augmentation therapy. Am J Respir Crit Care Med 1999;160:1468–72.

67. Sandhaus R. Alpha-1-antitrypsin deficiency : new and emerging therapies for alpha-1 antytripsin deficiency. Thorax 2004;59:904–9.

68. Nichol KL, Baken L, Nelson A. Relation between influenza vaccination and outpatient visits, hospitalization, and mortality in elderly persons with chronic lung disease. Ann Intern Med 1999;130:397–403.

69. Nichol KL, Mendelman PM, Mallon KP, et al. Effectiveness of live, attenuated intranasal influenza virus vaccine in healthy, working adults: a randomized controlled trial. JAMA 1999;282:137–44.

70. Reardon J, Awad E, Normandin E, et al. The effect of comprehensive outpatient pulmonary rehabilitation on dyspnea. Chest 1994;105:1046–52.

71. Goldstein RS, Gork EH, Stubbing D, et al. Randomized controlled trial of respiratory rehabilitation. Lancet 1994;344:1394–7.

72. Wijkstra PJ, Van Altens R, Kraan J, et al. Quality of life in patients with chronic obstructive pulmonary disease improves after rehabilitation at home. Eur Respir J 1994;7:269–73.

73. Bendstrup KE, Ingenman Jensen J, Holm S, Bengtsson B. Out-patient rehabilitation improves activities of daily living, quality of life, and exercise tolerance in chronic obstructive pulmonary disease. Eur Respir J 1997;10:2801–6.

74. Griffiths TL, Burr ML, Campbell IA, et al. Results at 1 year of outpatient multidisciplinary pulmonary rehabilitation: a randomized controlled trial. Lancet 2000;355:362–8.

75. Guell R, Casan P, Belda J, et al. Long-term effects of outpatient rehabilitation of COPD: a randomized trial. Chest 2000;117:976–83.

76. Wedzicha JA, Bestall JC, Garrod R, et al. Randomised controlled trial of pulmonary rehabilitation in severe chronic obstructive pulmonary disease patients, stratified with the MRC dyspnoea scale. Eur Respir J 1998;12:363–9.

77. Trooster T, Gosselink R, Decramer M. Short and long term effects of outpatients pulmonary rehabilitation in chronic obstructive pulmonary disease: a randomized trial. Am J Med 2000;109:207–12.

78. Maltais F., LeBlanc P, Simard C et al. Skeletal muscle adaptation to endurance training in patients with chronic obstructive pulmonary disease. Am J Respir Crit Care Med 1996;154:436–44.

79. Ries AL, Kaplan RM, Limberg TM, Prewitt LM. The effects of pulmonary rehabilitation on physiologic and psychosocial outcomes in patients with chronic obstructive pulmonary disease. Ann Intern Med 1995;122:823–32.

80. Ries A, Kaplan R, Myers R, Prewett L. Maintenance after rehabilitation in lung disease. A randomized trial. Am J Respir Crit Care Med 2003;167:880–8.

81. Belman MJ, Kendregan BA. Exercise training fails to increase skeletal muscle enzymes in patients with chronic obstructive pulmonary disease. Am Rev Respir Dis 1981;123:256–61.

82. Casaburi, R. Exercise training in chronic obstructive lung disease. In: Casaburi R, Petty TL (eds). Principles and practice of pulmonary rehabilitation. Philadelphia: WB Saunders, 1993.

83. O'Hara WJ, Lasachuk, BP, Matheson P, et al. Weight training and backpacking in chronic obstructive pulmonary disease. Respir Care 1984;29:1202–10.

84. Maltais F, Simard A, Simard J, et al. Oxidative capacity of the skeletal muscle and lactic acid kinetics during exercise in normal subjects and in patients with COPD. Am J Respir Crit Care Med 1995;153:288–93.

85. Casaburi R, Patessio A, Ioli F, et al. Reductions in exercise lactic acidosis and ventilation as a result of exercise training in patients with obstructive lung disease. Am Rev Respir Dis 1991;143:9–18.

86. ZuWallack R, Patel K, Reardon J, et al. Predictors of improvement in the 12-minute walking distance following a six-week outpatient pulmonary rehabilitation program. Chest 1991;99:805–8.

87. Celli B, Criner G, Rassulo J. Ventilatory muscle recruitment during unsupported arm exercise in normal subjects. J Appl Physiol 1988;64:1936–41.

88. Celli B, Rassulo J, Make B. Dyssynchronous breathing associated with arm but not leg exercise in patients with COPD. N Engl J Med 1986;314:1485–90.

89. Criner G, Celli B. Effect of unsupported arm exercise on ventilatory muscle recruitment in patients with severe chronic airflow obstruction. Am Rev Respir Dis 1988;138:856–67.

90. Ries A, Ellis B, Hawkins R. Upper extremity exercise training in chronic obstructive pulmonary disease. Chest 1988;93:688–92.

91. Martinez F, Vogel P, DuPont D, et al. Supported arm exercise vs. unsupported arm exercise in the rehabilitation of patients with chronic airflow obstruction. Chest 1993;103:1397–1402.

92. Keens T, Krastins I, Wannamaker E, et al. Ventilatory muscle endurance training in normal subjects and patients with cystic fibrosis. Am Rev Respir Dis 1977;116:853–60.

93. Couser J, Martinez F, Celli B. Pulmonary rehabilitation that includes arm exercise, reduces metabolic and ventilatory requirements for simple arm elevation. Chest 1993;103:37–8.

94. Epstein S, Celli B, Martinez F, et al. Arm training reduces the VO_2 and VE cost of unsupported arm exercise and elevation in chronic obstructive pulmonary disease. J Cardiopulm Rehabil 1997;17:171–7.

95. Roa J, Epstein S, Breslin E, et al. Work of breathing and ventilatory muscle recruitment during pursed lip breathing. Am Rev Respir Dis 1991;143:A77.

96. Leith D, Bradley M. Ventilatory muscle strength and endurance training. J Appl Physiol 1976;4:508–16.

97. Roussos C, Macklem P. The respiratory muscles. N Engl J Med 1982;307:786–97.

98. American Thoracic Society/European Respiratory Society. ATS/ERS statement on respiratory muscle testing. Am J Respir Crit Care Med 2002;166:518–624.

99. Gething AD, Williams M, Davies B. Inspiratory resistive loading improves cycling capacity: a placebo controlled trial. Br J Sports Med 2004;38:730–6.

100. Weiner P, Azgad Y, Ganam R, et al. Inspiratory muscle training in patients with bronchial asthma. Chest 1992;102:1357–61.

101. Sawyer EH, Clanton TL. Improved pulmonary function and exercise tolerance with inspiratory muscle conditioning in children with cystic fibrosis. Chest 1993;104:1490–7.

102. Cahalin LP, Semigran MJ, Dec GW. Inspiratory muscle training in patients with chronic heart failure awaiting cardiac transplantation: results of a pilot clinical trial. Phys Ther 1997;77:830–8.

103. Rutchik A, Weissman AR, Almenoff PL, et al. Resistive inspiratory muscle training in subjects with chronic cervical spinal cord injury. Arch Phys Rehabil 1998;79:293–7.

104. Wanke T, Toifl K, Merkle M, et al. Inspiratory muscle training in patients with Duchenne muscular dystrophy. Chest 1994;105:475–82.

105. Nomori H, Kobayashi R, Fuyuno G, et al. Preoperative respiratory muscle training: assessment in thoracic surgery patients with special reference to postoperative pulmonary complications. Chest 1994;105:1782–8.

106. Belman MJ, Botnick WC, Nathan SD, et al. Ventilatory load characteristics during ventilatory muscle training. Am J Respir Crit Care Med 1994;149:925–9.

107. Levine S, Weiser P, Gillen J. Evaluation of a ventilatory muscle endurance training program in the rehabilitation of patients with chronic obstructive pulmonary disease. Am Rev Respir Dis 1986;133:400–6.

108. Scherer TA, Spengler CM, Owassapian D, et al. Respiratory muscle endurance training in chronic obstructive pulmonary disease. Am J Respir Crit Care Med 2000;162:1709–14.

109. Pardy RL, Rivington RN, Despas PJ, et al. Inspiratory muscle training compared with physiotherapy in patients with chronic airflow limitation. Am Rev Respir Dis 1981;123:421–5.

110. Larson JL, Kim MJ, Sharp JT, et al. Inspiratory muscle training with a pressure threshold breathing device in patients with chronic obstructive pulmonary disease. Am Rev Respir Dis 1988;138:689–96.

111. Harver A, Mahler DA, Daubenspeck JA. Targeted inspiratory muscle training improves respiratory muscle function and reduces dyspnea in patients with chronic obstructive pulmonary disease. Ann Intern Med 1989;111:117–24.

112. Guyatt G, Keller J, Singer J, et al. Controlled trial of respiratory muscle training in chronic airflow limitation. Thorax 1992;47:598–602.

113. Lisboa C, Munoz V, Beroiza KT, et al. Inspiratory muscle training in chronic airflow limitation: comparison of two different training loads with a threshold device. Eur Respir J 1994;7:1266–74.

114. Preusser BA, Winningham ML, Clanton TL. High-vs low-intensity inspiratory muscle interval training in patients with COPD. Chest 1994;106:110–7.

115. Lisboa C, Villafranca C, Leiva A, et al. Inspiratory muscle training in chronic airflow limitation: effect on exercise performance. Eur Respir J 1997;10:537–42.

116. Riera HS, Rubio TM, Ruiz FO, et al. Inspiratory muscle training in patients with COPD. Chest 2001;120:748–56.

117. Covey MK, Larson JL, Wirtz SE, et al. High-intensity inspiratory muscle training in patients with chronic obstructive pulmonary disease and severely reduced function. J Cardiopulm Rehabil 2001;21:231–40.

118. Weiner P, Magadle R, Beckerman M, et al. Comparison of specific expiratory, inspiratory, and combined muscle training program in COPD. Chest 2003;124:1357–64.

119. Weiner P, Magadle R, Beckerman M, et al. Maintenance of inspiratory muscle training in COPD patients: one year followup. Eur Respir J 2004;23:61–5.

120. Beckerman M, Magadle R, Weiner M, Weiner P. The effects of 1 year of specific inspiratory muscle training in patients with COPD. Chest 2005;128:3177–82.

121. Koppers RJH, Vos PJE, Boot CRL, Folgering HTM. Exercise performance improves in patients with COPD due to respiratory muscle endurance training. Chest 2006;129:886–92.

122. Hill K, Jenkins SC, Phillippe DL, et al. High-intensity inspiratory muscle training in COPD. Eur Respir J 2006;27:1119–28.

123. Belman MJ, Mittman C. Ventilatory muscle training improves exercise capacity in chronic obstructive pulmonary disease patients. Am Rev Respir Dis 1980;121:273–80.

124. Ries A, Moser K. Comparison of isocapneic hyperventilation and walking exercise training at home in pulmonary rehabilitation. Chest 1986;90:285–9.

125. Belman MJ. Respiratory failure treated by ventilatory muscle training (VMT): a report of two cases. Eur J Respir Dis 1981;62:391–3.

126. Aldrich TK, Karpel JP, Uhrlass RM. Weaning from mechanical ventilation: adjunctive use of inspiratory muscle resistive training. Crit Care 1989;17:143–7.

127. Bellemare F, Grassino A. Evaluation of diaphragmatic fatigue. J Appl Physiol 1982;53:1196–206.

128. Brochard L, Mancebo J, Wysocki M, et al. Noninvasive ventilation for acute exacerbation of chronic obstructive pulmonary disease. N Engl J Med 1995;333:817–22.

129. Bott J, Carroll P, Conway J. Randomised controlled trial of nasal ventilation in acute ventilatory failure due to chronic obstructive airways disease. Lancet 1993;341:1555–7.

130. Kramer N, Meyer T, Meharg J, et al. Randomized prospective trial of non-invasive positive pressure ventilation in acute respiratory failure. Am J Respir Crit Care Med 1995;151:1799–806.

131. Braun N, Marino W. Effect of daily intermittent rest of respiratory muscles in patients with severe chronic airflow limitation. Chest 1984;85:59–62.

132. Zibrak J, Hill NS, Federman E, et al. Evaluation of intermittent long-term negative pressure ventilation in patients with severe chronic obstructive pulmonary disease. Am Rev Respir Dis 1988;138:1515–20.

133. Celli, B, Lee H, Criner G, et al. Controlled trial of external negative pressure ventilation in patients with severe chronic airflow limitation. Am Rev Respir Dis 1989;140:1251–7.

134. Shapiro S, Ernst P, Gray-Donald K, et al. Effect of negative pressure ventilation in severe pulmonary disease. Lancet 1992;340:1425–8.

135. Meecham-Jones J, Paul E, Jones P, Wedzicha J. Nasal pressure support ventilation plus oxygen compared with oxygen therapy alone in hypercapnic COPD. Am J Respir Crit Care Med 1995;152:538–44.

136. Strumpf D, Millman RP, Carlisle C, et al. Nocturnal positive-pressure ventilation via nasal mask in patients with severe chronic obstructive pulmonary disease. Am Rev Respir Dis 1991;144:415–20.

137. Casanova C, Celli BR, Tost L, et al. Long-term controlled trial of nocturnal nasal positive pressure ventilation in patients with severe COPD. Chest 2000;118:1582–90.

138. Clinic E, Sturani C, Rossi A, et al. The Italian multicenter study on non-invasive ventilation in chronic obstructive pulmonary disease patients. Eur Respir J 2002;20:529–38.

139. Schols AM, Slangen J, Volovics L, Wouters EF. Weight loss is a reversible factor in the prognosis of chronic obstructive pulmonary disease. Am J Respir Crit Care Med 1998;157:1791–7.

140. Cote C, Zilberberg M, Modym S, Celli B. Hemoglobin level and its clinical impact in a cohort of patients with COPD. Eur Respir J 2007;29:923–9.

141. Petty TL, Finigan MM. Clinical evaluation of prolonged ambulatory oxygen therapy in chronic airway obstruction. Am J Med 1968;45:242–52.

142. Weitzenblum E, Sautegeau A, Ehrhart M, et al. Long-term oxygen therapy can reverse the progression of pulmonary hypertension in patients with chronic obstructive pulmonary disease. Am Rev Respir Dis 1985;131:493–8.

143. Lopez-Majano V, Dutton RE. Regulation of respiratory drive during oxygen breathing in chronic obsructive lung disease. Am Rev Respir Dis 1973;108:232–40.

144. Krop AD, Block AJ, Cohen E. Neuropsychiatric effects of continuous oxygen therapy in chronic obstructive pulmonary disease. Chest 1973;64:317–22.

145. Tarpy S, Celli B. Long-term oxygen therapy. N Engl J Med 1995;333:710–4.

146. O'Donohue WJ. Effect of oxygen therapy on increasing arterial oxygen tension in hypoxemia patients with stable chronic obstructive pulmonary disease while breathing ambient air. Chest 1991;100:968–72.

147. Criner G, Celli BR. Ventilatory muscle recruitment in exercise with O_2 in obstructed patients with mild hypoxemia. J Appl Physiol 1987;63:195–200.

148. West GA, Primeau P. Nonmedical hazards of long-term oxygen therapy. Respir Care 1983;8:906–12.

149. Dunn WF, Nelson SB, Hubmayr RD. Oxygen-induced hypercarbia in obstructive pulmonary disease. Am Rev Respir Dis 1991;144:526–30.

150. Aubier M, Murciano D, Milic-Emili M, et al. Effects of the administration of oxygen therapy on ventilation and blood gases in patients with chronic obstructive pulmonary disease during acute respiratory failure Am Rev Respir Dis 1980;122:747–52.

151. Jackson RM. Pulmonary oxygen toxicity. Chest 1985;88:900–5.

152. Tiep BL, Christopher KL, Spofford BT, et al. Pulsed nasal and transtracheal oxygen delivery. Chest 1990;97:364–8.

153. Christopher KL, Spofford BT, Petrun MD, et al. A program for transtracheal oxygen delivery: assessment of safety and efficacy. Ann Intern Med 1987;107:802–6.

154. Hoffman LA, Wesmiller SW, Sciurba FC, et al. Nasal cannula and transtracheal oxygen delivery: comparison of patient response after six months use of each technique. Am Rev Respir Dis 1992;145:827–31.

155. Benditt J, Pollock M, Celli B. Transtracheal delivery of gas decreases the oxygen cost of breathing. Am Rev Respir Dis 1993;147:1207–10.

156. Donaldson GC, Seemungal TA, Bhowmik A, Wedzicha JA. Relationship between exacerbation frequency and lung function decline in chronic obstructive pulmonary disease. Thorax 2002;57:847–52.

157. Connors AF Jr, Dawson NV, Thomas C, et al. Outcomes following acute exacerbation of severe chronic obstructive lung disease. The SUPPORT investigators (Study to Understand Prognoses and Preferences for Outcomes and Risks of Treatments). Am J Respir Crit Care Med 1996;154:959–67.

158. Dewan NA, Rafique S, Kanwar B, et al. Acute exacerbation of COPD: factors associated with poor treatment outcome. Chest 2000;117:662–71.

159. Wedzicha JA. Role of viruses in exacerbations of chronic obstructive pulmonary disease. Proc Am Thorac Soc 2004;1:115–20.

160. Stockley RA, Bayley D, Hill SL, et al. Assessment of airway neutrophils by sputum colour: correlation with airways inflammation. Thorax 2001;56:366–72.

161. Davies L, Angus RM, Calverley PM. Oral corticosteroids in patients admitted to hospital with exacerbations of chronic obstructive pulmonary disease: a prospective randomised controlled trial. Lancet 1999;354:456–60.

162. Sayiner A, Aytemur ZA, Cirit M, Unsal I. Systemic glucocorticoids in severe exacerbations of COPD. Chest 2001;119:726–30.

163. Niewoehner DE, Erbland ML, Deupree RH, et al. Effect of systemic glucocorticoids on exacerbations of chronic obstructive pulmonary disease. N Engl J Med 1999;340:1941–7.

164. Aaron SD, Vandemheen KL, Hebert P, et al. Outpatient oral prednisone after emergency treatment of chronic obstructive pulmonary disease. N Engl J Med 2003;348:2618–25.

165. Maltais F, Ostinelli J, Bourbeau J, et al. Comparison of nebulized budesonide and oral prednisolone with placebo in the treatment of acute exacerbations of chronic obstructive pulmonary disease: a randomized controlled trial. Am J Respir Crit Care Med 2002;165:698–703.

166. Groenewegen KH, Wouters EF. Bacterial infections in patients requiring admission for an acute exacerbation of COPD; a 1-year prospective study. Respir Med 2003;97:770–7.

167. Ellis DA, Anderson IM, Stewart SM, et al. Exacerbations of chronic bronchitis: exogenous or endogenous infection? Br J Dis Chest 1978;72:115–21.

168. Wilson R, Jones P, Schaberg T, et al. Antibiotic treatment and factors influencing short and long term outcomes of acute exacerbations of chronic bronchitis. Thorax 2006;61:337–42.

169. Allegra L, Blasi F, de Bernardi B, et al. Antibiotic treatment and baseline severity of disease in acute exacerbations of chronic bronchitis: a re-evaluation of previously published data of a placebo-controlled randomized study. Pulm Pharmacol Ther 2001;14:149–55.

170. Celli BR. Chronic obstructive pulmonary disease: from unjustified nihilism to evidence-based optimism. Proc Am Thorac Soc 2006;3:58–65.

CHAPTER 27

SURGICAL THERAPY FOR CHRONIC OBSTRUCTIVE PULMONARY DISEASE

MARTIN R. ZAMORA, MD

EMPHYSEMA is characterized by airspace destruction and loss of the pulmonary capillary bed, resulting in the loss of elastic recoil, airflow limitation, hyperinflation, and ventilation-perfusion mismatching. These, in turn, lead to increased work of breathing, respiratory muscle fatigue, and the sensation of dyspnea. In chronic severe disease, dyspnea and exercise intolerance become very disabling for patients with emphysema. The lack of effective medical therapy to reverse these physiologic changes has prompted the development of surgical intervention for the treatment of emphysema. A variety of operative techniques aimed at correcting the underlying pathophysiology and/or alleviating symptoms and dyspnea in patients with chronic obstructive pulmonary disease (COPD) have been reported throughout the surgical literature. Thorough reviews of the history of surgery for emphysema were published by Knudson and Gaensler in 1965,[1] Deslauriers in 1995,[2] and Cooper in 1997[3] and in the first edition of this book.[4]

Initially, operations were designed to correct the anatomic deficiencies that were presumed to be the cause of the disease. The techniques of costochondrectomy and transverse sternotomy were designed to increase the mobilization of the chest wall to permit further hyperinflation of the lungs, whereas thoracoplasty and phrenic nerve interruption were designed to decrease lung volume. These operations were quickly abandoned as it was recognized that they decreased the motion of the hemidiaphragm and of the opposite hemithorax. Laforet commented on these early procedures, writing that "The alleged benefits of those maneuvers were frequently lost on patients whose worsened dyspnea left them little energy with which to debate their surgeons."[5]

Attempts to restore the normal diaphragmatic contour and motion included the use of abdominal belts, intermittent abdominal compression, and pneumoperitoneum. Although reported to improve symptoms and diaphragmatic excursion, these procedures were abandoned as being too impractical. Vagotomy, sympathectomy, and total lung denervation were all proposed for relieving dyspnea, bronchial reactivity, and excessive secretions, but these early procedures did not withstand the test of time. Glomectomy, or resection of the carotid body to relieve dyspnea, was initially reported by Nakayama in 1961 (involving almost 4,000 patients)[6] and later by Overholt (involving 800 patients)[7] and was one of the most controversial procedures in the history of surgical therapy for emphysema. The physiologic principle forming the rationale for this procedure was unclear. Although the majority of patients reported that they benefited from the procedure, it took several randomized double-blind studies (including control patients who received sham operations) to prove the lack of efficacy of this procedure.

Three procedures have been shown to significantly improve postoperative physiologic function and quality of life. Reduction pneumoplasty for giant bullous emphysema has been used for more than four decades and remains useful in patients with that form of emphysema. The technique of multiple wedge resections or lung volume reduction surgery (LVRS) was performed by Brantigan and colleagues in 1959,[8] and although patients reported a decrease in their sensation of dyspnea, little objective improvement was seen in postoperative studies, and this procedure was abandoned until recently. Cooper and colleagues reported preliminary findings in 20 patients undergoing bilateral volume reduction via median sternotomy, showing improvement in dyspnea, quality of life, and pulmonary function.[9] The renewed enthusiasm for and widespread expansion of LVRS led to the development of the landmark National Emphysema Treatment Trial (NETT). Immunosuppressive therapy, advances in surgical technique, and the realization of the critical importance of patient selection have resulted in the widespread use of lung transplantation for the treatment of emphysema.

One must remember that surgical therapy for emphysema is usually an elective procedure, and as such, all efforts should be taken to instruct the patient in the techniques of coughing, deep breathing, and chest physiotherapy. Smoking cessation is an absolute in the selection of appropriate candidates for these procedures. Medical therapy should be optimized to reverse airway obstruction, bronchospasm, and intercurrent pulmonary infections prior to surgery. Cessation of or a reduction in corticosteroids should be achieved as they may be associated with poor tissue healing and prolonged air leaks. Intensive pulmonary rehabilitation prior to the planned procedure is critical to successful outcomes following bullectomy, LVRS, or lung transplantation.

Reduction Pneumoplasty for Giant Bullous Emphysema
Rationale and Indications for Surgery

Bullectomy is performed to (1) relieve compressive changes in normal lung adjacent to a giant bulla, (2) increase compliance and airway diameter in the remaining lung, (3) improve ventilation-perfusion matching, (4) decrease dead-space ventilation, (5) decrease elevated intrathoracic pressure, and (6) treat complications related to the bulla.[10] The decision to operate on symptomatic patients with giant bullae (Figure 1) and otherwise normal lung function is not difficult. More

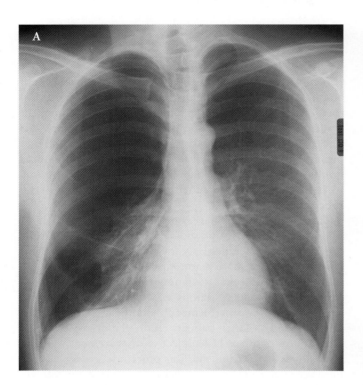

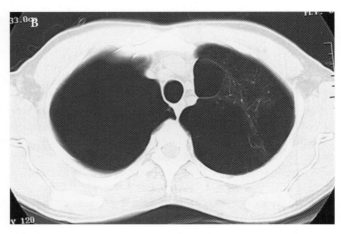

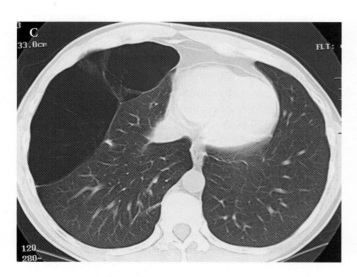

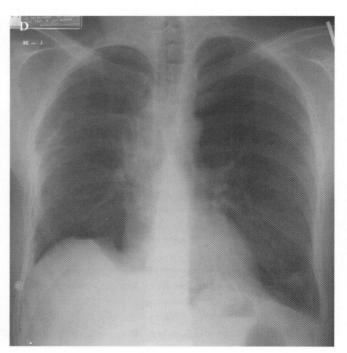

FIGURE 1. *A,* Imaging of a 36-year-old man who was a heavy smoker with an abnormal chest radiograph and dyspnea on exertion noted prior to elective orthopedic surgery. Preoperative posteroanterior chest radiography demonstrates a right upper lobe giant bulla with right middle and lower lobe compression. Note the evidence of hyperinflation of the left hemithorax owing to concomitant emphysema. *B,* Computed tomographic scan of the right upper lobe bullae. *C,* Computed tomographic scan of the right upper lobe bulla with compression of the right middle lobe and evidence of diffuse emphysema in the underlying left upper lobe parenchyma but with relatively normal lower lobes bilaterally. *D,* Postoperative posteroanterior chest radiography shows reexpansion of the right middle and lower lobes and a change in the contour of the hemidiaphragm following a stapled right upper lobe bullectomy.

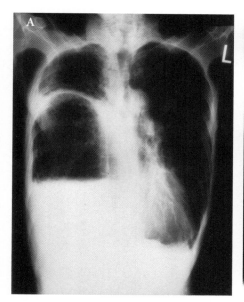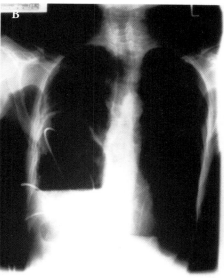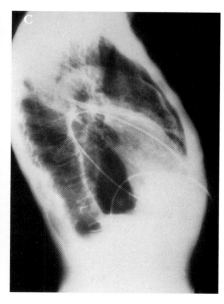

FIGURE 2. *A*, Posteroanterior chest radiograph of a patient with an infected bulla demonstrated by the presence of an air-fluid level. *B*, Posteroanterior chest radiograph shows tube thoracostomy drainage of the infected bulla. *C*, Lateral chest radiography shows tube thoracostomy drainage of the infected bulla.

problematic is the decision to operate on asymptomatic patients or on dyspneic patients with generalized emphysema.

In asymptomatic patients, surgery is indicated primarily for complications related to the bulla.[11] Bullae predispose patients to spontaneous pneumothoraces, which may be difficult to manage owing to further physiologic impairment of already limited patients, difficulty in diagnosing the pneumothorax in the presence of diffuse bullous disease, prolonged air leaks, and a high rate of recurrence. Chest pain occurring at rest or with exertion is related to overdistention of the bulla and to mediastinal shift. Infection of the bullae (Figure 2A) is uncommon and typically responds to conservative therapy; however, medical therapy may be unsuccessful owing to poor communication between the bronchial tree and the bulla. Surgical indications include infected fluid in the bulla, rupture into the pleural space, failure to respond to 4 to 6 weeks of antibiotic therapy, and hemoptysis. Bronchoscopy should be performed to rule out airway obstruction owing to bronchial carcinoma. Severely debilitated or high-risk patients may respond to percutaneous drainage by pigtail catheter (Figure 2, B and C). Hemoptysis owing to erosion of the bulla into an adjacent blood vessel is rare and should prompt a search to preoperatively rule out the possibility that the bleeding is from another lesion. Surgery is also indicated for lung cancer in scar tissue around the wall of the bulla. Rarely, surgery may be recommended to an asymptomatic patient with a giant bulla seen by chest radiography. Given that the natural history of untreated asymptomatic bullae is unpredictable and poorly documented,[12,13] it is generally agreed that surgery is indicated only if the bulla occupies more than half of the hemithorax or in patients with

high-risk occupations to reduce the risk of spontaneous pneumothorax.

In emphysema patients, it is critical to estimate the potential improvement in the function of the nonbullous lung and the effects of the bulla on the lung. Since the rationale for surgery is the restoration of elastic recoil and the reduction in airway and pulmonary vascular resistance, reexpansion of a previously compressed lung may increase vital capacity and forced expiratory volume in 1 second (FEV$_1$). Pulmonary vascular resistance may decrease, and a decrease in total lung volume may restore the normal curvature of the diaphragm, resulting in improved length-tension relationships and improved function. If the patient's symptoms are due primarily to emphysema, surgery is unlikely to help.

Selection for Surgery
CLINICAL AND PHYSIOLOGIC EVALUATION

Although no single preoperative variable is an absolute predictor of outcome, several variables (as determined by clinical, physiologic, and radiographic means) have been postulated to predict a favorable outcome (Table 1). Therefore, patients should undergo a thorough evaluation of their overall physical conditioning, pulmonary function and reserve, and cardiac status. This preoperative evaluation is designed to determine a patient's overall medical condition and his or her ability to withstand the risks of thoracotomy. Age, medical and surgical history (particularly of thoracic trauma or surgery), comorbid diseases, chronic bronchitis, cardiac status, smoking history, and unexplained weight loss are all important predictors of outcome.[14,15]

Clinical Parameter	Outcome Predictors	
	Good Outcome	Poor Outcome
Age	< 50 Yr	> 50 Yr
Comorbid disease	None	Present
Cardiac status	Normal	Right ventricular failure
Weight loss	< 10%	> 10%
Dyspnea	Rapidly progressive	Slowly progressive
PFTs		
FVC	Normal, or mild decrease	Markedly decreased
FEV$_1$	> 40%	< 35%
DL$_{CO}$	Normal	Decreased
PaO$_2$	Normal	Hypoxemia at rest or with exercise
PaCO$_2$	Normal	Increased
Imaging		
CXR	Bulla > 1/3 hemithorax; vascular crowding	Diffuse multiple small bullae; "vanishing lung" syndrome
CT	Large localized bullae with vascular crowding, normal-appearing lung adjacent to bulla	Multiple bilateral bullae; emphysema in lung
Angiography	Vascular crowding; normal distal vascular pattern	No crowding; "pruning" of distal vessels
V/Q scan	Localized matched defect; normal ventilation-perfusions in underlying lung	Diffuse defects; poor function in adjacent lung

Table 1 Selection Criteria for Bullectomy: Predictors of Outcomes

CT = computed tomography; CXR = chest radiography; DL$_{CO}$ = diffusion capacity for carbon monoxide; FEV$_1$ = forced expiratory volume in 1 second; FVC = forced vital capcity; PaCO$_2$ = partial pressure of arterial carbon dioxide; PaO$_2$ = partial pressure of arterial oxygen; PFTs = pulmonary-function tests; V/Q = ventilation-perfusion.

No single physiologic parameter will identify the patients who will benefit from bullectomy. Rather, a panel of pulmonary function tests may be associated with improved function postoperatively. Symptomatic and functional improvement is more likely in patients with an FEV$_1$ > 35% of predicted values,[16] those with a normal diffusing capacity,[17] or the absence of significant exercise hypoxemia. Although hypoxemia, hypercapnia, and pulmonary hypertension are not absolute contraindications to surgery, patients with these conditions should be considered with caution and carefully selected.[18] Patients requiring mechanical ventilation are rarely candidates for bullectomy. Pride and colleagues found that patients with low diffusing capacity or with higher compliance and larger total lung volume as measured by body plethysmo-graphy were more likely to have diffuse emphysema and unpredictable outcomes.[19] Gaensler and colleagues demonstrated that there is a good correlation between the size of localized bullae and FEV$_1$.[15] If the bulla occupies less than one-third of the hemithorax, severe dyspnea and a significant reduction in FEV$_1$ suggest that the symptoms are due to emphysema rather than the bulla. With large bullae, a discrepancy between the functional residual capacity as measured by plethysmography and gas dilution techniques suggests air trapping and a predominant effect of the bulla on overall pulmonary function.

IMAGING EVALUATION

Imaging studies are obtained to assess the underlying lung for its potential for reexpansion and improved function following removal of the bulla. Chest radiography serves as a valuable screening tool and provides important information on the size and progression of bullae. Bullae occupying more than 50% of the hemithorax are associated with better postoperative outcomes.[20] Typically, surgery is not indicated for bullae occupying less than 30% of the hemithorax.[21] Comparison with previous chest radiography can help determine the anatomic progression of the bulla, and in rapidly expanding bullae, surgery may be indicated rather than continued follow-up.[15] Complications of bullae, such as spontaneous pneumothorax, infection (see Figure 2A), or bleeding, may also be seen by chest radiography.

Angiography provides anatomic and functional information about the lung adjacent to a bulla. If the vasculature surrounding the bulla is crowded but intact (Figure 3), there is a high likelihood of reexpansion and improved function postoperatively. Thinning (or "pruning") of the vasculature or the lack of crowding suggests severe emphysema and poor outcomes after surgery.

Ventilation-perfusion scanning is effective in assessing vascular and parenchymal lung function and is the only technique that provides quantitative data on regional lung function. Bullae are depicted by matched ventilation and perfusion defects. Although the results of xenon 133 washout have been reported to predict a good surgical outcome,[16] most physicians use ventilation-perfusion scanning as a subjective estimate of lung function in the tissue adjacent to bullae.

Computed tomography (CT) has become the procedure of choice for evaluating patients for possible bullectomy as it is very sensitive for detecting the size and number of bullae, determining compression of the adjacent lung, and assessing the underlying lung tissue.[22] It is also useful for differentiating between large bullae and pneumothoraces. CT may show the presence of concomitant fibrotic lung disease not detected by chest radiography[20] and can also assess attenuation and displacement of the vasculature (see Figure 1, B and C) and the degree of lung destruction owing to emphysema.

Surgical Techniques

For a complete description of the various operative techniques of bullectomy, the reader is referred to reviews by Dartevelle and colleagues[23] and by Deslauriers.[2] In general, the bullectomy procedure aims to relieve compression while preserving all vascularized and potentially functioning lung tissue. This is best accomplished by limited resections such as local excision, plication of the bulla, or both.[24] Wakabayashi described the technique of thoracoscopic bullectomy using a neodymium:yttrium-aluminum-garnet (Nd:YAG) laser to cut or contract the bullae.[25] Lobectomies or segmentectomies are rarely necessary as bullous disease is seldom confined to segmental anatomy and as the hilum typically contains functioning lung tissue.[11] A variety of approaches have been described, including unilateral thoracotomy (Figure 4) or video-assisted thoracoscopic surgery (VATS). For patients with bilateral disease, exposure is gained via bilateral posterolateral thoracotomy or bilateral anterolateral thoracotomy (with or without transverse sternotomy) or through a median sternotomy.[26] All have been advocated, and each has its own advantages and disadvantages. Other surgeons prefer a two-stage bilateral procedure, which allows functional assessment of the first procedure before proceeding with the contralateral procedure.[24] In general, bilateral procedures should be limited to patients without severe emphysema, with the bullectomy done first on the lesser-functioning lung as determined by preoperative physiologic and imaging studies.[23] However, with the reemergence of LVRS, unilateral bullectomy with contralateral LVRS is becoming more common and can achieve acceptable outcomes in patients with bullae and severe emphysema. The final operative results may be adversely affected by persistent postoperative airspaces and prolonged air leaks, which may be limited by the use of pleural tents or buttressed staple lines with bovine pericardium (Peri-strips, Bio-Vascular, Inc., St. Paul, MN) or other materials.[12,27] The use of pleural abrasion by mechanical or chemical means may be necessary to achieve pleural symphysis,[23] but consideration of these measures must be evaluated in light of whether younger patients may require lung transplantation in the future.

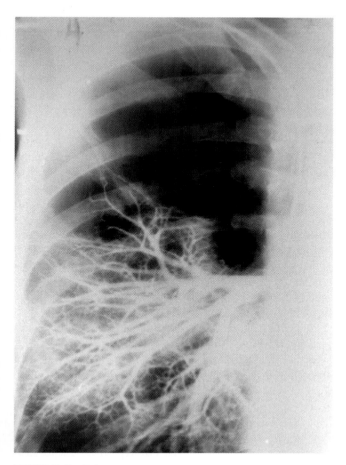

FIGURE 3. Pulmonary angiography demonstrates the preserved vascular pattern in the lung adjacent to a left upper lobe bulla.

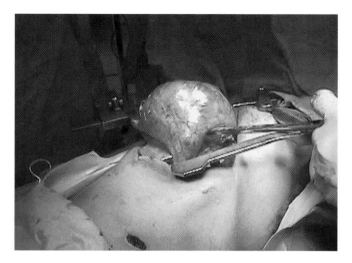

FIGURE 4. Intraoperative bullectomy of the patient shown in Figure 1. Exposure was obtained via a lateral thoracotomy.

An alternative to surgical excision is intracavitary drainage of bullae by tube thoracostomy, as originally described by Monaldi.[28] This technique was later modified by the Brompton group,[29] who employed CT to allow the optimal incision for a minithoracotomy and placement of the intracavitary drain; this obviates the need for removal of adjacent functional lung. Talc is then insufflated into the cavity to hasten sclerosis and to reduce air leaks around the intracavitary drain. The talc pleurodesis also allows subsequent bullae to be drained percutaneously. Using the "Brompton technique," this group reported significant improvements in pulmonary function that were durable for a mean of 2.5 years and for as long as 11 years. The operative mortality was 8.9%, and 6.7% of patients developed recurrent bullae, which were successfully treated by percutaneous drainage.

Outcomes

Although successfully performed for over four decades, bullectomy remains an option for the limited number of patients with this form of emphysema. A recent review of the 22 published series since 1950 included only 476 patients who have undergone this procedure.[30] There have undoubtedly been many more patients who have undergone this operation. Operative mortality appears to be approximately 0 to 8%.[26,31–34] Morbidity owing to prolonged air leaks can be significant, ranging from 5 to 20%. Subjective and objective results have been excellent in carefully selected patients, and symptoms improve within a few months postoperatively.

Improvement in FEV_1 ranges from 10 to 500%, but for the majority of patients, FEV_1 improves by 10 to 30%.[30] Increases in partial pressure of arterial oxygen (PaO_2) and forced vital capacity and decreases in partial pressure of arterial carbon dioxide ($PaCO_2$) and symptom scores have also been reported. Although long-term follow-up is not described in most reports, approximately 30 to 50% of patients maintained the improvement in FEV_1 for 5 or more years.[31,33–37] These series were retrospective in nature and did not contain control groups. Nonetheless, surgical experience with these patients suggests that acceptable candidates have bullae that occupy more than one-third of the hemithorax, CT evidence of compressed lung tissue, and an FEV_1 of < 50% of the predicted value.[22] Other predictors of physiologic improvement include a large volume of trapped gas, preservation of the diffusing capacity, and a near-normal $PaCO_2$.

Summary

In appropriately selected patients, bullectomy is associated with modest increases in pulmonary function and significant improvement in dyspnea. In general, the size of the bulla with evidence of lung compression is predictive of successful outcome postoperatively. Laros and colleagues (and other groups) have shown that bullae must occupy more than 30 to 50% of the hemithorax and must show definite compression of an adjacent lung.[32] Furthermore, there should be no evidence of "vanishing lung" syndrome or

chronic bronchitis. Regardless of the technique and approach, as much normal lung as possible should be preserved to facilitate reexpansion, limit air leaks, and optimize postoperative function. More experience with VATS may establish it as the procedure of choice rather than thoracotomy.

Lung Volume Reduction Surgery
History and Early Outcomes

In the 1950s, Brantigan and Mueller proposed the technique of multiple wedge resections for patients with nonbullous emphysema.[38] They theorized that decreasing the volume of the lung could increase traction on the distal airways, enlarging them and improving airflow. Since hyperinflation of the lung forces the diaphragm down in the thorax, changing its length-tension relationships, Brantigan and Mueller further speculated that decreasing the lung volume would restore the shape of the dome of the diaphragm and restore the diaphragm's efficiency as the respiratory pump. They emphasized that the operation was "directed at the restoration of a physiologic principle, not the removal of pathologic tissue" since the entire lung is involved with emphysema to varying degrees. Despite improved pulmonary symptoms, the procedure was soon abandoned because there was no objective measurement of improved pulmonary function and because the procedure was associated with significant morbidity and a mortality of 16%. With improved surgical techniques and insights gained during lung transplantation, surgical therapy for emphysema has undergone a resurgence. In the early 1990s, Wakabayashi reported success using laser bullectomy for patients with diffuse bullous emphysema.[39] Reporting on 296 video-assisted laser ablation procedures, Wakabayashi found an operative mortality of 4.7% and an improvement in ventilatory capacity in a majority of patients. The reintroduction of multiple wedge resections occurred when Cooper and colleagues, using a modification of Brantigan's technique, reported their results in 20 patients undergoing the procedure.[9] The operation was performed via a median sternotomy with a linear stapler and bovine pericardium to minimize air leaks along the staple lines. They reported no operative or late mortality, a mean improvement in FEV_1 of 82%, increased PaO_2, and an increase in 6-minute walking distance, along with improved dyspnea and quality of life scores.

Following Cooper and colleagues' report, many centers started performing LVRS in an uncontrolled fashion, making it difficult to assess entry criteria and outcomes. These centers reported their outcomes following bilateral LVRS.[40–46] This combined experience included 738 patients and found a mean improvement of 61% in FEV_1 and a mean improvement of 45.7% in 6-minute walking distance. Sixty-two percent of the oxygen-dependent patients became oxygen independent. Operative mortality ranged from 2.5 to 10%, and the mean hospital length of stay was 10.9 to 17 days.[47] A survey of European centers revealed similar results.[48]

Few studies compared LVRS with maximal medical therapy. Meyers and colleagues compared 22 Medicare patients, who were selected for but denied LVRS, with 65 contemporaneous patients who received surgery.[49] Patients who were denied the operation had a continued decline in pulmonary function, whereas patients who underwent LVRS were improved by the procedure. Survival was 82% in the surgical group versus 64% in the medical group. Geddes and colleagues performed a randomized controlled trial involving 48 patients and comparing maximal medical therapy and rehabilitation with LVRS and without LVRS.[50] They found a modest improvement in the surgical group in FEV_1 of 9.5% at 6 months, a 40% increase in the 6-minute walking distance, and improved quality of life. The mortality rate was 21% for the surgical group versus 12% for the medical group. The entry criteria of this study were amended during the trial after the death (in each study arm) of several patients whose diffusing capacities were < 30% or whose 6-minute walking distances were < 150 m. Despite this limitation and the small population size, this study confirmed the findings of Meyers and colleagues[49] and was the only early randomized controlled trial comparing medical therapy with LVRS with medical therapy without LVRS.

The results of these previously published series contrasted with data collected from Medicare claims by using the LVRS billing code.[51] In a cohort of 722 patients, mortality was 14.4% and 23% at 3 and 12 months postsurgery, respectively. Acute care hospitalization, the use of long-term care and rehabilitation services, and the average number of days in hospital, for the surgical group as a whole, were also greater postsurgery. These conflicting results led Medicare to refuse payment for the procedure and led to the collaboration of the Health Care Financing Administration (HCFA) and the National Heart, Lung, and Blood Institute in organizing a national registry and a controlled clinical trial, the NETT. This trial serves as a landmark study evaluating a surgical procedure to best medical therapy.

National Emphysema Treatment Trial

The NETT was a 5-year multicenter trial that randomly assigned 1,218 patients with severe emphysema who underwent pulmonary rehabilitation to undergo LVRS or to receive ongoing medical therapy.[52] The intent was to compare bilateral LVRS via median sternotomy or VATS with each other and with maximal medical therapy following intensive pulmonary rehabilitation and education. The trial was designed to (1) provide information on the role of LVRS in the management of emphysema, (2) define patient selection criteria and identify a subset of patients (if any) likely to benefit from LVRS, and (3) provide a basis on which the HCFA can determine reimbursement for LVRS. The trial was conducted at 18 academic medical centers in the United States. Following enrolment and completion of pulmonary rehabilitation, patients were randomized to continued medical therapy or to LVRS and medical therapy. At centers performing LVRS by both VATS and median sternotomy, patients randomized to surgery were randomized between the two approaches.

The inclusion criteria were developed to enrol patients with emphysema with diverse patterns of distribution, to determine whether anatomic emphysema distribution affects the response to therapy. Mandatory inclusion criteria include radiographic evidence of emphysema, evidence of severe airflow obstruction and hyperinflation on pulmonary function tests, and the ability to participate in and achieve preset goals of pulmonary rehabilitation. The exclusion criteria were designed to exclude patients at risk for perioperative morbidity and mortality, patients with obstructive disease not suitable for LVRS (eg, bronchiolitis), and patients with comorbid conditions that would prevent those patients from completing the trial. For a complete list of inclusion and exclusion criteria, the reader is referred to the NETT Research Group's statement on the rationale and development of the NETT.[47]

The primary outcome measures were survival and maximal exercise capacity. A number of secondary measures were used to assess outcomes. Quality of life was assessed by the Medical Outcomes Study short-form 36-item questionnaire and the Quality of Well-Being Scale. Disease-specific quality of life was assessed using the St. George's Respiratory Questionnaire, which was developed and validated for use in COPD patients. The degree of dyspnea was measured by the University of California, San Diego, Shortness-of-Breath Questionnaire and the modified Borg Dyspnea Scale. Cost efficacy was determined by dividing the incremental costs by the incremental quality-adjusted life-years. Pulmonary function and gas exchange measures included spirometry, lung volume assessment by plethysmography, diffusing capacity, arterial blood gases at rest, and maximal inspiratory and expiratory mouth occlusion pressures. Selected centers performed complete pulmonary mechanics and arterial blood gas analysis with maximal exercise. To determine whether the pattern or severity of emphysema influences outcome, patients were studied with chest radiography, CT, and ventilation-perfusion scanning. Oxygen requirements and 6-minute walking distance were assessed in all patients, and psychomotor testing was done as well. Cardiac evaluation included echocardiography at baseline and at least once postoperatively. Patients with evidence of pulmonary hypertension underwent right heart catheterization. Selected centers performed right heart catheterization at rest and with exercise, at baseline and postoperatively.

Results of the NETT

Overall, there was no difference in mortality between medical and surgical groups. After 2 years, exercise capacity had improved by > 10 Watts in 15% of the surgical patients compared with 3% of the medical group. Subgroup analysis revealed a high risk of mortality following LVRS in patients with a postbronchodilator FEV_1 < 20% predicted and either homogeneously distributed emphysema or a diffusion capacity of carbon monoxide (DL_{CO}) < 20% predicted.[53]

When this high-risk group was excluded, overall mortality was still no different between medical and surgical groups. Among patients with predominantly upper lobe disease and low exercise capacity, mortality was lower in the surgical group than in the medical group (relative risk [RR] for death = 0.47; p = .005). Among those with non-upper lobe disease and high exercise capacity, mortality was higher in the surgical group (RR = 2.06, p = .02). LVRS did confer an increase in exercise capacity, FEV_1, dyspnea scores, and quality of life scores after exclusion of the high-risk population. These changes were most striking in the upper lobe-predominant and high-exercise capacity group. These findings were questioned by the statistical issues related to post hoc review[54] but overall provide evidence-based recommendations for application of LVRS to patients with severe emphysema. The initial results of the trial have been shown to be durable to 5 years postoperatively based on stratification of the four identified subgroups.[55] Similar results have now been reported from randomized, controlled trials in Canada.[56]

Preoperative Evaluation

The preoperative evaluation of the potential LVRS candidate should include pulmonary function tests, with assessment of lung volume and diffusing capacity, inspiratory and expiratory chest radiography, CT scan of the chest, assessment of arterial blood gases, a 6-minute walk test, quantitative ventilation-perfusion lung scanning, and cardiac and psychosocial evaluations.

Pulmonary function testing should be the initial screening test for evaluating candidates for LVRS. Spirometry determines the degree of airflow limitation and whether there is a significant reversible component consistent with reactive airway disease. Lung volumes should be measured by body plethysmography rather than by helium dilution to accurately assess the volume of trapped gas and the residual volume (RV) as these may be underestimated by dilutional techniques. Diffusing capacity evaluates the severity of the destruction of the capillary bed. Arterial blood gases are indicative of the level of pulmonary reserve, with either severe hypoxemia or hypercapnia representing severe parenchymal destruction. The 6-minute walk test provides insight into the level of functional reserve.

Inspiratory and expiratory chest radiography (Figure 5A; see legend on next page) provides useful information about the degree of hyperinflation, the position of the diaphragm, and the presence of chest wall abnormalities such as kyphoscoliosis. CT provides information on the degree of heterogeneity, the location of so-called target areas, and the severity of parenchymal destruction (Figure 5B). Quantitative ventilation-perfusion lung scintigraphy also provides information on heterogeneity and the function of the remaining lung parenchyma (Figure 5C). Cardiac evaluation typically consists of a history, physical examination, and electrocardiography and echocardiography to assess left and right ventricular function and to estimate pulmonary artery pressures (PAPs). Right heart catheterization is performed in patients with evidence of pulmonary hypertension on echocardiography. In patients with multiple coronary risk factors or a previous history of coronary artery disease, a thallium stress test or left heart catheterization is indicated.

Patient Selection and Prediction of Outcome

Selection criteria may vary somewhat between institutions, but an absolute requirement is that the patient must have (1) emphysema and hyperinflation as determined by CT and pulmonary function tests and (2) disabling dyspnea despite

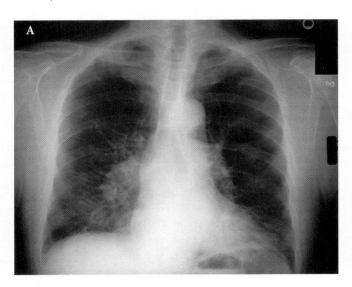

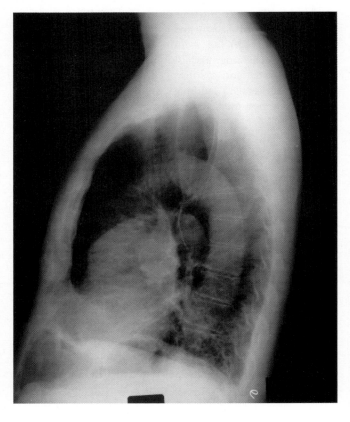

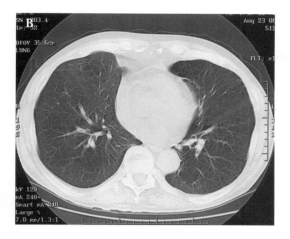

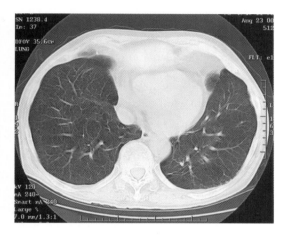

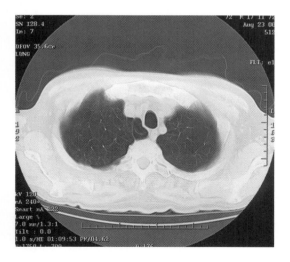

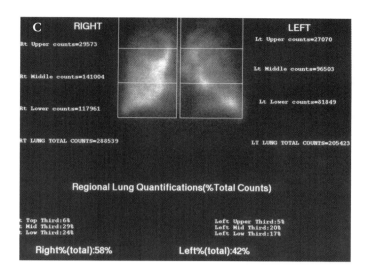

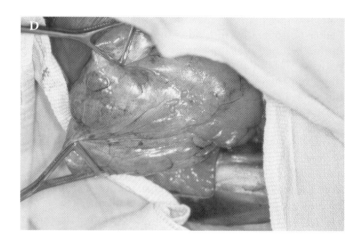

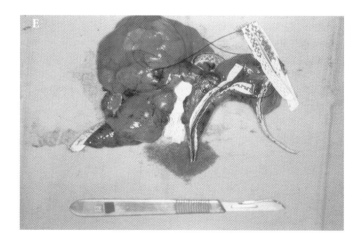

FIGURE 5. *A* (on previous page), Preoperative posteroanterior and lateral chest radiographs reveal hyperinflation and flattened hemidiaphragms. *B*, computed tomographic scans reveal upper lobe emphysema "target lesions" (top) and relatively preserved parenchyma in the middle lung (middle) and lower lung zones bilaterally (bottom). *C*, Quantitative ventilation-perfusion lung scan revealing a lack of perfusion to the upper lobes. *D*, Intraoperative view of an emphysematous lung during a lung volume reduction surgery procedure via a median sternotomy. *E*, Excised lung tissue, with staple lines reinforced with bovine pericardium.

maximal medical therapy. Suitable candidates should have abstained from smoking for at least 3 to 6 months, should have localized areas of emphysema (particularly in the upper lobes), and should have the physical ability to participate in a pulmonary rehabilitation program. Contraindications include older age (75–80 years), diffuse disease or a lack of surgical target areas, diffusing capacity < 20 to 25%, pulmonary hypertension (mean PAP > 35 mm Hg or systolic pressure > 45 mm Hg), the presence of reactive airway disease or asthma, significant bronchiectasis or chronic bronchitis, and severe anxiety disorders. General guidelines for the selection for LVRS candidates and contraindications for LVRS are outlined in Tables 2 and 3. Following proper screening, only 10 to 20% of patients referred for LVRS are found to be suitable candidates for the procedure.[40]

A variety of patient characteristics, physiologic parameters, and imaging patterns have been reported to predict outcomes following LVRS. Miller and colleagues reported that patients older than 70 years of age were more likely to suffer higher postoperative morbidity and mortality and had suboptimal functional outcomes compared with younger patients.[41] Similar age-related differences in functional improvement were reported by McKenna and colleagues,[57] but since there were no operative deaths in the older patients, no absolute upper age limit could be identified. However, Glaspole and colleagues confirmed the observation of Miller and colleagues that age greater than 70 years was associated with a significant risk of perioperative morbidity, mortality, and prolonged hospital stays.[58] Most centers employ an upper age limit of 70 years; however, in the absence of adverse physiologic predictors (hypercapnia or pulmonary hypertension) and in the presence of a heterogeneous disease pattern, successful outcomes following LVRS may be seen in carefully selected patients of up to 80 years of age.

A number of groups have reported that the morphology of the lung as determined by chest radiography, CT, or ventilation-perfusion scintigraphy is highly correlated with physiologic improvement following LVRS.[57,59–67] Heterogeneous disease, specifically upper lobe predominance, was identified as the strongest indicator of postoperative physiologic

improvement in the NETT[52] and identifies the "ideal" candidate. For patients with α_1-antitrypsin (A1AT) deficiency, who have predominantly lower lobe disease, LVRS has been controversial. Cooper and colleagues initially reported that the physiologic improvement seen in patients after LVRS was less than that seen in patients with upper lobe disease.[40] Despite this, these authors believed that this group of patients experienced significant functional improvement. Cassina and colleagues and Gelb and colleagues reported similar levels of improvement.[68,69] Cassina and colleagues also found that these modest improvements were short-lived and that patients returned to baseline or lower levels of performance within 2 years. The duration of benefit was more variable in the Gelb and colleagues' report. My own experience has been that patients with A1AT deficiency ($n = 10$) attained an increase of 40 to 100% in FEV_1 and retained this level for 2 to 6 years (unpublished data, 2000). Two patients returned to baseline at 3 and 6 years, respectively, and have undergone lung transplantation. My program offers LVRS as an alternative or bridge to lung transplantation in younger A1AT-deficient patients with an FEV_1 as low as 13%, as long as they have adequate surgical targets and a retained $DL_{CO} > 25\%$ and do not have significant additional risk factors or significant bronchiectasis.

Spirometry and gas exchange have also been reported to predict improvement after LVRS. Most investigators believe that an FEV_1 of between 20 and 35% of predicted values and a total lung capacity of greater than 130% of predicted values are associated with good outcomes. Miller and colleagues reported that patients who did not have an $FEV_1 > 0.5$ L or a diffusing capacity < 20% had increased postoperative morbidity and mortality and were probably better candidates for lung transplantation or continued maximal medical therapy.[41] However, Eugene and colleagues reported that patients with an $FEV_1 < 0.5$ L and with hypercarbia and pulmonary hypertension could undergo successful LVRS.[70] Similarly,

Table 2 Inclusion Criteria for Lung Volume Reduction Surgery

End-stage emphysema, refractory to maximal medical therapy

Severe dyspnea

FEV_1, 15 to 35%

Lung hyperinflation detected by body plethysmography or chest radiography

Ambulatory, with rehabilitation potential

Age < 75 years

FEV_1 = forced expiratory volume in 1 second.

Table 3 Exclusion Criteria for Lung Volume Reduction Surgery

Age > 75 years

Cigarette use within previous 3 months

Severe cachexia or obesity (ideal body weight 80 to 130% of predicted)

Severe or rapidly fatal comorbid medical illness

Severe pulmonary hypertension (mean PA pressure > 35 mm Hg or systolic PA pressure > 45 mm Hg)

Inability to complete pulmonary rehabilitation program

Severe hypercapnia ($PaCO_2 > 50$ mm Hg)

Ventilator dependence

PA = pulmonary artery; $PaCO_2$ = partial pressure of arterial carbon dioxide.

Argenziano and colleagues reported successful outcomes in patients with an $FEV_1 < 0.5$ L and concluded that this should not be an absolute contraindication to surgery.[71] Despite the apparent success of these two groups, most surgeons and physicians do not routinely advocate LVRS for patients with this degree of severe emphysema. Hypercarbia ($PaCO_2 > 50$ mm Hg or > 45 mm Hg at the altitude of Denver, Colorado) and pulmonary hypertension (mean PAP > 35 mm Hg or systolic PAP > 45 mm Hg) are generally held to predict poor outcomes. In their series, Miller and colleagues reported 50% mortality and 100% major morbidity in four patients with hypercapnia.[41] However, Wisser and colleagues and O'Brien and colleagues reported successful outcomes in patients with hypercapnia ($PaCO_2 > 45$ mm Hg), although the latter group found that the degree of physiologic improvement was less than that seen in normocapnic patients.[72,73] These authors concluded that hypercapnia alone should not be considered a contraindication to LVRS. However, both groups cautioned that in the presence of other risk factors (such as homogeneous disease, severe parenchymal destruction, or pulmonary hypertension), hypercapnia should be considered a contraindication to surgery.

Another physiologic preoperative predictor is inspiratory lung resistance. Ingenito and colleagues showed that preoperative lung resistance during inspiration predicted changes in expiratory flow rates after LVRS.[74] This measure correlated inversely with improvement in postoperative FEV_1 and may be a useful measure for the selection of patients with emphysema for LVRS. A less conventional explanation for the improvement following LVRS was postulated by Fessler and Permutt.[75] Using mathematical analysis and a graphic model of the mechanism of improvement in vital capacity and expiratory airflow and the mechanical properties of the lung in patients with emphysema, A1AT deficiency, or asthma, they determined that the ratio of RV to total lung capacity (TLC) determines the degree of improvement in lung function after LVRS. Thus, decreased airflow appears to result from the mismatch between the size of the lung and the size of the chest wall, and LVRS improves this mismatch. These authors argue that the RV to TLC ratio may be used to select patients who are likely to respond to LVRS. Those with the highest RV to TLC ratios are likely to have the greatest increase in FEV_1.

Other variables reported to predict poor outcomes are a short 6-minute walking distance, male gender, ventilator dependence, severe hypoxemia, steroid dependence, and a short time since smoking cessation.[76,77]

Operative Techniques and Choice of Procedure

The overall goal of LVRS is to decrease the volume of one or both lungs by 20 to 30%. This has been accomplished by laser ablation, stapled resection, or both. Operative mortality, duration of air leaks, and improved pulmonary function were found to be similar between these techniques.[78–80] However, delayed pneumothoraces were seen in up to 18% of the patients undergoing the laser procedure, and the stapled procedure produced superior physiologic results. The use of bovine pericardial strips to buttress the staple line has been shown to decrease the incidence, duration, and severity of air leaks.[9,81] Most authorities now consider the stapled procedure, with or without buttressing, to be the technique of choice for LVRS.

A number of approaches for stapled resections have been advocated, including median sternotomy, thoracotomy, clamshell incision, and VATS. Prior to the NETT, the choice of one procedure over another was generally a matter of the personal preference of the surgeon. As part of the NETT, randomized and nonrandomized comparisons of the median sternotomy and VATS approaches were performed. Mortality rates and postoperative complications were similar; however, hospital length of stay and the time required to return to independent living were longer in the median sternotomy group. Functional outcomes were similar between groups, but costs were lower for the VATS group.[82] Similar results were found in the early LVRS reports.[42,83-85]

Several groups also compared unilateral stapled resection with bilateral procedures.[43,44,86-88] In general, bilateral LVRS produced better physiologic results than unilateral procedures. Operative mortalities with the two procedures were similar, but there have been contradictory reports in the published literature. Long-term survival has been reported to be greater with bilateral procedures.[86,89] This has prompted most centers and the NETT investigators to consider bilateral LVRS to be the procedure of choice and to reserve the unilateral procedure for patients who are not candidates for bilateral procedures because of previous thoracic surgery or trauma, tumor location, or unilateral disease as seen by screening radiography.

Intraoperative and Postoperative Management

Intraoperatively, care must be taken to avoid overdistention of the lungs owing to positive pressure ventilation. This may result in impaired venous return, decreased cardiac output, and hypotension. Excessive hyperinflation may also result in tension pneumothorax owing to rupture of a bleb, bulla, or emphysematous tissue. Despite the presence of hypercarbia and hypoxemia, I request that the anesthesiologist allows permissive hypercapnic ventilation and, if necessary, removes the patient from the ventilator circuit to allow adequate exhalation and decompression. Peak airway pressure should be limited to < 30 mm Hg, and the inspiratory to expiratory ratio should be as long as possible. Patients are intubated with double-lumen endotracheal tubes, and the use of long-acting narcotics or anesthetics is avoided to facilitate early extubation at the end of the procedure. Prior to extubation, patients undergo fiberoptic bronchoscopy to remove blood and secretions and to obtain material for cultures. Almost all patients are extubated at the end of the procedure or shortly thereafter in the postanesthesia care unit. This limits the exposure to positive pressure and decreases the severity of any air leaks. Routine chest tube suction is not employed except in the case of large pneumothoraces or persistent large air leaks. With this protocol, the incidence of prolonged air leaks (> 7 days) is approximately 10% in my LVRS program. In the case of prolonged air leaks, the technique of blood patching is used at postoperative day 7, and the majority of leaks close soon after. Rarely has it been necessary to discharge a patient with a Heimlich valve in place, as described by McKenna and colleagues.[90]

Adequate pain control is initially achieved by the use of a thoracic epidural catheter; later, the patients receive patient-controlled anesthesia with morphine. This approach may decrease the gastrointestinal complications reported previously[41] and allows aggressive respiratory therapy, chest physiotherapy, and physical therapy. Respiratory care includes breathing exercises, inhaled bronchodilators, and early mobilization on a bedside treadmill. Instruction in these techniques is given preoperatively to all patients. Routine monitoring of oxygen saturation, blood pressure, heart rate, temperature, and urine output is performed for the first few postoperative days. Arterial blood gases are not assessed except when there is a change in clinical status or when (in the case of confusion or lethargy) severe hypercarbia must be ruled out. A stress dose of corticosteroids is given to those patients who were steroid dependent preoperatively. Antibiotic prophylaxis directed against *Haemophilus influenzae* and gram-positive organisms (pending bronchoscopic cultures), histamine$_2$ blockers for ulcer prophylaxis, and subcutaneous heparin or pneumatic stockings for deep venous thrombosis prophylaxis are used in all patients.

Postoperative mortality has been reported to be from 5 to 10% and to be primarily due to acute respiratory failure, pneumonia, or cardiac events. Typical complications include prolonged air leaks (in 10 to 50% of cases), pneumonia, respiratory insufficiency requiring invasive or noninvasive ventilation, colonic perforation or overdistention, and panic attacks.[41] A longer-term complication that has been increasingly reported is that of "metalloptysis" or expectoration of surgical staples and bovine pericardium, which may result in postobstructive pneumonia.[91] Careful attention to preoperative selection criteria, perioperative respiratory therapy, the use of epidural catheters for pain control, and care in an active center that performs LVRS and/or lung transplantation regularly most likely limit the incidence and severity of these complications.

Proposed Mechanisms of Improvement

The improvements in pulmonary function reported after LVRS have been attributed to increased elastic recoil, correction of ventilation-perfusion mismatching, improved respiratory muscle efficiency, and improved right ventricular performance.[92] These mechanisms are not mutually exclusive, and it is likely that one or more are operative to varying degrees in individual patients. The amount and characteristics of the removed and remaining lung have been reported to positively affect outcomes following LVRS.[93] Patients with compressed normal lung would be expected to have increased elastic recoil and perfusion after surgery. Those with a predominantly emphysematous lung may see little improvement in these measures but may have improved respiratory muscle function and cardiac performance owing to the decrease in static and dynamic hyperinflation. If areas of abnormal ventilation and perfusion are removed with more areas of normal ventilation-perfusion matching remaining, dead-space ventilation will be decreased, and PaO$_2$ at rest and during exercise will improve. Small airway pathology and morphometry have also been reported to correlate with outcome. Increased airway thickness[94] and an increase in luminal content[95] were associated with a lesser degree of improvement in FEV$_1$.

A number of reports have examined the effects of LVRS on certain parameters. Sciurba and colleagues demonstrated significant improvement in elastic recoil and FEV$_1$ and decreases in RV, TLC, and functional residual capacity.[96] Despite these changes, there were no changes in oxygenation, diffusing capacity, or the requirement for supplemental oxygen, but PaCO$_2$ was decreased. Gelb and colleagues and other groups confirmed the improvement in elastic recoil and suggested that this is the primary mechanism for the improvement in airflow limitation.[97-99] An increase in global respiratory muscle strength[100] and diaphragmatic function[101-104] and a decrease in the inspiratory elastic load imposed by the chest wall[105] have been shown by a number of groups. These effects resulted in reduced work of breathing and increased maximal ventilation, leading to improved exercise tolerance, gas exchange, and reduced dyspnea following LVRS. It has also been shown that LVRS improves maximal exercise performance through improvements in maximal ventilation, decreased dead-space ventilation, and decreased dynamic hyperinflation.[106-109] However, Albert and colleagues reported variable effects of LVRS on arterial blood gases and reported that some patients' hypoxemia and hypercapnia were made worse by LVRS.[110] Central respiratory drive and the ventilatory response to carbon dioxide have also been reported to improve after LVRS, and this may partly account for the symptomatic improvement in dyspnea reported by patients.[111] Cardiac dysfunction can limit exercise capacity in patients with emphysema.[112] Hypoxic pulmonary vasoconstriction and a reduction in the area of the pulmonary capillary bed can lead to elevated pulmonary vascular resistance and subsequent pulmonary hypertension and right ventricular failure. Further, dynamic hyperinflation has been postulated to cause increased intrathoracic pressure leading to functional cardiac tamponade, which limits right ventricular filling and decreases left ventricular ejection fraction, by the principle of ventricular interdependence.[113] The results of LVRS on pulmonary hemodynamics and cardiac function have been contradictory. Sciurba and colleagues reported a postoperative increase in right ventricular fractional shortening (suggesting improved cardiac output) but did not measure pulmonary hemodynamics.[96] Oswald-Mammosser and colleagues and Thurnheer and colleagues reported little or no change in PAPs and pulmonary vascular resistance (at rest or with exercise) after surgery.[114,115] However, Weg and colleagues reported a significant increase in PAP, pulmonary vascular resistance, and pulmonary artery occlusion pressure after LVRS.[116] This study contained a greater number of patients with resting pulmonary hypertension than the previous studies. These patients also had elevated pulmonary artery occlusion pressures at rest, suggesting left ventricular systolic or diastolic dysfunction. Kubo and colleagues also reported increased PAPs at rest and with exercise, which were unchanged after LVRS.[117] However, postoperatively, there was a significant decrease in the pulmonary artery occlusion pressure and an increase in cardiac index at rest and with exercise. Dynamic hyperinflation or intrinsic positive end-expiratory pressure (PEEP) has been shown to decrease postoperatively, suggesting that the cardiac limitation of the exercise capacity in emphysema patients is due to abnormal pulmonary mechanics.

Costs

The costs related to LVRS were assessed during the NETT.[118] For the entire cohort, the cost was $190,000 per quality-adjusted life-year. In the group most likely to benefit (upper lobe disease with low exercise capacity), the cost was $98,000 per quality-adjusted life-year. By comparison, the cost of coronary artery bypass surgery is $64,000 per quality-adjusted life-year gained. If one assumes that 10 to 20% of patients screened for LVRS will be ideal and suitable candidates and that 2 million Americans have emphysema, then 200,000 to 400,000 patients will be eligible for LVRS, and the costs of the procedure would be approximately $20 to 40 billion. If the procedure is extended to patients with less than ideal diffuse disease, costs could easily exceed $50 billion. Given limited health care resources, it is critical to apply LVRS to appropriately selected patients.

Alternative Applications

The LVRS procedure has been applied to patients in a number of clinical settings outside the standard emphysema surgery indication. Several groups have reported the use of LVRS as an adjunct to lobectomy or wedge resection for stage I or II lung cancer or for suspicious pulmonary nodules.[119–123] Although this may allow resection in previously unresectable patients, 3 of 10 patients in one series had early recurrences of their cancers.[124] LVRS has also been used to wean ventilator-dependent emphysema patients,[125] to reduce hyperinflation of the native lung during or after single-lung transplantation (SLT),[126-130] and as a bridge or alternative to lung transplantation.[131,132]

Bronchoscopic LVRS

Bronchoscopic LVRS is a recently developed technique designed to decrease lung volume without the need for a thoracotomy. For a thorough review of this topic, the reader is referred to a review by Hopkinson.[133] Most series to date consist of small numbers of patients who had one-way valves (Emphasys Endobronchial Valve, Redwood City, CA) placed bronchoscopically in the upper lobes of the treated subsegment. In patients developing atelectasis, small improvements in lung function and exercise tolerance were seen.[134,135] In a recent trial of 98 patients using a second generation one-way valve, improvements in FEV$_1$, RV, and 6-minute walking distance were seen.[136] However, three patients developed pneumothoraces, four had prolonged air leaks, and there was one death. Another trial using a different device, the Spiration Implantable Intrabronchial Valve (Spiration, Inc. Redmond, WA), found no deaths, improvements in quality of life, but no change in physiologic parameters or exercise capacity.[137] It is likely that collateral ventilation between subsegments prevented the development of atelectasis or collapsed or hyperinflated lung segments.[138] Alternative techniques include airway bypass, in which a stent is placed under ultrasound guidance from the cartilaginous airway directly into the lung to create new pathways for expiration.[139] Although unproven, these early trials provide encouraging results for nonsurgical approaches to LVRS. Other potential uses for bronchoscopic LVRS have included persistent airleak closure in ventilated patients,[140] and they also have been used to decrease acute native lung hyperinflation (ANLH) following SLT for COPD.[141]

Summary

LVRS is now of proven efficacy in a selected group of patients with emphysema. The greatest functional improvement appears to occur in patients with marked hyperinflation, airflow obstruction secondary to the loss of elastic recoil, and heterogeneous disease distributed in the upper lobes as determined by chest radiography, CT, or ventilation-perfusion scanning and low exercise capacity. It has been applied successfully to other conditions complicated by concomitant emphysema and appears to offer durable functional improvement to patients with severe emphysema.

Lung Transplantation

Any physician who has had the sad task of caring for a patient suffering from advanced pulmonary emphysema must on occasion have wished that human lung transplantation could offer some hope to these unfortunate patients.[142]

History and Background

Lung transplantation has proven to be more difficult than transplantation of the kidney, liver, or heart. The lungs are the only organs transplanted that are exposed to the environment, with its airborne pollutants and pathogens. The lungs are thus prone to infection and rejection and may be particularly susceptible to reperfusion injury. Despite these issues, approximately 16,000 lung transplantation procedures have been performed since the late 1980s, with approximately 50% for COPD or A1AT deficiency.[143]

Early attempts at lung transplantation were complicated by acute respiratory failure, rejection, pneumonia, and ischemic airway complications.[144,145] In addition, SLT in emphysema patients was complicated by ANLH and graft compression. In such cases, ventilation-perfusion lung scanning revealed progressive perfusion but decreasing ventilation to the graft.[146] This led to the conclusion that SLT for COPD was not possible and that bilateral or double-lung transplantation (DLT) would be required.

With the development of cyclosporine, solid-organ transplantation (and lung transplantation in particular) began to be performed successfully. Heart-lung transplantation was successfully applied by the Stanford group to patients with pulmonary vascular disease,[147] and SLT was performed for idiopathic pulmonary fibrosis in 1983.[148] Given the previous poor results of SLT for COPD, the en bloc DLT technique was developed in 1986 for patients with COPD.[149] Early results with this procedure were excellent. However, its application to diverse pulmonary diseases such as cystic fibrosis was met with the complications of cardiopulmonary bypass, namely, hemorrhage and cardiovascular instability. The en bloc DLT procedure was also associated with significant ischemic airway complications, which were sometimes fatal. Therefore, the bilateral sequential lung transplantation procedure was developed by the Washington University group in 1989.[150] In most patients, this procedure did not require cardiopulmonary bypass and lessened the perioperative morbidity and mortality. This procedure has now become the standard operation for DLT at most centers worldwide.

At about the same time, Mal and colleagues successfully performed SLT for COPD[151]; shortly thereafter, reports of success appeared in North America.[152,153] Ventilation-perfusion mismatching was not seen, and the functional results were excellent. SLT has now become the most frequently performed operation for lung transplantation, and many centers have reported excellent short- and long-term results.[154–157]

Recipient Selection

Each lung transplantation center has developed its own set of general recipient selection criteria felt to be critical for successful outcomes of lung transplantation (Table 4). Patients must have clinically or physiologically severe disease or disabling dyspnea that has not responded to maximal medical therapy and that is not amenable to conventional surgical therapy. The risks of surgery and the actuarial survival following lung transplantation must be weighed against the natural history of COPD. Therefore, patients should have a limited life expectancy (< 18–24 months). The relief of dyspnea and the improvement in exercise tolerance must likewise

Table 4 Lung Transplant Recipient Selection Criteria

Clinically or physiologically severe disease
Medical or surgical therapy ineffective or unavailable
Limited life expectancy (<18 to 24 months)
Limitation of activities of daily life
Ambulatory, with rehabilitation potential
Adequate cardiac function without significant coronary artery disease
Acceptable nutritional status (ideal body weight 75 to 120% of predicted)
Adequate support system and psychological status
Age ≤65 years for SLT or ≤60 years for DLT

DLT = double-lung transplantation
SLT = single-lung transplantation

be weighed against the surgical risks and the risks of long-term immunosuppression. Patients should be limited in the activities of daily life but must be ambulatory and have rehabilitation potential. Patients must also have adequate cardiac function without significant coronary artery disease, an acceptable nutritional status (as defined by a preoperative weight within 75 to 120% of ideal body weight), and an adequate support system and psychological status. In general, most centers employ age limitations of ≤65 years for SLT and ≤60 years for DLT.

Absolute contraindications to lung transplantation (Table 5) are not specific to emphysema and include active pulmonary or extrapulmonary infection, current cigarette smoking (candidates must have quit 3 to 6 months prior to evaluation and must undergo random drug screening for urine cotinine or blood carboxyhemoglobin levels), significant left ventricular dysfunction or coronary artery disease, current high-dose corticosteroid therapy (>3.0 mg/kg/d), severe osteoporosis, coexistent systemic disease with extrapulmonary organ involvement, significant psychosocial problems, alcohol or drug abuse, and a history of noncompliance with medical therapy. In evaluating patients with a history of previous malignancy, a period of at least 2 years without recurrence is recommended; this period may need to be longer in patients with malignant melanoma, breast or colorectal cancer, or hematologic malignancies.

Several former absolute contraindications are now considered to be relative contraindications. Preoperative corticosteroids (< 20 mg/d) have now been shown to have no adverse impact on posttransplantation airway healing.[158,159] In fact, corticosteroids may improve donor bronchial blood flow.[160] Ventilator dependence increases the morbidity and mortality of lung transplantation, but in carefully selected patients who were already on the waiting list and who developed respiratory failure, successful outcomes have been reported.[161] Previous thoracic surgery was felt to be a contraindication to lung transplantation; however, with currently available techniques

Table 5 Absolute Contraindications to Lung Transplantation
Current cigarette smoking
Active pulmonary or extrapulmonary infection
Recent or uncured malignancy
Significant left ventricular dysfunction or coronary artery disease
Current high-dose corticosteroid therapy (>0.3 mg/kg/d)
Severe osteoporosis
Coexistent systemic disease with significant extrapulmonary organ dysfunction
Significant psychosocial problems, alcohol or drug abuse, or history of noncompliance with medical therapy

Table 6 Lung Transplantation Selection Criteria for Patients with Chronic Obstructive Pulmonary Disease
Postbronchodilator FEV_1 <25% of predicted value
Not a candidate for lung volume reduction surgery
Resting hypoxemia
Hypercapnia
Secondary pulmonary hypertension
Progressive or rapid decline in FEV_1
Life-threatening exacerbations

FEV_1 = forced expiratory volume in 1 second.

and in the absence of cardiopulmonary bypass, bleeding is only rarely a postoperative problem. Therefore, pneumothoraces treated by tube thoracostomy (with or without pleurodesis), open lung biopsy, or uncomplicated lobectomy do not preclude lung transplantation. However, pleurodesis or pleurectomy significantly increases the technical difficulty of lung transplantation. With the advent of LVRS for emphysema, this may be a problem in the future. However, at our center and others, a number of patients have undergone subsequent lung transplantation without significant pleural bleeding.

The American Society of Transplantation, in conjunction with the American Thoracic Society, recently outlined recipient selection criteria specifically for patients with COPD, as shown in Table 6.[162] The development of the Lung Allocation Scoring (LAS) system has changed the way lungs are allocated in the United States from a system that was time based to one that is need based. Emphysema patients, who tend not to die on the waiting list, tend to have intermediate scores that lead to longer waiting times on the waiting list than for other diseases. It is anticipated that future iterations of the LAS that take elevations in $PaCO_2$ into account will allow emphysema patients with more severe disease to attain higher LAS scores and compete more favorably for available donor lungs.

Donor Selection

Donor selection, preoperative management, and procurement techniques are not specific to emphysema. They are discussed briefly as they are reviewed in detail elsewhere.[163,164] Acceptable lung donors should have (a) no history of underlying lung or systemic disease, (b) no evidence of acute lung injury (particularly owing to aspiration), (c) an alveolar PaO_2 to inspired fraction of oxygen (FIO_2) ratio of >300 mm Hg on 100% oxygen $\pm$ 5 cm PEEP, (d) a clear chest radiograph, (e) no evidence of pneumonia by bronchoscopy (ie, purulent secretions from a lobar or segmental bronchus that does not clear with aspiration), and (f) a smoking history of less than 30 pack-years. The use of the "marginal donor lung," which may not meet all of the ideal donor criteria, may not com-

promise early or late allograft function. Sundaresan and colleagues reported excellent postoperative results with the use of marginal donor lungs in emphysema patients.[165]

One donor issue that is specific to lung transplantation for emphysema is that of appropriate size matching. Donor lungs are matched to the recipient on the basis of height, body weight, and the vertical, horizontal, and circumferential measurements. The use of lungs too small for the thoracic cavity can lead to pleural space complications or hyperinflation of the contralateral native lung, leading to graft compression. In a retrospective analysis, Park and colleagues found that the ideal size match occurred at a donor to recipient inframammary chest wall circumference ratio of 0.89.[166] The implantation of lungs larger than the hemithorax can, after chest closure, result in cardiac tamponade, which manifests as hypotension or increased airway pressures. This may require nonanatomic stapled wedge resections or lobectomy to tailor the lung to the size of the hemithorax. In general, size matching within 25% of the recipient's predicted values results in acceptable postoperative lung function.

Choice of Procedure

Although SLT has become the most frequently performed operation for lung transplantation, controversy still remains regarding the choice of SLT versus DLT for patients with COPD. According to the International Society of Heart and Lung Transplantation (ISHLT) Registry, the vast majority of patients with COPD have undergone SLT[143]; however, this has been changing over the last 5 years. Of the patients transplanted for emphysema, approximately 70% have undergone SLT and only 30% DLT. Reports on the results of the efficacy of each procedure have been conflicting to date. Many programs have achieved success with their approach and have advocated it as the procedure of choice. Factors to consider when choosing a procedure include surgical risk and long-term mortality, functional outcomes and quality of life, "functional reserve" in the face of chronic rejection, and the waiting-list time and mortality rate of patients on the list.

The preference of our center is to perform SLT for emphysema patients in general, with DLT reserved for patients under the age of 50 years or for patients with A1AT deficiency. However, several large centers advocate a preference for the bilateral sequential lung transplantation procedure.[167,168] DLT offers a number of potential advantages over SLT. Replacement of a full complement of normal lung tissue would be expected to restore normal lung function. DLT would also prevent hyperinflation of the contralateral lung. It has also been suggested that DLT recipients may tolerate chronic rejection better than SLT recipients since they have increased "functional pulmonary reserve." This could potentially translate into improved long-term survival. Early reports noted the expected superior pulmonary function test results obtained in bilateral versus single-lung recipients.[169,170] However, these differences have not translated into a significant difference in exercise tolerance between groups unless the tests were performed under conditions of maximal exercise.[171] These early reports also found that the superior pulmonary function came at the expense of decreased early survival in the DLT recipients. The majority of these cases were performed with the older en bloc technique rather than the bilateral sequential technique. However, in more recent reports, Bavaria and colleagues and Sundaresan and colleagues found improved early and medium-term survival in DLT recipients.[172,173] Bavaria and colleagues also found that DLT was associated with decreased primary graft failure.[172] It is important to note, however, that these were not prospective trials comparing the two procedures and that the patients were not age matched. In both series, the SLT recipients were significantly older than the DLT recipients.

SLT is a technically simpler procedure with less operative risk. As such, it may offer advantages to older or higher-risk patients. As discussed earlier, as long as the donor lung is appropriately sized, there is minimal mediastinal shift and graft compression. However, in the face of severe ischemia reperfusion injury and graft dysfunction, the development of ANLH (Figure 6) has been reported to be a significant cause of morbidity and mortality. Yonan and colleagues reported an incidence of severe symptomatic ANLH of 30% in their cohort of 27 patients.[174] These patients required cardiopressor agents and independent lung ventilation and had an associated mortality rate of 42.6%. The authors identified risk factors for the development of ANLH, including an FEV_1 of < 15%, the presence of secondary pulmonary hypertension, a small donor to recipient TLC ratio, and significant reperfusion injury in the allograft. Based on these results, they advocated the routine use of independent lung ventilation, DLT, or right-sided SLT with or without contralateral LVRS for this subgroup of high-risk patients. However, these approaches have several disadvantages. Independent lung ventilation can result in increased morbidity owing to the inability to perform adequate pulmonary toilet with prolonged use of a dual-lumen endotracheal tube. Longer ischemic times during

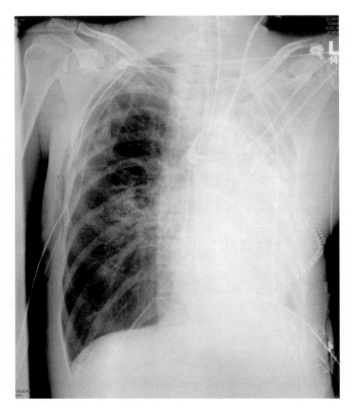

FIGURE 6. Anteroposterior chest radiography reveals acute native lung hyperinflation with graft reperfusion injury.

DLT may lead to increased operative risk, and reliance on DLT may decrease the number of available donor lungs. Excellent results have been reported for LVRS at the time of transplantation.[126,127]

My colleagues and I recently reviewed the results of SLT for emphysema patients ($N = 51$) and found that ANLH was indeed common radiographically, occurring in 31% of the patients; however, only half of these patients were symptomatic, and only 2 were severely so.[175] A high-risk group could not be identified on the basis of pulmonary function tests, predicted donor to recipient TLC ratio, PAPs, or the side transplanted. There was a trend toward an increased incidence of symptomatic ANLH in patients with bullous emphysema owing to A1AT deficiency (4 of 13 with A1AT vs 4 of 38 with COPD). No patient required cardiopulmonary bypass or inhaled nitric oxide intraoperatively. Patients with ANLH did not have evidence of severe ischemia reperfusion injury as determined by chest radiography scores or PaO_2 to FIO_2 ratio. Symptomatic patients did have longer ventilator times and hospital lengths of stay, but 30-day survival was 100% for these patients. Two patients' ANLH required independent lung ventilation and inhaled nitric oxide, but the majority were managed with decreased minute ventilation, cardiopressor agents, or early extubation. No patient required early LVRS or retransplantation. ANLH had no effect on FEV_1 or 6-minute walking distance at 1 year; survival at 1, 2, or 3 years; or the rate of acute rejection, infection, or bronchiolitis obliterans syndrome. Patients with bullous changes tended to have an increased incidence of late native lung hyperinflation (Figure 7). Although three of the patients required LVRS several years after lung transplantation, the results do not support routine use of DLT, exclusive use of right-sided SLT, simultaneous LVRS, or independent lung ventilation for patients with emphysema. These results were confirmed by Mal and colleagues, who found that acute hyperinflation was indeed common but rarely responsible for mortality following lung transplantation for emphysema.[176] Finally, although the incidence of chronic rejection is similar for the two procedures, it has been suggested that DLT recipients may tolerate chronic rejection better than SLT recipients (ie, they have greater "functional reserve" than single-lung recipients). Double-lung recipients maintain a higher functional level without oxygen dependency for longer periods of time, and this may translate into improved long-term survival compared with SLT recipients.[171,175] There does indeed appear to be a trend developing for superior long-term survival in DLT recipients. Sundaresan and colleagues showed that 5-year survival was 53% in DLT recipients versus 41% in SLT recipients.[173] However, al-Kattan and colleagues found a 5-year survival rate of 67% in SLT recipients versus 60% in heart-lung recipients.[177] The results of my group revealed a 5-year survival of 76% in DLT recipients ($n = 22$) versus 63% in SLT recipients ($n = 84$) (Figure 8). However, the small number of DLT recipients precludes statistical significance. In summary, although DLT achieves superior improvements in pulmonary function without increased operative morbidity and mortality and possibly improves long-term survival, one must balance this against the availability of donor lungs. SLT maximizes the use of available donor lungs. One must also compare the increase in total patient-years of survival versus

individual survival rates. Two SLT recipients surviving 5 years have more combined survival-years than one DLT recipient. The exclusive use of DLT may trade longer waiting times and more deaths on the waiting list for potentially increased long-term survival.

Technique
DONOR LUNG PROCUREMENT

The technique of donor lung procurement has been described previously.[163,178] Briefly, the donor is heparinized and given 500 mg of prostaglandin E_1 directly into the pulmonary artery. The lung circulation is then flushed with 3 to 4 L of 4°C low-potassium dextran (Perfudex) solution. The bilateral lung bloc is then removed subsequent to the heart and separated at the donor hospital or the recipient transplant center. The lungs are then transported, inflated, and immersed in iced low-potassium dextran solution. Acceptable ischemic times are up to 6 to 8 hours.

ANESTHESIA AND OPERATIVE TECHNIQUE
IN THE RECIPIENT

Recipients undergo intensive hemodynamic monitoring with arterial and pulmonary arterial catheters. Many centers routinely employ transesophageal echocardiography to assess cardiac function and the need for cardiopulmonary bypass. A left-sided double-lumen endotracheal tube is placed in most patients. Given the overly compliant nature of the emphysematous lung, care must be taken to avoid the development of auto-PEEP or overdistention of the native lung during single-lung ventilation. Progressive air trapping may result in progressive increased intrathoracic pressure, leading to decreased venous return and hypotension. If unrecognized, this may lead to barotrauma with

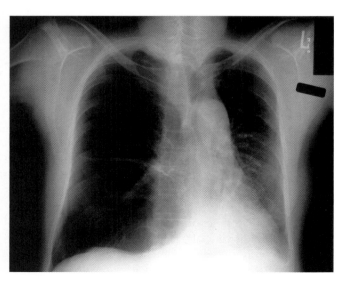

FIGURE 7. Posteroanterior chest radiography reveals chronic native lung hyperinflation in a patient with emphysema, 3 years post transplantation.

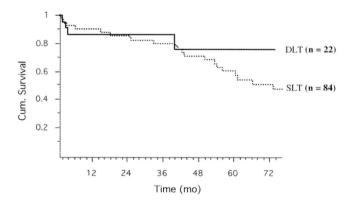

FIGURE 8. University of Colorado Health Sciences Center actuarial survival following lung transplantation for emphysema, by transplantation procedure. Single-lung transplant (SLT) recipients are depicted by the dotted line, and double-lung transplant (DLT) recipients are represented by the solid line. Kaplan-Meier analysis showed no significant difference between groups, but there does appear to be a trend developing for superior survival in DLT recipients after 5 years. Cum. = cumulative.

pneumothorax or bradycardia and cardiovascular collapse. This condition can be instantly corrected or prevented by intermittently opening the endotracheal tube to atmospheric pressure to allow slow decompression of the lung. Exposure for the single-lung procedure is attained via a posterolateral thoracotomy. The choice of the side for SLT is determined by quantitative ventilation-perfusion lung scanning during the evaluation process. Exposure for the bilateral sequential procedure is via bilateral anterolateral fourth or fifth intercostal thoracotomies connected by a transverse sternotomy. Recently, some have advocated a sternum-sparing approach. The side with the least perfusion is explanted and transplanted first. In the absence of pleural adhesions and a large thoracic cavity, as seen in patients with emphysema, the extraction of the native lungs and implantation of the donor lungs are technically straightforward. The anastomoses are constructed as follows: bronchus, main pulmonary artery, and left atrium. Cardiopulmonary bypass is rarely required for SLT or DLT in patients with emphysema.

POSTOPERATIVE MANAGEMENT

The routine postoperative management of lung transplant recipients has been described in detail elsewhere[179] but is described here specifically for emphysema patients. Following the exchange of the dual-lumen endotracheal tube used during the transplantation procedure for a standard single-lumen tube, patients undergo fiberoptic bronchoscopy to remove blood and secretions and to assess bronchial anastomotic integrity and viability. Some centers advocate extubation in the operating room; however, our center prefers to monitor the patient for 6 to 12 hours to determine whether they will develop significant reperfusion injury. Patients are transported to the surgical intensive care unit and remain paralyzed and sedated while requiring mechanical ventilation, which is maintained until standard weaning and extubation criteria are met (typically within 12 to 24 hours postoperatively). Single-lung and bilateral lung recipients require different ventilatory strategies. Single-lung recipients may develop air trapping and ANLH, particularly in the face of significant reperfusion injury. These patients are ventilated with low tidal volumes and respiratory rates, pending resolution of the allograft injury. In the absence of significant graft injury, ANLH can be alleviated by extubation. Bilateral lung recipients are ventilated with standard volumes and rates and with 5 cm of PEEP. Immunosuppressive regimens vary among institutions, but typical triple-drug therapy includes cyclosporine or tacrolimus, azathioprine or mycophenolate mofetil, and corticosteroids. The use of induction lympholytic therapy with antithymocyte globulin or OKT3 remains controversial. Antibacterial prophylaxis is employed in all patients to cover gram-positive and gram-negative organisms, or it may be used on the basis of the results of the donor Gram stain or cultures if available. Application of antiviral strategies to prevent cytomegalovirus (CMV)

infections are controversial, but most centers use ganciclovir prophylaxis, particularly in the case of CMV-seronegative recipients receiving lungs from seropositive donors. Herpesvirus prophylaxis is achieved with acyclovir, and *Pneumocystis carinii* prophylaxis is done with trimethoprim-sulfamethoxazole or monthly inhaled pentamidine in "sulfa-allergic" individuals.

Complications
ALLOGRAFT DYSFUNCTION

Despite improved organ preservation techniques, early allograft dysfunction owing to ischemia-reperfusion injury remains an important cause of early postoperative morbidity and mortality. Such injury occurs in 15 to 20% of recipients. Patients typically manifest pulmonary edema, increased PAPs, and progressive hypoxemia. Reperfusion injury is typically self-limited and resolves over a period of 2 to 5 days. A variety of strategies have been devised to attenuate ischemia-reperfusion injury, including antineutrophil adhesion strategies[180] and (recently) the prophylactic use of inhaled nitric oxide.[181] For patients with established severe reperfusion injury, inhaled nitric oxide has been shown to increase oxygenation and to lower PAPs.[155] Independent lung ventilation and extracorporeal membrane oxygenation may be required for life-threatening episodes.[182] In this situation, ANLH with graft compression is likely after SLT for emphysema.

AIRWAY COMPLICATIONS

Early reports of lung transplantation revealed that donor bronchial ischemia resulting in dehiscence or stenosis was a frequent cause of perioperative morbidity and mortality. Fatal episodes were seen primarily with the older en bloc technique, which employed a tracheal anastomosis. Bronchial dehiscence is treated by pleural drainage, antibiotics, and adequate nutrition; it occasionally requires surgical repair of the anastomosis. Treatment of a bronchial stenosis typically involves débridement, dilatation, or stent placement. Surgical therapy or retransplantation is rarely necessary.

INFECTION

Bacterial pneumonia remains the most common infectious complication following lung transplantation. Most infectious complications represent nosocomial infections owing to gram-negative organisms, and many are of donor origin. The use of prophylactic broad-spectrum antibiotics directed at both gram-positive and gram-negative organisms has significantly decreased the incidence of early pneumonia. Viral infections are usually not fatal but may have long-term effects on allograft function. CMV infection remains a major cause of morbidity after lung transplantation and has been associated with the development of chronic rejection. Prophylaxis with intravenous ganciclovir with or without CMV hyperimmune globulin has significantly decreased the incidence and severity of CMV infections. Herpesvirus infections have been virtually eliminated with the routine use of acyclovir prophylaxis. Fungal infections are unusual in the early postoperative period. Late infections owing to *Aspergillus* species can be significant causes of morbidity and mortality. These infections are seen less frequently owing to the availability of antifungal agents such as ketoconazole and itraconazole.

REJECTION

Most patients will suffer at least one or two episodes of rejection within the first 6 months posttransplantation. Acute rejection episodes are suspected in patients with new infiltrates on chest radiography, a fall of greater than 10% in FEV_1, or arterial oxygen desaturation at rest or with exercise. The diagnosis is confirmed by histologic analysis of transbronchial biopsy specimens, which typically reveal a perivascular lymphocytic infiltrate. Treatment consists of daily intravenous methylprednisolone boluses (10 mg/kg) for 3 successive days. Steroid-resistant episodes of rejection may require the use of cytolytic agents such as antithymocyte globulin or OKT3. Chronic rejection or bronchiolitis obliterans is manifested by a progressive decline in FEV_1, which is not reversible and (histologically) by a fibroproliferative lesion that obliterates the small airways. Most patients will have a progressive decline in pulmonary function despite enhanced immunosuppressive therapy. Bronchiolitis obliterans syndrome remains the leading cause of late mortality in lung transplant recipients, usually owing to allograft infections. Approximately 50% of long-term survivors will develop chronic rejection, which remains the major limitation to the long-term success of lung transplantation.

Outcomes

The outcomes of lung transplantation can be measured in several ways: physiologic function, actuarial survival, quality of life, and cost efficacy. Operative mortality for either SLT or DLT at most experienced centers ranges from 5 to 10%. According to ISHLT Registry data,[143] emphysema patients have a superior survival compared with patients with other indications for lung transplantation. Examination of the survival curves reveals that this is mainly due to a decrease in early postoperative mortality when compared with patients with pulmonary hypertension or idiopathic pulmonary fibrosis. There does not appear to be a difference in survival between patients transplanted for COPD and those transplanted for A1AT deficiency. As discussed previously, there does appear to be a trend developing for improved long-term survival in DLT recipients. Despite the high incidence of chronic rejection, functional results have been excellent. Not surprisingly, FEV_1 has been greater in DLT recipients than in SLT recipients. Exercise performance is also significantly improved after either procedure. Measures of quality of life have documented significant improvement in overall and health-related quality of life. The cost efficacy of lung transplantation has not been well characterized. One study from the University of Washington reported that the lifetime cost for the care of a lung transplant recipient was $424,853 and that the incremental cost per quality-adjusted life-year gained was $176,817.[183] Wage effects were not included in this analysis, but the Registry reports that only 30% of recipients were working full time.[143]

LVRS versus Lung Transplantation

Given the lack of adequate donor lungs suitable for transplantation, there is a need for alternatives to lung transplantation for the treatment of emphysema. Since LVRS has proven efficacy in emphysema patients with predominantly upper lobe disease, hyperinflation, and low exercise capacity, it may be offered to these patients in lieu of a transplant. Several studies have shown that LVRS provides durable results in patients otherwise meeting criteria for transplantation.[184] The advantage of this approach is physiologic improvement without the need for immunosuppressive therapy or transplant-related complications.[185] LVRS does not appear to adversely affect the outcomes of subsequent lung transplantation.[186] Therefore, a previous LVRS should not influence a patient's candidacy for lung transplantation, nor should the future need for lung transplantation impact the decision to undergo LVRS. These reports suggest that LVRS (1) is an alternative to lung transplantation in selected patients, (2) offers an earlier treatment option as a bridge to lung transplantation, and (3) provides treatment for patients with COPD who are not otherwise candidates for lung transplantation.

Conclusion

COPD has become the fourth most common cause of death in the United States. Options for the care of patients with end-stage COPD include continued medical management or pulmonary rehabilitation. With the exception of continuous oxygen therapy, few medical interventions improve survival in this disease. For patients with end-stage emphysema who have failed maximal medical therapy, the number of surgical options has grown; as a result, the selection of the appropriate timing for surgical intervention and the choice of procedure have become more complex. Knowledge of the advantages and disadvantages of the various surgical procedures for COPD and the indications and outcomes of LVRS or lung transplantation are critical for the treating physician to be able to adequately counsel the COPD patient. An algorithm for the approach to surgical treatment at the University of Colorado Health Sciences Center is presented in Figure 9. The optimal surgical approach to patients with end-stage emphysema continues to evolve. Data continue to accumulate on the efficacy of these procedures, and careful analysis of the LVRS procedure in ongoing multicenter trials will determine the optimal selection criteria and long-term outcomes of this group of patients.

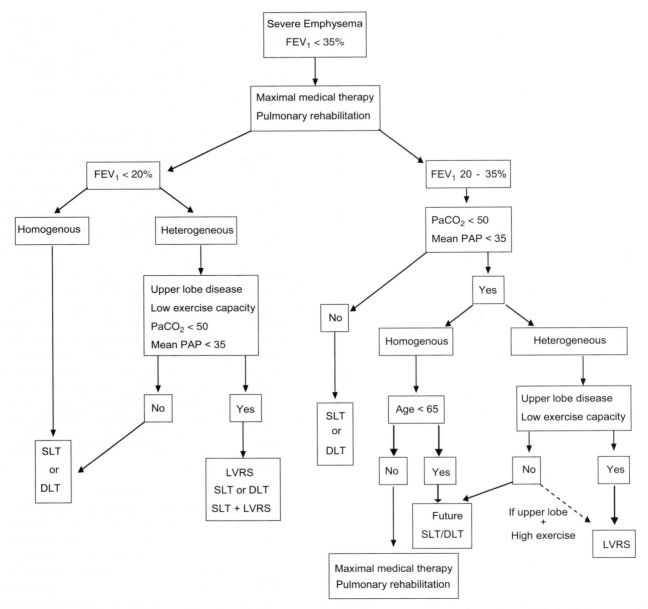

FIGURE 9. Treatment algorithm for patients with severe emphysema at the University of Colorado Health Sciences Center. DLT= double-lung transplant; FEV_1= forced expiratory volume in 1 second; LVRS = lung volume reduction surgery; $PaCO_2$ = partial pressure of carbon dioxide; PAP = pulmonary artery pressure; SLT = single-lung transplant.

References

1. Knudson RJ, Gaensler EA. Surgery for emphysema. Ann Thorac Surg 1965;1:332–62.
2. Deslauriers J. A perspective on the role of surgery in chronic obstructive lung disease. Chest Surg Clin N A 1995;5:575–602.
3. Cooper JD. The history of surgical procedures for emphysema. Ann Thorac Surg 1997;63:312–9.
4. Zamora MR. Surgical therapy for chronic obstructive lung disease. In: Voelkel NF, MacNee W, editors. Chronic obstructive lung diseases. Hamilton (ON): BC Decker; 2002. p. 377–402.
5. Laforet EG. Surgical management of chronic obstructive lung disease. N Engl J Med 1972;287:175–8.
6. Nakayama K. Surgical removal of the carotid body for bronchial asthma. Dis Chest 1961;40:595–604.
7. Overholt RH. Glomectomy for asthma. Dis Chest 1961;40:605-10.
8. Brantigan OC, Mueller E, Kress MB. A surgical approach to pulmonary emphysema. Am Rev Respir Dis 1959;80:194–206.
9. Cooper JD, Trulock EP, Triantafillou AN, et al. Bilateral pneumectomy (volume reduction) for chronic obstructive pulmonary disease. J Thorac Cardiovasc Surg 1995;109:106–19.
10. Mehran RJ, Deslauriers J. Indications for surgery and patient work-up for bullectomy. Chest Surg Clin N Am 1995;5:717–34.
11. Gaensler EA, Cugell DW, Knudson RJ, et al. Surgical management of emphysema. Clin Chest Med 1983;4:443–63.

12. Boushy SF, Billig DM, Lohen R. Changes in pulmonary function after bullectomy. Am J Med 1969;47:916–23.

13. Spear HG, Daughty DC, Chesney JG, et al. The surgical management of large pulmonary blebs and bullae. Am Rev Respir Dis 1961;84:186.

14. Hughes JA, MacArthur AM, Hutchinson DCS, et al. Longterm changes in lung function after surgical treatment of bullous emphysema in smokers and ex-smokers. Thorax 1984;39:140–2.

15. Gaensler EA, Jederlinic PJ, Fitzgerald MX. Patient workup for bullectomy. J Thorac Imaging 1986;1:75–93.

16. Nakahara KM, Nakaoka K, Ohno K, et al. Functional indications for bullectomy of giant bulla. Ann Thorac Surg 1983;35:480–7.

17. Hugh-Jones P, Whimster W. The etiology and management of disabling emphysema. Am Rev Respir Dis 1978;117:343–78.

18. Harris J. Severe bullous emphysema. Chest 1976;70:658–60.

19. Pride NB, Barter CE, Hugh-Jones P. The ventilation of bullae and the effect of their removal on thoracic gas volume and tests of pulmonary function. Am Rev Respir Dis 1973;107:83–98.

20. Morgan MDL, Denison DM, Strickland B. Value of computed tomography for selecting patients with bullous disease for surgery. Thorax 1986;41:855–62.

21. Ogilvie C, Catterall M. Patterns of disturbed lung function in patients with emphysematous bullae. Thorax 1959;14:216.

22. Sakai F, Gamsu D, Im J, et al. Pulmonary function abnormalities in patients with CT-determined emphysema. J Comput Assist Tomogr 1987;11:963–8.

23. Dartevelle P, Macchiarini P, Chapelier A. Operative technique of bullectomy. Chest Surg Clin N Am 1995;5:735–49.

24. Deslauriers J, Leblanc P, McClish A. Bullous and bleb diseases in the lung. In: Shields TW, editor. General thoracic surgery. 3rd ed. Philadelphia: Lea and Febiger; 1989. p. 1168–86.

25. Wakabayashi A. Thoracoscopic technique for the management of giant bullous lung disease. Ann Thorac Surg 1993;56:708–12.

26. Lima O, Ramos L, Biasi PD, et al. Median sternotomy for bilateral resection of emphysematous bullae. J Thorac Cardiovasc Surg 1981;82:892.

27. Cooper JD. Technique to reduce air leaks after resection of emphysematous lung. Ann Thorac Surg 1994;57:1038.

28. Monaldi V. Endocavitary aspiration: its practical application. Tubercle 1946;28:223–8.

29. Shah SS, Goldstraw P. The surgical treatment of bullous emphysema: experience with the Brompton technique. Ann Thorac Surg 1994;58:1452–6.

30. Snider GL. Reduction pneumoplasty for giant bullous emphysema. Implication for surgical treatment of nonbullous emphysema. Chest 1996;109:540–8.

31. Connolly J, Wilson S. The current status of surgery for bullous emphysema. J Thorac Cardiovasc Surg 1989;97:351–61.

32. Laros C, Gelissen H, Bergstein J, et al. Bullectomy for giant bullae in emphysema. J Thorac Cardiovasc Surg 1986;91:63–70.

33. Nickoladze G. Results of surgery for bullous emphysema. Chest 1992;101:119–22.

34. Pearson M, Ogilvie C. Surgical treatment of emphysematous bullae: late outcome. Thorax 1983;38:134–7.

35. Fitzgerald M, Keelan P, Angell D, et al. Long-term results of surgery for bullous emphysema. Surgery 1974;68:566–82.

36. Foreman S, Weill H, Duke R, et al. Bullous disease of the lung. Ann Intern Med 1968;69:757–67.

37. Sung D, Payne W, Black L. Surgical management of giant bullae associated with obstructive airway disease. Surg Clin North Am 1973;53:913–20.

38. Brantigan OC, Mueller E. Surgical treatment of emphysema. Am Surg 1957;23:789–804.

39. Wakabayashi A. Video-assisted laser resection is the best treatment for bullous emphysema. In: Proceedings of the 79th Annual Clinical Congress of the American College of Surgeons. Thoracic Surgery Postgraduate Course; 1993; San Francisco. p. 46–8.

40. Cooper JD, Patterson GA, Sundaresan RS, et al. Results of 150 consecutive bilateral lung volume reduction procedures in patients with severe emphysema. J Thorac Cardiovasc Surg 1996;112:1319–30.

41. Miller JI Jr, Lee RB, Mansour KA. Lung volume reduction surgery: lessons learned from emphysema. Ann Thorac Surg 1964;61:1464.

42. Wisser W, Tschernko E, Senbaklavaci O, et al. Functional improvement after volume reduction: sternotomy versus videoendoscopic approach. Ann Thorac Surg 1997;63:822–7.

43. McKenna RJ Jr, Brenner M, Fischel RJ, Gelb AF. Should lung volume reduction for emphysema be unilateral or bilateral? J Thorac Cardiovasc Surg 1996;112:1331–8.

44. Argenziano M, Thomashow B, Jellen PA, et al. Functional comparison of unilateral versus bilateral lung volume reduction surgery. Ann Thorac Surg 1997;64:321–6.

45. Bingasser R, Zollinger A, Hauser M, et al. Bilateral lung volume reduction surgery for diffuse pulmonary emphysema by video-assisted thoracoscopy. J Thorac Cardiovasc Surg 1996;112:875–82.

46. Daniel TM, Chan BK, Bhaskar V, et al. Lung volume reduction surgery. Case selection, operative technique and clinical results. Ann Surg 1996;223:526–33.

47. National Emphysema Treatment Trial Research Group. Rationale and design of lung volume reduction surgery: a prospective randomized trial of lung volume reduction surgery. Chest 1999;116:1750–61.

48. Hamacher J, Russi EW, Weder W. Lung volume reduction surgery: a survey on the European experience. Chest 2000;117:1560–7.

49. Meyers BF, Yusen RD, Lefrak SS, et al. Outcome of Medicare patients with emphysema selected for, but denied, a lung volume reduction operation. Ann Thorac Surg 1998;66:331–6.

50. Geddes D, Davies M, Koyama H, et al. Effect of lung volume reduction surgery in patients with severe emphysema. N Engl J Med 2000;343:239–45.

51. Health Care Financing Administration (US). Report to Congress: lung volume reduction surgery and Medicare coverage policy; implication of recently published evidence. Washington (DC): Department of Health and Human Services; 1998.

52. National Emphysema Treatment Trial Research Group. A randomized trial comparing lung-volume-reduction surgery with medical therapy for severe emphysema. N Engl J Med 2003;348:2059–73.

53. National Emphysema Treatment Trial Research Group. Patients at high-risk of death after lung volume reduction surgery. N Engl J Med 2001;345:1075–83.

54. Ware JH. The National Emphysema Treatment Trial-how strong is the data? N Engl J Med 2003;348:2055–6.

55. National Emphysema Treatment Trial Research Group. Long-term follow-up of patients receiving lung volume reduction surgery versus medical therapy for severe emphysema by the National Emphysema Treatment Trial Research Group. Ann Thorac Surg 2006;82:431–43.

56. Miller JD, Malthaner RA, Goldsmith CH, et al. A randomized clinical trial of lung volume reduction surgery versus best medical therapy for patients with advanced emphysema: a two-year study from Canada. Ann Thorac Surg. 2006;81:314–20.

57. McKenna RJ Jr, Brenner M, Fischel RJ, et al. Patient selection criteria for lung volume reduction surgery. J Thorac Cardiovasc Surg 1997;114:957–64.

58. Glaspole IN, Gabbay E, Smith JA, et al. Predictors of perioperative morbidity and mortality in lung volume reduction surgery. Ann Thorac Surg 2000;69:1711–6.

59. Maki DD, Miller WT Jr, Aronchick JM, et al. Advanced emphysema: preoperative chest radiographic findings as predictors of outcome following lung volume reduction surgery. Radiology 1999;212:49–55.

60. Date H, Goto K, Souda R, et al. Predictors of improvement in FEV1 (forced expiratory volume in 1s) after lung volume reduction surgery. Surg Today 2000;30:328–32.

61. Slone RM, Pilgram TK, Gierada DS, et al. Lung volume reduction surgery: comparison of preoperative radiologic features and clinical outcome. Radiology 1997;204:685–93.

62. Gierada DS, Slone RM, Bae KT, et al. Pulmonary emphysema: comparison of preoperative quantitative CT and physiologic index values with clinical outcome after lung volume reduction surgery. Radiology 1997;205:235–42.

63. Hamacher J, Bloch KE, Stammberger U, et al. Two years' outcome of lung volume reduction surgery in different morphologic emphysema types. Ann Thorac Surg 1999;68:1792–8.

64. Wang SC, Fischer KC, Slone RM, et al. Perfusion scintigraphy in the evaluation for lung volume reduction surgery: correlation with clinical outcome. Radiology 1997;205:243–8.

65. Mas JC. The lung scan in patient selection for lung volume reduction surgery. J Nucl Med Technol 1998;26:26–9.

66. Sugi K, Matsuoka T, Tanaka T, et al. Lung volume reduction surgery for pulmonary emphysema using dynamic xenon-133 and Tc-99m-MAA SPECT images. Ann Thorac Cardiovasc Surg 1998;4:149–53.

67. Thurnheer R, Engel H, Weder W, et al. Role of lung perfusion scintigraphy in relation to chest computed tomography and pulmonary function in the evaluation of candidates for lung volume reduction surgery. Am J Respir Crit Care Med 1999;159:301–10.

68. Cassina PC, Teschler H, Konietzko N, et al. Two-year results after lung volume reduction surgery in alpha-1-antitrypsin deficiency versus smoker's emphysema. Eur Respir J 1998;12:1028–32.

69. Gelb AF, McKenna RJ, Brenner M, et al. Lung function after bilateral lower lobe lung volume reduction surgery for alpha-1-antitrypsin emphysema. Eur Respir J 1999;14:928–33.

70. Eugene J, Dajee A, Kayaleh R, et al. Reduction pneumoplasty for patients with a forced expiratory volume in 1 second of 500 milliliters or less. Ann Thorac Surg 1997;63:186–90.

71. Argenziano M, Moazami N, Thomashow B, et al. Extended indications for lung volume reduction surgery in advanced emphysema. Ann Thorac Surg 1996;62:1588–97.

72. Wisser W, Klepetko W, Senbaklavaci O, et al. Chronic hypercapnia should not exclude patients from lung volume reduction surgery. Eur J Cardiothorac Surg 1998;14:107–12.

73. O'Brien GM, Furukawa S, Kuzma AM, et al. Improvements in lung function, exercise and quality of life in hypercapneic COPD patients after lung volume reduction surgery. Chest 1999;115:75–84.

74. Ingenito EP, Evans RB, Loring SH, et al. Relation between preoperative inspiratory lung resistance and the outcome of lung volume reduction surgery for emphysema. N Engl J Med 1998;338:1181–5.

75. Fessler HE, Permutt S. Lung volume reduction surgery and airflow limitation. Am J Respir Crit Care Med 1998;157:715–22.

76. Szekely LA, Oelberg DA, Wright C, et al. Preoperative predictors of operative morbidity and mortality in COPD patients undergoing bilateral lung volume reduction surgery. Chest 1997;111:550–8.

77. Naunheim KS, Hazelrigg SR, Kaiser LR, et al. Risk analysis for thoracoscopic lung volume reduction: a multi-institutional experience. Eur J Cardiothorac Surg 2000;17:673–9.

78. Wakabayashi A, Brenner M, Kayaleh RA, et al. Thoracoscopic carbon dioxide laser treatment of bullous emphysema. Lancet 1991;337:881–3.

79. Little AG, Swain JA, Nino JJ, et al. Reduction pneumoplasty for emphysema: early results. Ann Surg 1995;222:365–74.

80. McKenna RJ Jr, Brenner M, Gelb AF, et al. A randomized, prospective trial of stapled lung reduction versus laser bullectomy for diffuse emphysema. J Thorac Cardiovasc Surg 1996;111:317–21.

81. Hazelrigg SR, Boley TM, Naunheim KS, et al. Effect of bovine pericardial strips on air leak after stapled pulmonary resection. Ann Thorac Surg 1997;63:1573–5.

82. McKenna RJ, Benditt JO, DeCamp M, et al. Safety and efficacy of median sternotomy versus video-assisted thoracic surgery for lung volume reduction surgery. J Thorac Cardiovasc Surg 2004;127:1350–60.

83. Kotloff RM, Tino G, Bavaria JE, et al. Bilateral lung volume reduction surgery for advanced emphysema. A comparison of median sternotomy and thoracoscopic approaches. Chest 1996;110:1399–406.

84. Ko CY, Waters PF. Lung volume reduction surgery: a cost and outcomes comparison of sternotomy versus thoracotomy. Am Surg 1998;64:1010–3.

85. Roberts JR, Bavaria JE, Wahl P, et al. Comparison of open and thoracoscopic bilateral volume reduction surgery: complications analysis. Ann Thorac Surg 1998;66:1759–65.

86. Serna DL, Brenner M, Osana KE, et al. Survival after unilateral versus bilateral lung volume reduction surgery for emphysema. J Thorac Cardiovasc Surg 1999;118:1101–9.

87. Lowdermilk GA, Keenan RJ, Landreneau RJ, et al. Comparison of clinical results for unilateral and bilateral thoracoscopic lung volume reduction. Ann Thorac Surg 2000;69:1670–4.

88. Kotloff RM, Tino G, Palevsky HI, et al. Comparison of short term functional outcomes following unilateral and bilateral lung volume reduction surgery. Chest 1998;113:890–5.

89. Naunheim KS, Kaiser LR, Bavaria JE, et al. Long-term survival after thoracoscopic lung volume reduction: a multiinstitutional review. Ann Thorac Surg 1999;68:2026–31.

90. McKenna RJ Jr, Fischel RJ, Brenner M, Gelb AF. Use of a Heimlich valve to shorten hospital stay after lung volume reduction surgery for emphysema. Ann Thorac Surg 1996;61:1115–7.

91. Provencher S, Deslauriers J. Late complication of bovine pericardium patches used for lung volume reduction surgery. Eur J Cardiothorac Surg. 2003;23:1059–61.

92. Fein AM. Lung volume reduction surgery: answering the crucial questions. Chest 1998;113:277S–82S.

93. Brenner M, McKenna RJ Jr, Chen JC, et al. Relationship between amount of lung resected and outcome after lung volume reduction surgery. Ann Thorac Surg 2000;69:388–93.

94. Kim V, Criner GJ, Abdallah HY, et al. Small airway morphometry and improvement in pulmonary function after lung volume reduction surgery. Am J Respir Crit Care Med 2005;171:40–7.

95. Sciurba FC, Martinez FJ, Rogers RM, et al. Relationship between pathologic characteristics of peripheral airways and outcome after lung volume reduction surgery in severe chronic obstructive pulmonary disease. Proc Am Thorac Soc 2006;3:533–4.

96. Sciurba FC, Rogers RM, Keenan RJ, et al. Improvement in pulmonary function and elastic recoil after lung reduction surgery for diffuse emphysema. N Engl J Med 1996;334:1095–9.

97. Gelb AF, Brenner M, McKenna RJ Jr, et al. Serial lung function and elastic recoil 2 years after lung volume reduction surgery for emphysema. Chest 1998;113:1497–506.

98. Scharf SM, Rossoff L, McKeon K, et al. Changes in pulmonary mechanics after lung volume reduction surgery. Lung 1998;176:191–204.

99. Norman M, Hillerdal G, Orre L, et al. Improved lung function and quality of life following increased elastic recoil after lung volume reduction surgery in emphysema. Respir Med 1998;92:653–8.

100. Martinez FJ, de Oca MM, Whyte RI, et al. Lung volume reduction improves dyspnea, dynamic hyperinflation and respiratory muscle function. Am J Respir Crit Care Med 1997;155:1984–90.

101. Tschernko EM, Wisser W, Wanke T, et al. Changes in ventilatory mechanics and diaphragmatic function after lung volume reduction surgery in patients with COPD. Thorax 1997;52:545–50.

102. Keller CA, Ruppel G, Hibbett A, et al. Thoracoscopic lung volume reduction surgery reduces dyspnea and improves exercise capacity in patients with emphysema. Am J Respir Crit Care Med 1997;156:60–7.

103. Bloch KE, Li Y, Zhang J, et al. Effect of surgical lung volume reduction on breathing patterns in severe pulmonary emphysema. Am J Respir Crit Care Med 1997;156:553–60.

104. Criner G, Cordova FC, Leyenson V, et al. Effect of lung volume reduction surgery on diaphragmatic strength. Am J Respir Crit Care Med 1998;157:1578–85.

105. Barnas GM, Gilbert TB, Krasna MJ, et al. Acute effects of bilateral lung volume reduction surgery on lung and chest wall mechanical properties. Chest 1998;114:61–8.

106. Ferguson GT, Fernandez E, Zamora MR, et al. Improved exercise performance following lung volume reduction surgery for emphysema. Am J Respir Crit Care Med 1998;157:1195–203.

107. Benditt JO, Lewis S, Wood DE, et al. Lung volume reduction surgery improves maximal O_2 consumption, maximal minute ventilation, O_2 pulse and deadspace-to-tidal volume ratio during leg cycle ergometry. Am J Respir Crit Care Med 1997;156:561–6.

108. Stammberger U, Bloch KE, Thurnheer R, et al. Exercise performance and gas exchange after bilateral video-assisted thoracoscopic lung volume reduction for severe emphysema. Eur Respir J 1998;12:785–92.

109. Tschernko EM, Gruber EM, Jaksch P, et al. Ventilatory mechanics and gas exchange during exercise before and after lung volume reduction surgery. Am J Respir Crit Care Med 1998;158:1424–31.

110. Albert RK, Benditt JO, Hildebrandt J, et al. Lung volume reduction surgery has variable effects on blood gases in patients with emphysema. Am J Respir Crit Care Med 1998; 158:71–6.

111. Celli BR, Montes de Oca M, Mendez R, Stetz J. Lung reduction surgery in severe COPD decreases central drive and ventilatory response to CO_2. Chest 1997;112:902–6.

112. Belman MJ. Exercise in patients with chronic obstructive pulmonary disease. Thorax 1993;48:936–46.

113. Butler J, Schrijen F, Henriquez A, et al. Cause of the raised wedge pressure on exercise in chronic obstructive pulmonary disease. Am Rev Respir Dis 1988;138:350–4.

114. Oswald-Mammosser M, Kessler R, Massard G, et al. Effect of lung volume reduction surgery on gas exchange and pulmonary hemodynamics at rest and during exercise. Am J Respir Crit Care Med 1998;158:1020–5.

115. Thurnheer R, Bingisser R, Stammberger U, et al. Effect of lung volume reduction surgery on pulmonary hemodynamics in severe pulmonary emphysema. Eur J Cardiothorac Surg 1998;13:253–8.

116. Weg IL, Rossoff L, McKeon K, et al. Development of pulmonary hypertension after lung volume reduction surgery. Am J Respir Crit Care Med 1999;159:552–6.

117. Kubo K, Koizumi T, Fujimoto K, et al. Effects of lung volume reduction surgery on exercise pulmonary hemodynamics in severe emphysema. Chest 1998;114:1575–82.

118. National Emphysema Treatment Trial Research Group. Cost effectiveness of lung volume reduction surgery for patients with severe emphysema. N Engl J Med 2003;348:2092–102.

119. McKenna RJ Jr, Fischel RJ, Brenner M, Gelb AF. Combined operations for lung volume reduction surgery and lung cancer. Chest 1996;110:885–8.

120. Ojo TC, Martinez F, Paine R III, et al. Lung volume reduction surgery alters management of pulmonary nodules in patients with severe COPD. Chest 1997;112:1494–500.

121. DeMeester SR, Patterson GA, Sundaresan RS, Cooper JD. Lobectomy combined with lung volume reduction for patients with lung cancer and advanced emphysema. J Thorac Cardiovasc Surg 1998;115:681–8.

122. Sinjan EA, Van Schil PE, Ortmanns P, et al. Improved ventilatory function after combined operation for pulmonary emphysema and lung cancer. Int Surg 1999;84:185–9.

123. Mentzer SJ, Swanson SJ. Treatment of patients with lung cancer and severe emphysema. Chest 1999;116:477S–9S.

124. Hayashi K, Fukushima K, Sagara Y, Takeshita M. Surgical treatment for patients with lung cancer complicated by severe pulmonary emphysema. Jpn J Thorac Cardiovasc Surg 1999;47:583–7.

125. Criner GJ, O'Brien G, Furukawa S, et al. Lung volume reduction surgery in ventilator-dependent COPD patients. Chest 1996;110:877–84.

126. Khagani A, al-Kattan KM, Tadjkarimi S, et al. Early experience with single lung transplantation for emphysema with simultaneous volume reduction on the contralateral lung. Eur J Cardiothorac Surg 1997;11:604–8.

127. Todd TR, Perron J, Winton TL, Keshavjee SH. Simultaneous single-lung transplantation and lung volume reduction. Ann Thorac Surg 1997;63:1468–70.

128. Schulman LL, O'Hair DP, Cantu E, et al. Salvage by volume reduction of chronic allograft rejection in emphysema. J Heart Lung Transplant 1999;18:107–12.

129. Kroshus TJ, Bolman RM III, Kshettry VR. Unilateral volume reduction after single lung transplantation for emphysema. Ann Thorac Surg 1996;62:363–8.

130. Le-Pimpec-Barthes F, Debrosse D, Cuenod CA, et al. Late contralateral lobectomy after single-lung transplantation for emphysema. Ann Thorac Surg 1996;61:231–4.

131. Wisser W, Deviatko E, Simon-Kupilik N, et al. Lung transplantation following lung volume reduction surgery. J Heart Lung Transplant 2000;19:480–7.

132. Zenati M, Keenan RJ, Courcoulas AP, Griffith BP. Lung volume reduction or lung transplantation for end-stage pulmonary emphysema? Eur J Cardiothorac Surg 1998;14:31.

133. Hopkinson NS. Bronchoscopic lung volume reduction: indications, effects and prospects. Curr Opin Pulm Med 2007; 13:125–30.

134. Snell GI, Holsworth L, Borrill ZL, et al. The potential for bronchoscopic lung volume reduction using bronchial prosthesis: a pilot study. Chest 2003;124:1073–80.

135. Hopkinson NS, Toma TP, Hansell DM, et al. Effect of bronchoscopic lung volume reduction on dynamic hyperinflation and exercise in emphysema. Am J Respir Crit Care Med 2005;171:453–60.

136. Wan IY, Toma TP, Geddes DM, et al. Bronchoscopic lung volume reduction for end-stage emphysema: report on the first 98 patients. Chest 2006;129:518–26.

137. Wood DE, McKenna RJ, Yusen RD, et al. A multicenter trial of an intrabronchial valve for the treatment of severe emphysema. J Thorac Cardiovasc Surg 2007;133:65–73.

138. Fessler HE. Collateral ventilation, the bane of bronchoscopic volume reduction. Am J Respir Crit Care Med. 2005;171:423–5.

139. Lausberg HF, Chino K, Patterson GA, et al. Bronchial fenestration improves expiratory flow in emphysematous human lungs. Ann Thorac Surg 2003;75:393–7.

140. Feller-Kopman D, Bechara R, Garland R, et al. Use of a removable endobronchial valve for the treatment of bronchopleural fistula. Chest 2006;130:273–5.

141. Crespo MM, Johnson BA, McCurry KR, et al. Use of endobronchial valves for native lung hyperinflation associated with respiratory failure in a single-lung transplant recipient for emphysema. Chest 2007;131:214–6.

142. Bates D. The other lung [editorial]. N Engl J Med 1970;282:605–10.

143. The Registry of the International Society of Heart and Lung Transplantation: sixteenth official report - 1999. J Heart Lung Transplant 1999;18:611–25.

144. Veith FJ, Koerner SK. Problems in the management of human lung transplant patients. Vasc Surg 1974;8:273–82.

145. Veith FJ, Koerner SK. The present status of lung transplantation. Arch Surg 1974;109:734–40.

146. Stevens PM, Johnson PC, Bell RL, et al. Regional ventilation and perfusion after lung transplantation in patients with emphysema. N Engl J Med 1970;282:245–9.

147. Reitz BA, Walwork J, Hunt SA, et al. Heart-lung transplantation: successful therapy for patients with pulmonary vessel disease. N Engl J Med 1982;306:557.

148. Toronto Lung Transplant Group. Unilateral lung transplantation for pulmonary fibrosis. N Engl J Med 1986;314:1140–5.

149. Patterson GA, Cooper JD, Dark JH, et al. Experimental and clinical lung double lung transplantation. J Thorac Cardiovasc Surg 1988;95:70–4.

150. Pasque MK, Cooper JD, Kaiser LR, et al. Improved technique for bilateral lung transplantation: rationale and initial clinical experience. Ann Thorac Surg 1990;49:785–91.

151. Mal H, Andreassian B, Pamela F. Unilateral lung transplantation in end stage pulmonary emphysema. Am Rev Respir Dis 1989;140:797–802.

152. Patterson GA, Maurer JR, Williams TJ, et al. Comparison of outcomes of single and double lung transplantation for obstructive lung disease. The Toronto Lung Transplant Group. J Thorac Cardiovasc Surg 1991;101:623–31.

153. Calhoon JH, Grover FL, Gibbons WJ, et al. Single lung transplantation: alternative indications and technique. J Thorac Cardiovasc Surg 1991;101:816–25.

154. Marinelli WA, Hertz MI, Shumway SJ, et al. Single lung transplantation for severe emphysema. J Heart Lung Transplant 1992;11:577–83.

155. Mal H, Sleiman C, Jebrak G, et al. Functional results of single-lung transplantation for chronic obstructive lung disease. Am J Respir Crit Care Med 1994;149:1476–81.

156. Levine SM, Anzueto A, Peters JI, et al. Medium term functional results of single-lung transplantation for endstage obstructive lung disease. Am J Respir Crit Care Med 1994;150:398–402.

157. Brunsting LA, Lupinetti FM, Cascade PN, et al. Pulmonary function in single-lung transplantation for chronic obstructive pulmonary disease. J Thorac Cardiovasc Surg 1994;107:1337–45.

158. Schafers HJ, Wagner TOF, Demertzis S, et al. Preoperative corticosteroids: a contraindication to lung transplantation? Chest 1992;102:1522–5.

159. Miller JD, DeHoyos A. An evaluation of the role of omentopexy and of earlier perioperative corticosteroid administration in lung transplantation. J Thorac Cardiovasc Surg 1993;105:247–52.

160. Inui K, Schafers HJ, Aoki M, et al. Bronchial circulation after experimental lung transplantation: the effect of long-term administration of prednisolone. J Thorac Cardiovasc Surg 1993;105:474–8.

161. Flume PA, Egan TA, Westerman JH, et al. Lung transplantation for mechanically ventilated patients. J Heart Lung Transplant 1994;13:15–23.

162. Maurer JR, Frost AE, Glanville AR, et al. International guidelines for the selection of lung transplant candidates. Am J Respir Crit Care Med 1998;158:335–9.

163. Keshavjee S, Todd TRJ. Excision and storage of the donor lungs. In: Cooper DKC, Miller LW, Patterson GA, editors. The transplantation and replacement of thoracic organs. Dordrecht: Kluwer Academic Publishers; 1996. p. 445–9.

164. Frost AE. Donor criteria and evaluation. Clin Chest Med 1997;18:231–7.

165. Sundaresan S, Semenkovich J, Ochoa L, et al. Successful outcome of lung transplantation is not compromised by the use of marginal donor lungs. J Thorac Cardiovasc Surg 1995;109:1075–80.

166. Park SJ, Hauck J, Pifarre R, et al. Optimal size matching in single lung transplantation. J Heart Lung Transplant 1995;14:671–5.

167. Patterson GA, Cooper JD. Lung transplantation for emphysema. Chest Surg Clin N Am 1995;5:851–68.

168. Waddell TK, Keshavjee S. Lung transplantation for chronic obstructive pulmonary disease. Semin Thorac Cardiovasc Surg 1998;10:191–201.

169. Low DE, Trulock EP, Kaiser LR, et al. Morbidity, mortality and early results of single versus bilateral lung transplantation for emphysema. J Thorac Cardiovasc Surg 1992; 103:1119–26.

170. Bando K, Paradis IL, Keenan RJ, et al. Comparison of outcomes after single and bilateral lung transplantation for obstructive lung disease. J Heart Lung Transplant 1995;14:692–8.

171. Howard DA, Iademarco E, Trulock EP, et al. The role of cardiopulmonary exercise testing in lung and heart-lung transplantation. Clin Chest Med 1994;15:405–20.

172. Bavaria JE, Kotloff R, Palevsky H, et al. Bilateral versus single lung transplantation for chronic obstructive pulmonary disease. J Thorac Cardiovasc Surg 1997;113:520–8.

173. Sundaresan RS, Shiraishi Y, Trulock EP, et al. Single or bilateral lung transplantation for emphysema? J Thorac Cardiovasc Surg 1992;103:1119–26.

174. Yonan NA, El-Gamel A, Egan J, et al. Single lung transplantation for emphysema: predictors for native lung hyperinflation. J Heart Lung Transplant 1998;17:192–201.

175. Weill D, Torres F, Hodges TN, et al. Acute native lung hyperinflation is not associated with poor outcomes after single lung transplant for emphysema. J Heart Lung Transplant 1999;18:1080–7.

176. Mal H, Brugiere O, Sleiman C, et al. Morbidity and mortality related to the native lung in single lung transplantation for emphysema. J Heart Lung Transplant 2000;19:220–3.

177. al-Kattan K, Tadjkarimi S, Cox A, et al. Evaluation of the long-term results of single lung versus heart-lung transplantation for emphysema. J Heart Lung Transplant 1995; 14:824–31.

178. Sundaresan S, Trachiotis GD, Aoe M, et al. Donor lung procurement: assessment and operative technique. Ann Thorac Surg 1993;56:1409–13.

179. Simpson KP, Garrity ER. Perioperative management in lung transplantation. Clin Chest Med 1997;18:277–84.

180. DeMeester SR, Molinari MA, Shiraishi T, et al. Attenuation of rat isograft reperfusion injury with anti-adhesion molecule monoclonal antibodies. Surg Forum 1994;XLV:291–4.

181. Okabayashi K, Triantafillou AN, Yamashita M, et al. Inhaled nitric oxide reduces lung allograft reperfusion injury. Surg Forum 1994;XLV:276–8.

182. Badesch DB, Zamora MR, Jones S, et al. Independent ventilation and ECMO for severe unilateral pulmonary edema following SLT for primary pulmonary hypertension. Chest 1995;107:1766–70.

183. Ramsey SD, Patrick DL, Albert RK, et al. The cost-effectiveness of lung transplantation: a pilot study. Chest 1995; 108:1594–601.

184. Tutic M, Lardinois D, Imfeld S, et al. Lung volume reduction surgery as an alternative or bridging procedure to lung transplantation. Ann Thorac Surg. 2006;82:208–13.

185. Gaissert HA, Trulock EP, Cooper JD, et al. Comparison of early functional results after volume reduction or lung transplantation for chronic obstructive pulmonary disease. J Thorac Cardiovasc Surg 1996;111:296–307.

186. Nathan SD, Edwards LB, Barnett SD, et al. Outcomes of COPD lung transplant recipients after lung volume reduction surgery. Chest 2004;126:1569–74

CHAPTER 28

REHABILITATION

Andrew L. Ries, MD, MPH, and Smita Desai, DO

REHABILITATION PROGRAMS for patients with chronic lung diseases are well established as a means of enhancing standard therapy to control and alleviate symptoms and optimize functional capacity.[1–3] The primary goal is to restore the patient to the highest possible level of independent function. This goal is accomplished by helping patients and significant others learn more about their disease, treatment options, and coping strategies. Patients are encouraged to become actively involved in providing their own health care, more independent in daily activities, and less dependent on health professionals and expensive medical resources. Rather than focusing solely on reversing the disease process, rehabilitation attempts to improve disability from disease.

Many rehabilitation strategies have been developed for patients with disabling chronic obstructive pulmonary disease (COPD). Pulmonary rehabilitation has also been applied successfully to patients with other chronic lung conditions, such as bronchiectasis, cystic fibrosis, interstitial lung diseases, and chest wall diseases, among others.[2] In addition, it has been used successfully as part of the evaluation and preparation for surgical treatments such as lung transplantation and lung volume reduction surgery (LVRS).[4–7] Pulmonary rehabilitation is appropriate for any patient with stable chronic lung disease who is disabled by respiratory symptoms. Even patients with advanced disease can benefit, if they are selected appropriately and if realistic goals are set.

In 2006, the American Thoracic Society (ATS) and European Respiratory Society (ERS) adopted the following definition of pulmonary rehabilitation:

Pulmonary rehabilitation is an evidence-based, multidisciplinary, and comprehensive intervention for patients with chronic respiratory diseases who are symptomatic and often have decreased daily life activities. Integrated into the individualized treatment of the patient, pulmonary rehabilitation is designed to reduce symptoms, optimize functional status, increase participation, and reduce health care costs through stabilizing or reversing systemic manifestations of the disease.[1]

This definition focuses on three important features of successful rehabilitation:

1. *Multidisciplinary.* Pulmonary rehabilitation programs use expertise from various health care disciplines that is integrated into a comprehensive, cohesive program tailored to the needs of each patient.
2. *Individualized.* Patients with disabling lung disease require individual assessment of needs, individual attention, and a program designed to meet realistic individual goals.
3. *Multidimensional outcomes.* To be successful, pulmonary rehabilitation pays attention to goals focused on areas such as physical and psychological symptoms, physical activity, social interaction, and health care use.

The interdisciplinary team of health care professionals in pulmonary rehabilitation may include physicians, nurses, respiratory and physical therapists, psychologists, exercise specialists, and/or others with appropriate expertise. The specific team makeup depends on the resources and expertise available but usually includes at least one full-time staff member.[8]

Patient Selection

Any patient with symptomatic chronic lung disease is a candidate for pulmonary rehabilitation (Table 1). Appropriate patients are aware of disability from their disease and are motivated to be active participants in their own care to improve their health status. Patients with mild disease may not perceive their symptoms to be severe enough to warrant a comprehensive care program. On the other hand, patients with severe disease who are bed bound may be too limited to benefit greatly.

Criteria based on arbitrary lung function parameters or age alone should not be used in selection.[3] Pulmonary function is not a good predictor of symptoms, function, or improvement after rehabilitation in individuals.[9] Older patients with chronic lung diseases may live many years with pulmonary disability. In general, selection should be based on disability and functional limitation from respiratory symptoms, potential for improvement, and motivation to participate actively in a comprehensive self-care program.

Table 1   Patient Selection for Pulmonary Rehabilitation

Symptomatic chronic lung disease

Stable on standard therapy

Functional limitation and disability from disease

Relationship with primary care provider

Motivation to be actively involved in and take responsibility for own health care

No interfering or unstable medical conditions

No arbitrary lung function or age criteria

Other factors are also important in evaluating candidates. Pulmonary rehabilitation is not a primary mode of therapy. Patients should be evaluated and stabilized on standard therapy before beginning a program. They should not have other disabling or unstable conditions that might limit their ability to participate fully and to concentrate.

The ideal patient for pulmonary rehabilitation, then, is one with functional limitation from moderate to severe lung disease who is stable on standard therapy, not distracted or limited by other serious or unstable medical conditions, willing and able to learn about his or her disease, and motivated to devote the time and effort necessary to benefit from a comprehensive care program.

Patient Evaluation

The initial step in pulmonary rehabilitation is screening to ensure appropriate selection and set realistic individual and program goals (Figure 1). The evaluation process includes the following components: interview, medical evaluation, diagnostic testing, psychosocial assessment, and goal setting.

Interview

The screening interview is an important first step. It serves to introduce the patient to the program, as well as to review the medical history and identify psychosocial problems and needs. Significant others should be included. Communication with the primary care physician is also important, establishing the vital link for the rehabilitation staff in clarifying questions prior to the program and facilitating recommendations during and after treatment. Care and attention in this initial evaluation help in setting goals compatible with everyone's expectations and appropriate to program objectives.

Medical Evaluation

Reviewing the medical history helps identify the patient's lung disease and assess its severity. Other medical problems that might preclude or delay participation may be identified. Available laboratory data should be reviewed, including pulmonary function and exercise tests, rest and exercise arterial blood gas measurements, chest radiographs, electrocardiogram, and pertinent blood tests. Program staff can then determine the need for additional information or action before the program.

Diagnostic Testing

Planning an appropriate rehabilitation program requires accurate, current information. The complexity of the testing procedures performed depends on individual patient and program goals, as well as the facilities and expertise available.

Pulmonary function testing is used to characterize lung disease and quantify impairment. Spirometry and lung volume measurements are most useful; other tests, such as diffusing capacity, airway resistance, and maximal respiratory pressures to assess muscle strength, can be added as needed.

Exercise testing helps to assess the patient's exercise tolerance and to evaluate blood gas changes (hypoxemia or hypercapnia) with exercise.[10,11] This may also uncover coexisting diseases (eg, heart disease). The exercise test is also used to establish a safe and appropriate prescription for subsequent training.

Maximal exercise of patients with chronic lung disease is limited largely by their breathing reserve. Simple pulmonary function tests such as spirometry can be used to estimate a patient's capacity for sustained breathing (maximum ventilation) during exercise. However, an individual patient's maximum work capacity can be estimated only from lung function. Exercise tolerance also depends on the patient's perception and tolerance of the subjective symptom of breathlessness. Therefore, it is important to exercise patients to assess their physical function and symptom tolerance.

Exercise evaluation for rehabilitation is most easily performed with the type of activity planned for training (eg, a treadmill for a walking training program); however, test results from one type of exercise (eg, cycle) can be translated to related activities (eg, walking).[12] Variables measured or monitored during testing should include workload, heart rate, electrocardiogram, arterial oxygenation, and symptoms (eg, breathlessness). Other measures, such as ventilation or expired gas analysis to calculate oxygen uptake (VO_2) and related variables, may be obtained depending on the interest and expertise of the program staff and laboratory.[13,14]

Measurement of arterial oxygenation at rest and during exercise is important because of the frequent but unpredictable occurrence of exercise-induced hypoxemia.[15] Blood gas sampling during exercise makes testing more complex. A noninvasive estimate of arterial oxygen saturation by cutaneous oximetry is useful for continuous monitoring but has limited accuracy (eg, 95% confidence limits for cutaneous oximetry ± 4 to 5% saturation).[16]

Psychosocial Assessment

Successful rehabilitation requires attention not only to physical problems but also to psychological, emotional, and social ones. Patients with chronic illnesses experience psychosocial difficulties as they struggle to deal with symptoms they may not fully

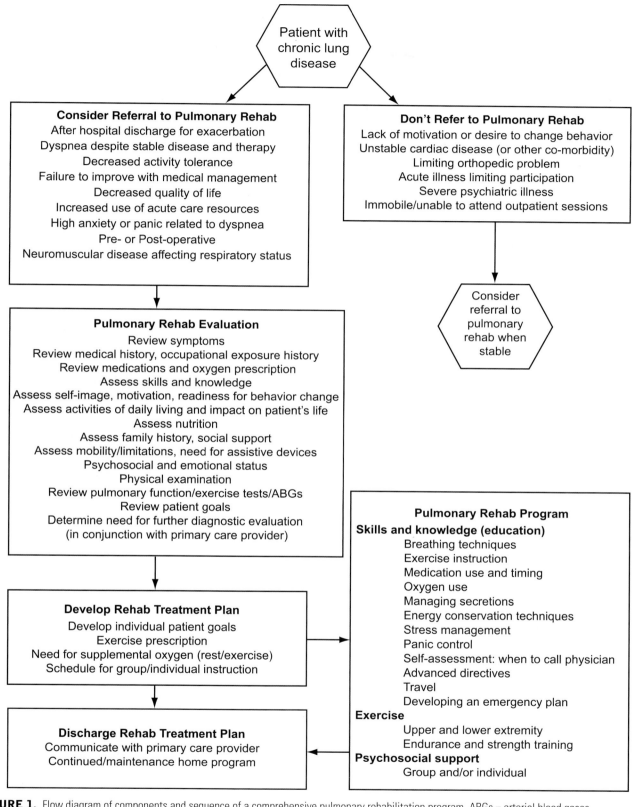

FIGURE 1. Flow diagram of components and sequence of a comprehensive pulmonary rehabilitation program. ABGs = arterial blood gases.

understand.[17] Neuropsychological impairment is common in patients with chronic lung disease and cannot be accounted for solely on the basis of age, depression, and physical disease.[18] Commonly, such patients become depressed, frightened, anxious, and more dependent on others to care for their needs. Progressive dyspnea is a frightening symptom and may lead to a vicious "fear-dyspnea" cycle: with progressive disease, less exertion results in more dyspnea, which produces more fear and anxiety, which, in turn, leads to more dyspnea. Ultimately, the patient avoids any physical activity associated with both of these unpleasant symptoms.

To address these problems, the initial evaluation should include an assessment of the patient's psychological state and close attention to psychosocial clues during screening interviews (eg, family and social support, living arrangement, activities of daily living, hobbies, employment potential). Important clues in initial interviews may be obtained by paying attention to nonverbal communication such as facial expression, physical appearance, handshake, and "body space." Cognitive impairment that may limit the ability to participate fully can be identified. Significant others may provide valuable insight and should be included in the screening process and program whenever possible.

Goals

After evaluating a patient's medical, physiologic, and psychosocial state, it is important to set specific goals that are compatible with each individual's disease, needs, and expectations. Goals should be realistic given the objectives of the program. Significant others should be included in this process so that everyone understands what can, and cannot, be expected.

Program Content

Comprehensive pulmonary rehabilitation programs typically include several key components: education, respiratory and chest physiotherapy instruction, psychosocial support, and exercise training. Often the various components are provided simultaneously; for example, during an exercise session, a patient may learn and practice breathing techniques for symptom control while being encouraged and supported by staff or other patients.

Education

Successful pulmonary rehabilitation depends on the understanding and active involvement of patients and those important for their social support. Education is an integral component; even patients with severe disease can gain a better understanding of their disease and learn specific means to deal with problems.[19] Instruction can be provided individually or in small groups but should be adapted to different learning abilities. Typical topics covered include how normal lungs work; what chronic lung disease is; medications; nutrition; travel; stress reduction and relaxation; when to call your doctor; and planning a daily schedule. Individual instruction and coaching may be provided on the use of respiratory therapy equipment and oxygen, breathing techniques, bronchial drainage, chest percussion, energy-saving techniques, and self-care tips. The general philosophy is to encourage patients to assume responsibility for and become partners with their physician in providing their own care.[20]

Respiratory and Chest Physiotherapy Techniques

Patients with chronic lung disease use, abuse, and are confused about respiratory and chest physiotherapy techniques. In pulmonary rehabilitation, each patient's needs for respiratory care techniques can be assessed and instruction provided in proper use. These may include chest physiotherapy techniques to control secretions; breathing retraining techniques to relieve and control dyspnea and improve ventilatory function (eg, pursed lips breathing); and proper use of respiratory care equipment, including nebulizers, metered-dose inhalers, and oxygen.[21]

Exercise

Exercise is important in pulmonary rehabilitation.[22,23] There is considerable evidence of favorable responses to exercise training in patients with chronic lung diseases.[2,24] The benefits are both physiologic and psychological. Patients may increase their maximum capacity and/or endurance for physical activity, even though lung function does not usually change. Patients may also benefit from learning to perform physical tasks more efficiently. Exercise training provides an ideal opportunity for patients to learn their capacity for physical work and to use and practice methods for controlling dyspnea (eg, breathing and relaxation techniques). Of all of the components in a comprehensive pulmonary rehabilitation program, exercise is probably the most difficult in terms of personnel, equipment, and expertise. Principles of exercise testing and training for patients with lung disease differ from those derived in normal individuals or other patient populations because of differences in the limitations to exercise and the problems encountered in training.[22]

Many approaches have been used in rehabilitation to train the person with chronic lung disease. To be successful, the program should be tailored to the individual's physical abilities, interests, resources, and environment. For general application, techniques should be simple and inexpensive. As in normal individuals and other patients, benefits are largely specific to the muscles and tasks involved in training. Patients tend to do best on activities and exercises for which they are trained. Walking programs are particularly useful. They have the added benefit of encouraging patients to expand social horizons. In inclement weather, many can walk indoors (eg, shopping malls). Other types of exercise (eg, cycling, swimming) are also effective. Patients should be encouraged to incorporate regular exercise into daily activities they enjoy (eg, golf, gardening). Since many persons with chronic lung disease have limited exercise tolerance, emphasis during training should be placed on increasing endurance. Changes in endurance are often greater than changes in maximal exercise tolerance.[25] This allows patients to become more functional within their physical limits. An increase in maximum exercise is also possible as patients gain experience and confidence with their exercise program.

A problem in planning a safe exercise program for patients with lung disease is the potential worsening of hypoxemia with exercise. Patients who may not be hypoxemic at rest can develop changes in arterial oxygenation that cannot be predicted reliably from resting measurements of pulmonary function or gas exchange.[15] Therefore, it is important to evaluate rest and exercise oxygenation. Such testing is also used to prescribe oxygen therapy at rest and with physical activity. With the availability of convenient, portable systems for ambulatory oxygen delivery, hypoxemia is not a contraindication to safe exercise training.

Exercise programs for pulmonary patients typically emphasize lower extremity training (eg, walking). However, many persons with chronic lung disease report disabling dyspnea for daily activities involving the upper extremities (eg, lifting, grooming) at work levels much lower than those for the lower extremities. Upper extremity exercise is accompanied by a higher ventilatory demand for a given level of work than for lower extremity exercise. Since training is generally specific to the muscles and tasks used in training, upper extremity exercises may be important in helping pulmonary patients cope better with common daily activities.[2,24]

Psychosocial Support

An essential component of pulmonary rehabilitation is psychosocial support, provided to help patients combat symptoms reflecting progressive feelings of hopelessness and inability to cope with a chronic, progressive disease. Psychosocial support is provided best by warm and enthusiastic staff who can communicate effectively with patients and devote the time and effort necessary to understand and motivate them. Significant others should be included in activities so that they can understand and cope better with the patient's disease. Support groups are also effective. Patients with severe psychological disorders may benefit from individual counseling and therapy. Psychotropic drugs should generally be reserved for patients with more severe psychological dysfunction.

Benefits of Pulmonary Rehabilitation

There is a growing body of evidence that supports the expected results and benefits of pulmonary rehabilitation in the management of patients with chronic lung disease. Evidence-based guidelines were published by a joint effort of the American College of Chest Physicians (ACCP) and the American Association of Cardiovascular and Pulmonary Rehabilitation (AACVPR) in 1997[24] and were updated in 2007.[2] Recommendations from the 2007 guideline are summarized in Table 2. The breadth of the topics covered highlights the significant increase in the published literature over the decade between the two guideline documents and the expanded scope of the evidence base.

For the 2007 guideline, the panel used a systematic approach to identify and review 928 articles on pulmonary rehabilitation in COPD published from 1996 through 2004. From these, 202 articles were selected for formal grading and review by the panel. Ultimately, 81 clinical trials were included in

Table 2 Summary of Recommendations from 2007 ACCP/AACVPR Evidence-Based Guidelines for Pulmonary Rehabilitation.

Evidence Grade*	Recommendation
1A	A program of exercise training of the muscles of ambulation is recommended as a mandatory component of pulmonary rehabilitation for patients with COPD
	Pulmonary rehabilitation improves the symptom of dyspnea in patients with COPD
	Pulmonary rehabilitation improves health-related quality of life in patients with COPD
	Six to 12 weeks of pulmonary rehabilitation produces benefits in several outcomes that decline gradually over 12 to 18 months
	Both low- and high-intensity exercise training produce clinical benefits for patients with COPD
	Addition of a strength training component to a program of pulmonary rehabilitation increases muscle strength and muscle mass
	Unsupported endurance training of the upper extremities is beneficial in patients with COPD and should be included in pulmonary rehabilitation programs
1B	Lower extremity exercise training at higher exercise intensity produces greater physiologic benefits than lower intensity training in patients with COPD
	The scientific evidence does not support the routine use of inspiratory muscle training as an essential component of pulmonary rehabilitation
	Education should be an integral component of pulmonary rehabilitation. Education should include information on collaborative self-management and prevention and treatment of exacerbations.
	Pulmonary rehabilitation is beneficial for some patients with chronic respiratory diseases other than COPD

(Continued)

Table 2 (Continued) Summary of Recommendations from 2007 ACCP/AACVPR Evidence-Based Guidelines for Pulmonary Rehabilitation	
1C	Some benefits, such as health-related quality of life, remain above control at 12 to 18 months Supplemental oxygen should be used during rehabilitative exercise training in patients with severe exercise-induced hypoxemia
2A	None
2B	Pulmonary rehabilitation reduces the number of hospital days and other measures of health care use in patients with COPD There are psychosocial benefits from comprehensive pulmonary rehabilitation programs in patients with COPD As an adjunct to exercise training in selected patients with severe COPD, noninvasive ventilation produces modest additional improvements in exercise performance
2C	Pulmonary rehabilitation is cost effective in patients with COPD Longer pulmonary rehabilitation programs (beyond 12 weeks) produce greater sustained benefits than shorter programs Maintenance strategies following pulmonary rehabilitation have a modest effect Current scientific evidence does not support the routine use of anabolic agents in pulmonary rehabilitation for patients with COPD on long-term outcomes There is minimal evidence to support the benefits of psychosocial interventions as a single therapeutic modality Administering supplemental oxygen during high-intensity exercise programs in patients without exercise-induced hypoxemia may improve gains in exercise endurance
Statement/No recommendation	There is insufficient evidence to determine if pulmonary rehabilitation improves survival in patients with COPD Although no recommendation is provided since scientific evidence is lacking, current practice and expert opinion support the inclusion of psychosocial interventions as a component of comprehensive pulmonary rehabilitation programs for patients with COPD There is insufficient evidence to support the routine use of nutritional supplementation in pulmonary rehabilitation of patients with COPD Although no recommendation is provided since scientific evidence is lacking, current practice and expert opinion suggest that pulmonary rehabilitation for patients with chronic respiratory diseases other than COPD should be modified to include treatment strategies specific to individual diseases and patients in addition to treatment strategies common to both COPD and non-COPD patients

Adapted from ACCP-AACVPR Pulmonary Rehabilitation Guidelines Panel.[2]
AACVPR = American Association of Cardiovascular and Pulmonary Rehabilitation; ACCP = American College of Chest Physicians; COPD = chronic obstructive pulmonary disease.
*Evidence Grades:

		Balance of Benefits to Risks and Burdens			
		Benefits Outweigh Risks/Burdens	Risks/Burdens Outweigh Benefits	Evenly Balanced	Uncertain
Strength of Evidence	High	1A	1A	2A	
	Moderate	1B	1B	2B	
	Low or Very Low	1C	1C	2C	2C

1A: Strong Recommendation   2A: Weak Recommendation
1B: Strong Recommendation   2B: Weak Recommendation
1C: Strong Recommendation   2C: Weak Recommendation

evidence-based tables and formed the basis of the recommendations. The assignment of evidence grades for the recommendations followed the ACCP system and is based on the relationship between the strength of evidence and the balance of benefits to risk and burden.[26] In this system, the recommendations are rated based on two characteristics: (1) strength of the scientific evidence (A, B, C, representing high, moderate, and low/very low, respectively) and (2) balance of benefits to risks and burdens (1 = imbalance when benefits outweigh risks/burdens or vice versa; 2 = equal balance between benefits and risks/burdens).

Ultimately, the 2007 ACCP/AACVPR panel made and rated 26 recommendations and statements regarding pulmonary rehabilitation. Of these, seven were given the highest rating of 1A, representing strong evidence and documented benefits. These included improvements from comprehensive pulmonary rehabilitation in lower extremity exercise training, dyspnea, and health-related quality of life and the decline in benefits over 12 to 18 months from a 6- to 12-week intervention. They also felt that there was high-quality evidence supporting exercise in pulmonary rehabilitation regarding both high- and low-intensity training, increase in muscle strength and muscle mass from strength training, and upper extremity training. Other benefits with moderate level evidence (1B) included greater physiologic benefits from higher exercise training intensity, incorporation of education in pulmonary rehabilitation, and benefits for some patients with chronic respiratory diseases other than COPD. As in 1997, the 2007 panel again did not recommend the routine use of inspiratory muscle training (1B). Weaker recommendations (1C) were made concerning maintenance of long-term benefits at 12 to 18 months and use of supplemental oxygen in patients with exercise-induced hypoxemia.

In addition to the ACCP/AACVPR guidelines, several other reviews support the benefits of pulmonary rehabilitation. The ATS/ERS statement on pulmonary rehabilitation provides a systematic review that complements the ACCP/AACVPR guidelines and concludes that there is strong and growing evidence for improvement in exercise endurance, dyspnea, functional capacity, and quality of life and reduced health care use from pulmonary rehabilitation.[1] In a 2006 Cochrane Review, Lacasse analyzed 31 randomized trials in patients with COPD and concluded that rehabilitation forms an important component of the management of COPD.[27] The author reported statistically and clinically significant improvement in important domains of quality of life (dyspnea, fatigue, emotions, and patients' control over disease). Improvement in measures of exercise capacity were slightly below the threshold for clinical significance. Similarly, after a systematic review, Cambach and colleagues reviewed 18 controlled studies evaluating the long-term effects of pulmonary rehabilitation in patients with asthma and COPD.[28] They found significant improvements for exercise measures of maximal exercise capacity, endurance time, and walking distance and for health-related quality of life measures in all dimensions of the Chronic Respiratory Disease Questionnaire (dyspnea, fatigue, emotion, and mastery). Improvements in maximal exercise capacity and walking distance were sustained for up to 9 months after rehabilitation.

Benefits and cost savings associated with pulmonary rehabilitation have been demonstrated not only in highly specialized centers but also in community-based practice settings. A collaborative study of 647 patients in 10 centers in California reported significant improvements in dyspnea and health-related quality of life along with a substantial reduction in measures of health care use over 18 months of follow-up.[29] Similar findings with a reduction in hospital and intensive care unit days in the year after compared with the year before pulmonary rehabilitation were reported by a consortium of 11 centers in Connecticut and New York in 128 patients.[30]

Rehabilitation Before and After Lung Surgery
Lung Transplantation

Pulmonary rehabilitation is recommended and used commonly in both the preoperative and postoperative phases of lung transplantation programs.[4,5,31] Although the general strategies of rehabilitation may be similar, the individual and program goals and specific program components differ. The efficacy of pre- and postoperative pulmonary rehabilitation in improving clinical outcomes in lung transplant patients, however, has not been evaluated in clinical trials. Such studies are needed.

PRETRANSPLANTATION REHABILITATION

Patients with advanced lung diseases who are candidates for lung transplantation are typically evaluated by the transplant team and then may be referred for pulmonary rehabilitation after acceptance. Rehabilitation staff can evaluate the patients to assess their needs and plan an appropriate program that can be maintained throughout a waiting period that can last months to years. Since these patients have advanced disease with limited life expectancy, the goals in this preoperative period differ from those that typically apply to chronic lung disease rehabilitation.

The overall goals are to maintain function, monitor disease progression, prevent complications, provide education about both the underlying lung disease and lung transplantation, and provide psychosocial support for patients and families in coping with the stresses of waiting for a potentially lifesaving procedure. Although patients may have some initial improvement in exercise tolerance or endurance as they begin rehabilitation, the primary goal for these patients with advanced, progressive lung disease is to maintain mobility and exercise capacity. Exercise sessions also provide an excellent means to monitor disease progression and to detect problems early, which may be associated with increased breathlessness or reduced arterial oxygenation with exercise.

The goals of education in the pretransplant period are to teach patients about their underlying lung diseases, as well as the transplantation procedures and what to expect after transplantation. Patients can also be taught techniques for self-care and self-assessment that will be useful before and after surgery.

The psychosocial stresses of waiting for transplantation are considerable. Many patients feel as if their life is on hold. Some may have moved away from family and their usual social support network to live close to the transplant center. Providing support for patients and family members during this time, whether through formal group support sessions or through informal contact with supportive staff and other patients, helps patients cope better with these problems.

POSTTRANSPLANTATION REHABILITATION

After undergoing lung transplant surgery, patients must learn to cope with a new level of function, new expectations, and a new set of problems. Rehabilitation in this phase can facilitate physical reconditioning, help implement self-care and assessment techniques, and help patients cope with the psychosocial adaptations to a new lifestyle.

Goals of exercise training after rehabilitation are to improve physical work tolerance and to continue to assess symptoms and oxygenation as early warning signs of complications such as rejection and infection. Educational goals are focused on self-care and assessment and the importance of compliance with a new medical regimen. Psychosocial support can assist with adaptation to a new set of stresses related to new demands and expectations of themselves and their significant others. Patients used to being "sick," disabled, and cared for by others may now be expected to be "well," be independent, return to work, and provide support for others.

Lung Volume Reduction Surgery

Recently, there has been a resurgence of interest in LVRS in the treatment of patients with severe emphysematous obstructive lung disease.[32] Pulmonary rehabilitation has been recommended as an important modality in the evaluation for and preparation of patients for this procedure and in the postoperative recovery phase.[6,7,33,34] Since these patients have severe, disabling chronic lung disease, they are typically good candidates for pulmonary rehabilitation. Enrolling patients in rehabilitation prior to surgery has the advantage of optimizing their functional status, improving physical and psychological symptoms, helping them learn more about their disease and alternative treatment options, and improving their skills for coping with and actively comanaging their disease. Patients can then make an informed decision about surgical treatment based on their optimal level of baseline function. After surgery, similar to the posttransplantation period, rehabilitation helps patients adapt to new levels of function and reassess symptoms and oxygenation needs. Prospective studies are still needed, however, to evaluate the efficacy of this practice in improving outcomes in the context of LVRS. The National Emphysema Treatment Trial (NETT), a multicenter, randomized clinical trial of medical therapy versus medical therapy plus LVRS, evaluated the benefits and risks of LVRS in patients with severe bilateral emphysema.[34] All patients enrolled in the NETT completed 6 to 10 weeks of pulmonary rehabilitation prior to randomization into medical therapy or medical therapy plus LVRS and participated in a maintenance program of additional rehabilitation after randomization. Significant improvements after pulmonary rehabilitation were observed in exercise capacity, dyspnea, and health-related quality of life in these patients with severe emphysema.[7]

Summary

Pulmonary rehabilitation has been well established as a means of improving symptoms and functional status and reducing disability and economic burden for patients with chronic lung diseases. These programs incorporate broad interdisciplinary expertise from a variety of health care disciplines that can be coordinated and directed toward the needs of individual patients. Although much of the experience in pulmonary rehabilitation to date has been with patients with COPD, it is clear that similar benefits can result for persons with other chronic pulmonary conditions. Pulmonary rehabilitation may also play an important role in the preoperative evaluation and preparation and postoperative recovery of patients undergoing surgical procedures such as lung transplantation, LVRS, and lung resection.

References

1. American Thoracic Society, European Respiratory Society. ATS/ERS statement on pulmonary rehabilitation. Am J Respir Crit Care Med 2006;173:1390–413.
2. Ries AL, Bauldoff GS, Carlin BW, et al. Pulmonary rehabilitation: joint ACCP/AACVPR evidence-based clinical practice guidelines. Chest 2007;131:4S–42S.
3. American Association of Cardiovascular and Pulmonary Rehabilitation. Guidelines for pulmonary rehabilitation programs. 3rd ed. Champaign (IL): Human Kinetics;2004.
4. Palmer SM, Tapson VF. Pulmonary rehabilitation in the surgical patient: lung transplantation and lung volume reduction surgery. Respir Care Clin North Am 1998;4:71–83.
5. Biggar DG, Malen JF, Trulock EP, et al. Pulmonary rehabilitation before and after lung transplantation. In: Casaburi R, Petty TL, editors. Principles and practice of pulmonary rehabilitation. Philadelphia: WB Saunders; 1993. p. 459–67.
6. Ries AL. Pulmonary rehabilitation and lung volume reduction surgery. In: Fessler HE, Reilly JJ Jr, Sugarbaker DJ, editors. Lung volume reduction surgery for emphysema. New York: Marcel Dekker; 2004. p. 123–48.
7. Ries AL, Make BJ, Lee SM, et al. The effects of pulmonary rehabilitation in the National Emphysema Treatment Trial. Chest 2005;128:3799–809.
8. Ries AL, Squier HC. The team concept in pulmonary rehabilitation. In: Fishman A, editor. Pulmonary rehabilitation. New York: Marcel Dekker; 1996. p. 55–65.
9. Niederman MS, Clemente PH, Fein AM, et al. Benefits of a multi-disciplinary pulmonary rehabilitation program: improvements are independent of lung function. Chest 1991;99:798–804.
10. American Thoracic Society-American College of Chest Physicians. ATS/ACCP statement on cardiopulmonary exercise testing. Am J Respir Crit Care Med 2003; 167:211–77.
11. Ries AL. The role of exercise testing in pulmonary diagnosis. Clin Chest Med 1987;8:81–9.
12. Ries AL, Moser KM. Predicting treadmill/walking speed from cycle ergometry exercise in chronic obstructive pulmonary disease. Am Rev Respir Dis 1982;126:924–7.
13. Jones NL. Clinical exercise testing. 4th ed. Philadelphia: WB Saunders; 1997.

14. Wasserman K, Hansen JE, Sue DY, et al. Principles of exercise testing and interpretation. 3rd ed. Philadelphia: Lippincott Williams & Wilkins; 1999.

15. Ries AL, Farrow JT, Clausen JL. Pulmonary function tests cannot predict exercise-induced hypoxemia in chronic obstructive pulmonary disease. Chest 1988;93:454–9.

16. Ries AL, Farrow JT, Clausen JL. Accuracy of two ear oximeters at rest and during exercise in pulmonary patients. Am Rev Respir Dis 1985;132:685–9.

17. Glaser EM, Dudley DL. Psychosocial rehabilitation and psychopharmacology. In: Hodgkin JE, Petty TL, editors. Chronic obstructive pulmonary disease: current concepts. Philadelphia: WB Saunders; 1987. p. 128–53.

18. Prigatano GP, Grant I. Neuropsychological correlates of COPD. In: McSweeny AJ, Grant I, editors. Chronic obstructive pulmonary disease: a behavioral perspective. New York: Marcel Dekker; 1988. p. 39–57.

19. Neish CM, Hopp JW. The role of education in pulmonary rehabilitation. J Cardiopulm Rehabil 1988;11:439–41.

20. Ries AL, Bullock PJ, Larsen CA, et al. Shortness of breath, a guide to better living and breathing. 6th ed. St. Louis: Mosby; 2001.

21. Rochester DF, Goldberg SK. Techniques of respiratory physical therapy. Am Rev Respir Dis 1980;122 Suppl:133–46.

22. Ries AL. The importance of exercise in pulmonary rehabilitation. Clin Chest Med 1994;15:327–37.

23. Casaburi R. Exercise training in chronic obstructive lung disease. In: Casaburi R, Petty TL, editors. Principles and practice of pulmonary rehabilitation. Philadelphia: WB Saunders; 1993. p. 204–24.

24. ACCP-AACVPR Pulmonary Rehabilitation Guidelines Panel. Pulmonary rehabilitation: Joint ACCP/AACVPR evidence based guidelines. Chest 1997;112:1363–96.

25. Ries AL, Kaplan RM, Limberg TM, et al. Effects of pulmonary rehabilitation on physiologic and psychosocial outcomes in patients with chronic obstructive pulmonary disease. Ann Intern Med 1995;122:823–32.

26. Guyatt G, Gutterman D, Baumann MH, et al. Grading strength of recommendations and quality of evidence in clinical guidelines: report from an American College of Chest Physicians task force. Chest 2006;129:174–81.

27. Lacasse Y. Pulmonary rehabilitation for chronic obstructive pulmonary disease. Cochrane Database of Systematic Reviews 2006; Issue 4. Art. No.: CD003793. DOI: 10.1002/14651858.CD003793.pub2.

28. Cambach W, Wagenaar RC, Koelman TW, et al. The long-term effects of pulmonary rehabilitation in patients with asthma and chronic obstructive disease: a research synthesis. Arch Phys Med Rehabil 1999;80:103–11..

29. California Pulmonary Rehabilitation Collaborative Group. Effects of pulmonary rehabilitation on dyspnea, quality of life and health care costs in California. J Cardiopulm Rehabil 2004;24:52–62.

30. Raskin J, Spiegler P, McCusker C, et al. The effect of pulmonary rehabilitation on healthcare utilization in chronic obstructive pulmonary disease: the Northeast Pulmonary Rehabilitation Consortium. J Cardiopulm Rehabil 2006;26:231–6.

31. Craven JL, Bright J, Dear CL. Psychiatric, psychosocial, and rehabilitative aspects of lung transplantation. Clin Chest Med 1990;11:247–57.

32. National Emphysema Treatment Trial Research Group. A randomized trial comparing lung-volume-reduction surgery with medical therapy for severe emphysema. N Engl J Med 2003;348:2059–73.

33. Celli BR. Pulmonary rehabilitation and lung volume reduction surgery in the treatment of patients with chronic obstructive pulmonary disease. Monaldi Arch Chest Dis 1998;53:471–9.

34. National Emphysema Treatment Trial Research Group. Rationale and design of the National Emphysema Treatment Trial (NETT): a prospective randomized trial of lung volume reduction surgery. Chest 1999;116:1761.

CHAPTER 29

STEM CELLS

VICTOR I. PEINADO, PhD, AND JOAN ALBERT BARBERÀ, MD

THE IDEA OF A MAINTENANCE PROGRAM in the adult lung has emerged in recent years.[1] This program may be defective in some chronic diseases, such as chronic obstructive pulmonary disease (COPD), in which emphysematous destruction of lung parenchyma takes place.[2] Usually, the lung copes with external challenges by inhaled particles, toxic gases, and invading microorganisms. The defense against this external injury depends on different mechanisms (antioxidants, antiproteases, immune response) and an efficient system to remove and replace apoptotic cells. Critical to lung homeostasis is the role of stem cells that retain their ability to replicate and differentiate into structural cells. Both resident and bone marrow–derived stem cells (BMSCs) may play such a role in the lung. Failure of stem cells to cope with external injury or cell apoptosis may underlie the pathogenesis of emphysema in COPD. On the other hand, excessive repair by stem cells may result in tissue hyperplasia and remodeling.

In this chapter, we review some basic concepts on stem cells, their origin and location in the lung, their contribution to lung tissue repair, and, finally, the potential for cell therapy in COPD.

Definition and Concepts

Stem cells are primordial cells that retain the ability to renew themselves through frequent cycles of cell division (clone) while maintaining the undifferentiated state and, under certain conditions, are able to differentiate into a wide range of specialized cell types, forming tissues and organs. Cellular differentiation is a strongly regulated process that involves activation and deactivation of different genes, resulting in the acquisition of a new morphology and functional specialized structure.

There are three broad categories of stem cells in mammals: embryonic, fetal, and adult stem cells. Stem cells can also be classified according to their potential for differentiation into totipotent, pluripotent, and multipotent cells. A *totipotent* stem cell possesses the capacity to form a complete organism. A *pluripotent* stem cell cannot form a complete organism but harbors the capacity to generate cells of any of the three embryonic layers (ectoderm, mesoderm, or endoderm). A *multipotent* stem cell can only differentiate into cells of the same germ layer. In the most developed animals, embryonic stem cells derive from the cellular internal mass of the embryo

in the blastocyst stage (7–14 days) and are *multipotential* cells. Adult stem cells are undifferentiated cells that belong to a differentiated (specialized) tissue and possess the capacity to yield any of the specialized cell types in the tissue. Adult stem cells can make identical copies of themselves for the lifetime of the organism (self-renewal). Adult stem cells usually divide to generate *progenitor* or *precursor* cells, which then differentiate into "mature" cell types, with characteristic shapes and specialized functions (Figure 1).

Progenitor cells are in an advanced stage of differentiation in the fetus and adult tissues and possess limited potential for self-renewal, being able to generate two totally specialized cells. Progenitor cells preserve a certain degree of *plasticity* and can replace damaged or dead cells, thus contributing to maintain the integrity and functionality of the tissues. Owing to this plasticity, adult stem cells from a certain tissue can generate one or more specialized cellular types of another tissue.

The behavior of stem cells in tissues is controlled by the local microenvironment (cells and extracellular matrix proteins), also known as the *niche*. The specific niche of each lineage determines in a precise way both how a stem cell will divide and the fate of the descendant cells by interactions with extracellular matrix proteins and cell–cell interactions, likely mediated by growth factors.

Origin of Stem Cells in the Lung

The mammalian lung develops between the fourth and fifth week of gestation as an outgrowth of the embryonic gut that in humans originates from a diverticulum of the ventral wall of the primitive esophagus. From then on, the nascent epithelium undergoes dichotomous branching into the surrounding splanchnic mesenchyme in a highly ordered process called branching morphogenesis.[3] The mature human lung has distinct anatomic regions lined by different types of epithelial cells (see also Chapter 2, "Lung Development").[4,5]

Tissue-Specific Adult Stem Cells

Compared with other organs, the adult lung has a much reduced level of regeneration. Despite that, some subsets of cells are clonogenic and capable of self-renewal and multilineage differentiation,[6–8] although their identification has been hampered by the difficulty of isolating them (Table 1).

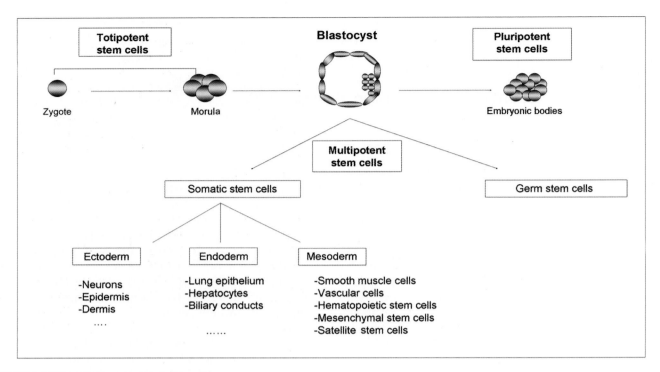

FIGURE 1. Differentiation potential of stem cells.

PROXIMAL AIRWAYS

The trachea and major bronchi are lined with a pseudostratified epithelium. The main phenotypes present in proximal airways are ciliated and mucous secretory (or goblet) cells. Less frequently, neuroendocrine cells and poorly differentiated basal cells are found in a basal position. Some studies have reported that the tracheal epithelium is repopulated from stem cells present in the epithelial lining,[9–11] whereas others suggest that tracheal gland duct cells may harbor repopulating cells.[12] Basal and parabasal cells may contain a pluripotent cell reserve since these cells show great resistance to injury.[13,14] *In-vitro* studies that involve denudation of the trachea have demonstrated that basal cells can produce all of the major cell phenotypes found in the trachea, including basal, ciliated, goblet, and granular secretory cells.[15–17] Basal and parabasal cells also have a high rate of proliferation.[9]

BRONCHIOLES

Clara cells, nonciliated cells present in the bronchiolar wall, have the ability to renew themselves and act as progenitors of ciliated cells.[10,18] There is a variant of Clara cells that expresses Clara cell secretory protein (CCSP) that shows multipotent differentiation capacity and is resistant to airway pollutants, such as naphthalene.[19–23] These cells are located in discrete pools in neuroepithelial bodies and at the bronchoalveolar duct junction.

ALVEOLI

The alveoli are lined by flattened squamous (type I) and cuboidal (type II) alveolar cells. Type II cells in the alveolus are considered progenitor lung cells on the basis of their capacity for self-renewal and give rise to differentiated type I alveolar cells. Type II alveolar cells also have a relatively high proliferation rate, are relatively resistant to injury, and have

Table 1 Lung Tissue—Specific Stem Cells	
Epithelial Precursor Cell	*Specialized Cells*
Tracheal basal cell	Mucous, ciliated, neuroendocrine
Tracheal mucus-gland duct cell	Mucous, ciliated, neuroendocrine
Tracheal secretory cell	Mucous, ciliated, neuroendocrine
Bronchiolar Clara cell	Mucous, ciliated (type I/II pneumocyte?)
Alveolar type II pneumocyte	Type I and II pneumocytes (Clara cells?)
Neuroendocrine	Pulmonary neuroendocrine cells (Clara cells?)

high telomerase activity.[24] Proliferation of type II alveolar cells is induced by injury to type I alveolar cells and inflammatory infiltrates.[24,25] Type II cell injury and apoptosis seem to be important early features in the pathogenesis of pulmonary fibrosis.[26]

MICROVASCULATURE

Endothelial cells (and, presumably, smooth muscle cells) of large and small vessels appear to derive from distinct embryologic origins. Endothelial cells in small vessels seem to derive from the lung mesenchyme through vasculogenesis, whereas in large vessels, they derive from the pulmonary truncus through angiogenesis.[27]

Clinical and experimental observations suggest that pericytes contribute to the regulation of microvascular growth and function. Pericytes have properties of multipotential stem cells that are fully capable of differentiating into different cell types, including fibroblasts, connective tissue cells, and vascular smooth muscle cells, providing the endothelial cells with a balanced cellular microenvironment.[28,29] Pericytes contain actin and myosin proteins and exhibit contractile properties, suggesting that they may contribute to modulate blood flow.[30]

Circulating Stem Cells

There is some evidence that progenitor cells can give rise to some subsets of pulmonary cells and may originate outside of the lung. Those cells might home the lung and contribute to the lung maintenance program.

BONE MARROW-DERIVED STEM CELLS

Adult bone marrow contains pluripotent stem cells that have the capacity for self-renewal and give rise to hematopoietic and mesenchymal cell lineages.[31] BMSCs can serve as precursors for differentiated cells of multiple organs, including the lung.[32–36] In fact, it has been shown that donor bone marrow cells can give rise to bronchial epithelial cells, as well as type I and type II alveolar epithelial cells (Figure 2).[33,5,36] In humans, cells with bone marrow origin have been found sputtering the adult lung after hematopoietic stem cell transplantation, suggesting that these cells might play some role in lung tissue repair.[37] The exact mechanisms by which BMSCs are selectively recruited and differentiate in specific tissues are not known, although recruitment is enhanced by tissue injury, suggesting that the process might be regulated by inflammatory cytokines.[33,38,39] The role of bone marrow–derived progenitor cells has been intensely evaluated in vascular biology. Asahara and colleagues observed that purified CD34+ hematopoietic progenitor cells from adults can differentiate *ex vivo* to an endothelial phenotype.[40] These cells, named endothelial progenitor cells (EPCs), show expression of various endothelial markers and are incorporated into new vessels at sites of ischemia.

SIDE POPULATION

Side population cells were recently identified in multiple species and isolated from various tissues, including bone marrow, liver, skeletal muscle, and lung.[41,42] These cells exhibit a potent capacity to locally reconstitute damaged tissues. In the lung, side population cells comprise 0.03 to 0.07% of total lung cells and are evenly distributed in proximal and distal lung regions. It remains to be determined whether these cells have a bone marrow origin or are resident cells in the lung.

Phenotypical Characterization of Stem Cells in the Lung

Stem cells are difficult to identify because (1) cells with long-term replicative ability are rare; (2) there are multiple types of stem cells; (3) surface antigens used to identify them are downregulated as cells differentiate, making them difficult to track; and (4) the appearance of stem cells is similar to that of other tissue cells. In addition, there are no specific markers for each stem cell. Accordingly, the most common approach to identify and characterize stem cells is through the combined expression of several markers. The most common antigens used to identify stem cells are listed in Table 2.

The quantification of EPCs can be performed by flow cytometric analysis of unfractionated bone marrow or peripheral blood cells, purified mononuclear cells, or cultured mononuclear cells. A combination of markers such as CD34/CD133/KDR or CD45/CD34/CD133 may be used in these approaches to identify a specific subset of progenitor cells (EPCs in this case) (Figure 3).[43]

Lung Tissue Injury and Repair in COPD

The airway epithelium is a primary interface with the external environment and a potential target for cigarette smoke compounds and other environmental agents that are the main cause of COPD. The pathologic changes underlying COPD are destruction of the lung parenchyma owing to emphysema, thickening of small airways, and luminal obstruction by inflammatory mucoid secretions. Emphysema is also remarkable for the relative paucity of blood vessels, suggesting that the preservation of the capillary network may be essential to avoid the progression of parenchymal destruction.[44,45] All of these features are relevant in the pathogenesis of COPD since they may indicate defective mechanisms for tissue repair.

Several factors, including inflammation, cigarette smoking, hypoxia, and cellular senescence, may contribute to the pathogenesis of COPD through mechanisms involving stem cells.

Inflammation

Inflammatory processes involve the active recruitment and differentiation of bone marrow–derived hematopoietic and non-hematopoietic progenitor cells. These cells have the potential to differentiate into several cell types found in normal tissues and

Marker	Alternative Name	Function/Cell Type
Table 2 Main Stem Cell Markers		
	Lung resident precursor cells	
Cytokeratin 5	—	Basal and parabasal cells
Cytokeratin 14	—	Basal and parabasal cells
Thomsen-Friedenreich	—	Type II pneumocyte
	Hematopoietic stem cells	
CD7	Gp40	Expressed on pluripotent hematopoietic cells, T cells, and thymocytes
CD11	—	Early immature EPCs
CD13	Gp150, aminopeptidase N	Expressed on pluripotent granulocytes and monocytes and bone marrow stroma
CD14	Lipopolysaccharide receptor (LPS-R)	Expressed on monocytes and macrophages and early immature EPCs
CD34	GP105–120, ligand for CD62 (L-selection)	Expressed on pluripotent hematopoietic cells, capillary endothelium, and early immature EPCs
CD38	T-10, ADP-ribosylcyclase	Augments B-cell proliferation and expressed on lymphoid progenitors
CD45	Leukocyte common antigen (LCA), B220, T200	Expressed on leukocytes, side population cells (in bone marrow–derived cells), and early immature EPCs
CD71	T9, transferring receptor	Expressed on proliferating cells
CD90	Thymus cell antigen-1 (Thy-1)	Expressed on hematopoietic stem cells, mesenchymal stem cells, NK cells
CD117	c-kit, stem cell factor receptor (SCFR)	Expressed on hematopoietic progenitors and mast cells and early immature EPCs, and "side population" cells
CD123	Interleukin-3 receptor (IL-3Rα)	Expressed on bone marrow stem cells, granulocytes, monocytes, and megakaryocytes
CD124	Interleukin-4 receptor (IL-4Rα)	Expressed on hematopoietic precursors and mature B and T cells
CD133	AC133, PROML1, hematopoietic stem cell antigen	Expressed on hematopoietic stem cells and early EPCs
CXCR-4	Stroma-derived factor 1 receptor (SDF-1R)	Role in attracting stem cells
Flk-1	Vascular endothelial growth factor receptor 2 (VEGFR2), KDR	Expressed on early hematopoietic progenitor cells and EPCs
Flt-1	Vascular endothelial growth factor receptor 1 (VEGFR1)	Expressed on early hematopoietic progenitor cells and monocytes and megakaryocyte precursors
Lin	Lineage marker	A combination of markers of hematologic or lymphoid differentiation
OX44	CD53	Expressed on myeloid and peripheral lymphoid cells
Sca-1	Stem cell antigen 1, lymphocyte activation protein 6A (Ly-6A)	Expressed on hematopoietic progenitor cells and "side population" cells

ADP = adenosine diphosphate; EPC = endothelial progenitor cell; KDR = kinase insert domain receptor; NK = natural killer.

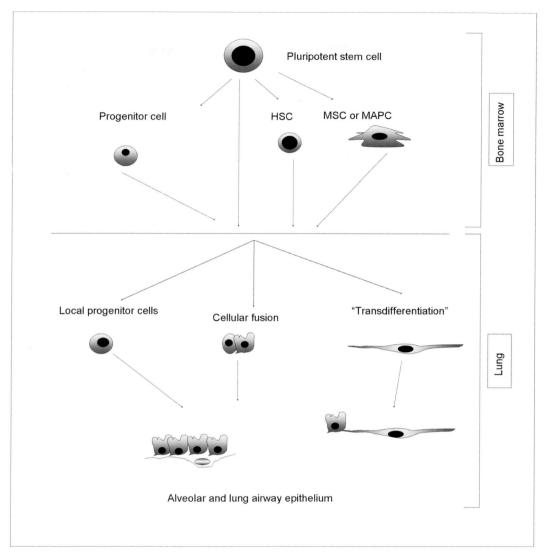

FIGURE 2. Pluripotent bone marrow stem cells, hematopoietic stem cells (HSC), mesenchymal stem cells (MSC), multipotent adult progenitor cells (MAPC), or lung-commited progenitor cells can be the source of lung epithelial cells. Bone marrow–derived progenitor cells can engraft the lung epithelium by mechanisms that include trafficking to a local progenitor niche, fusion with differentiated epithelial cells, or transdifferentiation into lung epithelial cells.

to contribute to repair and remodeling following lung injury. In the injured tissue, these cells can differentiate into inflammatory effector cells (such as neutrophils, eosinophils, basophils, mast cells, and monocytes) or nonhematopoietic cells that are able to promote structural and functional tissue repair.

Some inflammatory mediators, such as granulocyte-macrophage colony-stimulating factor, granulocyte colony-stimulating factor (G-CSF), monocyte colony-stimulating factor, interleukin (IL)-5, IL-6, IL-8, IL-12, and macrophage inflammatory protein 1α, are critical in the regulation of BMSC trafficking and differentiation when they are spread systemically during acute and chronic airway inflammation.

Mediators such as stromal cell–derived factor 1α (SDF-1α) have been shown to promote homing of stem cells from bone marrow.[46] Its receptor, the CXC chemokine receptor 4, expressed in mesenchymal stem cells, is thought to be involved

in the homing of these cells to tissues.[47] SDF-1α, vascular endothelial growth factor (VEGF) A and fibroblast growth factor 2 are enhanced following tissue injury, and it has been postulated that these cytokines promote homing of EPCs into damaged tissues. In an animal model, lung injury induced by irradiation and elastase digestion increased the recruitment of BMSCs into the lung, suggesting that local production of homing factors in the lung promotes the recruitment of BMSCs into damaged lung tissues, contributing to the modulation of airway inflammatory responses (Figure 4).[48]

Cigarette Smoke

Information on the direct effects of cigarette smoke on the biology of resident stem cells in the lung is scarce. Cigarette smoke causes injury of alveolar epithelial cells, suppressing their proliferation, attenuating their attachment, and

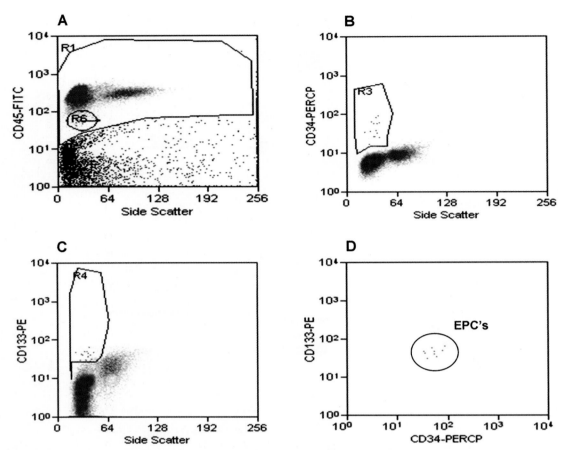

FIGURE 3. Representative flow cytometry analyses of an endothelial progenitor cell (EPC) subpopulation. EPCs were detected with the combination of markers CD133, CD34, and CD45. Peripheral blood mononuclear cells have been labeled with fluorescein isothiocyanate (FITC)-conjugated anti-CD45 (*A*), peridinin-chlorophyll-protein complex (PERCP)-conjugated anti-CD34+ (*B*), and phycoeritrin (PE)-conjugated CD133 (*C*). Triple-positive cells for CD45, CD133, and CD34 are considered EPCs (*D*).

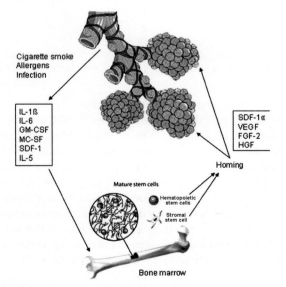

FIGURE 4. Schematic diagram of main inflammatory stimuli inducing bone marrow stem cell release and incorporation (homing) into the lung. FGF = fibroblast growth factor; GM-CSF = granulocyte-macrophage colony-stimulating factor; HGF = hepatocyte growth factor; IL = interleukin; M-CSF = macrophage colony-stimulating factor; SDF = stromal cell–derived factor; VEGF = vascular endothelial growth factor.

augmenting their detachment.[49,50] It can also cause deoxyribonucleic acid (DNA) single-strand breaks in the cells, suppress surfactant secretion, and induce collagen production.[49,51] Some *in-vitro* observations have revealed that cigarette smoke extract induces at low concentrations apoptosis of type II alveolar cells, suggesting that this mechanism might be involved in the development of COPD.[52] Cigarette smoke extract also affects the proliferative capacity of fibroblasts. Nyunoya and colleagues showed that cigarette smoke extract inhibits the proliferation of lung fibroblasts and induces their senescence.[53] Interestingly, patients with COPD exhibit a reduced growth rate of lung fibroblasts, suggesting that tobacco consumption might result in a defective repair by lung fibroblasts after lung injury, thus promoting the development of emphysema.[54,55]

In addition, cigarette smoking is a well-established risk factor for vascular damage. Numerous reports indicate that nicotine and cigarette smoking cause endothelial injury and impair neovascularization.[56–59] Polycyclic aromatic hydrocarbons, contaminants generated through the incomplete combustion of organic materials, can markedly alter cell expansion and differentiation of human progenitor CD34+ cell cultures by inducing their apoptosis.[60] It has been postulated that an insufficient number of circulating vascular progenitor cells could compromise both vessel repair and endothelial function.[61] These findings are in agreement with observations in subjects chronically exposed to cigarette smoke or in patients with severe COPD who show reduced circulating levels of bone marrow–derived endothelial and hematopoietic progenitors.[62,63] A potential explanation for these observations is the depletion of stem cells from bone marrow storages, and, as a consequence, the reduced number of circulating progenitor cells might indicate defective tissue repair capacity. Alternatively, the reduced number of circulating progenitor cells may be a consequence of their sequestration in injured organs. Indeed, short exposure to cigarette smoke or air pollutants stimulates a rapid release of immature cells as part of the response for tissue repair.[64–67] Of note, some studies have shown that nicotine increases the endothelial cell number, reduces apoptosis, and increases capillary network formation *in-vitro*, as well as enhances neovascularization in different murine models.[68–70]

Hypoxia

Tissue hypoxia is a common feature of many diseases, including heart failure, cerebral ischemia, COPD, and cancer.[71–74] A common feature in hypoxic tissues is that following ischemic injury, growth of new blood vessels (neovascularization) is critical to maintain tissue reperfusion and homeostasis. Indeed, ischemia is a stimulus for the mobilization of stem cells from the bone marrow into the circulation, differentiation into circulating EPCs, and homing to sites of ischemia, thus contributing to the formation of new blood vessels.[75] VEGF and the chemokine SDF-1, which are produced by ischemic tissues, seem to have important roles in the mobilization of EPCs from the bone marrow.[76–78] Recently, a molecular link between hypoxia and bone marrow cell mobilization, involving the transcription factor hypoxia-inducible factor 1α and SDF-1, has been reported.[78]

Because most animal models of ischemia involve inflammation in addition to hypoxia, it is unclear to what extent hypoxia alone is capable of recruiting BMSCs to the vessels.

Cellular Senescence

Emphysematous changes in the lungs are associated with increased levels of apoptosis in alveolar epithelial and endothelial cells.[79,80] To maintain the integrity of the alveolar structure, the alveolar cells lost by apoptosis must be replaced by proliferation of new cells. However, similarly to other somatic cells, the ability of alveolar cells to proliferate is limited because repeated cell cycles may cause cell senescence. Once alveolar cells reach the senescence stage, the ability to proliferate and compensate for apoptosis diminishes and lost alveolar cells are not replaced, thus promoting the development of emphysema.[81,82]

Cellular senescence is induced by telomere shortening and by telomere-independent signals, such as DNA damage and oxidative stress.[83] The repeated cell cycles of alveolar cells in emphysematous lungs may shorten telomere length, resulting in replicative senescence. Furthermore, environmental stress associated with emphysema, such as that caused by exposure to cigarette smoke and oxidants, may induce alveolar cells to undergo premature senescence without telomere shortening.[84]

Hematopoietic stem cells from young and aged individuals differ in their activity. Some evidence has shown that there is an age-dependent functional decline in hematopoietic stem cells.[85–87] Given that stem cell activity is necessary to replenish differentiated cells that are lost, it has been hypothesized that aging of hematopoietic stem cells leads to reduced stem cell renewal and hence reduced tissue homeostasis in aged animals.[85–90] This process is enhanced by age-associated anemia and a decline in immune cell function in elderly persons.[91–95] It is interesting to point out that hematopoietic stem cell aging is intrinsic to the aged cell and cannot be reversed by exposing hematopoietic stem cells from aged animals to a young microenvironment.[94–96]

Tissue Repair by Stem Cells in COPD

The current view on the pathogenesis of COPD is that cigarette smoke induces the recruitment of inflammatory cells, which then release reactive oxygen species and proteolytic enzymes, causing the degradation of lung matrix and the death of structural cells. However, recent data from both animal models and studies in human subjects suggest that disruption of the balance between apoptosis and replenishment of structural cells in the lung might also contribute to the destruction of lung tissue in response to cigarette smoke, leading to emphysema.[2] In these studies, emphysema was induced, despite a remarkable lack of pulmonary inflammation, by directly targeting the alveolar cells or by inactivating VEGF or its receptor (VEGFR).[85,97–100] These findings suggest that apoptosis is in equilibrium with proliferation and differentiation of alveolar stem cells and plays a role in the maintenance of normal tissue homeostasis. Examination of lung tissue from patients with COPD reveals the presence of apoptotic cells in greater numbers than in control lungs or those from smokers without COPD.[79,80,82,101–104] At this point, the progression of emphysema may depend on the susceptibility of tissue repair mechanisms to cigarette smoke exposure. In fact, loss of fibroblasts owing to smoke-induced apoptosis may represent a potential mechanism for the development of COPD and emphysema.[105] Interestingly, apoptotic cells persist in patients with COPD even after quitting smoking.

The age-dependent increase in the prevalence of COPD suggests an intimate relationship between the pathogenesis of COPD and aging.[106] Indeed, there is the concept that emphysema is the manifestation of premature aging of the lung. Cellular senescence contributes to the physiologic aging process since tissue regenerative capacity may be compromised. However, the role of cellular senescence in the etiology of COPD is unknown. Senescence of alveolar epithelial and endothelial cells is accelerated in patients with emphysema.[107] Interestingly, the senescence of fibroblasts in patients with emphysema has also been related to a reduced proliferation rate.[54,85]

In addition to lung-resident stem cells, there is evidence indicating that bone marrow is a source of EPCs, which are mobilized into the peripheral blood in response to cytokines or tissue injury and recruited to the lung.[33,35] Several data in animal models have shown that incorporation and differentiation of circulating BMSCs into lung parenchymal cells are limited. However, when the lung is injured, the dynamics of stem cells become quite different.[108] Yamada and colleagues showed that in mice, stem cells are required for the normal repair of lung tissue following pneumonia induced by lipopolysaccharide.[109] Intra-airway lipopolysaccharide induces the release of bone marrow–derived progenitor stem cells and their accumulation within the lungs, where they adopt an endothelial cell phenotype. In elastase-induced emphysema, cells derived from the bone marrow develop characteristics of endothelial cells and seem to contribute to repair of the alveolar capillary wall.[109,110] Differentiation of BMSCs toward epithelial cell phenotypes also occurs in this region.[109–111]

Palange and colleagues evaluated the number of circulating hematopoietic cells and EPCs in patients with moderate to severe COPD.[63] The study showed that in COPD patients with moderate to severe respiratory impairment, blood cell counts were normal, whereas circulating hematopoietic and endothelial progenitor counts were greatly decreased, compared with control subjects. Interestingly, the reduction in the number and function of circulating progenitors correlated with airway obstruction, severity of hypoxemia, and exercise capacity. The reduced number of circulating hematopoietic progenitors in COPD might suggest insufficient hematopoietic function or stimulation. However, the hemoglobin concentration was normal in the majority of these COPD patients, blood cell counts were not reduced, and there were no differences in the plasma concentration of cytokines normally involved in the survival and proliferation of hematopoietic progenitors compared with control subjects. The investigators suggested a potential link between systemic inflammation and reduced circulating progenitors and that the bone marrow might be a systemic target of COPD.[63]

Long-term hypoxemia may induce depletion of circulating EPCs by exhaustion of the stored precursor pools. In a study performed in restrictive and obstructive patients with long-term hypoxemia, Fadini and colleagues observed that patients with chronic hypoxemia and severe lung disease showed lower levels of circulating progenitors than controls, which were associated with an increase in apoptotic cell death.[112] In both restrictive and obstructive patients, the reduction in EPCs was related to diminished lung volumes concluding that depletion of circulating EPCs may be involved in altered endothelial homeostasis of the pulmonary circulation in these disorders.[112] An alternative interpretation for the decreased number of EPCs is that it resulted from an ongoing recruitment into and sequestration in inflamed lung tissue.

Consistent with the recruitment hypothesis of circulating EPCs in injured tissues, the authors identified vascular progenitor cells in the endothelium and in the intima of pulmonary arteries from COPD patients (Figure 5).[113] Interestingly, the number of vascular progenitor cells was greater in patients with COPD than in control subjects and correlated with the thickness of the arterial wall, as well as with the expression of VEGF and VEGFR2 messenger ribonucleic acid in the arterial wall. These findings suggest that vascular progenitor cells could be involved in the pathogenesis of intimal hyperplasia in COPD. Indeed, in a preliminary study, the authors also observed that CD133+ cells are able to migrate into remodeled intimas of pulmonary arteries from COPD patients and differentiate into smooth muscle cells.[114]

Some types of circulating progenitor cells have myogenic potential *in-vitro*.[115] Interestingly, compromised skeletal muscle performance and muscle wasting are frequent features of patients afflicted with chronic disorders. Recent work from several laboratories supports the idea that bone marrow–derived stem cells, possibly hematopoietic or

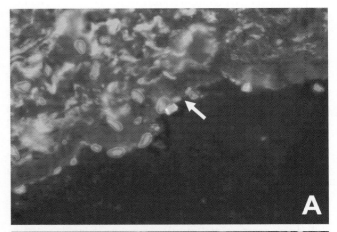

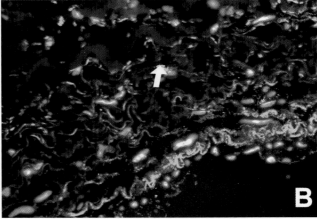

FIGURE 5. Transverse sections of a pulmonary artery obtained from a patient with chronic obstructive pulmonary disease immunostained with an antibody against CD133. Positive cells (arrows) were localized either adhered to the endothelium (*A*) or infiltrating the arterial wall (*B*) (×600 original magnification).

angioblastic in nature, can reach the sites of muscle regeneration and contribute to muscle repair and replenishment of the satellite cell pool.[116,117] In this context, cigarette smoke might contribute to defective muscle repair by diminishing circulating progenitors in severe COPD. In addition, transient and repeated oxidative imbalance might modulate myogenesis of satellite cells (see also Chapter 21).

Cell-Based Therapy

Major lung diseases likely involving stem cells may be broadly classified according to whether they involve stem cell deficiency, hyperproliferation, or, possibly, a combination of both. For instance, toxic destruction of the alveolar epithelium suggests a stem cell deficiency in emphysema. By contrast, fibrotic reaction and scarring in response to epithelial injury may be viewed as hyperproliferation of mesenchymal stem cells. The general concept is that augmentation of stem cells may minimize lung injury, enhance repair, and, possibly, regenerate lost tissue. However, inhibition of excessive growth of stem cells may also be a valid therapeutic goal when hyperproliferation contributes to the pathophysiology, as in fibrosis, smooth muscle hyperplasia, or lung cancer.

Emphysema

Emphysema is a complex entity because of the need for structural regeneration of basement membrane and replacement of alveolar and endothelial cells. In a model of elastase-induced pulmonary emphysema in rabbits, autologous bone marrow mononuclear cell transplantation ameliorated the progression of the disease.[118] The mechanisms that mediated such a response were related to the attenuation of inflammation, metalloproteinase 2 expression, and apoptosis, while enhancing alveolar cell proliferation. Furthermore, intravenous administration of bone marrow–derived mesenchymal stem cells protected mouse lungs against the injury induced by bleomycin, as suggested by the reduction in inflammation.[119]

Transplantation of adipose tissue-derived stromal cells into elastase-treated emphysema models induced a significant increase in endogenous hepatocyte growth factor (HGF) expression in lung tissue, with the maximal levels reached after 4 weeks of transplantation. Further, alveolar and vascular regeneration were significantly enhanced via inhibition of alveolar cell apoptosis, enhancement of epithelial cell proliferation, and promotion of angiogenesis in pulmonary vasculature, leading to the improvement in pulmonary function. These data suggest that autologous adipose tissue-derived stromal cell therapy may have potential for pulmonary emphysema by inducing the selective expression of HGF in injured lung tissue.[120]

As an alternative treatment for pulmonary emphysema, it has been suggested that the administration of hematopoietic cytokines, such as G-CSF, should be able to mobilize bone marrow cells.[121] However, systemic administration of such cytokines does not produce lung regeneration, whereas it may aggravate emphysematous lung destruction in a model of elastase injury.[122] Administration of adrenomedullin, a potent vasodilator peptide that regulates cell growth and survival, appears to improve elastase-induced emphysema in mice, at least in part, via mobilization of bone marrow-derived cells.[123]

Other studies have suggested a role for retinoic acid in alveolar regeneration when used alone or in combination with G-CSF.[110,124] In mice with elastase-induced emphysema, the combination of retinoic acid and G-CSF promoted lung regeneration and possibly increased the number of bone marrow–derived cells in the alveoli.[110]

Vascular Remodeling

In COPD, endothelial cell destruction and dysfunction may contribute to the development of pulmonary hypertension.[113,125,126] For this reason, repopulation of the pulmonary circulation with normally functioning endothelial cells by means of EPCs is theoretically attractive.

The beneficial effects of EPCs to vascular lesions were first investigated in mechanical vascular injury experiments. Griese and colleagues demonstrated that autologous transplantation of EPCs into balloon-injured carotid arteries and into bioprosthetic grafts in rabbits resulted in rapid endothelialization of denuded vessels and graft segments.[127] Kong and colleagues reported that transplantation of autologous EPCs, overexpressing endothelial nitric oxide synthase (eNOS), into balloon-injured rabbit carotid arteries led to the inhibition of neointimal hyperplasia.[128] He and colleagues showed a significant improvement in endothelium-dependent relaxation and accelerated endothelialization 4 weeks after transplantation of autologous EPCs into the lumen of denuded rabbit carotid arteries.[129] All of these reports showed the potential benefit of the use of EPCs in preventing vascular remodeling.

EPCs have been used in the treatment of pulmonary hypertension in animal models.[86,130,131] Intravenous administration of bone marrow cells significantly attenuated pulmonary hypertension induced by administration of monocrotaline in mice.[86] In contrast, chronically hypoxic mice subjected to the same procedure failed to show improvement in pulmonary hypertension.[86] Animals receiving EPCs transduced with human eNOS exhibited significant reversal of pulmonary hypertension in rats treated with monocrotaline.[131] Transplantation of autologous EPCs into the lung can improve pulmonary vascular resistance in dehydromonocrotaline-induced pulmonary hypertension in dogs.[130] Furthermore, transplantation of EPCs expressing adrenomedullin was associated with a greater improvement in monocrotaline-induced pulmonary hypertension in rats than transplantation of EPCs alone.[132] Taken together, these results suggest that the administration of EPCs can inhibit pulmonary hypertension and pulmonary arterial remodeling in animal models by accelerating endothelial healing in damaged pulmonary arterioles. Nevertheless, despite the beneficial role in tissue repair, given the potential of progenitor cells in terms of plasticity, they might also participate in the progression of lesion injury.[113,133–136] In fact, Werner and colleagues demonstrated in an animal model that after induction of endothelial damage in the carotid artery, a prominent intimal vascular lesion was initiated by bone marrow–derived progenitor cells.[113,133–136] Interestingly, treatment with rosuvastatin, a 3-hydroxy-3-methylglutaryl coenzyme A reductase inhibitor, promoted bone marrow-dependent reendothelialization and diminished vascular lesion development. These studies suggest that the use of bone marrow-derived progenitors as cell-based therapy requires therapeutic strategies combined with other drugs since they could contribute not only to vascular healing but also to lesion formation under certain pathologic conditions.

Summary

The expanding clinical applications of BMSCs, along with a better understanding of the biopathology of tissue repair, will offer novel treatment strategies for lung regeneration in COPD. However, great caution must be taken with the eventual therapeutic use of stem cells owing to their potential for carcinogenic transformation or, less dramatically, their contribution to hyperplasia and tissue remodeling.

References

1. Voelkel N, Taraseviciene-Stewart L. Emphysema: an autoimmune vascular disease? Proc Am Thorac Soc 2005;2:23–5.
2. Tuder RM, Yoshida T, Fijalkowka I, et al. Role of lung maintenance program in the heterogeneity of lung destruction in emphysema. Proc Am Thorac Soc 2006;3:673–9.
3. Hogan BL. Morphogenesis. Cell 1999;96:225–33.
4. Breeze RG, Wheeldon EB. The cells of the pulmonary airways. Am Rev Respir Dis 1977;116:705–77.
5. McDowell EM, Barrett LA, Glavin F, et al. The respiratory epithelium. I. Human bronchus. J Natl Cancer Inst 1978; 61:539–49.
6. Blau HM, Brazelton TR, Weimann JM. The evolving concept of a stem cell: entity or function? Cell 2001;105:829–41.
7. Fuchs E, Segre JA. Stem cells: a new lease on life. Cell 2000;100:143–55.
8. Weissman IL. Stem cells: units of development, units of regeneration, and units in evolution. Cell 2000;100:157–68.
9. Boers JE, Ambergen AW, Thunnissen FB. Number and proliferation of basal and parabasal cells in normal human airway epithelium. Am J Respir Crit Care Med 1998;157:2000–6.
10. Boers JE, Ambergen AW, Thunnissen FB. Number and proliferation of Clara cells in normal human airway epithelium. Am J Respir Crit Care Med 1999;159:1585–91.
11. Delplanque A, Coraux C, Tirouvanziam R, et al. Epithelial stem cell-mediated development of the human respiratory mucosa in SCID mice. J Cell Sci 2000;113 (Pt 5):767–78.
12. Duan D, Sehgal A, Yao J, et al. Lef1 transcription factor expression defines airway progenitor cell targets for in utero gene therapy of submucosal gland in cystic fibrosis. Am J Respir Cell Mol Biol 1998;18:750–8.
13. Emura M, Ochiai A, Singh G, et al. In vitro reconstitution of human respiratory epithelium. In Vitro Cell Dev Biol Anim 1997;33:602–5.
14. Emura M. Stem cells of the respiratory epithelium and their in vitro cultivation. In Vitro Cell Dev Biol Anim 1997;33:3–14.
15. Inayama Y, Hook GE, Brody AR, et al. In vitro and in vivo growth and differentiation of clones of tracheal basal cells. Am J Pathol 1989;134:539–49.
16. Liu JY, Nettesheim P, Randell SH. Growth and differentiation of tracheal epithelial progenitor cells. Am J Physiol 1994;266:L296–307.
17. Nettesheim P, Jetten AM, Inayama Y, et al. Pathways of differentiation of airway epithelial cells. Environ Health Perspect 1990;85:317–29.
18. Evans MJ, Cabral-Anderson LJ, Freeman G. Role of the Clara cell in renewal of the bronchiolar epithelium. Lab Invest 1978;38:648–53.
19. Hong KU, Reynolds SD, Giangreco A, et al. Clara cell secretory protein-expressing cells of the airway neuroepithelial body microenvironment include a label-retaining subset and are critical for epithelial renewal after progenitor cell depletion. Am J Respir Cell Mol Biol 2001;24:671–81.
20. Mahvi D, Bank H, Harley R. Morphology of a naphthalene-induced bronchiolar lesion. Am J Pathol 1977;86:558–72.
21. Plopper CG, Suverkropp C, Morin D, et al. Relationship of cytochrome P-450 activity to Clara cell cytotoxicity. I. Histopathologic comparison of the respiratory tract of mice, rats and hamsters after parenteral administration of naphthalene. J Pharmacol Exp Ther 1992;261:353–63.
22. Reynolds SD, Giangreco A, Power JH, et al. Neuroepithelial bodies of pulmonary airways serve as a reservoir of progenitor cells capable of epithelial regeneration. Am J Pathol 2000;156:269–78.
23. Stripp BR, Maxson K, Mera R, et al. Plasticity of airway cell proliferation and gene expression after acute naphthalene injury. Am J Physiol 1995;269:L791–9.
24. Reddy R, Buckley S, Doerken M, et al. Isolation of a putative progenitor subpopulation of alveolar epithelial type 2 cells. Am J Physiol Lung Cell Mol Physiol 2004;286:L658–67.
25. Adamson IY, Bowden DH. The pathogenesis of bloemycin-induced pulmonary fibrosis in mice. Am J Pathol 1974;77:185–97.
26. Maeyama T, Kuwano K, Kawasaki M, et al. Upregulation of Fas-signalling molecules in lung epithelial cells from patients with idiopathic pulmonary fibrosis. Eur Respir J 2001;17:180–9.
27. Stenmark KR, Gebb SA. Lung vascular development: breathing new life into an old problem. Am J Respir Cell Mol Biol 2003;28:133–7.
28. Hirschi KK, DíAmore PA. Pericytes in the microvasculature. Cardiovasc Res 1996;32:687–98.
29. Schor AM, Canfield AE, Sutton AB, et al. Pericyte differentiation. Clin Orthop Relat Res 1995;313:81–91.
30. Kelley C, DíAmore P, Hechtman HB, et al. Microvascular pericyte contractility in vitro: comparison with other cells of the vascular wall. J Cell Biol 1987;104:483–90.
31. Pittenger MF, Mackay AM, Beck SC, et al. Multilineage potential of adult human mesenchymal stem cells. Science 1999;284:143–7.

32. Jiang Y, Jahagirdar BN, Reinhardt RL, et al. Pluripotency of mesenchymal stem cells derived from adult marrow. Nature 2002;418:41–9.

33. Kotton DN, Ma BY, Cardoso WV, et al. Bone marrow-derived cells as progenitors of lung alveolar epithelium. Development 2001;128:5181–8.

34. Kotton DN, Fine A. Derivation of lung epithelium from bone marrow cells. Cytotherapy 2003;5:169–73.

35. Krause DS, Theise ND, Collector MI, et al. Multi-organ, multi-lineage engraftment by a single bone marrow-derived stem cell. Cell 2001;105:369–77.

36. Theise ND, Henegariu O, Grove J, et al. Radiation pneumonitis in mice: a severe injury model for pneumocyte engraftment from bone marrow. Exp Hematol 2002;30:1333–8.

37. Suratt BT, Cool CD, Serls AE, et al. Human pulmonary chimerism after hematopoietic stem cell transplantation. Am J Respir Crit Care Med 2003;168:318–22.

38. Ferrari G, Cusella-De Angelis G, Coletta M, et al. Muscle regeneration by bone marrow-derived myogenic progenitors. Science 1998;279:1528–30.

39. Okamoto R, Yajima T, Yamazaki M, et al. Damaged epithelia regenerated by bone marrow-derived cells in the human gastrointestinal tract. Nat Med 2002;8:1011–7.

40. Asahara T, Murohara T, Sullivan A, et al. Isolation of putative progenitor endothelial cells for angiogenesis. Science 1997;275:964–7.

41. Goodell MA, Brose K, Paradis G, et al. Isolation and functional properties of murine hematopoietic stem cells that are replicating in vivo. J Exp Med 1996;183:1797–806.

42. Summer R, Kotton DN, Sun X, et al. Side population cells and Bcrp1 expression in lung. Am J Physiol Lung Cell Mol Physiol 2003;285:L97–104.

43. Keeney M, Chin-Yee I, Weir K, et al. Single platform flow cytometric absolute CD34+ cell counts based on the ISHAGE guidelines. International Society of Hematotherapy and Graft Engineering. Cytometry 1998;34:61–70.

44. Wiebe BM, Laursen H. Lung morphometry by unbiased methods in emphysema: bronchial and blood vessel volume, alveolar surface area and capillary length. APMIS 1998;106:651–6.

45. Voelkel NF, Douglas IS, Nicolls M. Angiogenesis in chronic lung disease. Chest 2007;131:874–9.

46. To LB, Haylock DN, Simmons PJ, et al. The biology and clinical uses of blood stem cells. Blood 1997;89:2233–58.

47. Honczarenko M, Le Y, Swierkowski M, et al. Human bone marrow stromal cells express a distinct set of biologically functional chemokine receptors. Stem Cells 2006;24:1030–41.

48. Hashimoto N, Jin H, Liu T, et al. Bone marrow-derived progenitor cells in pulmonary fibrosis. J Clin Invest 2004;113:243–52.

49. Lannan S, Donaldson K, Brown D, et al. Effect of cigarette smoke and its condensates on alveolar epithelial cell injury in vitro. Am J Physiol 1994;266:L92–100.

50. Wollmer P, Evander E. Biphasic pulmonary clearance of 99mTc-DTPA in smokers. Clin Physiol 1994;14:547–59.

51. Leanderson P, Tagesson C. Cigarette smoke-induced DNA damage in cultured human lung cells: role of hydroxyl radicals and endonuclease activation. Chem Biol Interact 1992;81:197–208.

52. Hoshino Y, Mio T, Nagai S, et al. Cytotoxic effects of cigarette smoke extract on an alveolar type II cell-derived cell line. Am J Physiol Lung Cell Mol Physiol 2001;281:L509–16.

53. Nyunoya T, Monick MM, Klingelhutz A, et al. Cigarette smoke induces cellular senescence. Am J Respir Cell Mol Biol 2006;35:681–8.

54. Holz O, Zuhlke I, Jaksztat E, et al. Lung fibroblasts from patients with emphysema show a reduced proliferation rate in culture. Eur Respir J 2004;24:575–9.

55. Noordhoek JA, Postma DS, Chong LL, et al. Different proliferative capacity of lung fibroblasts obtained from control subjects and patients with emphysema. Exp Lung Res 2003;29:291–302.

56. Folts JD, Gering SA, Laibly SW, et al. Effects of cigarette smoke and nicotine on platelets and experimental coronary artery thrombosis. Adv Exp Med Biol 1990;273:339–58.

57. Krupski WC. The peripheral vascular consequences of smoking. Ann Vasc Surg 1991;5:291–304.

58. Pittilo RM, Bull HA, Gulati S, et al. Nicotine and cigarette smoking: effects on the ultrastructure of aortic endothelium. Int J Exp Pathol 1990;71:573–86.

59. Powell JT. Vascular damage from smoking: disease mechanisms at the arterial wall. Vasc Med 1998;3:21–8.

60. van Grevenynghe J, Bernard M, Langouet S, et al. Human CD34-positive hematopoietic stem cells constitute targets for carcinogenic polycyclic aromatic hydrocarbons. J Pharmacol Exp Ther 2005;314:693–702.

61. Hill JM, Zalos G, Halcox JP, et al. Circulating endothelial progenitor cells, vascular function, and cardiovascular risk. N Engl J Med 2003;348:593–600.

62. Kondo T, Hayashi M, Takeshita K, et al. Smoking cessation rapidly increases circulating progenitor cells in peripheral blood in chronic smokers. Arterioscler Thromb Vasc Biol 2004;24:1442–7.

63. Palange P, Testa U, Huertas A, et al. Circulating haemopoietic and endothelial progenitor cells are decreased in COPD. Eur Respir J 2006;27:529–41.

64. Nakagawa M, Terashima T, D'yachkova Y, et al. Glucocorticoid-induced granulocytosis: contribution of marrow release and demargination of intravascular granulocytes. Circulation 1998;98:2307–13.

65. Terashima T, Wiggs B, English D, et al. Phagocytosis of small carbon particles (PM10) by alveolar macrophages stimulates the release of polymorphonuclear leukocytes from bone marrow. Am J Respir Crit Care Med 1997;155:1441–7.

66. Terashima T, English D, Hogg JC, et al. Release of polymorphonuclear leukocytes from the bone marrow by interleukin-8. Blood 1998;92:1062–9.

67. van Eeden SF, Kitagawa Y, Sato Y, et al. Polymorphonuclear leukocytes released from the bone marrow and acute lung injury. Chest 1999;116:43S–6S.

68. Heeschen C, Jang JJ, Weis M, et al. Nicotine stimulates angiogenesis and promotes tumor growth and atherosclerosis. Nat Med 2001;7:833–9.

69. Heeschen C, Weis M, Aicher A, et al. A novel angiogenic pathway mediated by non-neuronal nicotinic acetylcholine receptors. J Clin Invest 2002;110:527–36.

70. Heeschen C, Weis M, Cooke JP. Nicotine promotes arteriogenesis. J Am Coll Cardiol 2003;41:489–96.

71. Borden CW, Ebert RV, Wilson RH. Anoxia in myocardial infarction and indications for oxygen therapy. J Am Med Assoc 1952;148:1370–1.

72. Brown AW, Brierley JB. Evidence for early anoxic-ischaemic cell damage in the rat brain. Experientia 1966;22:546–7.

73. Raguso CA, Guinot SL, Janssens JP, et al. Chronic hypoxia: common traits between chronic obstructive pulmonary disease and altitude. Curr Opin Clin Nutr Metab Care 2004;7:411–7.

74. Kaur B, Khwaja FW, Severson EA, et al. Hypoxia and the hypoxia-inducible-factor pathway in glioma growth and angiogenesis. Neurooncology 2005;7:134–53.

75. Aicher A, Zeiher AM, Dimmeler S. Mobilizing endothelial progenitor cells. Hypertension 2005;45:321–5.

76. Asahara T, Takahashi T, Masuda H, et al. VEGF contributes to postnatal neovascularization by mobilizing bone marrow-derived endothelial progenitor cells. EMBO J 1999; 18:3964–72.

77. Askari AT, Unzek S, Popovic ZB, et al. Effect of stromal-cell-derived factor 1 on stem-cell homing and tissue regeneration in ischaemic cardiomyopathy. Lancet 2003; 362:697–703.

78. Ceradini DJ, Kulkarni AR, Callaghan MJ, et al. Progenitor cell trafficking is regulated by hypoxic gradients through HIF-1 induction of SDF-1. Nat Med 2004;10:858–64.

79. Yokohori N, Aoshiba K, Nagai A. Increased levels of cell death and proliferation in alveolar wall cells in patients with pulmonary emphysema. Chest 2004;125:626–32.

80. Kasahara Y, Tuder RM, Cool CD, et al. Endothelial cell death and decreased expression of vascular endothelial growth factor and vascular endothelial growth factor receptor 2 in emphysema. Am J Respir Crit Care Med 2001;163:737–44.

81. Aoshiba K, Yokohori N, Nagai A. Alveolar wall apoptosis causes lung destruction and emphysematous changes. Am J Respir Cell Mol Biol 2003;28:555–62.

82. Imai K, Mercer BA, Schulman LL, et al. Correlation of lung surface area to apoptosis and proliferation in human emphysema. Eur Respir J 2005;25:250–8.

83. Hayflick L, Moohead PS. The serial cultivation of human diploid cell strains. Exp Cell Res 1961;25:585–621.

84. Muller KC, Welker L, Paasch K, et al. Lung fibroblasts from patients with emphysema show markers of senescence in vitro. Respir Res 2006;7:32.

85. Geiger H, Van Zant G. The aging of lympho-hematopoietic stem cells. Nat Immunol 2002;3:329–33.

86. Raoul W, Wagner-Ballon O, Saber G, et al. Effects of bone marrow-derived cells on monocrotaline- and hypoxia-induced pulmonary hypertension in mice. Respir Res 2007;8:8.

87. Van Zant G, Liang Y. The role of stem cells in aging. Exp Hematol 2003;31:659–72.

88. Geiger H, True JM, de Haan G, et al. Age- and stage-specific regulation patterns in the hematopoietic stem cell hierarchy. Blood 2001;98:2966–72.

89. Sharpless NE, DePinho RA. Telomeres, stem cells, senescence, and cancer. J Clin Invest 2004;113:160–8.

90. Torella D, Rota M, Nurzynska D, et al. Cardiac stem cell and myocyte aging, heart failure, and insulin-like growth factor-1 overexpression. Circ Res 2004;94:514–24.

91. Butcher SK, Chahal H, Nayak L, et al. Senescence in innate immune responses: reduced neutrophil phagocytic capacity and CD16 expression in elderly humans. J Leukoc Biol 2001;70:881–6.

92. Kim M, Moon HB, Spangrude GJ. Major age-related changes of mouse hematopoietic stem/progenitor cells. Ann NY Acad Sci 2003;996:195–208.

93. Lipschitz DA. Age-related declines in hematopoietic reserve capacity. Semin Oncol 1995;22:3–5.

94. Rossi DJ, Bryder D, Zahn JM, et al. Cell intrinsic alterations underlie hematopoietic stem cell aging. Proc Natl Acad Sci U S A 2005;102:9194–9.

95. Sudo K, Ema H, Morita Y, et al. Age-associated characteristics of murine hematopoietic stem cells. J Exp Med 2000;192:1273–80.

96. Geiger H, Rennebeck G, Van Zant G. Regulation of hematopoietic stem cell aging in vivo by a distinct genetic element. Proc Natl Acad Sci USA 2005;102:5102–7.

97. Tang K, Rossiter HB, Wagner PD, et al. Lung-targeted VEGF inactivation leads to an emphysema phenotype in mice. J Appl Physiol 2004;97:1559–66.

98. Kasahara Y, Tuder RM, Taraseviciene-Stewart L, et al. Inhibition of VEGF receptors causes lung cell apoptosis and emphysema. J Clin Invest 2000;106:1311–9.

99. Petrache I, Natarajan V, Zhen L, et al. Ceramide upregulation causes pulmonary cell apoptosis and emphysema-like disease in mice. Nat Med 2005;11:491–8.

100. Tuder RM, Zhen L, Cho CY, et al. Oxidative stress and apoptosis interact and cause emphysema due to vascular endothelial growth factor receptor blockade. Am J Respir Cell Mol Biol 2003;29:88–97.

101. Hodge S, Hodge G, Scicchitano R, et al. Alveolar macrophages from subjects with chronic obstructive pulmonary disease are deficient in their ability to phagocytose apoptotic airway epithelial cells. Immunol Cell Biol 2003;81:289–96.

102. Hodge S, Hodge G, Holmes M, et al. Increased airway epithelial and T-cell apoptosis in COPD remains despite smoking cessation. Eur Respir J. 2005;25:447–54.

103. Majo J, Ghezzo H, Cosio MG. Lymphocyte population and apoptosis in the lungs of smokers and their relation to emphysema. Eur Respir J 2001;17:946–53.

104. Vandivier RW, Fadok VA, Hoffmann PR, et al. Elastase-mediated phosphatidylserine receptor cleavage impairs apoptotic cell clearance in cystic fibrosis and bronchiectasis. J Clin Invest 2002;109:661–70.

105. Ishii T, Matsuse T, Igarashi H, et al. Tobacco smoke reduces viability in human lung fibroblasts: protective effect of glutathione S-transferase P1. Am J Physiol Lung Cell Mol Physiol 2001;280:L1189–95.

106. Pauwels RA, Rabe KF. Burden and clinical features of chronic obstructive pulmonary disease (COPD). Lancet 2004;364:613–20.

107. Tsuji T, Aoshiba K, Nagai A. Alveolar cell senescence in patients with pulmonary emphysema. Am J Respir Crit Care Med 2006;174:886–93.

108. Yamada M, Kubo H, Ishizawa K, et al. Increased circulating endothelial progenitor cells in patients with bacterial pneumonia: evidence that bone marrow derived cells contribute to lung repair. Thorax 2005;60:410–43.

109. Yamada M, Kubo H, Kobayashi S, et al. Bone marrow-derived progenitor cells are important for lung repair after

lipopolysaccharide-induced lung injury. J Immunol 2004;172:1266–72.

110. Ishizawa K, Kubo H, Yamada M, et al. Bone marrow-derived cells contribute to lung regeneration after elastase-induced pulmonary emphysema. FEBS Lett 2004;556:249–52.

111. Ishizawa K, Kubo H, Yamada M, et al. Hepatocyte growth factor induces angiogenesis in injured lungs through mobilizing endothelial progenitor cells. Biochem Biophys Res Commun 2004;324:276–80.

112. Fadini GP, Schiavon M, Cantini M, et al. Circulating progenitor cells are reduced in patients with severe lung disease. Stem Cells 2006;24:1806–13.

113. Peinado VI, Ramirez J, Roca J, et al. Identification of vascular progenitor cells in pulmonary arteries of patients with chronic obstructive pulmonary disease. Am J Respir Cell Mol Biol 2006;34:257–63.

114. Díez M, Barberà JA, Ferrer E, et al. Plasticity of CD133+ cells: Role in pulmonary vascular remodelling. Cardiovasc Res 2007;76:517-527.

115. Torrente Y, Belicchi M, Sampaolesi M, et al. Human circulating AC133(+) stem cells restore dystrophin expression and ameliorate function in dystrophic skeletal muscle. J Clin Invest 2004;114:182–95.

116. Bhatia M, Bonnet D, Murdoch B, et al. A newly discovered class of human hematopoietic cells with SCID-repopulating activity. Nat Med 1998;4:1038–45.

117. LaBarge MA, Blau HM. Biological progression from adult bone marrow to mononucleate muscle stem cell to multinucleate muscle fiber in response to injury. Cell 2002;111:589–601.

118. Yuhgetsu H, Ohno Y, Funaguchi N, et al. Beneficial effects of autologous bone marrow mononuclear cell transplantation against elastase-induced emphysema in rabbits. Exp Lung Res 2006;32:413–26.

119. Rojas M, Xu J, Woods CR, et al. Bone marrow-derived mesenchymal stem cells in repair of the injured lung. Am J Respir Cell Mol Biol 2005;33:145–52.

120. Shigemura N, Okumura M, Mizuno S, et al. Autologous transplantation of adipose tissue-derived stromal cells ameliorates pulmonary emphysema. Am J Transplant 2006;6:2592–600.

121. Orlic D, Kajstura J, Chimenti S, et al. Mobilized bone marrow cells repair the infarcted heart, improving function and survival. Proc Natl Acad Sci U S A 2001;98:10344–9.

122. Ishikawa T, Aoshiba K, Yokohori N, et al. Macrophage colony-stimulating factor aggravates rather than regenerates emphysematous lungs in mice. Respiration 2006;73:538–45.

123. Murakami S, Nagaya N, Itoh T, et al. Adrenomedullin regenerates alveoli and vasculature in elastase-induced pulmonary emphysema in mice. Am J Respir Crit Care Med 2005;172:581–9.

124. Hind M, Maden M. Retinoic acid induces alveolar regeneration in the adult mouse lung. Eur Respir J 2004;23:20–7.

125. Dinh-Xuan AT, Higenbottam TW, Clelland CA, et al. Impairment of endothelium-dependent pulmonary-artery relaxation in chronic obstructive lung disease. N Engl J Med 1991;324:1539–47.

126. Peinado VI, Barberá JA, Ramírez J, et al. Endothelial dysfunction in pulmonary arteries of patients with mild COPD. Am J Physiol Lung Cell Mol Physiol 1998;18:L908–13.

127. Griese DP, Ehsan A, Melo LG, et al. Isolation and transplantation of autologous circulating endothelial cells into denuded vessels and prosthetic grafts: implications for cell-based vascular therapy. Circulation 2003;108:2710–5.

128. Kong D, Melo LG, Mangi AA, et al. Enhanced inhibition of neointimal hyperplasia by genetically engineered endothelial progenitor cells. Circulation 2004;109:1769–75.

129. He T, Smith LA, Harrington S, et al. Transplantation of circulating endothelial progenitor cells restores endothelial function of denuded rabbit carotid arteries. Stroke 2004;35:2378–84.

130. Takahashi M, Nakamura T, Toba T, et al. Transplantation of endothelial progenitor cells into the lung to alleviate pulmonary hypertension in dogs. Tissue Eng 2004;10:771–9.

131. Zhao YD, Courtman DW, Deng Y, et al. Rescue of monocrotaline-induced pulmonary arterial hypertension using bone marrow-derived endothelial-like progenitor cells: efficacy of combined cell and eNOS gene therapy in established disease. Circ Res 2005;96:442–50.

132. Nagaya N, Kangawa K, Kanda M, et al. Hybrid cell-gene therapy for pulmonary hypertension based on phagocytosing action of endothelial progenitor cells. Circulation 2003;108:889–95.

133. Saiura A, Sata M, Hirata Y, et al. Circulating smooth muscle progenitor cells contribute to atherosclerosis. Nat Med 2001;7:382–3.

134. Sata M. Circulating vascular progenitor cells contribute to vascular repair, remodeling, and lesion formation. Trends Cardiovasc Med 2003;13:249–53.

135. Shimizu K, Sugiyama S, Aikawa M, et al. Host bone-marrow cells are a source of donor intimal smooth-muscle-like cells in murine aortic transplant arteriopathy. Nat Med 2001;7:738–41.

136. Werner N, Priller J, Laufs U, et al. Bone marrow-derived progenitor cells modulate vascular reendothelialization and neointimal formation—effect of 3-hydroxy-3-methylglutaryl coenzyme a reductase inhibition. Arterioscler Thromb Vasc Biol 2002;22:1567–72.

CHAPTER 30

PSYCHOSOCIAL ASPECTS OF CHRONIC OBSTRUCTIVE PULMONARY DISEASE

RACHEL NORWOOD, MD

As a chronic, progressive disease, chronic obstructive pulmonary disease (COPD) is the fourth leading cause of death in the United States, currently afflicting up to 24 million patients, with that number certain to grow as the population ages.[1] In spite of these growing numbers, the morbidity and mortality associated with COPD have not significantly decreased in the past 20 years, placing the focus of treatment on symptom management, reduction of exacerbations, and maximizing patients' quality of life. An important part of the latter is the recognition and management of the psychosocial impacts of COPD, in particular the psychiatric diagnoses of depression and panic/anxiety, both of which occur in COPD patients at rates well above those of community populations.

Depression
Epidemiology

Arriving at a reliable prevalence rate for depression in COPD is challenging. Several factors contribute to this difficulty, including studies that employ small sample sizes, variation in diagnostic instruments (self-report instruments typically result in lower rates than those that are examiner driven), different levels of COPD severity, and variable rigor in separating the symptoms of depression from pulmonary illness. A review of epidemiologic studies finds a prevalence rate for comorbid depression in COPD covering a wide range, with the majority of the strongest studies averaging 40 to 45%. This compares with a rate of 15% in the general population.[2–6] In a cluster of studies comparing rates of depression across diverse chronic illnesses, COPD patients are repeatedly found to suffer from depression with greater frequency and with a greater chronicity of the mood symptoms.[7–10] Applying the conservative estimated prevalence of 40% to the COPD population means that 10 million COPD patients in the United States alone suffer from a significant level of clinical depression that is directly associated with their COPD. Evidence suggests, however, that the depression experienced by COPD patients is not a homogeneous entity.

Etiology of Depression in COPD

The relationship between COPD and depression is neither exclusively linear nor unidirectional. Multiple contributors that come into influence at different life stages drive the development of depression in patients with COPD. Chronologically, the earliest risk may be a genetic predisposition to depression, followed by the environmental assaults imposed by the symptoms of the respiratory illness and, finally, the direct neuropsychiatric effects of chronic respiratory disease.

GENETICS

In the psychiatric literature, the heritability of a vulnerability to depression has been well established. In community samples, first-degree relatives of individuals with major depression are two to three times more likely to develop depression when compared with the first-degree relatives of controls.[11–13] The age at which this increased risk manifests varies widely from individual to individual but is often already evident in adolescence.[14] This vulnerability plays a role in the eventual development of COPD in that adolescents and young adults who are depressed or have a history of depression are more vulnerable to developing an addiction to nicotine than children who are not depressed,[15–17] and smoking is the greatest single risk factor for the later development of COPD. The genetic underpinning of this vulnerability is being fleshed out with the recent finding that the likelihood of an adolescent's smoking progressing from initial nicotine exposure to regular smoking was doubled by each additional copy of an identified allele (DRD2A1) for a subtype of a dopamine receptor. When this genetic vulnerability was identified in children who were also depressed, the risk for regular use of nicotine was magnified.[18]

Smoking, COPD, and depression are interrelated in a trinity (Figure 1), with depression playing a role in the initiation and maintenance of smoking, smoking leading to the development of COPD and COPD, in turn, contributing to the genesis of depression. Because of depression's role in the development of nicotine dependence, it can be considered a risk factor for COPD. In adults, continued smoking increases the morbidity and mortality experienced in COPD, and a history of either recent or distant depression decreases an individual's success in smoking cessation, causes more persistent withdrawal symptoms, and increases the likelihood of recurrence of the depression if nicotine is discontinued.[19–21] Taken to the next step, prescription of antidepressants has been found to be useful in helping smokers achieve abstinence.[22–25] The benefits from the application of antidepressants may not exclusively derive from the relief of depressive symptoms but potentially because the vulnerability to

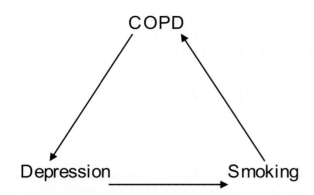

FIGURE 1. Interrelationship between chronic obstructive pulmonary disease, depression, and smoking.

nicotine dependence and the vulnerability to depression share a common genetic source, possibly one that defines some characteristic of the dopamine pathways.[26]

IMPACT OF CHRONIC ILLNESS

Early theory held that depression in chronic illness was a reaction to the losses imposed by the illness—an understandable grief response.[27] Since that time, both the reactions and the losses have been more clearly defined. Loss of function in terms of decreased mobility, loss of occupation, shifted family roles, and decreased ability to participate in recreational activities are all increased in chronic illnesses, including COPD.[28] COPD patients struggle with another common insult to self-image, the use of supplemental oxygen. They are often so self-conscious about appearing "sick" and alienating others that they are nonadherent.[29]

A second factor in any patient's ability to adjust to the burden of illness is the patency of internal coping mechanisms such as self-efficacy and a sense of mastery. The stronger patients' sense of mastery or ability to impact the daily experience of their illness, the lower is their risk for depression.[30] In a cohort of severe COPD patients, their level of perceived self-efficacy and functionality had a stronger association with their subjective quality of life than either spirometry measures or subjective assessments of pulmonary function.[31]

A third influence on patients' resilience in dealing with a chronic illness is their perceived level of social support. Generally, the greater the level of perceived social support, the less likely it is that a patient will report symptoms of depression.[32] In one group of subjects with lung disease (asthma, chronic bronchitis, or emphysema), "diffuse" relationships, those that were defined as less intimate, community-based relationships, were most helpful in "buffering" the negative effects of the illness.[33] Associated with higher reports of depressive symptoms across all groups was patients' receipt of "instrumental support"—tangible assistance with disease management. One interpretation of this effect is that receiving high levels of instrumental support reinforces feelings of dependence and helplessness, countermanding feelings of

self-efficacy and mastery.[33] Among COPD patients, there is an increased risk of depression noted for subjects who live alone or are socially isolated, who have poor reversibility of forced expiratory volume in 1 second (FEV_1) on spirometry, or who suffer severe functional impairment.[34] These studies suggest that educating patients and caregivers in strategies that maximize independence, encourage patients to develop and nurture their support systems and to participate in effective rehabilitation, can help with both the physical and the psychosocial aspects of COPD.

Losses are common to most chronic illnesses, yet COPD patients demonstrate higher rates of depression than patients with other chronic illnesses, including cardiovascular disease, most forms of cancer, and human immunodeficiency virus (HIV). The explanations for this disparity include the early vulnerability posited by genetics studies and the longitudinal, physiologic effects of chronic respiratory disease.

COPD'S EFFECTS ON THE CENTRAL NERVOUS SYSTEM

Magnetic resonance imaging (MRI) is a nonradiologic imaging technique that offers detailed study of soft tissues. In T_2-weighted MRI scans, cerebrospinal fluid and areas of acute anoxia or elevated fluid content, such as that seen with edema, appear white. These sites of increased signal are termed hyperintensities.[35] Multiple studies have noted an increased prevalence of these hyperintensities in subcortical areas in the brains of elderly subjects, collectively called subcortical hyperintensities (SHs). The concentration of these subcortical lesions increases with advancing age (by approximately 5% per additional year of age), but they are not universally associated with clinical pathology.[36–38] When present, SHs are typically seen in the "watershed" or border zones of vascular supply. As such, one pathologic association is that the prevalence and severity of SH increase with cardiovascular risk factors.[39,40] Other pathologies in the differential diagnosis for the lesions include malignancies, infarcts, and multiple sclerosis, as well as arteriosclerosis and the diminution of autoregulation of blood pressure and subsequent aberrations in blood flow.[41]

The fundamental insult in ischemia is a failure to deliver sufficient oxygen to the site of involvement, and that insufficiency can be caused by either hypoperfusion or hypoxemia. By the very nature of the disease process COPD is associated with chronic, if often subclinical, hypoxemia. The consequences of chronic hypoxemia include both impaired cognitive function and depression, although the evidence supporting the latter is less robust.[42,43] When the cognitive function of healthy subjects, COPD patients, and patients with Alzheimer disease (AD) with mild hypoxemia is compared, the AD patients had the worst performance, with the COPD patients showing significant impairment relative to the normals.[44] In a COPD population, greater SH burden is associated with lower FEV_1 and a positive smoking history.[45]

Drawing together the cause-and-effect relationship between COPD and depression, it has been found that the concentration of SH is also elevated in elderly patients with depression, particularly among the subset of patients whose depression developed after their fifth decade.[46–52] Although not consistent across studies, there is evidence that when compared with individuals who developed depression prior to 40 years of age, a higher concentration of SH is seen in older depressed subjects.[53] One explanation for this increased vulnerability to depression with age is the concept of "vascular depression."

The vascular depression theory states that chronic exposure to compromised circulation of sufficiently oxygenated blood contributes to the development of depression. The "chronicity" qualifier suggests that the risk for this damage would be expected to increase with increasing age. The theory as a whole is supported by findings that cerebrovascular disease often predates the onset of the depression, that there is an increased prevalence of depression in individuals who also suffer from hypertension or coronary artery disease, and that patients with vascular dementia manifest increased concentrations of depressive symptoms when compared with those with nonvascular AD. Additionally, accumulating MRI evidence shows a high concentration of SH in elderly depressed patients and the localization of those lesions in areas at increased risk for vascular compromise.[54,55]

There are strong relationships between COPD, SHs, and the onset and severity of late-life depression.[56] Lastly, there is the relationship of smoking to SH lesions. Smoking has been shown to be cytotoxic to endothelial cells, and this intravascular damage is a likely contributor to the observed SH.[57] Smoking has also been shown to increase the risk for permanent brain injury following exposure to what might, in the absence of a smoking history, have been a transient ischemic insult.[58]

Finally, there is growing evidence that depression and COPD impose similar microvascular and biochemical insults that would be expected to contribute to the accumulation of SH. Both depression and chronic respiratory disease have been associated with processes that jeopardize the microvasculature of the brain. In depression, this has been evidenced by significantly elevated biomarkers of oxidative damage. Levels of 8-hydroxy-2′-deoxyguanosine were directly correlated with the severity of the depression, and the level of the resultant oxidative damage was correlated with the chronicity of the depression.[59] Oxidative stress has also been associated with biochemical alterations in cell membranes. In patients with mental illness, these cell membrane aberrations are thought to interfere with effective transduction of neurotransmitter signaling.[60] In a treatment study, depressed patients were noted to have deranged oxidant and antioxidant defense systems at baseline. After treatment with antidepressants, depression measures improved and oxidative stress was reduced.[61]

In both COPD and depression, there is evidence that increased platelet activation may lead to thrombotic insult to the microvasculature, the type of injury to which the narrow

perforating arteries of the brain are particularly vulnerable. In COPD, the synthesis of a marker of platelet activation was significantly elevated and inversely related to arterial oxygen tension.[62] In a comparison of depressed patients and controls, the patients demonstrated increased platelet activation at baseline and increased platelet reactivity.[63] In a small study of depressed patients, treatment with the antidepressant sertraline diminished a pretreatment elevation in platelet activation.[64]

Diagnosis and Differentiation of Depression

Depression, like most psychiatric disorders, is diagnosed by matching patient and corroborating sources' reports of symptoms against a list of criteria for the disorder. In the United States, those lists are compended in the *Diagnostic and Statistical Manual of Mental Disorders*, currently in its fourth incarnation (*DSM-IV*), whereas the *International Classification of Diseases*, tenth revision (*ICD-10*), is the standard in Europe. By *DSM-IV* criteria, the diagnosis of a major depressive episode requires a subjective report of depressed mood or significant loss of interest or pleasure in usual activities. Then, if either of these criteria is met, the patient must also experience at least four additional complaints for at least a 2-week period. Table 1 outlines the symptoms used to diagnose a depressive episode. Examination of Table 1 also shows that there is significant overlap between the signs and symptoms of depression and common patient complaints in COPD. Both are associated with increased fatigue, sleep and appetite disruption, difficulties with concentration, and seeming "slowed down"—psychomotor slowing. In addition, some of the psychological symptoms of depression may represent normal reactions to the medical illness. When queried about anhedonia, the decreased ability to enjoy previously pleasurable activities, COPD patients will often answer in the affirmative. With further questioning, it emerges that what they're communicating is that the pulmonary illness has eroded their ability to participate in favorite activities, and they may not have found satisfying alternatives. Finally, patients nearing the end of their lives owing to chronic illness often think about death and its meaning to them, some of which may be attractive, that is, an end to suffering and a very effortful existence. These thoughts are not the same as suicidal ideation, which is clearly associated with depression, but that differentiation requires unhurried and thoughtful interviewing.[65] To make the differentiation, two criteria appear to be fairly reliably associated with depression and not with COPD. These are diminished self-esteem and an inability to emotionally brighten in the face of environmental pleasures. Asking directly how a patient feels about himself or herself as a person ("How's your self-esteem?") addresses the first. The second can be evaluated by asking the patient to gauge response to a favorite event—a visit from a grandchild, or attending a special outing. If they are genuinely able to enjoy it to its fullest, depression becomes less likely.

Table 1 DSM-IV Criteria for a Major Depressive Episode
Five (or more) of the following symptoms have been present during the same 2-week period and represent a change from previous functioning; at least one of the symptoms is either (1) depressed mood or (2) loss of interest or pleasure.
1. Depressed mood most of the day, nearly every day, as indicated by either subjective report or observations made by others
2. Markedly diminished interest or pleasure in all, or almost all, activities most of the day, nearly every day (as indicated either by subjective account or observation made by others)
3. Significant weight loss when not dieting or weight gain (a change of more than 5% of body weight in a month) or decrease or increase in appetite nearly every day
4. Insomnia or hypersomnia nearly every day
5. Psychomotor agitation or retardation nearly every day (observable by others, not merely subjective feelings of restlessness or being slowed down)
6. Fatigue or loss of energy nearly every day
7. Feelings of worthlessness or excessive or inappropriate guilt nearly every day
8. Diminished ability to think or concentrate, or indecisiveness, nearly every day
9. Recurrent thoughts of death, recurrent suicidal ideation without a specific plan, or a suicide attempt or a specific plan for committing suicide

Adapted with permission from the American Psychiatric Association.[80]

Impact of Depression on COPD Patients

Multiple studies have demonstrated that when the severity of respiratory symptoms is controlled for, COPD patients with comorbid depression report lower quality of life and demonstrate greater objective impairment in functional performance compared with nondepressed patients.[5,66] In fact, depression accounts for more of the variance in the functional performance of subjects than does disease burden or COPD severity. Furthermore, attempts to address functional deficits with pulmonary rehabilitation demonstrate improved exercise tolerance but no significant improvement in mood measures.

Depression, by decreasing motivation and increasing hopelessness, can decrease adherence to COPD treatment. Depressed patients are often less willing and less able to participate in prescribed rehabilitation programs, and, as noted above, their fragile self-esteem can intrude on their adherence to supplemental oxygen use.

There is also an interaction between the depression and the COPD wherein the depression is aggravated by worsening dyspnea, fatigue, and perceived poor health, while depression, in turn, diminishes functional performance and exercise tolerance.[67] As patients increasingly limit their activities, they become more deconditioned, leading to an even greater reduction in their functionality. Lastly, recent research has shown that depressed patients are slower to recruit medical assistance in the course of an emerging exacerbation, allowing the exacerbation to progress to a more virulent stage, potentially worsening their outcomes.[68] For both improved quality of life and improved disease management, treatment of depression is a critical step in the care of COPD patients.

Management of Depression in COPD

In spite of the prevalence and deleterious impact of comorbid depression in COPD, only a limited number of good quality studies have addressed its management. The pharmacologic studies that have been done have been plagued by low power, too short durations of treatment, insufficient dosing, and variable rigor in diagnostic and outcome measures. Because of these deficiencies, formal guidelines have been necessarily general although typically supportive of a multidisciplinary approach.[69]

Once a diagnosis of depression is made, it is useful to attempt to clarify if the patient is more likely suffering from an "early-" or a "late-onset" depression. To the extent that late-onset depression is correlated with greater global central nervous system dysfunction, it might be expected that these patients will manifest with more associated cognitive dysfunction, functional disability, limited insight, and psychomotor retardation. In turn, patients with early-onset depression are likely to have a more "classic" presentation of depression but, in the context of COPD, perhaps greater difficulty with smoking cessation. For those patients with primarily a late-onset picture, increasing support networks and taking steps to protect against vascular damage will be especially important, whereas early-onset patients may especially benefit from increased structure and support in smoking cessation programs. For both groups, another important element is the inclusion of pulmonary rehabilitation. Pulmonary rehabilitation, among other benefits, improves quality of life by increasing patients' perception of available social supports, as well as improving their ability to participate in stress-reducing activities and increasing their sense of self-mastery.

In addition to the supportive elements of the treatment plan, a physician working with a depressed COPD patient will want to consider the prescription of an antidepressant. The best study of an antidepressant intervention was conducted in the early 1990s but is now of somewhat limited benefit because it used a tricyclic antidepressant that has fallen out of first-line status because of difficult side effects. However, the study did demonstrate that application of the antidepressant did improve both mood and subjective functionality.[70] More recent studies have used selective serotonin reuptake inhibitors (SSRIs), the current first-line medications for the management of depression in community populations, but have suffered from the flaws noted above. Among those studies, there does appear to be support for the usefulness of SSRIs in the COPD population, but the data need to be subjected to the scrutiny of peer review and then replicated. In the absence of strong, evidence-based guidance, an algorithm parallel to that used for non-COPD-depressed patients is the best clinical strategy (Figures 2 and 3). Figure 2 outlines the strategies for initial trial and selection of an antidepressant, whereas Figure 3 outlines the longer-term maintenance protocol for antidepressant use. In applying this algorithm, it is important to remember that the COPD population has a greater number of medical comorbidities, increased risk for medicine–medicine interactions, and greater physical debilitation than the community population for which the algorithm was originally designed. So although it is a useful guide, it is imperative to recognize the above limitations in treatment planning. Additionally, available research does not support the use of any particular medication over others in terms of significantly improved response. As SSRIs are the first-line treatment for primary depression, it is reasonable to start with them in this scenario as well. Selection among the SSRIs is made based on side-effect profiles, comorbid diagnoses that may benefit from secondary indications, medication interactions, and the impact of half-life. Table 2 provides a comparison of the SSRIs (and two serotonin-norepinephrine reuptake inhibitors) that may help with the selection of an antidepressant.

The side effects potentially common to all SSRIs include start-up difficulties with gastrointestinal upset, diarrhea, headaches, tremors, and either psychomotor activation or sedation. This latter continuum, that is, from sedation to agitation, is frequently problematic for COPD patients in that their dyspnea tends to impose a baseline level of anxiety that can be aggravated by SSRIs, leading to impaired adherence. Over time, the SSRIs also carry a risk for sexual dysfunction, in particular diminished libido and delayed or inhibited climax. Some side effects that are more unique to individual agents are shown in Table 2. A full discussion of

Table 2   Comparison of Various Serotoninergic Antidepressants

Medication	Approved Indications	Most Common Side Effects	Half-Life (Metabolite)	Usual Daily Dosing	Common Interactions
Fluvoxamine (Luvox)	OCD	Significant GI upset; requires bid/tid dosing	15 h	50–150 mg bid	Inhibits CYP1A2, 2C9, 2C19, 3A4 Substrate for 2D6
Fluoxetine (Prozac)	Depression, OCD, bulimia	Minimum weight gain	2–3 d (7–9 d)	20–40 mg daily; higher doses in eating disorders (80 mg)	Inhibits 2C9, 2C19, 2D6, 3A4 Substrate for 2D6
Sertraline (Zoloft)	Depression, OCD, PMDD, PTSD, panic		26 h	50–200 mg daily	Inhibits 2C19 Substrate for 2D6, 3A4
Paroxetine (Paxil)	Depression, OCD, panic	Intense discontinuation syndrome + weight gain	21 h	20–50 mg daily	Inhibits 2C19, 2D6 Substrate for 2D6
Citalopram (Lexapro, Celexa)	Depression, GAD	Minimal weight gain; occasional tremors		Celexa: 20–60 mg daily Lexapro: 10–40 mg daily	Inhibits 2D6 Substrate for 2C19, 3A4
Venlafaxine (Effexor)	Depression, GAD	Agitation at start-up and at discontinuation	Varies by formulation: immediate release vs extended release	75–300 mg daily	—
Duloxetine (Cymbalta)	Depression, GAD, pain associated with diabetic neuropathy	Agitation at discontinuation	12 h	30–60 mg daily	Substrate for 1A2, 2D6 Inhibits 2D6

bid = two times daily; GAD = generalized anxiety disorder; GI = gastrointestinal; OCD = obsessive-compulsive disorder; PMDD = premenstrual dysphoric disorder; PTSD = posttraumatic stress disorder; tid = three times daily.

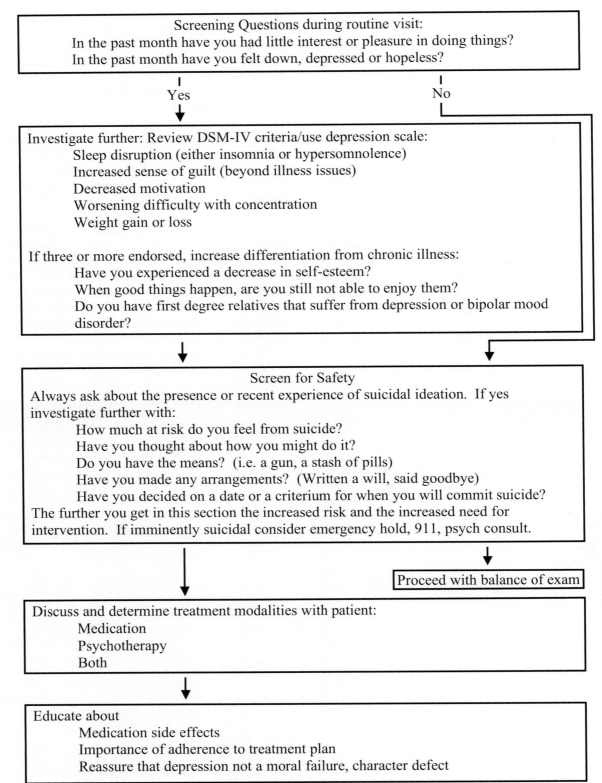

Screening Questions during routine visit:
In the past month have you had little interest or pleasure in doing things?
In the past month have you felt down, depressed or hopeless?

Yes   No

Investigate further: Review DSM-IV criteria/use depression scale:
    Sleep disruption (either insomnia or hypersomnolence)
    Increased sense of guilt (beyond illness issues)
    Decreased motivation
    Worsening difficulty with concentration
    Weight gain or loss

If three or more endorsed, increase differentiation from chronic illness:
    Have you experienced a decrease in self-esteem?
    When good things happen, are you still not able to enjoy them?
    Do you have first degree relatives that suffer from depression or bipolar mood disorder?

Screen for Safety
Always ask about the presence or recent experience of suicidal ideation. If yes investigate further with:
    How much at risk do you feel from suicide?
    Have you thought about how you might do it?
    Do you have the means? (i.e. a gun, a stash of pills)
    Have you made any arrangements? (Written a will, said goodbye)
    Have you decided on a date or a criterium for when you will commit suicide?
The further you get in this section the increased risk and the increased need for intervention. If imminently suicidal consider emergency hold, 911, psych consult.

Proceed with balance of exam

Discuss and determine treatment modalities with patient:
    Medication
    Psychotherapy
    Both

Educate about
    Medication side effects
    Importance of adherence to treatment plan
    Reassure that depression not a moral failure, character defect

FIGURE 2. Strategies for initial trial of antidepressant.

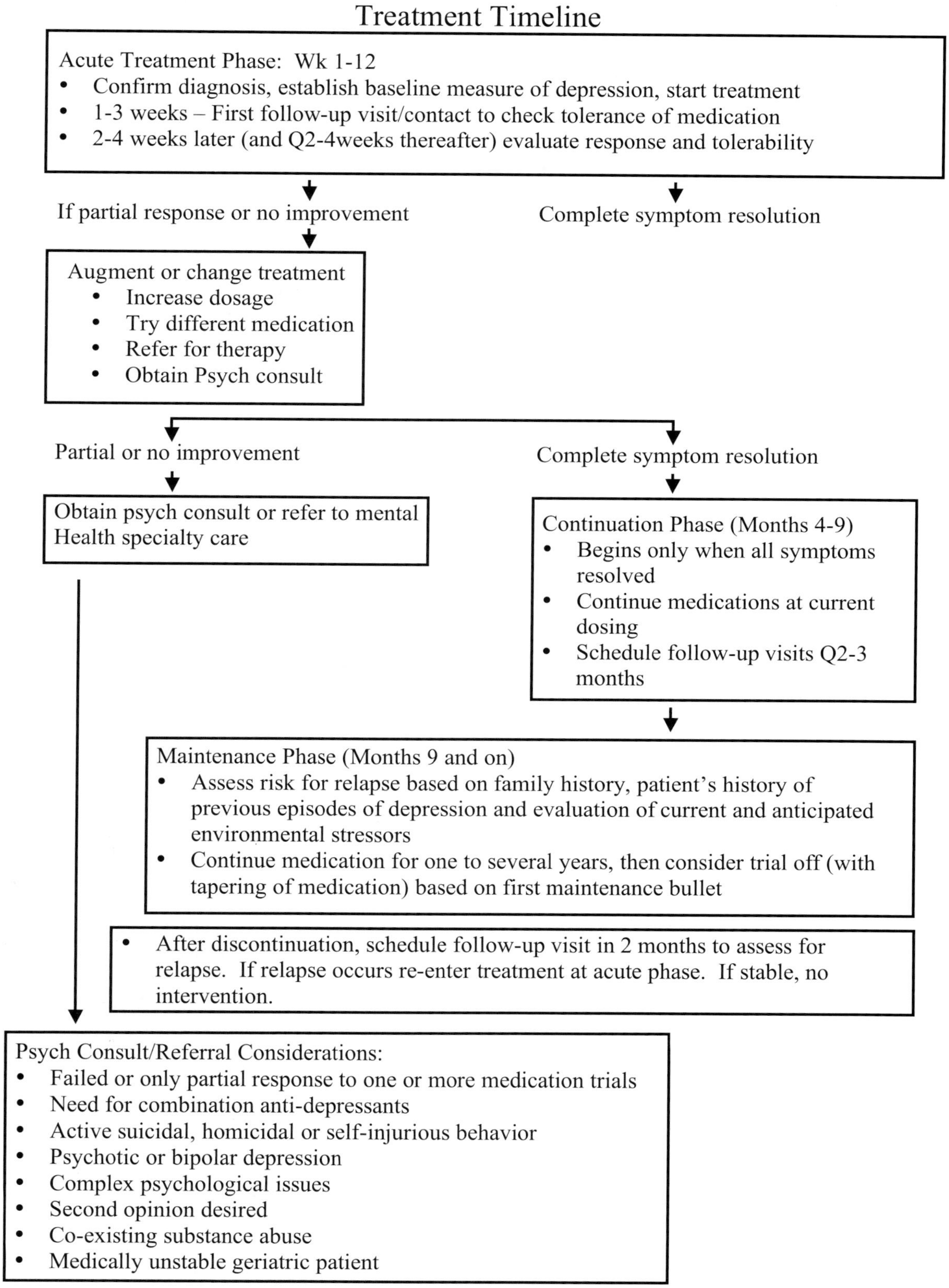

Treatment Timeline

Acute Treatment Phase: Wk 1-12
- Confirm diagnosis, establish baseline measure of depression, start treatment
- 1-3 weeks – First follow-up visit/contact to check tolerance of medication
- 2-4 weeks later (and Q2-4weeks thereafter) evaluate response and tolerability

If partial response or no improvement   Complete symptom resolution

Augment or change treatment
- Increase dosage
- Try different medication
- Refer for therapy
- Obtain Psych consult

Partial or no improvement   Complete symptom resolution

Obtain psych consult or refer to mental
Health specialty care

Continuation Phase (Months 4-9)
- Begins only when all symptoms resolved
- Continue medications at current dosing
- Schedule follow-up visits Q2-3 months

Maintenance Phase (Months 9 and on)
- Assess risk for relapse based on family history, patient's history of previous episodes of depression and evaluation of current and anticipated environmental stressors
- Continue medication for one to several years, then consider trial off (with tapering of medication) based on first maintenance bullet

- After discontinuation, schedule follow-up visit in 2 months to assess for relapse. If relapse occurs re-enter treatment at acute phase. If stable, no intervention.

Psych Consult/Referral Considerations:
- Failed or only partial response to one or more medication trials
- Need for combination anti-depressants
- Active suicidal, homicidal or self-injurious behavior
- Psychotic or bipolar depression
- Complex psychological issues
- Second opinion desired
- Co-existing substance abuse
- Medically unstable geriatric patient

FIGURE 3. Long-term and maintenance strategies for antidepressants. Adapted from Colorado *Clinical Guidelines* Collaborative Practice. Guideline: Major Depression Disorder in Adults, 5/7/2003.

all possible medication interactions involving SSRIs and the range of medications that are used for COPD patients is beyond the scope of this chapter, but we can draw some general outlines. The SSRIs as a group are substrates of cytochrome P-450 2D6 primarily and 3A4 and 2C19 secondarily. In addition, they are also mild inhibitors of 2D6 and 2C19. As such, the SSRIs are typically not very problematic with the majority of bronchodilators or steroids. An exception is theophylline, which is notorious for its tendency to interact with other medications, in this case, particularly with fluvoxamine, a rarely used SSRI. The pharmacokinetic interaction between fluvoxamine and theophylline can decrease the clearance of theophylline by up to 80%, increasing the steady-state serum concentrations of the bronchodilator two to three times.[71] The risk for interaction should be a factor in selecting both the bronchodilator and the antidepressant. Antibiotics also present a potential risk for interaction with the SSRIs, particularly the macrolides and the fluoroquinolones. These two groups of antibiotics both block potassium channels, leading to possible Q–Tc prolongation.[72] SSRIs have also been found to have potential for the same cardiotoxicity.[73] As is the usual case with this phenomenon, the risk associated with a single medication may be marginal, but prescribers must be attentive to amplifying this risk by combining offending agents. Finally, the macrolides tend to inhibit the cytochrome P-450 3A4 enzymes with varying degrees of potency. Since the SSRIs are substrates of these enzymes, logic would suggest that this interaction might be a source of increasing antidepressant concentration, although the literature does not report this happening or, at least, as being problematic.

In addition to medication trials, patients may also benefit from the addition of appropriate psychotherapy. Cognitive behavioral therapy allows for a very problem-focused approach to managing the daily challenges these patients face. Other options include supportive or psychodynamic therapy depending on the needs and interests of the patient. It is also critically important to recognize the impact that both COPD and depression have on family and friends around a patient and to include "support for the support group." Finally, for patients whose depression is refractory to all other interventions, electroconvulsive therapy can be lifesaving.

The complexity of effectively managing depression in COPD patients raises the question of when a patient should be referred to a psychiatrist. Some clear indications that such a consultation would be useful include a patient with multiple comorbid psychiatric diagnoses, a patient with manic-depressive illness or other types of bipolar depression, and a patient with depression that has shown itself to be largely refractory to treatment options with which the primary physician is comfortable. Of course, the most appropriate answer to the question of when to request a consultation is whenever the treating physician feels it would be useful. Because depression is so common in COPD patients, a psychosocial evaluation should be included in the initial workup of the patient, and mood symptoms should be monitored regularly throughout treatment. Because the risks for refractory illness, side-effect complications, and patient difficulties can be so great in COPD patients, pulmonary physicians should have a low threshold for involving their psychiatric colleagues.

Anxiety

The inability to breathe is a frightening experience faced daily by people with severe COPD. Frequently, that fear begins to encroach on the patient's baseline experience, so he or she develops a heightened level of anxiety regardless of immediate respiratory status. During an episode of dyspnea, the patient becomes vulnerable to even more intensified levels of anxiety, which can eventually progress to full-blown panic events.

Epidemiology

There are data establishing that patients with COPD have a disproportionately high prevalence of panic disorder (between 11% and 24%) compared with a community level of less than 5%.[74,75] Similarly, these patients have more baseline anxiety, with a prevalence of approximately twice that seen in individuals without respiratory disease.[76] This high degree of comorbidity likely is the result of multiple contributing factors, including cognitive accommodation, or learning, as patients endure and try to manage repeated events, as well as physiologic responses to a compromised respiratory system.

Etiology
LEARNING

As with depression, the longest standing explanation for increased rates of panic and anxiety in COPD patients revolves around cognitive explanations. As patients experience repeated bouts of dyspnea, they are less able to apply clear reasoning skills to the event, leading to difficulty in accurately assessing the danger posed by an episode of dyspnea. This results in disproportionate fear and mounting anxiety. Each subsequent attack augments the patient's fear of being unable to breathe, heightening anxiety and often leading to panic. Soon symptoms of anxiety are present even in the absence of a respiratory trigger, and symptoms of panic can set in early during a respiratory event, when respiratory symptoms are still mild and would otherwise be manageable. Thus, elevated anxiety becomes a baseline condition, and panic is triggered or exacerbated by the patient's perception of impending dyspnea rather than the actual, biologic characteristics of the respiratory event.

FALSE SUFFOCATION

Papp and colleagues proposed that these subjects have a "biologic vulnerability" manifested as an increased sensitivity to CO_2 levels and subsequent susceptibility to panic owing to an abnormally sensitive chemoreceptor in the brainstem responsible for monitoring respiratory function.[77] When this sensor detects signs of impending suffocation (ie, increasing CO_2 or elevated lactate levels), it triggers an increased ventilation rate and inspiratory drive in panic-susceptible patients and ultimately leads to symptoms of panic. Klein referred to this as the "false suffocation alarm."[78]

A confusing diagnostic picture emerges. Is the dyspnea caused by anxiety and panic? Or are anxiety and panic the result of dyspnea? Both are possible, and resolving this conundrum is essential to choosing the correct pharmaceutical agents for management.

Differential Diagnosis: Anxiety versus Dyspnea

As clinicians, we are faced with the challenge of ascertaining what portion of a patient's presentation is primarily respiratory (ie, dyspnea) and what portion is primarily due to anxiety symptoms, either generalized anxiety or panic. This discrimination is critical for directing the management of symptoms because the pharmacologic approaches to dyspnea can exacerbate anxiety and vice versa.

GENERALIZED ANXIETY DISORDER

According to the most recent edition of the *DSM-IV*, generalized anxiety disorder (GAD) is characterized by "at least six months of persistent and excessive anxiety and worry."[79] The worry is difficult to control and is associated with at least three symptoms, such as irritability, impaired concentration, or muscle tension. The anxiety causes significant clinical distress or impairment in function.[80] The full set of criteria is presented in Table 3.

Again in parallel with depression, anxiety disorders are frequently present even before the patient develops symptoms of COPD. Typically, patients with GAD have struggled with heightened anxiety for much of their lives and may have been diagnosed with some form of anxiety disorder as early as their twenties or thirties.[81]

Additionally, it is important to realize that not all anxiety is pathologic. Some anxiety is a normal and an understandable response to the challenges posed by a chronic illness such as COPD. Assessing the degree and duration of anxiety can be key in discriminating between GAD and the normal adjustment to respiratory illness. The *DSM-IV* distinguishes between GAD and "adjustment disorder with anxiety," in which the stressor may be a serious general medical condition. The distinction is subtle: COPD patients have a highly debilitating progressive and incurable illness that generates a high level of stress in their lives. It is, therefore, adaptive for them to be more attentive to a variety of issues (availability of oxygen, level of exertion, risk of infection, impact of the illness on family, end-of-life planning) to effectively manage their daily experience. This degree of attention and illness management can trigger some anxiety but may not be considered a pathologic level of anxiety. That level becomes pathologic when illness-related stress becomes a defining experience of patients' lives. Anxiety should not cause significant impairment in concentration and mood or physical symptoms, such as muscle tension and insomnia. These would be signs of GAD rather than an appropriate level of illness-induced anxiety.

The following set of questions can help differentiate GAD from appropriate attentiveness to disease management or from the milder diagnosis of "adjustment disorder with anxiety":

1. Is the anxiety usually present at an uncomfortable baseline level, regardless of immediate health status?
2. Is the content of the anxiety general and wide-ranging or specific to the realistic challenges posed by the COPD? Does it extend beyond health concerns to the well-being of family members, to social interactions, to impoverishment (especially in the face of financial stability), or to excessive concern about news stories and world events that have no apparent immediate relevance to the patient's life?

Table 3 *DSM-IV* Symptoms Criteria for Generalized Anxiety Disorder

A. Excessive anxiety and worry (apprehensive expectation), occurring more days than not for at least 6 months, about a number of events or activities

B. The person finds it difficult to control the worry

C. The anxiety and worry are associated with three or more of the following six symptoms:

  1. Restlessness or feeling keyed up or on edge

  2. Being easily fatigued

  3. Difficulty concentrating or mind going blank

  4. Irritability

  5. Muscle tension

  6. Sleep disturbance (difficulty falling or staying asleep or restless unsatisfying sleep)

D. The anxiety, worry, or physical symptoms cause clinically significant distress or impairment in social, occupational, or other important areas of functioning

Adapted with permission from the American Psychiatric Association.[80]

3. Has the patient been a "worrier" much of his or her life, even before developing COPD?
4. Does the patient feel the level of worry is excessive?
5. Is the anxiety (rather than the direct effects of the COPD) causing significant impairment in other areas of health, social functioning, or employment?

Affirmative responses to these questions are more likely to be associated with GAD than with adjustment disorder with anxiety or anxiety owing to a medical condition.

PANIC DISORDER

Panic disorders and anxiety disorders are closely related because a panic attack is often associated with a baseline state of elevated anxiety. To qualify for a diagnosis of panic disorder, a patient must experience recurrent panic attacks and interepisode anxiety related to the attacks. That anxiety may take the form of fear of having a future attack or fear that the attack signifies underlying mental illness.[75] The *DSM-IV* defines a panic attack as "a discrete period of intense fear or discomfort in the absence of real danger." The attack is accompanied by symptoms that may include nausea, abdominal distress, palpitations, sweating, trembling, shortness of breath or choking, chest pain, and dizziness.

Even a cursory review of these symptoms reveals the diagnostic confusion that may arise in cases of patients with COPD and comorbid panic because of the significant overlap between symptoms associated with dyspnea and those associated with panic attack. Despite the striking similarities, however, it is important to note that dyspnea is not the same as primary panic disorder. Dyspnea occurs when the demand placed on the respiratory systems exceeds the ability of the respiratory system to efficiently meet that demand. In people with COPD, this respiratory dysfunction with accompanying reduction in oxygen exchange results from the damage to the alveoli and airways caused by the disease process. Panic, on the other hand, is a cognitive identification of threat and a cognitive, emotional, and physiologic response to that perceived threat. Moreover, anxiety must be present not only during the acute event (which is a physiologic response to the inability to breathe) but also between attacks.

Thus, the key to distinguishing between primary panic disorder and the temporary panic caused by COPD-induced dyspnea lies in a thorough understanding of the patient's emotional state both during and after the attack. An additional clue is provided by the presence or absence of typical panic attack symptoms not associated with COPD, such as gastrointestinal distress or a fear of "going crazy."

Clinicians may evaluate the situation using the following series of questions:

1. Are the episodes accompanied by nausea or abdominal distress? (not requisite but a possible point of discrimination)
2. During the episode, is the patient afraid of dying owing to suffocation or of "going crazy?" Does the patient worry about his or her mental stability between attacks as well?
3. Are the episodes typically associated with increased exertion (more likely respiratory), or do they sometimes occur when the patient is sitting quietly (more likely panic)?

Some patients may not have immediate answers to these questions. Asking them to keep a log of dyspneic events and any identified triggers (environmental and emotional) for those events; activity at the time of onset; duration of the event; how they felt before, during, and after the event; and steps taken to manage the event can help clarify their experience. In addition, the patient and family members can offer important data about family history since both panic disorder and GAD are known to have a genetic component.[82] If there are first-degree relatives with these disorders, it increases the likelihood that the patient has primary GAD or panic disorder rather than dyspnea.

Pharmacologic Management of Anxiety

The recognition of a comorbid anxiety or panic disorder in a patient with COPD impacts the pharmacologic management of both the psychiatric and pulmonary complaints. The medications used to treat dyspnea often aggravate the symptoms of anxiety, whereas some of the agents for the management of anxiety can worsen respiratory symptoms.

Because poorly managed dyspnea has more irrevocable consequences than poorly managed anxiety, targeting the respiratory symptoms first is the recommended protocol. However, if the presenting symptoms worsen—as can happen if the dyspnea is actually a symptom of panic—or if significant anxiety symptoms remain after implementation of the

Table 4 Psychiatric Impacts of Dyspnea Medications

Medication	Impact on Psychiatric Symptoms
β_2-Agonists (eg albuterol)	Increased heart rate, sleep disturbance*
Anticholinergics (eg, ipratropium)	Increased heart rate†
Theophylline	Increased risk for hyperactivity, anxiety, mania*
Glucocorticoids	Agitation, hyperactivity, sleep/mood disturbance, psychosis‡

*See Hardman JG, editor. Goodman & Gilman's the pharmacological basis of therapeutics. 10th ed. McGraw Hill; New York 2001.
†See Papiris S, Kotanidou A, Malagari K et al. Clinical Review: Severe Asthma. Critical Care 2002;6(1):30–44.
‡See Drugs that may cause psychiatric symptoms. The Medical Letter on Drugs and Therapeutics. The Medical Letter, Inc. (publisher), New York 2002;44:59–61.

Table 5 Anxiety Medications

Medication	Indications (FDA Approved)	Clinical Considerations
Benzodiazepines	Panic, GAD	Risk for respiratory depression at high doses or in combination with another CNS depressant. Risk for abuse/dependence.
Tricyclic antidepressants	Panic, MDD	Must be taken for 4–6 weeks before benefits realized. High rate of problematic side effects: weight gain, anticholinergic, sedation, tachycardia/orthostasis, cardiac conduction irregularities.
SSRIs	Panic, MDD, GAD, PTSD (sertraline, paroxetine)	Must be taken for 4–6 weeks before benefits realized. Common sexual side effects. Small group of case studies suggest potential benefit in dyspnea.
Venlafaxine, duloxetine	MDD, GAD (pain for duloxetine)	Must be taken for 4–6 weeks before benefits realized. May be helpful for panic. Side effects similar to SSRIs; risk for hypertension with higher doses (>300 mg of venlafaxine).
Buspirone	GAD	Good choice for patients with history of substance abuse (other than nicotine). Must be taken for 4–6 weeks before benefits realized.
Gabapentin	Chronic pain	Good tolerability; side effects include sedation, dizziness

Adapted from Schatzberg AF, Cole JO, DeBattista D. Manual of clinical psychopharmacology. 4th ed. Washington (DC): American Psychiatric Publishing; 2003.
CNS = central nervous system; FDA = US Food and Drug Administration; GAD = generalized anxiety disorder; MDD = major depressive disorder; Panic = panic disorder; PTSD = posttraumatic stress disorder; SSRI = selective serotonin reuptake inhibitor.

dyspnea treatment, then the treatment must be modified to target the anxiety symptoms.

Medications routinely used for the management of chronic dyspnea in patients with COPD include bronchodilators (β_2-agonists and anticholinergics), theophylline and its derivatives, and, potentially, glucocorticoids. Table 4 discusses these drugs with reference to their effect on psychiatric symptoms.

Although these medications may improve patients' respiratory status, if patients experience an actual worsening of dyspnea while using these agents, taking a more "anxiolytic-oriented" approach may be helpful. Table 5 lists the psychiatric medications used to manage anxiety diagnoses, their uses, any known impact on dyspnea, and considerations for the clinician to keep in mind when prescribing them. There are very limited data suggesting any direct benefit from these medications in terms of relieving dyspnea. What they do offer is management of panic or generalized anxiety, with little detriment to patients' respiratory status in most cases.

In summary, overlapping symptoms can make the distinction between dyspnea and anxiety elusive. However, by listening to the details of the patient's experience and combining that understanding with a reasonable risk/benefit approach to symptom control, clinicians can provide more comprehensive, targeted, and effective care.

References

1. Manino DM. COPD surveillance US. Morb Mortal Rep 2002;51(6):1–16.
2. van Ede L, Yzermans CJ, Brouwer HJ. Prevalence of depression in patients with chronic obstructive pulmonary disease: a systematic review. Thorax 1999;54:688–92.
3. Light RW, Merrill EJ, Despars JA, et al. Prevalence of depression and anxiety in patients with COPD. Relationship to functional capacity. Chest 1985;87:35–8.
4. Yohannes A. Mood disorders in elderly patients with COPD. Rev Clin Gerontol 2000;10:193–202.
5. Aydin IO, Ulusahin A. Depression, anxiety comorbidity, and disability in tuberculosis and chronic obstructive pulmonary disease patients: applicability of GHQ-12. Gen Hosp Psychiatry 2001;23:77–83.
6. Kunik ME, Roundy K, Veazey C, et al. Surprisingly high prevalence of anxiety and depression in chronic breathing disorders. Chest 2005;127:1205–11.
7. Kurosawa H. The relationship between mental disorders and physical severities in patients with acute MI. Jpn Circ J 1983;47:723–5.
8. Evans DL, Staab JP, Petitto JM, et al. Depression in the medical setting: biopsychological interactions and treatment considerations. J Clin Psychiatry 1999;60 Suppl 4:40–55.
9. Katon W, Sullivan MD. Depression and chronic medical illness. J Clin Psychiatry 1990;51(6 Suppl):3–11; discussion 2–4.
10. Cruess DG, Evans LE, Repetto MJ, et al. Prevalence, diagnosis, and pharmacological treatment of mood disorders in HIV disease. Biol Psychiatry 2003;54:307–16.
11. Kaplan HI, Sadock BJ, Grebb JA, eds. Kaplan and Sadock's Synopsis of psychiatry, 8th ed. Baltimore: Lippincott, Williams & Wilkins; 1988. p. 543.
12. Sullivan PF, Nealt MC, Kendler S. Genetic epidemiology of major depression: review and meta-analysis. Am J Psychiatry 2000;157:1552–62.
13. Kendler KS, Gatz M, Gardner CO, et al. A Swedish national twin study of lifetime major depression. Am J Psychiatry 2006;163:109–14.
14. Elely TC, Liang H, Plomin R, et al. Parental familial vulnerability, family environment, and their interactions as predictors of

depressive symptoms in adolescents. J Am Acad Child Adolesc Psychiatry 2004;43:298–306.

15. Ferguson DM. Comorbidity between depressive disorders and nicotine dependence in a cohort of 16 year olds. Arch Gen Psychiatry 1996;53:1043–7.

16. Patton GC, Hibbert M, Rosier MJ, et al. Is smoking associated with depression and anxiety in teenagers? Am J Public Health 1996;86:225–30.

17. Breslau N, Kilbey MM, Andreski P. Nicotine dependence and major depression. New evidence from a prospective investigation. Arch Gen Psychiatry 1993;50:31–5.

18. Audrain-McGovern J, Lerman C, Wileyto EP, et al. Interacting effects of genetic predisposition and depression on adolescent smoking progression. Am J Psychiatry 2004; 161:1224–30.

19. Covey LS, Glassman AH, Stetner F. Cigarette smoking and major depression. J Addict Dis 1998;17:35–46.

20. Covey LS. Tobacco cessation among patients with depression. Prim Care 1999;26:691–706.

21. Covey LS, Glassman AH, Stetner F. Major depression following smoking cessation. Am J Psychiatry 1997;154:263–5.

22. Hitsman B, Pingitore R, Spring B, et al. Antidepressant pharmacotherapy helps some cigarette smokers more than others. J Consult Clin Psychol 1999;67:547–54.

23. Hall SM, Reus VI, Munoz RF, et al. Nortriptyline and cognitive-behavioral therapy in the treatment of cigarette smoking. Arch Gen Psychiatry 1998;55:683–90.

24. Hurt RD, Sachs DP, Glover ED, et al. A comparison of sustained-release bupropion and placebo for smoking cessation. N Engl J Med 1997;337:1195–202.

25. Niaura R, Britt DM, Shadel WG, et al. Symptoms of depression and survival experience among three samples of smokers trying to quit. Psychol Addict Behav 2001;15:13–7.

26. Lerman C, Berrettini W. Elucidating the role of genetic factors in smoking behavior and nicotine dependence. Am J Med Genet B Neuropsychiatr Genet 2003;118:48–54.

27. Agle DP, Baum GL. Psychological aspects of chronic obstructive pulmonary disease. Med Clin North Am 1977;61:749–58.

28. Dunlop DD, Lyons JS, Manheim LM, et al. Arthritis and heart disease as risk factors for major depression: the role of functional limitation. Med Care 2004;42:502–11.

29. Earnest MA. Explaining adherence to supplemental oxygen therapy: the patient's perspective. J Gen Intern Med 2002;17:749–55.

30. Brown GW, Andrews B, Harris T et al. Social support, vulnerability and depression. Psychol Med 1986;16(4):813–31.

31. Kohler CL, Fish L, Greene PG. The relationship of perceived self-efficacy to quality of life in chronic obstructive pulmonary disease. Health Psychol 2002;21:610–4.

32. McCathie HC, Spence SH, Tate RL. Adjustment to chronic obstructive pulmonary disease: the importance of psychological factors. Eur Respir J 2002;19:47–53.

33. Penning MJ, Strain LA. Gender differences in disability, assistance, and subjective well-being in later life. J Gerontol 1994;49(4):S202–8.

34. van Manen JG, Bindels PJ, Dekker FW, et al. Risk of depression in patients with chronic obstructive pulmonary disease and its determinants. Thorax 2002;57:412–6.

35. Yudofsky SC, Hales RE. Textbook of neuropsychiatry. 2nd ed. Washington (DC): American Psychiatric Press; 1992.

36. Coffey CE, Willkinson WE, Parashos LA, et al. Quantitative cerebral anatomy of the aging human brain: a cross-sectional study using magnetic resonance imaging. Neurology 1992;42:527–36.

37. Guttmann CR, Jolesz FA, Kikinis R, et al. White matter changes with normal aging. Neurology 1998;50:972–8.

38. Grafton ST, Sumi SM, Stimac GK, et al. Comparison of post-mortem magnetic resonance imaging and neuropathologic findings in the cerebral white matter. Arch Neurol 1991;48:293–8.

39. Brown FW, Lewine RJ, Hudgins PA, et al. White matter hyperintensity signals in psychiatric and nonpsychiatric subjects. Am J Psychiatry 1992;149:620–5.

40. Awad IA, Spetzler RF, Hodak JA, et al. Incidental subcortical lesions identified on magnetic resonance imaging in the elderly. I. Correlation with age and cerebrovascular risk factors. Stroke 1986;17:1084–9.

41. Campbell JJ 3rd, Coffey CE. Neuropsychiatric significance of subcortical hyperintensity. J Neuropsychiatry Clin Neurosci 2001;13:261–88.

42. Ozge C, Ozge A, Unal O. Cognitive and functional deterioration in patients with severe COPD. Behav Neurol 2006;17:121–30.

43. El-Ad B, Lavie P. Effect of sleep apnea on cognition and mood. Int Rev Psychiatry 2005;17:277–82.

44. Kozora E, Filley CM, Julian LJ, et al. Cognitive functioning in patients with chronic obstructive pulmonary disease and mild hypoxemia compared with patients with mild Alzheimer disease and normal controls. Neuropsychiatry Neuropsychol Behav Neurol 1999;12:178–83.

45. Longstreth WT Jr, Manolio TA, Arnold A, et al. Clinical correlates of white matter findings on cranial magnetic resonance imaging of 3301 elderly people. The Cardiovascular Health Study. Stroke 1996;27:1274–82.

46. Coffey CE, Wilkinson WE, Weiner RD, et al. Quantitative cerebral anatomy in depression: a controlled magnetic resonance imaging study. Arch Gen Psychiatry 1993;50:7–16.

47. Krishnan KR, Goli V, Ellinwood EH, et al. Leukoencephalopathy in patients diagnosed as major depressive. Biol Psychiatry 1988;23:519–22.

48. Krishnan KR, McDonald WM, Doraiswamy PM, et al. Neuroanatomical substrates of depression in the elderly. Eur Arch Psychiatry Clin Neurosci 1993;243:41–6.

49. Figiel GS, Krishnan KR, Doraiswamy PM, et al. Subcortical hyperintensities on brain magnetic resonance imaging: a comparison between late age onset and early onset elderly depressed subjects. Neurobiol Aging 1991;12:245–7.

50. Lesser IM, Boone KB, Mehringer CM, et al. Cognition and white matter hyperintensities in older depressed patients. Am J Psychiatry 1996;153:1280–7.

51. Howard RJ, Beats B, Forstl H, et al. White matter changes in late onset depression: a magnetic resonance imaging study. Int J Geriatr Psychiatry 1993;8:183–5.

52. Videbech P. MRI findings in patients with affective disorder: a meta-analysis. Acta Psychiatr Scand 1997;96:157–68.

53. Salloway S, Malloy P, Kohn R, et al. MRI and neuropsychological differences in early- and late-life-onset geriatric depression. Neurology 1996;46:1567–74.

54. Alexopoulos GS, Meyers BS, Young RC, et al. 'Vascular depression' hypothesis. Arch Gen Psychiatry 1997;54:915–22.
55. Alexopoulos GS, Meyers BS, Young RC, et al. Clinically defined vascular depression. Am J Psychiatry 1997;154:562–5.
56. van Dijk EJ, Vermeer SE, de Groot JC, et al. Arterial oxygen saturation, COPD, and cerebral small vessel disease. J Neurol Neurosurg Psychiatry 2004;75:733–6.
57. Blann AD, McCollum CN. Adverse influence of cigarette smoking on the endothelium. Thromb Haemost 1993;70:707–11.
58. Wang L, Kittaka M, Sun N, et al. Chronic nicotine treatment enhances focal ischemic brain injury and depletes free pool of brain microvascular tissue plasminogen activator in rats. J Cereb Blood Flow Metab 1997;17:136–46.
59. Forlenza MJ, Miller GE. Increased serum levels of 8-hydroxy-2'-deoxyguanosine in clinical depression. Psychosom Med 2006;68:1–7.
60. Ponizovsky AM, Barshtein G, Bergelson LD. Biochemical alterations of erythrocytes as an indicator of mental disorders: an overview. Harv Rev Psychiatry 2003;11:317–32.
61. Khanzode SD, Dakhale GN, Khanzode SS, et al. Oxidative damage and major depression: the potential antioxidant action of selective serotonin re-uptake inhibitors. Redox Report 2003;8:365–70.
62. Davi G, Basili S, Vieri M, et al. Enhanced thromboxane biosynthesis in patients with chronic obstructive pulmonary disease. Am J Respir Crit Care Med 1997;156:1794–9.
63. Musselman DL, Tomer A, Manatunga AK, et al. Exaggerated platelet reactivity in major depression. Am J Psychiatry 1996;153:1313–7.
64. Markovitz JH, Shuster JL, Chitwood WS, et al. Platelet activation in depression and effects of sertraline treatment: an open-label study. Am J Psychiatry 2000;157:1006–8.
65. Levensen JL. Depression in the medically ill. Prim Psychiatry 2005;12:22–4.
66. Felker B, Katon W, Hedrick SC, et al. The association between depressive symptoms and health status in patients with chronic pulmonary disease. Gen Hosp Psychiatry 2001;23:56–61.
67. Yeh M-L, Chen H-H, Liao Y-C, et al. Testing the functional status model in patients with chronic obstructive pulmonary disease. J Adv Nurs 2004;48:342–50.
68. Dowson CA, Town GI, Frampton C, et al. Psychopathology and illness beliefs influence COPD self-management. J Psychosom Res 2004;56:333–40.
69. National Collaborating Centre for Chronic Conditions. National clinical guidelines on management of chronic obstructive pulmonary disease in adults in primary and secondary care. Thorax 2004;59 Suppl 1:1–232.
70. Borson S, McDonald GJ, Gayle T, et al. Improvement in mood, physical symptoms, and function with nortriptyline for depression in patients with chronic obstructive pulmonary disease. Psychosomatics 1992;33:190–201.
71. Rasmussen BB, Jeppesen U, Gaist D, et al. Griseofulvin and fluvoxamine interactions with the metabolism of theophylline. Ther Drug Monit 1997;19:56–62.
72. Iannini PB. Cardiotoxicity of macrolides, ketolides and fluoroquinolones that prolong the QTc interval. Expert Opin Drug Saf 2002;1:121–8.
73. Varriale P. Fluoxetine (Prozac) as a cause of QT prolongation. Arch Intern Med 2001;161:612.
74. Smoller JW, Pollack MH, Otto MW, et al. Panic anxiety, dyspnea, and respiratory disease. Theoretical and clinical considerations. Am J Respir Crit Care Med 1996;154:6–17.
75. Yellowlees PM, Alpers JH, Bowden JJ, et al. Psychiatric morbidity in patients with chronic airflow obstruction. Med J Aust 1987;146:305–7.
76. Agle DP, Baum GL, Chester EH, et al. Multidiscipline treatment of chronic pulmonary insufficiency. 1. Psychologic aspects of rehabilitation. Psychosom Med 1973;35:41–9.
77. Papp LA, Klein DF, Gorman JM. Carbon dioxide hypersensitivity, hyperventilation, and panic disorder. Am J Psychiatry 1993;150:1149–57.
78. Klein DF. False suffocation alarms, spontaneous panics, and related conditions. An integrative hypothesis. Arch Gen Psychiatry 1993;50:306–17.
79. American Psychatric Association. Diagnostic and statistial manual of mental disorders. 3rd ed. Washington (DC): American Psychiatric Association; 1994.
80. American Psychiatric Association. Diagnostic and statistical manual of mental disorders. 4th ed. Washington (DC): American Psychiatric Association; 2004.
81. Kaplan HI, Sadock BJ, Grebb JA. Synopsis of psychiatry. Baltimore: Williams & Willkins; 1994.
82. Gorwood PH. [Is anxiety hereditary?]. Encephale 1998;24:252–5.

CHAPTER 31

TELEMEDICINE AND CHRONIC OBSTRUCTIVE PULMONARY DISEASE

PATRICIA B. KOFF, MEd, RRT, AND JOHN M. WESTFALL, MD

THE RISE OF CHRONIC OBSTRUCTIVE PULMONARY DISEASE (COPD) to the fourth leading cause of death in the United States and anticipated third leading cause worldwide has highlighted the economic burden of the problem and increased awareness that current management of patients with COPD is often less than optimal. Telemedicine holds the potential to address both the economic issues and the need for more effective standardized evidence-based care.

Telemedicine is a rapidly evolving method for delivering medical care over large geographic areas and in a synchronous (real time) or asynchronous manner. Numerous terms are used to describe the process, including *telehealth, eHealth* (with Internet involvement), *mHealth* (with mobile phone technology), *telehomecare,* and *telemonitoring.* The term used is most closely associated with the type of telemedicine employed. Generally, there are three main categories of telemedicine: education, consultation, and direct patient care. They often are interrelated (Figure 1).

Education via telemedicine may be oriented toward patients, medical students or residents in training, or continuous medical education for practicing physicians or other health care providers. The term *telehealth* is often used to focus on patient education for improved self-care of conditions.

Consultation use of telemedicine in radiology and other medical specialties involves transmission of test results that are interpreted from off-site locations. Radiology has one of the best records of success, has been rapidly adopted, and

is almost universally reimbursed.[1] Consultations can be synchronous, such as the primary care provider (PCP) contacting the specialist while the patient is present. The viability of such exchanges for COPD was demonstrated in a Japanese report in which noninvasive patient monitoring was shared in real time with the respiratory specialist and the attending physician.[2] Consultations may also be asynchronous, for example, e-mail that is sent for interpretation and response at a later time. Szot and colleagues documented the usefulness and reliability of e-mail interpretations of chest radiographs.[3]

Patient care is one of the most useful and potentially cost-beneficial types of telemedicine, especially with regard to rural, remote, or isolated settings. Programs can vary from simple telephone line–based medication reminders or emergency devices that provide an alert to a remote switchboard if, for example, a patient falls to interactive voice recognition programs that query the patient as to today's health status. An integrated care program using a Web-based call center for COPD patients has demonstrated the potential to use information technology to create health care savings.[4] The terms *telemonitoring* and *telehealth* are often used for these types of programs. Diagnostic testing is possible with telemedicine, as is case management. Evaluation of patients by telemedicine was as effective as traditional face-to-face meetings in a study by Pacht and colleagues.[5] Synchronous or "real-time" designs are employed, as well as asynchronous or "store-and-forward" forms. Nobel and Norman stated that information technologies have already begun to offer quantifiable benefits to disease management.[6]

Security for transmission of patient information is always an ongoing concern. Data management systems often use encrypted, firewall-protected approaches. Multiuse hardware equipment can be employed (such as the telephone, fax, or computer) with certain considerations for security; dedicated telemedicine equipment may be necessary in some cases. Regardless of the equipment used, privacy and security must be incorporated into any design.[7,8]

In employing telemedicine, one can also address the need for an improved model of care for chronic conditions in contrast to our current crisis-oriented care. A *New England Journal of Medicine* study highlighted the fact that adherence to quality indicators for chronic conditions is provided in about 56% of the cases. COPD scored 58%, meaning that

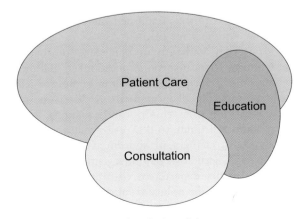

FIGURE 1. General categories of telemedicine.

recommended care was being received in just over half of the COPD cases reviewed.[9] Significant improvement in implementing evidence-based guidelines is needed and is further documented in the Swiss study, which demonstrated major gaps in the core elements of COPD management.[10] The model developed by the Institute for Healthcare Improvement (IHI) emphasizes an integrated approach to care, and Casas and colleagues have highlighted this approach for COPD patients.[4,11] The IHI promotes having patients become active, informed participants in their care while at the same time encouraging the health care system to approach care through more collaborative, integrated designs. Decision support with closer ties between specialists and primary care providers is a key feature. Information systems such as telemedicine can play a vital role in this redesigning of chronic disease management.

The US Centers for Medicare and Medicaid Services developed the Medicare Health Support pilot programs to address chronic illness using a form of telemedicine termed health information technology (HIT). These programs were established under provisions of the *Medicare Prescription Drug Improvement and Modernization Act of 2003.* Programs specific to managing congestive heart failure and diabetes are now in the pilot phase.[12] The programs use a disease management approach, and statute-required elements include the areas outlined in Table 1. Chronic care for Medicare recipients is decidedly complicated and a revision is needed as demonstrated by this quote: "Given that the *average* Medicare recipient sees seven physicians and fills upwards of twenty prescriptions each year, a revised, integrated, collaborative approach to care is critical."[12] The pilot programs are likely to expand to other conditions, such as COPD, pending positive outcomes. Based on 2002 planning documents for the Medicare programs, the COPD cohort of over 1 million patients had several comorbidities (Table 2). Addressing as many aspects as possible through telemedicine and integrating the results with primary care practice holds promise for an improved management approach.

This chapter focuses on the use of telemedicine for direct patient care with COPD management and patient education and monitoring. It attempts to strike a balance between the key clinical decisions related to the use of telemedicine systems with COPD patients, the practicality in relationship to the available technology, staffing implications, and the logistical realities of introducing telemedicine into daily practice.

COPD Considerations

Management of pulmonary conditions in general by telemedicine approaches has had a slow start compared with radiology department use and management of cardiac problems and diabetes. The fact that upward of 60% of the costs associated with COPD are related to exacerbations makes the prevention of exacerbations a ready target for telemedicine.[13] Several

Table 1 Medicare Prescription Drug, Improvement, and Modernization Act of 2003, Title VII SEC.701 Update in Home Health Services, Subtitle C—Chronic Care Improvement SEC. 721 Elements
1. Individualized, goal-oriented care management plan
2. Designated point of contact
3. Self-care education
4. Education for physicians and other providers and collaboration to enhance communication of relevant clinical information
5. Use of monitoring technologies that enable patient guidance through the exchange of pertinent clinical information, such as vital signs, symptomatic information, and health self-assessment
6. The provision of information about hospice care, pain and palliative care, and end-of-life care

Centers for Medicare and Medicaid Services, US Department of Health and Human Services.[41]

Table 2 Comorbidities Associated with COPD	
Description	*Total Patients (%)*
Essential hypertension	47
Angina pectoris	41
Other pneumonias	27
Diabetes mellitus	26
Asthma	20
Cancer of lungs, bronchi, or mediastinum	6

Adapted from Medicare Health Support Programs.[12]

groups have begun investigating telemedicine applications oriented to reducing exacerbations (Table 3).[4,14–26] COPD can also influence the length of stay of patients after orthopedic, abdominal, and other surgical procedures. If COPD can be well managed according to established guidelines, other problems become more manageable.[27]

The day-to-day variation in the status of the COPD patient is similar to most chronic conditions in that the term *stable* generally describes a functioning range.[28] Ideally, telemedicine can help determine when a drop in stability is detected and early interventions can be planned. By monitoring patients' cardinal COPD exacerbation symptoms (dyspnea, cough, changes in sputum characteristics) and determining the need for early intervention, exacerbations requiring emergency department visits and hospital admissions can potentially be reduced. Patient education can also be provided and can be beneficial in improving patient stability and avoidance of exacerbations.[29,30]

A philosophical decision must be made during the planning phase of telemedicine programs. (The planning and organization phase may require upward of 6 months.) Should data be automatically transmitted, or should the patient be responsible for entering the data? Our program has opted for patient ownership and responsibility; we have selected equipment with patient ease of use in mind but require that the patient enter his or her self-assessed parameters.

Pulmonary Assessment Devices

Simple, easily used monitoring devices can help patients in their home with the early identification of exacerbations. The use of peak flow monitoring devices for asthma patients has become almost routine. Given that the COPD population is often older and may be suffering from comorbidities such as arthritis and cardiac problems, the specific equipment must be tailored to this population. This may or may not be

Table 3 Telemedicine COPD-Related Studies and Reports

Study	N	Type of Study/Report	Outcome
Casas et al.[4]	155	RCT	Decreased hospitalization rate and fewer readmissions with use of integrated care and Web-based call center
Dale et al.[23]	55	Survey	Approximately 50% decrease in rates of hospital admissions with home monitoring
Dang et al.[14]	17	Survey	Telecare with home messaging may reduce resource use
Demiris et al.[26]	3 of 10	Survey	Videophones received 95% average rating for technical quality and visit themes were identified
Finkelstein et al.[15]	7 of 53 completing	RCT	Virtual visits can improve outcomes at lower costs
Johnston et al.[16]	49 of 212	RCT	Remote technology has cost-savings potential and can improve access to home health care
Koff et al.[22]	40	RCT	eHealth improved quality of life and indicated health care savings may be possible
Koizumi et al.[2]	2	Informational	Successfully tested a multistation system for communication between patient, specialist, and primary care provider
Lamothe et al.[24]	Not reported	Survey	Work organization changes based on ad hoc patients' needs and alerts
Maiolo et al.[42]	30 with 23 completions	Survey	Hospital admissions for exacerbations decreased 50% with twice-weekly monitoring of saturation and heart rate
Mair et al.[43]	Not reported	Informational; RCT planned	Difficult to procure equipment, and staff training has proven to be a barrier
Mair et al.[19]	22 patients 14 nurses	RCT	Patients had consistently more positive views of telecare encounters than their health care providers did
Pacht et al.[15]	40	Comparison of videoconferencing and face-to-face evaluations	Evaluations were equally effective between the two methods
Pfeifer et al.[21]	Not reported	Review	"Flying visits" determine right time for seeing patients
Ryan et al.[25]	911 total COPD not separately identified	Survey	Medication compliance increased nearly 50%; technology was easy to use and understand
Vontetsianos et al.[18]	18	Survey	Hospitalizations, emergency department visits, and health care services decreased with home monitoring
Young et al.[17]	Not reported	Informational only	Describes the telephone process used for routine calls, exacerbation calls, and exacerbation follow-up calls
Zarakovitis et al.[20]	Not reported	Informational	Describes e-Vital monitoring at home

COPD = chronic obstructive pulmonary disease; RCT = randomized controlled trial.

possible with any given technology system. Generally, for COPD patients, the following equipment can be incorporated into many technology platforms. In some cases, a platform for data transfer may not even be required.

Pulse oximeters, especially for patients on oxygen therapy, are probably the key piece of home monitoring equipment. In addition to providing an objective assessment of the patient's status and presumably an early indicator of change, use of an oximeter seems to reduce the anxiety and apprehension related to patients' experience of shortness of breath.[2] Several models have been used in various studies (Table 4). Some are chosen for their ability to link directly to technology platforms and others for their simplicity and ease of use. Some are offering blue tooth connections to the technology platforms so that cables are unnecessary for direct links. The cost of the oximeter becomes one of the most significant expenses of the home monitoring package. In our experience, the oximeter appears to be one of the most valuable equipment items and definitely worth the investment for COPD patients.

Table 4 Technology Used with COPD Telemedicine Programs						
Study	*Oximeter*	*Spirometer*	*End-Tidal Capnography*	*ECG*	*Blood Pressure*	*Platform Elements*
Casas et al.[4]	—	—	—	—	—	Web-based call center
Dang et al.[14]	—	—	—	—	—	Health Buddy®
Demiris et al.[26]	—	—	—	—	—	Videophones
Finkelstein et al.[15]	Nonin Onyx	SpiroCard, QRS Diagnostic LLC	—	—	Not described	Via TV Video camera Web-based messaging
Johnston et al.[16]	—	—	—	—	—	American Telecare Video system
Koff et al.[22]	Datex Ohmeda TuffSat	Microlife PF 100	—	—	—	Health Buddy®
Koizumi et al.[2]	TX-001T Nihon Kohden	—	NPB-75, Mallinckrodt	TX-001T Nihon Kohden	TX-001T Nihon Kohden	TMS 5002 Nihon Kohden FMV 6400 Fujitsu Videophone Picsend-R Docomo
Lamothe et al.[24]	Yes	Yes	—	Yes	Yes	HomMed Sentry comprehensive system
Mair et al.[19]	Yes, saturations and pulse	—	—	—	Yes	Videophone using plain old telephone system (POTS)
Maiolo et al.[42]	Nocturnal saturations and pulse	—	—	—	—	Hospital processing center contact via POTS
Pacht et al.[5]	—	—	—	—	—	Videoconferencing for assessment and chest auscultation
Pfeifer et al.[21]	—	—	Viasys			
Ryan et al.[25]	Aviva combination unit	—	—	—	Aviva combination unit	Aviva Telev-You, Health Buddy®
Vontetsianos et al.[18]	Yes	Yes	—	Yes	Yes	Videoconference camera and bandwidth added to home
Young et al.[17]	—	—	—	—	Yes	Computer-controlled voice telephone contact
Zarakovitis et al.[20]	?	?	?	Yes	?	Ongoing e-Vital Program

COPD = chronic obstructive pulmonary disease; ECG = electrocardiography.

Forced expiratory volume in 1 second (FEV_1) as a daily measurement is possible at home with several different devices, and more are expected on the market. We have employed a small handheld spirometer that offers both peak flow and FEV_1 measurements and can serve as a trend monitor. Some groups have opted for more sophisticated devices that provide detailed reporting. We have found that simplicity and reliability are keys to successful patient use. We also have considered the cost of each piece of equipment and the relative value in the scheme of monitoring. The FEV_1 monitor may be the key piece of equipment for the COPD patient who is not being treated with supplemental oxygen therapy. Our pilot study identified a possible trend toward early recognition of exacerbations using the monitor with this group.[22] Although the oximeter is especially helpful and nearly essential for oxygen-dependent patients, someone with moderate or borderline severe COPD may only see changes from 96 to 92% with an oximeter during an impending exacerbation, although their FEV_1 may decrease from 1.0 to 0.75 L and the degree of airflow limitation can be quantified.

End-tidal CO_2 monitors have been incorporated into at least one pilot study.[2] The possibility exists, albeit remote at present, that as more exhaled monitors assessing nitric oxide or other exhaled markers of respiratory change become available in mainstream use, they may also find a place in home monitoring.

Blood pressure monitors have often been incorporated into home monitoring pilot programs, and for good reason.[2,25] According to Medicare detail, hypertension is present in nearly 50% of COPD patients.[12] Attention to comorbidities of COPD patients can create more stability and potentially alter the likelihood of exacerbation risk.

Body weight scales are also often used, especially if the patient is diagnosed with congestive heart failure. Some systems use a digitally connected scale so that they have the patient step on the scale, perhaps apply a blood pressure cuff, insert a finger in an oximeter, and transmit the full data set in one simple maneuver. These full-service systems represent some of the more expensive options in home care monitoring and potentially continue the paternalistic or maternalistic approach to health care management. If one of the goals of a telemedicine program is to provide education and encourage self-care, providers must consider how this can best be accomplished with the available technology.

Pedometers are part of our self-assessment package. The emphasis is placed on a daily 6-minute walk during which the steps are monitored and reported. Many patients will walk more than the 6-minute walking distance each day, but some find it a challenge to meet that goal. Based on the research of Pitta and colleagues, the request to walk 6 minutes may be nearly doubling some of the most severe COPD patients' activity levels.[31,32] Pedometers are the least expensive pieces of equipment in comparison with the other items we use, but they seem to be one of the trend monitors most valuable in detecting early changes. If a patient is feeling poorly on a particular day, foregoing the walk is one of the first things that seems to happen. Caution is needed in regard to the accuracy of the pedometers. The patient's gait (eg, shuffling or off-center) and excess abdominal weight can make accurate recording difficult.

Technology Platform Selection

The means of communicating the monitored parameters to health care providers or third-party reimbursement sites depends on the selected technology platform. Some systems allow for automatic transmission; others require patient entry of parameters. The choice of technology can be influenced by the literacy level required by the patient, as well as vision and dexterity requirements.[25] The incorporation of monitoring related to comorbidities can also be helpful. An "open" platform, one in which additional self-monitoring equipment can be added, will be valuable as we learn more about the home management of COPD patients.

Synchronous systems may require more time for the patient and health care providers but may address problems at their earliest occurrence. Some examples of real-time delivery include the use of a plain old telephone systems (POTS) to establish a set telephone call consultation. A videoconference system becomes a more elaborate example and may involve installation of bandwidth technology into a patient's home prior to use.[2,4,16,18] The same is true for a video-Internet program. The benefit of synchronous systems may be the ability to link the PCP, patient, and pulmonologist at the same time. Whether funding for such elaborate approaches will become available remains questionable .

Once an Internet connection is introduced into the system, several asynchronous methods become possible. The simplest, e-mail, allows patients to forward self-monitored parameters, which the health care provider reviews at a later time. Transmission of peak flow data for asthma patients has been accomplished in this manner, but the relatively limited use of e-mail by the current senior COPD population does not seem to make it a valuable approach. Partridge described a 21% e-mail use rate by patients in a chest clinic, and e-mail use was more common in younger age groups.[33]

Creation of software programs using an extended mark-up language (XML) approach that walks a patient through a series of questions can be asynchronous and yet provide detailed patient assessments.

We have used an asynchronous approach (less expensive, less technology dependent) with the patient using a POTS and our care coordinators retrieving information from a secured Internet site via laptop computers the following day. Although the immediacy of information is slightly sacrificed, the ability to monitor on a daily basis offers greater information than scheduled outbound calls that may perhaps occur during stable periods. As many practitioners will agree, COPD patients often begin to have a general sense that they are feeling poorly and may wait for days to seek medical attention. In all fairness, the opposite may also be true, especially for the most severe patients; deterioration can escalate between morning and evening, and it is necessary to communicate as quickly as possible. We have found that through the value-added education component of the asynchronous platform we have chosen, patients begin to understand their cardinal symptoms of exacerbation and monitor themselves more closely during times of respiratory distress.

Staffing Issues

Identifying and hiring staff for a telemedicine program can be challenging. An information technology staff member may need to be identified. Clinical staff must possess strong skills, embrace technology, and be open to problem solving–related issues.[34] Staff members (or care coordinators, as we identify our staff) must also possess the interest and willingness to "go the extra mile" for their patients. They must have an ability to assess a patient's self-monitored parameters and with a brief telephone call determine the urgency related to a problem. For our COPD program, we have found registered nurses and registered respiratory therapists with 5 or more years of experience to be generally well suited. Originally, we required intensive care unit (ICU) experience but found that extensive physician office experience or pulmonary rehabilitation experience is also beneficial.

The care coordinator will be the problem-solving agent while miles away from the equipment and user. A low tolerance for frustration related to technology will rapidly sink an otherwise enthusiastic coordinator's attitude. Again, ICU experience may be a helpful background, and a track record demonstrating problem solving in a positive manner is a plus. According to Ryan and others, "Staff acceptance of the technology has been a major hurdle."[8,19,24,25]

The degree of medical oversight for the program may vary depending on the type of program and technology platform selected. We have a pulmonologist on call for clinical questions, and coordinators are encouraged to dis-

cuss case issues with the on-call person or the program medical director. An algorithm for handling typical issues (such as medication issues, equipment problems, missed reports, alarming self-monitored parameters, or psychosocial issues) is helpful. Depending on the level of responsibility given to the coordinators for intervention activities, various protocols can be developed from the algorithms. Also, individualized patient care plans or "action plans" are essential in the effective home management of patients.[35] Communication between the PCP, care coordinator, and pulmonologist is often needed for development of these plans.

Education and training of a care coordinator team for telemedicine require several phases. Initially, a solid understanding of the evidence-based guidelines for COPD is needed. Second, an introduction to telemedicine in general is helpful. (This can help reinforce the idea that the coordinators are not alone in this developing area and can encourage brainstorming problem-solving sessions.) Once the introductory phase is complete, training in all related self-monitoring equipment is essential. The staff must know the equipment in detail to problem-solve from a distance. Regardless of the particular monitoring equipment chosen, an understanding of home oxygen delivery is also needed since many COPD patients will have both stationary and portable systems. Coordinators may also need to become involved with the patients' home care providers. Several training sessions are needed related to the specific technology platform that will be used for transferring and retrieving the self-monitored data. The actual initial enrollment process of patients (especially if a consent process is also involved) should be observed first before starting enrollments. The patient evaluation involved during enrollment can be extensive and the paperwork requirements tedious. Data collection may be essential, although for future evaluation of the program, coordinators must be thoroughly trained in those aspects.

Table 5 Telemedicine Cost Factors	
Aspect	*Considerations*
Technology platform	Synchronous/asynchronous
Monitoring equipment	Oximetry, spirometry, blood pressure, electrocardiogram, pedometers, weight scales
Staffing	Medical direction Medical oversight and support Care coordinator requirements (COPD clinical experience and abilities, attitude, problem-solving abilities, start-up experience) Call center needed? Information technology specialist needed?
Coordinator space and technology	Telephones, computers, demonstration equipment
Education materials	Staff, patient, other health care providers
Evaluation	Instruments, statistical support staff

COPD = chronic obstructive pulmonary disease.

Economic Realities

The financing of the telemedicine systems remains an open question. Costs must be calculated for many factors (Table 5). In determining the support available for a program, an initial evaluation of the needs of the COPD patients in the health care facility can be helpful. (For example, how many COPD exacerbation admissions occur each year? How many individuals had repeated admissions? What is the average length of stay in the hospital? How often is COPD listed as a secondary diagnosis on admission? What are the other comorbidities? Which medical groups are providing care for these patients?)

The Veterans' Administration has adopted some telemedicine programs, and the central governments for some of the European nations are seriously considering such programs. The European Union has funded specific pilot programs to encourage the wider use of technology in health care.[4,18,20,35] The Medicare Health Support pilot programs are setting the stage for possible widespread use in the United States. Currently, some third-party payers are exploring telemedicine use in conjunction with in-house disease or case management programs. In some instances, these programs have been directed to patients without any integration into primary care. This has led to confusion on the patient's part and concern on the PCP's part when medications or care plans have been changed with no knowledge shared with the PCP. Organizing telemedicine programs with a patient-centered focus and communication across all participants remains a key goal.

Our approach to providing telemedicine has been to seek grant support and keep capital equipment investments as low as possible. Initially, we incorporated multiuse equipment for the coordinators (hospital-based personal computers and office telephones) and now have laptops and cellphones for coordinators. Goal setting for the program can also help focus the patient-monitoring equipment to key instruments. Determining if real-time (synchronous) systems are necessary for the goals or if asynchronous systems will be sufficient can have a major impact on the costs of the program.

Outcome Assessments

The St. George's Respiratory Questionnaire (SGRQ) is one of the standard instruments available for the assessment of pre and post responses to changes in respiratory care.[36] We are using the SGRQ with our COPD programs to assess quality-of-life changes. Our initial pilot study with eHealth demonstrated a 10-unit average improvement of the SGRQ with the application of telemedicine.[22] Patients improved symptom scores, increased exercise ability, and reduced the impact of the condition on their everyday life.

Assessment of the financial impact of telemedicine is critical to the future sustainability of telemedicine programs.[37] Reducing health care costs while providing care according to

evidence-based guidelines and striving to improve patients' quality of life is a realistic goal of telemedicine. Financial outcomes require assessment from several perspectives relative to the potential cost savings generated from reduced exacerbations and health care costs. Puig-Junoy and colleagues have documented a reduced direct cost for COPD home hospitalization using the Web-based call center detailed in Casas and colleagues' study.[4,38] Ideally, more randomized controlled trials are needed to fully evaluate these aspects. Our pilot study using home monitoring, a study conducted through Kaiser Permanente with video equipment used for chronically ill patients; the Casas and colleagues' study, which used a Web-based call center; and Finkelstein and colleagues' virtual visits are the only COPD studies that have used this approach.[4,15,16,22] Many studies are presently being designed to compare health care costs pre- and postintervention.

Specific Rural Considerations

Telemedicine has the potential to expand access to health care in rural, remote, or isolated locations. Resources, personnel, and geographic barriers often limit health care in these areas. Telemedicine can be a "value-added" feature to the existing primary care structure. Development of telemedicine has been promoted in several Scandinavian countries for these reasons, as well as the access available to leading telecommunication companies.[24,39,40] Patients can be remotely monitored and communication provided back to the primary caregiver. PCPs can obtain decision support and/or distant consultation from specialists. Continuing medical education can be structured as part of this process.

Potential Disadvantages and Barriers to Telemedicine

The current limited funding for telemedicine is a distinct disadvantage and/or barrier.[15,40] Another potential disadvantage is that the patient cannot be directly observed; even with good video systems, there is some barrier. Nonspecific problems may be missed if examinations or "vitual visits" are not comprehensive or are solely focused on one medical problem. Routine primary care may be impacted, and there have been concerns that routine care could be replaced by telemedicine visits. Medical practice across state lines creates medicolegal questions that become magnified with the easy availability to cover widespread areas with telemedicine.

These concerns should not deter one from implementing telemedicine initiatives. Awareness and vigilance are needed to avoid some of the problems. Front-end planning with these concerns in mind can also minimize a negative impact. Most importantly, as mentioned frequently in this chapter, the potential pitfalls can be overcome by closely working with patients, specialists, existing primary care services, and available community support to integrate care across all levels.

Summary

Telemedicine can potentially improve our ability to intervene early and reduce COPD exacerbations and the need for emergency department and hospital admissions. In addition, telemedicine can help ensure the consistent application of evidence-based guidelines for care. It can also expand the delivery of that care to rural, remote, or isolated settings.

Currently, we know that telemedicine is possible for COPD patients, and patients are well satisfied with its use. It may also help improve the quality of life for patients with COPD. Staff acceptance of telemedicine can be problematic. Education and training on the application of telemedicine are required and can lead to better acceptance. The addition of telemedicine technology to an already overburdened staff coupled with minimal instruction is a setup for failure.

The business aspect or cost-benefit analysis of telemedicine requires additional attention. More randomized controlled trials are needed, with careful review of the technology expenses and the staffing requirements compared with the cost savings generated by reduced emergency department visits and hospital admissions. In addition, a determination of the duration of a telemedicine program is required, as well as the degree and intensity of monitoring that is beneficial relative to the cost savings. Third-party payers and government-financed programs may help lead the way in this important aspect of telemedicine evaluation.

Acknowledgments

P. Koff would like to thank Dr. Josep Roca and the CHRONIC program staff of the University of Barcelona for the leadership provided regarding telemedicine applications with COPD, as well as Dr. Norbert Voelkel for his vision in applying this within a US patient population.

References

1. Field MJ, Grigsby J. Telemedicine and remote patient monitoring. JAMA 2002;288:423–5.
2. Koizumi T, Takizawa M, Nakai K, et al. Trial of remote telemedicine support for patients with chronic respiratory failure at home through a multistation communication system. Telemed J E Health 2005;11:481–6.
3. Szot A, Jacobson FL, Munn S, et al. Diagnostic accuracy of chest x-rays acquired using a digital camera for low-cost teleradiology. Int J Med Inform 2004;73:65–73.
4. Casas A, Troosters T, Garcia-Aymerich J, et al. Integrated care prevents hospitalisations for exacerbations in COPD patients. Eur Respir J 2006;28:123–30.
5. Pacht ER, Turner JW, Gailiun M, et al. Effectiveness of telemedicine in the outpatient pulmonary clinic. Telemed J 1998;4:287–92.
6. Nobel JJ, Norman GK. Emerging information management technologies and the future of disease management. Dis Manag 2003;6:219–31.
7. Nazi KM. The journey to e-Health: VA Healthcare Network Upstate New York (VISN 2). J Med Syst 2003 27:35–45.
8. Harnett B. Telemedicine systems and telecommunications. J Telemed Telecare 2006;12:4–15.
9. McGlynn EA, Asch SM, Adams J, et al. The quality of health care delivered to adults in the United States. N Engl J Med 2003;348:2635–45.
10. Rutschmann OT, Janssens JP, Vermeulen B, Sarasin FP. Knowledge of guidelines for the management of COPD: a survey of primary care physicians. Respir Med 2004;98:932–7.
11. Institute for Healthcare Improvement. Available at: http://www.ihi.org (accessed April 1, 2007).
12. Medicare Health Support Programs. Available at: http://www.cms.hhs.gov/CCIP/02_Highlights.asp#TopOfPage; http://www.cms.hhs.gov/CCIP/03_Data%20Analysis.asp#TopOfPage (accessed April 1, 2007).
13. Chapman KR, Mannino DM, Soriano JB, et al. Epidemiology and costs of chronic obstructive pulmonary disease. Eur Respir J 2006;27:188–207.
14. Dang S, Ma F, Nedd N, et al. Differential resource utilization benefits with Internet-based care coordination in elderly veterans with chronic diseases associated with high resource utilization. Telemed J E Health 2006;12:14–23.
15. Finkelstein SM, Speedie SM, Demiris G, et al. Telehomecare: quality, perception, satisfaction. Telemed J E Health 2004; 10:122–8.
16. Johnston B, Wheeler L, Deuser J,. Sousa KH. Outcomes of the Kaiser Permanente Tele-Home Health Research Project. Arch Fam Med 2000;9:40–5.
17. Young M, Sparrow D, Gottlieb A, et al. A telephone-linked computer system for COPD care. Chest 2000;119:1565–75.
18. Vontetsianos T, Giovas P, Katsaras T, et al. Telemedicine-assisted home support for patients with advanced chronic obstructive pulmonary disease: preliminary results after nine-month follow-up. J Telemed Telecare 2005;11 Suppl 1:86–8.
19. Mair FS, Goldstein P, May C, et al. Patient and provider perspectives on home telecare: preliminary results from a randomized controlled trial. J Telemed Telecare 2005;11 Suppl 1:95–7.
20. Zarakovitis K, Angelidis P, Kourtidou-Papadeli C, Psymarnou M. Ambulatory monitoring for chronic cardiac and pulmonary patients. Stud Health Technol Inform 2004; 103:362–7.
21. Pfeifer M, Werner B, Magnussen H. Telecare of patients with chronic obstructive airway diseases. Med Klin (Munich) 2004;99:106–10.
22. Koff PB, Stevens CS, Cashman J, et al. Telemonitoring/eHealth management improves quality of life and healthcare expenditures in COPD. Am J Respir Crit Care Med 2006;3:A123.
23. Dale J, Connor S, Tolley K. An evaluation of the west Surrey telemedicine monitoring project. J Telemed Telecare 2003;9 Suppl 1:S39–41.
24. Lamothe L, Fortin JP, Labbe F, et al. Impacts of telehomecare on patients, providers, and organizations. Telemed J E Health 2006;12:363–9.
25. Ryan P, Kobb R, Hilsen P. Making the right connection: matching patients to technology. Telemed J E Health 2003;9:81–8.
26. Demiris G, Speedie S, Finkelstein S, Harris I. Communication patterns and technical quality of virtual visits in home care. J Telemed Telecare 2003;9:210–5.

27. Executive summary: global strategy for the diagnosis, management, and prevention of COPD. Revised 2006. Available at: http://www.goldcopd.com/GuidelinesResources.asp?l1=2&l2=0 (accessed April 1, 2007).

28. Rodriguez-Roisin R. Toward a consensus definition for COPD exacerbations. Chest 2000;117(5 Suppl 2):398S–401S.

29. Bourbeau J, Julien M, Maltais F, et al. Reduction of hospital utilization in patients with chronic obstructive pulmonary disease: a disease-specific self-management intervention. Arch Intern Med 2003;163:585–91.

30. Gadoury MA, Schwartzman K, Rouleau M, et al. Self-management reduces both short- and long-term hospitalisation in COPD. Eur Respir J 2005;26:853–7.

31. Pitta F, Troosters T, Spruit MA, et al. Characteristics of physical activities in daily life in chronic obstructive pulmonary disease. Am J Respir Crit Care Med 2005;171:972–7.

32. Pitta F, Troosters T, Probst VS, et al. Physical activity and hospitalization for exacerbation of COPD. Chest 2006;129:536–44.

33. Partridge MR. An assessment of the feasibility of telephone and email consultation in a chest clinic. Patient Educ Couns 2004;54:11–3.

34. Pelligrino L, Kobb R. Skill sets for the home telehealth practitioner: a recipe for success. Telemed J 2005;11:151–6.

35. Hernandez C, Casas A, Escarrabill J, et al. Home hospitalisation of exacerbated chronic obstructive pulmonary disease patients. Eur Respir J 2003;21:58–67.

36. Jones PW, Quirk FH, Baveystock CM, Littlejohns P. A self-complete measure of health status for chronic airflow limitation. The St. George's Respiratory Questionnaire. Am Rev Respir Dis 1992;145:1321–32.

37. Seemungal TA, Wedzicha JA. Integrated care: a new model for COPD management? Eur Respir J 2006;28:4–6.

38. Puig-Junoy J, Casas A, Font-Plannells J, et al. The impact of home hospitalization on healthcare costs of exacerbations in COPD patients. Eur J Health Econ 2007 [Epub ahead of print].

39. Omenaas E, Dahl R, Bakke PS, Lehmann S. Nordic physicians' management of asthma and chronic obstructive pulmonary disease. Respir Med 2006;Suppl A:S31–7.

40. Bauer JC, Ringel MA. Telemedicine and the reinvention of healthcare; the seventh revolution in medicine. New York: McGraw-Hill;1999. p.148–9,157.

41. Centers for Medicare and Medicaid Services, US Department of Health and Human Services. Available at: http://www.cms.hhs.gov/CCIP/ (accessed January 19, 2007).

42. Maiolo C, Mohamed EI, Fiorani CM, De Lorenzo A. Home telemonitoring for patients with severe respiratory illness: the Italian experience. J Telemed Telecare 2003;9:67–71.

43. Mair F, Boland A, Angus R, et al. A randomized controlled trial of home telecare. J Telemed Telecare 2002;8 Suppl 2:58–60.

CHAPTER 32

CHRONIC OBSTRUCTIVE PULMONARY DISEASE, THE FINAL CHAPTER—LUNG CANCER

ROBERT L. KEITH, MD, STEINN JONSSON, MD, AND YORK E. MILLER, MD

LUNG CANCER IS OFTEN THE LAST CHAPTER in the medical history of patients with chronic obstructive pulmonary disease (COPD). There is a remarkable increase in risk for lung cancer in patients with COPD compared with smokers with similar tobacco exposure but normal pulmonary function.[1–3] The two disorders share a common environmental cause—tobacco smoke, have long latencies before disease expression, and almost certainly share common genetic susceptibilities and pathogenetic mechanisms.[4]

Lung cancer is the leading cause of cancer death and accounts for more cancer deaths in the United States than the combination of breast, prostate, colon, and rectal cancers.[5] COPD is the fourth leading cause of death in the United States. In proportion to their societal burden in terms of morbidity and mortality, research for both lung cancer and COPD remains grossly underfunded. Both disorders are eminently preventable, but current trends in smoking by young people virtually ensure that they will remain prominent for the next 50 years.

Research on these two disorders has been parallel and separate, without as much cross-fertilization as would be optimal. Now it is becoming clear that many basic disease mechanisms are shared (Table 1). The protease/antiprotease imbalance that has been a central hypothesis of COPD causation is now being appreciated as relevant to many aspects, including angiogenesis, tissue invasion, and metastasis, of the development and progression of cancer. Dysregulation of growth factors has been initially studied in neoplasia, and for over a decade, growth factors have been appreciated as important in tissue remodeling. Inflammation has been linked to the development of lung cancer in murine models[6,7] and is a highly plausible common factor in COPD and lung cancer. Although cigarette smoking in humans increases inflammatory cells in the lungs, it has been difficult to demonstrate that individuals with either COPD or lung cancer have more inflammation than smokers without disease. Oxidant stress is another consequence of cigarette smoking that could plausibly lead to both tissue damage and genetic mutations. To date, strategies of administering antioxidants have not been effective in preventing lung cancer or COPD. Alterations in gene expression, either through mutational or epigenetic mechanisms, have yielded insight into cancer cell biology for many years, and a similar understanding for COPD is at a much earlier stage. The high

frequency at which somatic mutations are found in the respiratory epithelial cells of all smokers has only recently been appreciated. The relevance of expansion of mutated or methylated clones of respiratory epithelial cells to lung carcinogenesis is obvious, but this phenomenon may also lead to some of the persistent abnormalities in gene expression and tissue function seen in COPD. Deoxyribonucleic acid (DNA) methylation and histone deacetylation are other mechanisms of gene silencing that have now been demonstrated in both lung cancer and premalignant respiratory epithelium.[8] As predicted in the previous version of this chapter, epigenetic alterations in gene expression have become a focus of interest in COPD; mutational mechanisms have proved more difficult to explore but are also likely to be of importance.

Table 1 Potential Shared Mechanisms of Pathogenesis in Chronic Obstructive Pulmonary Disease and Lung Cancer	
COPD	Lung Cancer
Protease/antiprotease imbalance	—
Inflammation	—
Oxidant/antioxidant imbalance	—
Latent viral infection	—
Increased apoptosis	Decreased apoptosis
Decreased angiogenesis	Increased angiogenesis
—	Growth control dysregulation
—	Gene mutation
—	Chromosomal instability
—	Expansion of genetically altered clones
—	Epigenetic gene silencing
—	Gene promoter methylation
Histone acetylation	Histone deacetylation

COPD = chronic obstructive pulmonary disease.
The mechanisms are listed under the disease in which they have been most prominently associated; however, they are likely shared by both.

Epidemiology

Environmental exposures are critical in the causation of lung cancer. Tobacco smoking accounts for approximately 90% of lung cancer cases, with small cell lung cancer (SCLC) having the highest attributability to smoking, squamous cell cancer the next highest, and adenocarcinoma the lowest.[9,10] Nonetheless, approximately 80 to 85% of adenocarcinomas are caused by tobacco smoking. Passive exposure to environmental tobacco smoke causes additional cases, and exposure during childhood is more strongly associated with development of lung cancer than exposure as an adult.[11] Additional agents have been implicated in the development of lung cancer; typically, the risk for development of lung cancer increases synergistically when more than one pulmonary carcinogen is involved. Asbestos, radon, nitrogen mustard gas, plutonium, beryllium, arsenic, cadmium, chromium, nickel, chloromethyl ethers, acrylonitrile, and vinyl chloride are well-established lung carcinogens; chronic silica exposure is more controversial.

Smoking cessation results in a reduction in the risk for lung cancer that improves for more than 10 years. Owing to the large number of ex-smokers in the US population, slightly more cases of lung cancer are currently diagnosed in ex-smokers than in smokers.[12] This finding should not obscure the benefits of smoking cessation, which were recently demonstrated to decrease lung cancer mortality in a randomized controlled study.[13] Additional strategies, including the administration of chemopreventive agents for prevention of lung cancer development in ex-smokers, are under intense investigation.[14]

Second to smoking cessation, diet appears to be a major modifiable risk for lung cancer.[15–19] A diet high in fruits and vegetables is consistently associated with lower lung cancer risk in epidemiologic studies, with approximately a 50% risk reduction when smoking history is controlled for. There have been no prospective controlled studies to determine whether dietary modification does cause a lowering of risk for lung cancer, however. Attempts at chemoprevention with retinoids (ie, β-carotene) have been unsuccessful, actually resulting in an increase in lung cancer.[20–25]

Only a minority of smokers exhibit accelerated loss of pulmonary function.[26] It is remarkable that these same individuals are at a significantly increased risk for lung cancer. Several studies have demonstrated a two- to fourfold increased incidence of lung cancer in current or ex-smokers with airflow obstruction.[2,27,28] The increased risk is proportional to the degree of airflow obstruction. In simple terms, the lower the forced expiratory volume in 1 second (FEV$_1$), the higher the risk for development of lung cancer. Lung cancer is a major cause of death in individuals with airflow obstruction, the magnitude of which is increasingly being appreciated. The Lung Health Study has provided interesting data as to the incidence of lung cancer in a cohort of patients with mild airflow obstruction who are being followed prospectively.[29] In the first 5 years of the Lung Health Study,

lung cancer was the single most common cause of death, accounting for 57 of 149 deaths in 5,887 individuals enrolled. Lung cancer deaths even exceeded deaths from heart disease and stroke in this population. More recent follow-up data have shown that this trend has continued, with over 250 lung cancer deaths in this cohort.[30] Again, in this susceptible population of smokers with airflow obstruction, lung cancer exceeds cardiovascular disease as a cause of death. In the most high-risk populations of COPD patients, the annual rate of lung cancer incidence approaches 2%.[31]

Lung cancer risk can be estimated from a number of the demographic characteristics described above, all of which are easily assessable by taking a history. Airflow obstruction on spirometry is a useful biomarker of risk that can be easily obtained. Additional biomarkers in blood, sputum, and bronchial epithelium are being assessed, but only a few have been validated, and these are not in widespread clinical use. Table 2 summarizes risk assessment for lung cancer.

Genetic Susceptibility to COPD and Lung Cancer
Shared Genetic Susceptibility to COPD and Lung Cancer

Although 90% of lung cancer develops in smokers, only about 12% of lifetime smokers develop lung cancer, suggesting that underlying host factors are important in determining lung cancer risk. A number of studies have shown that lung cancer risk increases with declining lung function as measured by the FEV$_1$.[28] These observations are based on longitudinal studies in smokers and individuals with airway obstruction and seem to persist after adjustment for the amount smoked and other determinants of lung function.[2] The possibility of a common genetic link between lung cancer and COPD was first suggested by Cohen and colleagues based on epidemiologic data.[4] With the ability to map the human genome using high-throughput techniques, analysis

Table 2 Risk Assessment for Lung Cancer	
Demographic	*Biomarker*
Smoking history	Airflow obstruction
Previous history of tobacco-induced cancer (eg, head and neck, lung, bladder)	Sputum cytologic atypia, especially severe or worse
Other carcinogens (eg, asbestos, radon, arsenic)	Multiple gene promoters methylated in sputum
Diet low in fruits and vegetables	Chromosomal aneusomy in sputum
Family history, especially for early-onset lung cancer, lung cancer with minimal smoking history, or multiply affected relatives	—

of genetic variability in complex diseases such as cancer and COPD using deoxyribonucleic acid (DNA) from patients and their relatives is now possible. The experimental tools may therefore be available to unravel the suspected genetic relationship between lung cancer and COPD. Despite the inherent difficulties in controlling for smoking history and carcinogen exposure, there is now new evidence to support the notion that the increased risk for lung cancer in COPD patients, independent of smoking intensity, may be caused by a common genetic predisposition.[32]

Attention to familial and genetic factors in lung cancer and COPD has long been overshadowed by the dominant common risk factor of smoking. In 1963, Tokuhata and Lilienfeld first observed a more than twofold increase in the development of lung cancer in first-degree relatives of lung cancer patients in a case-control study that was adjusted for smoking, age, and gender and suggested a familial or genetic predisposition to lung cancer.[33] Twin studies demonstrate that the relative risk for lung cancer of an identical twin who smokes is 1.4 to 2.0; this supports a genetic susceptibility that is not highly determinant.[34]

More recently, a study involving all 2,756 cases of lung cancer diagnosed within the Icelandic population from 1955 to 2002 showed that familial risk was not limited to first-degree relatives but extended to second- and third-degree relatives and was strongest in early-onset cases.[35] This was the first study that demonstrated that the familial risk of lung cancer extends beyond the immediate family and thus a shared environment. A large cohort study from Japan showed a similar familial predisposition and found the relationship to be stronger in women than in men and among nonsmokers than smokers.[36] Racial differences in familial risk have also been reported.[37] This consistent evidence indicates that there is indeed a genetic predisposition to the development of lung cancer that is strongest in early-onset patients and that this predisposition is not only present among first-degree relatives but also extends to second- and third-degree relatives, with declining risk ratios with further distance from the proband. A segregation study carried out in a population in which smoking is highly prevalent has suggested that a gene carried by approximately 10% of the population causes increased susceptibility to lung cancer, but this gene has not been mapped or identified.[38]

In a recent report, a major lung cancer susceptibility locus was mapped to chromosome 6q23–25.[39] Among 52 families with three or more individuals with lung, throat, or laryngeal cancer, a logarithm of the odds score (LOD—score) of 2.79 was found at 155 cM on chromosome 6q. In a further subset of 23 families with five or more affected individuals, an LOD score of 4.26 was seen, which achieves genome-wide significance. Several candidate genes in the region may have tumor suppressor effects, and the sequencing of exons in the affected families is under way. The genetic defect mapped to chromosome 6q is likely quite rare in the general population. Even small exposures to tobacco smoke lead to an overwhelming risk for lung cancer in these individuals. Evidence for a different human adenocarcinoma susceptibility locus has also been found on chromosome 12 with an orthologous locus in mice on chromosome 6q near the K-*ras* locus.[40]

In linkage studies of familial COPD in patients who do not have α_1-antitrypsin deficiency, a locus on chromosome 6q at 184.5 cM reached genome-wide significance with a LOD score of 5.0.[41] Additional evidence for linkage in COPD has been found on chromosome 12 but with weaker signals.[42]

Although these results are promising and may lead to the identification of shared susceptibility genes for lung cancer and COPD, much work remains to be done to elucidate the factors that affect genetic risk. Information gained from these new epidemiologic and genetic studies may prove important in allowing for more accurate risk assessment for both early detection and prevention. The combination of family history, smoking history, and lung function tests may, in the future, provide better information on lung cancer risk, with implications for early detection and chemoprevention.

Genetic Susceptibility to Lung Cancer

Certain neoplasms with a major genetic component, such as retinoblastoma, Wilms tumor, or breast cancer, result from the effects of high-penetrance genes that are relatively rare in the population.[43] Lung cancer is thought to most commonly result from the additive or synergistic effects of multiple low-penetrance genes that are common in the population,[44] although the recently described chromosome 6q locus appears to be a highly penetrant but low-frequency susceptibility gene.[35]

Genes affecting susceptibility to lung cancer can be divided into three classes: gatekeepers, housekeepers, and landscapers.[45,46] Gatekeepers include classic growth control genes such as *P53*, *Rb*, *P16^{INK}*, and *ras*. Housekeepers include DNA repair genes, such as *XPB*, *ATM*, *MSH2*, and *MLH1*. Genes controlling the metabolism of carcinogens also fall into the housekeeper class. The third class of cancer susceptibility genes, landscapers, includes genes that control the milieu that carcinogenesis occurs in by affecting processes such as inflammation, tissue remodeling, and cell–cell interaction. These three classes are not mutually exclusive, nor do they encompass all genes affecting cancer susceptibility. As an example, genes that affect the susceptibility to nicotine addiction are now being sought and have clear relevance to both COPD and lung cancer.[47]

Germline mutations in gatekeeper genes do not appear to be responsible for a significant proportion of lung cancer. Acquired somatic mutations in *P53* and *Rb* genes are common in lung tumors. Individuals with inherited mutations in *P53* and *Rb* are probably more likely to develop lung cancer if they smoke, but only a tiny fraction of lung cancer patients have germline mutations in either *P53* or *Rb*. Mice develop lung adenomas that have many similarities to human adenocarcinoma.[48] Genetic susceptibility to these tumors varies considerably between inbred mouse strains.[49–51] One of the loci determining variation in murine susceptibility to lung adenomas is within an intron of the K-*ras* gene, with the polymorphism conferring increased susceptibility also determining increased K-*ras* expression. Whether an analogous polymorphism exists in humans is not known.

The housekeeper class of cancer susceptibility genes includes genes involved in mutation repair and carcinogen metabolism. Polymorphisms in known DNA repair genes have not been associated with significant risk for the development of lung cancer. The ability of lymphocytes to repair DNA damage varies between individuals, and low repair capability has been associated with the development of lung cancer, particularly in low-intensity smokers.[52] However, the assays that measure DNA repair detect a phenotype, not a genotype, the genetic determination of which is incompletely understood.

Much attention has been directed toward the analysis of genes controlling the metabolism of carcinogens contained within tobacco smoke.[44] These genes are classified into two groups: phase I genes encode enzymes involved in the metabolic activation of carcinogens, and phase II genes encode enzymes that inactivate carcinogens. *CYP1A1* encodes a member of the cytochrome P-450 enzyme superfamily.[53,54] Polymorphic variants conferring increased activity of cytochrome P-450 are associated with increased risk for lung cancer. This relationship has been most readily demonstrated in Oriental populations and is most striking in low-intensity smokers. Presumably, for individuals with a high-intensity smoke exposure, the genetic variation in susceptibility is less important. Phase II genes that have been extensively studied include *GSTM1*, encoding glutathione *S*-transferase M1, and *NAT2*, encoding *N*-acetyltransferase 2.[55,56] The null variant of *GSTM1* is characterized by a deletion polymorphism, resulting in no *GSTM1* activity. This polymorphism has been associated with an increased risk for lung cancer, particularly in light or nonsmokers. Combinations of phase I and phase II genes that both increase carcinogen activation and decrease inactivation have been reported to result in large (10- to 20-fold) changes in the relative risk for lung cancer.[53] However, these reports are from relatively small association studies and should not be considered to be definitive.

Landscaper genes affect the microenvironment in which cancers arise.[46] Juvenile polyposis syndrome (JPS) is in some cases caused by an inactivating mutation in *SMAD4*, which encodes a signaling molecule in the transforming growth factor β signal transduction pathway.[57] JPS is characterized by multiple hamartomas of the gastrointestinal tract, some of which give rise to epithelium-derived carcinomas. It is postulated that the abnormal epithelial-stromal cell–cell interactions within the hamartomas are responsible for the development of cancer. Although the landscaper class of cancer susceptibility gene is less well studied than gatekeepers or housekeepers, it may have particular relevance to the development of lung cancer in COPD patients. α_1-Antitrypsin deficiency might be a common landscaper defect, resulting in an abnormal microenvironment, linking genetic susceptibility to COPD and lung cancer. One recent study has suggested an increased risk for

lung cancer in carriers of mutant α_1-antitrypsin alleles.[58] However, caution needs to be used in interpreting this report as it is an unreplicated association study.

Genes controlling growth factor–activated signal transduction pathways are intuitively attractive for determining susceptibility to neoplasia but also may be important in determining susceptibility to COPD. Morphologic studies have demonstrated a correlation between airway wall thickness and airflow obstruction.[59] Airway remodeling could easily be a growth control–related response. Elevated serum levels of insulinlike growth factor I (IGF-I) obtained from 7 to 10 years earlier in a retrospective longitudinal study have been linked to an increased risk for the development of prostate cancer.[60] In subsequent reports, elevated IGF-I levels have been associated with breast, prostate, colon, and lung cancer.[61] The question arises as to whether elevated IGF-I levels are a cause or result of neoplasia, but the recent development of a transgenic mouse with the IGF-I gene expressed in prostatic epithelium has demonstrated that increases in IGF-I production cause epithelial carcinogenesis. Similar development of spontaneous lung tumors in transgenic mice expressing IGF-I under the control of the human surfactant apoprotein C (SPC) promoter has been described.[62] The underlying basis of variation in serum IGF-I levels in humans is multifactorial, with a well-documented genetic component.[63] Thus, it is well established that variation in IGF-I levels, which is partly genetically determined, causes variation in susceptibility to neoplasia.

Inflammation has been postulated as an important condition in the development of COPD and lung cancer.[64] Studies in inbred strains of mice with varying susceptibility to lung carcinogenesis have shown a good correlation between inflammatory response to injected butylated hydroxytoluene and lung tumor susceptibility.[7,65] In humans, the support for this attractive theory is less robust. Although cigarette smoking reproducibly leads to an increase in the number of inflammatory cells in the lungs, it has been difficult to consistently demonstrate that pulmonary inflammation is increased in smokers with lung cancer or COPD compared with smokers without disease. A more refined approach to inflammation, beyond simple cell counts, may clarify this area. Administration of the anti-inflammatory corticosteroid budesonide, either systemically or by inhalation, has been demonstrated to result in chemoprotection of mice from lung tumors.[66,67] Two small observational studies in humans also support a chemopreventive role for corticosteroids, although the data are by no means definitive.[68–70]

Cigarette smoking increases the level of oxidants in the lung. Oxidative damage may plausibly contribute to both COPD and lung carcinogenesis through tissue damage and mutation. A diet high in fruits and vegetables, which provides antioxidants, has consistently been associated with decreased risk for COPD and lung cancer in epidemiologic studies, even among smokers.[71] Unfortunately, attempts to chemoprevent lung cancer in humans with antioxidant treatment have either had no effect or have led to an increased incidence of lung cancer.[72] Antioxidant treatment has not been demonstrated to be beneficial in COPD. Given the intense interest in oxidant/antioxidant balance in the pathogenesis of lung cancer, the paucity of reports linking genetic polymorphisms in antioxidant enzymes and lung cancer risk is surprising.[73–76]

Premalignant Respiratory Epithelial Biology

It is important to define the alterations in respiratory epithelium that lead to lung cancer for several reasons:

1. High-risk individuals may be identified by the presence of specific histologic, genetic, and gene expression patterns in their respiratory epithelium. As a better understanding of premalignant bronchial epithelial changes emerges, the translation of findings from airway biopsies to other specimens (ie, sputum or buccal smears) is potentially feasible.
2. Alterations in respiratory epithelium that reflect progression toward lung cancer may serve as intermediate end-point biomarkers in the evaluation of various chemoprevention strategies.
3. Finally, further understanding of the carcinogenic process may lead to rationally designed chemopreventive strategies.

The understanding of the genetic mutations and alterations in gene expression that commonly precede lung cancer, particularly squamous cell carcinoma, is advancing rapidly.

Histologic Abnormalities Preceding Lung Cancer

A well-defined progression of smoking-associated pathologic changes occurs in the respiratory epithelium of the central airways prior to the development of squamous cell carcinoma, including basal cell hyperplasia, squamous metaplasia, squamous dysplasia (mild, moderate, severe), and squamous carcinoma in situ (Figure 1).[77,78] If colon cancer is to be used as a paradigm, the histologic changes preceding lung cancer will also contain key genetic and cellular changes that ultimately result in the malignant phenotype. Some of the mutational defects that coincide with increasing levels of histologic dysplasia are listed in Table 3. The degree of dysplasia on sputum cytology has been demonstrated to vary with the risk for development of lung cancer. Moderate dysplasia has an approximately 10% risk over 10 years, whereas severe dysplasia or carcinoma in situ on sputum cytology has approximately a 50% risk of lung cancer over 2 years.[31]

The study of premalignant airway lesions has been aided through the use of autofluorescence bronchoscopy, a technology based on the observation that atypical or neoplastic epithelium emits a different spectrum of fluorescent light compared with normal respiratory epithelium.[79] Our group described a lesion characterized by reduced fluorescence in the airways of high-risk current and former smokers (with airflow limitation on spirometry) termed angiogenic squamous dysplasia (ASD).[80] ASD consists of projections of

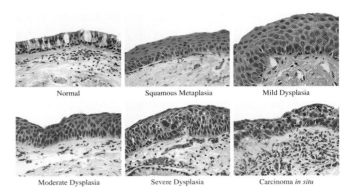

FIGURE 1. Progressive stages of endobronchial preneoplasia (hematoxylin-eosin stain).

capillary loops into overlying metaplastic or dysplastic epithelium and may represent a distinct "angiogenic phenotype" (Figure 2). ASD lesions have been characterized as containing increased levels of vascular endothelial growth factor (VEGF) and VEGF receptor messenger ribonucleic acids.[81] Coupling the reliance of tumor development and growth on angiogenesis with the observation of angiogenic changes in these lesions provides evidence of angiogenesis occurring prior to malignant transformation. Based on the current intense interest in targeted therapy using angiogenesis inhibition, this may prove to be an attractive target for chemoprevention, particularly in patients with COPD.

We and others have hypothesized that increased bronchial epithelial proliferation would be a biomarker of risk for central squamous cell lung cancer.[82–84] We studied this by assessing the Ki-67 index, reflective of proliferation, in bronchial biopsies taken from never-, current, or ex-smokers with normal spirometry and no lung cancer; current or ex-smokers with airflow obstruction on spirometry; and current, ex-, or never-smokers with lung cancer.[84] We found that current smoking and male gender are highly associated with increases in the Ki-67 index in the bronchial epithelium and that ex-smokers quickly revert to a lower Ki-67 index that is indistinguishable from never-smokers. After adjustment for smoking and gender, there was no relationship between either lung cancer or airflow obstruction and increased bronchial epithelial proliferation as measured by the Ki-67 index. Although increased bronchial epithelial proliferation is a hypothetically attractive biomarker of risk for either lung cancer or COPD, there appears to be no such relationship after adjustment for the confounding variable of current smoking.

Precursor lesions for adenocarcinoma and SCLC are much less well established than for squamous cell carcinoma. Atypical adenomatous hyperplasia (AAH) has been proposed to be a precursor for adenocarcinoma.[85] The lesion of AAH consists of cuboidal cells lining alveoli. These cells usually exhibit cytologic dysplasia, and the lesions are not

Table 3 Progressive Genetic Changes in Premalignant Bronchial Epithelial Tissue

Histologic Lesion	Genetic Changes
Normal epithelium	3p LOH
—	Telomeric deletions
—	Microsatellite instability
Reserve cell hyperplasia	9p, 17p LOH
—	Telomerase dysregulation
Squamous metaplasia (neoangiogenesis; ASD)	*myc* overexpression
Squamous dysplasia (neoangiogenesis; ASD)	8p LOH Loss of *FHIT* (3p14), RAR-β
—	p53 (17p13) protein accumulation
EGFR overexpression	Aneuploidy
—	Promoter hypermethylation
Carcinoma in situ (neoangiogenesis; ASD)	*P53* mutation 2q, 18q LOH
Cyclin D₁ overexpression	
5q LOH	
—	K-*ras* mutation

ASD = angiogenic squamous dysplasia; *EGFR* = epidermal growth factor receptor; *FHIT* = fragile histidine triad; LOH = loss of heterozygosity; RAR = retinoic acid receptor.

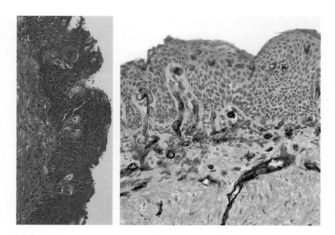

FIGURE 2. Angiogenic squamous dysplasia lesion. *Left*: Hematoxylin-eosin-stained section; note the multiple capillaries containing red blood cells within the bronchial epithelium. *Right*: A CD31-immunostained section demonstrating endothelial cells.

accompanied by inflammation or reactive hyperplasia of multiple cell types. The borders of AAH lesions are typically well circumscribed.[86] Although AAH has been most extensively described in the Japanese literature, it has also been described in other geographic regions and genetic populations.[87] Evidence supporting the premalignant nature of AAH is steadily increasing and includes a monoclonal epithelial population, preferential association with adenocarcinoma, and multiple genetic mutations mirroring those found in lung adenocarcinoma.[88–90]

No histologic precursor lesion for SCLC has been described. Idiopathic diffuse hyperplasia of pulmonary neuroendocrine cells can be mistaken for metastatic SCLC but has not been associated with the development of SCLC.[91] Peripheral bronchial carcinoids are frequently associated with idiopathic diffuse hyperplasia of pulmonary neuroendocrine cells, and the latter has been proposed as a precursor lesion to carcinoid.[92]

Carcinoid tumors of the lung have traditionally been thought of as closely related to SCLC. Gene expression profiling has demonstrated that SCLC has more in common with the gene expression patterns of normal bronchial epithelial cells and non–small cell lung cancer cell (NSCLC) lines than carcinoids.[93] Carcinoids are more similar to tumors arising from the central nervous system.

Premalignant Mutation

Chromosomal instability has been studied in a group of subjects who have had bronchial epithelial cells cultured from endobronchial biopsies, which were then subjected to spectral karyotyping (SKYFISH). Chromosomal aneusomy was rare in never-smokers. Smokers with and without lung cancer had high rates of chromosomal aneusomy by SKYFISH, which was then documented as occurring in the endobronchial biopsies and cultures by conventional fluorescence in situ hybridization.[94] These studies also confirmed the concept of mutant clonal expansion and dispersal as identical chromosomal rearrangements were often seen at widely separated sites in a given individual. Chromosomal aneusomy in sputum is a promising test for lung cancer risk assessment and early diagnosis.[95]

Extensive genetic alterations have been described in both non–small cell and small cell tumors using a variety of techniques, and these studies have been extended to bronchial epithelium samples obtained during bronchoscopy or at autopsy from patients with COPD and/or lung cancer.[96–99] Mutational analysis of premalignant bronchial epithelial changes in patients with COPD has been performed and has included examination for loss of heterozygosity (LOH) and microsatellite instability (MSI). LOH is characterized by the loss of one allele and suggests that a chromosomal deletion has occurred in the amplified region of interest. These deletions are most commonly heterozygous; in more rare instances, in which both copies of a gene are lost, the deletion is termed homozygous. In current and former smokers, bronchial epithelial LOH is most often seen in chromosomes 3p, 9p, 17p, and 13q.[96] Similar changes are found in lung cancers. Nonmalignant bronchial epithelium (including normal epithelium, metaplasia, and dysplasia) contains genetic changes (both LOH and MSI) that persist for years following smoking cessation. Furthermore, it has been difficult to demonstrate a correlation between these mutations and smoking intensity. Thus, although these mutations are intuitively very attractive as reflecting risk for lung cancer, the dissociation between their frequency and smoking intensity and cessation, which are well known to be related to lung cancer risk, raises some questions as to whether they can be used as risk markers. It is more likely that as our understanding of the molecular alterations in preneoplasia increases, specific mutations will be more strongly associated with cancer risk than others.

When DNA repair enzymes are inactivated, the number of tandem repeats may increase or decrease to create MSI. Microsatellites can be amplified with polymerase chain reaction, and MSI is represented by alterations in band size on gel electrophoresis. For example, chromosome 3p21 contains a mismatch repair gene and is a site of MSI in NSCLC.[100,101] To date, formal LOH and MSI analysis of the bronchial epithelium of COPD and lung cancer patients shows similar alterations, suggesting an overlap in the acquired genetic alterations that accompany each illness. Table 1 contains well-documented genetic changes in premalignant bronchial lesions that have relevance to observed changes in COPD and squamous cell lung cancer.

One gene of particular interest has been P53, a tumor suppressor gene located on chromosome 17p, a region frequently exhibiting LOH in premalignant epithelium. P53 activation can initiate either apoptosis or cell-cycle arrest, and loss of P53 can result in defects in apoptosis and cell-cycle control. A role for P53 in suppressing inflammation was recently documented.[102] The exact timing of P53 mutations during tumorigenesis depends on the tumor type, and loss or mutation of P53 is commonly seen in lung cancers. To date, most evidence points to P53 mutation being a late event in lung carcinogenesis. P53 protein accumulation may or may not reflect mutation. However, many studies in the past have incorrectly equated P53 detection by immunohistochemistry with P53 mutation. P53 overexpression has been documented in preoplastic epithelium adjacent to lung cancers.[103,104] The effect of P53 protein accumulation on cellular physiology is incompletely understood.

Epigenetic Mechanisms of Gene Inactivation

The inheritance of information on the basis of gene expression is known as epigenetics, as opposed to genetics, which refers to information transferred on the basis of gene sequence. Epigenetic silencing refers to nonmutational gene inactivation that can be faithfully propagated to clones of daughter cells.[105–107] Epigenetic gene silencing can occur by methylation of cytosines and deacetylation of histones, two processes that appear to act synergistically. These epigenetic patterns can also be reversed through DNA methylation inhibitors, such as 5-azacytidine, and histone deacetylase inhibitors, such as trichostatin A. Histone deacetylase has been described as decreased in COPD and postulated to play a role in the increased expression of nuclear factor

κB-controlled inflammation.[108,109] Histone deacetylase inhibitors are being evaluated for cancer treatment and considered for chemoprevention. If decreased histone deacetylase activity is critical in the pathogenesis of COPD, these therapies could possibly lead to accelerated loss of lung function.

Epigenetic silencing of tumor suppressor genes by methylation of promoter CpG islands is a common mechanism of inactivation in cancer.[110] Hypermethylation of normally unmethylated CpG islands in the promoter regions of many tumor suppressor genes, including P16, P15, VHL, E-cadherin, and hMLHI, correlates well with loss of transcription in human cancer. Furthermore, most of these genes can be reactivated by the addition of 5-aza-2'-deoxycytidine (5-aza), a demethylating agent. Trichostatin A, a histone acetylator, rarely reactivates genes by itself, but, in general, it appears that most inactivated genes need pretreatment with 5-aza to induce substantial reexpression.[111] The potential reversibility of these epigenetic changes in tumor cells makes them an attractive target for pharmacologic interventions with demethylating and deacetylating agents.

Knowledge derived from the study of methylated tumor suppressor genes may be useful in the diagnosis, early detection, and treatment of lung cancer and precursor lesions. Methylation assays can be performed with a small amount of DNA from small pathologic specimens. Several studies exploring methylation detection for early identification of lung cancer appear promising. In one study, methylation of the P16 tumor suppressor gene was associated with loss of expression in precursor lesions of lung cancer. The P16 gene was coordinately methylated in 75% of the carcinoma in situ lesions adjacent to the squamous cell carcinomas harboring this change.[8] Moreover, the frequency of P16 methylation increased during disease progression from basal cell hyperplasia (17%) to squamous metaplasia (24%) to carcinoma in situ (50%). Furthermore, methylation of the P16 was associated with loss of expression in both tumors and precursor lesions, demonstrating that both alleles were inactivated. These data link aberrant methylation of the P16 gene to early stages of lung cancer and suggest a potential use of this epigenetic change as a biomarker for early detection of patients with lung cancer or those at risk for lung cancer. Increased promoter methylation of multiple genes in DNA isolated from sputum has been demonstrated to be a risk biomarker for lung cancer.[112]

We do not currently know whether specific epithelial genes are silenced in COPD by epigenetic mechanisms or whether these genes may be involved in the pathogenesis of either COPD or lung cancer.

Field Carcinogenesis

Smokers with one aerodigestive cancer have a risk for a second independent primary aerodigestive tumor of from 15 to 45%. This phenomenon has been recognized for approximately 50 years and has given rise to the term "field carcinogenesis."[113] The most frequently cited mechanism for this high incidence of second primary tumors is that the aerodigestive epithelium is exposed to high concentrations of carcinogens. An additional potential mechanism is that the affected individuals are genetically susceptible to the development of lung and other aerodigestive cancers. Recently, an alternative mechanism has been suggested by the demonstration of two potentially related phenomena: allele-specific mutation and mutant clonal expansion.

Molecular studies of LOH in airway epithelium by several groups have demonstrated that when multiple sites are examined for LOH at the same locus, the allele that is lost does not appear to be randomly determined, but the same allele is most commonly lost at multiple sites.[114,115] This is termed allele-specific mutation. The two most likely mechanisms for allele-specific mutation are as follows: (1) one allele is more susceptible to loss, so loss at the more susceptible allele occurs more often, and (2) after mutation by LOH or some other mechanism, a mutated epithelial cell has a survival advantage. This cell then divides and multiplies, colonizing increasingly larger regions of the respiratory mucosa.

The latter possibility has been termed mutant clonal expansion. A case report in which a dominant negative *P53* point mutation, accompanied by wild-type *P53*, was found in multiple sites, including both airway and alveolar surfaces, of the lung epithelium of a smoker with COPD but without lung cancer demonstrates that mutant clonal expansion can occur in principle.[113] How commonly this does occur is unknown, but we have now observed a second individual with a similar pattern of *P53* mutation in widely separated regions of the bronchial epithelium. If this is a frequent occurrence, then COPD patients may often harbor abnormal epithelial clones. If specific mutations did have a survival or proliferative advantage (as the dominant negative *P53* mutation would be expected to have), then it is possible that they would be relatively commonly found. And if specific mutations with survival advantage resulted in altered structure or function of the airway, then they might also contribute to the pathogenesis of COPD. Although this schema has not been proven, similar clonal expansion has been demonstrated to occur in vascular pathology, specifically atheromatous and plexiform lesions.[116,117]

Intervention in the Progression of COPD to Lung Cancer

It is now being increasingly appreciated that individuals with COPD are at an extremely high risk for the development of lung cancer.[31] Smoking cessation is an important first step in interdicting this process but does not reduce risk to that of a never-smoker. Although there are administrative difficulties in combining efforts between different organizations focused on cancer research and lung research, there is much to be gained from communication and cooperation between these groups, particularly in the realm of large clinical studies.

Screening

Screening for lung cancer is currently not recommended, based on several studies conducted over a quarter of a century ago.[118] At the time that these studies were designed, the increased incidence of lung cancer in COPD was not appreciated and airflow obstruction was not used to define a high-risk population. More recently, we used airflow obstruction to define a high-risk group for intermediate end-point marker studies and found that the yield of moderate dysplasia increased from approximately 1% (in the Mayo Lung Project) to 20%.[119] In our studies of current or ex-smokers with airflow obstruction, we found a 1% incidence of lung cancer using cytology, compared with 0.1% in the Mayo Lung Project. Thus, the entry criteria of the old screening studies certainly can now be improved on in new screening studies. The use of helical computed tomography (CT) for lung cancer screening has recently been popularized and is currently highly controversial.[120,121] Widely divergent views are held of the desirability of instituting CT screening programs; one camp regards it as unethical to subject the question of efficacy to randomized trials, whereas others believe that screening will lead to increased cost and mortality owing to workup and treatment of many nodules, only a small percentage of which are malignancies. The only means to settle this controversy is to conduct prospective randomized controlled trials; the National Lung Screening Trial is such a trial and has now enrolled 50,000 subjects into CT screening and control chest radiograph arms. Initial analysis of the results will begin in 2009.

Chemoprevention

The most potent intervention known to decrease the risk of developing lung cancer is smoking cessation.[13] Advances in nicotine biology have afforded a greater understanding of the effects of nicotine in the human brain and have allowed for the development of a new class of smoking cessation drugs, the $\alpha_4\beta_2$ nicotinic acetylcholine receptor partial agonists.[122] However, the majority of lung cancer in the United States is diagnosed in former smokers, so there is an impetus for discovery of chemopreventive agents that would further decrease risk. Multiple steps in the carcinogenic process could potentially be targeted, as illustrated in Figure 3. To date, effective agents for the chemoprevention of lung cancer have not been identified, but basic and clinical research continues.

Historically, epidemiologic studies revealed an association between increased dietary intake of fruits and vegetables, and the resultant increase in vitamins A, E, and β-carotene, to be associated with a decreased incidence of human lung cancer.[22] Retinoids, derivatives of vitamin A, are a family of compounds that control gene expression by binding to retinoic acid receptors (RARs), which then bind to retinoic acid response elements of DNA and activate transcription of specific genes. Loss of specific RARs may be associated with lung cancer promotion, as evidenced by the finding of decreased RAR expression in NSCLC.[123] Several clinical trials have examined the chemopreventive effects of retinoids. The combination of β-carotene and vitamin A was extensively

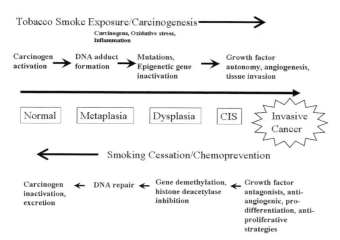

FIGURE 3. Multiple stages of carcinogenesis, including mechanisms thought to be most important at each stage, with potential chemopreventive strategies for reversing or slowing the carcinogenic process.

examined in the Alpha-Tocopherol, Beta Carotene Cancer Prevention Trial (ATBC) and the Beta-Carotene and Retinol Efficacy Trial (CARET), with the results showing no benefit (ATBC) or an increased lung cancer incidence (CARET).[20,21] Subset analysis of the ATBC focusing on the cohort of patients with COPD failed to show any improvement in symptoms among the treatment group.[124] Thus, although retinoids were the most attractive class of potential chemopreventive agents, the trials to date suggest that intake of high doses may actually promote the development of lung cancer. All-*trans* retinoic acid has also been evaluated in COPD, and a preliminary feasibility study did not show clinical benefit.[125] Large health care system databases have been used to examine whether other commonly prescribed medications may have an effect on lung cancer incidence. The results of analysis of lung cancer risk associated with use of statins (3-hydroxy-3-methylglutaryl coenzyme A reductase inhibitors) have been conflicting, with a recent study suggesting a risk reduction in US veterans.[126] This is in direct contrast to a previously published study and a meta-analysis.[127,128]

More recent studies have continued to examine whether inhaled corticosteroids may modify lung cancer risk and improve survival in COPD. Preclinical research in mice supports the potential for a chemopreventive effect of inhaled corticosteroids.[67] A recent study by Parimon and colleagues reported on a cohort study in outpatient clinics of the Department of Veterans' Affairs, and in those highly compliant subjects on high-dose inhaled corticosteroids (5% of the total population studied), there was a decreased lung cancer risk.[68,70] Although the use of inhaled corticosteroids in COPD has been shown to decrease all-cause mortality in a meta-analysis, a recent study summarizing the results of the TORCH (Towards a Revolution in COPD Health) study failed to show improved survival in the inhaled steroid groups.[69,129] Inhaled budesonide was also evaluated to determine the effect on endobronchial dysplasia, which may be a histologic

biomarker of central squamous cell carcinoma. Again, no effect on bronchial epithelial dysplasia was observed when inhaled budesonide was compared with placebo.[130] Overall, the use of inhaled steroids for lung cancer chemoprevention can not be endorsed at this time, but further study is warranted.

Medications that alter arachidonic acid metabolism have also been examined as chemopreventive agents. This includes nonselective inhibitors of cyclooxygenase-1 (COX-1) and COX-2 or COX-2 selective inhibitors. In one large US cohort, 32% fewer lung cancers developed in frequent aspirin users.[131] However, epidemiologic studies of COX inhibitors and lung cancer incidence have not been consistently positive.[132] Nonselective COX inhibitors have shown positive results in murine models of lung cancer chemoprevention.[133–135] The selective COX-2 inhibitor celecoxib was not chemopreventive, although it did reduce lung inflammation.[136] Human trials involving COX-2 inhibition are in progress.[137] The results of these trials will need to be balanced against a better understanding of the biology leading to elevated cardiovascular event risk in subjects on long-term COX-2 inhibitors.[138]

Manipulation of prostaglandin metabolism distal to the COX enzymes in murine models of lung tumorigenesis is an area of active interest as different prostaglandin H_2 metabolites could have either pro- or anticarcinogenic properties, as illustrated in Figure 4. Our group has shown that lung-specific overexpression of prostacyclin synthase decreases tumor incidence and multiplicity in multiple tumorigenesis models, including tobacco smoke exposure.[139,140] This effect is secondary to increased lung levels of prostacyclin, and alternative mechanisms, such as depletion of prostaglandin H_2 and its metabolites (prostaglandin E_2 and thromboxane), have not proven to be critical. Prostacyclin classically acts through a G protein–coupled seven-transmembrane spanning receptor but also activates peroxisome proliferator–activated receptor γ

Regulation of Prostaglandin Production

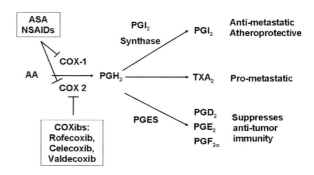

FIGURE 4. Pathways of arachidonic acid metabolism illustrating that the downstream metabolites have differing biologic activities. Cyclooxygenase (COX) inhibition depresses levels of both pro- and anticarcinogenic compounds. ASA = acetylsalicylic acid, aspirin; NSAID = nonsteroidal anti-inflammatory drugs; AA = arachidonic acid; PGI_2 = prostacyclin; PGES = prostaglandin E_2 synthase; PGE_2 = prostaglandin E_2; PGD_2 = prostaglandin D_2; $PGF_{2\alpha}$ = prostaglandin F_2 alpha.

(PPARγ), and overexpression of PPARγ selectively inhibits invasive metastasis of NSCLC cell lines and promotes a more differentiated phenotype.[141] A recent epidemiologic report on PPAR agonists (rosiglitazone and pioglitazone) showed a 33% decrease in lung cancer rates.[142] However, this must be balanced against concerns of a significantly increased myocardial infarction rate in subjects taking rosiglitazone.[143] Newer pharmaceutical agents currently under development, such as the long-acting oral prostacyclin analog iloprost, may prove effective in preventing the development of lung cancer in high-risk individuals. One attractive feature of prostacylin analogues is an atheroprotective role in mice.[144] Iloprost is currently being evaluated at multiple sites in the Lung Cancer Biomarkers and Chemoprevention Consortium in a phase 2 chemoprevention trial with endobronchial dysplasia as the primary end point.

Conclusion

Lung cancer and COPD share many common elements of pathogenesis: genetic predisposition, exposure to inflammation and oxidative stress, dysregulation of growth factor expression and cell-cycle control, somatic mutation, and epigenetic alterations leading to aberrant gene expression. The close relationship of these two tobacco-induced diseases should be exploited for both basic and clinical investigations. It is tragic that tobacco smoking is so preventable, yet most societies lack the motivation to take effective steps to decrease its inception.

Drs. Miller and Keith are collaborators on a pending patent application for the use of prostaglandin analogs for the prevention of cancer.

References

1. Petty TL. Are COPD and lung cancer two manifestations of the same disease? Chest 2005;128:1895–7.
2. Tockman MS, Anthonisen NR, Wright EC, Donithan MG. Airways obstruction and the risk for lung cancer. Ann Intern Med 1987;106:512–8.
3. Skillrud DM, Offord KP, Miller RD. Higher risk of lung cancer in chronic obstructive pulmonary disease. A prospective, matched, controlled study. Ann Intern Med 1986;105:503–7.
4. Cohen BH, Diamond EL, Graves CG, et al. A common familial component in lung cancer and chronic obstructive pulmonary disease. Lancet 1977;2:523–6.
5. Greenlee RT, Murray T, Bolden S, Wingo PA. Cancer statistics, 2000. CA Cancer J Clin 2000;50:7–33.
6. Malkinson AM, Bauer A, Meyer A, et al. Experimental evidence from an animal model of adenocarcinoma that chronic inflammation enhances lung cancer risk. Chest 2000;117:228S.
7. Malkinson AM, Radcliffe RA, Bauer AK. Quantitative trait locus mapping of susceptibilities to butylated hydroxytoluene-induced lung tumor promotion and pulmonary inflammation in CXB mice. Carcinogenesis 2002;23:411–7.
8. Belinsky SA, Nikula KJ, Palmisano WA, et al. Aberrant methylation of p16(INK4a) is an early event in lung cancer and a

9. MillerYE, Franklin WA. Molecular events in lung carcinogenesis. Hematol Oncol Clin North Am 1997;11:215–34.
10. Wynder EL, Graham EA. Landmark article May 27, 1950: Tobacco smoking as a possible etiologic factor in bronchiogenic carcinoma. A study of six hundred and eighty-four proved cases. JAMA 1985;253:2986–94.
11. Janerich DT, Thompson WD, Varela LR., et al. Lung cancer and exposure to tobacco smoke in the household. N Engl J Med 1990;323:632–6.
12. Tong L, Spitz MR, Fueger JJ, Amos CA. Lung carcinoma in former smokers. Cancer 1996;78:1004–10.
13. Anthonisen NR, Skeans MA, Wise RA, et al. The effects of a smoking cessation intervention on 14.5-year mortality: a randomized clinical trial. Ann Intern Med 2005;142:233–9.
14. Keith RL, Miller YE. Lung cancer: genetics of risk and advances in chemoprevention. Curr Opin Pulm Med 2005;11:265–71.
15. Feskanich D, Ziegler RG, Michaud DS, et al. Prospective study of fruit and vegetable consumption and risk of lung cancer among men and women. J Natl Cancer Inst 2000;92:1812–23.
16. Virtamo J. Vitamins and lung cancer. Proc Nutr Soc 1999;58:329–33.
17. Lee BW, Wain JC, Kelsey KT, et al. Association between diet and lung cancer location. Am J Respir Crit Care Med 1998;158:1197–203.
18. Mathers JC, Burn J. Nutrition in cancer prevention. Curr Opin Oncol 1999;11:402–7.
19. Menkes MS, Comstock GW, Vuilleumier JP, et al. Serum beta-carotene, vitamins A and E, selenium, and the risk of lung cancer. N Engl J Med 1986;315:1250–4.
20. The effect of vitamin E and beta carotene on the incidence of lung cancer and other cancers in male smokers. The Alpha-Tocopherol, Beta Carotene Cancer Prevention Study Group. N Engl J Med 1994;330:1029–35.
21. Omenn GS, Goodman GE, Thornquist MD, et al. Effects of a combination of beta carotene and vitamin A on lung cancer and cardiovascular disease. N Engl J Med 1996;334:1150–5.
22. Koo LC. Diet and lung cancer 20+ years later: more questions than answers? Int J Cancer Suppl 1997;10:22–9.
23. Hennekens CH, Buring JE, Manson JE, et al. Lack of effect of long-term supplementation with beta carotene on the incidence of malignant neoplasms and cardiovascular disease. N Engl J Med 1996;334:1145–9.
24. Goodman GE. Prevention of lung cancer. Crit Rev Oncol Hematol 2000;33:187–97.
25. Vainio H. Chemoprevention of cancer: lessons to be learned from beta-carotene trials. Toxicol Lett 2000;112-3:513–7.
26. Lebowitz MD, Holberg CJ, Knudson RJ, Burrows B. Longitudinal study of pulmonary function development in childhood, adolescence, and early adulthood. Development of pulmonary function. Am Rev Respir Dis 1987;136:69–75.
27. Islam SS, Schottenfeld D. Declining FEV1 and chronic productive cough in cigarette smokers: a 25-year prospective study of lung cancer incidence in Tecumseh, Michigan. Cancer Epidemiol Biomarkers Prev 1994;3:289–98.
28. Kuller LH, Ockene J, Meilahn E, Svendsen KH. Relation of forced expiratory volume in one second (FEV1) to lung

potential biomarker for early diagnosis. Proc Natl Acad Sci U S A 1998;95:11891–6.

cancer mortality in the Multiple Risk Factor Intervention Trial (MRFIT). Am J Epidemiol 1990;132:265–74.

29. Anthonisen NR, Connett JE, Kiley JP, et al. Effects of smoking intervention and the use of an inhaled anticholinergic bronchodilator on the rate of decline of FEV1. The Lung Health Study. JAMA 1994;272:1497–505.

30. Anthonisen NR, Connett JE, Enright PL, Manfreda J. Hospitalizations and mortality in the Lung Health Study. Am J Respir Crit Care Med 2002;166:333–9.

31. Prindiville SA, Byers T, Hirsch FR, et al. Sputum cytological atypia as a predictor of incident lung cancer in a cohort of heavy smokers with airflow obstruction. Cancer Epidemiol Biomarkers Prev 2003;12:987–93.

32. Schwartz AG, Ruckdeschel JC. Familial lung cancer: genetic susceptibility and relationship to COPD. Am J Respir Crit Care Med 2006;173:16–22.

33. Tokuhata GK, Lilienfeld AM. Familial aggregation of lung cancer in humans. J Natl Cancer Inst 1963;30:289–312.

34. Lichtenstein P, Holm NV, Verkasalo PK, et al. Environmental and heritable factors in the causation of cancer—analyses of cohorts of twins from Sweden, Denmark, and Finland. N Engl J Med 2000;343:78–85.

35. Jonsson S, Thorsteinsdottir U, Gudbjartsson DF, et al. Familial risk of lung carcinoma in the Icelandic population. JAMA 2004;292:2977–83.

36. Nitadori J, Inoue M, Iwasaki M, et al. Association between lung cancer incidence and family history of lung cancer: data from a large-scale population-based cohort study, the JPHC study. Chest 2006;130:968–75.

37. Cote ML, Kardia SL, Wenzlaff AS, et al. Risk of lung cancer among white and black relatives of individuals with early-onset lung cancer. JAMA 2005;293:3036–42.

38. Sellers TA, Bailey-Wilson JE, Elston RC, et al. Evidence for mendelian inheritance in the pathogenesis of lung cancer. J Natl Cancer Inst 1990;82:1272–9.

39. Bailey-Wilson JE, Amos CI, Pinney SM, et al. A major lung cancer susceptibility locus maps to chromosome 6q23-25. Am J Hum Genet 2004;75:460–74.

40. Yanagitani N, Kohno T, Sunaga N, et al. Localization of a human lung adenocarcinoma susceptibility locus, possibly syntenic to the mouse Pas1 locus, in the vicinity of the D12S1034 locus on chromosome 12p11.2-p12.1. Carcinogenesis 2002;23:1177–83.

41. Joost O, Wilk JB, Cupples LA, et al. Genetic loci influencing lung function: a genome-wide scan in The Framingham Study. Am J Respir Crit Care Med 2002;165:795–9.

42. Silverman EK, Palmer LJ, Mosley JD, et al. Genomewide linkage analysis of quantitative spirometric phenotypes in severe early-onset chronic obstructive pulmonary disease. Am J Hum Genet 2002;70:1229–39.

43. Shields PG. Molecular epidemiology of lung cancer. Ann Oncol 1999;10 Suppl 5:S7–11.

44. Shields PG, Harris CC. Cancer risk and low-penetrance susceptibility genes in gene-environment interactions. J Clin Oncol 2000;18:2309–15.

45. Kinzler KW, Vogelstein B. Cancer-susceptibility genes. Gatekeepers and caretakers. Nature 1997;386:761, 763.

46. Kinzler KW, Vogelstein B. Landscaping the cancer terrain. Science 1998;280:1036–7.

47. Lerman C, Caporaso NE, Bush A, et al. Tryptophan hydroxylase gene variant and smoking behavior. Am J Med Genet 2001;105:518–20.

48. Stearman RS, Dwyer-Nield L, Zerbe L, et al. Analysis of orthologous gene expression between human pulmonary adenocarcinoma and a carcinogen-induced murine model. Am J Pathol 2005;167:1763–75.

49. Malkinson AM. Inheritance of pulmonary adenoma susceptibility in mice. Prog Exp Tumor Res 1999;35:78–94.

50. Festing MF, Lin L, Devereux TR, et al. At least four loci and gender are associated with susceptibility to the chemical induction of lung adenomas in A/J x BALB/c mice. Genomics 1998;53:129–36.

51. Horio Y, Chen A, Rice P, et al. Ki-ras and p53 mutations are early and late events, respectively, in urethane-induced pulmonary carcinogenesis in A/J mice. Mol Carcinog 1996;17:217–23.

52. Qingyi W, Lie C, Amos CI, et al. Repair of tobacco carcinogen-induced DNA adducts and lung cancer risk: a molecular epidemiologic study. J Natl Cancer Inst 2000;92:1764–72.

53. Bartsch H, Nair U, Risch A, et al. Genetic polymorphism of CYP genes, alone or in combination, as a risk modifier of tobacco-related cancers. Cancer Epidemiol Biomarkers Prev 2000;9:3–28.

54. Bennett WP, Alavanja MC, Blomeke B, et al. Environmental tobacco smoke, genetic susceptibility, and risk of lung cancer in never-smoking women. J Natl Cancer Inst 1999;91:2009–14.

55. Seow A, Zhao B, Poh WT, et al. NAT2 slow acetylator genotype is associated with increased risk of lung cancer among non-smoking Chinese women in Singapore. Carcinogenesis 1999;20:1877–81.

56. Stucker I, de Wazier I, Cenee S, et al. GSTM1, smoking and lung cancer: a case-control study. Int J Epidemiol 1999;28:829–35.

57. Woodford-Richens K, Williamson J, Bevan S, et al. Allelic loss at SMAD4 in polyps from juvenile polyposis patients and use of fluorescence in situ hybridization to demonstrate clonal origin of the epithelium. Cancer Res 2000;60:2477–82.

58. Yang P, Wentzlaff KA, Katzmann JA, et al. Alpha1-antitrypsin deficiency allele carriers among lung cancer patients. Cancer Epidemiol Biomarkers Prev 1999;8:461–5.

59. Hogg JC, Chu F, Utokaparch S, et al. The nature of small-airway obstruction in chronic obstructive pulmonary disease. N Engl J Med 2004;350:2645–53.

60. Chan JM, Stampfer MJ, Giovannucci E, et al. Insulin-like growth factor I (IGF-I), IGF-binding protein-3 and prostate cancer risk: epidemiological studies. Growth Horm IGF Res 2000;10 Suppl A:S32–3.

61. Pollak M. Insulin-like growth factor physiology and cancer risk. Eur J Cancer 2000;36:1224–8.

62. Frankel SK, Moats-Staats BM, Cool CD, et al. Human insulin-like growth factor-IA expression in transgenic mice promotes adenomatous hyperplasia but not pulmonary fibrosis. Am J Physiol Lung Cell Mol Physiol 2005;288:L805–12.

63. Harrela M, Koistinen H, Kaprio J, et al. Genetic and environmental components of interindividual variation in circulating levels of IGF-I, IGF-II, IGFBP-1, and IGFBP-3. J Clin Invest 1996;98:2612–5.

64. Brody JS, Spira A. State of the art. Chronic obstructive pulmonary disease, inflammation, and lung cancer. Proc Am Thorac Soc 2006;3:535–7.

65. Malkinson AM, Koski KM, Evans WA, Festing MF. Butylated hydroxytoluene exposure is necessary to induce lung tumors in BALB mice treated with 3-methylcholanthrene. Cancer Res 1997;57:2832–34.

66. O'Shaughnessy JA, Kelloff GJ, Gordon GB, et al. Treatment and prevention of intraepithelial neoplasia: an important target for accelerated new agent development. Clin Cancer Res 2002;8:314-46.

67. Wattenberg LW, Wiedmann TS, Estensen RD, et al. Chemoprevention of pulmonary carcinogenesis by aerosolized budesonide in female A/J mice. Cancer Res 1997;57:5489–92.

68. Parimon T, Chien JW, Bryson CL, et al. Inhaled corticosteroids and risk of lung cancer among patients with chronic obstructive pulmonary disease. Am J Respir Crit Care Med 2007;175:712–9.

69. Sin DD, Wu L, Anderson JA, et al. Inhaled corticosteroids and mortality in chronic obstructive pulmonary disease. Thorax 2005;60:992–7.

70. Miller YE, Keith RL. Inhaled corticosteroids and lung cancer chemoprevention. Am J Respir Crit Care Med 2007;175:636–7.

71. Meyskens FL Jr, Szabo E. Diet and cancer: the disconnect between epidemiology and randomized clinical trials. Cancer Epidemiol Biomarkers Prev 2005;14:1366–9.

72. Omenn GS. Chemoprevention of lung cancer: the rise and demise of beta-carotene. Annu Rev Public Health 1998;19:73–99.

73. Yamada N, Yamaya M, Okinaga S, et al. Microsatellite polymorphism in the heme oxygenase-1 gene promoter is associated with susceptibility to emphysema. Am J Hum Genet 2000;66:187–95.

74. Ho JC, Mak JC, Ho SP, et al. Manganese superoxide dismutase and catalase genetic polymorphisms, activity levels, and lung cancer risk in Chinese in Hong Kong. J Thorac Oncol 2006;1:648–53.

75. Liu G, Zhou W, Wang LI, et al. MPO and SOD2 polymorphisms, gender, and the risk of non-small cell lung carcinoma. Cancer Lett 2004;214:69–79.

76. Wang LI, Neuberg D, Christiani DC. Asbestos exposure, manganese superoxide dismutase (MnSOD) genotype, and lung cancer risk. J Occup Environ Med 2004;46:556–64.

77. Franklin WA. Diagnosis of lung cancer: pathology of invasive and preinvasive neoplasia. Chest 2000;117:80S–9S.

78. Franklin WA. Pathology of lung cancer. J Thorac Imaging 2000;15:3–12.

79. Hirsch FR, Prindiville SA, Miller YE, et al. Fluorescence versus white-light bronchoscopy for detection of preneoplastic lesions: a randomized study. J Natl Cancer Inst 2001;93:1385–91.

80. Keith RL, Miller YE, Gemmill RM, et al. Angiogenic squamous dysplasia in bronchi of individuals at high risk for lung cancer. Clin Cancer Res 2000;6:1616–25.

81. Merrick DT, Haney J, Petrunich S, et al. Overexpression of vascular endothelial growth factor and its receptors in bronchial dypslasia demonstrated by quantitative RT-PCR analysis. Lung Cancer 2005;48:31–45.

82. Lee JJ, Liu D, Lee JS, et al. Long-term impact of smoking on lung epithelial proliferation in current and former smokers. J Natl Cancer Inst 2001;93:1081–8.

83. Szabo E. Lung epithelial proliferation: a biomarker for chemoprevention trials? J Natl Cancer Inst 2001;93:1042–3.

84. Miller YE, Blatchford P, Hyun D, et al. Bronchial epithelial-Ki-67 is related to histology, smoking and gender but not lung cancer or chronic obstructive pulmonary disease. Cancer Epidemiol Biomarkers Prev 2007;16:2425–31.

85. Miller RR, Nelems B, Evans KG, et al. Glandular neoplasia of the lung. A proposed analogy to colonic tumors. Cancer 1988;61:1009–14.

86. Ritter JH. Pulmonary atypical adenomatous hyperplasia. A histologic lesion in search of usable criteria and clinical significance [editorial]. Am J Clin Pathol 1999;111:587–9.

87. Chapman AD, Kerr KM. The association between atypical adenomatous hyperplasia and primary lung cancer. Br J Cancer 2000;83:632–6.

88. Niho S, Yokose T, Suzuki K, et al. Monoclonality of atypical adenomatous hyperplasia of the lung. Am J Pathol 1999;154:249–54.

89. Yokozaki M, Kodama T, Yokose T, et al. Differentiation of atypical adenomatous hyperplasia and adenocarcinoma of the lung by use of DNA ploidy and morphometric analysis. Mod Pathol 1996;9:1156–64.

90. Kitamura H, Kameda Y, Ito T, Hayashi H. Atypical adenomatous hyperplasia of the lung. Implications for the pathogenesis of peripheral lung adenocarcinoma. Am J Clin Pathol 1999;111:610–22.

91. Aguayo SM, Miller YE, Waldron JA Jr, et al. Brief report: idiopathic diffuse hyperplasia of pulmonary neuroendocrine cells and airways disease. N Engl J Med 1992;327:1285–8.

92. Miller RR, Muller NL. Neuroendocrine cell hyperplasia and obliterative bronchiolitis in patients with peripheral carcinoid tumors. Am J Surg Pathol 1995;19:653–8.

93. Anbazhagan R, Tihan T, Bornman DM, et al. Classification of small cell lung cancer and pulmonary carcinoid by gene expression profiles. Cancer Res 1999;59:5119–22.

94. Varella-Garcia M, Chen L, Powell RL, et al. Spectral karyotyping detects chromosome damage in bronchial cells of smokers and cancer patients. Am J Respir Crit Care Med 2007;176:505–12.

95. Varella-Garcia M, Kittelson J, Schulte AP, et al. Multi-target interphase fluorescence in situ hybridization assay increases sensitivity of sputum cytology as a predictor of lung cancer. Cancer Detect.Prev 2004;28:244–51.

96. Wistuba II, Lam S, Behrens C, et al. Molecular damage in the bronchial epithelium of current and former smokers. J Natl Cancer Inst 1997;89:1366–73.

97. Wistuba II, Behrens C, Milchgrub S, et al. Sequential molecular abnormalities are involved in the multistage development of squamous cell lung carcinoma. Oncogene 1999;18:643–50.

98. Sato M, Shames DS, Gazdar AF, Minna JD. A translational view of the molecular pathogenesis of lung cancer. J Thorac Oncol 2007;2:327–43.

99. Virmani AK, Fong KM, Kodagoda D, et al. Allelotyping demonstrates common and distinct patterns of chromosomal loss in human lung cancer types. Genes Chromosomes Cancer 1998;21:308–19.

100. Bronner CE, Baker SM, Morrison PT, et al. Mutation in the DNA mismatch repair gene homologue hMLH1 is associated with hereditary non-polyposis colon cancer. Nature 1994;68:258–61.

101. Wieland I, Ammermuller T, Bohm M, et al. Microsatellite instability and loss of heterozygosity at the hMLH1 locus on chromosome 3p21 occur in a subset of nonsmall cell lung carcinomas. Oncol Res 1996;8:1–5.

102. Komarova EA, Krivokrysenko V, Wang K, et al. p53 is a suppressor of inflammatory response in mice. FASEB J 2005;19:1030–2.

103. Bennett WP, Colby TV, Travis WD, et al. p53 protein accumulates frequently in early bronchial neoplasia. Cancer Res 1993;53:4817–22.

104. Rusch V, Klimstra D, Linkov I, Dmitrovsky E. Aberrant expression of p53 or the epidermal growth factor receptor is frequent in early bronchial neoplasia and coexpression precedes squamous cell carcinoma development. Cancer Res 1995;55:1365–72.

105. Tycko B. Epigenetic gene silencing in cancer. J Clin Invest 2000;105:401–7.

106. Wigler M, Levy D, Perucho M. The somatic replication of DNA methylation. Cell 1981;24:33–40.

107. Pollack Y, Stein R, Razin A, Cedar H. Methylation of foreign DNA sequences in eukaryotic cells. Proc Natl Acad Sci U S A 1980;77:6463–7.

108. Szulakowski P, Crowther AJ, Jimenez LA, et al. The effect of smoking on the transcriptional regulation of lung inflammation in patients with chronic obstructive pulmonary disease. Am J Respir Crit Care Med 2006;174:41–50.

109. Ito K, Ito M, Elliott WM, et al. Decreased histone deacetylase activity in chronic obstructive pulmonary disease. N Engl J Med 2005;352:1967–76.

110. Brock MV, Herman JG, Baylin SB. Cancer as a manifestation of aberrant chromatin structure. Cancer J 2007;13:3–8.

111. Cameron EE, Bachman KE, Myohanen S, et al. Synergy of demethylation and histone deacetylase inhibition in the re-expression of genes silenced in cancer. Nat Genet 1999;21:103–7.

112. Belinsky SA, Liechty KC, Gentry FD, et al. Promoter hypermethylation of multiple genes in sputum precedes lung cancer incidence in a high-risk cohort. Cancer Res 2006;66:3338–44.

113. Franklin WA, Gazdar AF, Haney J, et al. Widely dispersed p53 mutation in respiratory epithelium. A novel mechanism for field carcinogenesis [published erratum appears in J Clin Invest 1997;100:2639]. J Clin Invest 1997;100:2133–7.

114. Wistuba II, Behrens C, Virmani AK, et al. Allelic losses at chromosome 8p21-23 are early and frequent events in the pathogenesis of lung cancer. Cancer Res 1999;59:1973–9.

115. Mao L, Lee JS, Kurie JM, et al. Clonal genetic alterations in the lungs of current and former smokers. J Natl Cancer Inst 1997;89:857–62.

116. Lee SD, Shroyer KR, Markham NE, et al. Monoclonal endothelial cell proliferation is present in primary but not secondary pulmonary hypertension. J Clin Invest 1998;101:927–34.

117. Schwartz SM, Murry CE. Proliferation and the monoclonal origins of atherosclerotic lesions. Annu Rev Med 1998;49:437–60.

118. Patz EF Jr, Goodman PC, Bepler G. Screening for lung cancer. N Engl J Med 2000;343:1627–33.

119. Kennedy TC, Proudfoot SP, Franklin WA, et al. Cytopathological analysis of sputum in patients with airflow obstruction and significant smoking histories. Cancer Res 1996;56:4673–8.

120. Henschke CI, Yankelevitz DF, Libby DM, et al. Survival of patients with stage I lung cancer detected on CT screening. N Engl J Med 2006;355:1763–71.

121. Bach PB, Jett JR, Pastorino U, et al. Computed tomography screening and lung cancer outcomes. JAMA 2007;297:953–61.

122. Tonstad S, Tonnesen P, Hajek P, et al. Effect of maintenance therapy with varenicline on smoking cessation: a randomized controlled trial. JAMA 2006;296:64–71.

123. Hong WK. Chemoprevention of lung cancer. Oncology (Huntingt) 1999;13:135–41.

124. Rautalahti M, Virtamo J, Haukka J, et al. The effect of alpha-tocopherol and beta-carotene supplementation on COPD symptoms. Am J Respir Crit Care Med 1997;156:1447–52.

125. Roth MD, Connett JE, D'Armiento JM, et al. Feasibility of retinoids for the treatment of emphysema study. Chest 2006;130:1334–45.

126. Khurana V, Bejjanki HR, Caldito G, Owens MW. Statins reduce the risk of lung cancer in humans: a large case-control study of US veterans. Chest 2007;131:1282–8.

127. Setoguchi S, Glynn RJ, Avorn J, et al. Statins and the risk of lung, breast, and colorectal cancer in the elderly. Circulation 2007;115:27–33.

128. Bonovas S, Filioussi K, Tsavaris N, Sitaras NM. Statins and cancer risk: a literature-based meta-analysis and meta-regression analysis of 35 randomized controlled trials. J Clin Oncol 2006;24:4808–17.

129. Calverley PM, Anderson JA, Celli B, et al. Salmeterol and fluticasone propionate and survival in chronic obstructive pulmonary disease. N Engl J Med 2007;356:775–89.

130. Lam S, leRiche JC, McWilliams A, et al. A randomized phase IIb trial of pulmicort turbuhaler (budesonide) in people with dysplasia of the bronchial epithelium. Clin Cancer Res 2004;10:6502–11.

131. Schreinemachers DM, Everson RB. Aspirin use and lung, colon, and breast cancer incidence in a prospective study. Epidemiology 1994;5:138–46.

132. Wall RJ, Shyr Y, Smalley W. Nonsteroidal anti-inflammatory drugs and lung cancer risk: a population-based case control study. J Thorac Oncol 2007;2:109–14.

133. Castonguay A, Rioux N, Duperron C, Jalbert G. Inhibition of lung tumorigenesis by NSAIDS: a working hypothesis. Exp Lung Res 1998;24:605–15.

134. Rioux N, Castonguay A. Prevention of NNK-induced lung tumorigenesis in A/J mice by acetylsalicylic acid and NS-398. Cancer Res 1998;58:5354–60.

135. Moody TW, Leyton J, Zakowicz H, et al. Indomethacin reduces lung adenoma number in A/J mice. Anticancer Res 2001;21:1749–55.

136. Kisley LR, Barrett BS, Dwyer-Nield LD, et al. Celecoxib reduces pulmonary inflammation but not lung tumorigenesis in mice. Carcinogenesis 2002;23:1653–60.

137. Mao JT, Cui X, Reckamp K, et al. Chemoprevention strategies with cyclooxygenase-2 inhibitors for lung cancer. Clin Lung Cancer 2005;7:30–9.

138. Solomon SD, McMurray JJ, Pfeffer MA, et al. Cardiovascular risk associated with celecoxib in a clinical trial for colorectal adenoma prevention. N Engl J Med 2005;352:1071–80.

139. Keith RL, Miller YE, Hoshikawa Y, et al. Manipulation of pulmonary prostacyclin synthase expression prevents murine lung cancer. Cancer Res 2002;62:734–40.

140. Keith RL, Miller YE, Hudish TM, et al. Pulmonary prostacyclin synthase overexpression chemoprevents tobacco smoke lung carcinogenesis in mice. Cancer Res 2004;64:5897–904.

141. Bren-Mattison Y, Van Putten, V, Chan D, et al. Peroxisome proliferator-activated receptor-gamma (PPAR(gamma)) inhibits tumorigenesis by reversing the undifferentiated phenotype of metastatic non-small-cell lung cancer cells (NSCLC). Oncogene 2005;24:1412–22.

142. Govindarajan R, Ratnasinghe L, Simmons DL, et al. Thiazolidinediones and the risk of lung, prostate, and colon cancer in patients with diabetes. J Clin Oncol 2007;25:1476–81.

143. Nissen SE, Wolski K. Effect of rosiglitazone on the risk of myocardial infarction and death from cardiovascular causes. N Engl J Med 2007;356:2457–71.

144. Egan KM, Lawson JA, Fries S, et al. COX-2-derived prostacyclin confers atheroprotection on female mice. Science 2004;306:1954–7.

Epilogue

At the time of final editing of the second edition of this book, we have some concluding remarks. Overall, research in the field of chronic obstructive pulmonary disease (COPD) has taken clearer shape since we entered the twenty-first century. The importance of advancing research in COPD is no longer in doubt; COPD research on all levels now has a prominent place in international respiratory meetings, and is proceeding at a rapid pace all over the world. Large, multicenter trials are ongoing in many countries, and the Lung Division of the National Institutes of Health (HLB) has initiated two large population studies: the COPD gene initiative and the SubPopulations and InteRmediate Outcome Measures In COPD Study (SPIROMICS). The first initiative will enroll patients for a genome wide association study (GWAS), the second will be designed to phenotype patients with COPD. The expectations are that within the next 10 years we will have a better understanding of the genetic and epigenetic factors that determine both susceptibility to COPD and the factors that influence particular phenotypes. The field of gender-related issues in COPD will require closer attention, to determine (for example) whether there are female (hormonal) determinants of COPD/emphysema.[1]

In addition to understanding the genetics of the phenotypes, we will also need to advance our knowledge of the pathobiology of the COPD syndrome. To quote B. Celli: "We are witnessing a change in the COPD paradigm from a simple problem of airflow limitation to a multicomponent disease where other manifestations may become targets of interventions."[2] One would hope that individualized phenotype-oriented therapy will soon be part of the practice guidelines. To understand the pathobiology of COPD in its many manifestations, we believe, we will need to apply a system biology approach rather than a lung- or airway-centered[3] approach. It is already apparent that two such systems must be integrated. These are the vasculature (and perhaps more specifically, the endothelial cells), and the many interactions between the innate and the adaptive immune system. Such a 'biology of systems' approach will not entirely lead us away from the lung-mechanical-disease models but will be a necessary element in understanding autoimmune mechanisms and critical cell/cell interactions against the backdrop of a common inflammatory disease etiology. Such a common inflammatory disease etiology, together with inheritable epigenetic traits, would explain many of the systemic effects and consequent co-morbidities related to COPD.[4] All in all, the ground has been prepared for the development of COPD-specific, non-bronchodilator drugs.

Norbert F. Voelkel
William MacNee

1. Sin DD, Greaves L, Kennedy S. The tip of the "ICEBERGS": a national conference to combat the growing global epidemic of COPD in women. Proc Am Thorac Soc 2007;4:669–70.

2. Celli BR. Predicting mortality in chronic obstructive pulmonary disease: chasing the "Holy Grail." Am Respir Crit Care Med 2006;173:1298–9.

3. Hersh CP, Jacobson FL, Gill R, Silverman EK. Computed tomography phenotypes in severe, early-onset chronic obstructive pulmonary disease. COPD 2007;4:331–7.

4. Ekbom A, Brandt L, Granath F, et al. Increased risk of both ulcerative colitis and Crohn's disease in a population suffering from COPD. Lung 2008;Mar 11 [Epub ahead of print].

INDEX

Respiratory muscle resting
  nutritional evaluation, 385
  psychological support, 385
Respiratory syncytial virus (RSV), 207, 212
Respiratory virology, 205
Respiratory viruses
  airway inflammation in COPD exacerbations, 209
  bacterial interactions, 207
  clinical syndromes, 205
  innate immune response, 210–212
  studies on COPD exacerbations interactions, 205–206
  susceptibility of COPD patients, 205, 208
Reticular fibers, 2
Retinoblastoma, 471
Retinoic acid, 439
Retinoic acid receptors (RARs), 474t, 476
Retinoids, 470, 476, 477
Reversible restriction, 177
Rhesus monkeys. *See also* Small animal models of emphysema
  in asthma studies
    airway generation, 250
    airway nerves, 258
    airway physiology, 250
    airway wall/BMZ changes, 253–255
    bronchial vasculature changes, 256–258
    epithelial changes, 250–253
    fibroblast changes, 255–256
    smooth muscle changes, 256
    unique similarities to humans, 248–249
  in oxidant stress in COPD studies, 259–262
  postnatal airways development (comparison), 240–248
  tracheobronchial airways (comparison), 235–240
Rheumatoid arthritis, 338
RHF. *See* Right heart failure
Rhinovirus ribonucleic acid (RNA), 206
Rhinoviruses, 205–208, 210
  cytokines and inflammatory mediators induced by, 211t
Rho kinase inhibitors, 70
Right heart catheterization
  in diagnosis of PH, 305–306
  for pulmonary hypertension, 401, 402
  of pulmonary hypertension (PH) in COPD, 300
Right heart failure (RHF), 299, 303, 304
  from pulmonary hypertension to, 308–309
Right ventricular hypertrophy (RVH), 299
  pulmonary hypertension (PH) diagnosis, 299, 302, 305
Risedronate, 338, 339t
Risk assessment
  for lung cancer, 470
Risk factors
  for COPD exacerbations, 372
  for COPD patients, 20–26
  for osteoporosis, 331–334

RNA. *See* Rhinovirus ribonucleic acid
ROFA. *See* Residual oil fly ash
Roflumilast, 228, 379
ROS. *See* Reactive oxygen species
Rosiglitazone, 478
Rosuvastatin, 440
RP. *See* Relapsing polychondritis
RSV. *See* Respiratory syncytial virus
RV. *See* Residual volume
RVH. *See* Right ventricular hypertrophy

Saber-sheath trachea
imaging diagnosis of, 277
Saccular lung development, 9, 10
Saccule lumen, 10
Salmeterol, 295, 361, 376
SaO2. *See* Oxygen saturation
SAR. *See* Small airway remodeling
Sarcoidosis
  diagnosis and treatment, 163–164
  interstitial lung disease involving small airways (mimicking COPD), 169–170
Sarcomeres, 317, 318f
Sarcoplasmic reticulum, 317
Satellite stem cells, 319–321, 432f
Saturation, arterial, 385
SCFR. *See* Stem cell factor receptor
Scintigraphy. *See also* Ventilation-perfusion scanning, 402, 404
SCLC. *See* Small cell lung cancer
SDF-1α. *See* Stromal cell-derived factor 1α
SDF-1R. *See* Stroma-derived factor 1 receptor
Secondary pulmonary lobule, 169
Secondary septa, 10
Secretogogues, 55
Secretory products
  species comparison, 241f
Sedentarism
  as a muscle injury mechanism (in COPD), 321–322
Segmentectomies, 399
Selective serotonin reuptake inhibitors (SSRIs), 449, 452, 455t
Senescence
  in emphysema, 70, 70–71
  stem cell response in, 437
Senescence marker protein 30 (SMP-30), 70
Serine proteinase inhibitors
  α1-antitrypsin, 53
Serine proteinases, 56
Serotonin-norepinephrine reuptake inhibitors, 449
Serotoninergic antidepressants
  comparison chart, 449t
SERPINE2
  genetic determinant of COPD, 44